Alveolar Gas Exchange and Pulmonary Circulation

Main Symbols

C	concentration in a liquid
Cap	capacity
D	diffusing capacity
f	respiratory frequency
F	fraction
G	conductance
P	pressure, total or partial
Q	volume of liquid
$\dot{Q}$	flow of blood, perfusion
R	gas-exchange ratio
S	saturation
V	gas volume
$\dot{V}$	ventilation
β	slope of a dissociation curve
θ	reaction rate

Modifiers

a	arterial
A	alveolar
B	barometric
c	capillary
DS	dead space
e	effective
E	expired
I	inspired
la	left atrial
m	membrane
p	plasma
pa	pulmonary arterial
pc	pulmonary capillary
pc′	pulmonary end capillary
pv	pulmonary venous
pw	pulmonary wedge
s	shunt
t	time t
T	total
ti	tissue
v	venous
$\bar{v}$	mixed venous
va	venous admixture
0	(zero) initial value

Special Symbols

ATPD	ambient temperature and pressure, dry
ATPS	ambient temperature and pressure, saturated
BTPS	body temperature, ambient pressure, saturated with water vapor
STPD	standard temperature and pressure, dry

Examples of Combinations

$C\bar{v}_{O_2}$	concentration of O_2 in mixed venous blood
O_2Cap	O_2 capacity
Pa_{O_2}	partial pressure of O_2 in arterial blood
$PA_{O_2} - Pa_{O_2}$	alveolar-arterial difference in partial pressure of O_2
P_{O_2}	partial pressure of O_2
$\dot{Q}T$	cardiac output
Sa_{O_2}	saturation of hemoglobin with O_2 in arterial blood
$\dot{V}A/\dot{Q}$	ventilation-perfusion ratio
$\dot{V}E$	expired minute ventilation
$\dot{V}max_{O_2}$	maximum O_2 consumption (also $\dot{V}_{O_2 max}$)

Control of Breathing

$Pm_{0.1}$	mouth occlusion pressure 0.1 s after onset of inspiration
TE	expiratory time
TI	inspiratory time
TT	total respiratory cycle duration

See Symbols and Abbreviations, p. ix.

HANDBOOK OF PHYSIOLOGY

SECTION 3: The Respiratory System, VOLUME I

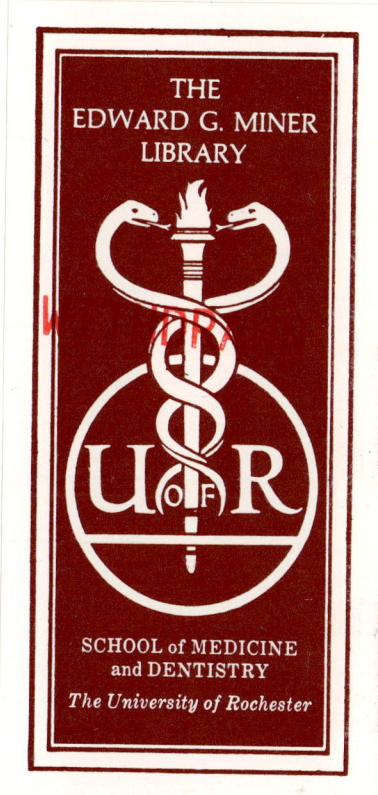

PUBLICATIONS COMMITTEE

HOWARD E. MORGAN, *Chairman*
WILLIAM F. GANONG
LEONARD R. JOHNSON
FRANKLYN G. KNOX
ERICH E. WINDHAGER

Laurie S. Chambers, Elizabeth M. Cowley,
Michael A. Edington, Susie P. Mann, *Editorial Staff*

Brenda B. Rauner, *Production Manager*

Constantine J. Gillespie, *Indexer*

HANDBOOK OF PHYSIOLOGY

A critical, comprehensive presentation of physiological knowledge and concepts

---

SECTION 3: ## The Respiratory System

Formerly SECTION 3: Respiration

VOLUME I.
Circulation and Nonrespiratory Functions

Section Editor: ALFRED P. FISHMAN

Volume Editors: ALFRED P. FISHMAN
                      ARON B. FISHER

Executive Editor: STEPHEN R. GEIGER

American Physiological Society, BETHESDA, MARYLAND, 1985

© Copyright 1964 (Volume I), American Physiological Society
© Copyright 1965 (Volume II), American Physiological Society

© Copyright 1985, American Physiological Society

Library of Congress Catalog Card Number 84-24381

International Standard Book Number 0-683-03244-5

Printed in the United States of America by Waverly Press, Inc., Baltimore, Maryland 21202

Distributed by The Williams & Wilkins Company, Baltimore, Maryland 21202

Preface to the Section on Respiration

The intent of this *Handbook* section is to provide a scholarly, comprehensive, and critical view of contemporary respiratory physiology within the framework of respiratory biology. This has been no simple task; in the 20 years since the first edition, respiratory physiology has extended far beyond its original bounds while becoming more deeply rooted within traditional confines. In large measure this flourishing of respiratory physiology is attributable to the biochemists, anatomists, pharmacologists, pathologists, and bioengineers who have entered the field and enriched it with their approaches, knowledge, concepts, and techniques. During this period the growth of ideas, advances in technology, and accumulation of facts has been steady, with occasional punctuation by scientific upheavals that have reoriented thinking and opened new directions for exploration. To accommodate the expanded body of knowledge and its conceptual framework requires four volumes instead of the three volumes originally planned.

The increase in content, the new direction, and the broader horizons are reflected in the title of this section. The 1964–1965 edition was simply designated *Respiration*; this edition is entitled *The Respiratory System*. This change is a reminder of the complexity, organization, and integration that make respiration possible. Other parts of the body have the same characteristics, but probably in no other component are these characteristics so striking because of the phasic nature of the breathing process, the automatic adjustments of breathing to changing metabolic states, and the many provisions for interruptions in the phasic process by episodic events, such as eating, talking, coughing, straining, and vomiting.

One fruitful way to regard the living organism is to view it as a system of interrelated functional hierarchies. From this vantage a hierarchy or its components can be probed in great detail, always within the larger framework of the whole animal. In this section, one large hierarchy—the respiratory system—and its component parts are put under the microscope, leaving other large and related units, such as the circulatory system, to be considered elsewhere.

The hierarchical approach has broad implications. First, the predominant concern is with function rather than anatomy; boundaries, orderliness, and self-containment are more a matter of feedback mechanisms than of structural restraints. Second, within the framework of the whole body a hierarchy may be involved in more than one function; a single hierarchy (such as the arachidonic acid cascade) generates some substances that act locally and others that behave as circulating hormones and exert their biological effects in remote corners of the body. Third, large systems (such as the respiratory and circulatory systems) are closely interlinked and interdependent; as a rule the larger systems modulate the activities of smaller hierarchies within them. Fourth, at the level of the cell and organelle, hierarchies are exceedingly minute, yet they retain complexity and integration as cardinal features; in this realm, structure gives way to molecular interactions as the basis for function. Finally, the living body could not operate effectively as a conglomeration of hierarchies without sophisticated methods for information transfer to ensure integrated performance.

Currently much physiological experimentation is concerned with information transfer and control mechanisms. Not very long ago this aspect of physiology dealt almost exclusively with nerves and neurohumoral transmitters. Visionaries such as Bernard, Cannon, Barcroft, Henderson, and Sherrington constructed grand schemes to explain the complicated biological interplays that automatically adjust the body at rest, during exercise, on exposure to unsettling environments, and during the fight-or-flight reaction. Their legacy is a body of monumental concepts epitomized by rubrics such as "Homeostasis," "The Architecture of Physiologic Function," and "The Wisdom of the Body."

Although the integrated responses of the whole body continue to be intensely researched, within the hierarchies of the body there is apparently much more to information transfer than nerves, neurohumoral substances, and feedback mechanisms. Individual cells could not do their job without self-replenishing receptors at their surfaces for signal transduction, which triggers biochemical events that activate and regulate the activities of the cells. Endothelial cells that line blood vessels communicate by elaborate biological machinery with smooth muscle cells in the vascular walls. Electrical stimuli conveyed by nerves link events at the cellular level with humors in the central nervous system. An elaborate system for maintaining acid-base balance ensures a background of stability in hydrogen ion concentration so that background noise does not interfere with message centers or media in a hierarchical system that relies so heavily on uninterrupted information transfer for its survival, operation, and propagation.

The respiratory system is currently being explored as a component of the entire organism and in terms of its constituent parts: the perspective of overall integration is exemplified by the exploration of the control of breathing; that of molecular biology is exemplified by the study of macromolecular transport across special domains on the plasma membrane of the pulmonary capillary endothelial cell. The broad sweep of research on the respiratory system and its components and the ways in which the system relates to other systems during rest, activity, stress, and adaptation are the mainstays of this *Handbook* section.

For convenience the section has been subdivided into four volumes: *Circulation and Nonrespiratory Functions*, *Control of Breathing*, *Mechanics of Breathing*, and *Gas Exchange*. The hierarchies vary from chapter to chapter in size, complexity, regulatory mechanisms, and machinery for information transfer. The volumes devoted to the circulation and nonrespiratory functions of the lungs and gas exchange give high priority to organization and operation at the cellular level. Those concerned with the control and mechanics of breathing are more inclined toward integrating mechanisms at the level of the whole body. Full understanding of the respiratory system requires reconciliation of its materials and design with its effectiveness in performance under ordinary and under trying conditions. No matter how meticulously and successfully each component of the system is probed, in the last analysis the responsibility of physiology is to restore the isolated component to its proper place in the operations of the respiratory system and to reconcile the respiratory system with the other inner workings of the entire organism.

My debt to the volume editors and authors is self-evident: without them there would be neither content, organization, nor style (in fact, no books). Less evident is my obligation to those in my organization, particularly Jayne Pickard, who managed—by prompting and cajoling authors and editors and by unremitting devotion to the cause—to ensure proper review in my office while maintaining an uninterrupted flow of manuscripts to the Society's publications office.

This was a large effort. One can only hope that the product lives up to the expectations and needs of the readers.

ALFRED P. FISHMAN
Section Editor

Preface

The previous edition of the *Handbook* section on respiration dealt primarily with the function of the lungs from the standpoint of traditional organ physiology. It included such familiar topics as lung volumes and ventilation, mechanical properties of the lungs and thorax, control of breathing, and respiratory gas exchange. This edition not only delves deeper into these aspects of respiratory physiology but also extends into the newer fields of respiratory biology. The broader sweep is exemplified by topics that had no previous counterparts: development and growth of the lungs, pulmonary circulation, pulmonary metabolism, and pulmonary defense mechanisms.

In large measure the extension into respiratory biology was effected by amalgamating into respiratory physiology the concepts and tools of other disciplines. One reflection of this merger is the designation "structure-function," a byword in contemporary respiratory physiology. Although the idea of relating function to structure is traditional, the term has taken on new meaning as physiology and morphology have evolved. No longer does "structure-function" merely signify a collaboration between morphologists and physiologists. It now also implies serious efforts to make comparative measurements under comparable conditions. This requirement is critical for the lungs, an inflatable organ, where distending and interstitial pressures strongly influence microscopic and macroscopic appearances.

Another refinement in anatomical approach of great significance to physiologists is the increasing reliance on morphometry. This emphasis on quantification, sampling, and reconstruction has added new dimensions to correlations between physiological behavior and anatomical structure. The fruitfulness of this approach is evident in the first two chapters of this volume, which deal with lung development and growth and lung cell biology.

The morphologic underpinnings of physiology are also evident in chapters 3 and 4, which deal with both pulmonary circulation and pulmonary interstitial spaces and lymphatics. For example, the pore theory of transcapillary exchange of macromolecules is a physiological concept seeking anatomical explanations. However, attempts to explain the movement of macromolecules through the interstitial space after traversing the alveolar-capillary barrier have made it increasingly clear that the full explanation cannot be found in anatomy. Macromolecular progress through the interstitium depends as much on biochemical interplay with the ground substance as on preformed channels. Indeed, lessons from cell biology indicate that function at the molecular level is more firmly anchored in biochemical events than in anatomical conduits, barriers, or sluices.

Ultrastructure and biochemistry permeate chapters 5–12, which deal with the metabolism of lung cells and the metabolic functions of the lungs. Chapters 5–7 describe oxygen utilization, intermediary metabolism, and protein synthesis by the lung. Chapters 8–12 turn to the special metabolic functions of the lungs: surfactant turnover, the handling of biologically active amines and peptides, and the involvement of the lungs in processing prostaglandins and lipoproteins. The distinction between substances produced within the lungs that act locally and others that act afar is of great physiological interest in these chapters. Also noteworthy is the recurring theme that without the intervention of the metabolically active expanse of pulmonary capillary endothelium at the gateway to the systemic circulation, vital organs (such as the brain and heart) would constantly face the threat of noxious agents returning to the heart from the peripheral tissues and of fluctuating levels of bioactive materials leaving the liver. Finally, these chapters on pulmonary metabolism place new significance on the composition of arterial blood: just as concentrations and partial pressures of the respiratory gases can be used to judge the overall efficiency of the lungs as a gas-exchanging organ, so also levels of biologically active materials can be used to judge the nonrespiratory functions of the lungs.

The final five chapters of this volume are concerned with the pulmonary defense mechanisms, from secretions and cilia in the conducting airways to macrophages in the respiratory tract. In these chapters, ultrastructure and molecular biology intertwine with physiological concepts of integration and regulation. Chapters 16 and 17 deal with events in the bloodstream: coagulation, fibrinolysis, and interactions between formed elements of the blood and the endothelial lining. In these chapters, the span of structure-function enlarges to draw on the lessons of cell biology, molecular genetics, and immunology.

Preoccupation with the individual components of the respiratory system should not obscure the dominant and pervasive concern of physiology with regulatory mechanisms. Feedback linkages operate endlessly and automatically; these linkages are often disclosed only by experimental or pathological disruptions of a predetermined sequence. Disturbances leading to oxygen toxicity highlight the self-adjusting mechanisms that enable life on earth in an oxygen-rich environment; experimental and clinical pulmonary edemas underscore normal regulatory mechanisms responsible for water exchange in the lungs; and abnormal behavior of cilia sheds light on normal pulmonary defense mechanisms. Undoubtedly the control mechanisms operating at the cellular level that are responsible for normal respiratory performance will occupy a central position in physiological research during the next decade. This line of research will continue to draw heavily on structure-function relationships for meaningful models and new lines of investigation. However, as respiratory physiology moves inevitably toward cell biology and integrative biology, the traditional meanings of structure and function will change and the boundaries of conventional physiology and other scientific disciplines—notably biochemistry, biophysics, molecular biology, pharmacology, and cell biology—will grow increasingly blurred.

ALFRED P. FISHMAN
ARON B. FISHER

Symbols and Abbreviations

In the summer of 1977 at the International Union of Physiological Sciences Congress in Paris, the Commission on Respiratory Physiology established a committee to improve the glossary of terms and symbols used in respiratory physiology. Shortly thereafter the American Physiological Society decided to publish the new *Handbook* series on respiratory physiology. To incorporate the IUPS symbols into these books, a committee consisting of one of the editors of each *Handbook* was established, namely Leon E. Farhi, Alfred P. Fishman, Peter T. Macklem (chairman), and Jonathan H. Widdicombe, along with Curt von Euler and Peter Scheid. The symbols and abbreviations chosen by this committee were approved by the Commission on Respiratory Physiology at the Budapest Congress in 1980 and subsequently approved for publication in the *Handbook of Physiology* by the Publications Committee of the American Physiological Society.

SYMBOLS IN RESPIRATORY PHYSIOLOGY

Main Symbols

The main symbol indicates the nature of the variable and usually appears in the form of a single large capital letter. More rarely it is denoted by a Greek letter, a lowercase letter, or a combination of capital and lowercase letters. Exceptions are the subdivisions of lung volume and symbols for measurements of forced respiratory maneuvers for which accepted usage has been followed.

The main symbol can be modified by a character that appears over the symbol itself (bar for a mean or average value, single dot for the first time derivative, two dots for the second time derivative).

Modifiers

Main symbols are further clarified by the addition of one or more modifiers, usually small capitals for the gas phase, standard chemical symbols for the chemical species, and lowercase letters in most other instances. Modifiers denote locations, anatomic structures, media in which the measurements are made, respiration phases, types of resistance to motion, chemical species, and so forth. The first modifier appears directly after the main symbol. Subsequent modifiers are either separated from the other modifiers by commas or more rarely appear as subscripts. Chemical species always appear as subscripts and follow all other modifiers used (the only exception is the symbol for capacity of a gas). Modifiers denoting time (t or 1.0 s) or numerical designations (0, 1, 2, 3, ...) appear as subscripts.

The symbols have been divided into three main groups: *1*) respiratory mechanics, *2*) alveolar gas exchange and pulmonary circulation, and *3*) control of breathing. Rather than introduce entirely new symbols to replace those that have gained widespread acceptance, the committee that prepared this guide feels that greater clarity is achieved by some symbols having different meanings and some words more than one symbol. Thus $\dot{V}$ in respiratory mechanics usually means flow, whereas in gas exchange it usually means ventilation. The symbol C can have one of three meanings: compliance in mechanics of breathing, capacity in the subdivisions of lung volume, and concentration in a liquid in gas exchange. In gas exchange, capacity is represented by the symbol Cap. The symbol R signifies respiratory exchange ratio or resistance. The meaning of the symbols should be clearly understood from the context. (*See* endpapers.)

PETER T. MACKLEM

Contents

1. Development and growth of the human lung
   PETER H. BURRI 1
2. Lung cell biology
   EWALD R. WEIBEL 47
3. Pulmonary circulation
   ALFRED P. FISHMAN 93
4. Pulmonary interstitial spaces and lymphatics
   AUBREY E. TAYLOR
   JAMES C. PARKER 167
5. Oxygen utilization and toxicity in the lungs
   ARON B. FISHER
   HENRY J. FORMAN 231
6. Glucose and intermediary metabolism of the lungs
   DONALD F. TIERNEY
   STEPHEN L. YOUNG 255
7. Protein turnover in the lungs
   DONALD MASSARO 277
8. Lipid synthesis and surfactant turnover in the lungs
   RICHARD J. KING
   JOHN A. CLEMENTS 309
9. 5-Hydroxytryptamine and other amines in the lungs
   ALAIN F. JUNOD 337
10. Processing of angiotensin and other peptides by the lungs
    UNA S. RYAN 351
11. Lung metabolism of eicosanoids: prostaglandins, prostacyclin, thromboxane, and leukotrienes
    Y. S. BAKHLE
    SERGIO H. FERREIRA 365
12. Lipoproteins and lipoprotein lipase
    MARGIT HAMOSH
    PAUL HAMOSH 387
13. Regulation of airway secretions, ion transport, and water movement
    JAY A. NADEL
    JONATHAN H. WIDDICOMBE
    ANTHONY C. PEATFIELD 419
14. Macrophages in the respiratory tract
    JOSEPH D. BRAIN 447
15. Function-structure correlations in cilia from mammalian respiratory tract
    PETER SATIR
    ELLEN ROTER DIRKSEN 473
16. Blood coagulation and fibrinolysis
    ROBERT W. COLMAN
    ANDREI Z. BUDZYNSKI 495
17. Platelet–blood vessel interactions
    RUSSELL ROSS
    STEPHEN M. SCHWARTZ 545

Index 561

CHAPTER 1

Development and growth of the human lung

PETER H. BURRI | *Department of Anatomy, University of Berne, Berne, Switzerland*

CHAPTER CONTENTS

Lung Morphology
    Gas-exchange region
    Airways
    Blood vessels
Structural Development of the Human Lung
    Embryonic development
        Airways
        Blood vessels
    Fetal period
        Pseudoglandular stage
        Canalicular stage
        Terminal sac stage
    Postnatal development of respiratory tissue—alveolar stage
        Experimental studies
        Observations in the human lung
Growth of the Lung
    Normal growth
        Postnatal growth of respiratory tissue
        Postnatal growth of conducting airways and blood vessels in the human lung
    Adaptive growth of gas-exchange apparatus
        General considerations
        Exposure to hypoxia
        Increased oxygen consumption
        Lung tissue resection
        Structural features of adaptive response
Final Dimensions of the Human Lung
Development of Pulmonary Surfactant System
    Historical background and function of pulmonary surfactant
    Biochemistry of pulmonary surfactant
        Composition
        Pathways of phosphatidylcholine and phosphatidylglycerol synthesis in the adult and fetal lung
        Surfactant turnover
    Type II cells and regulation of surfactant production
        Lamellar bodies and surfactant production
        Influence of corticosteroid hormones
        Influence of thyroid hormones

AT BIRTH THE LUNG IS SUDDENLY in charge of the O_2 supply for the organism. Fetal lung development is therefore programmed so that at this crucial moment the organ reaches a determined degree of morphological, physiological, and biochemical maturity. This does not mean, however, that lung development is complete at birth. The newborn lung undergoes further steps of differentiation to reach maturity.

The major function of the lung is gas exchange. In the last decade, however, it has been realized that this is not the only contribution of this organ to the general function of the organism. The lung fulfills important metabolic tasks, but its architecture is conceived to primarily accomplish the respiratory function. In other words, the leitmotiv of the structural design of the lung is the O_2 supply of the organism. This holds also for its morphogenesis. Therefore this chapter emphasizes the development of the lung as a respiratory organ.

For a better understanding of the developmental steps, one must first present the normal pulmonary architecture, the end result of pulmonary differentiation. A more detailed and comprehensive analysis of the mature lung and its cells is presented in the chapter by Weibel in this *Handbook*.

The organization of the lung is largely determined by the hierarchy of airways and blood vessels. Their function is dual: *1*) they contain and retain the two media, air and blood, in distinct compartments throughout the lung; and *2*) their wall structure is modified toward the periphery so that gases can rapidly diffuse between the two media. According to this double function (especially for the airways) the organ can be divided into three zones (Fig. 1). The conductive zone guides air from the trachea toward the sites of gas exchange. The respiratory zone is at the distal end of the airway tree where diffusion largely prevails. The transitional zone between these two areas contains conducting channels so intimately related to alveoli and capillaries that functionally they cannot be separated from the respiratory zone. Therefore the transitional and respiratory zones together make up the gas-exchange region of the lung, also called the pulmonary parenchyma.

LUNG MORPHOLOGY

Gas-Exchange Region

The gas-exchange region comprises three compartments: air, blood, and tissue. The latter provides a relatively stable supporting framework in which the two dynamic systems are enclosed; it ensures on the one hand a clear separation of air and blood and on the other hand a close enough contact between them to allow for rapid exchange of gases. For this function

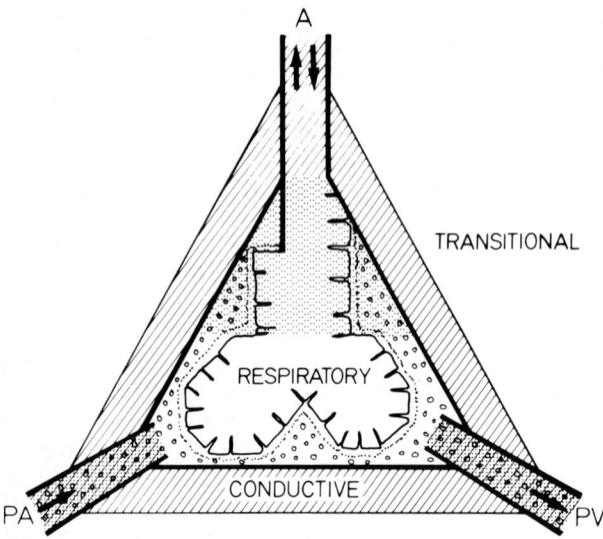

FIG. 1. Lung with 3 zones: conductive, transitional, and respiratory. A, airways; PA, pulmonary artery; PV, pulmonary vein.

140 m² of surface area are available in the mature lung. The respiratory portion of the lung resembles a sponge in structure and consistency and is made of delicate tissue septa containing capillaries. The septa subdivide the air spaces into morphological units, the alveoli (Fig. 2), that, considering their shape and dense packing, can be compared with the cells of a honeycomb. They are arranged around air-supplying channels, the alveolar ducts and alveolar sacs, and open into them (Fig. 3). The interalveolar septum is a tissue sheet covered on both sides by an epithelium and containing a dense capillary network. The latter is interlaced with a delicate skeleton of connective tissue fibers, forming a three-dimensional continuum throughout the lungs [Fig. 4; (371)]. Circular apertures (pores of Kohn or interalveolar pores) that are normally bridged (in vivo and in specimens fixed by vascular perfusion) by surfactant material (144) are commonly found in the interalveolar walls. In human alveoli fixed through the airways the weighted average number of pores was 9.2 per exposed alveolar surface, with a weighted mean pore diameter of 8.1 µm. In material fixed by vascular perfusion only 2 pores per alveolus were found open, each with a diameter of ~7 µm (336). At the free margins of the septa the fiber bundles are usually reinforced (Figs. 2 and 3) and may be associated with some smooth muscle cells to form the entrance rings of the alveolar mouths (351). The connective tissue framework also contains fibroblasts that are responsible for the formation and maintenance of the fibrous skeleton (Fig. 5). They also have contractile filaments and were considered to be potential regulators of capillary blood flow (202), according to the sheet-flow model of Fung and Sobin (131). However, Weibel and Bachofen (368) described these cells as anchoring together the lining epithelia of both sides or less frequently the epithelium to the capillary wall. Therefore they proposed that these myofibroblasts might restrict the compliance of the interstitial space and prevent the accumulation of fluid in the interalveolar septum. From the recent demonstration that they are coupled to each other by gap junctions, one can assume that they could behave as a functional syncytium (24). The interstitial space of the alveolar walls seems to be a compartment that is well secured against fluid accumulation. At the places of contact between the alveolar and extra-alveolar connective tissue spaces, exchange of fluid between the perivascular or peribronchial cuffs and the interstitium of the interalveolar septa seems to be restricted by specially placed interstitial cells (142).

Blood flowing through the capillaries intimately contacts the air of two adjacent alveoli, due to the special design of the septum. This tends to keep the air-blood barrier as thin as possible (0.3–0.6 µm over large parts) by hiding away the thicker barrier portions (e.g., epithelial type II cells) in clefts or niches

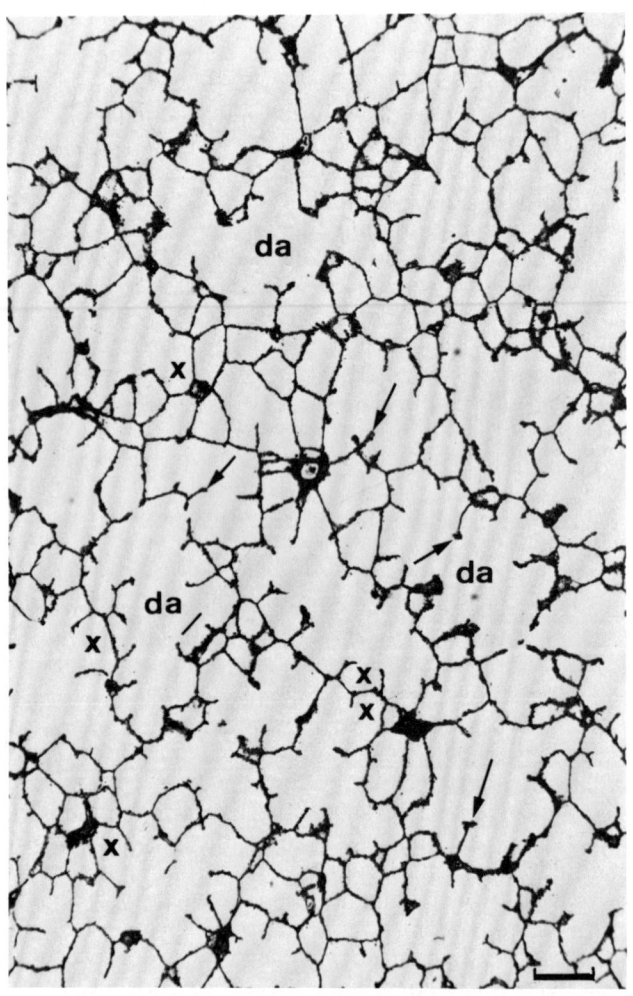

FIG. 2. Light micrograph of gas-exchanging parenchyma of adult human lung. Delicate tissue framework delineates air spaces; alveoli (x) open into alveolar ducts (da). Note sporadically thickened entrance rings (arrows). Scale, 200 µm; × 41.

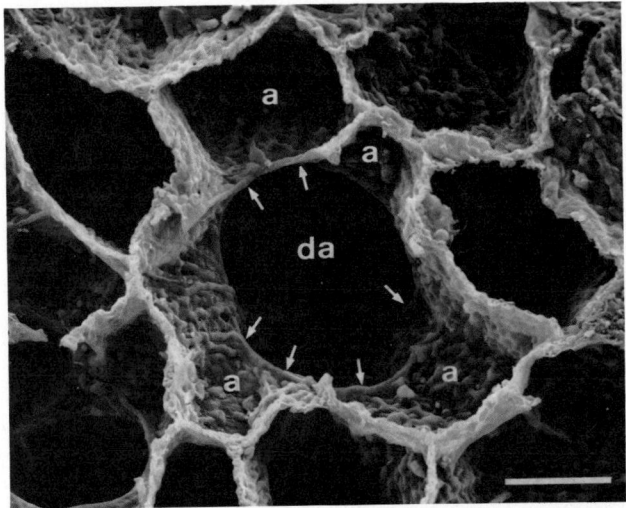

FIG. 3. Scanning electron micrograph of alveoli (*a*) arrangement around alveolar duct (*da*) of adult human lung. Capillary relief of interalveolar septa clearly visible due to fixation by instillation of glutaraldehyde into airways. Note alveolar entrance ring (*arrows*). Scale, 100 μm; × 150.

between the capillary segments. Morphologically the air-blood barrier is composed of four elements. Three of them form the tissue barrier: the epithelium, interstitium, and endothelium; the fourth one is a thin extracellular aqueous film carrying the surface-active material called pulmonary surfactant. Fixation by intratracheal instillation does not preserve the surfactant layer; perfusion is generally needed to fix it in situ (143, 369). Its morphological appearance may be polymorphic. Usually it consists of *1*) a fluid pool of moderate electron density, the hypophase that smoothes the pits and crevasses of the alveolar surface and *2*) an osmiophilic lining layer at the air-liquid interface (369, 370). Within the air spaces the surface-active material can also take the form of tubular myelin, osmiophilic lamellae arranged like a fingerprint or a filigree (372, 375). Sanders and co-workers (306) recently were able to directly prove that tubular myelin originated from the intracellular lamellar bodies by using refined procedures to isolate lamellar bodies.

Figure 6 illustrates the structure of the gas-exchange barrier at the functionally most efficient sites. It is extremely thin because both epithelial and endothelial cells form very flat cytoplasmic extensions and because the interstitial layer is reduced to its simplest expression, the apparently fused epithelial and endothelial basement laminae. Huang (191) recently showed, however, that the two basement laminae represent independent scaffold systems that retain their structural entity throughout the lung and hence do not really fuse where they merge. The epithelium of the gas-exchange region forms a continuous layer coating the septa. The major part of the alveolar surface [93%; (84)] is covered by a thin, squamous cell layer, the so-called type I pulmonary epithelial cells (Fig. 7*A*). Their thin cytoplasmic extensions reach far from the cell body even into neighboring alveoli, giving rise to the nonnucleated plates of the era before the electron microscope. Their complex topological properties have been elucidated (364) and may be the very practical reason why these cells probably do not divide.

The remaining small percentage of the gas-exchange surface is covered by the much smaller but more numerous granular pneumocytes or type II epithelial cells, which are typically located in niches (depressions) between capillaries (Fig.7*B*). Their free surface has short microvilli, but their most characteristic features are typical lamellated granular inclusions (lamellated or lamellar bodies), which represent the intracellular storage form of surface-active phospholipids (143). Type II cells are currently considered to represent the proliferative cells of the alveolar epithelium. After epithelial damage with cell desquamation, they were found to divide and subsequently transform into type I cells (14, 116, 366).

A rare, third cell type, the alveolar brush cell, has been described in the alveolar septum of rat lung (170, 248, 256). It has a small free surface covered with a densely packed group of squat cylindrical microvilli, thick bundles of microfibrils traversing the cytoplasm,

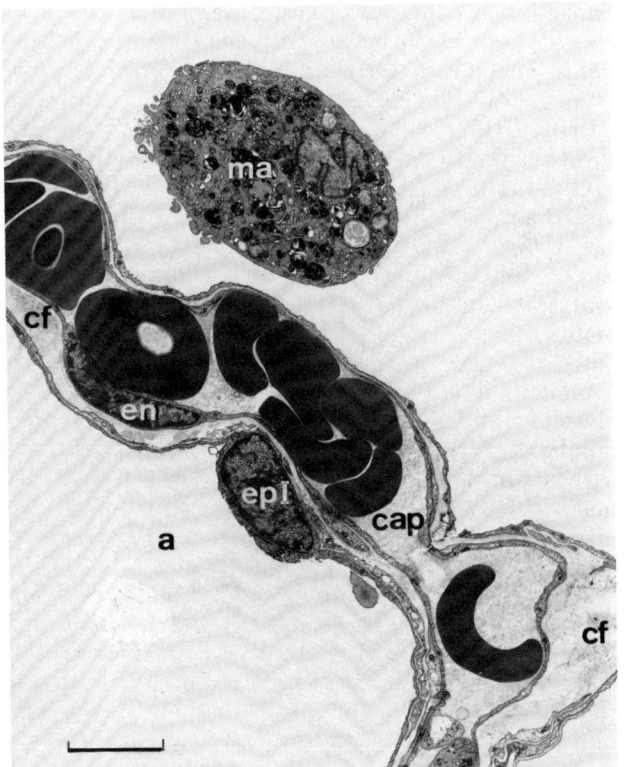

FIG. 4. Electron micrograph of portion of interalveolar septum of adult human lung. Pulmonary capillary (*cap*) containing plasma and erythrocytes interlaced with connective tissue fibers (*cf*). *a*, Alveolar space; *epI*, nucleus of epithelial type I cell; *en*, nucleus of endothelial cell; *ma*, alveolar macrophage. Scale, 5 μm; × 2,550.

and β-glycogen particles; it lacks lamellated bodies. In humans these brush cells have not been seen at the alveolar level; however, they were observed in the large airways (295, 358). In the rat they are easily found in the transitional regions between conducting and respiratory airways (Fig. 8). After treatment with bleomycin, which induces interstitial pneumonia, their number increases at all levels of the airways, including the alveolar wall (170). They seem to occur also in some other organs, e.g., the gallbladder, submaxillary gland, or rectum [for refs. see Luciano et al. (247) and Meyrick and Reid (258)]. Nerve fibers have been found close to brush cells in rat trachea, and it has therefore been suggested that they might represent a kind of receptor cell (247); however, no convincing evidence has been presented. Unmyelinated nerve fibers are rarely encountered in the interalveolar wall, although physiological studies suggest their presence (280). Meyrick and Reid (257) found a few axons in the alveolar septum of the rat. In mice, however, nerves were regularly seen in all examined samples of 18 lungs (193). Two types of nerve endings were observed: an enlarged terminal with many small mitochondria, located in the interstitium or related to type I cells, and a second one lying near type II pneumocytes and

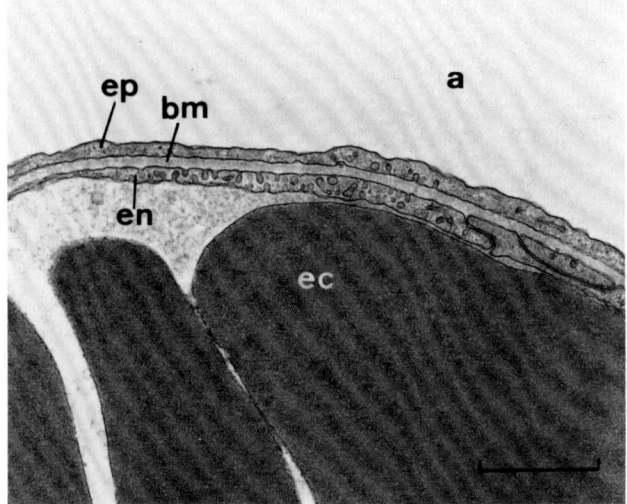

FIG. 6. Electron micrograph of thin portion of air-blood barrier of human lung showing 3-layered structure with epithelium (*ep*), basement membrane (*bm*), and endothelium (*en*). *a*, Alveolar space; *ec*, erythrocyte. Scale, 1 μm; × 16,000.

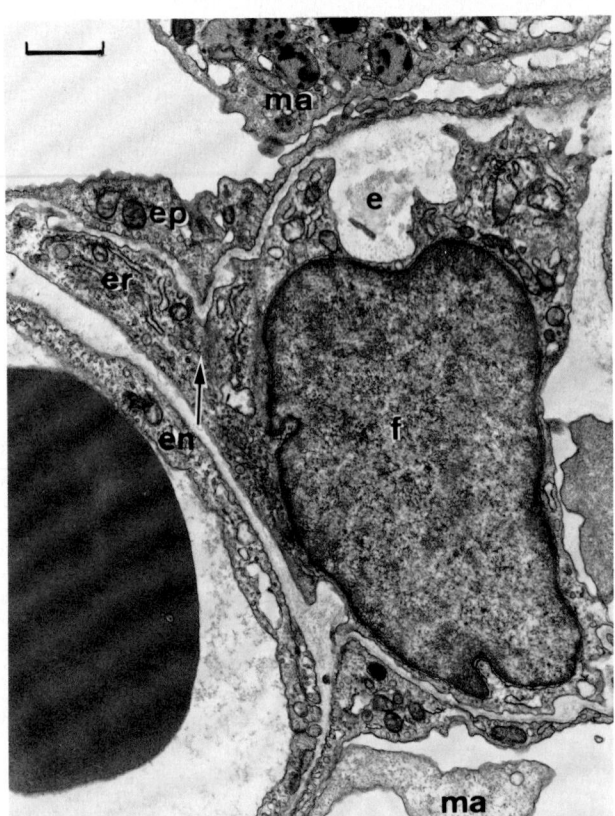

FIG. 5. Electron micrograph of fibroblast (*f*) in human interalveolar septum. Cell contains rough endoplasmic reticulum (*er*) as sign of active protein synthesis. In a bay elastic fibers (*e*) and collagen fibrils have been deposited. Note intracytoplasmic filaments anchoring epithelium (*arrow*). *ep*, Epithelial type I cell; *en*, endothelial cell; *ma*, macrophage. Scale, 1 μm; × 10,000.

containing large, dense-core vesicles. The authors speculated that the first type could correspond to the juxtacapillary (type J) receptors of Paintal (280) and the second one to an autonomic efference to type II cells. It is not known whether the mouse represents a special case or whether nerve fibers have often been missed in other species.

Alveolar macrophages are found on top of the epithelium. In vivo these large cells (15–20 μm diam) creep around on the alveolar surface in the liquid layer (Figs. 7C and 9) and clean from the alveolar walls foreign material that may have reached the alveoli and debris originating from cell damage or normal cell death. Lung macrophages are derived from blood monocytes (350). They migrate from the capillary into the pulmonary interstitium, where they divide and mature before entering the alveoli (40, 41). Undoubtedly a fraction of the macrophage population is normally able to divide within the alveoli; these cells, however, seem to be immature and their number is very low. It appears unlikely that they are responsible for the rapid proliferation of macrophages observed under phagocytotic stress, like the instillation into the airways of carbon particles (5).

Lung capillaries are lined by a continuous endothelium very similar to that in other parts of the body. Like type I epithelial cells, endothelial cells form very thin cytoplasmic sheets that help greatly to keep the air-blood barrier thin. Their cytoplasm is unobtrusive and contains only very few organelles, mostly in the perikaryon (Fig. 7D). Despite their paucity in organelles, the pulmonary endothelial cells are not limited to the membrane or barrier function for either gas or fluid and solute exchange (182). They assume a large number of metabolic functions (201), as is discussed further in later chapters in this *Handbook*. The pul-

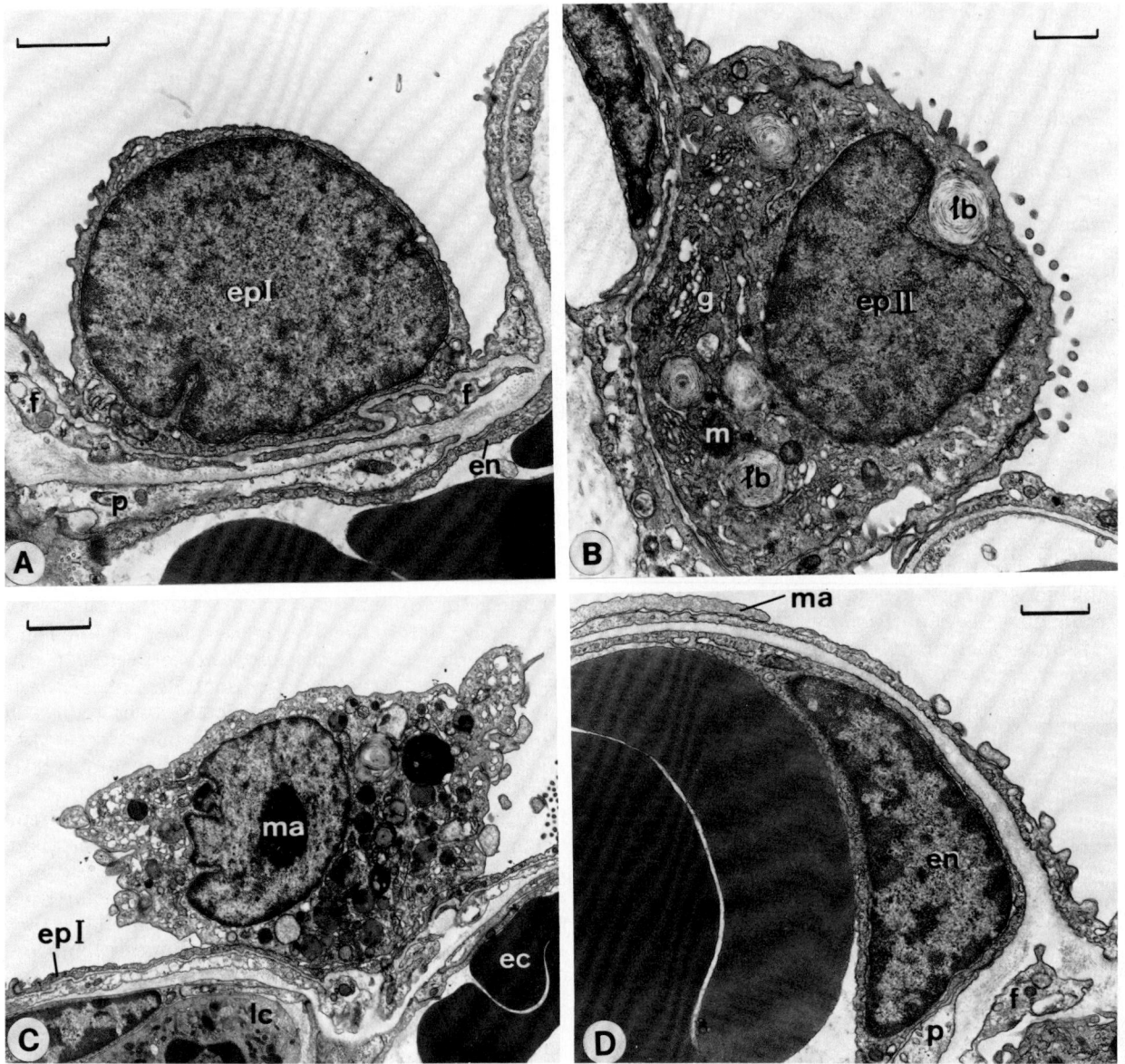

FIG. 7. *A*: electron micrograph of alveolar epithelial type I cell (*epI*) in human lung. Cell body consists merely of nucleus enclosed in very narrow cytoplasmic rim. Cell possesses long and thin cytoplasmic extensions. *en*, Endothelium; *f*, cytoplasmic process of fibroblast; *p*, process of pericyte. Scale, 2 μm; × 7,200. *B*: electron micrograph of alveolar epithelial type II cell (*epII*) in human lung. Cell edges are covered by type I cell extensions; free surface shows short microvilli. In cytoplasm, prominent Golgi apparatus (*g*), few small mitochondria (*m*), and characteristic lamellar bodies (*lb*). Scale, 1 μm; × 9,300. *C*: electron micrograph of alveolar macrophage (*ma*) attached to underlying epithelium of type I cell (*epI*) in human lung. In septum, capillaries with erythrocytes (*ec*) and a leukocyte (*lc*). Scale, 2 μm; × 4,500. *D*: electron micrograph of capillary endothelial cell (*en*) in human lung. As in epithelial type I cells, nucleus is enclosed in thin cytoplasmic rim with very few organelles. On one side, cell body connects neighboring cell with junction; on the other side it tapers into thin cytoplasmic process. *f*, Cytoplasmic process of fibroblast; *p*, pericytic process; *ma*, pseudopodium of macrophage. Scale, 1 μm; × 10,000.

monary capillaries are provided with pericytes (367). Their frequency seems to depend on the size of the lung; the smaller the lung, the rarer the pericytes. In the human lung, processes of pericytes are regularly observed (Fig. 7A, D).

Airways

The gas-exchanging function of the lung periphery would be meaningless if the lungs were not replenished continuously with air (i.e., ventilated) and if the O$_2$

taken up into the blood were not carried away to the sites of consumption (i.e., if lung capillaries were not continuously perfused). The airway system plays a dominant role during lung development; the degree of its morphological differentiation is used as a reference parameter for the classification of pulmonary development into distinct stages. Therefore it is necessary to review briefly the present concepts on the structural arrangement of the airway tree in the adult human lung.

The works of Weibel (360) and Horsfield and Cumming (187, 188) serve as a basis for the following general description. As shown in Figure 1, the airways can be divided into three portions: the proximal, purely conducting airways; the peripheral gas-exchanging or respiratory airways; and in between, the transitional passage where both functions merge. The conducting airways extend from the trachea, designated as generation zero, down to the terminal bronchioles, airways ~0.7–1 mm in diameter that correspond on average to generation 16 of the airway tree (Fig. 10). From here toward the periphery the gas-exchange function becomes gradually more important. The straight walls of the airway tubes are more and more frequently interrupted by alveolar outpouchings, and a growing portion of their lining is formed by a thin air-blood barrier. Therefore the first segments of these transitional airways are called respiratory bronchioles; they occupy on the average three generations in the airway tree. When only alveoli are found to line the airways, the respiratory function predominates largely and the segments are called alveolar ducts. After about three generations of alveolar ducts the airway system ends blindly with the alveolar sacs representing, on average, generation 23.

Clearly, the airway tree described terribly oversim-

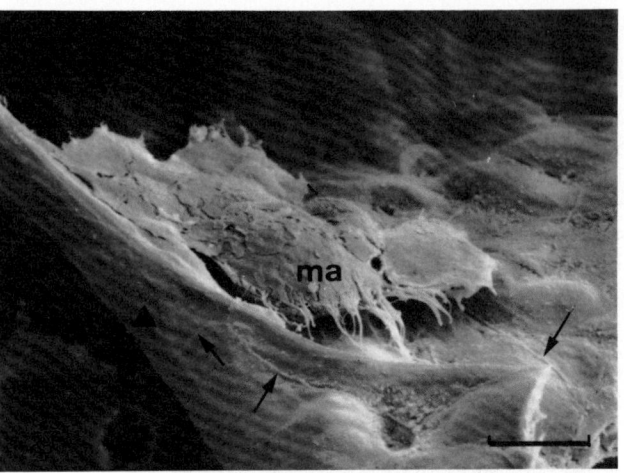

FIG. 9. Scanning electron micrograph of human alveolar macrophage (*ma*) close to edge of alveolar entrance ring (▲) and extending numerous filopodia. Note cell borders of epithelial type I cells (*arrows*). Scale, 1 µm; × 1,400.

plifies the real situation. The branching is in fact so complex and probably also variable that it cannot exactly be described. Therefore model assumptions are a prerequisite for the analysis of the design and function of this structure. It is generally accepted that the human lung branches according to the rules of irregular dichotomy. This means that each branch gives rise to two daughter branches that may greatly vary in length and diameter. Weibel (360) confirmed the irregular dichotomy based on the analysis of a single human lung. However, in addition to presenting an irregular dichotomy model, he also fitted his measurements to a symmetric branching pattern representing a regularized dichotomy. To this end Weibel applied the mean values of the measured lengths and diameters to each generation. Because of its accessibility to calculations, this so-called model A of Weibel has been used for theoretical and experimental work on airflow pattern (for review see ref. 288) and airway clearance (for reviews see refs. 190, 261). Another model, which is perhaps closer to reality because it takes into account the branching asymmetry (but is less easy to handle), has been worked out by Horsfield and Cumming (187). Applying analytical techniques employed by geographers to study river systems (378), they numbered the airways in reverse order, starting with generation zero at the lobular level and ending with generation 25 at the trachea. Asymmetry is taken care of by the possibility of a lower-ordered airway entering a higher-ordered one at any level, e.g., a tube of generation zero joining a tube of any order >1. This type of analysis has some advantages in the investigation of specific problems (187–189).

The structure of the airway wall at the different levels is best recapitulated by Figure 11. It explains how the fibrocartilaginous sheet of the trachea and bronchi is superseded by a simple peripheral connec-

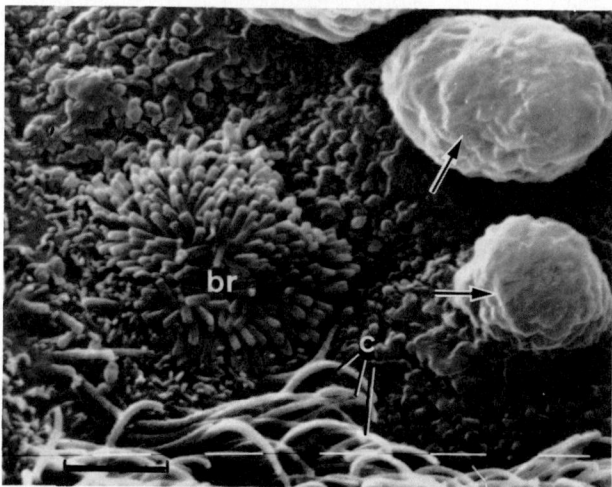

FIG. 8. Scanning electron micrograph of brush cell (*br*) in distal portion of rat terminal bronchiole. Numerous short microvilli are arranged like a bunch of flowers at top of cell. Neighboring cells are ciliated (*c*) or Clara cells (*arrows*). Scale, 2 µm; × 7,200. (Micrograph courtesy of G. Wandel.)

tive tissue layer and how the smooth muscle cells grouped in the wall at the backside of the trachea slowly form a distinct layer between mucosa and adventitia. The respiratory epithelium decreases in height toward the periphery (Fig. 11), and the frequent goblet cells are replaced at the bronchiolar level by the Clara cells. As opposed to the bronchus, the bronchiole is a small airway devoid of cartilage, seromucous glands, and goblet cells. Clara cells were a candidate for the production of the surface film or the hypophase of the pulmonary surfactant (92, 114, 269, 326) until this role was ascribed to the type II pneumocyte. Then this function was dropped and others proposed. It was suggested that Clara cells might produce the serouslike secretions forming the liquid layer of the airways in which the cilia beat (227, 258). It was also advanced that the secretions of Clara cells might participate in degradation of surfactant phospholipids (382). In addition to ciliated and Clara cells, brush cells and serous cells have been reported in the bronchioles (197). According to autoradiographic investigations by Evans and co-workers (115), the Clara cells represent (like the type II pneumocytes in the alveolar lining) the progenitor cells of the bronchiolar epithelium. After the cells of the terminal bronchioles were injured by NO_2 exposure the Clara cells were found to discharge their granules, synthesize DNA, and divide and

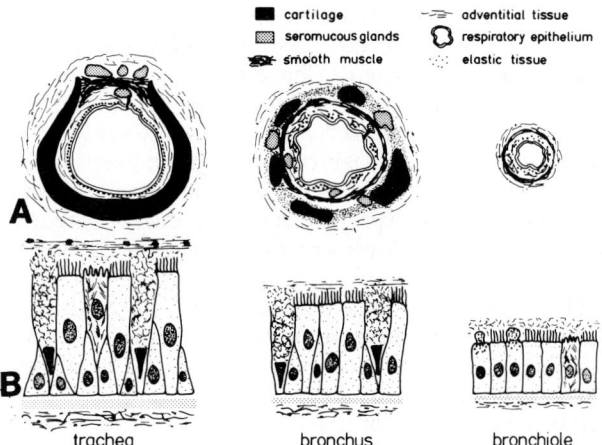

FIG. 11. Wall structure of large and small conducting airways (A) and their epithelial lining (B). B: basal cells, ciliated cells, goblet cells, and brush cell in trachea and bronchus. In bronchiole, goblet cells are replaced by Clara cells. Mucous blanket carrying particles lies on top of epithelium.

mature through serous cells to Clara cells or alternatively to ciliated or brush cells.

Endocrine cells belonging to the amine precursor uptake and decarboxylation (APUD) system (285), called Kultschitsky cells (alternatively Feyrter, argyrophil, argentaffin, enterochromaffin, or clear cells), are dispersed throughout the airway epithelium. They are found in various mammals including humans, either as single cells or in groups named neuroepithelial bodies (90, 152, 232, 233). They contain dense-core vesicles showing morphological variations related to species. The function of these cells is still debated; the single cells could represent storage and secretion sites for serotonin (166), whereas a receptor function has been postulated for the neuroepithelial bodies (234). The view that brush cells, single endocrine cells, and neuroepithelial bodies are different entities has been challenged recently. Taira and Shibasaki (335) proposed that these cells may all represent various functional states of a single cell type that should be simply described as a nonciliated cell. They showed that in mouse tracheal epithelium these cells share the same ultrastructural characteristics.

A serous fluid topped by a blanket of sticky mucus carrying intercepted particles is found at the surface of the cellular lining of the airway. These are moved outwardly due to the synchronized rhythmic beat of the cilia in the serous layer (for reviews see refs. 315, 357).

Blood Vessels

The lung is a complex organ as regards blood circulation, with two distinct though not completely separate vascular systems: a low-pressure pulmonary system and a high-pressure bronchial system. Whereas the pulmonary circulation is responsible for the O_2

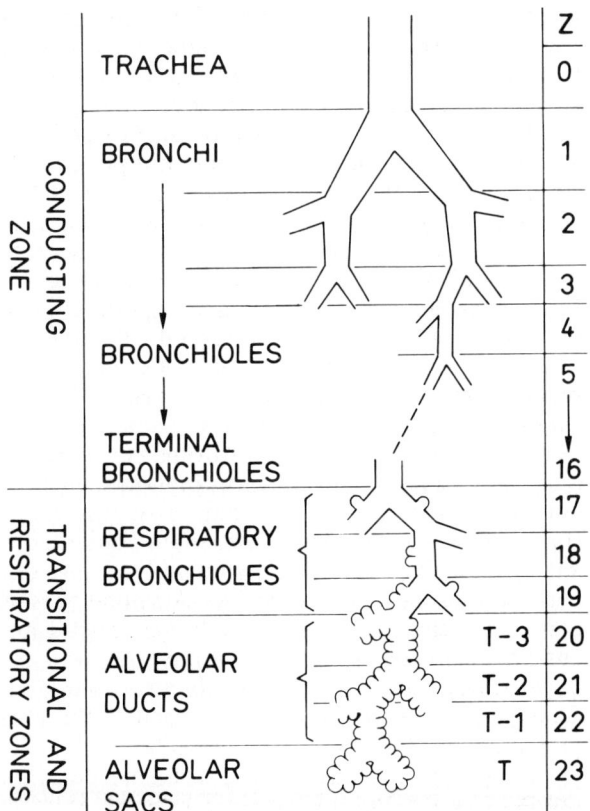

FIG. 10. Airway tree with subdivision in conducting, transitional, and respiratory zones. Z, branching order. [From Weibel (360).]

supply of the organism (vasa publica), the bronchial circulation assumes the maintenance of the walls of the bronchial tree and of the large pulmonary vessels, i.e., of the larger central structures of the lung (vasa privata). With a few exceptions the bronchial arteries do not reach the end of the conductive airway tree; they generally end several generations proximal to the terminal bronchioles by splitting into capillaries around the walls of bronchi and vessels that also supply adjacent air spaces (291). Their blood is then naturally collected by pulmonary veins. Structure and development of the two systems are completely different. Bronchial arteries develop late and their walls are typically systemic, i.e., comparable to other arteries of corresponding size in the body; pulmonary arteries develop early with the bronchial tree and generally branch with it. The branching pattern of the adult human pulmonary arteries has been analyzed by various techniques (105, 186, 317, 363, 372).

Because intravascular pressure determines the structure of the arterial walls, they are much flimsier than those in systemic vessels of corresponding size. Arterioles, a very important segment of the systemic vasculature, are virtually absent in the pulmonary circulation. The capillaries are much more compliant to an increase in blood pressure because they are practically exposed to air and not surrounded by supporting tissue. Pulmonary veins and venules are extremely thin walled (for review of pulmonary vascular structures see ref. 355).

Though the anlage of the two vascular systems is separate, they develop interconnections at many levels (359); these are summarized in Table 1. At the venous level the bronchial blood drains largely into the pulmonary veins and is responsible for a certain venous admixture to the arterialized blood.

STRUCTURAL DEVELOPMENT OF THE HUMAN LUNG

Pulmonary development proceeds through three distinct chronological periods: the embryonic, fetal, and postnatal. These periods encompass the phases of lung development commonly defined in the treatises on embryology. The phases are related to the morphological stages the airway system undergoes during development. Table 2 shows the timetable of pulmonary development and the temporal relationship be-

TABLE 1. *Anastomoses Between Blood Vessels of the Two Pulmonary Vascular Systems*

	Pulmonary Circulation	Bronchial Circulation	Bronchopulmonary Connections
Artery to artery	−	+	+
Vein to vein	−	+	+
Artery to vein	−	+	−

+, Existent; −, nonexistent. [Data from Weibel (359).]

TABLE 2. *Timetable of Pulmonary Development*

Stage	Prenatal Period — Embryonic	Prenatal Period — Fetal*	Postnatal Period
Embryonic	1–7 wk		
Pseudoglandular		5–17 wk	
Canalicular		16–26 wk	
Terminal sac (saccular)		24–38 wk	
Alveolar			36 wk or birth to 3–8 yr
Normal growth			Completion of alveolar formation to end of somatic growth

Because development is continuous, different stages overlap. * 5 wk to term.

tween the two classifications. Because lung development is continuous, it is evident that the descriptive stages of the morphological classification overlap.

Embryonic Development

AIRWAYS. In the human lung this period comprises the first 5–7 wk after fertilization (dating based on time of ovulation). In this phase embryoblastic cells segregate from trophoblastic ones and differentiate into the three germ layers. From the 4th wk to about the 8th wk the majority of the organs are laid down. The lung appears about day 26 as a ventral bud of the esophagus at the caudal end of the laryngotracheal sulci (Fig. 12). While the grooves deepen, ultimately joining each other and separating the prospective trachea from the esophagus, the bud rapidly divides into two branches that elongate and grow distally into the surrounding mesenchyme. These branches already represent the anlage of the two main bronchi. In this way the future airways continue growing, elongating and branching dichotomously, giving rise to a tubular tree preforming exactly the definitive branching pattern of the conductive airways. By day 37 these conducting airways are preformed to the lobar, by day 41 to the segmental, and by day 48 to the subsegmental bronchi. In agreement with the budding from the foregut, the epithelium of these tubes is derived from the endoderm; it is high columnar and rich in glycogen, which serves as energy source for the proliferation.

Experiments have shown that interaction between the endodermal epithelium and the mesodermal mesenchyme is needed for branching and cytodifferentiation. Indeed, removal of mesenchyme at the tip of a bud abolished further branching of the epithelial tube. Mesenchyme from the tip of a bud transplanted to the side of the prospective tracheal tube induced outgrowth of a further bronchial branch (8, 330, 374). In embryonic mouse lung, Bluemink and co-workers (37) observed intimate cell contacts between epithelial and mesenchymal cells along the distal outgrowths of the airway tubes. They thought that these contacts could trigger an influx of Ca^{2+} and hence induce cell con-

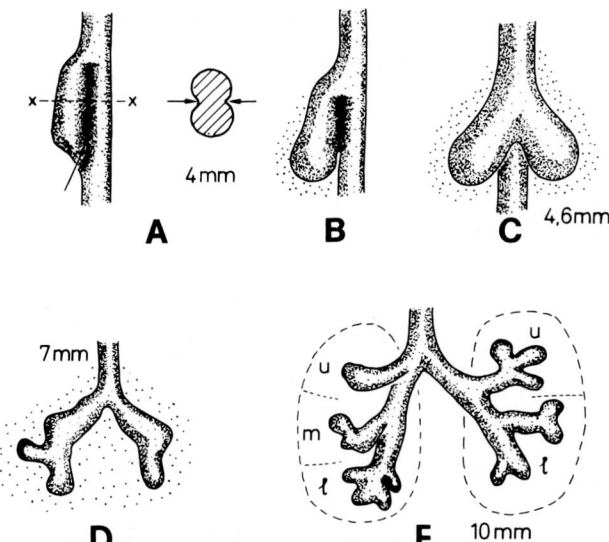

FIG. 12. Early development of human lung in side view (A, B) and ventral view (C–E); fetal age is indicated by crown-rump lengths. A: appearance of prospective lung as protrusion in foregut. B: formation of lung bud by distal-to-proximal segregation of prospective trachea from foregut by deepening of laryngotracheal grooves (arrows). C: dichotomous branching of lung bud, forming prospective main bronchi. D: prospective main bronchi growing into surrounding mesenchyme. E: left and right lungs formed with their lobar and partly segmental bronchi. u, Upper lobes; m, middle lobe; l, lower lobes.

traction; this again would initiate the bifurcation of the tubular sprouts. On the other hand, collagen in the interstitial space is apparently needed for proper branching morphogenesis, but inhibition of its extracellular cross-linking did not interfere with branching, a subtle difference (329). Taderera (334) showed that the type of lung mesoderm influenced the branching type of the bronchial buds; when chicken lung mesoderm was apposed to mouse lung epithelium the latter branched in avian fashion. Finally, the quantity of mesenchyme present around the epithelial tube seems to play a role in morphogenesis and cytodifferentiation of the epithelium (253). It has been advanced that branching of the growing epithelial tubes occurred because of the resistance to forward growth by the compressed mesenchyme. This mechanism would allow the filling in of bronchial divisions at places of lower resistance (196).

Toward the end of this first stage the mesenchymal cells around the trachea condense and differentiate focally to cartilage precursors. Distinct embryonic cartilage is found along the trachea at the end of the 7th wk (59).

BLOOD VESSELS. In this early organogenetic period the development of the pulmonary vasculature is closely linked to the development of the heart and the primitive systemic blood vessels. Figure 13A illustrates the origin of the pulmonary arteries. They branch off from the sixth pair of aortic arches and descend to the freshly formed lung buds, forming a vascular plexus in the surrounding mesenchyme. During further development the ventral (or proximal) part of the right aortic arch is incorporated into the right pulmonary artery, while the dorsal (or distal) part disappears. The dorsal part of the left arch, on the other hand, is maintained and eventually forms the ductus arteriosus connecting the pulmonary artery to the aortic arch. Due to differences in growth rates between the branches, the ventral part of the left sixth aorta forms the main pulmonary trunk that, after absorbing parts of the corresponding right aortic arch, gives rise to both the left and right pulmonary artery (Fig. 13B).

Pulmonary veins start to develop about the 5th wk as a single short evagination in the sinoatrial portion of the heart. This bud elongates, grows dorsad, divides many times, and finally connects to the pulmonary plexus, which at this time is already linked to systemic veins around the trachea and esophagus. When on the right side the sinus venosus is taken up into the right atrium of the heart, on the left side the wall of the single pulmonary vein stem is included into the left atrium. This process continues: the atrium progressively absorbs further branches of the venous tree, first the right and left lung veins and then the main tributaries of both lung veins. Eventually four separate pulmonary veins are found to open into the posterior part of the left atrium.

About day 50 the embryonic period is considered to terminate and merge into the fetal one. At this stage the lung very much resembles an acinar gland; this explains the term *pseudoglandular*, used to describe

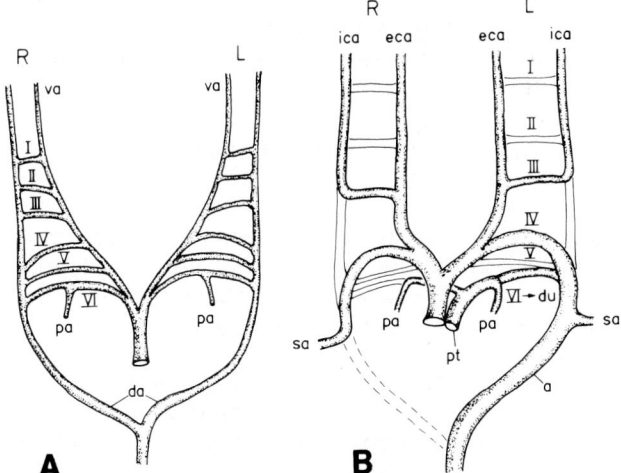

FIG. 13. Origin and development of pulmonary arteries. A: paired ventral (va) and dorsal (da) aortae interconnected by 6 pairs of aortic arches (I–VI). Pulmonary arteries (pa) branch off from 6th pair of aortic arches and connect to pulmonary mesenchyme. Diagram is simplified in the sense that the 6 aortic arches are never present simultaneously. B: further development of blood vessels. Some segments of arterial pathway regress and disappear (white areas), others develop further and show preferential growth (dotted areas). a, Aorta; du, ductus arteriosus; eca, external carotid artery; ica, internal carotid artery; pt, pulmonary trunk; sa, subclavian artery.

the following period of lung development, which lasts until about the 4th mo.

Fetal Period

During the fetal period proper, from the 5th–7th wk to term, the lung undergoes three phases of development to reach a degree of functional maturity, which enables the organism to survive at birth. The pseudoglandular, canalicular, and terminal sac stages are the successive periods, the terminology of which is purely descriptive.

PSEUDOGLANDULAR STAGE. Most publications describe this period as lasting from the 5th wk to the 16th wk (59, 178, 244). Boyden (45), whose careful reconstruction studies represent the most authoritative work on airway development performed so far, proposed the pseudoglandular period to start about day 52 and to last at least until the end of the 16th wk. He fixed the transition to the next stage at the moment when delineation of the pulmonary acinus first becomes visible (44). At this age the acinus is defined as the portion of lung parenchyma supplied by a prospective terminal bronchiole. Though this criterion provides a good reference point to assess the developmental stage of a given part of a lung, it does not allow one to extrapolate the age of the whole lung. Kikkawa and co-workers (210) found that upper lobes developed faster than lower lobes in the rabbit. A similar pattern was described in the lamb (309) and rhesus monkey (222). It is most likely that the lobes of the human lung also do not exhibit a synchronized differentiation pattern. In rabbits the difference was up to 1.5 days. With a total gestation period of 30 days for rabbits and 40 wk for humans, the difference in development between single lobes could amount to almost 2 wk in human development.

Through further growth and branching of the few bronchopulmonary segments present in the last week of the embryonic period, the future lung resembles more and more an acinar gland (Fig. 14). Growth and branching, however, are not uniform throughout this period. According to Bucher and Reid (59), growth is accelerated in the 10th–14th wk of gestation so that at the 16th wk there are 15–26 generations along the axial pathway, depending on the segment length. Virtually all the preacinar airways are formed at the end of the pseudoglandular stage, and at their uttermost periphery the prospective acinar airway portion has just been born. This presence of the prospective respiratory region observed by Boyden (45) seems to be supported by recent findings in mice. Using immunofluorescent techniques allowing identification of type II pneumocytes or their precursor cells, Ten Have-Opbroek (337, 338) found that the tubular tree of the pseudoglandular stage of mice contained fluorescent cells at the periphery. In other respects she strongly disagrees with present concepts of lung development.

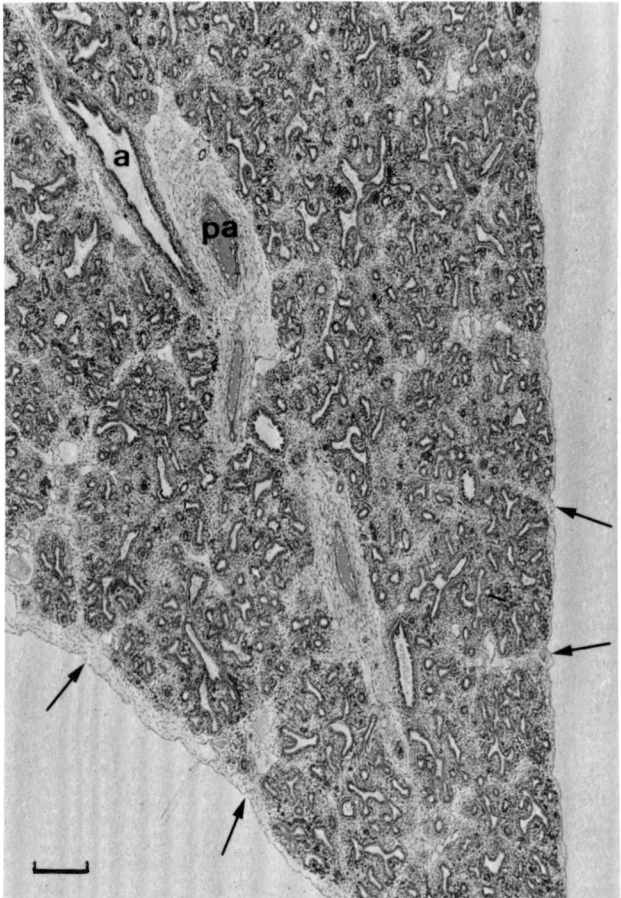

FIG. 14. Light micrograph of pseudoglandular stage of human fetal lung, gestational age ~15 wk. Airway tubes are embedded in loose mesenchyme and represent roughly the prospective conductive airways. From mesenchyme underlying the pleura, septa penetrate into pulmonary tissue (*arrows*); they contain venous vessels and delineate mostly prospective lobules. A broader layer of mesenchyme ensheathes larger aiways (*a*) and accompanying branches of pulmonary arteries (*pa*). Scale, 200 μm; × 35.

During this stage the airway tubes are lined proximally by high columnar cells that distally decrease in height and are simply cuboidal at the periphery. Their cytoplasm is poorly differentiated; it contains mitochondria, many free ribosomes, and a few cisternae of rough endoplasmic reticulum in addition to large patches of glycogen and some lipid droplets. The nuclei are oblong or spherical, depending on the shape of the cells, and contain one or two nucleoli. Mitotic figures are frequent. Early in this stage the first few scattered cilia can be observed in central airways (151). From the beginning the epithelium forms a closed cellular barrier because the cells are attached to each other by tight junctions. Small desmosomes bridging the intercellular cleft can easily be seen. Development of the junctional complexes between the pulmonary epithelial cells was beautifully demonstrated by Schneeberger (309) in the fetal lamb. She showed, as early as she was able to trace it (i.e., back to day 69 of gestation), that the epithelial lining was functionally tight. From day 76 the freeze-fracture morphology of the tight junctions was similar to that of full-term animals. From day 58 of gestation (i.e., ~2/3 of the pseudoglandular stage) to the end of the canalicular stage, gap junctions were associated with the tight junctions. After differentiation of the epithelium into type I and II cells they were no longer present (309), which could indicate that nexus are required for cellular differentiation.

In humans the epithelium of the proximal airways contains ciliated, nonciliated, and goblet cells by the 13th wk, whereas basal cells are found as early as the 10th wk of fetal life (60). However, as the epithelial differentiation proceeds centrifugally, the lining of the most peripheral tubules is always maintained in an undifferentiated state. This holds until the end of fetal development, when the last airway generations (but not the alveoli) have been formed. These caps of undifferentiated cells seem to be required for growth and branching of the airway tubes.

Early in this stage the airways are embedded in a loose network of mesenchymal cells, from which they are separated first by a patchy, later continuous, basal lamina. Primitive capillaries are randomly interspersed in the mesenchyme. Toward the end of this period, however, they start to arrange around the peripheral epithelial tubes.

Differentiation of the airway wall tissues, apparent first in the trachea during the embryonic phase, extends now toward the periphery. The mesenchyme condenses around the tubes and differentiates centrifugally into cartilage and smooth muscle cells. Cartilage is found in main bronchi about the 10th wk and in segmental bronchi in the 12th wk. However, new cartilage formation occurs far beyond the pseudoglandular stage, up to the 25th wk (178).

Mucous gland formation is also initiated in the second part of this stage. A cluster of epithelial cells first bulges into the mesenchyme, ruptures the basal lamina, and grows as a solid sprout downward into the future lamina propria (151). This is first detected in the trachea, then in bronchi in the 12th–13th wk of gestation. The sprouts later ramify and, developing a lumen, become primitive tubular glands. In the 14th wk active mucous production is found in the trachea (60, 178). Almost simultaneously with the glands, goblet cells develop in the airway epithelium. They show (as do cartilage, muscle cells, and glands) the same proximal-to-distal pattern of differentiation; i.e., they appear first in the trachea and extend to the periphery. Figure 15 summarizes the development of the bronchial tree and visualizes the timing of the appearance of its various components.

Blood vessels. As a rule, arteries develop and grow according to the pattern of the airways. Few data are available on arterial development in the early pseudoglandular stage. From the extensive analysis of blood vessel development after the 12th wk in the human fetus by Hislop and Reid (174, 175), it is known that the main arterial pathways are present in the 14th wk of gestation (178). In contrast to the airway system, which in the adult averages 23 generations, the arterial system has 28–30 generations. This means that additional branching occurs. Arteries following the divisions of the airways are called conventional arteries; the smaller vessels branching in between and supplying alveolar regions adjacent to airways are termed *supernumerary arteries*. At 12 wk of age these two types of arteries are already present; this means that supernumerary arteries develop simultaneously with conventional branches of the same level (174). Because there is very little blood flow through these vessels, they remain small and are much less conspicuous than the corresponding airways.

In principle the veins show a confluence pattern similar to the branching pattern of the arteries. They do not, however, follow the path of airways and arteries but run interaxially in the mesenchyme, demarcating segments and subsegments (Fig. 14). In addition to conventional veins there are two types of supernumerary veins. The type I supernumerary vein collects the blood from the immediate vicinity of the interaxial vein; the type II supernumerary vein is larger and runs

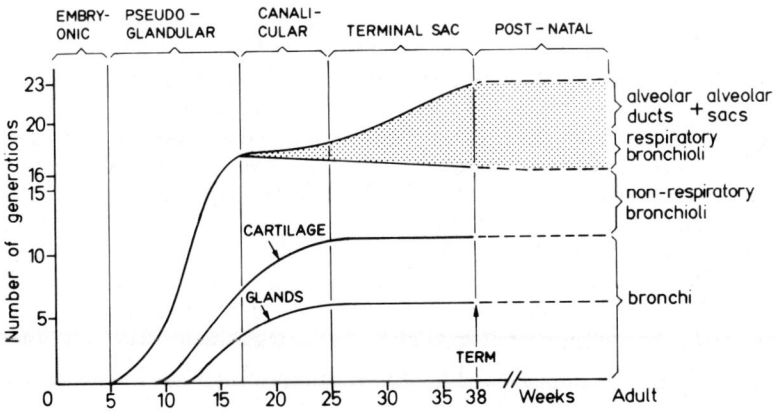

FIG. 15. Timetable for development of the airway tree, its generations, and typical wall structures. Generation numbers are fitted to the averaged airway tree of Weibel's dichotomous branching model [(360); see also Fig. 10]. *Dotted area*, respiratory portion of airway tree. Most of these respiratory airway generations develop between wk 16 and birth by peripheral branching and growth; a few may develop by centripetal transformation of nonrespiratory into respiratory bronchioles. [Adapted from Bucher and Reid (59).]

for a greater distance before usually entering the conventional vein at a right angle (176).

At the end of the pseudoglandular stage the preacinar veins, like the preacinar airways and arteries, are probably laid down in a pattern corresponding to that in adults.

CANALICULAR STAGE. Three major events characterize the canalicular stage: *1)* the birth of the acinus at the beginning of this stage; *2)* the differentiation of the pulmonary epithelium and the development of the typical air-blood barrier throughout this stage; and *3)* the start of surfactant synthesis toward the end of this stage.

Birth of acinus. According to Boyden (45) the transition of the pseudoglandular to the canalicular period of lung development is marked by delineation of the future acinus. The acinar boundary becomes visible due to thinning and rarefaction of the mesenchyme. Generally the acinus is defined as the portion of gas-exchange tissue that is supplied by a terminal bronchiole. As explained later (see EXPERIMENTAL STUDIES, p. 16), because of possible postnatal transformations of airways the parenchymal portion defined as fetal acinus may be supplied by a respiratory bronchiole in an adult lung. A model acinus of this stage as described by Boyden (44) consists of its root, formed by the actual last segment of the prospective conducting airways (i.e., by a terminal bronchiole), a number (2-4) of prospective respiratory bronchioles, and a cluster composed of short tubular branches and rounded buds that becomes the smooth-walled channels and saccules of the later terminal sac or saccular period. For detailed descriptions of adult human acini see references 161 and 310.

Differentiation of pulmonary epithelium and development of typical air-blood barrier. The most important developmental step regarding lung function is probably the transformation of the peripheral tubules lined by cuboidal epithelium into thin-walled and wide canaliculi lined by flat epithelial cells. During the canalicular stage the airway segments distal to the conductive zone not only grow in length but also widen at the expense of the intervening mesenchyme. In some branches the cells start to reduce their height and develop attenuated cytoplasmic extensions so that, except for the nuclear region, they become invisible in the light microscope. This is why it was debated for years whether or not the mature air spaces were lined by an epithelium; this question was rapidly and definitely solved with the first electron-microscopic investigations of the lung by Low (245, 246). These focal epithelial changes are accompanied by important vascular adaptations. In addition to a manifest increase in vascularization of the mesenchyme, the capillaries come to lie closer to the epithelial layer, forming a pericanalicular network. Underneath the regions covered by a thin epithelium the capillaries intimately contact the squamous cells, merely separated from them by a basal lamina. Whether the vicinity of capillaries induces the epithelial differentiation or vice versa remains unknown; the two processes are closely related. The first signs of the forthcoming epithelial attenuation can be detected at the intercellular junctions. The junctional complexes are shifted from the apical cell boundaries to the lower half of the intercellular clefts (Fig. 16). It is likely that cells that do not follow this pattern correspond to prospective secretory cells of the alveolar lining, the type II cells. Mercurio and Rhodin (254, 255) carefully studied the process of type I cell differentiation in the cat by examining serial sections with the electron microscope. According to these authors the first reliable criterion for the differentiation of the epithelium into a type I cell is the attenuation of a portion of its cytoplasm and not the lack of lamellar bodies. Indeed, both differentiated and undifferentiated type I cells contain lamellar bodies and cannot primarily be distinguished from type II cells. This latter fact supports the finding that type II cells are the progenitor cells of type I cells in [^{3}H]thymidine-labeling experiments in the developing rat (4). From this it must be concluded that the developing epithelial cells start to synthesize lamellar bodies before they differentiate further into either type I or actively secreting type II cells. A cell type resembling the future granular pneu-

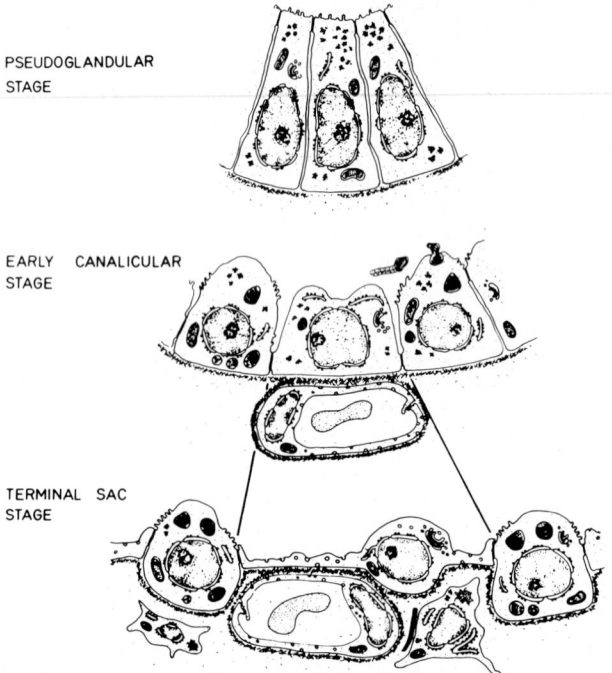

FIG. 16. Phases of epithelial transformation. Pseudoglandular stage: high columnar epithelium, cells rich in glycogen. Canalicular stage: epithelium begins to differentiate into 2 cell types, secretory cells and prospective lining cells, labeled by low position of junctional complex with neighboring cells and close contact with capillaries. Terminal sac stage: differentiation of type I and type II cells; increasing portions of air-blood barrier are thin. [Adapted from Burri and Weibel (72).]

mocyte is thus a kind of intermediary cell between the undifferentiated epithelium and the definitive type I and type II cells. The phenomenon that cells containing lamellar bodies can divide and transform to type I cells is confirmed in pulmonary development by means of cytokinetic studies (206, 207) and in adult lungs during repair of the damaged alveolar epithelium (3, 13–15, 83, 116–118, 203). It is still unclear, however, whether these dividing cells are fully differentiated secreting type II cells or some kind of immature or dedifferentiated cells.

Formation of the air-blood barrier does not start at the uttermost periphery, because the last airway generations are still growing and branching during the canalicular and saccular stages. Thus they maintain caps of cylindrical or cuboidal cells at their blind ends (Fig. 17). Formation of the air-blood barrier can be extremely rapid, as in rodents, whereas in the human lung it seems slow.

Start of surfactant synthesis. During the canalicular stage certain cuboidal cells with apically situated junctional complexes rich in glycogen and relatively rich in ribosomes (free and membrane bound) start to show more lamellar bodies in their cytoplasm. These appear in groups and are often associated with multivesicular bodies and with membrane-bounded granules containing a moderately electron-dense material resembling the cores of lamellar bodies. This conjunction supports the view that lamellated bodies develop from multivesicular organelles (328); their presence always precedes that of osmiophilic material in the air spaces. It has been established that lamellar bodies are the storage sites of the surface-active material present in alveolar surfactant (93, 143). They appear on day 18 in mice (61, 379), about day 20 in rats (62, 72), after day 24 in rabbits (212), between days 120 and 130 in lambs (211, 277), and in the 6th mo of fetal development in humans (73). This means that in most mammalian species investigated their first appearance is in late pregnancy, i.e., at ~80%–85% of gestation duration. In the human fetus, however, they are present at ~60% of gestation duration.

Appearance of surfactant in humans is hence well correlated with the formation of thin air-blood barrier segments. This early start of epithelial differentiation allows for slow propagation of the process through the prospective parenchyma until birth. The opposite is found in some other mammals, where this process sets in late and progresses very rapidly.

Blood vessels. After the 4th mo of gestation the newly born acinus grows rapidly. The new airway branches are accompanied by developing arterial pathways, both of the conventional and supernumerary types, while the preacinar vessels, present in their full complement, grow intensely (178).

TERMINAL SAC STAGE. At the end of the canalicular phase air spaces are assumed to be formed down to the so-called terminal sac region. This comprehends

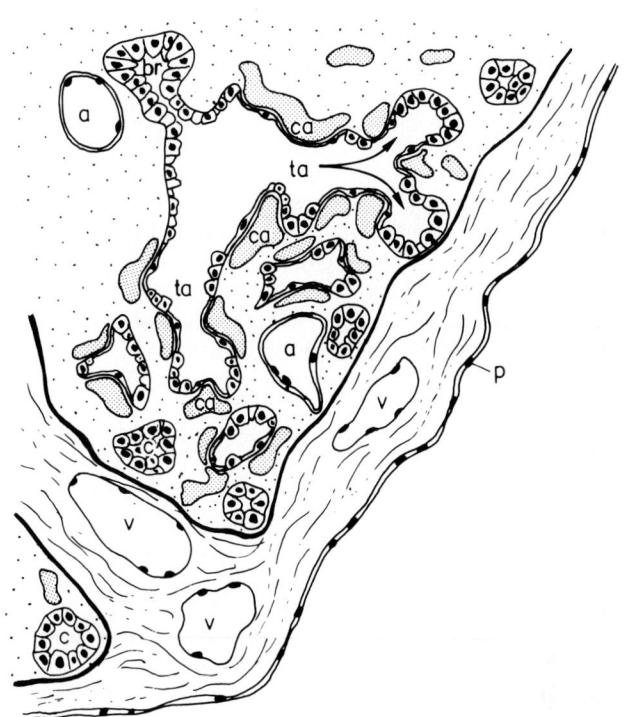

FIG. 17. Early saccular stage of human lung. Bronchiole (br) generates 2 transitory airways (ta). Upper branch produces at least 2 transitory saccules (*arrows*) that are lined by caps of cuboidal epithelium (c) that appear in transections either as tubules or cell clusters. Transitory airways are lined partly by cuboidal and partly by flat epithelium; the latter is present where capillaries (ca and *dotted areas*) are closely apposed to epithelial lining. p, Pleura with subpleural embryonal connective tissue; a, arteries; v, veins.

the airways down to the last prospective respiratory bronchioles and, attached to them, a cluster of wide, thin-walled, irregularly shaped saccules that have been called terminal sacs. These may be connected to the prospective last respiratory bronchiole by a short, straight airway lined by a flat epithelium, which Boyden (42, 47) called the transitional duct. Boyden used this term because he could not determine whether this segment was going to be incorporated into the preceding or the following generation, or whether it stood as a generation on its own.

Until term the terminal sacs are supposed to produce the last generations of air spaces, i.e., on the average three generations of alveolar ducts and the alveolar sacs. During their development these wide and thin-walled channels have been called *saccules* (43, 177). However, this name is inappropriate because the word *sac* or *saccule* implies a wide lumen closed at its distal end. Obviously, any airway distal to the last prospective respiratory bronchiole was a genuine saccule at a given time as long as it represented the last generation. With further development, however, as it branches and produces a new generation of airways, this saccule becomes a tube. The morphology of these channels and saccules changes until alveolization is completed after birth. Therefore they are better termed *transitory ducts*, and the actual last generation *transitory saccules*. This means that each transitory saccule transforms into a transitory duct as soon as it develops further branches, and this same transitory duct eventually turns into an alveolar duct when alveoli develop in its wall. The last transitory saccule formed on each pathway is a real terminal saccule that lastly develops into an alveolar sac after birth. Because it is often impossible on histological sections to determine whether one has a duct or a saccule, the neutral term *transitory airway* can also be used. This terminology allows adequate naming of peripheral airways at any stage during development, and is used in this chapter.

During this last period before birth the peripheral part of the airway tree, the prospective parenchyma, tremendously increases in size. This is due to lengthening and widening of all segments distal to the terminal bronchioles and also to the addition of the last air-space generations. A clue for the further branching ability of the transitory saccules is the presence of cuboidal cells where they terminate (Fig. 17). This configuration can be seen until nearly full term (230).

Widening of the respiratory air spaces during the canalicular and terminal sac stages leads to a drastic reduction in the amount of interstitial tissue and to a rearrangement of the capillary network surrounding the airways. The capillaries establish a close spatial relationship with the epithelial lining, and the airways approach each other. This process extends into the period after birth (65) and is discussed further in the section on alveolization (see EXPERIMENTAL STUDIES, p. 16). Nevertheless the intersaccular and interductal septa still remain rather broad. They are highly cellular and contain only a delicate network of collagen fibers. Elastic fibers start to be deposited at intervals underneath the epithelium of the transitory ducts and sacs. This material is first found extracellularly in bays of large interstitial cells, which show a well-developed organelle compartment (Fig. 18). Deposition of elastin plays an important role in preparing alveolar formation. As early as 1936 Dubreuil et al. (100) postulated that elastic material was laid down at those places where the future alveolar humps (French *bourrelets*) would appear—an absolutely correct statement, as shown later (see EXPERIMENTAL STUDIES, p. 16).

The human fetus born during this period, especially during the second half of it, has increasing chances of survival. To a certain extent the lung is already able to function as a gas exchanger, i.e., the air-blood barrier is thin enough over large enough portions of the internal surface to allow O_2 uptake. If the prematurely born infant is at risk it is mainly because of immaturity of the surfactant system. Whether this is due primarily to a quantitative deficiency (reduced number of type II cells or weak secretory activity), a

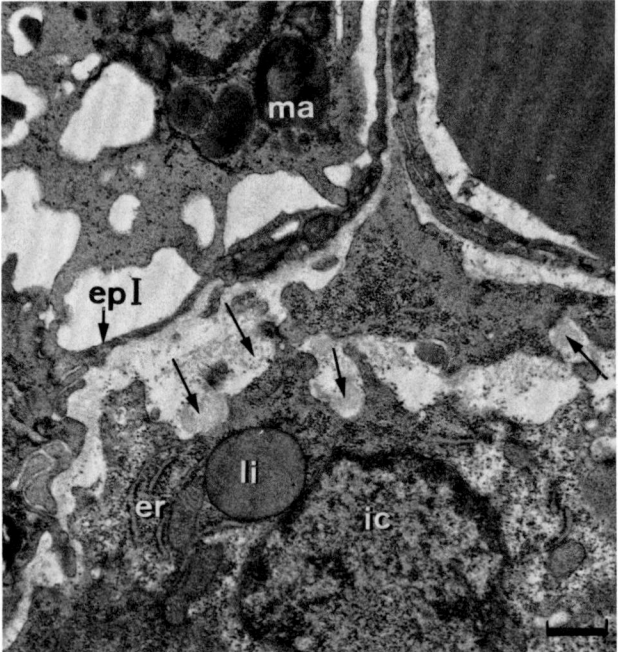

FIG. 18. Electron micrograph of interstitial cell (*ic*) in interalveolar septum of human lung. Cell is actively secreting collagen and elastin into extracellular bays (*arrows*). *er*, Rough endoplasmic reticulum; *li*, lipid droplet; *epI*, epithelial type I cell; *ma*, alveolar macrophage. Scale, 0.5 μm; × 16,000.

qualitative deficiency (chemical incompleteness of the product), or to a combination of these factors remains to be shown. No quantitative data on epithelial differentiation in the human lung are available.

Although it is clear that the cuboidal epithelium lining the fetal peripheral air spaces is the source of type I and type II cells, it has not been shown whether in the human lung it also gives rise to alveolar brush cells. In fetal rabbits and rats these cells have been detected on days 22 and 21 of gestation, respectively (198). It is likely that they also have an endodermal origin and are an additional path of differentiation of the primitive peripheral airway epithelium.

In larger airways, Kultschitsky-type cells and neuroepithelial bodies have been found both in fetal and infant human lung, respectively (91, 235). They have also been described in fetal rats (89), rabbits (88, 166, 167), and neonatal mice (194). Their function is still much disputed (88, 167, 232, 335). For further details about these structures and the development of the pulmonary innervation see the review by Loosli and Hung (243).

Shortly before birth the number of alveolar macrophages in the air spaces increases sharply, as has been demonstrated in rabbits (316, 385). Influx of new cells continues during the first postnatal month and is accompanied by morphological and biochemical maturation (266, 386). Bactericidal activity of macrophages in rabbits is low at birth and improves markedly in the first few postnatal weeks (33, 313, 386). There are no data of this kind for humans.

The processes characterizing the terminal sac stage can be summarized as follows: *1)* production of new peripheral air-space generations; *2)* differentiation of alveolar epithelium throughout the future parenchyma into type I and type II cells and establishment of wide areas with a thin air-blood barrier; *3)* growth of all generations of airways, especially those distal to the terminal bronchioles; *4)* widening of the parenchymal air spaces with massive reduction of interstitial tissue and rearrangement of the capillary networks; *5)* deposition of elastic tissue along the peripheral air-space walls, which prepares alveolar formation; *6)* maturation of the surfactant system; and *7)* influx of alveolar macrophages into the air spaces.

Blood vessels. During this stage the arterial pathways grow in size and length, and at the acinar level new vessels are formed. From the careful studies of Hislop (172; cited in 178) more is known about arterial size changes during fetal life and childhood. Measurements on arteriograms show that the diameter of an artery depends mainly on its distance from the end of the pathway, irrespective of fetal or postnatal age. This means that at a given distance from the end of the pathway the arterial diameter is more or less constant. In an early fetal lung such a vessel supplies a relatively large part of a lobe, whereas in a child it supplies merely an acinus. Figure 19 illustrates how arteries grow in diameter with increasing age at two points of the pathway, at the hilum and at 75% distance from the hilum to the periphery. Centrally the increase with age is steeper than in the periphery, and this is much more pronounced before birth than after birth. The most plausible explanation for this behavior is that the central supplying vessels have to grow faster while their distal generations multiply and increase in size. This may also be the reason why conventional arteries grow faster than supernumerary ones.

In later fetal life the structural differences along the

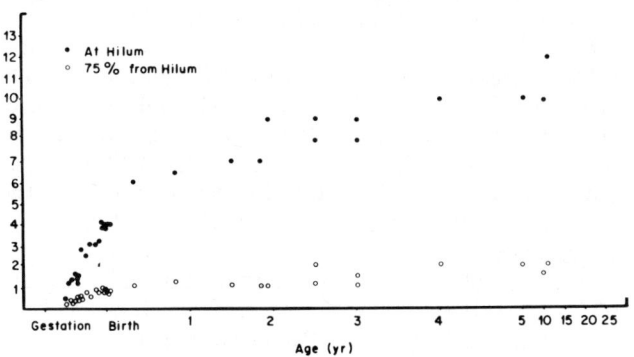

FIG. 19. Growth of intraluminal arterial diameters of human lung during fetal life and childhood. Data from measurements on arteriograms of lower lobe at hilum and at 75% distance from hilum to periphery. [From Hislop and Reid (178).]

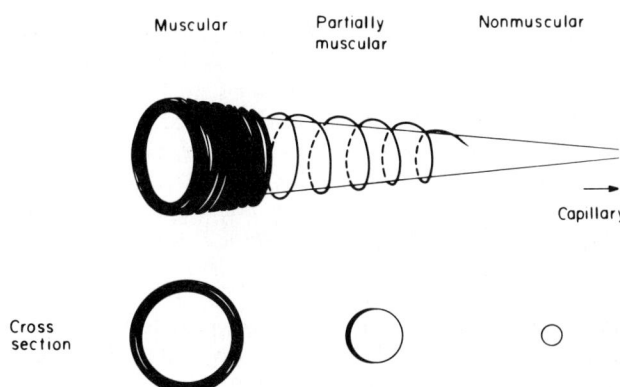

FIG. 20. Muscular structure of a pulmonary artery toward its distal end. Muscle coat ends in the form of a muscle spiral. In this segment the vessel appears as partially muscular in cross sections. [From Hislop and Reid (178).]

arterial pathway are similar to those of the adult lung. Proximally, the arteries are of the elastic type; their media is made of several elastic lamellae strutted to each other by smooth muscle cells. As diameter decreases, the number of elastic lamellae is reduced. Toward the periphery the vessels show a transitional structure. Apart from a few elastic membranes the muscular structure becomes more prominent, and eventually the media is completely muscular. Figure 20 shows the distal end of a pulmonary artery. The muscular media gets thinner and ends in a spiral configuration; on sections these vessels appear as partially muscular. In the most distal segments only intima is left with an endothelial sheet underlined by a fine elastic lamina. It is impossible to establish the diameters at which the character of the vessel walls changes, because they differ from one pathway to another.

Intrapulmonary veins have almost no muscle cells in their walls until the end of the canalicular period. At birth, however, a thin muscle layer is present that extends, as in the adult lung, down to vessels ~100 μm in diameter (176).

Because in the early fetal stage the vessels of the lung primordium form a plexus connected to the systemic and pulmonary circulations, it seems likely, as Weibel (359) postulated, that the number of anastomoses between vessels of various types is higher during development than in adult lungs. Wagenvoort and Wagenvoort's (354) investigation of the perinatal human lung seems to confirm this trend. The same types of anastomoses as in the adult lung were found (see Table 1), but venovenous pulmonary anastomoses not described by Weibel were also detected. Furthermore they found bronchopulmonary arteries (i.e., bronchial arteries supplying capillaries of the respiratory tissue) and also pulmobronchial arteries (i.e., pulmonary arteries connected directly to capillaries of the peribronchial or perivascular connective tissue). The first type was not found in older infants, whereas the occurrence of the latter type was independent of age.

Postnatal Development of Respiratory Tissue—Alveolar Stage

The lung at birth is far from being a miniaturized version of the adult lung. Most probably all of the airway generations are present; the peripheral ones, however, are short and greatly lengthen during childhood. The gas-exchange region is made of a few generations of wide and smooth-walled transitory ducts, of which the last ones open up into saccules with rounded contours. The arrangement and size of transitory ducts and saccules give the lung quite a normal aspect on light-microscopic sections. Therefore pathologists have for years disregarded the fact that the newborn lung has almost no alveoli. Postnatal alveolization allows the lung to drastically increase its internal surface area and to adequately supply the rapidly growing organism with O_2.

EXPERIMENTAL STUDIES. The alveolization process has been morphologically investigated in several mammalian species, e.g., the lamb (7), dog (46), cat (98), rabbit (314), rat (65, 109, 267, 268, 271, 361), and mouse (9, 109). Because it seems that postnatal pulmonary development in these species is comparable to the less well-studied human development, this topic is first discussed and illustrated on the basis of experiments in rats (65, 67, 207), and the human findings are presented in a separate section (see OBSERVATIONS IN THE HUMAN LUNG, p. 20). Figure 21 compares a rat lung on postnatal day 1 with one on postnatal day

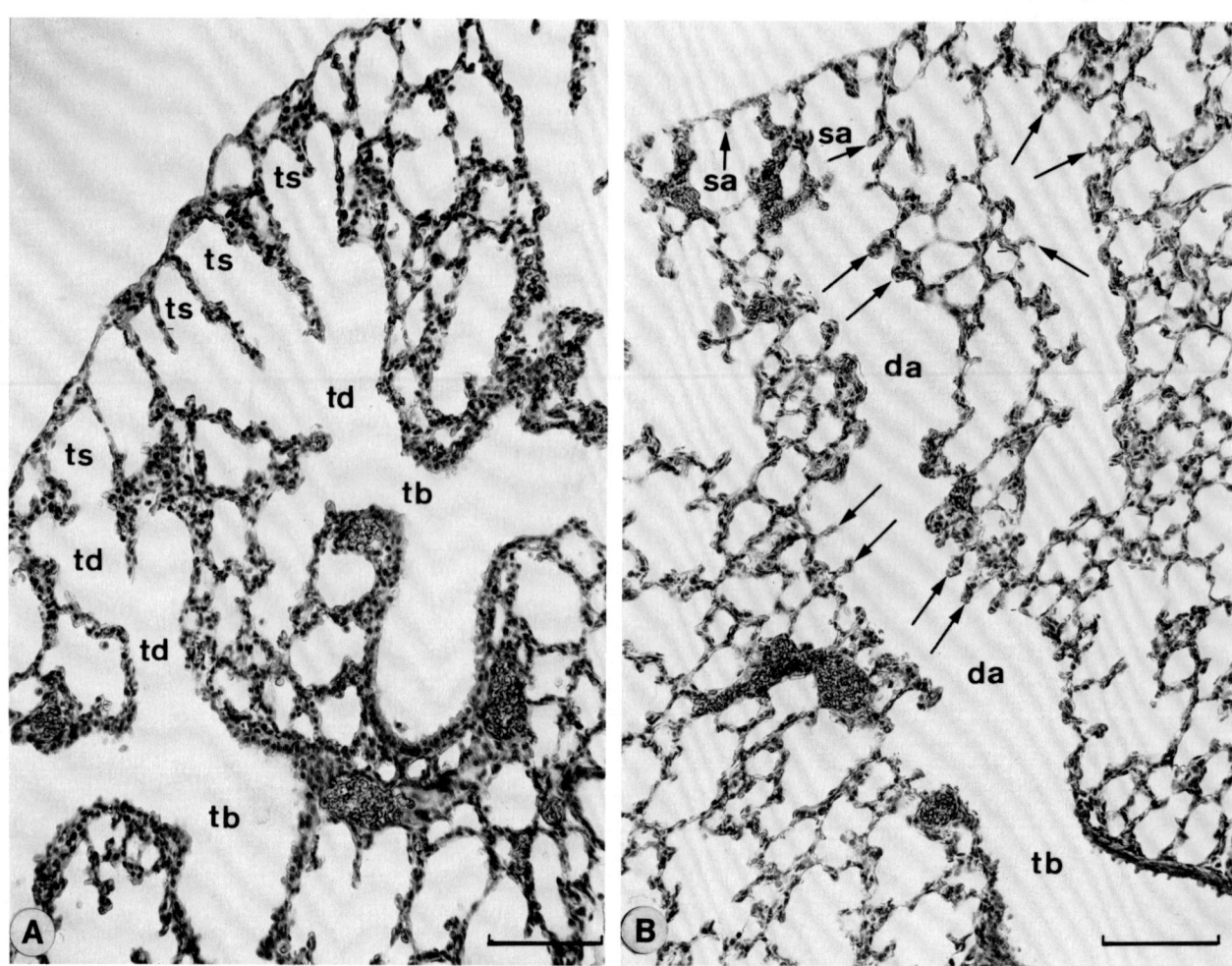

FIG. 21. *A*: light micrograph of paraffin section of rat lung 1 day old. Terminal bronchiole (*tb*) branches into smooth-walled channels (transitory ducts, *td*) opening into terminal saccules (*ts*). Air spaces are smoothly contoured; septa are thick. These terminal airways have often been mistaken as alveoli; direct comparison with an older lung (*B*), however, reveals their nature. *B*: light micrograph of paraffin section of rat lung 21 days old. Terminal bronchiole and its branches at the same magnification as in *A*. Terminal saccules have been partitioned by newly formed septa (secondary septa, *arrows*) and now represent alveolar sacs (*sa*). By the same process transitory ducts have been transformed into alveolar ducts (*da*). Scale, 100 μm; × 160.

21. In this short period dramatic structural transformations have occurred. At birth the parenchyma consists of smooth-walled channels (transitory ducts) and terminal saccules; the walls between ducts and saccules are relatively thick and straight. At 3 wk the septa are slender and show a zigzag pattern; the airways exhibit a crenated contour and have been incompletely partitioned into smaller units, the alveoli. This partitioning has been achieved by the formation of new septa (the so-called *secondary septa*) that develop from those present at birth, termed *primary septa* (65). At greater magnification one can detect another important difference in the structure of the two lungs. In the newborn the septa are thick and have a three-layered structure containing a central sheet of connective tissue and, on both sides of it, a network of capillaries (Fig. 22). This corresponds to the primitive or immature form of the parenchymal septum. The mature septum, however, is a delicate membrane containing a single capillary network interwoven with fine collagen fibers (Fig. 4). The capillary system

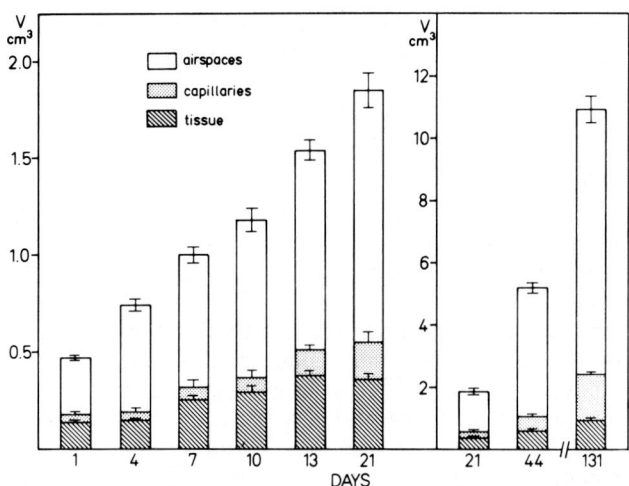

FIG. 23. Quantitative findings in growing rat lung showing volume changes of pulmonary parenchyma and its compartments. Note that increase in parenchymal volume between days 1 and 4 is brought about by the air-space compartment, the increase between days 4 and 7 by the tissue and blood compartments. The latter period corresponds to phase of most active septal outgrowth. [Data from Burri et al. (67).]

therefore has to be completely remodeled—an important step in postnatal lung development. Morphological observations corroborated by morphometric measurements of the parenchymal compartments and of the gas-exchange surfaces established the following sequence of events. In the first few days after birth the air spaces are simply enlarged (Fig. 23), and alveolization does not start before postnatal day 4 (Fig. 24A, B). Within the next three days an increase in tissue mass brings about most of the lung volume increase (Fig. 23). At the same time the air-space and capillary surface areas start to increase to the 1.6th power of lung volume (Fig. 25), i.e., at a very high rate that can only be achieved by structural alterations of the peripheral lung morphology. (With simple isotropic growth one would expect air-space surface area to grow at a two-thirds power function of lung volume.) The high rate of surface increase indicates that septation has started. On day 7 or 8 the walls of the peripheral air spaces are covered at more or less regular intervals by small crestlike protrusions of tissue (Fig. 24B). These secondary septa soon increase in height and subdivide the saccules and the transitory ducts into alveolar sacs and alveolar ducts, respectively. This process is so rapid in the rat that the bulk of alveoli is formed between days 4 and 13. Morphometric analysis of the subcellular changes in type II pneumocytes during this phase shows that the rapid formation of gas-exchange surface area is paralleled by an augmentation in the mass of lamellar bodies (347).

Figures 26 and 27 illustrate the mechanism and structure of septal outgrowth. Formation of the secondary septa can most likely be explained by the

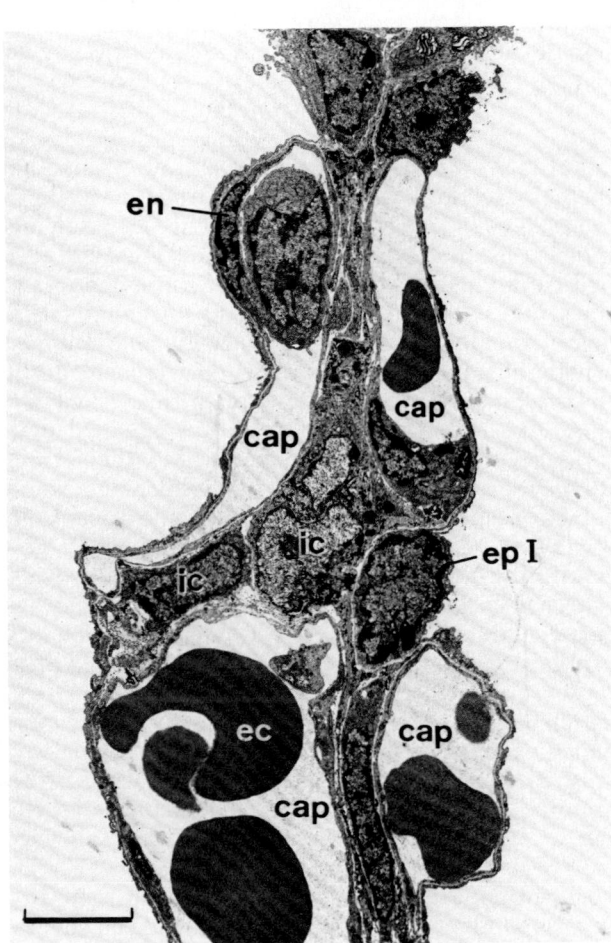

FIG. 22. Electron micrograph of ultrastructure of immature primary septum during early postnatal days. Capillary network (*cap*) is present on both sides of a highly cellular interstitial layer. *ic*, Nuclei of interstitial cells; *epI*, nucleus of epithelial type I cell; *en*, nucleus of endothelial cell; *ec*, erythrocytes. Scale, 5 μm; × 3,000.

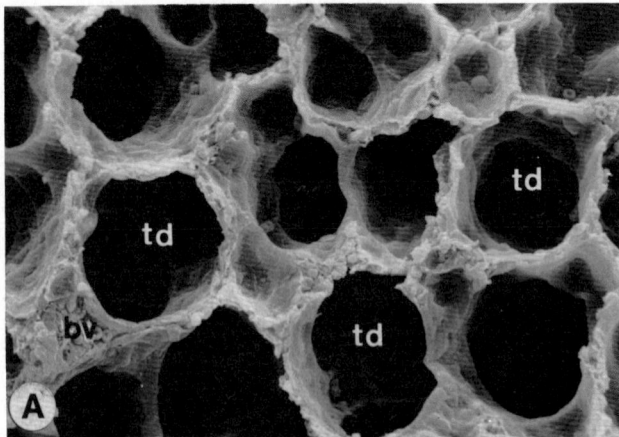
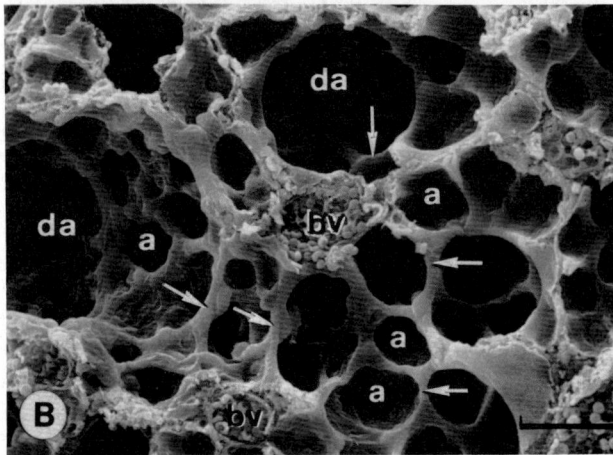

FIG. 24. *A*: scanning electron micrograph of gas-exchange tissue of rat lung 4 days old. Transitory ducts (*td*) and air spaces in general are rounded; septa are smooth. *bv*, Blood vessel. *B*: scanning electron micrograph of pulmonary parenchyma of rat lung 8 days old. Numerous secondary septa have appeared (*arrows*), dividing air spaces into alveoli (*a*) and transforming transitory ducts into alveolar ducts (*da*). Scale, 50 μm; × 280.

upfolding of one of the capillary networks from the primary septum, forming first only a low ridge, then by growth a crest, and finally an interalveolar wall. Invariably, due to the mode of formation, the secondary septa possess (like the primary ones) two capillary networks with a central core of connective tissue. This sheet contains interstitial cells of two types: a dormant type containing lipid droplets and an active myofibroblastic type involved in collagen and elastin synthesis (56, 346). Collagen fibrils and, at the tip of the crest, originally thin bundles of elastic fibers that grow in diameter as the septum heightens form the fibrous skeleton of these septa.

The appearance of elastic tissue seems closely linked with alveolar formation. Although no definite statement can be made from analysis of static pictures, these suggest that the elastic fibers or networks might represent kinds of anchoring cables for the formation of interalveolar septa. In this respect the investigation of the activity of lung lysyl oxidase, an enzyme responsible for initiating cross-linking of collagen and elastin, may provide new information (54).

Shortly before septal growth the DNA synthetic activity of septal cells increases preferentially in the region of the forming crest, as revealed by an autoradiographic study with [^{3}H]thymidine (207). On day 4, DNA synthesis was highest for the mesodermally derived cells, the interstitial and endothelial cells, whereas peak activity was reached on day 7 in the type II cells derived from the endoderm. Within 1 h of the thymidine injections not a single type I cell was labeled, confirming the assumption that these cells cannot divide. On day 13, incorporation of [^{3}H]thymidine had returned to lower levels in all cells. The decline was most pronounced for the interstitial cells, which might be explained by the differentiation of the myofibroblast population (206). Because the gas-exchange surface area still increased at a high rate during the 3rd wk, the increase was postulated to be achieved by a restructuring of the existing septa (65) rather than formation of additional ones. This restructuring comprises *1*) lengthening and thinning of the interalveolar septa, combined with a reduction or condensation of the interstitial tissue and *2*) remodeling of the capillary networks. The first step is easily detected by simple comparison of the septal morphology at 2 and 3 wk of age. The visual impression is confirmed by the quantitative findings. Whereas the lung volume and the gas-exchange surface area increase markedly in size (Figs. 23 and 25), tissue volume does not, and interstitial volume even decreases (67). Figure 28 schematically illustrates the impact of these changes on the septal structure. The narrowing of the interstitial layer probably initiates the capillary remodeling. A schematic summary of capillary development during the fetal period may help to explain this second step (Fig. 29). Primarily, vascular spaces are laid down irregularly in the mesenchyme around the forming tubular sprouts (Fig. 29*A*). In the canalicular stage the capillaries are rearranged and come to lie closer to the airways, especially in the periphery (Fig. 29*B*). They even line up closely with the epithelial cells, which flatten (Fig. 29*C*). Reduction of the mesenchymal layer between the canaliculi leads to the formation of a capillary bilayer in the intercanalicular and later interductular or intersaccular septa (Fig. 29*D*). Alveolization comprises the formation of the secondary septa, which are also supplied by a double capillary network (Fig. 29*E*). Finally, it is plausible that after birth the approximation of the capillary layers continues, ending in direct contact between capillaries and eventually in capillary fusions (Figs. 28 and 29*F*). The observation of capillaries on the left and right sides separated merely by a single endothelial cell suggests this process, though it is not a proof. Further investigations are needed to clarify this point.

In addition to the mode of alveolization described above, there seems to be another mechanism of alveolar formation in more central lung regions observed

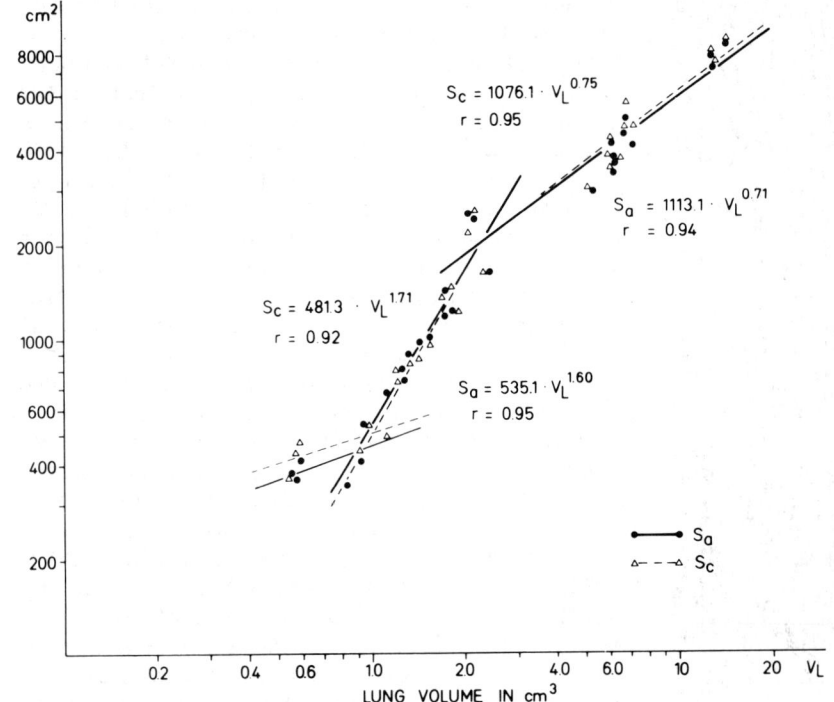

FIG. 25. Double logarithmic plot of alveolar (S_a) and capillary (S_c) surface areas against lung volume (V_L) in growing rat lung. Triphasic growth pattern with most intense increase in surface area between day 4 and wk 3. r, Correlation coefficient. [Data from Burri et al. (67).]

by Boyden and Tompsett in dogs (46) and humans (47). They found a centripetal extension of the gas-exchange region with transformation of respiratory bronchioles into alveolar ducts and of terminal bronchioles into respiratory bronchioles. This means that in peripheral conducting airways new alveoli can be formed by flattening of the cuboidal epithelium and subsequent local outpouching of the freshly created air-blood barrier, first forming shallow depressions and later true alveoli. The number of gas-exchanging airway generations may therefore increase centripetally before and after birth as shown in Figure 15. This shortening of the conducting airways is likely to affect the supplying airways of the acinus. If at birth an acinus is defined as the portion of lung parenchyma supplied by a terminal bronchiole, in the adult this "newborn acinus" may ultimately be supplied by a respiratory bronchiole.

In summarizing these observations in the rat lung, the postnatal period of lung development (the alveolar stage) can be divided into three phases: *1*) a short preparative phase of lung expansion; *2*) a phase of tissue proliferation with formation of interalveolar septa and alveoli; and *3*) a phase of remodeling of the parenchymal septa, involving their lengthening and thinning, and transformation of the septal capillary system from a double- to a single-network structure.

The results described for the rat are to a great extent corroborated by observations in other animal species. *1*) Nearly identical structural findings are documented in mice with a slightly different timing (9). *2*) The initial phase of lung expansion is found in cats and rabbits. In cats it is signaled by a drop in air-space surface density [i.e., air-space surface area per unit lung volume (V_L)] during the first days of life (98); in rabbits the percentage of air-space volume increases from 68.6% on day 1 to 80% on day 5 after birth (314). *3*) Postnatal alveolization by whatever means is postulated in the literature for all kinds of species, e.g., opossums, mice, rats, rabbits, cats, and dogs (46, 49, 57, 98, 109, 314). However, rhesus monkeys (208) and lambs (7) seem to be exceptions; in these species alveoli are already formed during fetal life. *4*) Tissue proliferation that accompanies this period has been ascertained in mice and hamsters by means of [^{3}H]-thymidine labeling (85). Low values of labeling at birth (comparable to those of adult lungs, where they represent cell renewal) increase within a few days to reach a peak on day 6 and return to approximately postpartum values on day 16. In hamsters the peak was measured on day 4, followed by a rapid decrease within 3 days.

Little information, however, is available on septal and capillary remodeling. Amy, Burri, et al. (9) confirmed the disappearance of the double capillary network during the 3rd wk in mice, proposing that in addition to capillary fusion, stretching of the septa may also contribute to the change. Septal restructuring is accompanied by a massive appearance of interalveolar pores. In mice, for example, pores of Kohn are occasionally found in the newborn lung. Yet after 2 wk of age they dramatically increase in number so that the interalveolar septa of the adult lungs appear fenestrated (9). Between 3 and 25 mo of age their number remains stable, with ~10 pores per alveolus in the subpleural and peribronchial regions versus ~6

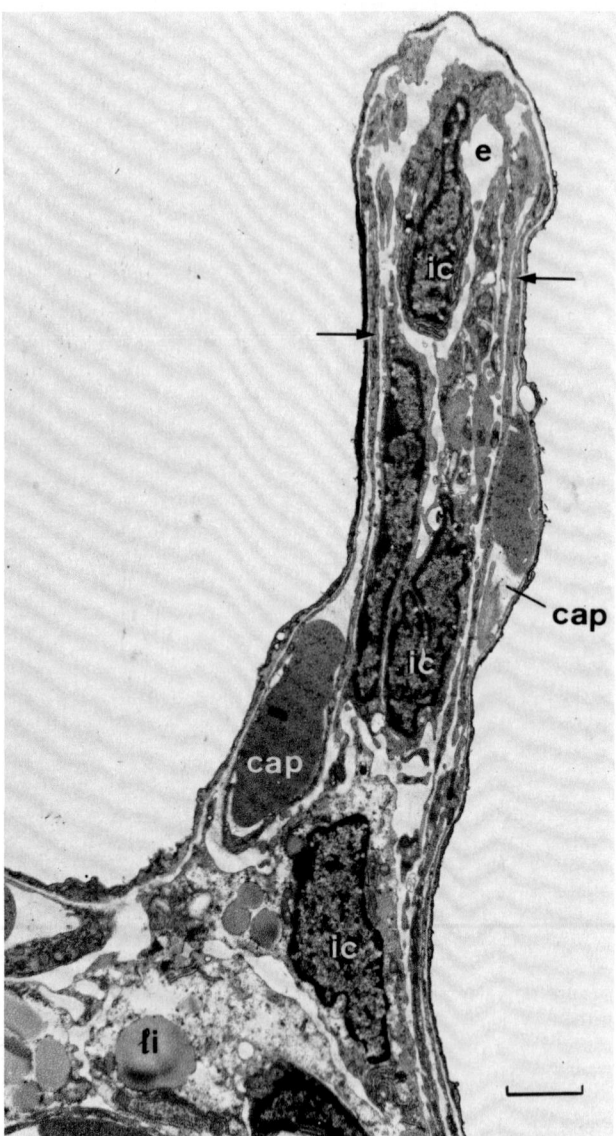

FIG. 26. Electron micrograph of secondary crest of rat lung 7 days old with capillaries (*cap*) on both sides. Central interstitial layer contains interstitial cells (*ic*) of 2 types: at base, interstitial cells contain lipid droplets (*li*); toward tip they contain no lipid but form slender cytoplasmic extensions enfolding connective tissue (*e*, elastin). Capillary walls form closed extensions toward tip of crest (*arrows*). Scale, 2 μm; × 5,200.

Whether or not the newborn child actually already has a limited number of alveoli is a controversial issue. Due to the formation of elastic tissue in the prospective gas-exchange region during the terminal sac stage (the step initiating septal outgrowth), rather shallow indentations lining the saccules and transitory ducts are present at birth. Whether these should be called alveoli is a matter of interpretation and definition. They represent alveoli in a nascent state; counting such alveoli is particularly problematic. Dunnill's (101) estimate of 24 million alveoli at birth is therefore seriously questioned by Boyden (45), who believes that Dunnill counted saccules. Regardless of who is right, it seems justified to place alveolar formation after birth because at least 280 million alveoli have to be formed postnatally. According to Dunnill, alveolar multiplication occurs up to 8 yr of age. However, from the great difference between values found in lungs of adults and children one can assume that alveolar formation could be completed before this. Yet Emery, Mithal, and Wilcock (106–108, 259) found an increase in alveolar number up to 20 yr of age by performing radial counts along a defined line in the periphery of the lung. Because of the different counting procedure their results cannot be compared numerically with the findings of others.

There are no studies on the postnatal alterations of the parenchymal ultrastructure in the human lung. Therefore morphological and quantitative informa-

pores in midzonal lung portions (293). Clearly this phenomenon is related to the drastic reduction in interstitial tissue and the thinning of the septa observed during the third phase of postnatal lung development.

OBSERVATIONS IN THE HUMAN LUNG. It is generally agreed that in the human lung the bulk of alveoli is formed during childhood. Table 3 presents data on alveolar counts obtained in humans at different ages by various authors. Starting with ~20 million at birth, the alveolar number is ~300 million in adulthood. Thereby it seems that alveolar number can vary greatly and is related to body size (11).

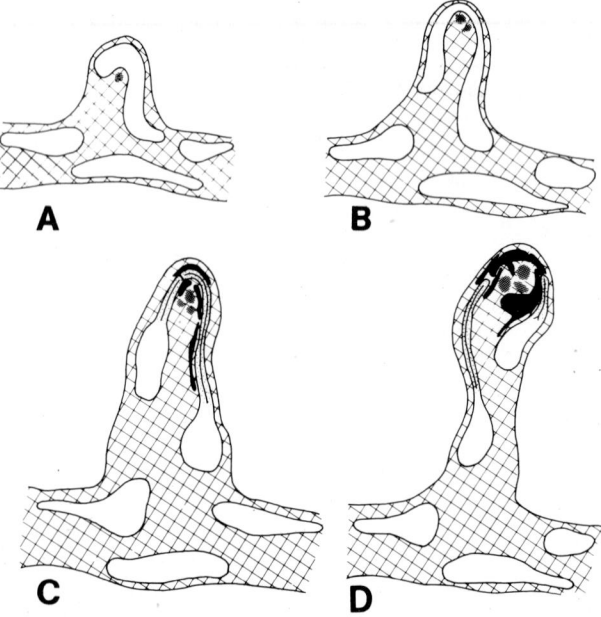

FIG. 27. Formation and capillarization of secondary septa. Capillary meshes are folded up from primary septum present at birth (*A*) and form secondary septum (*B*). This increases in height as new capillary segments are formed by sprouting (*C, D*). At tip of crests increasing amounts of elastic tissue are present. *Quadratic lattice*, septal tissue; *white spaces*, capillary lumina; *fine dots*, closed capillary segments; *coarse dots*, elastic fibers; *black spaces*, cells of unknown origin, which seem to participate in lengthening and sprouting of capillaries. [From Burri (65).]

FIG. 28. Model for structural transformation and maturation of immature interalveolar septum (*dotted area*, interstitial tissue). Through thinning of interstitium and lengthening of septum with expansion of capillary meshes (*arrows*), immature structure (*left*) is transformed into mature form (*right*). Capillary fusion may complete the picture so that blood flows, e.g., from *a* to *d* over *b* and *c*. [From Burri (65).]

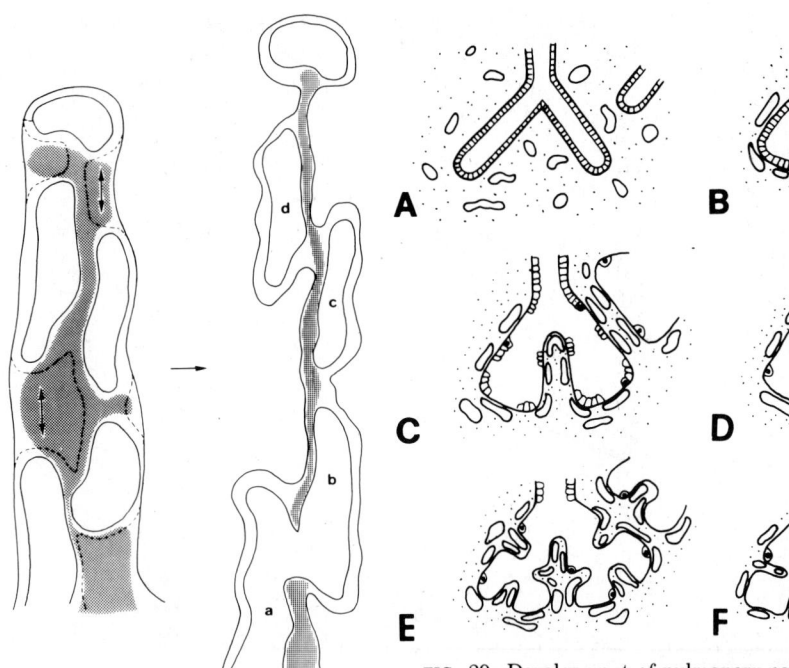

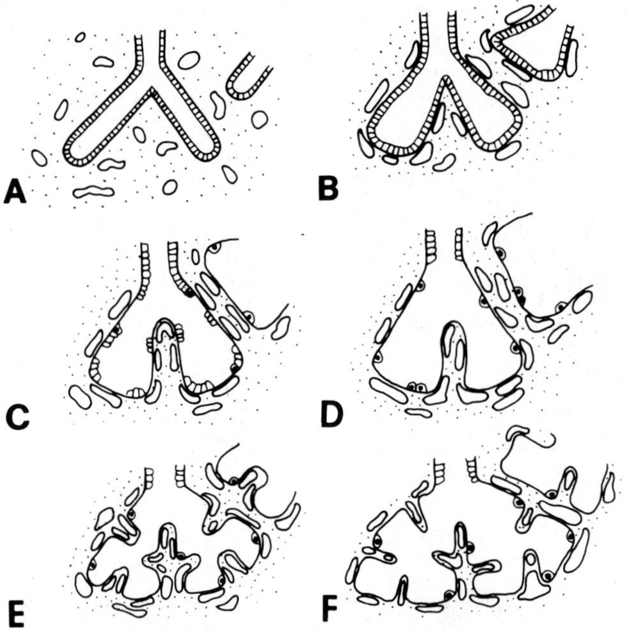

FIG. 29. Development of pulmonary capillaries. *A*: pseudoglandular stage, capillaries are randomly distributed in mesenchyme. *B*: beginning of canalicular stage, capillaries start to arrange around epithelial tubes, which enlarge to canaliculi. *C*: canalicular stage, capillaries establish close contact to lining epithelium, which flattens to form thin air-blood barriers. Widening of canaliculi reduces intervening interstitium so that capillary layers of adjacent air spaces lie closer to each other. *D*: end of saccular stage, epithelium differentiated in type I and type II cells, intersaccular walls with 2 capillary networks. *E*: alveolar stage, formation of secondary septa; all septa contain 2 capillary networks; further reduction of interstitial tissue. *F*: mature lung, capillary layers in primary and secondary septa have fused; at a few places double row may stay; septa have lengthened and narrowed.

TABLE 3. *Postnatal Growth of the Human Lung*

	Number of Alveoli, × 10⁶		Alveolar Surface Area, m²		
	Dunnill (101)	Davies and Reid (95)	Short (315)	Hieronymi (169)	Dunnill (101)
Stillborn		17			
Newborn			2.8	1	
3 mo	79			3.5	6.5
4 mo		77			
7 mo	112			4	8.4
10 mo			16		
12 mo				7	
13 mo	129				12.2
16 mo	127				12.8
22 mo	160				14.2
3 yr		196		9	
4 yr	257				22.2
5 yr				12	
8 yr	280				32
9 yr			50		
11 yr		336			
20 yr				25	
Adult	296		120	34	75

tion about alveolar formation is lacking, and nothing is known about possible capillary remodeling. From some encoded and vague comments by Dubreuil et al. (100) that the capillary system is immature at birth, one can assume that these authors realized a difference in the septal morphology between neonatal and adult human lungs. Because of the congruence of the findings in different species it is, however, very likely that the human lung undergoes the postnatal changes described above. This has been implied in a number of recent reviews (341, 342). Figure 30 compares the lung of a normal boy 1 mo of age who died from sudden infant death with the lung of a rat 7 days of age. Except for the size difference of the air spaces, the structural similarity is striking. In both lungs the primary septa are thick, very cellular, and have a large number of secondary septa of different heights projecting into the air spaces. Most septa exhibit the immature arrangement of two capillary layers (Fig. 31*A*, *B*). This observation gives confidence that the human lung does not essentially deviate during its postnatal development from the pattern described in animal species.

GROWTH OF THE LUNG

Normal Growth

POSTNATAL GROWTH OF RESPIRATORY TISSUE. *Animal studies.* In the 3rd wk the rat lung has a largely

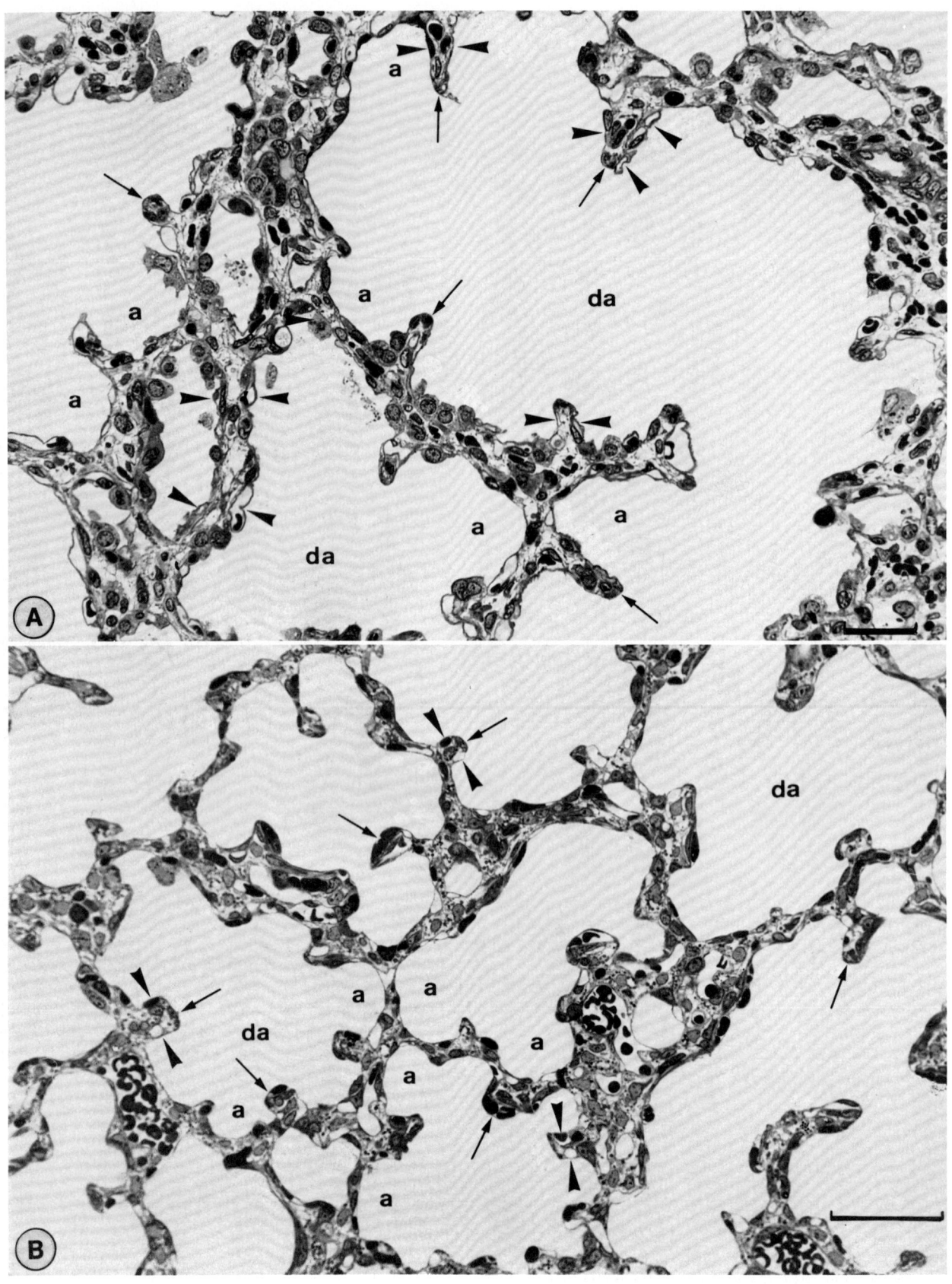

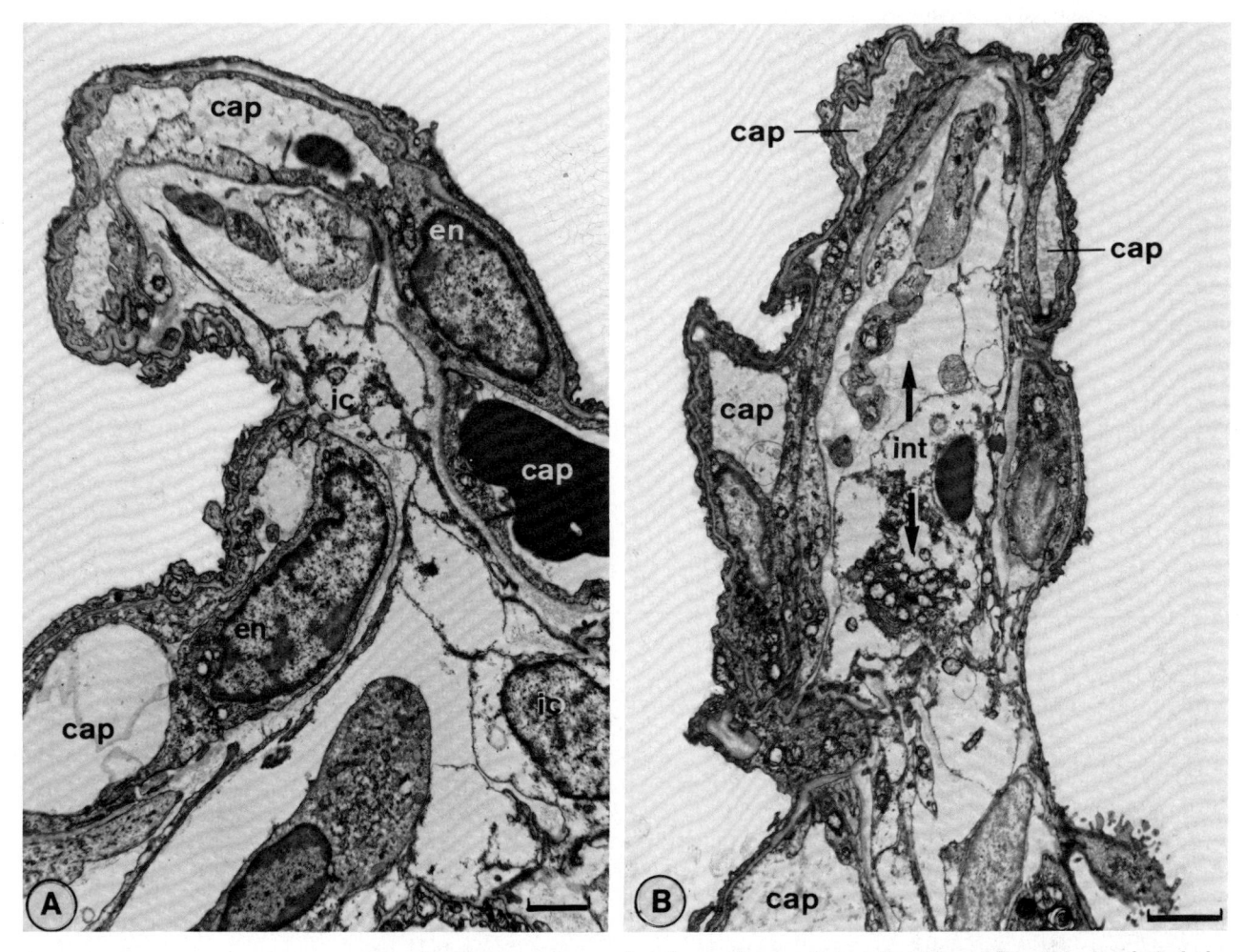

FIG. 31. Electron micrographs of secondary septa in infant lung of Fig. 30A. A: relatively low septum with capillary loop passing over edge of crest. *cap*, Capillaries; *en*, endothelial cells; *ic*, interstitial cells. Scale, 2 μm; × 5,200. B: higher secondary septum with double capillary networks (*cap*). Interstitial layer (*int* and *arrows*) swollen and not well preserved due to delay between death and fixation of lung. Scale, 2 μm; × 4,000. (Micrographs courtesy of A. Keller.)

mature structure and enters a period of normal growth. Whereas in interspecies comparisons lung volume increases in direct proportion to body weight (137, 365), in the growing rat it increases to the 0.73rd power of body weight (67). Between days 21 and 131 tissue volume augments by a factor of 2.6 and airspace volume by a factor of 6.2. On the other hand, capillary volume increases 7.6 times in the same period. These findings indicate that during normal, unperturbed growth, growth rates of the parenchymal components may vary. The older the lung the more air it contains relative to septal tissue; furthermore it also contains more blood (Fig. 23). Quantitative data of other authors confirm these observations. Most of these ratios—lung volume and alveolar surface area per gram body weight, alveolar surface area and tissue volume per gram or per milliliter lung volume—have been reported to fall with age (98, 267, 268, 314).

FIG. 30. Light micrographs of postnatal structure of gas-exchange tissue in human and rat, illustrating similarity of alveolization process in both species. A: lung of normal boy 1 mo old who died from sudden infant death. Alveolar ducts (*da*) show numerous secondary septa (*arrows*) defining alveoli (*a*). Secondary and rather thick primary septa possess 2 capillary networks (*arrowheads*). Epon section 1 μm thick; scale, 50 μm; × 260. B: parenchyma of rat lung 1 wk old. Alveolar ducts much smaller than in human lung (note different magnification) but show same structural pattern. Secondary septa (*arrows*) demarcating alveoli and double capillary networks (*arrowheads*) are also visible. Epon section 1 μm thick; scale, 50 μm; × 415. (Micrographs courtesy of A. M. Steiner.)

Normal growth often implies proportionate growth of all the compartments, but these findings show this is not correct. With age the gas-exchange tissue alters its quantitative composition, which obviously affects lung morphology. It is well known that alveoli increase in size with age. In the rat they enlarge about twofold between 3 and 7 wk of age (69).

Whether or not alveolar formation stops completely after the initial burst observed in the rat during the 2nd wk after birth cannot definitely be answered. After the 3rd wk the air-space surface area increased as a function of $V_L^{0.71}$, which is not significantly different from $V_L^{0.67}$ expected from proportional growth of the air spaces. For air-space surface area Weibel (361) and Bartlett (25) calculated allometric functions of $V_L^{0.94}$ and $V_L^{1.08}$, respectively, but their experiments contained animals younger than 3 wk of age. Development of new alveoli was described in rats of >200 g body wt (25, 184) and in rabbits between 12 wk of age and adulthood (312), periods far beyond the stage of initial alveolization. It was also postulated many times that further addition of alveoli occurred during adaptive or regenerative growth after the phase of alveolar formation (see *Adaptive Growth of Gas-Exchange Apparatus*, p. 26). These claims are, however, based either on alveolar counting, which is an unsafe procedure (160), or indirect estimates, e.g., the ratio of air-space surface area to air-space volume or the allometric relationship between alveolar surface and lung volume. But one has to bear in mind that a lengthening of the septa and/or a corrugation of the alveolar surface have the same quantitative effects on these parameters as alveolar formation. Therefore it is not settled whether the growing lung keeps the ability to form a sizable amount of alveoli after the period of alveolization.

Human lung. Limited knowledge about postnatal structural development of the human lung and the large difference between alveolar counting results make it impossible to determine when the human lung passes from the alveolar stage into the period of normal growth. Only a few publications present other quantitative data (in addition to alveolar counts) based on a stereologic approach (101, 169, 315). Short (315) was the first to apply modern morphometric techniques to the investigation of the human lung. In a first study on the rabbit lung (314) he had presented (in collaboration with C. A. Rogers, a mathematician at the University College in London) the stereological basis for the measurement of air-space surface density in the lung. Short probably was not aware that the linear-intercept method had already been published in 1945 by Tomkeieff (344). Subsequently he applied these methods to the study of the growing human lung and found the air-space surface area to increase from 2.8 m² at birth to 120 m² in adulthood (315). He particularly questioned when alveoli stopped forming, reasoning that if during growth lung volume increased by simple expansion, air-space surface density would be reduced in the enlarged lung by the cube root of the volume increase. If air-space surface density were larger than expected according to this reasoning, it would indicate further subdivision of air spaces. Short concluded that septal formation stopped (and hence normal growth started) during the second year of life.

More recently Thurlbeck (341) used the same correction technique on data of interalveolar wall distances measured in human lungs of various ages. He obtained gradually decreasing values until 15–25 yr of age; then the trend reversed to indicate cessation of alveolar multiplication and uptake of normal organ growth. The uncorrected interalveolar wall distances, however, increased continuously with age during childhood, despite alveolar formation. This was interpreted by Thurlbeck as a faster increase of lung volume than of alveolar number. Increasing alveolar diameters with age are confirmed by Short (315), Hieronymi (168, 169), and Dunnill (101).

POSTNATAL GROWTH OF CONDUCTING AIRWAYS AND BLOOD VESSELS IN THE HUMAN LUNG. *Airways*. The branching pattern and structure of conducting airways are mature at birth, so that except for the terminal bronchioles (where transformation into respiratory passages may occur) the adult bronchial tree is the enlarged replica of the newborn one. Indeed, measuring metal casts of the bronchial tree, Hieronymi (169) found a relatively constant growth factor for length and diameter of various segments. Between birth and adulthood the trachea and bronchi enlarged both in length and diameter by a factor of ~3. Assuming that a given volume of bronchial air supplies a constant amount of lung tissue, lung volume would be expected to increase 27-fold from birth to adulthood. Remarkably, Dunnill's data (101) exactly fit this assumption: lung volume (distended to the internal dimensions of the thorax) increased from 200 cm³ at birth to 5,500 cm³ in adulthood.

In a study principally aimed at establishing the quantitative morphological bases for understanding preacinar airway function during growth, Hislop and co-workers (173) measured the lengths and diameters of the branches on a single axial pathway from hilum to periphery at different postnatal ages. Because the number of generations between hilum and terminal bronchioles varied, branching points were expressed as percentages of the path length. It appeared from this study that the relationship between diameter and relative distance from the hilum was almost constant with age. The authors concluded that the conductive bronchial tree underwent a fully proportionate growth, an interpretation consistent with the findings of Cudmore et al. (86). The study suggested that the airway conductance (the inverse of resistance) expressed per gram lung tissue remained constant throughout the preacinar region and was independent of age (173). In a more recent analysis of resin casts of the bronchial tree in dogs, the postnatal proportionate growth of the conducting airway system was also established; mean diameters and mean lengths of the branches in each branching order grew in constant proportion to the cube root of body weight (185). Earlier, Hogg and coworkers (183) reported that growth of the bronchial tree was rather uniform with one exception. They observed disproportionately narrow peripheral airways (beyond generation 18) in children under 5 yr of age, suggesting that the small airways grew at a retarded rate. However, as Hislop et al. (173) commented, this conclusion was based on measurements of a single bronchial pathway and therefore has to be interpreted with caution.

Pulmonary arteries. The most important event for the pulmonary circulation at birth is the closure of the ductus arteriosus. During fetal life, blood flow to the lung is very limited, between 10% and 15% of the cardiac output. The transition to air breathing, accompanied by a shift of blood flow to the lung, is prepared for during the last three months of gestation by formation in the ductus arteriosus of muscular humps called endothelial cushions. Soon after birth muscular contraction closes the duct functionally, whereas the anatomical closure (organization of an intravascular clot by invading fibrous tissue) takes a few weeks. The ligamentum arteriosum is the remnant of this important prenatal structure.

Arterial wall structure is largely determined by the intravascular pressure. Until birth the pulmonary arteries are exposed to a high pressure; thus their thickness and wall structure resemble those of the aorta and the larger systemic arteries. After birth the relative wall thickness (often expressed as a percentage of the external diameter) decreases (95, 263, 264, 353). In small arteries (<200 μm diam) this happens within days and is probably due to dilatation of the vessels (by a drop in smooth muscle tone), whereas in larger arteries the adaptation is mainly structural and takes a few months (175).

According to Hislop and Reid (178) the larger proximal vessels grow without much structural change once they have reached the range of relative wall thickness corresponding to adult values (at ~10 mo of age). Others, however, have reported that the elastic type of artery extends toward the periphery between birth and 15 yr of age (238). Arguing that all vessels >800 μm in diameter would certainly be of the elastic type, the authors measured (on arteriograms of surgically removed lobes) the relative lengths of the elastic and muscular pathways (238). They found that at birth the elastic segment constituted 50%–60% of the total length, whereas in adulthood it occupied 80%–90%. These authors concluded that a given type of vessel functions optimally within a certain size range, and that consequently a growing vessel has to alter its structure.

In smaller arteries, pronounced shifts between the frequencies of the muscular, partially muscular, and nonmuscular types were detected (95, 175). During alveolar proliferation (and to at least 11 yr of age) there is a much higher percentage of partially muscular and nonmuscular arteries than in late fetal and adult age. Thus for a given diameter more vessels with less muscle are seen during childhood than before and after. This apparent paucity in muscle is not due to regression of muscle along the arterial wall but to an increase in vessel size with muscle formation lagging behind. Gradually muscle extends more into the periphery (Fig. 32). At 11 yr of age a media with muscle cells extends down to the level of the alveolar ducts. This process continues until adulthood, when muscular arteries have been reported at the level of the alveolar wall (175).

Whereas preacinar vessels simply grow, there is rapid development and growth of new intra-acinar arteries during the first 18 mo. This reflects the intense development of alveoli, and both types of arteries (conventional and supernumerary) are formed. After 18 mo the number of conventional arteries does not increase much, but supernumerary arteries continue to multiply up to 8 yr of age. During early childhood the small peripheral arteries (200 μm diam) increase markedly in number, both absolutely and per unit area of lung section. After 5 yr of age, however, their number per unit area of pulmonary tissue starts to fall. This was proposed to be related to the enlarging of the alveoli, because during this period the ratio between alveolar and arterial number remained constant (178). Regarding growth of the smaller vessels, these authors observed that proximal arteries in an acinus grew more than distal ones. This was caused

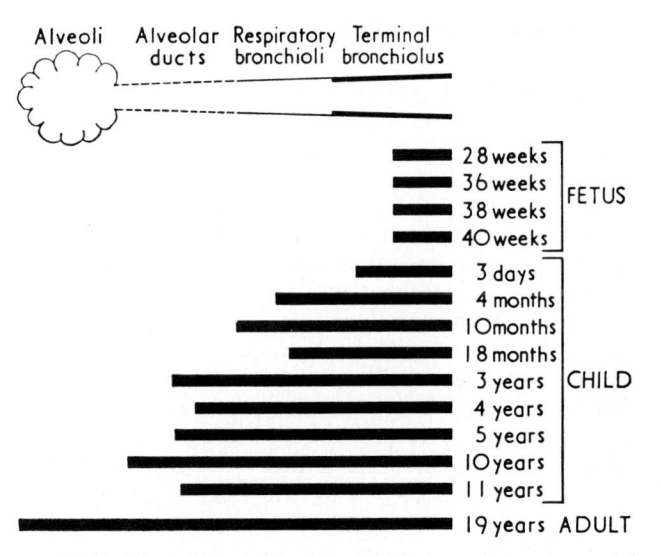

FIG. 32. Progressive extension with age of muscle coat in arterial walls. Within acinus, muscle is not found before birth. With increasing age muscle coat extends into parenchymal region. [From Hislop and Reid (178).]

(as found in the preacinar arteries before birth) by the formation of new peripheral vessels that they had to supply.

Pulmonary veins. Veins increase in size and number during childhood, very much like the arteries. It is obvious from hemodynamic considerations that veins, being approximately the same size as arteries, are more numerous per unit area of lung tissue than arteries in which the flow rate is higher. As mentioned at the beginning of this chapter (see *Blood Vessels*, p. 7), the amount of smooth muscle in veins is very low. As the veins grow in diameter, the muscle layer thickens and extends more toward the periphery (176). Pressure dependence of venous muscularization has been demonstrated in dogs, where the reversal of blood flow to a lung lobe transformed medium-size pulmonary veins into vessels with the histological appearance of pulmonary arteries (319).

Adaptive Growth of Gas-Exchange Apparatus

GENERAL CONSIDERATIONS. Assuming that the gas-exchange tissue is designed and dimensioned to adequately supply the organism with O_2, one may wonder whether lung size is genetically predetermined or whether it can be adapted to altered supply conditions. This question is addressed by presenting three types of experiments where the quantitative structure-to-function relationships (O_2 availability in ambient air, dimensions of gas-exchange tissue, O_2 needs of the organism) have been disturbed. The three topics are adaptive response of the lung to hypoxia, to exercise, and to lung tissue resection, respectively. This sequence is chosen because the last test of the hypothesis is by far the least physiological.

Problems of this type can only be solved by exact quantitation. The introduction into histology of morphometric techniques based on quantitative stereology has greatly facilitated this approach. The most interesting quantitative parameters in this context are those directly influencing the functioning of the lung: air-space and capillary surface areas, air-blood barrier thickness, and capillary volume. All of these parameters can be reliably measured on electron-microscopic sections and the results used to estimate the functioning of the lung. Indeed, some 10 years ago Weibel (363) published a model defining the diffusing capacity (39) based on the quantitative structural parameters noted above. [For details of the model see original publication (363) and its recent modifications (137, 369).] Clearly this morphometrically determined diffusion capacity is the most adequate parameter for the analysis of experiments on adaptive growth, but it is not always available. The air-space (or alveolar) surface area is assuredly the second-best parameter and the most widely used, but it informs only about one of the facets of the possible adaptive mechanisms.

EXPOSURE TO HYPOXIA. In view of the large number of people living at high altitude, humans seem able to adapt fairly well to a hypoxic environment. Physiologists have always been intrigued by the adaptive mechanisms allowing high-altitude natives to overcome the respiratory problems of hypoxia (128). A wealth of literature focusing on physiological parameters has been produced that is not discussed in this chapter. From their descriptions, however, one may retain that high-altitude natives usually have remarkable thoracic development in relation to their body size (16, 127, 195) and that they have larger lungs than lowlanders (10, 55, 127). In comparison with the physiological studies, there was rather little effort to elucidate whether hypoxia could influence the structure of the gas-exchange apparatus. Tenney and Remmers (339) were probably the first to try to tackle the problem by quantitative analysis of the respiratory tissue. They investigated the lungs of guinea pigs and sheep brought up in the Andes at an altitude of 4,500 m and compared them with those of animals raised at sea level. Using strict statistical evaluation, they concluded that the lungs of hypoxic animals were not different from those of the sea-level controls, although there was a trend toward larger values. A second investigation of rats kept 2 wk at a partial pressure of O_2 (P_{O_2}) of 75 mmHg (26) yielded similar results.

On the other hand, a morphometric investigation of the toxic effects of pure O_2 at 258 mmHg on the lungs produced interesting side results. Deficient growth of the alveolar surface area was shown in growing rats (after 2 wk) and young dogs (after 7 mo) in an O_2-enriched environment (220, 311). This growth retardation could reflect the toxic effects of O_2 on the lung cells, but one could also speculate that the pulmonary parenchyma had adapted quantitatively to the hyperoxic environment. The question was worth reexamining. We exposed rats to hypoxia at high altitude ($P_{O_2} \sim 100$ mmHg), hyperoxia in an O_2 chamber ($P_{O_2} \sim 290$ mmHg), and room air ($P_{O_2} \sim 150$ mmHg) from day 23 to day 44 of their lives (71). As expected, the rats that grew up under hyperoxia had significantly smaller lungs, with a normal quantitative distribution of the air space, tissue, and blood compartments in the parenchyma. Expressed in absolute values, all of these parameters and the gas-exchange surface areas were smaller than in controls. In the group exposed to hypoxia the results were the opposite: high-altitude rats had increased average lung volumes although they weighed 11% less than the controls. Quantitative lung parameters expressed in relation to body weight (so-called specific values) were all significantly larger in comparison to those of controls. Because the lung size but not its compartmental composition was altered, it was assumed that there were more alveoli per gram body weight. Figure 33 summarizes the results by presenting the specific pulmonary diffusing capacity for the three groups as calculated from the morphometric data. Bartlett and Remmers (28) subsequently confirmed these findings in rats placed for 3 wk in a simulated high-altitude environment with a P_{O_2} of 95

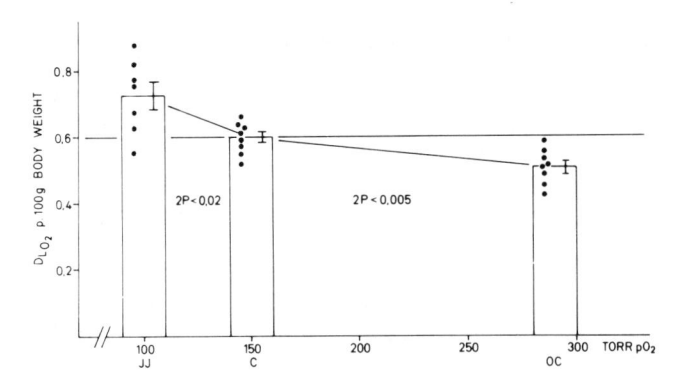

FIG. 33. Quantitative adaptation of rat parenchymal lung structures to altered P_{O_2}. Morphometrically determined specific diffusing capacity (DL) of rats in 3 groups: raised for 3 wk at high altitude (JJ), in room air as controls (C), and in O_2 chamber with 40% O_2 (OC). [From Burri and Weibel (71).]

mmHg. Furthermore comparing the lungs of a population of mice living at high altitude (4,660 m above sea level) with those of mice at sea level, Pearson and Pearson (287) found that the high-altitude animals not only had larger lungs with larger alveolar and capillary surface areas per gram body weight but also had a significantly increased volume proportion of tissue. The increase in tissue mass was due to larger cells rather than an increase in cell number. Pearson and Pearson deduced that the lungs of hypoxic mice not only had more respiratory units but also smaller ones. They suggested that alveolar size reduction is a further step in the adaptive response to hypoxia. A later study confirmed that the type II epithelial cells were significantly larger in mice native to high altitude than in sea-level controls, and that they also had more and larger lamellar bodies (286).

The characteristics of the adaptive response of the lung seem to depend on the age of the animals at exposure. In rats newly born and 3 wk of age exposed to hypoxia for 3 wk, the increase in the ratio of lung weight to body weight was due to an increase in the number and size of alveoli and alveolar ducts (87). In adult rats (9 wk of age) a similar exposure also produced an increase in specific lung weight, but this was due solely to an increase in size and not in the number of air spaces. Furthermore alveolar ducts were enlarged more than alveoli. In other experiments rats exposed to high altitude from birth to 3 wk of age (i.e., during the period of alveolar formation) did not show the expected increase in specific lung volume but seemed to suffer from a general growth depression (P. H. Burri, unpublished observations).

Lechner and Banchero's (237) recent morphometric study of lungs of growing guinea pigs acclimatized to hypoxia confirmed that within 3 wk of exposure lung volumes and surface areas increased by ~30% compared to weight-matched controls. However, with increasing exposure time and continuing growth, the differences were progressively reduced and finally leveled when the animals weighed >900 g. By extrapolating the slopes of the allometric growth curves for hypoxic and control animals to higher body weights, these authors concluded that chronic hypoxia simply accelerated lung growth toward normal adult dimensions. This interesting conclusion has to be considered with caution; at 900 g body wt the lung volumes of hypoxic animals were still significantly larger than those of the controls, and morphometric data for higher body weights were obtained by extrapolation only and not by comparison of measured values. Furthermore the control animals were raised in Denver, Colorado, at 1,600 m above sea level, an altitude that could already have enhanced lung growth. These remarks exemplify some of the difficulties faced in interpreting data of this type of experiment. After exposure to hyperoxia the results are clear: exposed animals have the same body weights as controls but much smaller lung volumes. During exposure to hypoxia, however, the animals usually have a slower increase in body weight. The slowing of growth is general, because all organs are affected except one—the lung. Is it correct in this case to relate lung volume to body weight? This and similar questions are discussed in detail in a review by Thurlbeck (341), in which he finally proposed that the skeletal length or preferably the length of a long bone might be a more adequate reference for lung parameters than body weight. He also suggested that a difference should be made between experiments performed under normobaric hypoxia and those performed under hypobaric conditions. Based on the findings published, however, such a differentiation does not shed more light on the situation.

Concerning humans, there is one morphometric investigation of the quantitative structural differences in lungs of people living at high altitude and at sea level, and the report is only available in abstract form. Lungs of the high-altitude group had more and larger alveoli with a larger alveolar surface area than those of the sea-level population (305). Certainly more investigations of this type are overdue (164). On the other hand, physiological measurements of pulmonary function performed in Peruvian high-altitude natives nicely fit the hypothesis that high-altitude lungs have increased volumes with increased alveolar numbers but also suggest that the bronchial tree does not participate in the adaptive response and is comparable to that of lowlanders (55).

INCREASED OXYGEN CONSUMPTION. Three procedures have been used repeatedly to increase O_2 consumption in experimental animals: physical exercise, cold exposure, and administration of thyroid hormones. The effect of physical training on lung size and parenchymal morphology was investigated repeatedly decades ago. With rather simple examinations of alveolar dimensions, it was postulated that physical training enlarged the lungs and increased the number of alveoli (138, 226, 343). Applying morphometric techniques to measure the alveolar surface area (among other parameters), Bartlett (25) investigated the influence of daily exercise and thyroid hormones on the growing rat lung. Neither depression of thyroid activity by treatment with thiouracil, nor daily administration of L-thyroxine, nor 30-min daily physical exercise affected lung growth. In 1971 Geelhaar and Weibel (134) investigated the lungs of Japanese waltzing mice (JWM) and compared them with those of normal white laboratory mice. The JWM suffer from a genetic defect of the brain and of the vestibular and cochlear systems. By 3 wk of age they are deaf and develop a hyperkinetic syndrome, the typical high-speed waltz (up to 3 turns per s) accompanied by chorea-athetotic movements during resting phases. The size of the gas-exchange apparatus matched their heavily increased O_2 consumption. The authors interpreted these findings as a functional adaptation to the increased rate of O_2 consumption ($\dot{V}_{O_2}$); they could not, however, exclude the possibility that lung size was determined by a genetic factor. Indeed, it seems that the latter is true, as Bartlett and Areson (27) recently showed by investigating JWM and comparing them with their nonwaltzing littermates. They found no differences in lung parameters between dancers and normal animals.

As it became possible to induce a waltzing syndrome very similar to that of JWM in normal laboratory mice, the hypothesis that increased O_2 demand could enhance lung growth was again tested (68). After three daily injections of the drug imino-$\beta\beta'$-dipropionitrile (IDPN) at 3 wk of age, normal mice developed within 5 days a pattern of locomotion resembling that of JWM and increased their O_2 consumption per gram body weight by 50%. Complete morphometric analysis of the lungs of these animals 3.5 mo later revealed larger specific lung volumes and especially a morphometric pulmonary O_2 diffusing capacity per gram body weight (Fig. 34) that was increased proportionally to specific $\dot{V}_{O_2}$ (192).

Because the IDPN-related substance β-aminopropionitrile (a lysyl oxidase inhibitor and lathyrogen) inhibits the cross-linking of collagen and elastin (23, 228), one might suspect that alterations in lung size were produced by increased lung compliance (209). In the morphometric data of IDPN-injected mice, however, air-space volume density (i.e., the percentage of V_L occupied by air) was smaller, not larger as one would expect with simple lung dilatation. Furthermore air-space surface density (surface area per unit V_L) was significantly enlarged, indicating a higher complexity of internal lung structure.

In a further experiment, the $\dot{V}_{O_2}$ increase was achieved by cold exposure. Growing rats exposed to an ambient temperature of 11°C had a $\dot{V}_{O_2}$ increase of 64% compared with controls kept at 24°C. After a 3-wk exposure the low-temperature rats had 24% larger lungs, morphometric analysis of the respiratory tissue

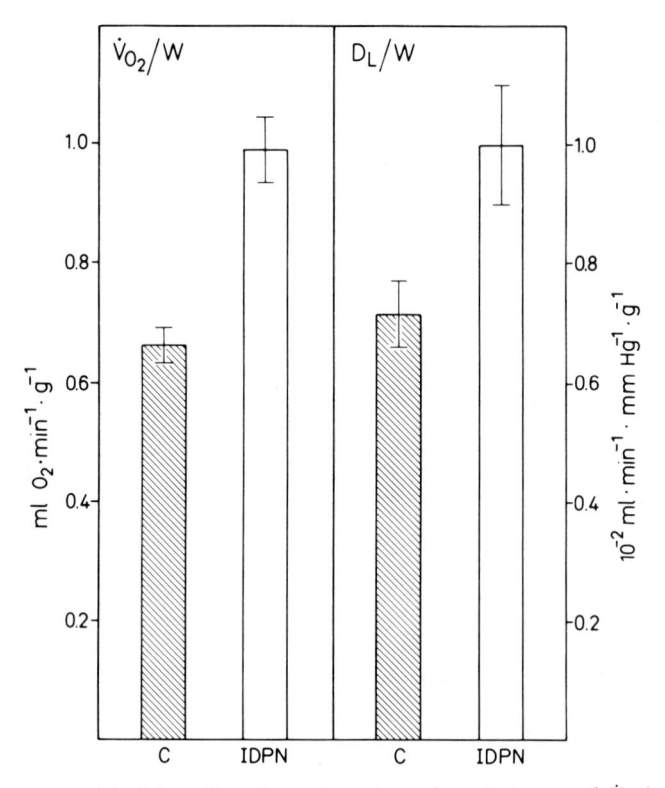

FIG. 34. Adaptation of growing mouse lung to increased $\dot{V}_{O_2}$/body weight (W). Drug-induced waltzing mice [imino-$\beta\beta'$-dipropionitrile (IDPN)] show a 50% increase in specific $\dot{V}_{O_2}$/W when compared to their nonwaltzing littermates (C). Specific morphometrically determined pulmonary diffusing capacity (DL/W) was correspondingly increased 3.5 mo after induction of the permanent waltzing syndrome. [From Hugonnaud, Burri, et al. (192).]

revealed 18% larger gas-exchange surface areas, and the calculated pulmonary diffusing capacity was increased more than 20% over control values (136). Unlike in experiments with low P_{O_2} or with IDPN, these experimental rats had the same body weights as controls. Figure 35 shows the results of an analogous experiment made in hamsters (340). By either cold exposure (5°C) or daily injections of triiodothyronine, $\dot{V}_{O_2}$ was increased by 26% over control values for 4 wk. A third experimental group was treated with methimazole, an antithyroid drug. As illustrated in Figure 35 the alveolar surface area was increased proportionally to the $\dot{V}_{O_2}$ change, whereas methimazole lowered $\dot{V}_{O_2}$ but did not affect lung size.

Lechner and Banchero (236) further confirmed this stimulation of lung growth by increased $\dot{V}_{O_2}$ in guinea pigs exposed to cold. In guinea pigs exposed to hypoxia, however, the differences became smaller as the experiments increased in duration. As for hypoxia, these authors concluded that chronic increase in O_2 consumption accelerated lung growth in young guinea pigs toward normal adult dimensions.

LUNG TISSUE RESECTION. The introduction to this section (see GENERAL CONSIDERATIONS, p. 26) briefly

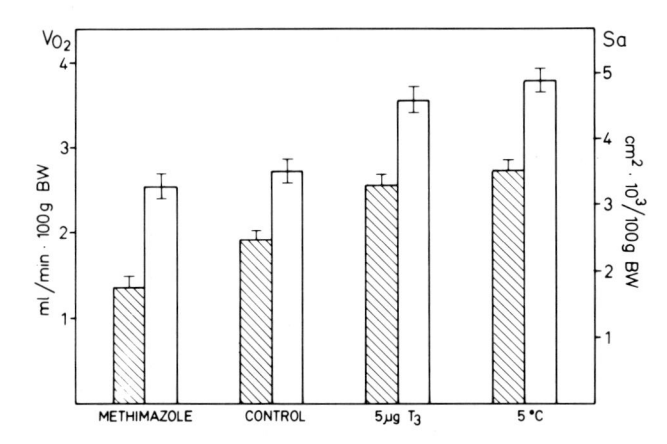

FIG. 35. The $\dot{V}_{O_2}$ per 100 g body wt (*shaded bars*) and corresponding alveolar surface area (Sa) per 100 g body wt (*open bars*) in 4 groups of hamsters under different treatments from postnatal wk 6 to 10. T_3, triiodothyronine. [Adapted from Thompson (340).]

mentioned that it was somehow problematic to compare the regenerative reactions of pulmonary tissue after pneumonectomy with the adaptive reactions to stress factors such as hypoxia, exercise, or cold. In investigating lung regeneration, one may be confronted with mechanisms relying more on the grounds of homeostatic regulations of tissue mass than on functional requirements. Nevertheless, considering particularly the morphological and quantitative aspects, it is interesting to analyze the results obtained in this type of experiment. They reflect the enormous plasticity of the pulmonary structure and its ability to recover from heavy insults.

The reaction of the lung remainders after pneumonectomy preoccupied researchers for nearly a century. Although the general facts are known, including many details about regenerative reactions in rats and rabbits, almost no information is available on the alterations of lung structure induced in humans by resection of pulmonary tissue. Detailed reviews of the literature are referred to in recent publications on this subject (51, 69, 70, 231, 341).

From my experiments with growing rats, integrated with findings of other authors obtained in rats or other species, the following response to lung tissue resection can be crystallized. After left-sided pneumonectomy (the most frequently practiced operation) or the removal of the upper and middle lobes of the right lungs (bilobectomy), the remaining parts of the lung increase in volume and weight within a few days. The marked volume increase of the first 24–48 h is brought about exclusively by dilatation of the air spaces, whereby alveolar ducts are first affected more than alveoli (day 1), which appear enlarged on postoperative day 4 (69). During this phase the first biochemical changes can be detected. In mice the activity of cAMP-related enzymes was elevated maximally during postoperative days 1–3 (270). In days 2–6 tissue proliferation begins, and the rate of both RNA and DNA synthesis increases rapidly to reach a maximum on postoperative days 4–6; it returns as rapidly to normal values within another week [Fig. 36; (53, 82, 298); P. H. Burri, unpublished observations]. Peaks in mitotic activity, as observed by the colchicine metaphase-arrest technique, fall about day 6 (125). In rabbits the reaction was slower; at the alveolar level maximal DNA synthesis was recorded 11 days after pneumonectomy (94). During the phase of intense cellular reaction, synthesis of collagen was increased in rabbits (82); in experiments with rats the interalveolar septa were slightly thickened, and the dilatation of the air spaces appeared to have regressed (69). A few days later, on postoperative day 9, lung morphology as seen in the scanning electron microscope was back to normal. This sequence of events was fully confirmed by morphometric analysis performed on the same animals (66), where on day 9 no parameters in the pulmonary parenchyma differed from those of the age-matched control rats.

These recent data confirm and specify the timing of previous observations that described the full recovery of all parenchymal compartments, including the gas-exchange surface area, 6.5 wk after bilobectomy (70). The only difference between lobectomized and control rats found in that study was the significantly smaller volume densities of the bronchial tree and the larger blood vessels in the former group. This indicates that the parenchymal structures have greater adaptive potential than nonparenchymal structures. Interestingly, Brody and co-workers (55) made an analogous observation regarding the lack of adaptation of the bronchial tree to hypoxia in the population of Peruvian high-altitude natives. This lagging behind of the supplying elements may have functional implications for the dynamics of ventilation and perfusion (70).

As may be expected, young animals show a better tolerance to pneumonectomy than older ones. Their rate of increase in DNA synthesis is greater (64), and lung weight increases faster and (unlike that in older rats) fully reaches the presurgery value (265). It has often been reported that sequelae are much more pronounced when pneumonectomy is performed in adult animals (22, 50, 149, 184, 242, 375).

On the other hand, morphometric investigation of the adaptive potential of the adult rat lung yielded (except for details) the same results as those obtained in young rats. In female rats of 240 g body wt, 6.5 wk after a 25% resection of lung volume the dimensions of the gas-exchange apparatus were fully restored (356). The animals investigated were adult but still growing—increasing on average from 240 to 320 g. It is possible that this remaining growth potential was still large enough to also cover the extra growth. In a study of pneumonectomized adult rats of 330 g body wt in which the lung weight–to–body weight ratio and lung cell size had stabilized, DNA synthesis increased (peak on postoperative day 4) and the ratio of lung

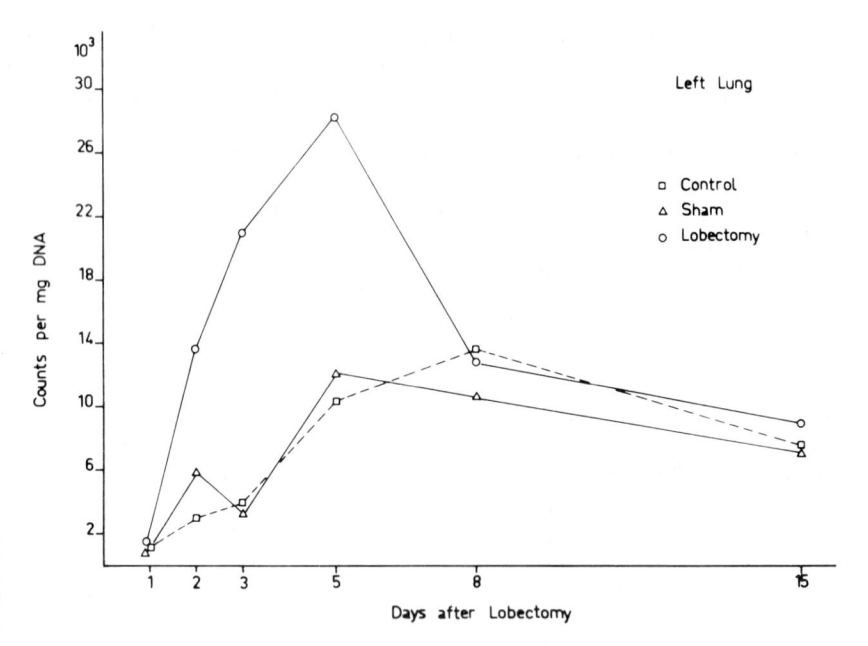

FIG. 36. Synthesis of DNA in left lung and right lower lobe of rats subjected to resection of upper and medium lobes of right lung at 3 wk of age. Incorporation of [^{3}H]thymidine into lung DNA expressed as disintegrations per min (or counts) per mg DNA by liquid-scintillation counting. Note high peaks in lobectomy group and quicker response in right lung. (P. H. Burri, unpublished data.)

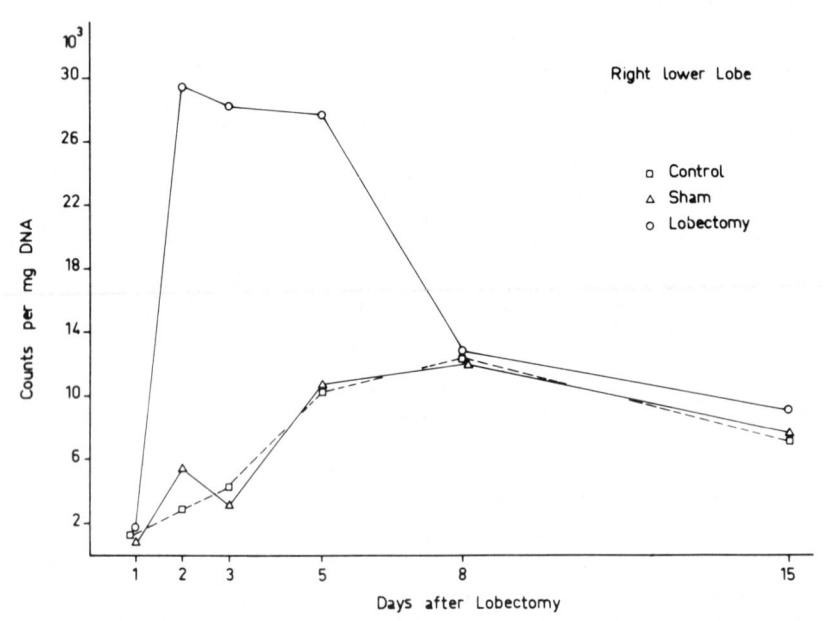

weight to body weight and the RNA and protein contents were restored within 7 days (294). These results let one assume that the ability to restore lung mass after significant tissue loss is not limited to the young rat. However, the adult rat may be a special case because portions of its thoracic cage are never ossified, allowing for temporally extended growth of the thorax and possibly of the lung (96).

Studies in humans indicate that the remaining lung increases in volume but never returns to the original dimensions as in animals. A follow-up study of children and adults, 5–25 yr after undergoing lung tissue resection, reported that the operation was remarkably well tolerated when performed at a young age (232).

In isolated cases exceptional changes in lung size were observed. A patient with extensive lung tissue resection showed a three- to fourfold increase of the uniquely remaining right upper lobe, as verified by radiology and lung function tests (32). The carbon monoxide diffusing capacity reached three-quarters of that calculated for the whole lung. These findings suggest that in addition to functional remodeling, a certain quantitative structural recovery was likely to have occurred. Morphometric analysis of the remaining lung after pneumonectomy has, to our knowledge, been performed once with no hints of alveolar multiplication (102). The air spaces were widened, but without signs of tissue destruction.

STRUCTURAL FEATURES OF ADAPTIVE RESPONSE. Whether or not new alveoli can be formed during the adaptive reaction of the lung to hypoxia, increased $\dot{V}_{O_2}$, or lung tissue resection deserves mention. Understandably morphologists want to know by what structural measures the lung is able to reactively increase its size and especially its gas-exchange surface. Due to the assumption that a lung is better equipped for O_2 uptake if it has more respiratory units (which is not necessarily correct), the number of alveoli in the lung has always received special attention. Among the three types of experimental stimulation of lung growth, the removal of lung tissue induces by far the largest quantitative and morphological changes. Therefore it is sensible to discuss the problem of alveolar formation on the basis of data obtained in resection experiments. However, if one is expecting an unambiguous response from these experiments the results are deceiving. Even in the case of heavy stimulation by removing two lobes of the right lung or, alternatively, the entire left lung (i.e., 25% or 35%, respectively, of total VL), the findings are controversial. Publications postulating formation of new alveoli (6, 80, 171, 184, 231) are counterbalanced by others denying this mechanism (38, 52, 64, 296, 312). Admittedly not all of these papers are based on solid quantitative analysis, because the techniques were not yet available, but even the more recent publications using a morphometric approach yield contradicting findings. This may be partly due to the problems inherent to the alveolar counting procedures—it is extremely difficult to properly define alveoli in histological sections. Three-dimensional reconstructions of lung parenchyma have proven that large errors could be made by misinterpretation of alveolar ducts and alveoli in light-microscopic sections (160). Also from a theoretical point of view alveolar counting is unreliable if alveoli alter their shape (67), which certainly happens during alveolar formation. The problem is further complicated because different regions of the pulmonary parenchyma may present dissimilar patterns of reaction. Nattie and co-workers (265) described enlarging of central alveoli and multiplication of subpleural ones after a left-sided pneumonectomy. Thus there is little hope to solve the problem by simply counting alveoli or air spaces.

From a structural point of view, given the mode of alveolar formation after birth, it is unlikely that a lung consisting of mature interalveolar septa could produce further alveoli unless one postulates a new way of alveolar formation. However, it cannot be excluded that after postnatal formation of the bulk of alveoli there are focally distributed areas that retain the primitive septal morphology and with it the ability to form new septa.

Scanning electron microscopy showed that after transient widening of the air spaces there was no difference in parenchymal morphology between operated animals and controls 9 days after a bilobectomy (69). However, scanning electron microscopy did not provide clues for alveolar formation.

Are there means other than alveolar formation allowing for such a complete recovery? We recently discussed two alternatives (69): *1*) a compensatory enlargement of the air spaces in certain lung regions or *2*) a masking of the original air-space dilatation by a growth in length of the interalveolar septa. Whereas no clues were found for the first alternative, a two-dimensional model was proposed that illustrated how the parenchymal morphology could apparently be restored (i.e., particularly how the widening of the air spaces could be masked to the observer's eye) by a lengthening of the interalveolar septa. Morphometric measurements of the model showed that standard parameters like volume density, surface density, and mean linear intercepts of air spaces were not discriminating enough to assess the differences between the normal and postrecovery states of the model. This study demonstrated that alveolar formation was not necessarily needed to explain the morphological recovery of the lung and stressed that sophisticated morphometric techniques are required to definitely answer this problem.

FINAL DIMENSIONS OF THE HUMAN LUNG

Alveolar counts and alveolar surface area were the parameters most often determined in human lungs (11, 95, 101, 163, 169, 315). Weibel and Gomez (360, 372) and Dunnill (101) published more extensive morphometric studies providing more detailed analyses of the parenchyma. All of these studies, however, are based on measurements performed under the light microscope (i.e., with relatively poor resolution and on a material that had undergone considerable shrinkage). Since then a large number of animal studies have been published using refined stereologic techniques in combination with the high resolution of the electron microscope. Yet only recently has it been possible to obtain comparable data for the human lung. Gehr and co-workers (135) analyzed the lungs of eight patients who died abruptly from nonrespiratory causes. Their measurements of the parenchymal compartments and the gas-exchange surface areas were subsequently completed by an analysis of the cellular composition of the gas-exchange tissue performed on the same lungs by Crapo and co-workers (84). Table 4 gives a synopsis of these results. From a quantitative point of view, these data reflect the end result at which pulmonary development was aimed. Therefore they are well suited to close the morphological section of this chapter.

DEVELOPMENT OF PULMONARY SURFACTANT SYSTEM

Biochemical functions of the lung encompass a wide spectrum of metabolic activities. It is sensible to clas-

TABLE 4. *Quantitative Structural Analysis of the Normal Human Lung*

Body wt, kg	74 ± 4
Volume, ml	
Lung	4,341 ± 285
Air space	3,386 ± 243
Parenchyma	3,907 ± 256
Parenchymal tissue	298 ± 36
Capillary	213 ± 31
Surface area, m^2	
Alveoli	143 ± 12
Capillary	126 ± 12
Total number of parenchymal cells, × 10^9	230 ± 25
Total cell number, %	
Alveolar type I cells	8.3 ± 0.6
Alveolar type II cells	15.9 ± 0.8
Endothelial cells	30.2 ± 2.4
Interstitial cells	36.1 ± 1.0
Macrophages	9.4 ± 2.2
Alveolar surface covered by, %	
Type I cells	92.9 ± 1.0
Type II cells	7.1 ± 1.0

Values are means ± 1 SE for 8 normal human lungs. [Data from Gehr et al. (135) and Crapo et al. (84).]

sify them into two groups: the respiration-related and the nonrespiration-related functions. The most important respiration-related biochemical function of the lung is the production of the surface-active material of the alveolar lining layer that protects the lung from atelectasis. At birth the presence of a qualitatively and quantitatively adequate surfactant system is a matter of life or death. Therefore a wealth of studies has investigated before and around birth the development of both the structural background and the enzymatic machinery needed for surfactant production. On the other hand, the nonrespiration-related or so-called nonrespiratory functions of the lung, which have received increasing interest in the past two decades, are not as directly involved in the perinatal readjustment of the life-supporting mechanisms. Therefore there was probably rather little urge to investigate their prenatal emergence. As a result, relatively little information is available on the development and maturation of these activities. Because of the multiplicity of nonrespiratory functions of the lung and of the scarcity of data available on their fetal development, it is not possible to efficiently review these topics within the scope of this chapter. They are addressed in detail in the chapters by Junod, Ryan, and Bakhle and Ferreira in this *Handbook*.

The last section of this chapter is therefore aimed at concisely surveying the development of the surfactant system and its perinatal functioning. For further information there are several recent review articles (29, 31, 159, 180).

Historical Background and Function of Pulmonary Surfactant

The surfactant system is designed to function as a stabilizer of the air spaces. In 1929 von Neergaard (352) suggested that the observed retractile forces of the lung were due two-thirds to the presence of an air-liquid interface producing relatively large surface forces. According to Laplace's law $P = 2\gamma/r$, relating the pressure (P) inside a bubble to the surface tension (γ) and to the reciprocal of the bubble radius (r), the surface forces would be greatest in small alveoli and/or at low inflation levels so that alveolar collapse would ensue. Von Neergard suggested that the alveolar surface film was composed of a surface tension–lowering layer. This was confirmed more than 25 years later by Pattle (283), who observed that lung fluid formed a very stable foam. Yet this confirmation of the presence of a surface-active material still did not solve the problem of why, in contradiction to Laplace's law, the small alveoli could exist next to the large ones. Clements and co-workers (78) elucidated this question by demonstrating on a modified Wilhelmy surface-tension balance that lung washings and saline extracts of whole lung had high surface tensions when spread over a large surface and very low surface tensions when the film was compressed. This signified that the surfactant material was able to maintain alveolar stability at end-expiratory volumes and also reduce the work when alveoli were to be opened (308). Finally, in 1968 the surfactant layer was demonstrated in situ with electron microscopy by Weibel and Gil (370).

Biochemistry of Pulmonary Surfactant

COMPOSITION. In 1961 Pattle and Thomas (284) suggested that the surface-active material was a lecithin-protein complex, and Klaus and co-workers (221) published a brief note that the foamy fluid isolated from beef lungs contained 50%–70% lipids, of which 74% were phospholipids, and that this phospholipid fraction was capable of lowering the surface tension to 1–5 dyn/cm when compressed on a Wilhelmy balance. Since then it has been shown that the surfactant material is a complex mixture of phospholipids, neutral lipids, proteins, and carbohydrates. Among the phospholipids, phosphatidylcholine (PC or lecithin) is by far the largest component (129, 162, 213, 215–217). The PCs of the pulmonary surfactant are unique in the sense that they contain two saturated fatty acyl constituents at carbon positions 1 and 2, whereas PCs from other sources usually have an unsaturated fatty acid chain in carbon position 2 (Fig. 37). The most frequent fatty acid constituent, palmitic acid, is found in both positions so that dipalmitoyl phosphatidylcholine (DPPC) is the most abundant component of surfactant and also greatly responsible for its surface tension–lowering property. The second phospholipid present in surfactant (7%–14%, depending on the authors) is phosphatidylglycerol (PG), a molecule greatly resembling DPPC, because again palmitic acyl groups are the most frequent fatty acid chains in the two carbon positions. Phosphatidylglycerols can also

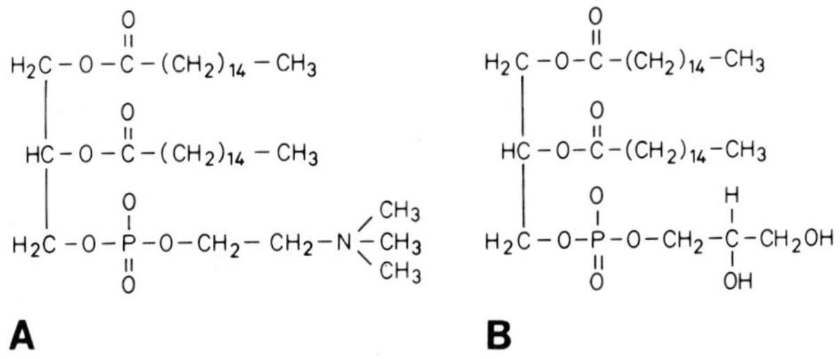

FIG. 37. Structure of the 2 most important phospholipids of pulmonary surfactant. A: dipalmitoyl phosphatidylcholine. B: dipalmitoyl phosphatidylglycerol.

lower surface tension, but because their concentration is relatively low alternative functions have been postulated. They could play a role in stabilizing the surfactant complex (150) and/or activate enzymes relevant to phospholipid synthesis (289). That proteins are associated with the phospholipids was suggested early and has been demonstrated many times (76, 81, 97, 143, 213, 214, 218, 219, 252, 281, 282). Present knowledge indicates that two probably specific nonserum proteins (34,000–36,000 and 10,000–11,000 daltons), called apoproteins of surfactant, are present in the surface-active material. Hitchcock (180) suggested that they could stabilize the surfactant after secretion and help the adsorption of the surface-active material at the air-liquid interface. On the basis of a kinetic study where the appearance of the 10,000-dalton protein moiety was delayed, King and co-workers (219) proposed that the smaller protein was a metabolic fragment of the 35,000-dalton molecule.

Much less is known about the association of carbohydrates with surfactant. In 1954 Macklin (249) proposed that the alveoli possess a mucoid film secreted by the granular pneumocytes. After this a number of histochemical studies demonstrated the presence of polysaccharides either related to the cell membrane (cell coat) or in the liquid layer (34, 35, 75, 77, 272). For a while the relationship between this material and the alveolar surfactant was rather unclear, but demonstration of the electron-microscopic characteristics of the surfactant material fixed in situ helped to clear the situation (144, 370). With the assessment of DPPC as the principal surface-active component, polysaccharides were dismissed from this role. It is likely, however, that surfactant carbohydrates are associated with the proteins (218, 281, 282). Recently it was proposed that they may take part in the transformation, within the alveolar space, of the material secreted from the lamellar bodies into the tubular myelin figures (333).

PATHWAYS OF PC AND PG SYNTHESIS IN THE ADULT AND FETAL LUNG. Biosynthesis of lung phospholipids was reviewed a few years ago (120, 122, 348, 349). Figure 38 illustrates the main steps of the pathways for PC and PG. In the lung, PC is produced de novo via the so-called cytidine diphosphate (CDP)-choline pathway. In short, glucose or glycerol is converted to dihydroxyacetone-phosphate, which is then esterified with a saturated fatty acid at carbon position 1 (or α). The resulting acylglycerol-3-phosphate is esterified at carbon position 2 (or β) with an unsaturated fatty acid. The resulting α-saturated, β-unsaturated phosphatidic acid plays a key role in both PC and PG synthesis. After hydrolyzation of phosphatidic acid to 1,2-diacylglycerol by the phosphatidic acid phosphohydrolase the molecule is ready for the incorporation of the energetic CDP-choline, a reaction catalyzed by the enzyme cholinephosphotransferase. The CDP-choline is generated from choline to cholinephosphate under the influence of choline kinase and ATP, and further to CDP-choline by the cholinephosphate cytidylyltransferase. All of the enzymes needed have been repeatedly demonstrated in adult and, importantly, fetal lungs (21, 121, 275, 304, 383, 384).

The product of these synthetic steps is an α-saturated, β-unsaturated PC that is a constituent of membranes but does not show particular surface activity. The type II cell may use it as a membrane component during phases of cell proliferation and as a precursor molecule in the fully differentiated and secreting cell (320). For surfactant production the cell transforms the monosaturated molecule to a disaturated molecule. Figure 38 (frame G) also describes the mechanism by which the fatty acid composition is remodeled. A pulmonary phospholipase A2 (133) located in the endoplasmic reticulum degrades preferentially PCs with an unsaturated fatty acid at carbon position 2, producing 2-lysophosphatidylcholine (LPC). Reacylation to a disaturated PC by the enzyme LPC acyltransferase follows (130, 229). Whether this enzyme shows a preference for a particular fatty acid (especially palmitic acid) is disputed (110, 130, 165). Alternatively, two LPC molecules condense in such a way that the palmitic acid in the α-position of one is transferred to the β-position of the other. The products of this reaction are one molecule of DPPC and one molecule of glycerophosphorylcholine. This mechanism, called the Marinetti pathway (250), is found in adult and fetal lungs and was first described by Abe and Akino (1). It has been suggested that the involved enzyme was responsible for both the deacylation and the transacylation steps of this reaction (58).

From the two mechanisms of conversion it seems that in the adult lung the LPC acyltransferase is more important than the Marinetti pathway (30). However, this may be different in the fetal and newborn lung. In fetal mouse lung (274) and fetal rat lung (273) the LPC–LPC acyltransferase was found to increase shortly before term.

Two groups of authors recently proposed that saturated PC molecules are selectively transported from their production site in the endoplasmic reticulum to their storage site (the lamellar body) by a phospholipid-exchange protein (111, 297). By this means sat-

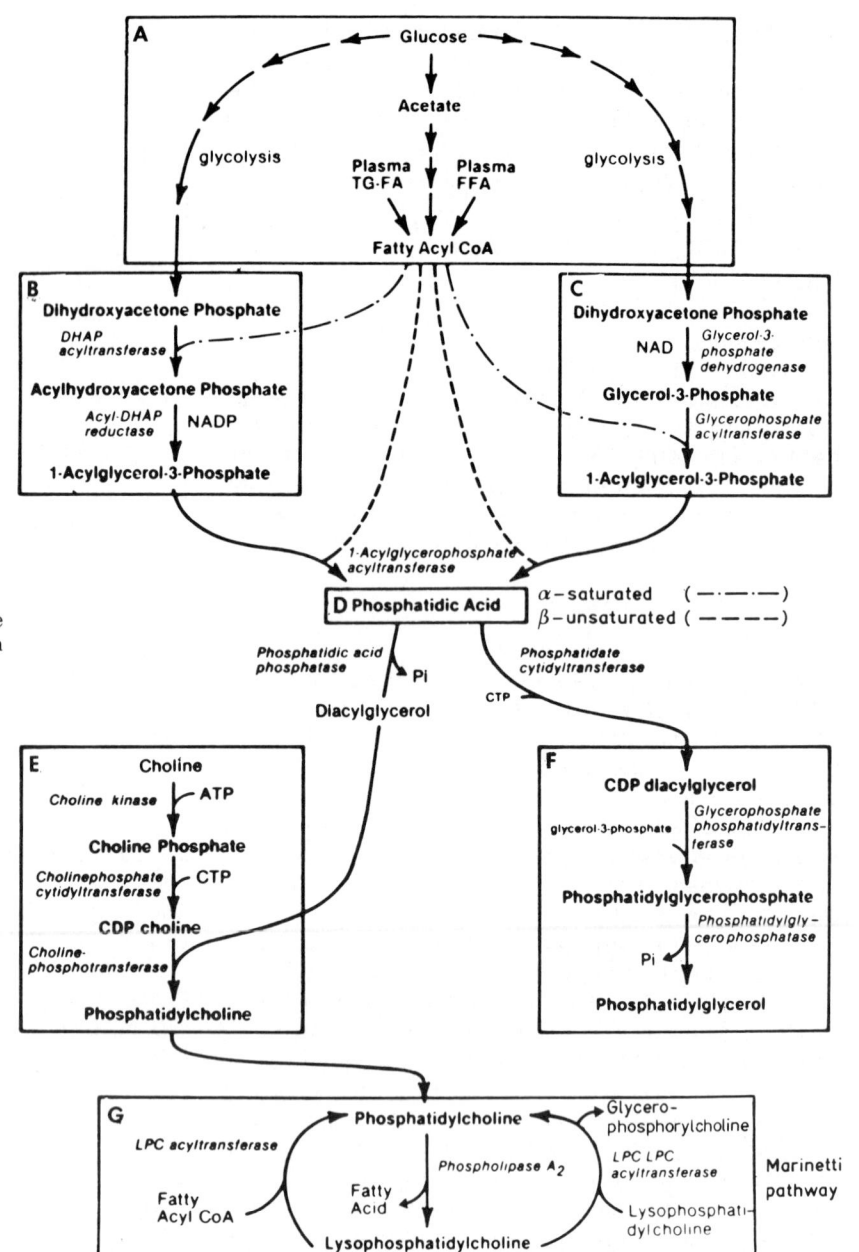

FIG. 38. Pathways of phosphatidylcholine and phosphatidylglycerol biosynthesis. [From Perelman et al. (289).]

urated PCs are specifically accumulated in the prospective surfactant material (345).

Phosphatidylcholine can be synthesized in many tissues by an alternative route—the methylation pathway. This involves phosphorylation of ethanolamine, linkage to diglyceride to form phosphatidylethanolamine, followed by a stepwise methylation. The most investigated key enzyme of this pathway (phosphatidylethanolamine methyltransferase) is present in the lung, but its activity is only a fraction of that in the liver. For a while it was assumed that the methylation pathway might be particularly important in the fetal lung (147, 148); however, recent studies have discounted its significance in the lung, particularly in the fetus (225, 302). This route seems to account for 5% of the total PC synthesis; thus it can be concluded that the CDP-choline pathway is the source of DPPC in surfactant (289).

Compared to that of PC synthesis, knowledge about the mechanism of PG production is poor. Presence of PG has been established in pulmonary surfactant and lamellar body fractions of adult (155, 157, 158, 199, 299, 303, 306, 307) and fetal specimens of various species including humans (153, 158). Despite activity in other subcellular fractions, particularly mitochondria, the site of synthesis has been placed in the lamellar body (303) or in the microsomal fraction (154, 156). Two of the enzymes involved in PG synthesis are phosphatidate cytidylyltransferase and glycerophosphate phosphatidyltransferase; both have been found in fetal and adult lungs (155, 156, 304). Whether remodeling of the fatty acyl constituents occurs in the formation of disaturated PGs, as has been observed for PCs, has not yet been investigated.

SURFACTANT TURNOVER. Clearly the synthesis of surface-active material must be a continuous process. Through pulse labeling of surfactant phospholipids Jobe et al. (199, 200) found a relatively high turnover. Interestingly, it seems that surfactant utilization is correlated with ventilation rate or possibly with ventilation depth. Hyperventilation was found to stimulate both surfactant production (103, 278, 279) and its degradation (103, 381). Furthermore Gail and co-workers (132) reported that intracellular and alveolar surfactant reserves were proportionately increased in animal species with higher respiratory rates.

Type II Cells and Regulation of Surfactant Production

LAMELLAR BODIES AND SURFACTANT PRODUCTION. The close coupling between the formation of type II cells, the development of intracytoplasmic lamellar bodies, and the appearance of surfactant material in the primitive air spaces has already been discussed (see *Start of surfactant synthesis*, p. 13). No doubts remain regarding the structure-function relationship between lamellar bodies and surface-active material [for review see Hitchcock (180)]. This author and her co-workers presented a surfactant marker system (unspecific esterases) that allows correlation of biochemical and morphological findings in all kinds of preparations: whole lung, surfactant-enriched lung fractions, lamellar body fractions, lung lavage fluid, and isolated type II cells (181). The enzymes have also been demonstrated in organotypic cultures from fetal rat lung (99). Unlike in humans, where surfactant already appears in the lung tissue (and in small quantities also in the alveoli) toward the end of fetal month 6 (73), surfactant production usually starts in most species investigated at 80%–85% of total gestation period (Fig. 39). A morphological feature of type II cell maturation is the appearance of lamellar bodies, which is accompanied by a progressive depletion of the glycogen stores. Glycogen in fetal tissues generally represents an energy store for cell proliferation and differentiation. This is also true in type II cells. However, the glucose produced by glycogenolysis can serve as a substrate for both the glyceride backbone and the fatty acid constituents of the surfactant phospholipids. Alveolar epithelial cells of fetal rat lung accumulated glycogen until 3 days before birth and were then depleted synchronously with the appearance of lamellar bodies, strongly suggesting that this material was used for phospholipid synthesis (377). Gilden and co-workers (145) investigated the effect of cortisol treatment on PC synthesis, found an increased incorporation of glucose into PC, and postulated that glycogen could be the source of the glucose. Although very little is known about the regulation of glycogen stores in the lung, it is likely that many hormones influencing the glycogen metabolism also influence type II cell differentiation and surfactant production at this stage.

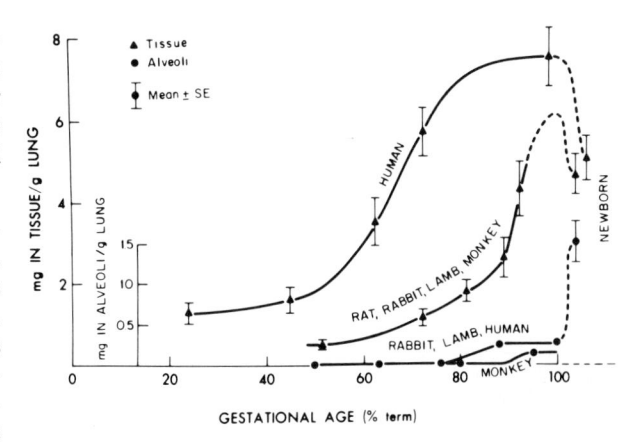

FIG. 39. Concentrations of disaturated phosphatidylcholine in lung tissue and alveoli plotted against relative gestational age for rat, rabbit, lamb, monkey, and human. Values are averaged over intervals of 10%–20% of gestation. [From Clements and Tooley (79), by courtesy of Marcel Dekker, Inc.]

It was not this idea, however, that triggered the wealth of investigations on the effects of drugs and hormones on lung maturation performed in the last 10–15 years. Ten years after Avery and Mead's (12) discovery that a deficiency of the surfactant system was at the origin of the respiratory distress syndrome, Buckingham and co-workers (63) proposed that the timing of lung maturation might be manipulated by hormonal treatment. In 1953 Moog (260) observed the influence of steroids on the differentiation of phosphatase in the duodenal epithelial cells of suckling mice. Buckingham and co-workers (63) therefore hypothesized that because the alveolar epithelium was derived from the endoderm of the foregut it might still be regulated by mechanisms similar to those functioning in the gut epithelium. This hypothesis rapidly gained support from Liggins (239), who observed that fetal lambs whose premature birth had been induced by dexamethasone injections showed advanced lung maturation with precocious appearance of surfactant. Since then many morphological, physiological, biochemical, and clinical studies have completed our knowledge of the effects of glucocorticoids. In addition interest has turned to other hormones, factors, and drugs. Table 5 lists the effects of the various agent compounds tested for activity. This chapter does not review the literature on this subject. Yet because of the close relationship of the matter with normal pulmonary maturation, this section briefly reviews the two most frequently tested groups of hormones, corticosteroid and thyroid hormones.

TABLE 5. *Drugs and Hormones Influencing Surfactant Biosynthesis*

	Effect
Steroids	
Glucocorticoids	Stimulate
Estrogens	Stimulate
11-Oxosteroids	Stimulate, after reduction to 11β-hydroxysteroids by lung fibroblasts
Thyroid hormones and analogues	
Thyroxine	Stimulates
Triiodothyronine	Stimulates
Reverse triiodothyronine	Unknown
3,5-Dimethyl-3′-isopropylthyronine (DIMIT)	Stimulates
Peptide hormones	
Adrenocorticotropic hormone	Stimulates
Fibroblast-pneumonocyte factor	Stimulates
Prolactin	Stimulates (?)
Epithelial growth factor	Stimulates
Thyrotropin-releasing hormone	Stimulates
Insulin	Inhibits
Other agents	
Heroin	Stimulates
Bisolvon (metabolite VIII)	Stimulates
cAMP, methylxanthines	Stimulate

From Smith and Bogues (322).

INFLUENCE OF CORTICOSTEROID HORMONES. There is a bulk of evidence that surfactant phospholipid synthesis is increased after in vivo or in vitro glucocorticoid treatment of various adult and fetal animals or tissue and cell cultures, respectively (104, 123, 223, 290, 300). According to Perelman and co-workers (289), enhanced incorporation of choline palmitate, glucose, acetate, and glycerol into pulmonary PC could be demonstrated after treatment with cortisol or cortisol analogues. Results were less homogeneous, however, as to which enzymes are particularly affected by the steroid hormones. Of the three main enzymes of the major pathway, the CDP-choline pathway—cholinephosphotransferase, cholinephosphate cytidylyltransferase, and choline kinase—only the first one seemed to be activated by 9-fluoroprednisolone acetate or dexamethasone treatment (123, 275). Yet these findings are contested by others. Another enzyme induced to increase its activity by corticosteroids was the phosphatidic acid phosphatase (PAPase) [see Fig. 38; (48, 300)]. In addition to PC synthesis, PG synthesis and the related enzyme glycerophosphate phosphatidyltransferase are reported to be increased (301). This list of enzymes is far from complete and the results are controversial.

In view of these conflicting data as to whether and which enzymes are activated, Gilden and co-workers (145) suggested an interesting alternative. They proposed that glucocorticoids enhance PC production by maturing the type II cells and increasing the substrate supply. Indeed, they observed an enhanced glycogenolysis in fetal rabbit lungs treated with cortisol and an increased flux of [^{14}C]glucose into PC. Regardless of the mechanisms of action, cytoplasmic and nuclear glucocorticoid receptors have often been demonstrated in fetal lungs (17–19, 139–141, 327) so that one can assume direct hormone action on the cells. The number of receptors varies with development, however; it is low early in fetal life, increases toward term, and decreases after birth (140, 327). Because the peak of this fluctuation correlates with surfactant production, it is postulated that pulmonary maturation is controlled physiologically by endogenous glucocorticoids. Smith and Bogues (322) have reviewed facts supporting this assumption. Smith has hypothesized that glucocorticoid action on type II cells could partly be mediated by pulmonary fibroblasts. He showed that under glucocorticoid treatment lung fibroblasts secreted a factor that stimulated type II cell maturation after injection into fetal rats (321). In this context it is interesting to note the influence exerted by the pulmonary mesenchyme on the growing and branching epithelial tube during development of the airways (see *Embryonic Development*, p. 8).

The morphological observations correspond to the expectations. Kikkawa and co-workers (210) observed accelerated morphological development of the fetal rabbit lung after cortisol treatment. Depletion of glycogen in the alveolar epithelium and cellular differentiation into type II and type I cells were more rapid, and the number of lamellar inclusions in type II cells was increased. Kauffman (205) recently made similar observations in mice. The decapitation experiments of fetal rats in utero by Blackburn and co-workers (36) give further evidence for the implication of glucocorticoids in normal type II cell development. Although the crude experimental design does not allow one to determine the responsible factor, the authors observed delayed type II cell maturation with a decreased number of lamellar bodies.

Normal differentiation and maturation require the equilibrated interaction of many factors, comparable to the harmonious playing of an orchestra. If glucocorticoids exert physiological control on the maturation process of type II cells and the surfactant system, it is not surprising that success of steroid therapy depends on its timing. This has indeed been observed. Liggins and Howie (240) found that glucocorticoid treatment in view of a premature birth was most effective in the 26th–32nd wk of gestation. Animal experiments also confirmed the variability of the effects of corticoids on PC synthesis, depending on the timing (292). In primary mixed monolayer cultures of fetal lung cells from rabbits, incorporation of [^{14}C]-palmitate into DPPC after incubation with cortisol increased when cells were harvested from fetuses 26–28 days of age (324) and simultaneously proliferation was reduced. In cultures from fetuses 20–22 days of age, however, cortisol stimulated cell growth (Figs. 40 and 41).

There are also possible deleterious consequences of

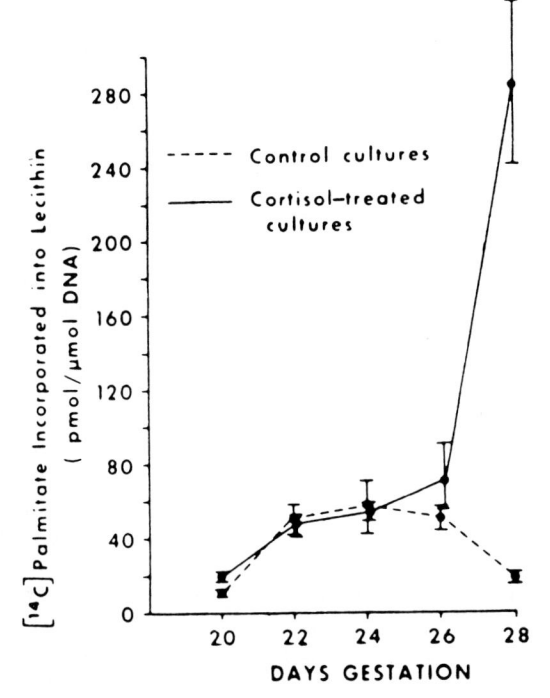

FIG. 40. Effect of cortisol on [1-^{14}C]palmitate incorporation into lecithin by primary mixed cultures of fetal rabbit lung prepared at gestation days 20–28. Solid line, cultures grown in the presence of cortisol at 5.5 µmol. [From Smith et al. (324), by copyright permission of The American Society for Clinical Investigation.]

steroid treatment. Motoyama and co-workers (262) reported that pregnant rabbits treated with cortisol had higher fetal death rates than controls and that their fetuses were smaller with lower lung weights. Obviously, differentiation accelerates at the expense of decreased growth (74, 204, 205). Adverse effects of steroid therapy on the nervous system have also been reported (119, 126). Therefore its routine use in premature labor is disputed and has even been strongly warned against (146). However, it has been reported that observed growth inhibition and retardation can be overcome after birth with adequate nutrition (224).

INFLUENCE OF THYROID HORMONES. As with glucocorticoids, thyroxine levels also increase during late gestation in the human fetus and thyroid hormones were also found to hasten lung maturation (180). In fetal rabbits the morphological effects of thyroxine treatment were very similar to those observed with steroids: quicker maturation of type II cells with accelerated glycogen depletion and a larger number of lamellar bodies (380). Because thyroxine does not cross the placental barrier, it had to be injected directly into the fetuses or the amniotic sac. Lindenberg and co-workers (241) recently presented an elegant method to bypass this difficulty. They used 3,5-dimethyl-3'-isopropylthyronine (DIMIT, a synthetic analogue of triiodothyronine), which freely crosses the placental barrier after maternal injection. Fetuses of treated mothers had less lung glycogen, exhibited a stimulated PC synthesis as measured by choline incorporation, and increased PAPase activity (20). The same trend was also manifest in experiments with organotypic or cell culture systems (2, 323).

Findings that thyroidectomized ovine fetuses had smaller lungs, lower lung protein concentrations, and lower ratios of protein to DNA than controls show that endogenous thyroid hormone is important for normal lung maturation. In addition, there was morphological evidence for delayed type II cell maturation (112, 113). Clinical investigations seem also to indicate a correlation between neonatal hypothyroidism and the occurrence of respiratory distress syndrome (124, 325). Encouraged by the promising results of many animal studies Mashiach and co-workers (251) injected thyroxine intra-amniotically into eight women with high-risk pregnancies with indicated or inevitable premature delivery. Although the infants were only 30–34 wk of age at delivery, none developed respiratory distress syndrome.

Lindenberg et al. (241) showed that fetal and adult lungs possess thyroxine receptors. The hormone can therefore directly interact with the binding site, a highly specific nuclear receptor. An intermediate cytoplasmic binder (as for steroids) has not been identified [see reviews by Sterling (331) and Oppenheimer (276)]. It is currently believed that the primary action of thyroid hormones is stimulation of messenger RNA and protein synthesis, and hence promotion of growth and development.

In summary, glucocorticoid and thyroid hormones both have a pronounced effect on the maturation of type II cells and the surfactant system. It is therefore not astonishing that the interaction between these hormones on lung development will be a topic of

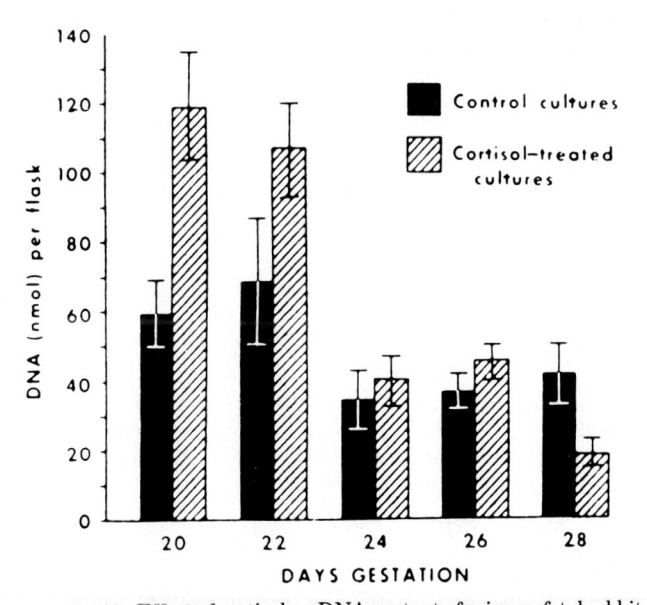

FIG. 41. Effect of cortisol on DNA content of primary fetal rabbit lung cell cultures prepared at gestation days 20–28. Bars, means; brackets, ± 1 SD. [From Smith et al. (324), by copyright permission of The American Society for Clinical Investigation.]

research. Hitchcock (179) recently provided an indication that, as has been observed in other organ systems, thyroxine and glucocorticoids are likely to potentiate each other's effect in the lung.

Research was supported by grants from the Swiss National Science Foundation (3.293.78 and 3.129-0.81). The technical assistance of Dr. L. Fischer, R. M. Fankhauser, and K. Babl in preparing this chapter is gratefully acknowledged.

REFERENCES

1. ABE, M., AND T. AKINO. The conversion of lysolecithin to lecithin in supernatant fractions of various rat tissues: on the distribution of the so-called Marinetti's enzyme. *Tohoku J. Exp. Med.* 110: 167–172, 1973.
2. ADAMSON, I. Y. R., AND D. H. BOWDEN. Reaction of cultured adult and fetal lungs to prednisone and thyroxine. *Arch. Pathol.* 99: 80–85, 1973.
3. ADAMSON, I. Y. R., AND D. H. BOWDEN. The type 2 cell as progenitor of alveolar epithelial regeneration. A cytodynamic study in mice after exposure to oxygen. *Lab. Invest.* 30: 35–42, 1974.
4. ADAMSON, I. Y. R., AND D. H. BOWDEN. Derivation of type 1 epithelium from type 2 cells in the developing rat lung. *Lab. Invest.* 32: 736–745, 1975.
5. ADAMSON, I. Y. R., AND D. H. BOWDEN. Role of monocytes and interstitial cells in the generation of alveolar macrophages. II. Kinetic studies after carbon loading. *Lab. Invest.* 42: 518–524, 1980.
6. ADDIS, T. Compensatory hypertrophy of the lung after unilateral pneumectomy. *J. Exp. Med.* 47: 51–56, 1928.
7. ALCORN, D. G., T. M. ADAMSON, J. E. MALONEY, AND P. M. ROBINSON. A morphologic and morphometric analysis of fetal lung development in the sheep. *Anat. Rec.* 201: 655–667, 1981.
8. ALESCIO, T., AND A. CASSINI. Induction in vitro of tracheal buds by pulmonary mesenchyme grafted on tracheal epithelium. *J. Exp. Zool.* 150: 83–94, 1962.
9. AMY, R. W. M., D. BOWES, P. H. BURRI, J. HAINES, AND W. M. THURLBECK. Postnatal growth of the mouse lung. *J. Anat.* 124: 131–151, 1977.
10. ANDERSON, H. R., J. A. ANDERSON, H. O. M. KING, AND J. E. COTES. Variations in the lung size of children in Papua, New Guinea: genetic and environmental factors. *Ann. Hum. Biol.* 5: 209–218, 1978.
11. ANGUS, G. E., AND W. M. THURLBECK. Number of alveoli in the human lung. *J. Appl. Physiol.* 32: 483–485, 1972.
12. AVERY, M. E., AND J. MEAD. Surface properties in relation to atelectasis and hyaline membrane disease. *Am. J. Dis. Child.* 95: 517–523, 1959.
13. BACHOFEN, M., H. BACHOFEN, AND E. R. WEIBEL. Lung edema in the adult respiratory distress syndrome. In: *Pulmonary Edema*, edited by A. P. Fishman and E. M. Renkin. Bethesda, MD: Am. Physiol. Soc., 1979, chapt. 18, p. 241–252.
14. BACHOFEN, M., AND E. R. WEIBEL. Basic pattern of tissue repair in human lungs following unspecific injury. *Chest* 65, Suppl.: 14S–19S, 1974.
15. BACHOFEN, M., AND E. R. WEIBEL. Alterations of the gas exchange apparatus in adult respiratory insufficiency associated with septicemia. *Am. Rev. Respir. Dis.* 116: 589–615, 1977.
16. BAKER, P. T. Human adaptation to high altitude. *Science* 163: 1149–1156, 1969.
17. BALLARD, P. L. Glucocorticoid receptors in the lung. *Federation Proc.* 36: 2660–2665, 1977.
18. BALLARD P. L., AND R. A. BALLARD. Cytoplasmic receptor for glucocorticoids in lung of the human fetus and neonate. *J. Clin. Invest.* 53: 477–486, 1974.
19. BALLARD, P. L., B. J. BENSON, AND A. BREHIER. Glucocorticoid effects in the fetal lung. *Am. Rev. Respir. Dis.* 115: 29–36, 1977.
20. BALLARD, P. L., B. J. BENSON, A. BREHIER, J. P. CARTER, B. M. KRIZ, AND E. C. JORGENSEN. Transplacental stimulation of lung development in the fetal rabbit by 3,5-dimethyl-3'-isopropyl-L-thyronine. *J. Clin. Invest.* 65: 1407–1417, 1980.
21. BARAŃSKA, J., AND L. M. G. VAN GOLDE. Role of lamellar bodies in the biosynthesis of phosphatidylcholine in mouse lung. *Biochim. Biophys. Acta* 488: 285–293, 1977.
22. BARNERIAS, M. J., A. H. PEYROT, L. J. HELMBRECHT, M. M. NEWMAN, AND A. A. SIEBENS. Changes in lung following early pneumonectomy (Abstract). *Federation Proc.* 24: 204, 1965.
23. BARROW, M. V., C. F. SIMPSON, AND E. J. MILLER. Lathyrism: a review. *Q. Rev. Biol.* 49: 101–128, 1974.
24. BARTELS, H. Freeze-fracture demonstration of communicating junction between interstitial cells of the pulmonary interalveolar septa. *Am. J. Anat.* 155: 125–129, 1979.
25. BARTLETT, D., JR. Postnatal growth of the mammalian lung: influence of exercise and thyroid activity. *Respir. Physiol.* 9: 50–57, 1970.
26. BARTLETT, D., JR. Postnatal growth of the mammalian lung: influence of low and high oxygen tensions. *Respir. Physiol.* 9: 58–64, 1970.
27. BARTLETT, D., JR., AND J. G. ARESON. Quantitative lung morphology in Japanese waltzing mice. *J. Appl. Physiol.: Respirat. Environ. Exercise Physiol.* 44: 446–449, 1978.
28. BARTLETT, D., JR., AND J. E. REMMERS. Effects of high altitude exposure on the lungs of young rats. *Respir. Physiol.* 13: 116–125, 1971.
29. BATENBURG, J. J. Isolated type II cells from fetal lung as model in studies on the synthesis and secretion of pulmonary surfactant. *Lung* 158: 177–192, 1980.
30. BATENBURG, J. J., W. J. LONGMORE, W. KLAZINGA, AND L. M. G. VAN GOLDE. Lysolecithin acyltransferase and lysolecithin:lysolecithin acyltransferase in adult rat lung alveolar type II epithelial cells. *Biochim. Biophys. Acta* 573: 136–144, 1979.
31. BATENBURG, J. J., AND L. M. G. VAN GOLDE. Formation of pulmonary surfactant in whole lung and in isolated type II alveolar cells. In: *Reviews in Perinatal Medicine*, edited by E. M. Scarpelli and E. V. Cosmi. New York: Raven, 1979, vol. 3, p. 73–114.
32. BATES, D. V., P. T. MACKLEM, AND R. V. CHRISTIE. *Respiratory Function in Disease: An Introduction to the Integrated Study of the Lung* (2nd ed.). Philadelphia, PA: Saunders, 1971.
33. BELLANTI, J. A., L. S. NERURKAR, AND B. J. ZELIGS. Host defenses in the fetus and neonate: studies of the alveolar macrophage during maturation. *Pediatrics* 64: 726–739, 1979.
34. BERNSTEIN, J., S. S. JANG, H. S. HAHN, AND J. KIKKAWA. Mucopolysaccharide in the pulmonary alveolus. I. Histochemical observations on the development of the alveolar lining layer. *Lab. Invest.* 21: 420–425, 1969.
35. BIGNON, J., F. JAUBERT, AND M. C. JAURAND. Plasma protein immunocyto-chemistry and polysaccharide cytochemistry at the surface of alveolar and endothelial cells in the rat lung. *J. Histochem. Cytochem.* 24: 1076–1084, 1976.
36. BLACKBURN, W. R., H. TRAVERS, AND D. M. POTTER. The role of the pituitary-adrenal-thyroid axes in lung differentiation. I. Studies on the cytology and physical properties of anencephalic fetal rat lung. *Lab. Invest.* 26: 306–318, 1972.
37. BLUEMINK, J. G., P. VAN MAURIK, AND K. A. LAWSON. Intimate cell contacts at the epithelial/mesenchymal interface in embryonic mouse lung. *J. Ultrastruct. Res.* 55: 257–270, 1976.
38. BOATMAN, E. S. A morphometric and morphological study of the lungs of rabbits after unilateral pneumonectomy. *Thorax* 32: 406–417, 1977.
39. BOHR, C. Ueber die spezifische Tätigkeit der Lungen bei der respiratorischen Gasaufnahme. *Scand. Arch. Physiol.* 22: 221–280, 1909.

40. BOWDEN, D. H., AND I. Y. R. ADAMSON. The pulmonary interstitial cell as immediate precursor of the alveolar macrophage. *Am. J. Pathol.* 68: 521–528, 1972.
41. BOWDEN, D. H., AND I. Y. R. ADAMSON. Adaptive responses of the pulmonary macrophagic system to carbon. I. Kinetic studies. *Lab. Invest.* 38: 422–429, 1978.
42. BOYDEN, E. A. The terminal air sacs and their blood supply in a 37-day infant lung. *Am. J. Anat.* 116: 413–427, 1965.
43. BOYDEN, E. A. The pattern of the terminal air spaces in a premature infant of 30–32 weeks that lived nineteen and a quarter hours. *Am. J. Anat.* 126: 31–40, 1969.
44. BOYDEN, E. A. The mode of origin of pulmonary acini and respiratory bronchioles in the fetal lung. *Am. J. Anat.* 141: 317–328, 1974.
45. BOYDEN, E. A. Development and growth of the airways. In: *Lung Biology in Health and Disease. Development of the Lung*, edited by W. A. Hodson. New York: Dekker, 1977, vol. 6, chapt. 1, p. 3–35.
46. BOYDEN, E. A., AND D. H. TOMPSETT. The postnatal growth of the lung in the dog. *Acta Anat.* 47: 185–215, 1961.
47. BOYDEN, E. A., AND D. H. TOMPSETT. The changing patterns in the developing lungs of infants. *Acta Anat.* 61: 164–192, 1965.
48. BREHIER, A., B. J. BENSON, M. C. WILLIAMS, R. J. MASON, AND P. L. BALLARD. Corticosteroid induction of phosphatidic acid phosphatase in fetal rabbit lung. *Biochem. Biophys. Res. Commun.* 77: 883–890, 1977.
49. BREMER, J. L. Postnatal development of alveoli in the mammalian lung in relation to the problem of the alveolar phagocyte. *Contrib. Embryol.* 147: 85–119, 1935.
50. BREMER, J. L. The fate of the remaining lung tissue after lobectomy or pneumonectomy. *J. Thorac. Surg.* 6: 336–343, 1936–37.
51. BRODY, J. S. Time course of and stimuli to compensatory growth of the lung after pneumonectomy. *J. Clin. Invest.* 56: 897–904, 1975.
52. BRODY, J. S., AND W. J. BUHAIN. Hormonal influence on postpneumonectomy lung growth in the rat. *Respir. Physiol.* 19: 344–355, 1973.
53. BRODY, J. S., R. BÜRKI, AND N. KAPLAN. Deoxyribonucleic acid synthesis in lung cells during compensatory lung growth after pneumonectomy. *Am. Rev. Respir. Dis.* 117: 307–315, 1978.
54. BRODY, J. S., H. KAGAN, AND A. MANALO. Lung lysyl oxidase activity: relation to lung growth. *Am. Rev. Respir. Dis.* 120: 1289–1295, 1979.
55. BRODY, J. S., S. LAHIRI, M. SIMPSER, E. K. MOTOYAMA, AND T. VELASQUEZ. Lung elasticity and airway dynamics in Peruvian natives to high altitude. *J. Appl. Physiol.: Respirat. Environ. Exercise Physiol.* 42: 245–251, 1977.
56. BRODY, J. S., AND C. VACCARO. Postnatal formation of alveoli: interstitial events and physiologic consequences. *Federation Proc.* 38: 215–223, 1979.
57. BROMAN, I. Zur Kenntnis der Lungenentwicklung. I. Wann und wie entsteht das definitive Lungenparenchym? *Anat. Anz.* 57: 83–96, 1923.
58. BRUMLEY, G., AND H. VAN DEN BOSCH. Lysophospholipase–transacylase from rat lung: isolation and partial purification. *J. Lipid Res.* 18: 523–532, 1977.
59. BUCHER, U., AND L. REID. Development of the intrasegmental bronchial tree: the pattern of branching and development of cartilage at various stages of intra-uterine life. *Thorax* 16: 207–218, 1961.
60. BUCHER, U., AND L. REID. Development of the mucus-secreting elements in human lung. *Thorax* 16: 219–225, 1961.
61. BUCKINGHAM, S., AND M. E. AVERY. Time of appearance of lung surfactant in the foetal mouse. *Nature London* 193: 688–689, 1962.
62. BUCKINGHAM, S., W. F. MCNARY, JR., AND S. C. SOMMERS. Pulmonary alveolar cell inclusions: their development in the rat. *Science* 145: 1191–1193, 1964.
63. BUCKINGHAM, S., W. F. MCNARY, S. C. SOMMERS, AND J. ROTHSCHILD. Is lung an analog of Moogs' developing intestine? I. Phosphatases and pulmonary alveolar differentiation in fetal rabbits (Abstract). *Federation Proc.* 27: 328, 1968.
64. BUHAIN, W. J., AND J. S. BRODY. Compensatory growth of the lung following pneumonectomy. *J. Appl. Physiol.* 35: 898–902, 1973.
65. BURRI, P. H. The postnatal growth of the rat lung. III. Morphology. *Anat. Rec.* 180: 77–98, 1974.
66. BURRI, P. H., L. C. BERGER, AND H. B. PFRUNDER. Early adaptive response of pulmonary parenchyma after bilobectomy in the rat. *Experientia* 36: 740, 1980.
67. BURRI, P. H., J. DBALY, AND E. R. WEIBEL. The postnatal growth of the rat lung. I. Morphometry. *Anat. Rec.* 178: 711–730, 1974.
68. BURRI, P. H., P. GEHR, K. MÜLLER, AND E. R. WEIBEL. Adaptation of the growing lung to increased V_{O_2}. I. IDPN as inducer of hyperactivity. *Respir. Physiol.* 28: 129–140, 1976.
69. BURRI, P. H., H. B. PFRUNDER, AND L. C. BERGER. Reactive changes in pulmonary parenchyma after bilobectomy: a scanning electron microscopic investigation. *Exp. Lung Res.* 4: 11–28, 1982.
70. BURRI, P. H., AND S. ŠEHOVIC. The adaptive response of the rat lung after bilobectomy. *Am. Rev. Respir. Dis.* 119: 769–777, 1979.
71. BURRI, P. H., AND E. R. WEIBEL. Morphometric estimation of pulmonary diffusion capacity. II. Effect of P_{O_2} on the growing lung, adaptation of the growing rat lung to hypoxia and hyperoxia. *Respir. Physiol.* 11: 247–264, 1971.
72. BURRI, P. H., AND E. R. WEIBEL. Ultrastructure and morphometry of the developing lung. In: *Lung Biology in Health and Disease. Development of the Lung*, edited by W. A. Hodson. New York: Dekker, 1977, vol. 6, chapt. 5, p. 215–268.
73. CAMPICHE, M. A., A. GAUTIER, E. I. HERNANDEZ, AND A. REYMOND. An electron microscope study of the fetal development of human lung. *Pediatrics* 32: 976–994, 1963.
74. CARSON, S. H., H. W. TAEUSCH, JR., AND M. E. AVERY. Inhibition of lung cell division after hydrocortisone injection into fetal rabbits. *J. Appl. Physiol.* 34: 660–663, 1973.
75. CHASE, W. H. The surface membrane of pulmonary alveolar walls. *Exp. Cell Res.* 18: 15–28, 1959.
76. CHEVALIER, G., AND A. J. COLLET. In vivo incorporation of choline-^{3}H, leucine-^{3}H and galactose-^{3}H in alveolar type II pneumocytes in relation to surfactant synthesis. A quantitative radioautographic study in mouse by electron microscopy. *Anat. Rec.* 174: 289–310, 1972.
77. CHRISTNER A., P. SCHAAF, C. MEYER, W. LINSS, AND G. GEYER. Ultrahistochemical study of the carbohydrate cell coat (glycocalyx) in the lung of the rat. *Acta Histochem.* 38: 121–126, 1970.
78. CLEMENTS, J. A., E. S. BROWN, AND R. P. JOHNSON. Pulmonary surface tension and the mucus lining of the lungs: some theoretical considerations. *J. Appl. Physiol.* 12: 262–268, 1958.
79. CLEMENTS, J. A., AND W. H. TOOLEY. Kinetics of surface-active material in the fetal lung. In: *Lung Biology in Health and Disease. Development of the Lung*, edited by W. A. Hodson. New York: Dekker, 1977, vol. 6, chapt. 8, p. 349–366.
80. COHN, R. Factors affecting the postnatal growth of the lung. *Anat. Rec.* 75: 195–205, 1939.
81. COLACICCO, G., A. R. BUCKELEW, JR., AND E. M. SCARPELLI. Protein and lipid-protein fractions of lung washings: chemical characterization. *J. Appl. Physiol.* 34: 743–749, 1973.
82. COWAN, M. J., AND R. G. CRYSTAL. Lung growth after unilateral pneumonectomy. Quantitation of collagen synthesis and content. *Am. Rev. Respir. Dis.* 111: 267–277, 1975.
83. CRAPO, J. D., B. E. BARRY, H. A. FOSCUE, AND J. SHELBURNE. Structural and biochemical changes in rat lungs occurring during exposures to lethal and adaptive doses of oxygen. *Am. Rev. Respir. Dis.* 122: 123–143, 1980.
84. CRAPO. J. D., B. E. BARRY, P. GEHR, AND M. BACHOFEN. Cell

numbers and cell characteristics of the normal human lung. *Am. Rev. Respir. Dis.* 126: 332–337, 1982.
85. CROCKER, T. T., A. TEETER, AND B. NIELSEN. Postnatal cellular proliferation in mouse and hamster. *Cancer Res.* 30: 357–361, 1970.
86. CUDMORE, R. E., J. L. EMERY, AND A. MITHAL. Postnatal growth of bronchi and bronchioles. *Arch. Dis. Child.* 37: 481–484, 1962.
87. CUNNINGHAM, E. I., J. S. BRODY, AND B. P. JAIN. Lung growth induced by hypoxia. *J. Appl. Physiol.* 37: 362–366, 1974.
88. CUTZ, E., W. CHAN, AND K. S. SONSTEGARD. Identification of neuro-epithelial bodies in rabbit fetal lungs by scanning electron microscopy: a correlative light, transmission and scanning electron microscopic study. *Anat. Rec.* 192: 459–466, 1978.
89. CUTZ, E., W. CHAN, V. WONG, AND P. E. CONEN. Endocrine cells in rat fetal lungs. Ultrastructural and histochemical study. *Lab. Invest.* 30: 458–464, 1974.
90. CUTZ, E., W. CHAN, V. WONG, AND P. E. CONEN. Ultrastructure and fluorescence histochemistry of endocrine (APUD-type) cells in tracheal mucosa of human and various animal species. *Cell Tissue Res.* 158: 425–437, 1975.
91. CUTZ, E., AND P. E. CONEN. Ultrastructure and cytochemistry of Clara cells. *Am. J. Pathol.* 62: 127–134, 1971.
92. CUTZ, E., AND P. E. CONEN. Endocrine-like cells in human fetal lungs: an electron microscopic study. *Anat. Rec.* 173: 115–122, 1972.
93. DARRAH, H. K., AND J. HEDLEY-WHYTE. Rapid incorporation of palmitate into lung: site and metabolic fate. *J. Appl. Physiol.* 34: 205–213, 1973.
94. DAS, R. M., AND W. M. THURLBECK. The events in the contralateral lung following pneumonectomy in the rabbit. *Lung* 156: 165–172, 1979.
95. DAVIES, G., AND L. REID. Growth of the alveoli and pulmonary arteries in childhood. *Thorax* 25: 669–681, 1970.
96. DAWSON, A. B. Further studies on the epiphyses of the albino rat skeleton, with special reference to the vertebral column, ribs, sternum and girdles. *Anat. Rec.* 34: 351–363, 1927.
97. DICKIE, K. J., G. D. MASSARO, V. MARSHALL, AND D. MASSARO. Amino acid incorporation into protein of a surface-active lung fraction. *J. Appl. Physiol.* 34: 606–614, 1973.
98. DINGLER, E. C. Wachstum der Lunge nach der Geburt. *Acta Anat.* 32: 1–86, 1958.
99. DOUGLAS, W. H. J., AND K. R. HITCHCOCK. Organotypic cultures of diploid type II alveolar pneumonocytes: surfactant associated esterase activity. *J. Histochem. Cytochem.* 27: 852–856, 1979.
100. DUBREUIL, G., A. LACOSTE, AND R. RAYMOND. Observations sur le développement du poumon human. *Bull. Histol. Appl. Tech. Microsc.* 13: 235–245, 1936.
101. DUNNILL, M. S. Postnatal growth of the lung. *Thorax* 17: 329–333, 1962.
102. DUNNILL, M. S. Quantitative observations on the anatomy of chronic non-specific lung disease. *Med. Thorac.* 22: 261–274, 1965.
103. EGAN, E. A., R. M. NELSON, AND B. MCINTYRE. Ventilation induced release of pulmonary surfactant in immature fetal goats (Abstract). *Pediatr. Res.* 12: 560, 1978.
104. EKELUND, L., G. ARVIDSON, H. EMANUELSSON, H. MYHRBERG, AND B. ÅSTEDT. Effect of cortisol on human fetal lung in organ culture. A biochemical, electron-microscopic and autoradiographic study. *Cell Tissue Res.* 163: 263–272, 1975.
105. ELLIOTT, F. M., AND L. REID. Some new facts about the pulmonary artery and its branching pattern. *Clin. Radiol.* 16: 193–198, 1965.
106. EMERY, J. L. The postnatal development of alveoli. In: *The Anatomy of the Developing Lung*, edited by J. Emery. Lavenham, UK: Lavenham, 1967, chapt. 2, p. 8–17.
107. EMERY, J. L., AND A. MITHAL. The number of alveoli in the terminal respiratory unit of man during late intrauterine life and childhood. *Arch. Dis. Child.* 35: 544–547, 1960.
108. EMERY, J. L., AND P. F. WILCOCK. The postnatal development of the lung. *Acta Anat.* 65: 10–29, 1966.
109. ENGEL, S. The structure of the respiratory tissue in the newly-born. *Acta Anat.* 19: 353–365, 1953.
110. ENGLE, M. J., R. L. SANDERS, AND W. J. LONGMORE. Phospholipid composition and acyltransferase activity of lamellar bodies isolated from rat lung. *Arch. Biochem. Biophys.* 173: 586–595, 1976.
111. ENGLE, M. J., L. M. G. VAN GOLDE, AND K. W. WIRTZ. Transfer of phospholipids between subcellular fractions of the lung. *FEBS Lett.* 86: 277–281, 1978.
112. ERENBERG, A., K. OMORI, J. H. MENKES, W. OH, AND D. A. FISHER. Growth and development of the thyroidectomized ovine fetus. *Pediatr. Res.* 8: 783–789, 1974.
113. ERENBERG, A., M. L. RHODES, M. M. WEINSTEIN, AND R. L. KENNEDY. The effect of fetal thyroidectomy on ovine fetal lung maturation. *Pediatr. Res.* 13: 230–235, 1979.
114. ETHERTON, J. E., D. M. CONNING, AND B. CORRIM. Autoradiographical and morphological evidence for apocrine secretion of dipalmitoyl lecithin in the terminal bronchiole of mouse lung. *Am. J. Anat.* 138: 11–36, 1973.
115. EVANS, M. J., L. J. CABRAL, R. J. STEPHENS, AND G. FREEMAN. Renewal of alveolar epithelium in the rat following exposure to NO_2. *Am. J. Pathol.* 70: 175–198, 1973.
116. EVANS, M. J., L. J. CABRAL, R. J. STEPHENS, AND G. FREEMAN. Transformation of alveolar type 2 cells to type 1 cells following exposure to NO_2. *Exp. Mol. Pathol.* 22: 142–150, 1975.
117. EVANS, M. J., L. J. CABRAL-ANDERSON, AND G. FREEMAN. Role of the Clara cell in renewal of the bronchiolar epithelium. *Lab. Invest.* 38: 648–655, 1978.
118. EVANS, M. J., N. P. DEKKER, L. J. CABRAL-ANDERSON, AND G. FREEMAN. Quantitation of damage to the alveolar epithelium by means of type 2 cell proliferation. *Am. Rev. Respir. Dis.* 118: 787–790, 1978.
119. EWERBECK, H., H. HELWIG, J. W. REYNOLDS, AND R. W. PROVENZANO. Treatment of idiopathic respiratory distress syndrome with large doses of corticoids (Letter to the editor). *Pediatrics* 49: 467–468, 1972.
120. FARRELL, P. M., AND M. HAMOSH. The biochemistry of fetal lung development. *Clin. Perinatol.* 5: 197–229, 1978.
121. FARRELL, P. M., D. W. LUNDGREN, AND A. J. ADAMS. Choline kinase and choline phosphotransferase in developing fetal rat lung. *Biochem. Biophys. Res. Commun.* 57: 696–701, 1974.
122. FARRELL, P. M., AND T. E. MORGAN. Lecithin biosynthesis in the developing lung. In: *Lung Biology in Health and Disease. Development of the Lung*, edited by W. A. Hodson. New York: Dekker, 1977, vol. 6, chapt. 7, p. 309–347.
123. FARRELL, P. M., AND R. D. ZACHMAN. Induction of choline phosphotransferase and lecithin synthesis in the fetal lung by corticosteroids. *Science* 179: 297–298, 1973.
124. FISCH, R. O., M. K. BILEK, L. D. MILLER, AND R. R. ENGEL. Physical and mental status at 4 years of age of survivors of the respiratory distress syndrome. Follow-up report from the collaborative study. *J. Pediatr.* 86: 497–503, 1975.
125. FISHER, J. M., AND J. D. SIMNETT. Morphogenetic and proliferative changes in the regenerating lung of the rat. *Anat. Rec.* 176: 389–396, 1973.
126. FITZHARDINGE, P. M., A. EISEN, C. LEJTENYI, K. METRAKOS, AND M. RAMSEY. Sequelae of early steroid administration to the newborn infant. *Pediatrics* 53: 877–883, 1974.
127. FRISANCHO, R. A. Human growth and pulmonary function of high altitude Peruvian Quechua population. *Hum. Biol.* 41: 366–379, 1969.
128. FRISANCHO, R. A. Functional adaptation to high altitude hypoxia. *Science* 187: 313–319, 1975.
129. FROSOLONO, M. F., B. L. CHARMS, P. PAWLOWSKI, AND S. SLIVKA. Isolation, characterization, and surface chemistry of a surface-active fraction from dog lung. *J. Lipid Res.* 11: 439–457, 1970.
130. FROSOLONO, M. F., S. SLIVKA, AND B. L. CHARMS. Acyl

transferase activities in dog lung microsomes. *J. Lipid Res.* 12: 96–103, 1971.
131. FUNG, Y. C., AND S. S. SOBIN. Theory of sheet flow in lung alveoli. *J. Appl. Physiol.* 26: 472–488, 1969.
132. GAIL, D. B., H. STEINKAMP, AND D. MASSARO. Interspecies variation in lung lavage and tissue saturated phosphatidylcholine. *Respir. Physiol.* 33: 289–297, 1978.
133. GARCIA, A., J. D. NEWKIRK, AND R. D. MAVIS. Lung surfactant synthesis: a Ca^{++}-dependent microsomal phospholipase A2 in the lung. *Biochem. Biophys. Res. Commun.* 64: 128–135, 1975.
134. GEELHAAR, A., AND E. R. WEIBEL. Morphometric estimation of pulmonary diffusion capacity. III. The effect of increased oxygen consumption in Japanese waltzing mice. *Respir. Physiol.* 11: 354–366, 1971.
135. GEHR, P., M. BACHOFEN, AND E. R. WEIBEL. The normal human lung: ultrastructure and morphometric estimation of diffusion capacity. *Respir. Physiol.* 32: 121–140, 1978.
136. GEHR, P., C. HUGONNAUD, P. H. BURRI, H. BACHOFEN, AND E. R. WEIBEL. Adaptation of the growing lung to increased $\dot{V}_{O_2}$. III. The effect of exposure to cold environment in rats. *Respir. Physiol.* 32: 345–353, 1978.
137. GEHR, P., D. K. MWANGI, A. AMMANN, G. M. O. MALOIY, C. R. TAYLOR, AND E. R. WEIBEL. Design of the mammalian respiratory system. V. Scaling morphometric pulmonary diffusing capacity to body mass: wild and domestic mammals. *Respir. Physiol.* 44: 61–86, 1981.
138. GEHRIG. H. Ueber tierexperimentelle Einwirkung von körperlicher Ueberanstrengung und sportlichem Training (Schwimmen) auf die Lungenmorphologie. Würzburg, West Germany: Universität Würzburg, 1951. Inaugural dissertation.
139. GIANNOPOULOS, G. Glucocorticoid receptors in lung. I. Specific binding of glucocorticoids to cytoplasmic components of rabbit fetal lung. *J. Biol. Chem.* 248: 3876–3883, 1973.
140. GIANNOPOULOS, G., S. MULAY, AND S. SOLOMON. Cortisol receptors in rabbit fetal lung. *Biochem. Biophys. Res. Commun.* 47: 411–418, 1972.
141. GIANNOPOULOS G., S. MULAY, AND S. SOLOMON. Glucocorticoid receptors in lung. II. Specific binding of glucocorticoids to nuclear components of rabbit fetal lung. *J. Biol. Chem.* 248: 5016–5023, 1973.
142. GIL, J., AND J. M. MCNIFF. Interstitial cells at the boundary between alveolar and extraalveolar connective tissue in the lung. *J. Ultrastruct. Res.* 76: 149–157, 1981.
143. GIL, J., AND O. K. REISS. Isolation and characterization of lamellar bodies and tubular myelin from rat lung homogenates. *J. Cell Biol.* 58: 152–171, 1973.
144. GIL, J., AND E. R. WEIBEL. Improvements in demonstration of lining layer of lung alveoli by electron microscopy. *Respir. Physiol.* 8: 13–36, 1969–70.
145. GILDEN, C., A. SEVANIAN, D. F. TIERNEY, S. A. KAPLAN, AND C. T. BARRETT. Regulation of fetal lung phosphatidyl choline synthesis by cortisol: role of glycogen and glucose. *Pediatr. Res.* 11: 845–848, 1977.
146. GLUCK, L. Administration of corticosteroids to induce maturation of fetal lung. *Am. J. Dis. Child.* 130: 976–978, 1976.
147. GLUCK, L., M. V. KULOVICH, A. I. EIDELMAN, L. CORDERO, AND A. F. KHAZIN. Biochemical development of surface activity in mammalian lung. IV. Pulmonary lecithin synthesis in the human fetus and newborn and etiology of the respiratory distress syndrome. *Pediatr. Res.* 6: 81–99, 1972.
148. GLUCK, L., M. SRIBNEY, AND M. V. KULOVICH. The biochemical development of surface activity in mammalian lung. II. The biosynthesis of phospholipids in the lung of the developing rabbit fetus and newborn. *Pediatr. Res.* 1: 247–265, 1967.
149. GNAVI, M., E. PANSA, AND G. ANSELMETTI. L'accrescimento e la rigenerazione del polmone (ricerche sperimentali). *Minerva Chir.* 25: 1491–1504, 1970.
150. GODINEZ, R. I., R. L. SANDERS, AND W. J. LONGMORE. Phosphatidylglycerol in rat lung. I. Identification as a metabolically active phospholipid in isolated perfused rat lung. *Biochemistry* 14: 830–834, 1975.

151. HAGE, E. The morphological development of the pulmonary epithelium of human foetuses studied by light- and electron microscopy. *Z. Anat. Entwicklungsgesch.* 140: 271–279, 1973.
152. HAGE, E., J. HAGE, AND G. JUEL. Endocrine-like cells of the pulmonary epithelium of the human adult lung. *Cell Tissue Res.* 178: 39–48, 1977.
153. HALLMAN, M., B. H. FELDMAN, E. KIRKPATRICK, AND L. GLUCK. Absence of phosphatidylglycerol (PG) in respiratory distress syndrome in the newborn. Study of the minor surfactant phospholipids in newborns. *Pediatr. Res.* 11: 714–720, 1977.
154. HALLMAN, M., AND L. GLUCK. Phosphatidylglycerol in lung surfactant. I. Synthesis in rat lung microsomes. *Biochem. Biophys. Res. Commun.* 60: 1–7, 1974.
155. HALLMAN, M., AND L. GLUCK. The biosynthesis of phosphatidylglycerol in the lung of developing rabbit (Abstract). *Federation Proc.* 34: 274, 1975.
156. HALLMAN, M., AND L. GLUCK. Phosphatidylglycerol in lung surfactant. II. Subcellular distribution and mechanism of biosynthesis in vitro. *Biochim. Biophys. Acta* 409: 172–191, 1975.
157. HALLMAN, M., AND L. GLUCK. Phosphatidylglycerol in lung surfactant. III. Possible modifier of surfactant function. *J. Lipid Res.* 17: 257–262, 1976.
158. HALLMAN, M., K. MIYAI, AND R. M. WAGNER. Isolated lamellar bodies from rat lung correlated ultrastructural and biochemical studies. *Lab. Invest.* 35: 79–86, 1976.
159. HALLMAN, M., K. TERAMO, K. KANKAANPÄÄ, M. V. KULOVICH, AND L. GLUCK. Prevention of respiratory distress syndrome: current view of fetal lung maturity studies. *Ann. Clin. Res.* 12: 36–44, 1980.
160. HANSEN, J. E., AND E. P. AMPAYA. Lung morphometry: a fallacy in the use of the counting principle. *J. Appl. Physiol.* 37: 951–954, 1974.
161. HANSEN, J. E., E. P. AMPAYA, G. H. BRYANT, AND J. J. NAVIN. Branching pattern of airways and air spaces of a single human terminal bronchiole. *J. Appl. Physiol.* 38: 983–989, 1975.
162. HARWOOD, J. L., R. DESAI, P. HEXT, T. TELEY, AND R. RICHARDS. Characterization of pulmonary surfactant from ox, rabbit, rat and sheep. *Biochem. J.* 151: 707–714, 1975.
163. HASLETON, P. S. The internal surface area of the adult human lung. *J. Anat.* 112: 391–400, 1972.
164. HEATH, D., AND D. R. WILLIAMS. The lung at high altitude. *Invest. Cell Pathol.* 2: 147–156, 1979.
165. HENDRY, A. T., AND F. POSSMAYER. Pulmonary phospholipid biosynthesis. Properties of a stable microsomal glycerophosphate acyltransferase preparation from rabbit lung. *Biochim. Biophys. Acta* 369: 156–172, 1974.
166. HERNANDEZ-VASQUEZ, A., J. A. WILL, AND W. B. QUAY. Quantitative characteristics of the Feyrter (APUD) cells of the neonatal rabbit lung in normoxia and chronic hypoxia. *Thorax* 32: 449–456, 1977.
167. HERNANDEZ-VASQUEZ, A., J. A. WILL, AND W. B. QUAY. Quantitative characteristics of the Feyrter cells and neuroepithelial bodies of the fetal rabbit lung in normoxia and short term chronic hypoxia. *Cell Tissue Res.* 189: 179–186, 1978.
168. HIERONYMI, G. Veränderungen der Lungenstruktur in verschiedenen Lebensaltern. *Verh. Dtsch. Ges. Pathol.* 44: 129–131, 1960.
169. HIERONYMI, G. Ueber den durch das Alter bedingten Formwandel menschlicher Lungen. *Ergeb. Allg. Pathol. Pathol. Anat.* 41: 1–62, 1961.
170. HIJIYA, K., Y. OKADA, AND H. TANKAWA. Ultrastructural study of the alveolar brush cell. *J. Electron Microsc.* 26: 321–329, 1977.
171. HILBER, H. Experimentell erzeugte Lungenregeneration. *Anat. Anz.* 78: 189–197, 1934.
172. HISLOP, A. *The Fetal and Childhood Development of the Pulmonary Circulation and its Disturbance in Certain Types of Congenital Heart Disease*. London: London Univ. Press, 1971. PhD thesis.

173. Hislop, A., C. P. Muir, M. Jacobsen, G. Simon, and L. Reid. Postnatal growth and function of the pre-acinar airways. *Thorax* 27: 265–274, 1972.
174. Hislop, A., and L. Reid. Intra-pulmonary arterial development during fetal life—branching pattern and structure. *J. Anat.* 113: 35–48, 1972.
175. Hislop, A., and L. Reid. Pulmonary arterial development during childhood: branching pattern and structure. *Thorax* 28: 129–135, 1973.
176. Hislop, A., and L. Reid. Fetal and childhood development of the intrapulmonary veins in man—branching pattern and structure. *Thorax* 28: 313–319, 1973.
177. Hislop, A., and L. Reid. Development of the acinus in the human lung. *Thorax* 29: 90–94, 1974.
178. Hislop, A., and L. Reid. Growth and development of the respiratory system—anatomical development. In: *Scientific Foundations of Paediatrics* (2nd ed.), edited by J. A. Davis and J. Dobbing. London: Heinemann, 1981, chapt. 20, p. 390–432.
179. Hitchcock, K. R. Hormones and the lung. I. Thyroid hormones and glucocorticoids in lung development. *Anat. Rec.* 194: 15–40, 1979.
180. Hitchcock, K. R. Lung development and the pulmonary surfactant system: hormonal influences. *Anat. Rec.* 198: 13–34, 1980.
181. Hitchcock-O'Hare, K., E. Meymaris, J. Bonaccorso, and S. B. Vanburen. Separation and partial characterization of surface-active fractions from mouse and rat lung homogenates. Identification of a possible marker system for pulmonary surfactant. *J. Histochem. Cytochem.* 24: 487–507, 1976.
182. Hogg, J. C., N. C. Staub, E. H. Bergofsky, and C. E. Vreim. Workshop on the pulmonary endothelial cell. *Am. Rev. Respir. Dis.* 119: 165–170, 1979.
183. Hogg, J. C., J. Williams, J. B. Richardson, P. T. Macklem, and W. M. Thurlbeck. Age as a factor in the distribution of lower-airway conductance and in the pathologic anatomy of obstructive lung disease. *N. Engl. J. Med.* 282: 1283–1287, 1970.
184. Holmes, C., and W. M. Thurlbeck. Normal lung growth and response after pneumonectomy in the rat at various ages. *Am. Rev. Respir. Dis.* 120: 1125–1136, 1979.
185. Horsfield, K. Postnatal growth of the dog's bronchial tree. *Respir. Physiol.* 29: 185–191, 1977.
186. Horsfield, K. Morphometry of the small pulmonary arteries in man. *Circ. Res.* 42: 593–597, 1978.
187. Horsfield, K., and G. Cumming. Morphology of the bronchial tree in man. *J. Appl. Physiol.* 24: 373–383, 1968.
188. Horsfield, K., and G. Cumming. Functional consequences of airway morphology. *J. Appl. Physiol.* 24: 384–390, 1968.
189. Horsfield, K., G. Dart, D. E. Olson, G. F. Filley, and G. Cumming. Models of the human bronchial tree. *J. Appl. Physiol.* 31: 207–217, 1971.
190. Hounam, R. F., and A. Morgan. Particle deposition. In: *Lung Biology in Health and Disease. Respiratory Defense Mechanisms*, edited by J. D. Brain, D. F. Proctor, and L. M. Reid. New York: Dekker, 1977, vol. 5, pt. 1, chapt. 5, p. 125–156.
191. Huang, T. W. Composite epithelial and endothelial basal laminas in human lungs. A structural basis for their separation and apposition in reaction to injury. *Am. J. Pathol.* 93: 681–692, 1978.
192. Hugonnaud, C., P. Gehr, E. R. Weibel, and P. H. Burri. Adaptation of the growing lung to increased oxygen consumption. II. Morphometric analysis. *Respir. Physiol.* 29: 1–10, 1977.
193. Hung, K. S., M. S. Hertweck, J. D. Hardy, and C. G. Loosli. Innervation of pulmonary alveoli of the mouse lung: an electron microscopic study. *Am. J. Anat.* 135: 477–495, 1972.
194. Hung, K. S., and C. G. Loosli. Bronchiolar neuro-epithelial bodies in the neonatal mouse lungs. *Am. J. Anat.* 140: 191–200, 1974.
195. Hurtado, A. Respiratory adaption in the Indian natives of the Peruvian Andes. Studies at high altitude. *Am. J. Phys. Anthropol.* 17: 137–165, 1932.
196. Hutchins, G. M., H. M. Haupt, and G. W. Moore. A proposed mechanism for the early development of the human tracheobronchial tree. *Anat. Rec.* 201: 635–640, 1981.
197. Jeffery, P. K., and L. M. Reid. The respiratory mucous membrane. In: *Lung Biology in Health and Disease. Respiratory Defense Mechanisms*, edited by J. D. Brain, D. F. Proctor, and L. M. Reid. New York: Dekker, 1977, vol. 5, pt. 1, chapt. 7, p. 193–245.
198. Jeffery, P. K., and L. M. Reid. Ultrastructure of airway epithelium and submucosal gland during development. In: *Lung Biology In Health and Disease. Development of the Lung*, edited by W. A. Hodson. New York: Dekker, 1977, vol. 6, chapt. 3, p. 87–134.
199. Jobe, A., E. Kirkpatrick, and L. Gluck. Labeling of phospholipids in the surfactant and subcellular fractions of rabbit lung. *J. Biol. Chem.* 253: 3810–3816, 1978.
200. Jobe, A., E. Kirkpatrick, and L. Gluck. Lecithin appearance and apparent biologic half-life in term newborn rabbit lung. *Pediatr. Res.* 12: 669–675, 1978.
201. Junod, A. F. Metabolism of vasoactive agents in lung. *Am. Rev. Respir. Dis.* 115: 51–57, 1977.
202. Kapanci, Y., A. Assimacopoulos, C. Irle, A. Zwahlen, and G. Gabbiani. Contractile interstitial cells in pulmonary alveolar septa: a possible regulator of ventilation/perfusion ratio? *J. Cell Biol.* 60: 375–392, 1974.
203. Kapanci, Y., E. R. Weibel, H. P. Kaplan, and F. R. Robinson. Pathogenesis and reversibility of the pulmonary lesions of oxygen toxicity in monkeys. II. Ultrastructural and morphometric studies. *Lab. Invest.* 20: 101–118, 1969.
204. Kauffman, S. L. Acceleration of canalicular development in lungs of fetal mice exposed transplacentally to dexamethasone. *Lab. Invest.* 36: 395–401, 1977.
205. Kauffman, S. L. Proliferation, growth and differentiation of pulmonary epithelium in fetal mouse lung exposed transplacentally to dexamethasone. *Lab. Invest.* 37: 497–501, 1977.
206. Kauffman, S. L. Cell proliferation in the mammalian lung. *Int. Rev. Exp. Pathol.* 22: 131–191, 1980.
207. Kauffman, S. L., P. H. Burri, and E. R. Weibel. The postnatal growth of the rat lung. II. Autoradiography. *Anat. Rec.* 180: 63–76, 1974.
208. Kerr, G. R., J. Couture, and J. R. Allen. Growth and development of the fetal rhesus monkey. VI. Morphometric analysis of the developing lung. *Growth* 39: 67–84, 1975.
209. Kida, K., and W. M. Thurlbeck. The effects of β-aminopropionitrile on the growing rat lung. *Am. J. Pathol.* 101: 693–710, 1980.
210. Kikkawa, Y., M. Kaibara, E. K. Motoyama, M. M. Orzalesi, and C. D. Cook. Morphologic development of fetal rabbit lung and its acceleration with cortisol. *Am. J. Pathol.* 64: 423–442, 1971.
211. Kikkawa, Y., E. K. Motoyama, and C. D. Cook. The ultrastructure of the lungs of lambs. The relation of osmiophilic inclusions and alveolar lining layer to fetal maturation and experimentally produced respiratory distress. *Am. J. Pathol.* 47: 877–903, 1965.
212. Kikkawa, Y., E. K. Motoyama, and L. Gluck. Study of the lungs of fetal and newborn rabbits. Morphologic, biochemical and surface physical development. *Am. J. Pathol.* 52: 177–209, 1968.
213. King, R. J. The surfactant system of the lung. *Federation Proc.* 33: 2238–2247, 1974.
214. King, R. J. Metabolic fate of the apoproteins of pulmonary surfactant. *Am. Rev. Respir. Dis.* 115: 73–79, 1977.
215. King, R. J., and J. Clements. Surface active materials from dog lung. I. Method of isolation. *Am. J. Physiol.* 223: 707–714, 1972.
216. King, R. J., and J. Clements. Surface active materials from dog lung. II. Composition and physiological correlations. *Am. J. Physiol.* 223: 715–726, 1972.
217. King, R. J., and J. Clements. Surface active materials from dog lung. III. Thermal analysis. *Am. J. Physiol.* 223: 727–733, 1972.

218. KING, R. J., D. J. KLASS, E. G. GIKAS, AND J. A. CLEMENTS. Isolation of apoproteins from canine surface active material. *Am. J. Physiol.* 224: 788–795, 1973.
219. KING, R. J., H. MARTIN, D. MITTS, AND F. M. HOLMSTROM. Metabolism of the apoproteins in pulmonary surfactant. *J. Appl. Physiol.: Respirat. Environ. Exercise Physiol.* 42: 483–491, 1977.
220. KISTLER, G. S., P. R. B. CALDWELL, AND E. R. WEIBEL. Pulmonary pathology of oxygen toxicity. II. Electron microscopic and morphometric study of rat lungs exposed to 97% O_2 at 258 torr (27,000 feet). *Aerosp. Med. Res. Lab.* 2: 1–14, 1966.
221. KLAUS, M. H., J. A. CLEMENTS, AND R. J. HAVEL. Composition of surface-active material isolated from beef lung. *Proc. Natl. Acad. Sci. USA* 47: 1858–1859, 1961.
222. KOTAS, R. V., P. M. FARRELL, R. E. ULANE, AND R. A. CHEZ. Fetal rhesus monkey lung development: lobar differences and discordances between stability and distensibility. *J. Appl. Physiol.: Respirat. Environ. Exercise Physiol.* 43: 92–98, 1977.
223. KOTAS, R. V., O. R. KLING, M. F. BLOCK, J. F. SOODSMA, R. D. HARLOW, AND W. M. CROSBY. Response of immature baboon fetal lung to intra-amniotic betamethasone. *Am. J. Obstet. Gynecol.* 130: 712–717, 1978.
224. KOTAS, R. V., C. M. LEROY, AND L. K. HART. Reversible inhibition of lung cell number after glucocorticoid injection into fetal rabbits to enhance surfactant appearance. *Pediatrics* 53: 358–361, 1974.
225. KOTAS, R. V., E. J. TRAINOR, C. M. LEROY, AND R. D. HARLOW. Discrepancies between the Brockerhoff and Gluck methods of lung lecithin fatty acid analysis. *Am. Rev. Respir. Dis.* 110: 669–671, 1974.
226. KUELBS. Ueber den Einfluss der Bewegung auf den wachsenden und erwachsenen Organismus. *Dtsch. Med. Wochenschr.* 38: 1916–1920, 1912.
227. KUHN, C., III, L. A. CALLAWAY, AND F. B. ASKIN. The formation of granules in the bronchiolar Clara cells of the rat. 1. Electron microscopy. *J. Ultrastruct. Res.* 49: 387–400, 1974.
228. KUHN, C., III, AND B. STARCHER. The effect of lathyrogens on the evolution of elastase-induced emphysema. *Am. Rev. Respir. Dis.* 122: 453–460, 1980.
229. LANDS, W. E. Metabolism of glycerolipids. 2. The enzymatic acylation of lysolecithin. *J. Biol. Chem.* 235: 2233–2237, 1960.
230. LANGSTON, C., K. KIDA, AND W. M. THURLBECK. Lung growth up to 1 month of postnatal age (Abstract). *Lab. Invest.* 40: 307, 1979.
231. LANGSTON, C., P. SACHDEVA, M. J. COWAN, J. HAINES, R. G. CRYSTAL, AND W. M. THURLBECK. Alveolar multiplication in the contralateral lung after unilateral pneumonectomy in the rabbit. *Am. Rev. Respir. Dis.* 115: 7–13, 1977.
232. LAUWERYNS, J. M., AND M. COKELAERE. Hypoxia-sensitive neuro-epithelial bodies. Intrapulmonary secretory neuroceptors, modulated by the CNS. *Z. Zellforsch. Mikrosk. Anat.* 145: 521–540, 1973.
233. LAUWERYNS, J. M., M. COKELAERE, AND P. THEUNYNCK. Neuro-epithelial bodies in the respiratory mucosa of various mammals. A light optical, histochemical and ultrastructural investigation. *Z. Zellforsch. Mikrosk. Anat.* 135: 569–592, 1972.
234. LAUWERYNS, J. M., M. COKELAERE, P. THEUNYNCK, AND M. DELEERSNYDER. Neuro-epithelial bodies in mammalian respiratory mucosa: light optical, histochemical and ultrastructural studies. *Chest* 65, Suppl.: 22S–29S, 1974.
235. LAUWERYNS, J. M., AND P. GODDEERIS. Neuroepithelial bodies in the human child and adult lung. *Am. Rev. Respir. Dis.* 111: 469–476, 1975.
236. LECHNER, A. J., AND N. BANCHERO. Lung morphometry in guinea pigs acclimated to cold during growth. *J. Appl. Physiol.: Respirat. Environ. Exercise Physiol.* 48: 886–891, 1980.
237. LECHNER, A. J., AND N. BANCHERO. Lung morphometry in guinea pigs acclimated to hypoxia during growth. *Respir. Physiol.* 42: 155–169, 1980.
238. LIBI-SYLORA, M., J. GRECO, AND C. FERENCZ. Postnatal growth of the pulmonary arterial tree. Morphologic characteristics. *Am. J. Dis. Child.* 115: 191–201, 1968.
239. LIGGINS, G. C. Premature delivery of foetal lambs infused with glucocorticoids. *J. Endocrinol.* 45: 515–523, 1969.
240. LIGGINS, G. C., AND R. N. HOWIE. A controlled trial of antepartum glucocorticoid treatment for prevention of respiratory distress syndrome in premature infants. *Pediatrics* 50: 515–525, 1972.
241. LINDENBERG, J. A., A. BREHIER, AND P. L. BALLARD. Triiodothyronine nuclear binding in fetal and adult rabbit lung and cultured lung cells. *Endocrinology* 103: 1725–1731, 1978.
242. LONGACRE, J. J., AND R. JOHANSMANN. An experimental study of the fate of the remaining lung following total pneumonectomy. *J. Thorac. Surg.* 10: 131–149, 1940.
243. LOOSLI, C. G., AND K. S. HUNG. Development of pulmonary innervation. In: *Lung Biology in Health and Disease. Development of the Lung*, edited by W. A. Hodson. New York: Dekker, 1977, vol. 6, chapt. 6, p. 269–306.
244. LOOSLI, C. G., AND E. L. POTTER. The prenatal development of the human lung. *Anat. Rec.* 109: 320–321, 1951.
245. LOW, F. N. Electron microscopy of the rat lung. *Anat. Rec.* 113: 437–443, 1952.
246. LOW, F. N. The pulmonary alveolar epithelium of laboratory mammals and man. *Anat. Rec.* 117: 241–246, 1953.
247. LUCIANO, L., E. REALE, AND H. RUSKA. Ueber eine "chemorezeptive" Sinneszelle in der Trachea der Ratte. *Z. Zellforsch. Mikrosk. Anat.* 85: 350–375, 1968.
248. LUCIANO, L., E. REALE, AND H. RUSKA. Bürstenzellen im Alveolarepithel der Rattenlunge. *Z. Zellforsch. Mikrosk. Anat.* 95: 198–201, 1969.
249. MACKLIN, C. C. The pulmonary alveolar mucoid film and the pneumocytes. *Lancet* 266: 1099–1104, 1954.
250. MARINETTI, G. V., J. ERBLAND, R. F. WITTER, J. PETIX, AND E. STOTY. Metabolic pathways of lysolecithin in a soluble rat liver system. *Biochim. Biophys. Acta* 30: 223–230, 1958.
251. MASHIACH, S., G. BARKAI, J. SACK, E. STERN, B. GOLDMAN, M. BRISH, AND D. M. SERR. Enhancement of fetal lung maturity by intra-amniotic administration of thyroid hormone. *Am. J. Obstet. Gynecol.* 130: 289–329, 1978.
252. MASSARO, G. D., AND D. MASSARO. Granular pneumocytes. Electron microscopic radioautographic evidence of intracellular protein transport. *Am. Rev. Respir. Dis.* 105: 927–931, 1972.
253. MASTERS, J. R. W. Epithelial-mesenchymal interaction during lung development: the effect of mesenchymal mass. *Dev. Biol.* 51: 98–108, 1976.
254. MERCURIO, A. R., AND J. A. G. RHODIN. An electron microscopic study on the type 1 pneumocyte in the cat: differentiation. *Am. J. Anat.* 146: 255–272, 1976.
255. MERCURIO, A. R., AND J. A. G. RHODIN. An electron microscopic study on the type 1 pneumocyte in the cat: pre-natal morphogenesis. *J. Morphol.* 156: 141–156, 1978.
256. MEYRICK, B., AND L. REID. The alveolar brush cell in rat lung—a third pneumonocyte. *J. Ultrastruct. Res.* 23: 71–80, 1968.
257. MEYRICK, B., AND L. REID. Nerves in rat intra-acinar alveoli: an electron microscopic study. *Respir. Physiol.* 11: 367–377, 1971.
258. MEYRICK, B., AND L. REID. Ultrastructure of alveolar lining and its development. In: *Lung Biology in Health and Disease. Development of the Lung*, edited by W. A. Hodson. New York: Dekker, 1977, vol. 6, chapt. 4, p. 135–214.
259. MITHAL, A., AND J. L. EMERY. The postnatal development of alveoli in premature infants. *Arch. Dis. Child.* 36: 446–450, 1961.
260. MOOG, F. The functional differentiation of the small intestine. III. The influence of the pituitary-adrenal system on the differentiation of phosphatase in the duodenum of the suckling mouse. *J. Exp. Zool.* 124: 329–346, 1953.
261. MORGAN, M. S., AND R. FRANK. Uptake of pollutant gases by the respiratory system. In: *Lung Biology in Health and Disease. Respiratory Defense Mechanisms*, edited by J. D. Brain, D. F. Proctor, and L. M. Reid. New York: Dekker, 1977, vol. 5, pt. 1, chapt. 6, p. 157–189.

262. MOTOYAMA, E. K., M. M. ORZALESI, Y. KIKKAWA, M. KAIBARA, B. WU, C. J. ZIGAS, AND C. D. COOK. Effect of cortisol on the maturation of fetal rabbit lungs. *Pediatrics* 48: 547–555, 1971.
263. NAEYE, R. L. Arterial changes during the perinatal period. *Arch. Pathol.* 71: 121–128, 1961.
264. NAEYE, R. L. Development of systemic and pulmonary arteries from birth through early childhood. *Biol. Neonate* 10: 8–16, 1966.
265. NATTIE, E. E., C. W. WILEY, AND D. BARTLETT, JR. Adaptive growth of the lung following pneumonectomy in rats. *J. Appl. Physiol.* 37: 491–495, 1974.
266. NERURKAR, L. S., B. J. ZELIGS, AND J. A. BELLANTI. Maturation of the rabbit alveolar macrophage during animal development. II. Biochemical and enzymatic studies. *Pediatr. Res.* 11: 1202–1207, 1977.
267. NEUHÄUSER, G. Beitrag zur Morphogenese der Lunge. *Anat. Anz.* 3, Suppl.: 277–284, 1962.
268. NEUHÄUSER, G., AND E. C. DINGLER. Lungenwachstum im Säuglingsalter (Untersuchungen an der Albinoratte). *Z. Anat. Entwicklungsgesch.* 123: 32–48, 1962.
269. NIDEN, A. H. Bronchiolar and large alveolar cell in pulmonary phospholipid metabolism. *Science* 158: 1323–1324, 1967.
270. NIJJAR, M. S., AND W. M. THURLBECK. Alterations in enzymes related to adenosine 3', 5'-monophosphate during compensatory growth of rat lung. *Eur. J. Biochem.* 105: 403–407, 1980.
271. NOACK, W., AND W. SCHWARZ. Elektronenmikroskopische Untersuchungen über die Entwicklung der Lunge bei Ratten (16. Tag a.p.–10. Tag p.p.). *Z. Anat. Entwicklungsgesch.* 134: 343–360, 1971.
272. O'HARE, K. H. Fine structural observations of ruthenium red binding in developing and adult rat lung. *Anat. Rec.* 178: 267–288, 1974.
273. OKANO, G., AND T. AKINO. Changes in the structural and metabolic heterogeneity of phosphatidylcholines in the developing rat lung. *Biochim. Biophys. Acta* 528: 373–384, 1978.
274. OLDENBORG, V., AND L. M. G. VAN GOLDE. Activity of cholinephosphotransferase, lysolecithin: lysolecithin acyltransferase and lysolecithin acyltransferase in the developing mouse lung. *Biochim. Biophys. Acta* 441: 433–442, 1976.
275. OLDENBORG, V., AND L. M. G. VAN GOLDE. The enzymes of phosphatidylcholine biosynthesis in the fetal mouse lung. *Biochim. Biophys. Acta* 489: 454–465, 1977.
276. OPPENHEIMER, J. H. Thyroid hormone action at the cellular level. *Science* 203: 971–979, 1979.
277. ORZALESI, M. M., E. K. MOTOYAMA, H. N. JACOBSON, Y. KIKKAWA, E. O. R. REYNOLDS, AND C. D. COOK. The development of the lungs of lambs. *Pediatrics* 35: 373–381, 1965.
278. OYARZÚN, M. J., AND J. A. CLEMENTS. Ventilatory and cholinergic control of pulmonary surfactant in the rabbit. *J. Appl. Physiol.: Respirat. Environ. Exercise Physiol.* 43: 39–45, 1977.
279. OYARZÚN, M. J., AND J. A. CLEMENTS. Control of lung surfactant by ventilation adrenergic mediators, and prostaglandins in the rabbit. *Am. Rev. Respir. Dis.* 117: 879–891, 1978.
280. PAINTAL, A. S. The mechanism of excitation of type J receptors, and the J reflex. In: *Breathing: Hering-Breuer Centenary Symposium*, edited by R. Porter. London: Churchill, 1970, p. 59–76. (Ciba Found. Symp.)
281. PASSERO, M. A., S. N. BHATTACHARYYA, AND W. S. LYNN. Origin of hydroxylated glycopeptides isolated from alveolar proteinosis material (Abstract). *Clin. Res.* 22: 571A, 1974.
282. PASSERO, M. A., R. W. TYE, K. H. KILBURN, AND W. S. LYNN. Isolation and characterization of two glycoproteins from patients with alveolar proteinosis. *Proc. Natl. Acad. Sci. USA* 70: 973–976, 1973.
283. PATTLE, R. E. Properties, function and origin of the alveolar lining layer. *Nature London* 175: 1125–1126, 1955.
284. PATTLE, R. E., AND L. C. THOMAS. Lipoprotein composition of the film lining the lung. *Nature London* 189: 844, 1961.
285. PEARSE, A. G. E. The cytochemistry and ultrastructure of polypeptide hormone-producing cells of the APUD series and the embryologic, physiological and pathologic implications of the concept. *J. Histochem. Cytochem.* 17: 303–313, 1969.
286. PEARSON, A. K., AND O. P. PEARSON. Granular pneumocytes and altitude: a stereological evaluation. *Cell Tissue Res.* 201: 137–144, 1979.
287. PEARSON, O. P., AND A. K. PEARSON. A stereological analysis of the ultrastructure of the lungs of wild mice living at low and high altitude. *J. Morphol.* 150: 359–368, 1976.
288. PEDLEY, T. J., R. C. SCHROTER, AND M. F. SUDLOW. Gas flow and mixing in the airways. In: *Lung Biology in Health and Disease. Bioengineering Aspects of the Lung*, edited by J. B. West. New York: Dekker, 1977, vol. 3, chapt. 3, p. 163–265.
289. PERELMAN, R. H., M. ENGLE, AND P. FARRELL. Perspectives on fetal lung development. *Lung* 159: 53–80, 1981.
290. POSSMAYER, F., G. DUWE, R. METCALFE, P. J. STEWART-DEHAAN, C. WONG, J. L. HERAS, AND P. G. R. HARDING. Cortisol induction of pulmonary maturation in the rabbit foetus. Its effects on enzymes related to phospholipid biosynthesis and on marker enzymes for subcellular organelles. *Biochem. J.* 166: 485–494, 1977.
291. PUMP, K. K. Distribution of bronchial arteries in the human lung. *Chest* 62: 447–451, 1972.
292. PYSHER, T. J., K. D. KONRAD, AND G. B. REED. Effects of hydrocortisone and pilocarpine on fetal rat lung explants. *Lab. Invest.* 37: 588–593, 1977.
293. RANGA, V., AND J. KLEINERMAN. Interalveolar pores in mouse lungs: regional distribution and alterations with age. *Am. Rev. Respir. Dis.* 122: 477–481, 1980.
294. RANNELS, D. E., D. M. WHITE, AND C. A. WATKINS. Rapidity of compensatory lung growth following pneumonectomy in adult rats. *J. Appl. Physiol.: Respirat. Environ. Exercise Physiol.* 46: 326–333, 1979.
295. RHODIN, J. Ultrastructure of the tracheal ciliated mucosa in rat and man. *Ann. Otol. Rhinol. Laryngol.* 68: 964–974, 1959.
296. RIENHOFF, W. F., F. L. REICHERT, AND G. E. HEUER. Compensatory changes in the remaining lung following total pneumonectomy. *Bull. Johns Hopkins Hosp.* 57: 373–383, 1935.
297. ROBINSON, M. E., L. N. Y. WU, G. W. BRUMLEY, AND R. H. LUMB. A unique phosphatidylcholine exchange protein isolated from sheep lung. *FEBS Lett.* 87: 41–44, 1978.
298. ROMANOVA, L. K., E. M. LEIKINA, K. K. ANTIPOVA, AND T. N. SOKOLOVA. The role of function in the restoration of damaged viscera. *Ontogenez* 2: 479–486, 1971.
299. ROONEY, S. A., P. M. CANAVAN, AND E. K. MOTOYAMA. The identification of phosphatidylglycerol in the rat, rabbit, monkey and human lung. *Biochim. Biophys. Acta* 360: 56–67, 1974.
300. ROONEY, S. A., L. J. GOBRAN, P. A. MARINO, W. M. MANISCALCO, AND I. GROSS. Effects of betamethasone on phospholipid content, composition and biosynthesis in the fetal rabbit lung. *Biochim. Biophys. Acta* 572: 64–76, 1979.
301. ROONEY, S. A., I. GROSS, L. N. GASSENHEIMER, AND E. K. MOTOYAMA. Stimulation of glycerolphosphate phosphatidyltransferase activity in fetal rabbit lung by cortisol administration. *Biochim. Biophys. Acta* 398: 433–441, 1975.
302. ROONEY, S. A., AND E. K. MOTOYAMA. Studies on the biosynthesis of pulmonary surfactant. The role of the methylation pathway of phosphatidylcholine biosynthesis in primate and non-primate lung. *Clin. Chim. Acta* 69: 525–531, 1976.
303. ROONEY, S. A., B. A. PAGE-ROBERTS, AND E. K. MOTOYAMA. Role of lamellar inclusions in surfactant production: studies on phospholipid composition and biosynthesis in rat and rabbit lung subcellular fractions. *J. Lipid Res.* 16: 418–425, 1975.
304. ROONEY, S. A., T. S. WAI-LEE, L. GOBRAN, AND E. K. MOTOYAMA. Phospholipid content, composition and biosynthesis during fetal lung development in the rabbit. *Biochim. Biophys. Acta* 431: 447–458, 1976.
305. SALDAÑA, M., AND E. GARCIA-OYOLA. Morphometry of the high altitude lung (Abstract). *Lab. Invest.* 22: 509, 1970.
306. SANDERS, R. L., R. J. HASSETT, AND A. E. VATTER. Isolation of lung lamellar bodies and their conversion to tubular myelin

figures in vitro. *Anat. Rec.* 198: 485–501, 1980.
307. SANDERS, R. L., AND W. J. LONGMORE. Phosphatidylglycerol in rat lung. II. Comparison of occurrence, composition, and metabolism in surfactant and residual lung fractions. *Biochemistry* 14: 835–840, 1975.
308. SANDERSON, R. J., G. W. PAUL, A. E. VATTER, AND G. F. FILLEY. Morphological and physical basis for lung surfactant action. *Respir. Physiol.* 27: 379–392, 1976.
309. SCHNEEBERGER, E. E. Barrier function of intercellular junctions in adult and fetal lungs. In: *Pulmonary Edema*, edited by A. P. Fishman and E. M. Renkin. Bethesda, MD: Am. Physiol. Soc., 1979, chapt. 2, p. 21–37.
310. SCHREIDER, J. P., AND O. G. RAABE. Structure of the human respiratory acinus. *Am. J. Anat.* 162: 221–232, 1981.
311. SCHWINGER, G., E. R. WEIBEL, AND H. P. KAPLAN. Pulmonary pathology of oxygen toxicity. Part III. Electron microscopic and morphometric study of dog and monkey lungs exposed to 98% O_2 at 258 torr for 7 months and followed by 1 month recovery in room air. *Aerosp. Med. Res. Lab. Interim Scientific Report, AF 61(052)-941, January 1967*, p. 1–21.
312. ŠERÝ, Z., E. KEPRT, AND M. OBRUČNÍK. Morphometric analysis of late adaptation of the residual lung following pneumonectomy in young and adult rabbits. *J. Thorac. Cardiovasc. Surg.* 57: 549–557, 1969.
313. SHERMAN, M., E. GOLDSTEIN, W. LIPPERT, AND R. WENNBERG. Neonatal lung defense mechanisms: a study of the alveolar macrophage system in neonatal rabbits. *Am. Rev. Respir. Dis.* 116: 433–440, 1977.
314. SHORT, R. H. D. Alveolar epithelium in relation to growth of the lung. *Philos. Trans. R. Soc. London* 235: 35–87, 1950.
315. SHORT, R. H. D. Aspects of comparative lung growth. *Proc. Soc. Biol.* 140: 432–441, 1952.
316. SIEGER, L. Pulmonary alveolar macrophages in pre- and postnatal rabbits. *J. Reticuloendothel. Soc.* 23: 389–395, 1978.
317. SINGHAL, S., R. HENDERSON, K. HORSFIELD, K. HARDING, AND G. CUMMING. Morphometry of the human pulmonary arterial tree. *Circ. Res.* 33: 190–197, 1973.
318. SLEIGH, M. A. The nature and action of respiratory tract cilia. In: *Lung Biology in Health and Disease. Respiratory Defense Mechanisms*, edited by J. D. Brain, D. F. Proctor, and L. M. Reid. New York: Dekker, 1977, vol. 5, pt. 1, chapt. 8, p. 247–288.
319. SMILEY, R. H., W. E. JAQUES, AND G. S. CAMPBELL. Pulmonary vascular changes in lung lobes with reversed pulmonary blood flow. *Surgery* 59: 529–533, 1966.
320. SMITH, B. T. Cell line A 549: a model system for the study of alveolar type 2 cell function. *Am. Rev. Respir. Dis.* 115: 285–293, 1977.
321. SMITH, B. T. Lung maturation in the fetal rat: acceleration by injection of fibroblast-pneumocyte factor. *Science* 204: 1094–1095, 1979.
322. SMITH, B. T., AND W. G. BOGUES. Effects of drugs and hormones on lung maturation in experimental animal and man. *Pharmacol. Ther.* 9: 51–74, 1980.
323. SMITH, B. T., AND J. TORDAY. Factors affecting lecithin synthesis by fetal lung cells in culture. *Pediatr. Res.* 8: 848–851, 1974.
324. SMITH, B. T., J. S. TORDAY, AND C. J. P. GIROUD. Evidence for different gestation-dependent effects of cortisol on cultured fetal lung cells. *J. Clin. Invest.* 53: 1518–1526, 1974.
325. SMITH, D. W., A. M. KLEIN, J. R. HENDERSON, AND N. C. MYRIANTHOPOULOS. Congenital hypothyroidism—signs and symptoms in the newborn period. *J. Pediatr.* 87: 958–962, 1975.
326. SMITH, P., D. HEATH, AND H. MOOSAVI. The Clara cell. *Thorax* 29: 147–163, 1974.
327. SOLOMON, S., AND D. K. H. LEE. Binding of glucocorticoids in fetal tissue. *J. Steroid Biochem.* 8: 453–461, 1977.
328. SOROKIN, S. P. A morphologic and cytochemical study on the great alveolar cell. *J. Histochem. Cytochem.* 14: 884–897, 1967.
329. SPOONER, B. S., AND J. M. FAUBION. Collagen involvement in branching morphogenesis of embryonic lung and salivary gland. *Dev. Biol.* 77: 84–102, 1980.
330. SPOONER, B. S., AND N. K. WESSELLS. Mammalian lung development: interactions in primordium formation and bronchial morphogenesis. *J. Exp. Zool.* 175: 445–454, 1970.
331. STERLING, K. Thyroid hormone action at the cell level. *N. Engl. J. Med.* 300: 117–123, 1979.
332. STILES, Q. R., B. W. MEYER, G. G. LINDESMITH, AND J. C. JONES. The effects of pneumonectomy in children. *J. Thorac. Cardiovasc. Surg.* 58: 394–400, 1969.
333. STRATTON, C. J. The periodicity and architecture of lipid retained and extracted lung surfactant and its origin from multilamellar bodies. *Tissue Cell* 9: 301–316, 1977.
334. TADERERA, J. V. Control of lung differentiation in vitro. *Dev. Biol.* 16: 489–512, 1967.
335. TAIRA, K., AND S. SHIBASAKI. A fine structure study of the non-ciliated cells in the mouse tracheal epithelium with special reference to the relation of "brush cells" and "endocrine cells." *Arch. Histol. Jpn.* 41: 351–366, 1978.
336. TAKARO, T., H. P. PRICE, AND S. C. PARRA. Ultrastructural studies of apertures in the interalveolar septum of the adult human lung. *Am. Rev. Respir. Dis.* 119: 425–434, 1979.
337. TEN HAVE-OPBROEK, A. A. W. Immunological study of lung development in the mouse embryo. II. First appearance of the great alveolar cell, as shown by immunofluorescence microscopy. *Dev. Biol.* 69: 408–423, 1979.
338. TEN HAVE-OPBROEK, A. A. W. The development of the lung in mammals: an analysis of concepts and findings. *Am. J. Anat.* 162: 201–219, 1981.
339. TENNEY, S. M., AND J. E. REMMERS. Alveolar dimensions in the lungs of animals raised at high altitude. *J. Appl. Physiol.* 21: 1328–1330, 1966.
340. THOMPSON, M. E. Lung growth in response to altered metabolic demand in hamsters: influence of thyroid function and cold exposure. *Respir. Physiol.* 40: 335–347, 1980.
341. THURLBECK, W. M. Postnatal growth and development of the lung. *Am. Rev. Respir. Dis.* 111: 803–844, 1975.
342. THURLBECK, W. M. Structure of the lungs. In: *Respiratory Physiology II*, edited by J. G. Widdicombe. Baltimore, MD: University Park, 1977, vol. 14, p. 1–36. (Int. Rev. Physiol. Ser.)
343. TIEMANN, F. Ueber die Sportlunge. *Muench. Med. Wochenschr.* 83: 1517–1520, 1936.
344. TOMKEIEFF, S. I. Linear intercepts, areas and volumes (Letter to the editor). *Nature London* 155: 24, 1945.
345. TSAO, F. H. C. Specific transfer of dipalmitoyl phosphatidylcholine in rabbit lung. *Biochim. Biophys. Acta* 601: 415–426, 1980.
346. VACCARO, C., AND J. BRODY. Ultrastructure of developing alveoli. I. The role of the interstitial fibroblast. *Anat. Rec.* 192: 467–480, 1978.
347. VAN FURTH, R. The origin and turnover of promonocytes, monocytes and macrophages in normal mice. In: *Mononuclear Phagocytes*, edited by R. Van Furth. Philadelphia, PA: Davis, 1970, p. 151–165.
348. VAN GOLDE, L. M. G. Metabolism of phospholipids in the lung. *Am. Rev. Respir. Dis.* 114: 977–1000, 1976.
349. VAN GOLDE, L. M. G. Metabolism of phospholipids in the lung. In: *Lung Disease: State of the Art, 1975–76*, edited by J. F. Murray. New York: Am. Lung Assoc., 1978, p. 375–398.
350. VIDIĆ, B., AND P. H. BURRI. Quantitative cellular and subcellular changes in the rat type II pneumocyte during early postnatal development. *Am. Rev. Respir. Dis.* 124: 174–178, 1981.
351. VON HAYEK, H. *Die menschliche Lunge* (2nd ed.). Berlin: Springer-Verlag, 1970.
352. VON NEERGAARD, K. Neue Auffassungen über einen Grundbegriff der Atemmechanik. Die Retraktionskraft der Lunge, abhängig von der Oberflächenspannung in den Alveolen. *Z. Gesamte Exp. Med.* 66: 373–394, 1929.
353. WAGENVOORT, C. A., AND N. WAGENVOORT. Age changes in muscular pulmonary arteries. *Arch. Pathol.* 79: 524–528, 1965.

354. WAGENVOORT, C. A., AND N. WAGENVOORT. Arterial anastomoses, bronchopulmonary arteries, and pulmobronchial arteries in perinatal lungs. *Lab. Invest.* 16: 13–24, 1967.
355. WAGENVOORT, C. A., AND N. WAGENVOORT. Pulmonary vascular bed: normal anatomy and responses to disease. In: *Lung Biology in Health and Disease. Pulmonary Vascular Diseases*, edited by K. M. Moser. New York: Dekker, 1979, vol. 14, chapt. 1, p. 1–109.
356. WANDEL, G., L. C. BERGER, AND P. H. BURRI. Quantitative changes in the remaining lung after bilobectomy in the adult rat. *Am. Rev. Respir. Dis.* 128: 968–972, 1983.
357. WANNER, A. Clinical aspects of mucociliary transport. *Am. Rev. Respir. Dis.* 116: 73–125, 1977.
358. WATSON, J. H. L., AND G. L. BRINKMAN. Electron microscopy of the epithelial cells of normal and bronchitic human bronchus. *Am. Rev. Respir. Dis.* 90: 851–866, 1964.
359. WEIBEL, E. R. Die Blutgefässanastomosen in der menschlichen Lunge. *Z. Zellforsch. Mikrosk. Anat.* 50: 653–692, 1959.
360. WEIBEL, E. R. *Morphometry of the Human Lung*. Heidelberg: Springer-Verlag, 1963.
361. WEIBEL, E. R. Postnatal growth of the lung and pulmonary gas-exchange capacity. In: *Development of the Lung*, edited by A. V. S. de Reuck and R. Porter. London: Churchill, 1967, p. 131–148. (Ciba Found. Symp.)
362. WEIBEL, E. R. Morphometry of pulmonary circulation. *Prog. Respir. Res.* 5: 2–12, 1970.
363. WEIBEL, E. R. Morphometric estimation of pulmonary diffusion capacity. I. Model and method. *Respir. Physiol.* 11: 54–75, 1970–71.
364. WEIBEL, E. R. The mystery of "non-nucleated plates" in the alveolar epithelium of the lung explained. *Acta Anat.* 78: 425–443, 1971.
365. WEIBEL, E. R. Morphometric estimation of pulmonary diffusion capacity. V. Comparative morphometry of alveolar lungs. *Respir. Physiol.* 14: 26–43, 1972.
366. WEIBEL, E. R. A note on differentiation and divisibility of alveolar epithelial cells. *Chest* 65, Suppl.: 19S–21S, 1974.
367. WEIBEL, E. R. On pericytes, particularly their existence on lung capillaries. *Microvasc. Res.* 8: 218–235, 1974.
368. WEIBEL, E. R., AND H. BACHOFEN. Structural design of the alveolar septum and fluid exchange. In: *Pulmonary Edema*, edited by A. P. Fishman and E. M. Renkin. Bethesda, MD: Am. Physiol. Soc., 1979, chapt. 1, p. 1–20.
369. WEIBEL, E. R., P. GEHR, L. M. CRUZ-ORIVE, A. E. MÜLLER, D. K. MWANGI, AND V. HAUSSENER. Design of the mammalian respiratory system. IV. Morphometric estimation of pulmonary diffusing capacity: critical evaluation of a new sampling method. *Respir. Physiol.* 44: 39–59, 1981.
370. WEIBEL, E. R., AND J. GIL. Electron microscopic demonstration of an extracellular duplex lining layer of alveoli. *Respir. Physiol.* 4: 42–57, 1968.
371. WEIBEL, E. R., AND J. GIL. Structure-function relationships at the alveolar level. In: *Lung Biology in Health and Disease. Bioengineering Aspects of the Lung*, edited by J. B. West. New York: Dekker, 1977, vol. 3, chapt. 1, p. 1–81.
372. WEIBEL, E. R., AND D. M. GOMEZ. Architecture of the human lung. *Science* 137: 577–585, 1962.
373. WEIBEL, E. R., G. S. KISTLER, AND G. TÖNDURY. A stereologic electron microscope study of "tubular myelin figures" in alveolar fluids of rat lungs. *Z. Zellforsch. Mikrosk. Anat.* 69: 418–427, 1966.
374. WESSELLS, N. K. Mammalian lung development: interactions in formation and morphogenesis of tracheal buds. *J. Exp. Zool.* 175: 455–466, 1970.
375. WILCOX, B. R., G. F. MURRAY, M. FRIEDMANN, AND R. PIMMEL. The effects of early pneumonectomy on the remaining pulmonary parenchyma. *Surgery* 86: 294–300, 1979.
376. WILLIAMS, M. C. Conversion of lamellar body membranes into tubular myelin in alveoli of fetal rat lungs. *J. Cell Biol.* 72: 260–277, 1977.
377. WILLIAMS, M. C., AND R. J. MASON. Development of the type II cell in the fetal rat lung. *Am. Rev. Respir. Dis.* 115: 37–47, 1977.
378. WOLDENBERG, M. J. Special order in fluvial systems: Horton's laws derived from mixed hexagonal hierarchy of drainage basin areas. *Geol. Soc. Am. Bull.* 80: 97–112, 1969.
379. WOODSIDE, G. L., AND A. J. DALTON. The ultrastructure of lung tissue from newborn and embryo mice. *J. Ultrastruct. Res.* 2: 28–54, 1958.
380. WU, B., Y. KIKKAWA, M. M. ORZALESI, E. K. MOTOYAMA, M. KAIBARA, C. J. ZIGAS, AND C. D. COOK. The effect of thyroxine on the maturation of fetal rabbit lungs. *Biol. Neonate* 22: 161–168, 1973.
381. WYSZOGRODSKI, I., K. KYEI-ABOAGYE, H. W. TAEUSCH, JR., AND M. E. AVERY. Surfactant inactivation by hyperventilation: conservation by end-expiratory pressure. *J. Appl. Physiol.* 38: 461–466, 1975.
382. YONEDA, K. Ultrastructural localization of phospholipases in the Clara cell of the rat bronchiole. *Am. J. Pathol.* 93: 745–752, 1978.
383. ZACHMAN, R. D. The enzymes of lecithin bio-synthesis in human newborn lungs. I. Choline kinase. *Biol. Neonate* 19: 211–219, 1971.
384. ZACHMAN, R. D. The enzymes of lecithin bio-synthesis in human newborn lungs. II. Methionine-activating enzyme and phosphatidyl methyltransferase. *Biol. Neonate* 20: 448–457, 1972.
385. ZELIGS, B. J., L. S. NERURKAR, AND J. A. BELLANTI. Maturation of the rabbit alveolar macrophage during animal development. I. Perinatal influx into alveoli and ultrastructure differentiation. *Pediatr. Res.* 11: 197–208, 1977.
386. ZELIGS, B. J., L. S. NERURKAR, AND J. A. BELLANTI. Maturation of the rabbit alveolar macrophage during animal development. III. Phagocytic and bactericidal functions. *Pediatr. Res.* 11: 1208–1211, 1977.

CHAPTER 2

Lung cell biology

EWALD R. WEIBEL | *Department of Anatomy, University of Berne, Berne, Switzerland*

CHAPTER CONTENTS

Basic Plan of the Cell
    Cell nucleus
    Cytoplasmic membrane systems and granules
    Mitochondria
    Ground substance and cytoskeleton
    Plasma membrane
Organization of Lung Cell Population
    Histogenetic origin of lung cells and tissues
    Differentiation of functional zones
    Morphometry of lung cell population
Epithelium
    Epithelium of conducting airways
        Ciliated cells
        Exocrine cells
        Endocrine and other cells
        Cell kinetics in conducting airway epithelium
    Alveolar epithelium
        Alveolar lining cells: type I pneumocytes
        Alveolar secretory cells: type II pneumocytes
        Alveolar brush cells: type III pneumocytes
        Cell kinetics in alveolar epithelium
Vascular Endothelium
    Structure of capillary endothelium
    Structure of arterial and venous endothelium
    Metabolic functions of endothelial cells
Interstitial Cells
    Cells related to connective tissue fibers
    Interstitial cells with contractile properties
        Smooth muscle cells
        Myofibroblasts and pericytes
    Lymphatics and free cells
    Nerves
Cells of Pulmonary Defense System
    Alveolar and interstitial macrophages
    Cells of immune defense system
    Granulocytes
Mesothelial Cells of Pleura

THE LUNG'S CARDINAL FUNCTION is to establish and maintain good conditions for gas exchange between air and blood. This requires a number of ancillary functions to be performed by cells, even though gas exchange occurs by diffusion and hence is a passive phenomenon. Adequate permeability barriers must be maintained between the blood space, interstitial fluid, and the surface lining layer of air spaces to keep the lung dry; this requires linings made of live cells. Maintaining a mechanically stable lung necessitates formation and upkeep of a fiber system and secretion of surfactant onto the surface of the air space. Air spaces exposed to our environment must be kept clean; cells intervene in this process as macrophages or as cells producing and propelling a mucous lining on the wall of conducting airways, allowing removal of particulate matter entering the lining with the inhaled air. Not all intruders are intercepted and removed by this process, however, and thus the lung needs to maintain an internal defense system of cells capable of fending off many kinds of potentially noxious elements. Ventilation and perfusion of respiratory units should be matched as closely as possible; this requires a potential for active regulation of airway and blood vessel caliber by smooth muscle sleeves, as well as cells capable of distributing information through either humoral or neural pathways.

These functions, served by a rather complex cell population, may be and are often called nonrespiratory, but in fact they are essential though ancillary for respiration; they serve no other purpose than to make gas exchange efficient. There may be a few functions performed by lung cells that are not directly related to gas exchange, such as the capacity of endothelial cells to metabolize certain compounds. However, these functions are generally not specific functions of lung cells and perhaps are only so conspicuous because the lung is the best-perfused organ of the body, traversed by full cardiac output.

This chapter first considers the basic plan of eukaryotic cells and the functional role played by their constituents and then discusses the particular differentiations characterizing the various cell types in relation to the specialized functions required by their location within a well-organized functional system.

BASIC PLAN OF THE CELL

A fundamental insight of modern cell biology is that all cells are built according to a basic plan and that differentiation is just a modulation on the same basic scheme. All cells are completely enwrapped by a plasma membrane that establishes and controls relations to the surrounding and neighboring cells. The cell interior is divided into two basic compartments: *1*) the nucleus containing the genetic control mechanism and *2*) the cytoplasm housing all the organelles by which the cell performs its specific functions. The properties of this basic organizational scheme are briefly reviewed before the differentiations encountered in the various lung cells are discussed, because reference is made repeatedly to many of these basic design features.

Cell Nucleus

The nucleus of the eukaryotic cell is bounded by a nuclear envelope made of two membranes (Fig. 1). This envelope is perforated by many nuclear pores ~80 nm in diameter that traverse both membranes and contain a highly organized pore structure. The function of these pores is not completely understood, but they appear to be the main gateways for exchange of matter between nucleus and cytoplasm, particularly for the transfer of ribosomal and messenger RNA from the nucleus to the cytoplasm (31).

Considerable knowledge has been gained about the organization of chromosomal DNA in the nucleus. The dense heterochromatin contains coiled up "silent" parts of the DNA, whereas those sequences that need to be transcribed to RNA are contained in unwound form in the lightly staining euchromatin. The relative amount of euchromatin and heterochromatin is therefore a rough sign of the level of synthetic activity because a cell with a light nucleus shows a wider spectrum of protein synthesis than a cell with a dense nucleus, where most of the DNA is in heterochromatic form. The DNA sequences that code for ribosomal RNA are contained in the nucleolus associated with ribonucleoprotein particles, the precursors of the ribosomes (89). A cell with a high level of protein synthesis contains one or more prominent nucleoli. The nucleus contains a number of additional granules whose function is poorly understood.

In preparation for cell division the nuclear DNA is first replicated during the S phase of the cell cycle (13, 89); at this time radioactively labeled nucleotides (e.g., tritiated thymidine) can be incorporated into the genome. At the onset of mitosis the chromatin filaments, made of the DNA and histones, are systematically coiled up to form chromosomes (13). The nuclear envelope then withdraws into the cytoplasm, the mitotic spindle is formed from the centrioles, and the two daughter nuclei are assembled at the poles of the spindle. The cytoplasm usually contracts into a spherical or ovoid shape without losing its differentiated features, and a cleavage furrow cuts the cell, organelles, and plasma membrane into two halves. As the chromosome halves are unraveled to re-form the chromatin structure of an interphase nucleus, the nuclear envelope is reconstructed; the cytoplasmic elements are redistributed to their normal position and proliferate to achieve the size necessary for cell function.

Cytoplasmic Membrane Systems and Granules

The cytoplasm contains in its matrix a set of particles, filaments, membrane-bounded compartments, and organelles that serve particular functions and are present in all cells, with very few exceptions (Figs. 1–3). The particle directly related to the cell's fundamental function, protein synthesis, which governs most other functions, is the ribosome (Fig. 2); the ribosome measures 20–25 nm in diameter and is built of two unequal subunits each made of RNA and proteins (21, 22, 141). Ribosomes are ancient cell constituents that occur in bacteria and eukaryotic cells and are so similar that even mammalian proteins can be synthesized on bacterial ribosomes under favorable in vitro conditions. The amino acid sequence of polypeptides is encoded on the filamentous messenger RNA molecule that attaches to the ribosome in a cleft formed between the two subunits. Because several ribosomes can attach in sequence to one messenger RNA molecule, ribosomes usually occur in groups called polyribosomes, and each ribosome of such a group is clearly engaged in making the same polypeptide. Depending on the final destination of the polypeptide, polyribosomes are either free in the cytoplasmic matrix, if the protein is to be used in the cytoplasm, or attached to membranes of the endoplasmic reticulum (ER), if the protein is made for export, i.e., for any function outside the cell (Fig. 2). Typical examples of the latter are fibroblasts (see Fig. 21) that synthesize tropocollagen or plasma cells (see Fig. 32) that make specific immunoglobulins, whereas muscle proteins are made on free polyribosomes.

The ER comprises a set of membrane-bounded compartments of differing shape and function. Their common feature is that a fine lipoprotein membrane separates the compartment space from the cytoplasmic ground substance (Figs. 2 and 3); anything entering this compartment is therefore removed from direct contact with the cytoplasm. The importance of this feature is evident in hydrolytic enzymes, which are made by virtually all cells: the membrane shields the cell proper against the enzyme's potentially destructive activity. Topologically the interior of the ER is an exterior space; anything contained in it can be extruded from the cell without traversing the cytoplasm proper, as convincingly demonstrated for enzymes of exocrine gland cells (94, 141) and for tropocollagen of fibroblasts (84, 154).

The ER occurs in three different forms that are partly interconnected (94, 135, 141). What is generally called the rough (or granular) endoplasmic reticulum (RER), because of its appearance on low-resolution electron micrographs, is a set of cisternae, flat membrane bags of narrow width but varying extension, to which polyribosomes are bound on the cytoplasmic side (Fig. 2). Ribosomes that make proteins for export are attached to the membrane to allow the nascent polypeptide chain to penetrate immediately into the cisternal space without ever coming into contact with the cytoplasmic matrix. The mechanisms allowing this function and controlling the release of such polypeptides have been studied extensively (21). Proteins destined to become constituents of any membrane of

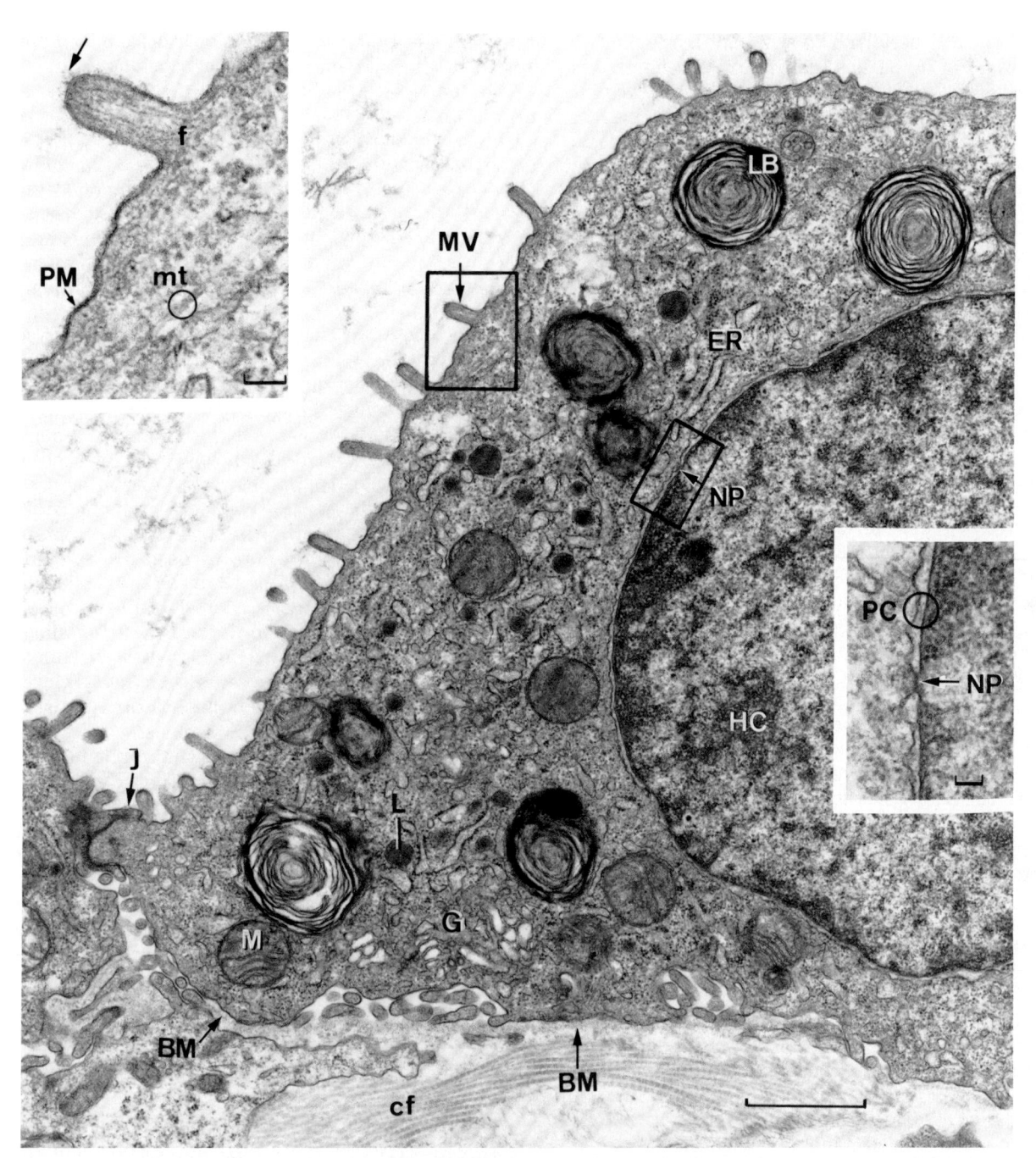

FIG. 1. Organization of half a type II epithelial cell from human lung (cf. Fig. 15B). Nucleus is enwrapped by a perinuclear cisterna (PC) made of 2 membranes, which is traversed by nuclear pores (NP), shown (inset, right) at greater magnification; nuclear content is divided into dense heterochromatin (HC) areas and karyoplasm, which contains euchromatin. Cell surface is made of the plasma membrane (PM) with a subjacent ectoplasmic layer of filaments (f) and a fuzzy coat or glycocalyx (arrow) on the outside (inset, left). Cells in epithelia are joined by junctional complexes (J) with terminal bars at the boundary between apical and lateral face; basal face is attached to the basement membrane (BM). Cytoplasm houses a variety of organelles. cf, Collagen fibrils; ER, endoplasmic reticulum; G, Golgi complex; L, lysosomes; LB, lamellar body; M, mitochondrion; mt, microtubule; MV, microvilli. Bars: 1 µm; 0.1 µm (insets).

the cell are formed in the same basic manner on membrane-bound ribosomes. The mechanisms by which they are inserted into the membrane and brought to their final destination (e.g., the plasma membrane) are less well understood. The nuclear envelope is an important part of the RER, because its outer membrane is studded with polyribosomes (Fig. 1); in addition the RER forms at least partly from the nuclear envelope in cells that undergo differentiation toward export protein synthesis.

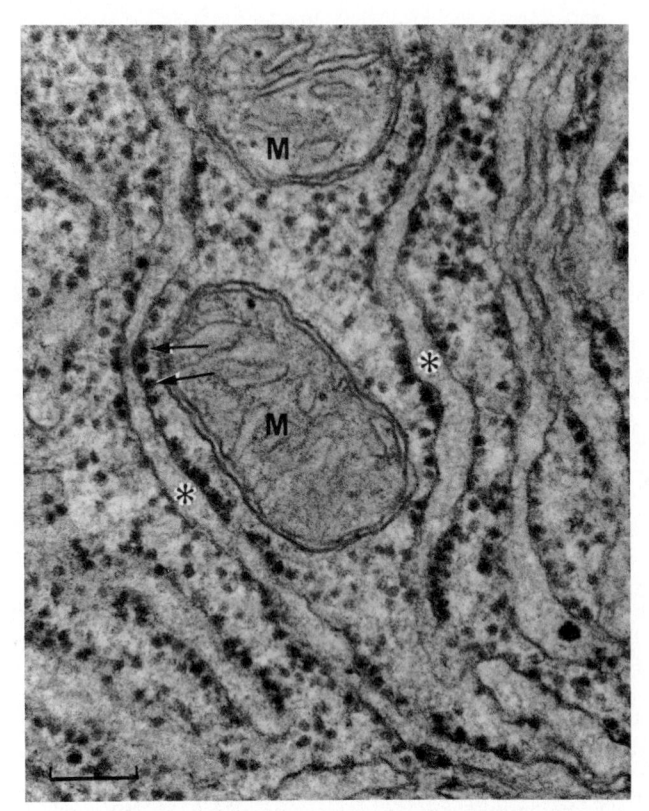

FIG. 2. Mitochondria (*M*) and rough endoplasmic reticulum with cisternal space (*asterisks*) bounded by fine membrane to which ribosomes (*arrows*) are attached. Some free ribosomes are not attached to membranes. Double membrane of mitochondria with formation of cristae. Plasma cell. *Bar*, 0.2 μm.

major site of synthesis in mucus-secreting cells such as goblet cells (134). The former function is also of great importance for many lung cells such as alveolar macrophages or type II alveolar cells.

The cell contains in the region of its Golgi complex a set of membrane-bounded granules of various sizes and compositions (Figs. 1 and 3); as a common feature they contain various hydrolytic enzymes, such as acid phosphatase and arylsulfatase, and are therefore called lysosomes. The RER is responsible for the synthesis of the enzymes, and the Golgi complex provides at least the container. Apparently the Golgi complex, RER, and lysosomes function as a coherent unit in many if not all cells (Fig. 3). Novikoff (135) therefore named this basic feature GERL (Golgi-associated endoplasmic reticulum and lysosomes). Lysosomes occur in at least two different states. Primary lysosomes simply store the enzymes and discharge them into secondary lysosomes containing some material that needs to be broken down by enzymatic digestion. This can be either foreign material picked up by phagocytosis or deteriorated cytoplasmic constituents that need to be removed in the course of cell turnover. In the latter instance the cytoplasmic constituents are first sequestered from the remaining cytoplasm by a membrane envelope in a process called autophagy; the resulting cytosegrosomes then receive hydrolytic enzymes from primary lysosomes, and their

The smooth (or agranular) endoplasmic reticulum (SER) is an entirely different structure, typically composed of a network of tubules, whose membrane contains a variety of different enzymes. The SER is particularly well developed in liver cells, where it carries mixed-function oxidases and other enzymes engaged in detoxification of foreign compounds such as drugs (181). Because the lung is also able to perform these functions, particularly on induction (54, 55), this organelle should also be found in lung cells, although it is generally not conspicuous. Type II cells of the alveolar epithelium may contain appreciable amounts of SER and are apparently capable of xenobiotic metabolism (54). Clara cells of bronchioles are known to be rich in SER in some species (53, 111, 147), although the specific function of SER in this cell type is unclear.

The Golgi complex, the third component of ER, is made of a stack of smooth-walled narrow cisternae surrounded by a maze of tubules and vesicles [Fig. 3; (135, 141, 192)]. It appears to have two basic functions: *1*) to serve as a pool of membrane "bags" for packaging proteins destined for export (141, 142) or lysosomes and *2*) to synthesize mucopolysaccharides (117, 189). The latter function is particularly important in lung cell biology because the Golgi complex becomes the

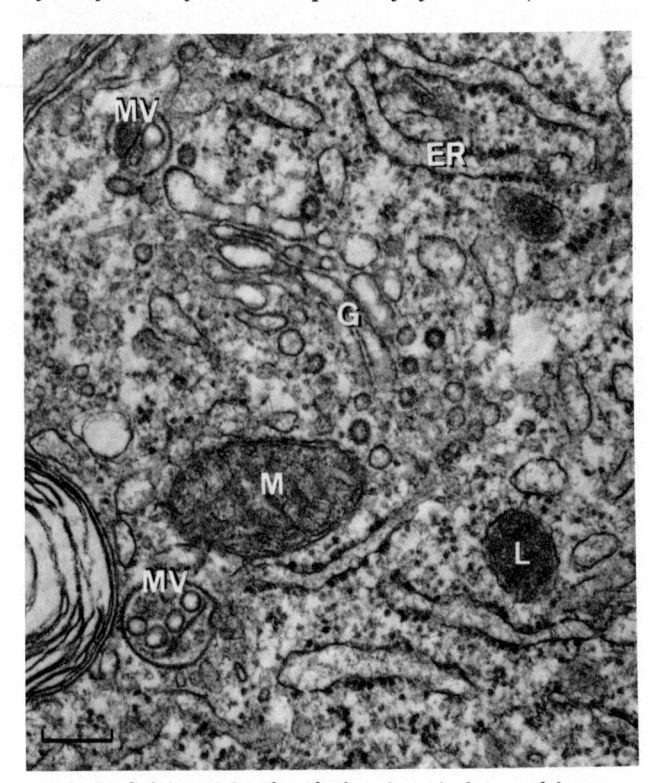

FIG. 3. Golgi-associated endoplasmic reticulum and lysosomes (GERL) from alveolar type II cell consists of Golgi complex (*G*) with a stack of cisternae surrounded by vesicles, rough endoplasmic reticulum (*ER*), and primary lysosomes (*L*). *M*, mitochondrion; *MV*, multivesicular bodies. *Bar*, 0.2 μm.

content can be digested intracellularly in a controlled manner. Autophagy probably occurs in all cells with a long life span. These cells undergo a continuous internal renewal and are adaptable to functional needs; autophagy is an important pathway for removing elements no longer needed. Heterophagy, more generally known as endocytosis (i.e., uptake of foreign material), is also a property of all cells, but only to a limited extent. In many cells it is restricted to an uptake of small macromolecules by micropinocytosis through small membrane vesicles, whereas macrophagy (i.e., uptake of larger particles) is limited to certain cell classes. In the lung the most prominent cell specialized in this respect is the alveolar macrophage, but histiocytes (tissue macrophages) and neutrophil granulocytes share this capability. There is another cytoplasmic granule belonging to the lysosomes: the residual body that stores—if need be as long as the cell and the organism live—indigestible residues. The best example from the lung is the anthracotic pigment (carbon) granules stored in histiocytes in pulmonary connective tissue or in peribronchial lymph nodes.

Thus the intracellular membrane system establishes a set of compartments that are potentially extracellular. This system must be closely associated with the group of vesicles and vacuoles that can connect with the plasma membrane and either discharge material originating in the cell to the outside by exocytosis (94, 141) or pick up extracellular material by endocytosis. This interconnection has been amply documented. The discharge of cell products via exocytosis by means of membrane-bounded vesicles is the common pathway for any type of cell secretion, whether it is enzymes from exocrine gland cells (94, 141) or tropocollagen from fibroblasts (84, 154); here the pathway goes from the RER through the Golgi complex to storage vacuoles whose membranes fuse with the plasma membrane in order to release only the content. However, this pathway is not totally reversible. Extracellular material brought into the cell by endocytosis is deposited in vacuoles of the lysosomal system but is blocked from penetrating further into elements of the Golgi complex or of RER.

Mitochondria

The mitochondria are also membrane-bounded organelles (Figs. 1 and 2), but they are essentially unrelated to the cytoplasmic membrane system discussed so far. Mitochondria are the organelles of oxidative phosphorylation. They are composed of two concentric membranes: *1*) the outer membrane, which forms a simple envelope, and *2*) the inner membrane, which forms a variable number of infoldings called cristae. This inner membrane separates the mitochondrion into two compartments: *1*) the matrix space containing the enzymes of the Krebs cycle and *2*) the so-called intermembrane space. The inner membrane carries the units of the respiratory chain and, on the matrix side, the enzyme ATPase, which phosphorylates ADP to make ATP. The current view of how this system functions can be summarized (see also refs. 150, 201). The Krebs cycle generates reducing equivalents (NADH) that are oxidized by the respiratory chain to produce H_2O at the end; the energy gained by this process establishes a proton gradient across the inner membrane. This proton gradient provides the energy required to add the energy-rich third phosphate group to ADP as protons flow back to the matrix space through appropriate channels associated with the mitochondrial ATPase (chemiosmotic theory). This process is well regulated because under optimal conditions there is a strict stoichiometric relation between the number of O_2 molecules consumed and the number of ATP molecules made, namely six ATP molecules for each O_2.

In many respects, mitochondria are most interesting elements. Their shape and size are highly variable; some cell types contain only two rather long and twisted mitochondria, so that the many mitochondrial profiles one observes on electron micrographs of sectioned cells may well belong to the same mitochondrion. Thus it is inappropriate to characterize the mitochondrial complement of a cell by the "mitochondrial number" because this parameter is undefinable. On the other hand, it has been shown repeatedly that the volume density of mitochondria or the surface area of their inner membrane is proportional to the cell's capacity to generate ATP by oxidative phosphorylation (201). Note, however, that an alternative pathway exists, namely anaerobic phosphorylation from glycolysis for which the enzymes are contained in the cytoplasmic matrix. Another interesting feature is that mitochondria apparently are not formed de novo but enlarge and multiply by division (136). Mitochondria contain their own ribosomes and their own circular DNA, which codes for only part of the mitochondrial proteins (136), however; the other part is supplied by cytoplasmic RER. There appears to be an active interchange between mitochondria and ER because the mitochondria furnish the heme components needed in some ER enzymes.

Ground Substance and Cytoskeleton

The cytoplasmic ground substance is mostly an unstructured sap. Besides stores such as glycogen granules and triglyceride droplets, it contains a host of filaments that have received increasing attention (148). The picture emerging from recent studies is that all cells contain an appreciable amount of actin that polymerizes to make fine filaments 6 nm thick. When these associate with myosin they become contractile and can actively move about cytoplasmic elements, such as vesicles, to which they are attached. The importance of such mechanisms of active intracellular movement is not fully appreciated. These actin filaments insert in the plasma membrane and thus perform movements of the cell periphery, such as those involved in the ameboid movement of cells and also phagocytosis (185, 186); clearly this system serves important functions in macrophages. The presence of actin and myosin in all or most cells is also important in view of the recent insight that fibroblasts may develop contractile properties and even transform to smooth muscle cells.

The cytoplasm contains two more types of fibrillar structures that appear to function as a cytoskeleton (Figs. 1 and 4): *1)* filaments 10 nm thick and *2)* microtubules 20 nm in diameter made of the protein tubulin (148). Microtubules derive partly from the centrioles; during cell division they form the mitotic spindle along which the chromosomes move to the two poles. The set of tubules that forms the skeleton of cilia is likewise derived from centrioles (160, 167); the ciliary contraction is not due to these tubules but rather to the protein dynein attached to them (see the chapter by Satir and Dirksen in this *Handbook*).

Plasma Membrane

Much could be said about the structure and function of the plasmalemma. Figure 5A shows a thin section of the plasma membrane of an erythrocyte with its typical appearance of two dark layers separated by a light space, which reflects the basic structure of a bimolecular layer of phospholipids with the hydrophobic fatty acid chains facing each other. This structure is often termed a *unit membrane*. If frozen cells are broken, the membranes split along their hydrophobic midplane, so that freeze-fracture replicas expose the two membrane leaflets seen from inside (Fig. 5B). These fracture surfaces appear studded with small particles that are now known to represent proteins that are inserted in and in fact span the entire thickness of the membrane; they are therefore termed *intramembrane particles*. The current view is that the basic structure of a membrane is that of a mosaic of different proteins embedded in a lipid phase of variable composition (208). The lipid layer forms a water barrier and the proteins constitute different functional units, some of which may establish selective pores for molecular exchanges between the cell and its surroundings.

On the outside the plasma membrane has a coat of polysaccharides (glycocalyx) that are anchored on membrane proteins and lipids (151, 189, 208). Toward the cytoplasm the membrane is underlaid by a network of proteins made of spectrin; this is apparently where the cytoplasmic filaments are anchored (148, 208). A zone of condensed cytoplasmic matrix usually underlies the plasma membrane (see Fig. 1, *inset*); this so-called ectoplasm contains fine filaments but is devoid of organelles or ribosomes, with the exception of microvesicles engaged in transport.

Basically the plasma membrane forms a tight barrier between cytoplasm and extracellular space; however, there are many leaks and gateways that allow a controlled transfer of ions or molecules. There are

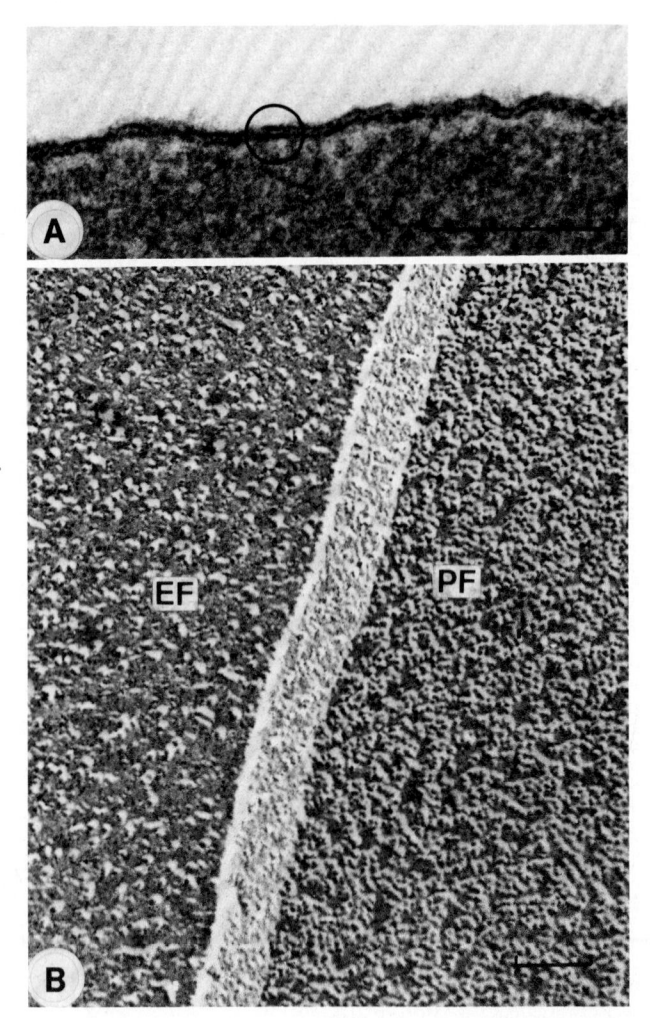

FIG. 5. *A*: thin section of cell membrane of erythrocyte with 2 dark staining leaflets (*circle*). *B*: freeze-fracture replica of cleaved membranes of 2 erythrocytes showing that intramembranous particles on inner protoplasmic leaflet (*PF*) facing the cytoplasm are denser than those on external leaflet (*EF*). Bars, 0.1 μm.

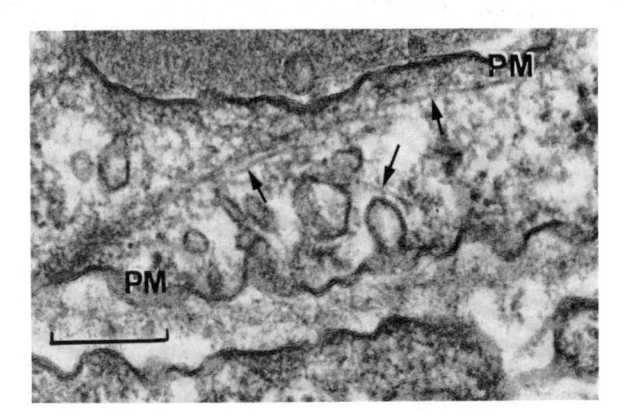

FIG. 4. Cytoskeletal 10-nm filaments (*arrows*) extend between 2 plasma membranes (*PM*) in alveolar type I cell. Bar, 0.2 μm.

even specialized regions in the cell membrane where two adjacent cells can be joined so that ions and small molecules can be directly exchanged from cytoplasm to cytoplasm, thus coupling the cells electrically and in part metabolically (11, 12, 75, 120). These intercellular junctions (nexus or gap junctions) are characterized by a regular array of intramembrane particles that function as intercellular pores (75). Other specializations of the plasma membrane in the region of cell-to-cell contact are desmosomes (macula adherens), small areas of mechanical connection between neighboring cells in which cytoskeletal filaments insert, and terminal bars or tight junctions (zonula occludens), which can seal intercellular spaces in epithelia and thus establish cell sheets that separate two tissue compartments (161, 164). The structure of tight junctions is best seen on freeze-fracture replicas (Fig. 6), where they appear as a band made of a network of strings of intramembrane particles, with the number and density of such strings proportional to the tightness of the intercellular junction (163).

By describing these junctions I have already referred to a fundamental property of some cells, namely the capability of epithelial cells to assemble into sheets at the interface between two tissue compartments, which derives directly from their development. These cells show a polar organization in that three different faces of the plasma membrane can be clearly distinguished (see Fig. 1): *1*) the apical face is in direct contact with the lumen bounded by the epithelium and is bordered by the terminal bar; *2*) the basal face is attached to the basal lamina (basement membrane) that bounds the interstitial space; and *3*) the lateral face is in contact with neighboring cells and extends from the terminal bar to the basal lamina. The membrane of these faces shows different properties. However, cell polarity is not limited to the plasma membrane; the organelles of the cytoplasm are often ordered in relation to this polarity as well.

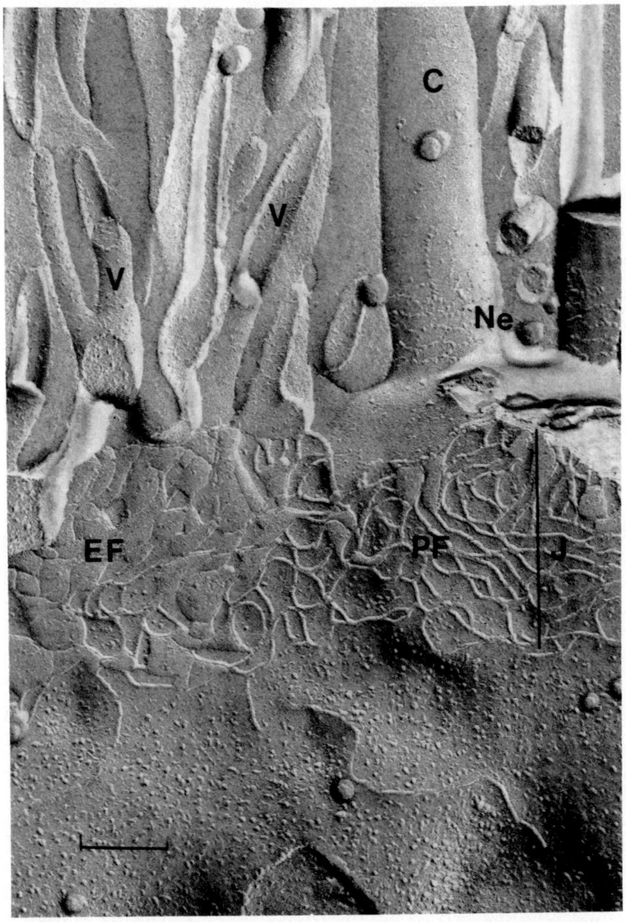

ORGANIZATION OF LUNG CELL POPULATION

The lung is organized according to two basic patterns that are relevant for the classification of the various differentiated cell types (26, 111, 202): *1*) the formation of cell or tissue layers that result from lung histogenesis and *2*) the formation of functional zones or compartments, notably the separation of the respiratory zone or lung parenchyma from those parts that merely distribute air and blood to the gas-exchange units and mechanically bind these units into a coherent structure (202, 203).

Histogenetic Origin of Lung Cells and Tissues

Histogenetically the lung's cell population evolves from a simple anlage made of an epithelial bud surrounded by a mesenchymal bed formed by the splanchnopleura. Note that the epithelial bud derives from the entoderm (for review see the chapter by Burri in this *Handbook* and refs. 38, 86, 139). In the foregut a long ventral groove gives rise to the trachea, whose caudal end bifurcates and grows laterally into the thickened pleural mesenchyme to form the anlage of the main stem bronchi. The airway tree is built from this epithelial anlage by sequential dichotomous branching; in the later fetal and early postnatal period this airway tube system differentiates into conducting and respiratory airways. Consequently the entire epithelial lining of all airways from the trachea to the alveoli is of identical histogenetic origin.

All other genuine lung structures are of mesodermal origin. Even before the tracheobronchial anlage forms, the gut is surrounded by a plexus of blood sinuses that originated in the angiogenetic tissue of the splanchnopleura. As the bronchial bud grows, this plexus is carried along into the lung anlage, where it sequen-

FIG. 6. Electron micrograph of human ciliated cells. Terminal bar or tight junction (*J*) appears as lacework of ~10 rows of densely aligned particles on fracture face of protoplasmic leaflet (*PF*) and as complementary grooves on external leaflet (*EF*) of adjacent cell. Tuft of microvilli (*V*) and base of cilium (*C*) with ciliary necklace of intramembrane particles (*Ne*). Bar, 0.2 μm. (Courtesy of E. E. Schneeberger.)

tially enlarges as the epithelial tubes grow and branch. The two pulmonary arteries arise from the sixth branchial arteries, whereas the pulmonary vein stem grows into the lung anlage from the dorsal wall of the left atrium; both connect with the pulmonary vascular plexus, and pulmonary circulation is established. The bronchial circulation derives from the same vascular plexus by retaining some of the branches that originally connected it to the aorta.

In early stages of lung development the mesenchyme, which is directly derived from the splanchnopleura, forms a loose bed of branched cells with some unstructured interstitial matter. As the epithelial tube begins to differentiate, the more central airways are enwrapped by a layer of condensed mesenchyme in which one can soon distinguish differentiated cells such as primitive smooth muscle cells and cartilage. Simultaneously, larger pulmonary arteries are enwrapped by a coat of differentiating smooth muscle cells. This mesenchymal differentiation gradually progresses peripherally, but the most distal airways, which will form the parenchymal units, remain embedded in a loose unstructured mesenchyme with the vascular plexus in close proximity to the epithelial tube (38).

All through this early stage of development a substantial part of the mesenchyme remains related to the pleura; it separates the forming parenchymal units and constitutes the elements of the bounding structures that extend from the hilum to the pleura, although they become much reduced in the course of further lung development and maturation. Histogenetically the lung is therefore made of three basic components or layers: *1*) airway epithelium of entodermal origin; *2*) vascular endothelium of mesodermal origin, specifically from angiogenetic tissue; *3*) mesenchymal tissues and pleura derived from the splanchnopleura, interposed between epithelium and endothelium. In addition, a number of cell types of different origin settle in the lung secondarily. Lymphocytes and plasma cells originate from lymphoid tissue and are brought in by the bloodstream, as are histiocytes and alveolar macrophages or granulocytes that come from bone marrow. Nerve fibers and some nerve cells grow in from nervous tissue. Some cells of the bronchial epithelium, the neuroendocrine or enterochromaffin cells, may be of ectodermal origin, deriving from the neural crest (45).

Differentiation of Functional Zones

In the later phases of lung development, the peripheral parts of the airway tubes and blood vessels differentiate into a gas-exchange apparatus by closely approximating blood capillaries and airways, reducing the mass of tissue while still maintaining the basic organization into the three layers—epithelium, interstitial tissue, and endothelium. Air spaces, blood vessels, and tissue form a functional unit to facilitate the diffusive exchange of O_2 and CO_2 between air and blood. Because this development of a respiratory structure involves several terminal generations of the branching airway tree, the structural unit of the gas-exchange apparatus is an acinus that consists of branching alveolar ducts on whose walls alveoli form postnatally (36). Each acinus receives air from one terminal bronchiole and blood through one branch of the pulmonary artery that enters next to the bronchiole, whereas the blood is drained into pulmonary veins at the periphery of the acinus. In most mammalian lungs the boundary between acini is not clearly marked, although the air passages and blood vessels are highly organized; the respiratory zone therefore forms a large mass of alveolated tissue, generally called lung parenchyma, characterized mainly by extreme thinning of all cell and tissue layers separating air and blood.

The central parts of the airway tubes and blood vessels form the structures of the conducting zone whose main function it is to distribute air and blood to the acini. In contrast to the respiratory zone, conducting airways and blood vessels remain clearly separated. Their wall structure is made of a variety of cell types differentiated toward specific functions, such as smooth muscle sleeves regulating the caliber of the passageway or an epithelial lining of bronchi cleansing inspired air. A connective tissue layer binds these conducting tubes together and houses part of the defense system of the lung.

The third functional compartment, quantitatively not very impressive, consists of the binding sheaths, the visceral pleura, bounded toward the pleural space by a mesothelium. The pleural connective tissue extends into the lung parenchyma with septa (202, 203), partially demarcating the units of the respiratory zone.

Morphometry of Lung Cell Population

Before considering the differentiated properties of each cell type in sequence, their relative importance in building a lung should be appreciated. Unfortunately the information available is scanty and fragmentary, with solid data only available for the respiratory zone. Furthermore rare cell types are usually not accounted for because they often elude the sampling strategies required to estimate morphometric parameters.

Table 1 gives provisional rough estimates of the volumes of different cell classes one may expect to encounter in mammalian lungs. The data used for this estimation were drawn from several sets of morphometric data obtained for different mammalian species (47–49, 82, 199); the numbers calculated are therefore no more than indications of approximate proportions. More realistic estimates would clearly be desirable, particularly in view of the increasing importance of cell-separation techniques for the study of the function of specific cell types (53, 79, 106).

TABLE 1. *Estimated Cell Volumes in Mammalian Lungs*

	Septal Tissue, %	Lung Volume, %*	Lung Weight, %†	Total Volume, Human Lung, ml‡
Total tissue§		7.56	44.5	284
Nonparenchyma		2.64	15.5	99
Alveolar septa		4.92	28.9	185
Total cell		5.67	33.4	213
Nonparenchyma		1.32	7.8	50
Alveolar septa		4.35	25.6	163
Parenchymal cell				
Alveolar epithelium				
Type I	12.6	0.62	3.6	23
Type II	9.7	0.48	2.8	18
Capillary endothelium	26.4	1.30	7.6	49
Interstitial cells	35.8	1.76	10.4	66
Alveolar macrophages	3.9	0.19	1.1	7

Cells are assumed to make up ~50% of nonparenchymal tissue. * 75% Total lung capacity (TLC). † With blood. ‡ TLC 6,000 ml. § Excluding blood. [Data from Crapo et al. (48), Haies et al. (82), and E. R. Weibel, unpublished observations.]

Probably the most important result of this estimation is the finding that ~75% of all lung cells, in terms of volume, are in the respiratory zone and that these make up ~25% of total lung weight. Considering the large number of different cell types that is described for nonparenchymatous structures, the total mass represented by each cell type is clearly rather small, at least for some. In terms of their function, however, the relative cell mass is not necessarily highly relevant for all cell types.

The cell population of lung parenchyma has been studied in several species. Table 2 summarizes some of the data obtained by different groups using a comparable approach. The most striking result is that there is little interspecies variation in the proportion of the various cell types or in their relative size; however, the human cells are about twice as large as the rat cells. In terms of volume (Table 1), both epithelial and endothelial cells apparently make up ~25% each of the parenchymal cells; interstitial cells are the largest cell population, whereas alveolar macrophages constitute a small fraction in the healthy lung.

EPITHELIUM

The lining of all airways and air spaces from the trachea to the alveoli is formed by a continuous epithelial cell sheet, whose main general properties are described as follows (Fig. 7).

1. The epithelial sheet forms an uninterrupted tight barrier between the subjacent interstitial (connective tissue) space and the air space, or rather the fine layer of free fluid that covers the epithelium toward the air space. This lining is tight because well-developed terminal bars or tight junctions seal the narrow intercellular clefts (80, 162). Even where the character of the epithelial sheet changes abruptly, for example, in progressing from bronchioles to alveolar walls, the epithelium is uninterrupted. The air-space epithelium is therefore appropriately described as a continuum with regionally modified differentiation (Fig. 7).

2. The epithelial cells are polarized (see Figs. 1 and 8A). They are all attached to the epithelial basement membrane (sometimes called basal lamina), which also forms a continuous sheet from the trachea to the alveoli. The part of the plasma membrane that is attached to the basal lamina, probably through its surface glycoproteins, is the basal face of the cell. Epithelial cells characteristically have an apical face that forms the actual surface of the epithelium and is delimited by the terminal bar. Epithelial cells are in immediate contact with their neighbors over the lateral face extending between the terminal bar and the attachment to the basal lamina (see Fig. 1). There is one notable exception to this rule: the basal cells of the pseudostratified epithelium of major airways are attached to the basal lamina but do not reach the epithelial surface (Fig. 8A), so they lack an apical face but are nonetheless polarized. This situation changes in squamous metaplasia of airway epithelia, because in a squamous epithelium only the basal cells are attached to the basal lamina and terminal bars are either lacking or incomplete in the apical cell layer; the epithelium itself is still polarized but not all of its individual cells.

3. At all levels the epithelium is a mosaic of cells

TABLE 2. *Morphometric Characteristics of Cell Population in Lung Parenchyma*

	Human (48)	Baboon (48)	Rat (47)	Rat (82)
Mean body weight, kg	74	29	0.36	0.25
Total cell number, $\times 10^9$	230	48	0.89	
Percent of total lung cells				
Alveolar epithelium				
Type I	8.3	11.8	8.9	7.5
Type II	15.9	7.7	14.2	14.5
Endothelium	30.2	36.3	46.2	43.0
Interstitial cells	36.1	41.8	27.7	31.8
Alveolar macrophages	9.4	2.3	3.0	3.2
Average cell volume, μm^3				
Alveolar epithelium				
Type I	1,764	1,224	2,042	915
Type II	889	539	443	366
Endothelium	632	365	387	336
Interstitial cells	637	227	331	615
Alveolar macrophages	2,492	1,059	1,058	665
Average apical cell surface, μm^2				
Alveolar epithelium				
Type I	5,098	4,004	5,320	4,518
Type II	183	285	123	62
Endothelium	1,353	1,040	1,105	946

Numbers in parentheses are references.

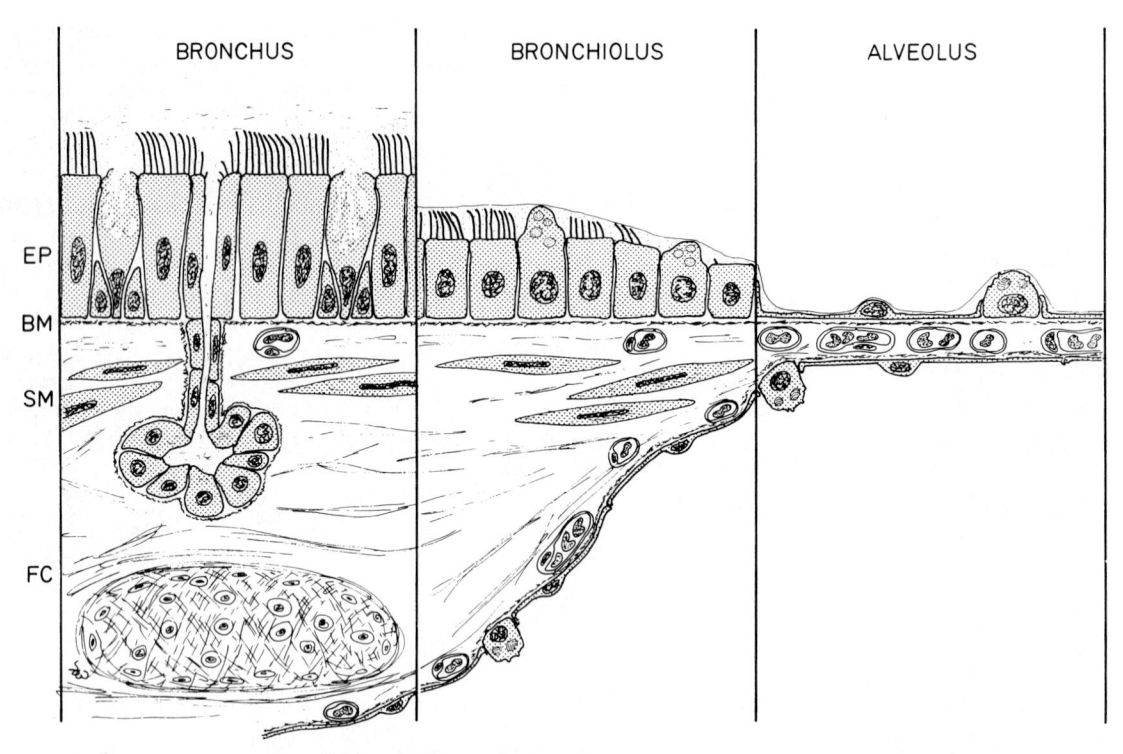

FIG. 7. Schematic representation of airway wall structure from bronchus to alveolus. EP, epithelial cells; BM, basement membrane; SM, smooth muscle cells; FC, fibrocartilaginous coat. [From Weibel (202).]

specialized for different functions. One can basically distinguish between cells that serve as a lining of the surface and secretory cells that produce essential constituents of the surface lining layer and hence belong to the class of exocrine cells. Some of these exocrine cells can be grouped in the form of small glands that are also continuous with the airway epithelium. Other cell types are also found interspersed in the epithelium, such as neuroendocrine cells and brush cells whose precise function has yet to be defined.

For a detailed description of these cells it is convenient to distinguish between two major regions: *1*) the conducting airways and *2*) the respiratory air spaces. The major difference between these regions is in the differentiation of the lining cells toward transport of the mucous blanket on the one hand and optimization of gas exchange on the other hand; this also has essential consequences for the kind of exocrine cells required.

Epithelium of Conducting Airways

The conducting airways play a major role in protecting the delicate respiratory tissue of lung parenchyma from potential impairments due to airborne noxious particles that may be inhaled. The surface of these airways has a thin film of a sticky mucus that can capture such particles. These particles are then removed with the mucus toward the larynx and pharynx, where they are either swallowed or coughed out. The epithelium of the conducting airways produces this surface blanket through its secretory cells, and the action of the ciliated lining cells propels it outward (196). Figure 8 shows the complex of major cell types that participate in this action in a medium-size bronchus from a human lung; a goblet cell is intercalated between ciliated cells and discharges a drop of mucus that spreads on top of the tufts of cilia of the ciliated cells.

The epithelium in these major airways is pseudostratified. Ciliated cells and goblet cells are slender high columnar cells that extend from the basal lamina to the surface; smaller basal cells that appear to be poorly differentiated are restricted to the lower part of the epithelium (Fig. 7). Farther down the airway tree the epithelium in smaller bronchioles is transformed to a simple columnar epithelium and the cell height is reduced until the ciliated and secretory cells are cuboidal (i.e., as high as they are wide). The height of the airway epithelium apparently is directly proportional to the absolute size of the airway, because in smaller species (e.g., rat or mouse) even the largest bronchi have a simple columnar epithelium of modest height or even cuboidal cells (140). Conversely the epithelium of major bronchi and trachea in humans is much higher than that shown in Figure 8.

The essential functional property of the epithelium of conducting airways is that it forms and maintains a continuous stream of fluid, partly covered by mucus, which moves from the airway periphery toward the

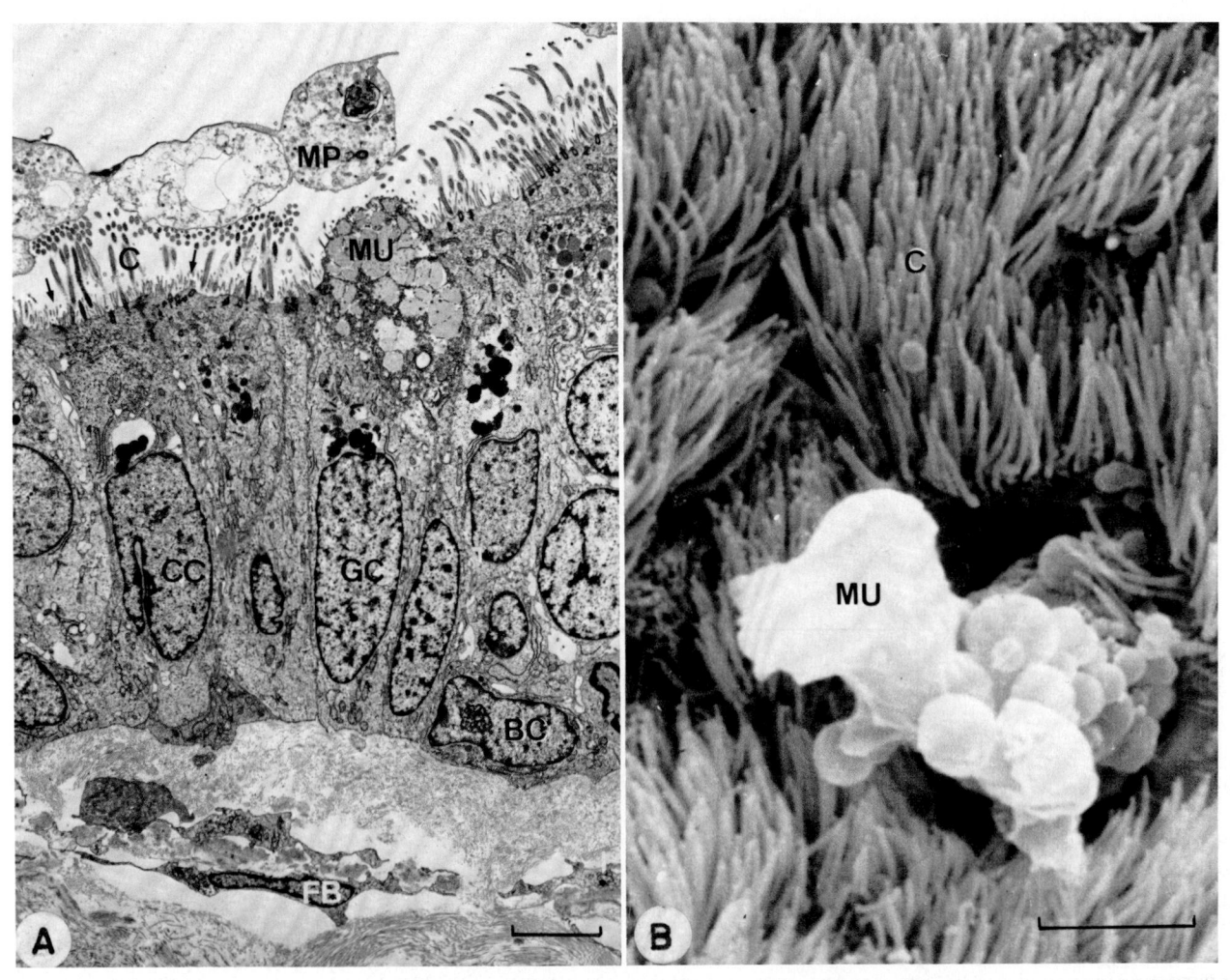

FIG. 8. Mucous membrane of small human bronchus. *A*: thin section showing ciliated cell (*CC*) with cilia (*C*) and microvilli (*arrows*), goblet cell (*GC*) with apical mucous plug (*MU*), and basal cell (*BC*). Fibers and fibroblasts (*FB*) in connective tissue. *MP*, macrophage. *B*: scanning electron micrograph of epithelial surface showing ciliary tufts (*C*) and mucous plug (*MU*) of goblet cell in process of extrusion. Bars, 5 μm.

center and up the trachea; this essential cleansing mechanism is often called the airway escalator.

The hierarchy of the airway tree has certain repercussions on the design properties of this escalator. As the airways branch, their diameter and length become systematically reduced, but their number doubles with each division so that the total airway surface increases appreciably in more peripheral generations (197). Consequently the pathway for mucus narrows as it is moved up the escalator. As under steady-state conditions, the flow rate of fluid across the entire perimeter (sum of perimeters of all airways in a given generation) must be the same for all generations, the flow rate in central airways must be greater, and the thickness of the mucous blanket must be larger. This is accentuated by the fact that mucus is being secreted all along the airway tract, perhaps in greater quantity in large than in small airways. Greater propulsive work is therefore required in larger airways; this is partly achieved by having a higher density of cilia on the surface of large than on the surface of small airways, mostly by increasing the relative number of ciliated cells.

CILIATED CELLS. To provide cells with cilia is a very archaic phylogenetic means of endowing them with the capacity of movement. Cilia or flagellae with their very characteristic structure occur on plant cells, on many forms of protozoa, and in several locations in all metazoan organisms. Cilia occur in embryos in virtually all derivatives of the entoderm as well as on parts of the ectoderm, and even in many fibroblasts spurious cilia are formed (176); the role of such transiently formed cilia is largely unknown. Even in the mature mammalian organism, cilia occur in many places, sometimes singly, as in the small biliary ducts or in the tail of spermatozoa. Single cilia are also found on the receptor cells of the vestibular apparatus

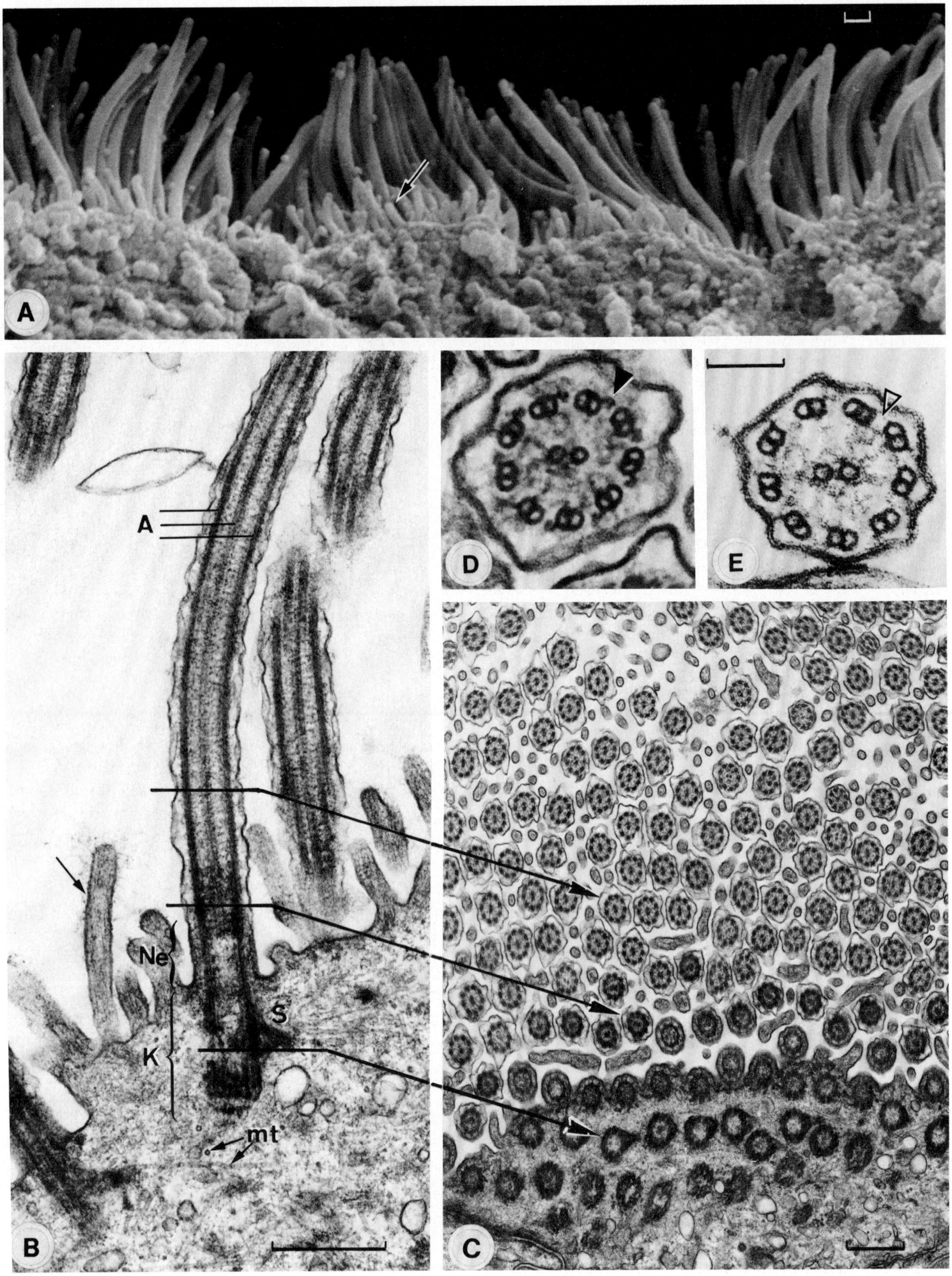
A
A
Ne
S
K
mt
B
C
D
E

and as the connecting stalk between inner and outer segments of the retinal rods and cones.

The cilium is a derivative of the centrioles, which are the organizers of cell division or rather of karyokinesis, that part of mitosis where the two halves of the chromosomes are split and divided to the two daughter cells in an orderly fashion, moving along the tubules of the mitotic spindle extending from one centriole to the other. Centrioles are able to replicate through a largely unknown mechanism; these replicas migrate toward the cell surface and act as organizers for the ciliary axoneme, giving rise to cilia by evaginating the cell membrane (see the chapter by Satir and Dirksen in this *Handbook* and ref. 167).

This digression into general cell biology is simply meant to show the widespread occurrence of this fundamental organelle of eukaryotic cells and the versatility of its use in forming specialized structures. In many instances the functional significance of these ciliary derivatives is unknown or at best speculative.

The cilia that occur on the mammalian respiratory tract epithelium, from the nasal cavity to the bronchioles, are a common type; they are also found in the buccal cavity of frogs, in mussels, and in protozoan ciliates such as paramecium. They are regular membrane-bounded protrusions of the apical cell surface (Fig. 9), ~5 μm long and 0.25 μm in diameter, with the ability to beat at a regular frequency of ~20 Hz. Because the chapter by Satir and Dirksen in this *Handbook* is dedicated to cilia (160), only a few of their important structural and functional properties are mentioned here.

The apical surface of each ciliated cell has a tuft of ~200 cilia; this number may be slightly lower in the smallest bronchioles. They are arranged in more or less regular rows with a center-to-center spacing of ~0.5 μm (Fig. 10).

The cilium is built of a set of highly characteristic tubules, but their structure and arrangement vary in the four parts of the cilium (167): *1*) the basal body, *2*) the neck, *3*) the shaft, and *4*) the tapering tip (Fig. 9). In the shaft, the part responsible for performing the ciliary beat, the complex of longitudinal tubules (axoneme) is most complete: a central pair of singlet tubules is surrounded by nine doublet tubules with a complex of fine radial spokes binding them together. Both types of tubules are built as complex polymers of the protein tubulin with a molecular weight of ~60,000, the same protein of which cytoplasmic mi-

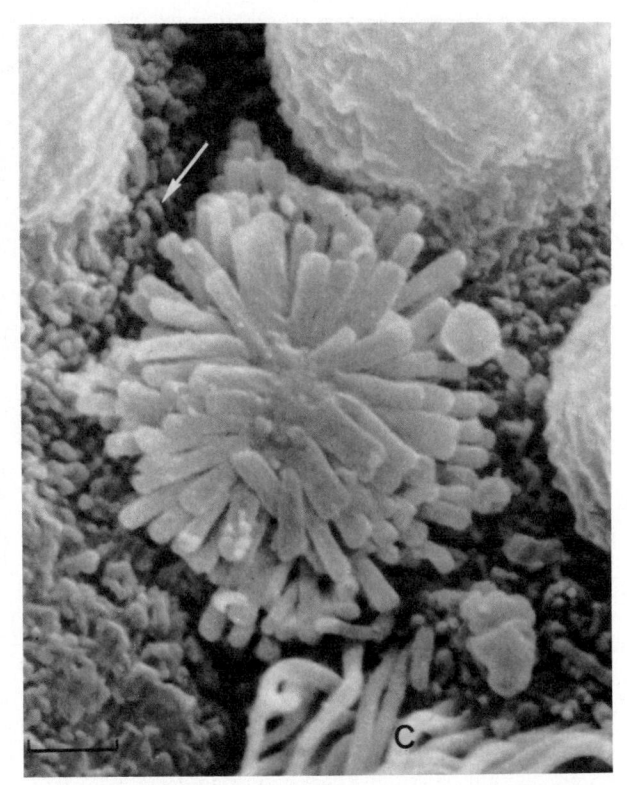

FIG. 10. Scanning electron micrograph of brush cell from small bronchiole of rat lung. Compare brush with cilia (C) and ordinary microvilli (*arrow*). Bar, 1 μm.

crotubules are made. In the shaft region, the outer doublet tubules have two "arms" (Fig. 9D) that have been identified as a characteristic protein called dynein; this molecule provides the cilium with its motility, whereas the microtubules appear to have a skeletal function. Separation of axonemal components has shown that the ATPase of the cilia is contained in the dynein. Furthermore it has recently been demonstrated that a hereditary absence of dynein arms (Fig. 9E) leads to immotile cilia (4, 155, 188), resulting in a syndrome of congenital respiratory infections due to a deficiency in clearing mucus from the airways and nasal cavity. This syndrome is associated with male sterility due to immotile spermatozoa and is found in 50% of patients with situs inversus (4), known for half a century as Kartagener's syndrome (4, 155).

This basic ciliary structure is modified toward the region of implantation in the cell surface. In the neck

---

FIG. 9. Scanning electron micrograph (A) and longitudinal (B) and transverse (C) thin sections of cilia of human bronchial epithelium. Microvilli (*arrows*) between cilia and axonemal complex (A) with its different structure in the shaft, neck (Ne), and basal body or kinetosome (K). *mt*, Microtubule; S, satellite of ciliary kinetosome. D: greater magnification of cross-sectioned shaft of a normal cilium with dynein arms (*arrowhead*). E: dynein arms are lacking in a cilium from a patient with immotile cilia syndrome. Bars: 0.5 μm (A–C); 0.1 μm (D, E). (E, courtesy of J. M. Sturgess.)

region the central pair of singlet tubules disappears and the outer doublets lose their dynein arms. Thus the axoneme appears somehow condensed and "stiff" in this region, where the cell membrane forms a straight cuff and shows a rather interesting regular arrangement of rows of intramembrane particles referred to as the "ciliary necklace" (see Fig. 6). The axoneme extends 0.5 µm into the cytoplasm in the form of basal bodies (Fig. 9B) that associate in various ways with microtubules and filaments, forming a dense web in the apical cytoplasm and perhaps extending, partly as characteristic striated rootlets, into deeper parts of the cells; however, there is great species variation in the disposition of these microtubules and filaments.

The cilia are asymmetrical structures (4): the pair of central tubules, the set of nine doublets with their one-sided attachments of dynein arms, and the satellite occurring on the basal body (Fig. 9B, C) give each cilium a well-defined orientation. This orientation determines the direction of the beat. All cilia of one cell show precisely the same orientation (Fig. 9C), and the orientation of neighboring cells differs usually only slightly. In the airway epithelium the average orientation of the cilia directs the effective stroke of the beat outward toward the larynx (or rather the pharynx). This is also true for cilia in the nasal epithelium, which beat in the opposite direction, moving the mucus inward, likewise toward the pharynx.

One intriguing and unsolved question is how this orientation of a large ciliary complex, extending from the trachea to the peripheral bronchioles, is manufactured and controlled. It is also not known how groups of cells are synchronized to allow a metachronal wave to move up the escalator. It is claimed that this is simply due to hydrodynamic or viscoelastic interaction between the moving cilia, which would tend to minimize energy dissipation by avoiding interference (167). Whether other mechanisms such as cell coupling through nexus connections (75) could also play a role is not established; it does not seem necessary because cilia can apparently react adequately to direct mechanical stimulation and are not influenced by nervous control, although hormonal stimulation does have some effects (167).

The propulsion of fluid through the ciliary beat involves essentially viscous forces (167): a cone of fluid surrounding the cilium is moved forward as the cilium, stretched to its full length, beats rapidly in the direction of the effective stroke. As the cilium recovers to its upright position, it bends and drags less fluid back than it propelled forward. This effect is greatly enhanced by the synchronized beat of neighboring cilia and by establishment of a metachronal wave of ciliary beat. However, in airways the cilia do not beat in mucus. The fluid lining is divided into two layers: 1) a layer of periciliary fluid of comparatively low viscosity and 2) a variable blanket of mucus, sometimes only disposed in patches. It has been suggested that the cilia perform most of their stroke in the serous periciliary fluid layer; when they straighten up in preparation for the effective stroke their tip may be inserted into the blanket of mucus and thus "claw" the mucus forward, withdrawing from the mucus as they bend down at the end of the stroke (167).

This mechanism clearly depends on tight regulation of the amount and composition of periciliary fluid. Although this has received much attention in recent years, it is not yet well understood. The apical surface of ciliated cells is endowed with a set of microvilli ~0.5 µm long and quite regularly interspersed between the cilia (Fig. 9). These microvilli have all the structural features of those occurring in brush borders; hence it is possible that they play a significant role in actively regulating ion and water exchange between the cells and the periciliary fluid.

Thus the ciliated cells show a very distinct polarity, with their special function organelles concentrated on the apical cell surface. The cytoplasmic organization accounts for this polarity. The nucleus, which has a loose chromatin structure, is contained in the lower half of the cells (Fig. 8A). The cytoplasm contains all organelles sparingly but shows a comparatively high density of microtubules and microfilaments (Fig. 9B) that possibly serve as cytoskeletal reinforcements in a cell whose apex must be under considerable mechanical stress. Mitochondria are frequent and often appear concentrated in the upper part of the cytoplasm, which is a good strategic location for providing the cilia with the fuel ATP, required for their beat. If microvilli are engaged in active ion transport, they too will require an appreciable flow of ATP.

EXOCRINE CELLS. The secretion of mucus and other fluids onto the airway surface involves their synthesis in the cytoplasm of specialized cells, their storage in an appropriate compartment of these cells, and their controlled extrusion. These basic mechanisms have been intensively studied in salivary glands, particularly in the pancreas and the parotid gland (41, 146), and in goblet cells of the intestinal epithelium (117, 134). They appear sufficiently general to allow extrapolation to the specific exocrine cells as they occur in the airways, although a detailed study of their function is not possible due to their low frequency and scattered occurrence.

Two basic types of exocrine cells are found in larger airways: 1) mucous cells and 2) serous cells (96). They occur mostly interspersed between ciliated cells in the epithelial lining, but in larger bronchi some are located in small mucosal glands that discharge their products to the epithelial surface through short slender ducts that sometimes end in widened epithelial pouches lined by ciliated cells.

Mucus-producing cells are the predominant exocrine cells of the epithelium of larger airways in humans and larger mammals, but they may be rare in smaller species, such as the rat (96) or mouse (140). The product of these cells, mucin, is a highly viscous solution consisting mainly of acid glycoproteins rich in sialic acid. Mucin is manufactured in the ER and in the Golgi complex, which is arranged in a characteristic pattern (187). The often small nucleus is located at the very base of these cells. Above the nucleus there are a few cisternae of RER, forming a sort of beaker in whose center large stacks of Golgi cisternae are arranged in a similar fashion. It is now well known that mucopolysaccharides are synthesized within the Golgi cisternae (134, 187), whereas the polypeptide moiety of glycoproteins is made in the ER and transferred to the Golgi cisternae. In the process of glycoprotein manufacture the Golgi cisternae gradually widen to form large membrane-bounded saccules whose content appears light and heterogeneous on electron micrographs and stains intensely with periodic acid–Schiff (PAS). They finally detach from the Golgi complex and move into the apical part of the cell. This process exhibits a distinct directionality, traversing the Golgi complex from its *cis* side (close to ER) to its *trans* side where the mucin saccules take off; thus the stack of Golgi cisternae exhibits a conspicuous polarity that can be demonstrated for all cells. As mucin synthesis progresses, the secretory saccules accumulate in the apical part of the cytoplasm, which then widens and often protrudes above the epithelial surface (Fig. 8A). The saccules lie close to each other so that their membranes can partly fuse, forming a large mucin droplet (Fig. 8A) enwrapped by a slim layer of cytoplasm that lies along the lateral membrane of the apical cell part. This gives the cell the appearance of a goblet, hence the term *goblet cell*. The mucin droplet is apparently discharged en bloc through a rupture in the apical cell membrane (Fig. 8B) and spreads as a thin patch on top of the periciliary fluid of low viscosity. The mucus-producing cell becomes narrow and the secretory cycle begins again.

The process of mucous synthesis is largely the same in mucous cells of the mucosal glands, but apparently the discharge occurs more continuously in the form of smaller droplets.

It is not entirely clear what kind of secretion is produced by the cells that have been called serous cells in analogy to similar cells occurring in salivary glands (96, 179). Considering the importance of RER and the relatively small Golgi complex, the product could be rich in protein, but histochemical stains suggest neutral glycoproteins as the main content of the round discrete secretion granules (179) whose membranes do not fuse as in goblet cells. The discharge occurs granule by granule through a fusion of the granule membrane with the apical plasma membrane. These cells seem to be the dominant exocrine cell in human fetal lungs and in major airways of rat (96) and mouse (140), but they are rare (if not missing) in the surface epithelium of adult human bronchi, where they occur only in mucosal glands.

The bronchiolar epithelium contains a mysterious cell, the Clara cell, which has attracted considerable attention, perhaps because it has so far consistently eluded the identification of its functional role (111, 147, 173). The description of Clara cells is partly inconsistent, perhaps because of large interspecies variations (147). In conventionally fixed preparations the apical part of the cell appears large and cone shaped, conspicuously protruding above the epithelial surface. In perfusion-fixed specimens, where the surface lining layer of bronchioles is preserved, this apical mound appears squashed down. The cell does seem to have a secretory function, as evidenced by the presence of some secretory granules in the apical part; however, these granules apparently are very heterogeneous, at least among species (111, 147). The cell is rich in mitochondria and ER, but the latter occurs in the form of smooth tubules devoid of ribosomes; therefore it cannot perform appreciable protein synthesis but might be the carrier of some membrane-bound enzymes serving some unrecognized metabolic function. The amount of SER again shows great interspecies variation, and SER is apparently missing in human Clara cells (147, 173). The question must be raised whether Clara cells are one cell type or whether this nondescriptive term is simply used as a label for different nonciliated cells of bronchioles whose functional role is unidentified. Recent successful attempts to isolate viable Clara cells from rat lungs should make it possible to clarify their function (53).

ENDOCRINE AND OTHER CELLS. The airway epithelium contains a variable number of cells that are neither ciliated nor exocrine. Some of these cells, sometimes called undifferentiated or intermediate (96, 111), lack identifying structural characteristics and may be precursors of ciliated or secretory cells. Basal cells of the pseudostratified epithelium of large bronchi may perhaps also be assigned to this class. These undifferentiated cells are particularly frequent in smaller bronchioles, where ciliated cells are scarce, and may simply constitute a plain cuboidal lining cell.

However, the airway epithelium does contain two rarer specialized cell types. The brush cell (122) is characterized by a narrow apical plate fitted with a dense tuft of broad, short microvilli with a flat end that appear arranged like the petals of an aster (Fig. 10). These microvilli contain a dense core of microfilaments that penetrate deep into the cytoplasm; some of these bundles extend to the basal portion of the cell. The function of this cell is unknown. It was first described in the tracheal epithelium and speculatively ascribed a chemoreceptive function (122) because of its similarity to taste bud cells and its apparent connections to afferent nerve fibers, although the latter property has not been convincingly established. The brush cell was simultaneously found as a scarce constituent of the alveolar epithelium (130), as discussed in ALVEOLAR BRUSH CELLS: TYPE III PNEUMOCYTES, p. 71.

In the epithelium of conducting airways, cells with an apparent neuroendocrine function are found; they are called either Feyrter or Kulchitsky cells (17, 50, 56, 60, 76, 81). The morphological characteristics of these cells, which span the epithelium from the surface to the basal lamina, include small dense-core vesicles in the basal portion of the cytoplasm, generally beneath the nucleus (Fig. 11). With light microscopy such cells can be identified either by staining with silver salts (argyrophilia) or by their fluorescence after formaldehyde treatment by the Falck-Hillarp technique (56, 143). This suggests the presence of amines. Some of the cells become visible only after incubation with L-dopa or 5-hydroxytryptophan, which they convert to dopamine or serotonin, suggesting that these cells belong to the class of APUD (amine precursor uptake and decarboxylation) cells (145). Their neuroendocrine nature, which suggests their ability to secrete serotonin or other biogenic amines, is further corroborated by the appearance of the dense-core vesicles in electron micrographs (Fig. 11). These cells, which may be secondary settlers derived from the neural crest (45, 46), are also found in all parts of the gastrointestinal tract, where they regulate intestinal functions. A well-known example is the regulation of gastric secretion by gastrin. In the mammalian airway epithelium these cells are found scattered singly or in small groups throughout the tracheobronchial tree (60, 81, 143) but apparently not in alveoli. Whether or not they are associated with nerve fibers is still debatable.

Note that these neuroendocrine cells are more frequent in fetal than in adult lungs. Particularly in fetal lungs they have been found to form larger complexes called neuroepithelial bodies (50, 92, 114, 115), which occur frequently in the region of bronchial bifurcations. In adult lungs these bodies are less conspicuous.

The epithelium of conducting airways may contain a variable amount of different cells in transit, such as granulocytes or lymphocytes, that traverse the epithelium through intercellular pathways to reach the surface lining layer. The airway epithelium is indeed intimately associated with cells of the defense system. Plasma cells, which occur in great numbers in the mucosal glands, are an important class of these cells, as described in *Cells of Immune Defense System*, p. 85.

CELL KINETICS IN CONDUCTING AIRWAY EPITHELIUM. Kauffman (103) recently reviewed the current knowledge of cell proliferation in the airways. The main tool for estimating cell kinetics in airway epithelium is to study the incorporation of [^{3}H]thymidine into the DNA of nuclei of various cell types by autoradiography. The evidence available is limited with respect to species, the bulk of the work having been done on rats, and with respect to location, with the trachea and peripheral bronchioles the focus of attention.

In normal rat trachea the turnover time for the entire epithelium apparently is 14-22 days (209). This time is prolonged up to 6 wk in cesarean-derived rats raised under pathogen-free conditions or may be shortened in diseased rats, indicating that the epithelium regulates its proliferative rate to the needs of repairing damages caused by various insults. In this pseudostratified epithelium the basal cells show the greatest proliferative capacity; their turnover time is only 9.5 days in conventionally raised rats (209). More recent evidence, however, shows that superficial cells (mostly mucous cells) also divide at a considerable rate and that their cycle time may be shorter than that of basal cells (25).

In bronchioles cell proliferation is apparently very

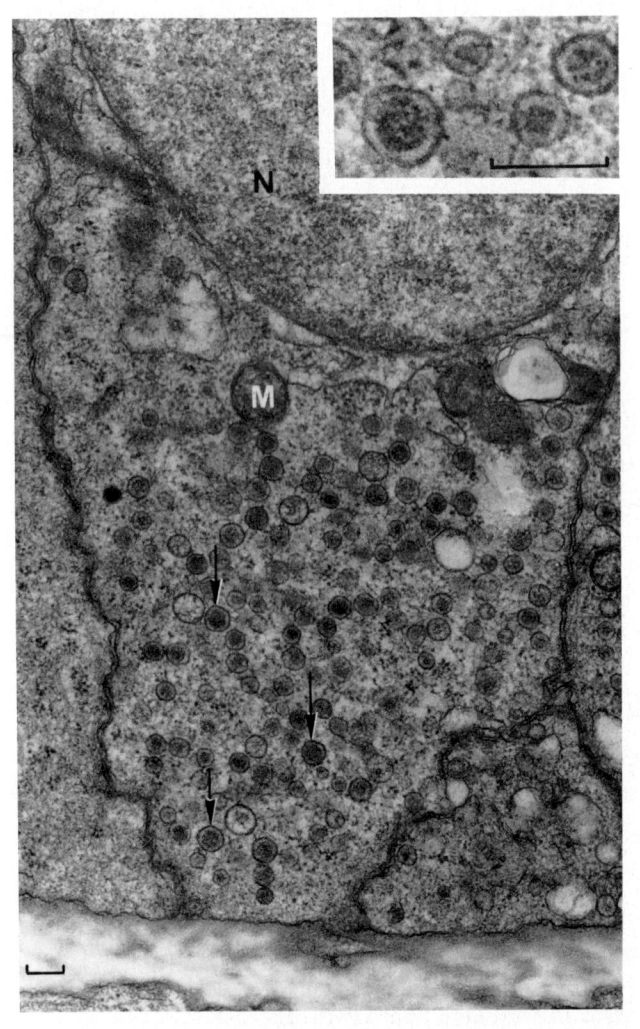

FIG. 11. Basal part of neuroendocrine cell of human bronchiolar epithelium showing part of nucleus (*N*), mitochondria (*M*), and secretory vesicles (*arrows*) with dark core, which are seen at greater magnification in *inset*. Bars, 0.2 μm.

low, with a labeling index (relative number of nuclei labeled with [³H]thymidine) generally well below 1% (103). Therefore there is little information on cell kinetics in the bronchioles. However, undifferentiated or Clara cells apparently may serve as progenitor cells for the renewal of bronchiolar epithelial cells (64), whereas most ciliated cells appear to be nondividing cells (103).

Alveolar Epithelium

The transition of epithelial structure from conducting bronchioles to alveolar surfaces is abrupt. The cuboidal cell lining of bronchioles yields to the very attenuated squamous epithelium of alveoli along a sharp demarcation line with no intermediates (see Fig. 7). However, the cell lining is complete, with alveolar epithelial cells forming tight junctions with bronchiolar cells. There is only one sort of transition: the alveolar secretory cells with their characteristic lamellar bodies occur in the epithelium of the most peripheral bronchioles, suggesting that they may be secreting surfactant onto the bronchiolar surface (74).

The general properties of the alveolar epithelium are determined by its role in minimizing the barrier between air and blood while simultaneously maximizing its surface. The two main cell types constituting the alveolar epithelial mosaic meet these requirements (Fig. 12): *1*) the alveolar lining cell is extremely thin but spreads out over a large surface, and *2*) the cuboidal secretory cell produces surfactant that allows the large surface between air and tissue to be maintained.

Although less numerous than the secretory cells (see Table 2), the lining cells cover ~97% of the alveolar surface. Despite the large difference in shape and thickness of these two cells, the terminal bars joining them form a continuous tight junction so that the epithelium acts as a semipermeable barrier between the alveolar lining fluid and the interstitium (10, 93, 161, 163, 164, 196).

ALVEOLAR LINING CELLS: TYPE I PNEUMOCYTES. In terms of cell biology the alveolar lining cell is very simple. It contains one usually small and compact nucleus surrounded by a slim rim of cytoplasm (Fig. 13*A*). In this perinuclear cytoplasm one finds a rather modest complement of the basic set of organelles: a few small mitochondria, some cisternae of ER with a few ribosomes, and a small Golgi complex with some associated vesicles. This is the picture of a quiescent cell with no great metabolic activity.

At the edge of the perinuclear region a very attenuated cytoplasmic leaflet emerges and spreads out broadly (Figs. 12 and 13*A*). This leaflet is essentially two plasma membranes with a very small amount of cytoplasmic ground substance containing microfilaments interposed (Fig. 14). The superficial membrane is part of the apical cell face and is richly endowed with a glycoprotein coat (7), whereas the deeper membrane attached to the basal lamina corresponds to the basal cell face. In this cytoplasmic leaflet, which appears to be made almost exclusively of ectoplasm, organelles are rarely found, with an occasional small mitochondrion or a cisterna of ER appearing here and

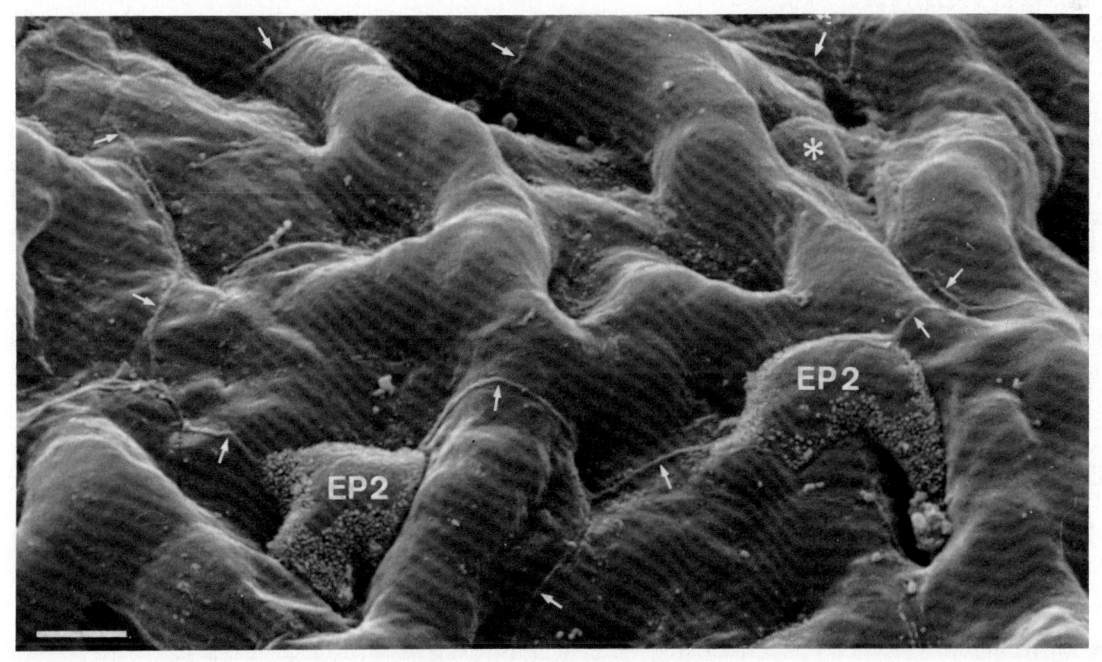

FIG. 12. Scanning electron micrograph of surface of alveolar epithelium of human lung with two type II epithelial cells (*EP2*). *Arrows*, boundary (terminal bar) of type I cell. *Asterisk*, nucleus of type I cell. *Bar*, 5 µm. [From Weibel (202).]

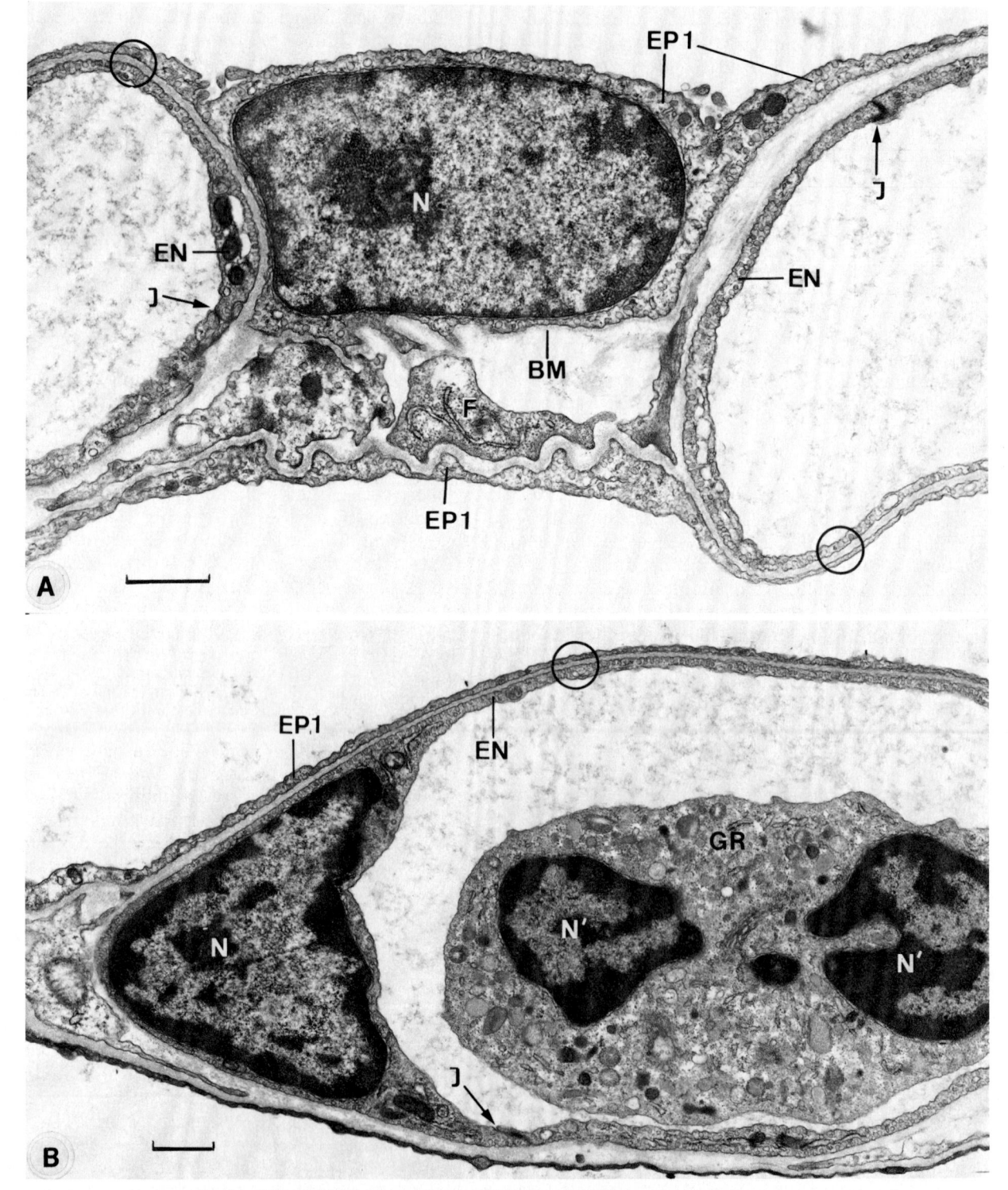

FIG. 13. *A*: squamous type I epithelial cell (*EP1*). *B*: capillary endothelial cell (*EN*) from human lung. Nuclei (*N*) are surrounded by little cytoplasm, which continues into squamous extensions. *Circles*, fused basement membranes (*BM*) in barrier parts. Capillary contains neutrophil granulocyte (*GR*) with 2 lobes of nucleus sectioned (*N′*). *F*, fiber; *J*, intercellular junction. *Bars*, 1 μm.

there. However, pinocytotic vesicles are found partly attached to one of the membranes as caveolae (Fig. 14).

Although this cell does not appear very impressive— indeed its existence was doubted until it was demonstrated by electron microscopy (121)—it is the largest cell in the alveolar septum (see Table 2). Its mean volume of ~900 μm^3 in the rat (49, 82) and ~1,800

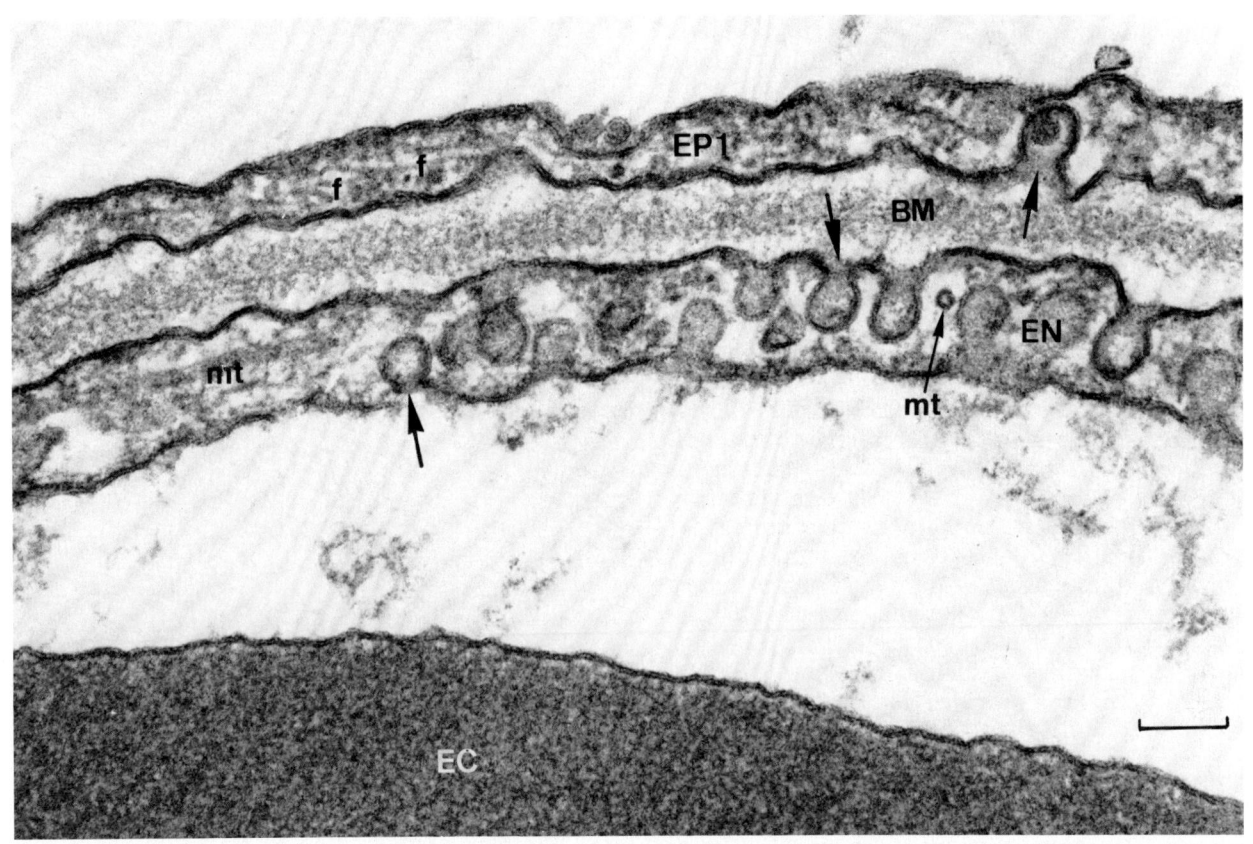

FIG. 14. Squamous extensions of endothelial cell (*EN*) and type I pneumocyte (*EP1*). Cytoplasm, bounded by plasma membrane similar to that of erythrocyte (*EC*), contains microfilaments (*f*), microtubules (*mt*), and pinocytotic vesicles (*arrows*). BM, basement membrane. Bar, 0.1 μm.

μm³ in humans (48) is more than twice that of an alveolar secretory cell. The common description of the lining cell as a "small" alveolar cell is certainly a misnomer.

The unique feature of the alveolar lining cell is its extraordinary broad extension (see Table 2). In the rat one cell covers ~4,500 μm² (82) and in the human lung ~5,000 μm² (48). On the other hand, the patches of alveolar surface covered by one lining cell are smaller, as evidenced by the terminal bars surrounding them. For example, the one large type I cell, as shown in Figure 12, has an area of ~1,400 μm², and there are not many that appear to be much larger. This apparent discrepancy is explained by the fact that alveolar lining cells are branched, forming several apical plates each completely bounded by terminal bars (198). Some of these plates appear devoid of a nucleus—Kölliker described them as nonnucleated plates (*kernlose Platten*)—but they are connected by cytoplasmic bridges to a nuclear region contained in another plate (198).

This complex shape of alveolar lining cells appears as an ingenious solution of the problem of optimizing maintenance pathways against the requirements of a very thin minimal barrier. The organizational and metabolic center of the cell is its nucleus with the perinuclear cytoplasm. Maintenance of cytoplasmic extensions with their high density of membranes requires a flow of metabolites such as ATP to drive ion pumps or information carriers such as messenger RNA for local protein synthesis. In view of the normal turnover of proteins or phospholipids for resealing leaky membranes, much of this material must originate in the perinuclear region. Because the cytoplasmic leaflets are arranged in the form of multiple plates, the distances for transfer of this matter from the nuclear region to any point in the periphery are considerably shorter than when the nucleus resides in the center of a simple squamous cell of large expanse. This advantage, however, has its price. The type I pneumocyte is incapable of self-reproduction by mitotic division (104); it is a terminal cell requiring division of a progenitor cell, in this case the type II cell, for renewal of the cell population. This is discussed in CELL KINETICS IN ALVEOLAR EPITHELIUM, p. 71.

The alveolar lining cell has some similarity to endothelial cells lining capillaries (Figs. 13*B* and 14). The latter are, however, simple squamous cells of much smaller volume and surface (see Table 2). Cytologically there are no greater differences in the structure of the perinuclear area and cytoplasmic leaflets of either cell (Figs. 13 and 14). Endothelial and type I epithelial cells contain a similarly large number of pinocytotic vesicles (73).

ALVEOLAR SECRETORY CELLS: TYPE II PNEUMOCYTES. The alveolar secretory cell is a conspicuous but comparatively small cell whose mean volume is ~400 μm^3 in the rat (47, 82) and ~900 μm^3 in the human (48), as shown in Table 2. Although they are numerically more frequent than the type I cell, they cover only ~3% of the alveolar surface. They are cuboidal cells and thus fairly thick; however, they are usually located in meshes of the capillary network (see Fig. 12) and do not severely obstruct the diffusion path for O_2 between air and blood.

Morphological features of type II pneumocyte. Figure 15 illustrates some of the essential structural features of this cell. In conventionally fixed preparations the apical surface of alveolar secretory cells bulges toward the lumen and has a dense tuft of short microvilli that are less frequent in the smooth central part of the cell. Microvilli are normally interpreted as surface membrane specializations endowed with active transport capabilities related to resorption. The alveolar surface lining layer usually accumulates in the cleft that forms between the bulge caused by an underlying capillary and the type II cell; the microvilli project into this pool of fluid. The "baldness" of the cell top is either related to the absence of such a fluid pool over the bulge or to membrane specialization toward release of the secretory product that occurs in this region.

The alveolar type II cell is richly endowed with cytoplasmic organelles (Figs. 1 and 15B) related to its main metabolic function: the synthesis and secretion of surfactant phospholipids and, perhaps, of some of the associated proteins. Figure 3 shows that ER associated with Golgi and GERL occurs in these cells. The protein-synthesis function performed by the RER is not quite certain: it produces either a protein for immediate secretion, or a set of enzymes required for the synthesis of surfactant phospholipids, or both. Compared with cells specifically differentiated for protein secretion the amount of ER of type II cells is relatively modest (Table 3). Nevertheless there is limited evidence in favor of active protein secretion by type II cells, which appear to traverse the lamellar bodies as storage granules (109, 123, 125). The SER is quantitatively more important than RER in type II cells of the rat (Table 3); this is possibly related to the recently demonstrated capacity of these cells to metabolize some foreign compounds (54, 55), which is known to occur in live cells (181).

The main metabolic functions of type II cells, well established by a large number of studies, are the synthesis, storage, and discharge of surfactant phospholipids, mainly of the disaturated dipalmitoyl phosphatidylcholine (43, 72). The storage site of this material is known: cell-fractionation studies have shown that the lamellar bodies contain these phospholipids in high concentration (72). These phospholipids cause the high osmiophilia and the frequent empty appearance of these storage granules in inadequately fixed material, due to extraction of the phospholipid by the solvents required for embedding the tissue in wax or

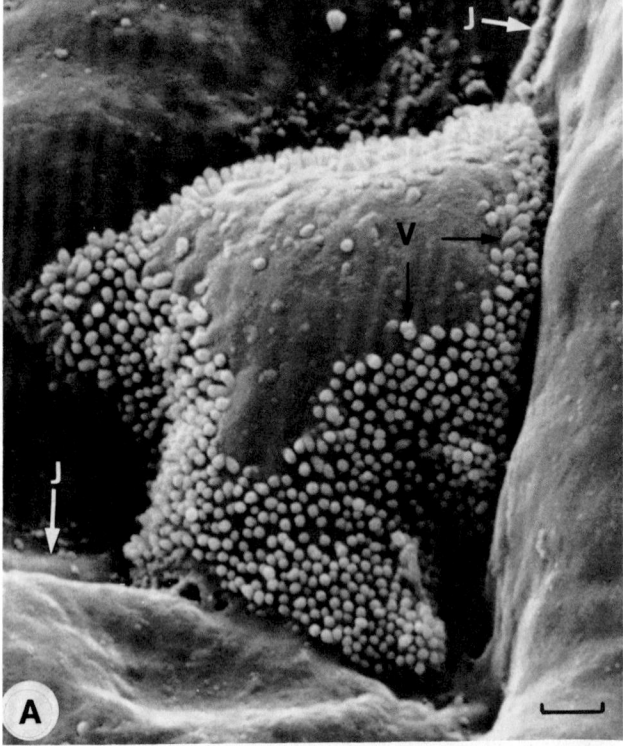

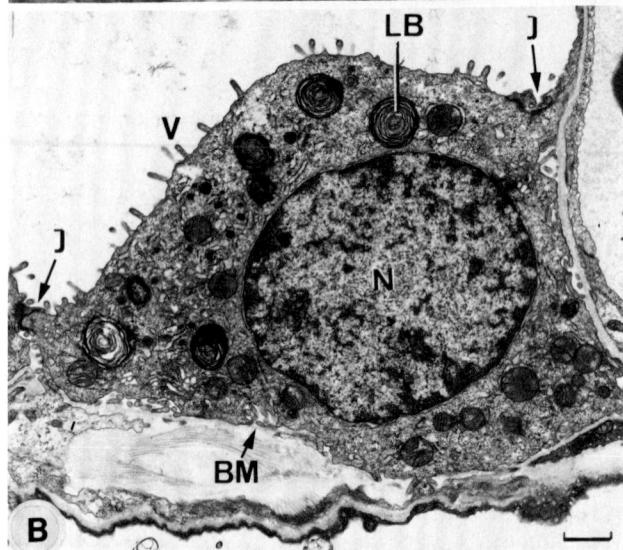

FIG. 15. Scanning electron micrograph (A) and thin section (B) of type II pneumocyte with microvilli (V) on peripheral zone of apical cell surface. BM, basement membrane; J, intercellular junction; LB, lamellar body; N, nucleus. Detail of this cell is shown in Fig. 1. Bars, 1 μm.

resins. Adequate preservation of these granules is only achieved by triple fixation with glutaraldehyde, osmium tetroxide, and uranyl acetate (Figs. 1, 15B, and 16A). Even then the preservation is incomplete; the irregular light clefts between lamellar packets are doubtless artifacts, as evidenced by the very regular total packing of lamellae observed in freeze-fracture

TABLE 3. *Morphometric Characteristics of Alveolar Type II Cells of Rat*

	Volume Density	
	% of cytoplasm	% of whole cell
Nucleus		24.8
Cytoplasm	100	75.2
Endoplasmic reticulum		
Total	12.4	9.3
Rough	4.0	3.0
Smooth	8.4	6.3
Multivesicular bodies	1.3	1.0
Lamellar bodies	20.3	15.2
Mitochondria	12.7	9.5
Ground substance	53.3	40.0

Data from D. M. Haies and E. R. Weibel, unpublished observations.

preparations [Fig. 16; (16, 157, 170, 211)]. The shape of these granules seems to show some interspecies variations. In the human lung (see Fig. 1), spherical granules with a concentric onionlike arrangement of the lamellae appear around a dense amorphous central core. In the rat lung (Fig. 16A, B) the granules are cone or bell shaped, with the lamellae arranged as stacks; an amorphous plug, with respect to which the lamellae are bent, is often at the tip of the cone. Sometimes the lamellae appear as flat stacks. These pictures must be interpreted cautiously because they are seen on section; on the other hand, such variations may not be very relevant. Other details of the electron-microscopic studies of lamellar bodies may be more important, such as the observation of a regular lattice on fracture faces of some phospholipid lamellae (170, 211). This lattice raises the question of whether *1*) the mixture of surfactant phospholipids is stored in a very precise composition and order or *2*) some additional product, such as surfactant apoproteins, is stored along with the phospholipids in a special spatial relationship. The relationship may be similar to that in the lipoprotein complex (tubular myelin) because it is in the surface lining layer (85, 206) but not in type II cells.

Less certain is the pathway through which lamellar bodies are formed. It has been claimed (77, 111, 128, 177) that the peculiar organelle called the multivesicular body is the progenitor of lamellar bodies. Morphological evidence suggests this. Figure 16C–E shows a sequence of multivesicular bodies containing stacks of osmiophilic lamellae of various sizes. There are clear-cut lamellar bodies that contain vesicles, particularly in the region of the amorphous plug. Furthermore both lamellar and multivesicular bodies are bounded by a similar membrane, characteristic for lysosomal granules. The nature of multivesicular bodies is not well established. Often found in the GERL area (see Fig. 3), they contain a number of lysosomal enzymes; thus they appear to be a special class of lysosomes perhaps equipped to perform lipid synthesis. However, they have eluded attempts to implicate them in the pathway for surfactant phospholipid synthesis; but with an isolated organelle of such small size the absence of autoradiographic labeling after palmitate or choline injection is not conclusive, particularly because the enzymes of multivesicular bodies may intervene at some other point of the complex synthesis pathway (43, 108). I conclude that the site of synthesis of surfactant phospholipids is not yet precisely localized and may (because the cells appear to have a certain versatility in that respect) occupy different organelles, depending on the substrate available (108).

The evidence for secretion of phospholipids onto the alveolar surface is essentially morphological (Fig. 17): in the center of the apical plasma membrane are open pockets that contain stacks of phospholipid lamellae identical to those in the lamellar bodies. Such pictures are ambiguous as to the direction of movement of the pocket content: potentially, endocytosis and exocytosis are equally likely. However, endocytosis is less likely in this case because of the clear difference in the disposition of osmiophilic lamellae in the surface lining layer and the lamellar bodies. Densely stacked lamellae occur only in lamellar bodies; they are disassembled and rearranged to tubular myelin, a lipoprotein complex of highly characteristic structure, in the lining layer (85, 206, 211). Endocytosis would require a restacking of these lamellae prior to engulfment into the pocket, which is not very likely in the extracellular fluid. If macrophages engulf surfactant material they take up whole tubular myelin (see *Alveolar and Interstitial Macrophages*, p. 82). Although firm evidence is still needed, pictures such as Figure 17 suggest surfactant exocytosis.

Cell biology of type II pneumocyte. One central postulate—perhaps even tacitly accepted dogma—of cell biology is that all metabolic events occur temporally and spatially in an orderly fashion. This specifically implies that these events occur in relation to spatial ordering principles, i.e., to certain of the cell's structural elements (e.g., membranes, granules, compartments), just as each cell type is equipped to perform a limited set of metabolic functions. Although it is now widely accepted that the type II pneumocyte and some of its characteristic organelles play the key role in the production of alveolar surfactant, specific questions must be asked. What metabolic functions are needed to produce surfactant, and what structural elements are involved at what step in this process?

The metabolic functions of surfactant production are not discussed in detail here; special chapters of this volume are devoted to these questions. This discussion reviews the approaches used to determine the spatial order of the metabolic events, i.e., their association with the type II cell and some of its organelles.

1. *Biochemistry of cell fractions.* The mechanical separation of individual cell components into different

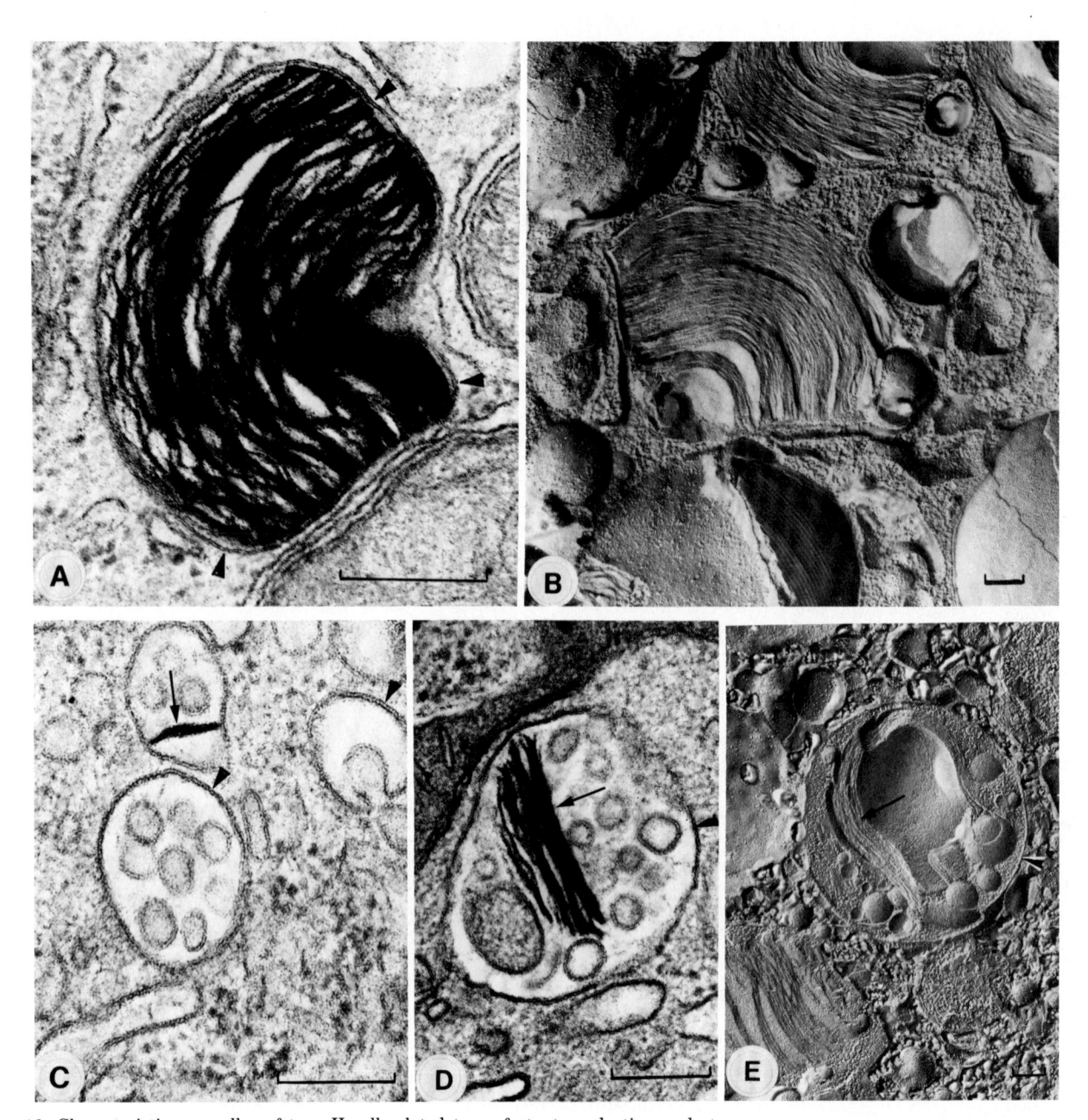

FIG. 16. Characteristic organelles of type II cell related to surfactant production and storage. Cone-shaped lamellar bodies from rat lung (A, B) and sequence of multivesicular bodies (C–E) with stacks of lamellae (*arrows*) and membrane envelope (*arrowheads*). A, C, D: thin sections. B, E: freeze-fracture preparation. Bars, 0.2 µm.

fractions that can then be subjected to detailed analytical studies (e.g., enzyme kinetics, substrate specificity studies) has produced deep insights in cell biology (141). This is the most widely used approach in biochemistry because it allows work with reasonably purified units of a complex system. Basically the material under study is homogenized and broken into different fractions by various procedures, such as differential or density-gradient centrifugation, elutriation, and affinity chromatography. Such methods, partly very elaborate, have been developed extensively for liver cells, in particular, and adapted for use on other tissues, such as the lung (83, 126, 153, 180).

It is difficult to identify the cellular origin of the fractions obtained (both with respect to cell type and organelle system) and estimate their purity. Often one finds the statement that a certain result could be explained by "contamination" from other fractions, indicating that the separation of cellular elements is often incomplete. Such contamination, for example, has led to the fallacious statement (since corrected) that surfactant originates in mitochondria, because

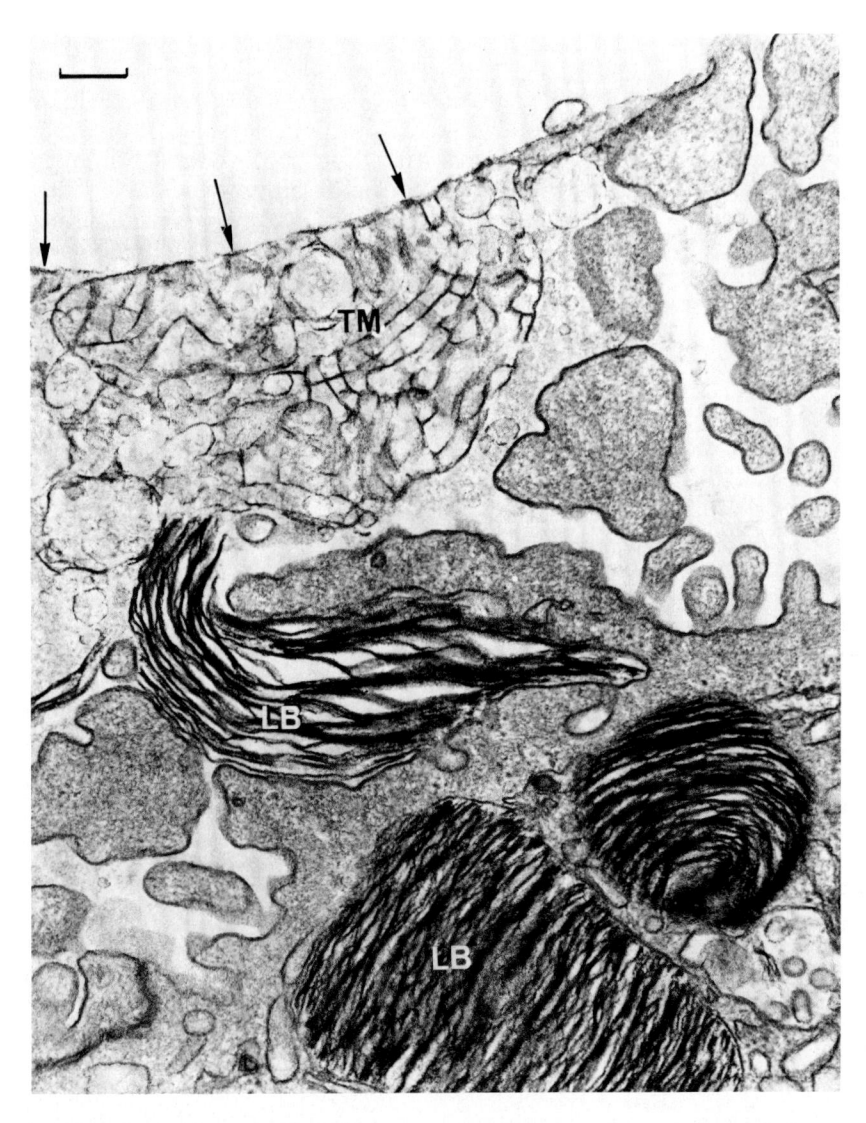

FIG. 17. Release of lamellar body (*LB*) from type II epithelial cell into surface lining layer, which contains tubular myelin (*TM*) continuous with the phospholipid surface film (*arrows*). Bar, 0.2 µm.

lamellar bodies would collect in the mitochondrial fractions of the older crude preparation procedures.

Characterizing the structural composition of the individual fractions is difficult. Electron microscopy is the most direct method of structural analysis, particularly when combined with morphometric methods (72, 181). This method, although possible, can also be fraught with considerable difficulties and uncertainties because homogenization tends to destroy the structural integrity of some components, which are then unidentifiable on electron micrographs (23). An indirect characterization with so-called marker enzymes for certain cell constituents apparently solves this difficulty. Thus glucose 6-phosphatase is a universally accepted marker for ER, and one assumes that the activity of this enzyme estimated in a fraction is an estimate of the amount of ER (*microsomes* in the biochemical terminology) in the fraction. Although this approach is well established and part of the state of the art in biochemistry, a critical attitude is still necessary, for it depends essentially on a demonstrated clear and quantitative association between the marker enzyme and the structural element to which it is supposedly bound. Too often this is not checked, particularly when methods well established for the liver are adopted for studies on the lung; we cannot be certain that the ER of lung cells is the same as that of liver cells.

In contrast to the predominance in mass of hepatocytes in the liver, type II cells make up only a small fraction of all the parenchymal lung cells (see Table 1); substantial contaminations from the other cells are therefore unavoidable, even if the homogenate is obtained from peripheral lung parenchyma by removing larger airways and blood vessels, as is the usual procedure (106, 108). Type II cells do not make up more than 15% in volume of the entire cell population, even in lung parenchyma (47, 48, 82). Considerable improvement of this situation is possible if methods for isolating type II cells are used; for a discussion of these methods see *Isolated type II cell preparations*, p. 70.

2. *Localization of metabolic effectors.* Methods are

available that make visible, by light or electron microscopy, the result of some enzyme activity. The approach of enzyme cytochemistry is to offer the cells a suitable substrate for a given enzyme or class of enzymes and to transform the reaction product into an insoluble and visible substance. The best known examples are various phosphatases where the phosphate cleaved from a substrate is converted, for example, to insoluble lead phosphate, which is electron dense (77, 128, 129, 177). Esterases, another example, are relevant for surfactant production (87, 138). The main problem with these methods is that they give only qualitative results, because it is difficult to control the process quantitatively.

In recent years good methods for localizing enzymes by immunocytochemistry have been developed. Antibodies against a certain purified enzyme or other protein are raised, reacted with the tissue, and rendered visible by labeling the tissue with a component that has high contrast in the electron microscope. One widely used method is to couple the antibody with a molecule of horseradish peroxidase; the reaction product can then be made visible (61, 190). Alternatively, an electron-dense particle such as ferritin or protein A–colloidal gold (156) is attached to the antibody; the advantage of this approach is that a quantitative analysis is possible because each particle corresponds to one antibody that labels one molecule of the antigen. This approach is promising, particularly when combined with morphometry, but refinements of all the methods are still needed. These methods have been used to some extent only in attempts to localize metabolic effectors of surfactant synthesis (61, 86, 129, 190, 212). Much can be gained by using monoclonal antibodies, which can now be obtained by the hybridoma method (110).

3. *Tracing the pathway of substrates and metabolites.* Autoradiography is a valuable approach for tracing the localization and the pathway of metabolites in tissue and cells (94, 141). If the cells are offered a radioactively labeled substrate, metabolites that can be fixed can then be made visible by exposing a section to a photosensitive emulsion. Protein synthesis can be traced with ^{3}H-labeled amino acids; DNA synthesis can be traced with [^{3}H]thymidine. Surfactant synthesis has been studied by incubating the lung with ^{3}H-labeled precursors of surfactant phospholipids (1, 6, 33, 42, 51, 97). The results thus obtained are probably the most direct evidence linking surfactant biosynthesis to the type II cell and some of its organelles, notably lamellar bodies and ER. Quantitative evaluation of the autoradiographs with a combination of substrates and careful control of the timing of tissue fixation with a pulse of labeled substrate application provide conclusive results (42, 51). The detailed quantitative study of Chevalier and Collet (42) with [^{3}H]-choline, [^{3}H]galactose, and [^{3}H]leucine indicates that phospholipids, carbohydrates, and proteins may use a slightly different pathway but end up eventually in the lamellar bodies. Such studies need to include other potential precursors of surfactant, particularly of phospholipids.

Some problems with this approach result from the difficulty of quantitatively retaining some metabolites in the cells during tissue preparation (51), which may make it necessary to resort to improved preparation procedures as they become available (207). The resolution of the method is also inherently limited, but advanced quantitative analysis can partially overcome this.

In conclusion, none of the three analytical methods by itself allows certain conclusions as to kinetics, localization, pathway, and control of surfactant production. If the three methods are combined in carefully designed and controlled experiments, considerable progress can be expected. Although the role of the type II cell in surfactant phospholipid production is undisputed on the basis of available evidence, a considerable number of uncertainties remain. For example, it still remains unknown where in the type II cells the various parts of the pathway for phospholipid synthesis take place, where surfactant apoproteins come from, and how specific the apoproteins are. The role of the substantial capacity of macrophages to synthesize phospholipids, though in some respects different from that in type II cells (171), also must be elucidated. Finally, the control of surfactant synthesis and turnover through hormonal factors requires an approach along several lines. One interesting approach is the study of metabolic events in isolated perfused lungs (15).

Isolated type II cell preparations. As mentioned above, a fundamental obstacle to obtaining clear results on the cell biology of type II cells is the fact that they comprise only a small fraction of all the lung cells. Considerable improvements could be expected if, in preparations for biochemical analysis, type II cells could be separated from the other cell types occurring in lung parenchyma. Kikkawa and Yoneda (106) described the first successful attempt in this direction; a number of similar reports followed (54, 79, 108). Basically these methods use the same sequence of procedures, differing more in detail than in principle. With the method of Kikkawa and Yoneda (106) as a reference, three steps are required: *1*) mechanical removal of free cells by sequential vascular perfusion and alveolar washing followed by vigorous shaking of a suspension of finely chopped lung tissue, all in physiological saline or another suitable medium; *2*) enzymatic dispersion of parenchymal cells by incubating the chopped lung tissue with trypsin and collecting the cells by filtration; and *3*) isolation of type II cells by centrifugation on a discontinuous density gradient. In the last step the separation of type II cells and macrophages is the most difficult because of their similar density. This difficulty can be overcome by exposing the chopped tissue to colloidal barium sulfate; the macrophages become loaded with these particles and their density increases. These methods can result in preparations that contain 90%–95% viable type II cells; the yield is, however, relatively small because only a fraction of the original cells are recovered. Nevertheless it is sufficient for many metabolic studies. Studies have shown that such cells perform the various steps of phospholipid synthesis observed in tissue preparations of the whole lung (107, 108, 171). The advantage of the isolated cell preparations is that the cells involved are well defined and relatively homogeneous; thus a comparison between different cell types, such as type II cells and macrophages or Clara cells, is possible (53, 171).

A durable cell that one can expose to some effects over a period of days would be an advantage for some metabolic studies. Type II cells isolated by one of the above procedures retain their morphological and functional properties in primary in vitro cultures reasonably well for ~3–5 days, after which they progressively deteriorate (14, 57, 58, 172). This deterioration is a difficulty with differentiated cells from adults. In their thorough review of type II cells in vitro, Douglas et al. (59) describe ways of overcoming this limitation so as to have long-term cultures available. They derived from an adult rat a clonal cell line L-2 that retains type II cell characteristics for a certain time but loses them after ~35 population doublings in vitro. Long-term in vitro cultures can be obtained starting with fetal tissue. Fetal lung cells are dissociated enzymatically; under suitable organotypic culture conditions they reaggregate to form histotypic elements resembling epithelial tubes in the fetal lung (58, 59). In such cultures alveolarlike structures are formed that are lined by cells resembling type II cells and by attenuated cells similar to type I cells (58, 59). These cultures perform the metabolic functions of surfactant biosynthesis and secrete the product into the internal alveolar spaces where it is transformed to tubular myelin. Thus it is likely that such cultures produce the complete surfactant, lipids and proteins alike, and that they furthermore mimic the cell kinetics of alveolar epithelium.

An alternative to fetal tissue for establishing long-term cultures are cell lines derived from tumors, which show a high and stable proliferative capacity in vitro and retain their differentiation characteristics. Lieber et al. (119) derived a continuous cell line A549 from a human pulmonary adenocarcinoma. This cell line is reasonably similar to the isolated type II cell, with respect both to morphological and biochemical properties; although there are certain differences the cell line can serve as a model for type II cells (133). Stoner et al. (183, 184) isolated and cloned similar cell line LA-4 from a mouse lung adenoma induced by urethan. More such cell lines may become available and are potentially very useful, but they must be made homogeneous by cloning.

ALVEOLAR BRUSH CELLS: TYPE III PNEUMOCYTES. Like the epithelium of conducting airways, the alveolar epithelium comprises a cell type that has been termed *brush cell* because of its conspicuous tuft of squat membrane-bounded microprocesses at the apical surface (Fig. 18). Meyrick and Reid (130) first described this brush cell in 1968. Characteristically the apical surface of this cone-shaped cell is rather narrow and completely occupied by the microprocesses; its lateral surfaces are either in contact with a type II cell or covered by a large cytoplasmic flap of a type I cell (Fig. 18A, B). The microprocesses have a flat end and taper toward their base; they contain a dense bundle of microfilaments that extends deep into the cytoplasm (Fig. 18C). Microfilament bundles are among the most conspicuous cytoplasmic elements that comprise a moderate number of mitochondria, some ER, and a fair amount of vesicles, particularly near the cell apex (Fig. 18C).

The brush cell is quite rare; the figures of 5%–10% sometimes given (111, 130) appear to be too generous; in several morphometric studies, in which random sampling methods were used on rat and human lung cells, this cell type could not be assessed (48, 49, 82). On the other hand the cell is apparently not homogeneously distributed throughout the alveolar surface but appears concentrated in central parts of the acinus, just beyond the terminal bronchiole (66), a finding we could recently confirm.

The function of this cell is unknown. Luciano et al. (122) and Meyrick and Reid (130) suggested a receptor function, but there is little positive evidence to support this. A connection to nerve fibers has not been established, and there is no evidence supporting a resorptive function (96).

CELL KINETICS IN ALVEOLAR EPITHELIUM. The aspects of cell kinetics and proliferation in the alveolar epithelium that need discussion are those that allow maintenance of a steady population of cells in the alveolar epithelium and repair of any epithelial damage that occurs because of cell destruction or death; Kauffman (103) lucidly reviewed these questions. Because there is no information on brush cells, this discussion is limited to type I and type II cells, which occur in the normal rat and human lung with a numerical frequency of ~1:2 (48, 49, 82).

Type I cells appear to be unable to undergo cell division. Labeling experiments with [^{3}H]thymidine, evaluated by autoradiography (25), indicate that type I cells do not, or at most rarely (2, 63, 103), synthesize DNA, even when the alveolar epithelium is proliferating as a whole, such as in growth (104), or when accentuated cell renewal must take place, such as after toxic injury (44, 63). In contrast, type II cells are able to go through the cell cycle, synthesize DNA, and divide by mitosis without giving up their differentiated state as secretory cells. During the phase of rapid expansion of the alveolar surface in the early postnatal rat lung, the proliferation of the type II cells alone could account for the numerical growth of the alveolar epithelial cell population (type I and type II cells together) (104). A similar conclusion was reached with respect to repair processes that occurred in rodent lungs after toxic injury (2, 63, 144). From this it was concluded that the type II pneumocyte is the stem or progenitor cell for the entire alveolar epithelium and that some of the newly formed cells differentiate into squamous type I cells. Whether all type II cells have the capacity to serve as progenitor cells or whether this is restricted to an unidentified subpopulation of these cells is not certain.

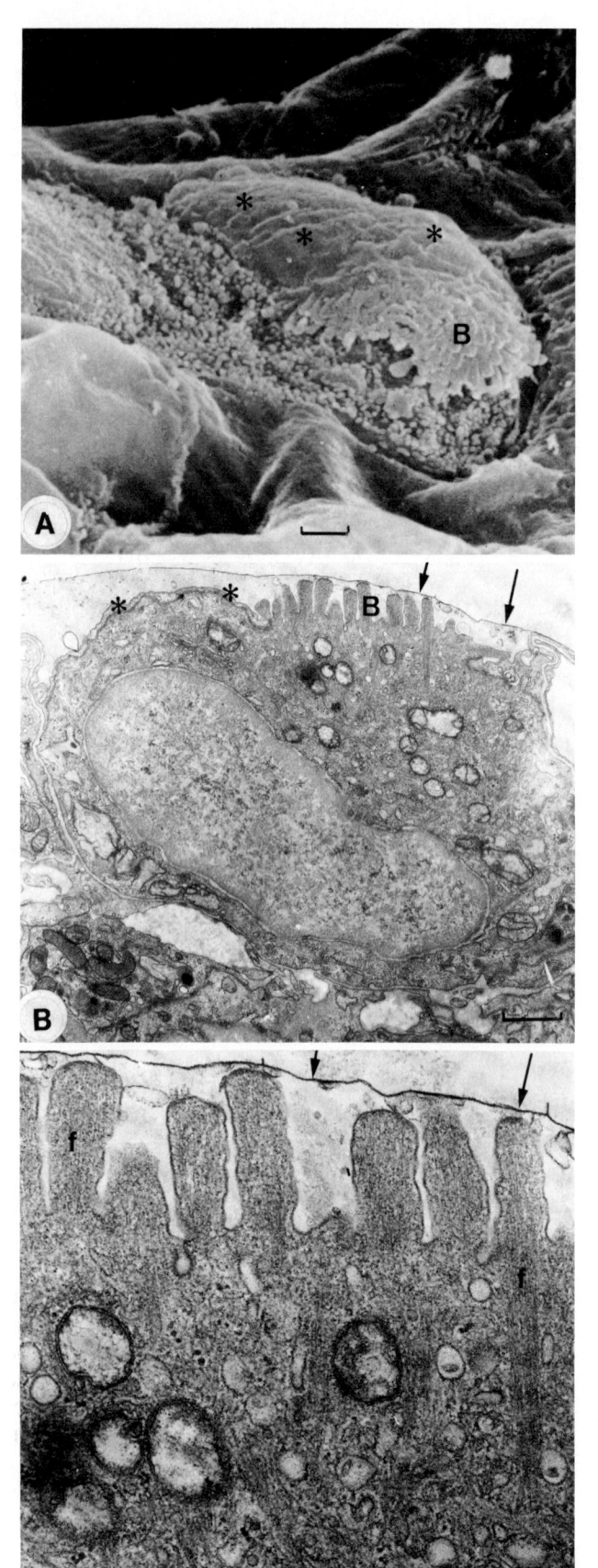

Evans et al. (63), who exposed rats to NO_2, thus inducing epithelial damage, carefully documented the transformation of type II into type I cells. Supplying these rats with [^{3}H]thymidine, they found about a third of all type II cells in the central part of the acinus with labeled nuclei, indicating a high rate of proliferative activity; labeling of type I cells was insignificant during this period. Figure 19 shows that type I cells became labeled to a significant proportion from the second day after withdrawal of the labeled thymidine; indeed, after that period half the labeled cells were type II cells and half were type I and "undetermined" cells. Although such long-term labeling experiments have many difficulties, mainly because of possible reutilization of label, this is rather strong evidence in support of the hypothesis that type II cells are progenitors for both type II and type I cells. The undetermined cells may, in part, be the intermediate stages in transformation; they may for some time retain a rich complement of organelles (including some osmiophilic granules) and form squamous cytoplasmic extensions similar to those characterizing the type I cell. The transformation of type II into type I cells appears to take ~2 days in the rat (63).

An intriguing question is why the type I cell is not able to undergo mitotic division. No conclusive evidence exists, so only speculations can be offered. The most conspicuous differentiation features of the type I cell are 1) its very vast expanse in surface and 2) the formation of multiple apical surfaces attached to cytoplasmic branches (198). Because of this second feature the cell may be topologically quite complex, so that the division of cytoplasm and plasma membrane into equal halves, as the cytokinesis phase of cell division requires, may be quite difficult. On the other hand, cells usually round off spherically prior to mitosis, without separating from their tissue. To do this the type I cell would have to withdraw its vast cytoplasmic flaps, which would either leave large areas of

FIG. 18. Alveolar brush cells from rat lung. *A*: scanning electron micrograph showing brush (*B*) on narrow apical surface bent to the side, whereas cell body is covered by smooth type I cell extension (*asterisks*). *B*: thin section shows brush beneath surface film (*arrows*) and covered by type I cell (*asterisks*). *C*: squat brush microvilli contain bundles of filaments (*f*) that extend deep into cell. *Bars*: 1 μm (*A*, *B*); 0.5 μm (*C*). [*B* from Weibel (199).]

alveolar septa denuded—an unlikely event—or require the entire septum to contract. It may therefore be preferable to recruit new cells from a cell type that can divide without endangering the integrity of the alveolar epithelial lining, for which the cuboidal type II cell is a good candidate. Interestingly, in conducting airways the ciliated lining cells also seem unable to divide (see CELL KINETICS IN CONDUCTING AIRWAY EPITHELIUM, p. 62).

These proliferative properties of the alveolar epithelium have considerable repercussions on the pattern of repair of epithelial damage. The type I cell, with its vast thin cytoplasmic extensions that are poor in organelles and far removed from the metabolic center of the cell, is very vulnerable. Under various effects (e.g., toxic injury by oxidants, sepsis, shock) focal or widespread destruction of the cytoplasmic lining of the alveolar surface is found (2, 8); repair by proliferation of type II cells ensues after a few days. The characteristic histological feature of such lungs is a lining of often contracted alveolar septa with a cuboidal epithelium that shows all the features of type II cells, in particular lamellar bodies and microvilli at the surface. For some time this image was associated with O_2 toxicity; now it is known that it is the result of a tissue-specific repair pattern after unspecific injury (8). If the patient or the experimental animal can survive the severe respiratory failure that is the consequence of both the original epithelial damage and the initial repair process, the cuboidal lining is transformed into a predominantly squamous lining again, and a well-functioning gas-exchange apparatus is restored (8).

VASCULAR ENDOTHELIUM

The vascular endothelium forms a continuous lining of all blood spaces in the greater and lesser circulation, including the heart, with a simple squamous epithelium that is of mesodermal origin. Two regions in the lung must be distinguished: the capillary endothelium in the gas-exchange region and the endothelial lining of conducting vessels (pulmonary arteries and veins).

Structure of Capillary Endothelium

Thin squamous cells line the alveolar capillaries (see Fig. 13B). They resemble in many respects the type I epithelial cells (see Figs. 13 and 14) with which they form the major part of the air-blood barrier, but they differ notably in size and cell shape. In contrast to the complex alveolar lining cells, the endothelial cells form simple sheets, each covering an average area of ~1,000–1,300 μm^2 [see Table 2; (48, 49, 82)]. This area is ~25% of the mean surface of type I cells and their number is ~4 times larger; thus endothelial cells constitute over 40% of the cells observed in lung parenchyma (see Table 2). Endothelial cells also appear to have a normal proliferative ability to expand the endothelial cell population during growth (103, 104) and to repair endothelial damage rapidly (8).

The cytoplasm of capillary endothelial cells forms a thin layer around the centrally located flattened nucleus and then extends into thin squamous sheets (see Fig. 13B). These cells have a modest set of organelles, a few small mitochondria, some ER with ribosomes, and a small but conspicuous Golgi complex. These organelles are usually concentrated in the perinuclear area, although some mitochondria and ER may occur in the cytoplasmic flaps, and often also in the cytoplasm adjacent to the cell junctions. Generally endothelial cells appear slightly thicker than type I epithelial cells; this is partly due to a greater number of nuclei per unit surface area. The major part of the cytoplasmic flaps is essentially the two plasma membranes and some intercalated cytoplasmic matrix with microfilaments and microtubules (see Fig. 14). They contain a variable amount of microvesicles, of which 30% each are attached as caveolae to either the luminal or abluminal plasma membrane; the remaining 40% are found free in the cytoplasm (73, 166). These vesicles have the characteristic structure of pinocytotic vesicles (32) and are thus interpreted as shuttle vehicles for transendothelial mass transport (142, 163, 166). Some part of the endothelial flaps are, however, free of vesicles; in these areas the two plasma membranes are separated by only a very thin layer of ectoplasm. The thickness and extent of such regions seem to depend on lung size; they are rare in human lungs but are prominent features in lungs of small mammals. The alveolar capillary endothelium of normal lungs does not have fenestrations and hence corresponds to the simple exchange-type endothelium, as observed also in muscle capillaries, for example; fenestrations may, however, develop in pulmonary fibrosis (191).

The junctions between neighboring endothelial cells are sealed by bandlike adhesions like those of tight

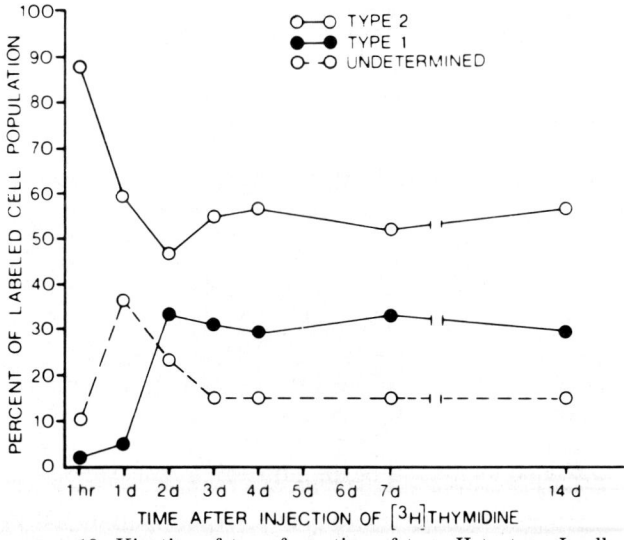

FIG. 19. Kinetics of transformation of type II to type I cells. Rats exposed to NO_2 to induce lung damage were injected with [^{3}H]thymidine at time 0 and killed from 1 h to 14 days later. [From Evans et al. (63).]

junctions, but on freeze-fracture preparations one finds only a small number of strands of intramembranous particles (161, 164). Accordingly these junctions are to some extent leaky; thus, at least under hemodynamic conditions that cause a certain degree of stretching of the endothelium, smaller macromolecules (e.g., horseradish peroxidase or hemoglobin) can traverse the fairly large intercellular pores, in contrast to the tight junctions of alveolar epithelium (161, 164). Consequently the blood plasma can rather freely exchange solutes with the interstitial fluid, and the endothelium does not form an osmotically active barrier (196). The degree of tightness does not seem uniform throughout the microvascular unit but shows, as in systemic microvascular units (142, 166), a gradient of decreasing tightness from the arteriolar to the venular side (161, 163, 164).

Finally, endothelial cells have a polarity similar to that of epithelial cells: the plasma membrane that faces the tissue side is attached to a basement membrane, whereas that facing the blood side has the normal "fuzzy" cell coat or glycocalyx of polysaccharides attached to membrane proteins and lipids. The basal side is furthermore in contact with pericytes (200), as described in MYOFIBROBLASTS AND PERICYTES, p. 79.

Structure of Arterial and Venous Endothelium

The endothelium of conducting blood vessels is thicker than that of capillaries and differs also in shape and cytoplasmic differentiation (Fig. 20). Endothelial cells of arterial vessels are elliptical disks with their long axis parallel to the direction of blood flow; in veins, however, endothelial cells form polygonal disks with equal dimensions in all directions. The surface membrane of these cells is not smooth but has many rugosities in the form of microvilli or lamellar protrusions, which greatly increase the surface area.

The cytoplasm of these endothelial cells is richly endowed with organelles that occur not only in the perinuclear area but also in the cytoplasmic flaps, which are thus considerably thicker than in the capillary endothelium (Fig. 20). Besides the usual organelles, the endothelial cells contain a peculiar organelle (206), a membrane-bounded rod-shaped granule with a matrix of small tubules (Fig. 20). This granule is a ubiquitous organelle of all noncapillary vascular endothelia in all vertebrates, from fish to human, one that is retained even in cell cultures of endothelial cells and does not occur in any other cell type. Unfortunately the function of this specific endothelial organelle is not known.

Metabolic Functions of Endothelial Cells

The endothelium of blood vessels apparently does not only function as a barrier between blood plasma and interstitial fluid. This is particularly true for pulmonary endothelia, capillary as well as arterial and venous. That certain biogenic amines and other substances are metabolized during their passage through the lung has long been known (9); this interesting topic is treated in detail in the chapter by Ryan in this *Handbook*. It has been suggested that the pulmonary vascular endothelia might have particular metabolic properties to serve these functions, mainly because the lung vasculature offers a very large surface of contact for blood plasma (9). One of the best known metabolic functions of this kind is the conversion of inactive angiotensin I to the active form angiotensin II, which is carried out by the so-called angiotensin-converting enzyme, a carboxydipeptidase that cleaves the terminal carboxydipeptide. With antibody-labeling techniques it is now possible to demonstrate the localization of such enzymes in the luminal plasma membrane of all pulmonary vascular endothelia (39, 158, 159). However, this is not a specific function of pulmonary endothelia; the same enzyme is found in similar concentrations in the endothelium of the aorta and other parts of the systemic circulation (39, 137). The role of the lung is special in that it confronts the entire blood flow in one cycle of the circulation over a large but spatially concentrated area. Often also maintained, but by no means demonstrated, is that the pulmonary vascular bed is strategically well situated for regulating the content of vasoactive substances in the blood because it screens the blood just prior to its delivery into the systemic circulation. However, for regulation to be diligently deployed the lung should be part of a regulatory circuit; this has not been demonstrated.

The pulmonary endothelium seems to display considerable specificity with respect to the substances it will metabolize. Serotonin and prostaglandins E and F are rapidly removed from the blood, whereas histamine and prostaglandin A pass through untouched (9). Fisher and Pietra (65) have also shown that serotonin uptake is a special ability of pulmonary vascular endothelium, in contrast to alveolar epithelium that can absorb only small amounts.

INTERSTITIAL CELLS

The interstitium of the lung can be broadly defined as the space intercalated between the airway epithelium, the vascular endothelium, and the pleural mesothelium, bounded toward these lining cell layers by basement membranes. One can ascribe two major functions to the interstitium: *1*) to mechanically join and support the different elements of the gas-exchange system of the lung and *2*) to establish a fluid space related to lymph. The first function is basically served by the system of connective tissue fibers that pervades the entire lung (203); however, this requires the intervention of various cell types (e.g., smooth muscle cells) in order to respond to short-term de-

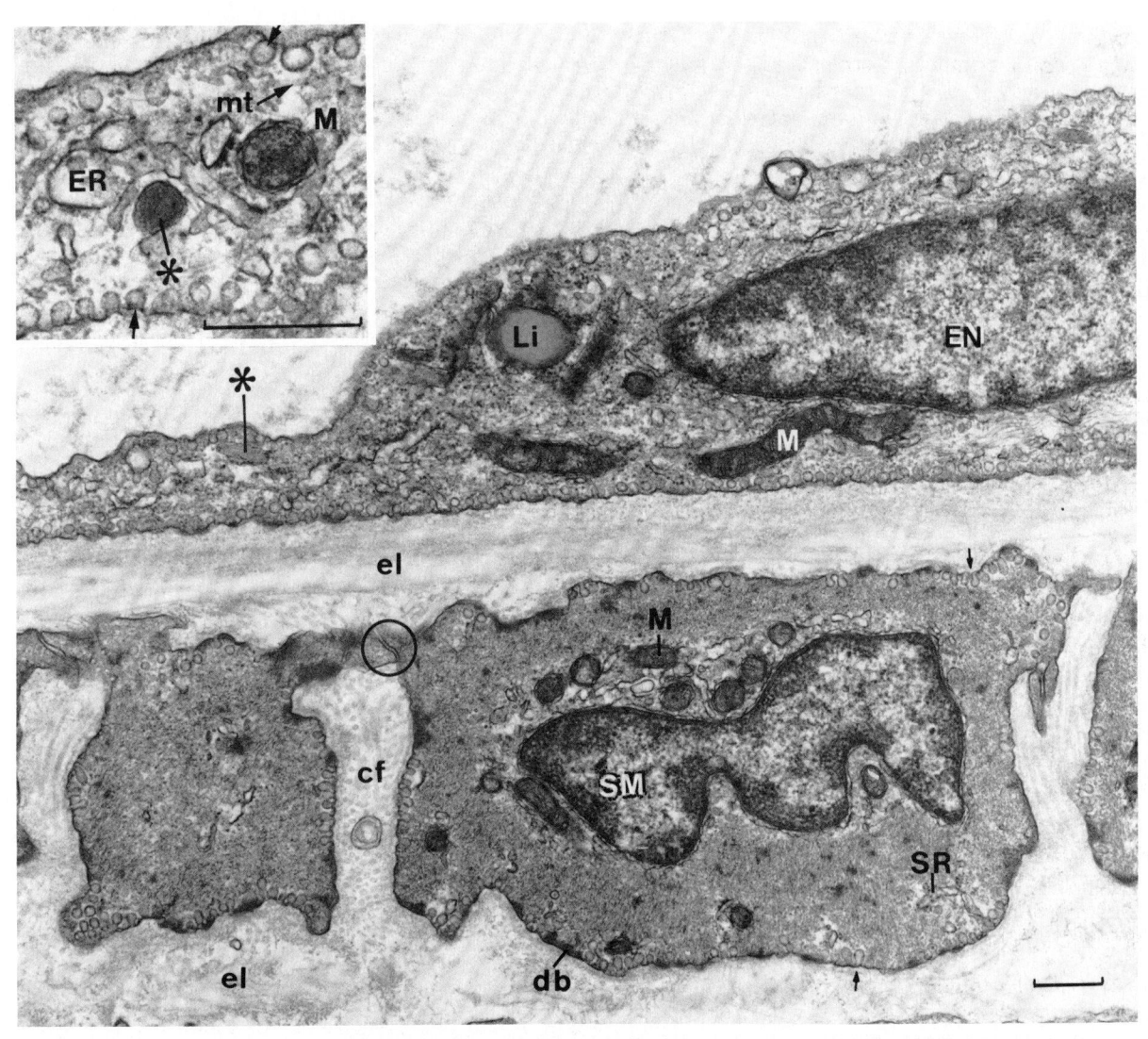

FIG. 20. Endothelium (*EN*) and single layer of smooth muscle (*SM*) from small pulmonary artery of human lung. Thick endothelial cytoplasm and wealth of organelles (*inset*) comprising mitochondria (*M*), endoplasmic reticulum (*ER*), lipid droplet (*Li*), specific granules (*asterisks*), microtubules (*mt*), and many vesicles (*arrows*). Cross-sectioned smooth muscle cells show central nucleus, mitochondria, sarcoplasmic reticulum (*SR*), membrane-bounded caveolae (*arrows*), filamentous matter with dense bodies (*db*), and cell-to-cell contacts (*circle*). *cf*, Collagen fibrils; *el*, elastic fibers. Bars, 0.5 μm.

mands on modified mechanical properties (27) or the intervention of fibroblasts to maintain the fiber system. The second function offers the opportunity to house an important part of the cells of the defense system in close proximity to the pathways for draining tissue fluids out of the respiratory tissue. The interstitial structures, in particular the interstitial cells, have different features depending on their location in either the alveolar septa or the walls of conducting tubes, airways, or blood vessels.

Cells Related to Connective Tissue Fibers

Wherever there are connective tissue fibers there are fibroblasts associated with them, because these cells are responsible for the synthesis of the building blocks of the fibers both during fibrogenesis and during maintenance of an established fiber system. A fibroblast engaged in active fibrogenesis (Fig. 21) has a well-developed ER capable of synthesizing proteins (e.g., tropocollagen or elastin) (84, 90) and a large Golgi complex involved in producing proteoglycans, which are important constituents of connective tissue fibers (149). The high level of metabolic activity of the cell is also reflected by a large volume of mitochondria and by an often prominent nucleolus, the site of ribosome formation. All these components are also present in fibroblasts engaged simply in fiber maintenance, but in much smaller amounts (Fig. 22).

The major constituent of connective tissue is colla-

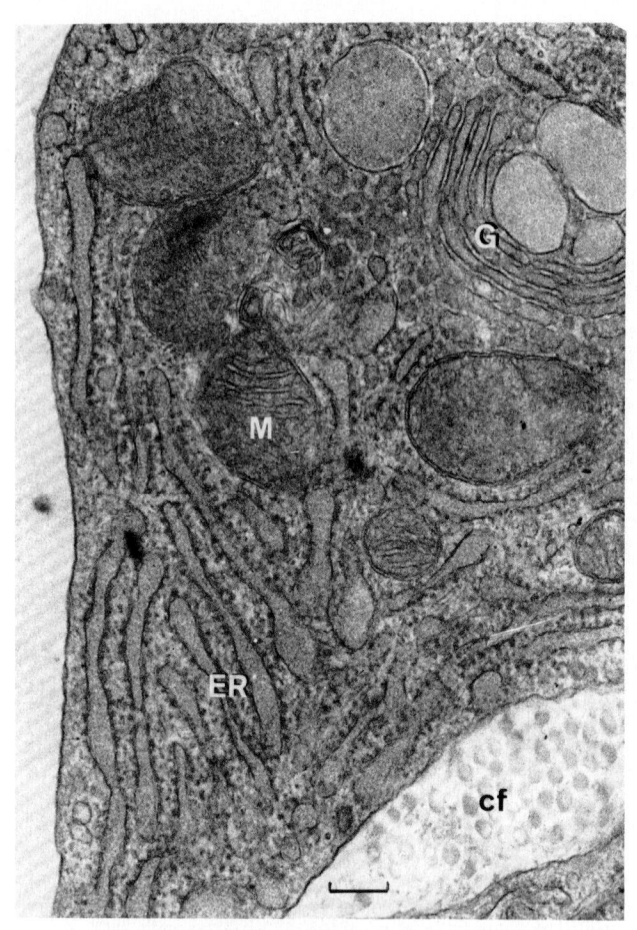

FIG. 21. Fibroblast engaged in fibrogenesis contains much endoplasmic reticulum (*ER*) with ribosomes and large Golgi complex (*G*), as well as mitochondria (*M*). *cf*, Collagen fibrils. *Bar*, 0.2 µm.

fibers are also formed by fibroblasts that are probably special.

Fibroblasts are shaped to fit the fiber system to which they are attached. Generally their central nucleus is enwrapped by a narrow rim of cytoplasm; multiple slim extensions emanate from this rim to follow the course of the fibers (Fig. 22). In larger connective tissue structures (e.g., peribronchial and perivascular sheaths) or in pleural septa these extensions are thin lamellae that are loosely apposed to the rather coarse fiber bundles and sometimes interca-

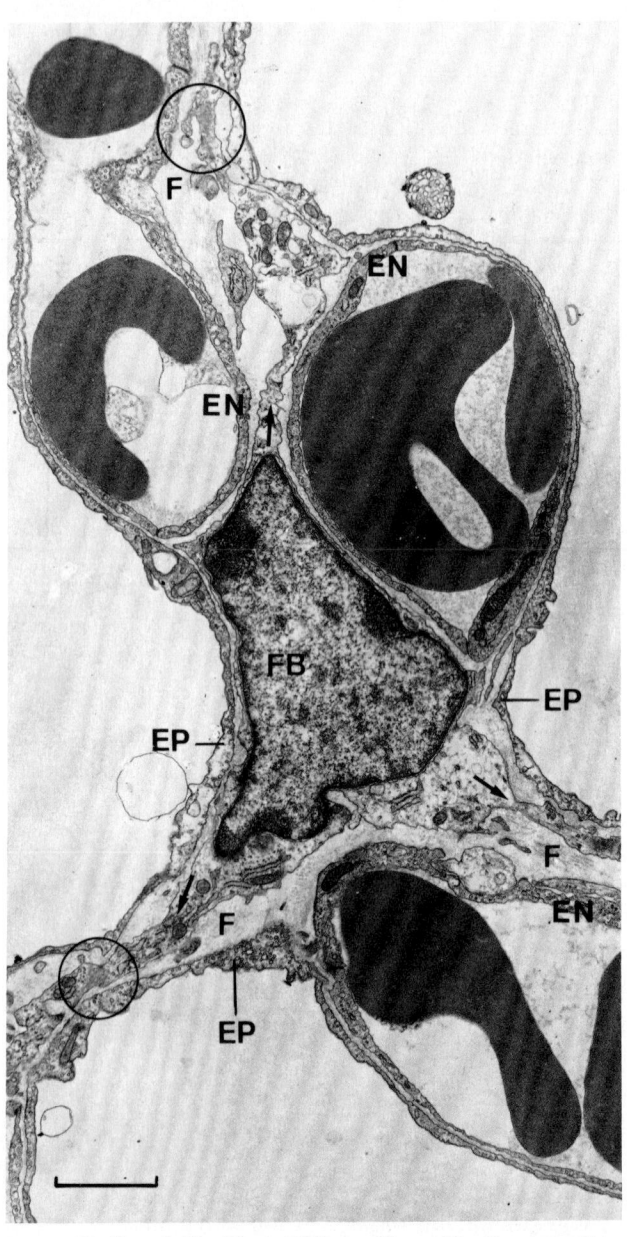

FIG. 22. Septal fibroblast (*FB*) ramifies with slim extensions (*arrows*) into interstitial spaces between capillary endothelium (*EN*) and alveolar epithelium (*EP*), following the fiber strands (*F*). *Circles*, cytoplasmic areas with condensed filaments spanning the interstitial space crosswise. *Bar*, 2 µm.

gen, a protein of which four types can be distinguished by their chemical nature (84). Only type I collagen appears to be responsible for the formation of collagen fibers. This protein is manufactured and secreted by the fibroblasts (154) in the form of tropocollagen, a triple helix of two different collagen molecules ~1.5 nm thick and ~300 nm long (84). In the extracellular space such units are assembled to form long fibrils 40–200 nm thick; their high tensile strength is achieved by establishing multiple cross-links within and between the tropocollagen units. How far fibroblasts intervene in this process of extracellular assembly is not known. Other connective tissue fibrils, such as reticulin fibers or anchoring fibrils, are also built of collagen, although some are different chemically. Basement membranes comprise type IV collagen and are apparently synthesized by the cells to which they are attached (i.e., epithelial and endothelial cells, or muscle fibers, rather than fibroblasts) (84). Elastic fibers, however, are made predominantly of elastin, a highly insoluble protein whose biochemical nature and synthetic pathways are poorly understood (90); elastic lated between fiber strands (see Fig. 8). In the alveolar septa, where the fibers form a network of fiber strands, the fibroblasts are highly ramified cells with apparently very long extensions (Fig. 22). The average total cell volume of the fibroblasts is estimated at ~600 μm^3 (see Table 2); thus they are the second largest cell type in lung parenchyma (82). The cytoplasmic extensions of fibroblasts vary in composition from mere cytoplasmic matrix to elaborate systems of ER with mitochondria.

Fibroblasts appear to be rather versatile cells that are able to assume functions other than those of fibrogenesis generally attributed to them (29, 71). Many of them, if not all, appear to have contractile properties, as is discussed next. This property plays an important role in wound healing, for example, by contracting the gap in the connective tissue caused by the injury, in preparation for scar tissue formation (68). Whether this property is also operative in some pulmonary diseases where repair processes may entail scar formation after contraction of interstitial cells is not known. Fibroblasts also appear to compartmentalize interstitial fluid into different spaces. Thus lymphatic capillaries seem to form from fibroblasts; recently Gil and McNiff (71) described a special arrangement of sheetlike fibroblasts as a potential boundary between the fluid spaces in the alveolar septa and larger connective tissue beds.

The chondrocyte, as it occurs in the cartilage associated with larger bronchi, is a special connective tissue cell with the ability to form fibers. This cell is highly specialized and is not discussed here.

Interstitial Cells With Contractile Properties

Recent studies have shown that many cells have contractile properties based on actomyosin complexes. This is particularly true of interstitial cells, which include smooth muscle cells and fibroblasts (with a variable degree of contractility).

SMOOTH MUSCLE CELLS. True smooth muscle cells are found in three locations in the lung: *1*) in the wall of conducting blood vessels; *2*) in the wall of all branches of the tracheobronchial tree down to the terminal bronchioles, disposed according to a different pattern in the largest bronchi and trachea than in the peripheral bronchi and bronchioles; and *3*) in the free edge of alveolar septa as fiber strands that engender the alveolar mouths in the form of a so-called entrance ring. The latter smooth muscle fibers are, in essence, parenchymal extensions of the bronchiolar muscle sheaths (203).

The current knowledge of smooth muscle cells has recently been reviewed rather extensively (34, 69, 168, 182). A short summary of some of the most important features follows. Smooth muscle cells are generally elongated, sometimes branched cells with a single centrally located nucleus (Figs. 20 and 23). They are

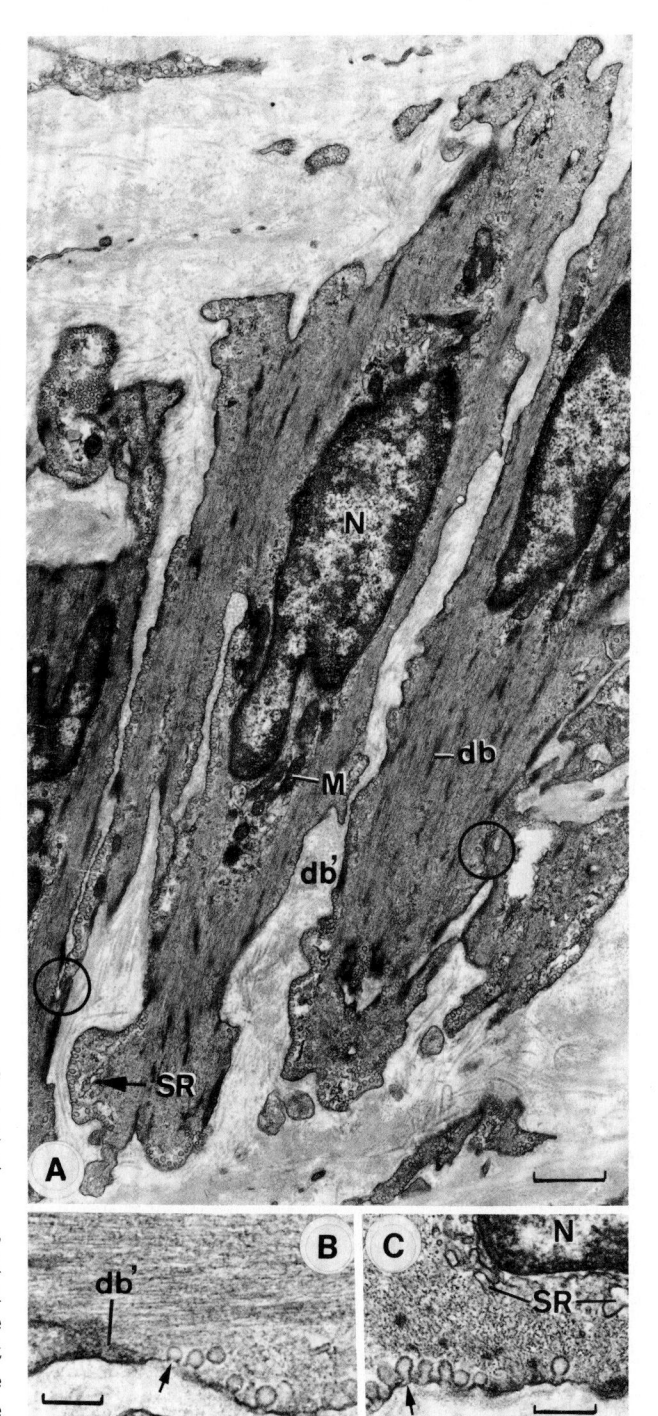

FIG. 23. *A*: smooth muscle cells from small pulmonary artery of human lung cut longitudinally. *db*, Dense bodies of filamentous matter; *db'*, dense bands on plasma membrane; *M*, mitochondria; *N*, central elongated nucleus; *SR*, sarcoplasmic reticulum. Greater magnification shows filaments on longitudinal (*B*) and transverse (*C*) sections together with caveolae (*arrows*) of plasma membrane, which is coated by basement membrane. Bars: 1 μm (*A*); 0.2 μm (*B*, *C*).

enwrapped by a plasma membrane and by a basement membrane that is interrupted only where neighboring cells establish direct contact. Their cytoplasm is, for the major part, occupied by actomyosin filaments that do not show the cross-striation of skeletal or heart muscle due to the organization of the contractile proteins into sarcomeres. In addition, they contain mitochondria, glycogen granules, and a set of membrane tubules referred to as sarcoplasmic reticulum. Most of the detailed knowledge about these cells has been obtained from organs where smooth muscle cells make up the bulk of the mass, such as the uterus, the urinary bladder, some blood vessels, and the intestine (particularly the taeniae in the colon); extrapolation to pulmonary smooth muscles must be done cautiously, because not all smooth muscles appear to be alike in every respect (69).

Considering first the organization of the filamentous matter one finds three types of filaments plus a patchlike electron-dense component called dense body (not to be confused with lysosomes, which are sometimes also called dense bodies). The three types of filaments are distinguished by their size and structural characteristics. The bulk of the filamentous matter consists of thin filaments 6–7 nm in diameter; they are normally arranged in the form of bundles, sometimes closely packed into a triangular lattice (Fig. 23B, C). These thin filaments, whose length is not yet determined, have long been recognized as structural units of smooth muscle cells; there is little doubt that they are actin filaments, probably associated with tropomyosin and troponin, just as in striated muscle (69). It is now clear that all smooth muscle cells contain thick filaments, although these filaments have not been found for a long time, perhaps because they are rather labile structures. These thick filaments are 14–16 nm in diameter, ~2 μm in length (69), and are myosin filaments; smooth muscle myosin differs somewhat from striated muscle myosin, both immunologically and physically, as it is more soluble and hence labile. The third class of filaments are 10 nm in diameter and appear to be built of four subunits; they are sometimes called intermediate filaments and appear to be related (though perhaps not totally identical) to the cytoskeletal filaments that occur as tonofilaments in many cells or as neurofilaments in nerve fibers.

The dense bodies are somehow related to the filamentous matter (44, 69, 169, 175). They appear on electron micrographs as condensed areas of comparatively high contrast (Fig. 23); their shape and size is very variable and their outline unsharp. Similar condensations occur beneath the plasma membrane in the form of dense bands. The nature of these dense structures is not well defined. They could correspond to Z lines in striated muscle, and studies have shown that the thin actin filaments are inserted in the dense bodies and dense bands; the latter could therefore correspond to the dense patches that occur in the intercalated disks of heart muscle where the myofibrils insert with their actin filaments. Cooke (44) made an interesting observation after the extraction of actin and myosin: the dense bodies appear to be part of the cytoskeletal system established by the intermediate filaments.

The contractile properties of smooth muscle cells are clearly due to their actomyosin complex, which is notably different from that of striated muscles. The relative amounts of actin and myosin are different (69, 169): in mammalian striated muscles the weight ratio of actin:myosin is 0.35; in smooth muscles it is 2–3. The numerical ratio of thin to thick filaments is also different, although the estimates vary considerably, partly because of methodological problems: whereas this ratio is 2 in mammalian striated muscle, it is of the order of 8–15 in smooth muscle.

In smooth muscles of the portal vein, the thick myosin filaments are arranged in a rather regular lattice and connect to the actin filaments with cross bridges like those in the A band of sarcomeres of striated muscle (5). This suggests that the contraction mechanism is similar to the sliding-filament model generally accepted for sarcomeres, but the evidence is not conclusive. No acceptable alternative model of the mechanism of smooth muscle contraction has been proposed.

A number of interesting differences between smooth and striated muscles are important. On the one hand the actomyosin filaments of smooth muscle are not arranged parallel to the long axis of the cell (169). In the stretched cell these filaments assume an angle of ~10° to this axis, but on contraction the angle increases considerably. Because of this arrangement, contraction of a smooth muscle cell leads to important shape changes: a contracted cell tends to be almost spherical at the end of the contraction. On the other hand, and related to this geometric property, smooth muscle fibers can undergo greater changes in length than striated muscle fibers.

It is well established that in striated muscle the contraction of actomyosin is controlled by the release and capture of Ca^{2+} by the sarcoplasmic reticulum; myosin binds to actin under high Ca^{2+} concentrations and detaches as Ca^{2+} concentration falls. Whether a similar mechanism is effective in smooth muscle is not known. Smooth muscle cells do have a set of cytoplasmic tubules and cisternae, which are called sarcoplasmic reticulum [Figs. 20 and 23C; (69)]. Part of these are studded with ribosomes and thus involved in protein synthesis of some sort, but most of the tubules are smooth and narrow. Characteristically such tubules course along the plasma membrane for rather long distances, often with caveolae, which abound on the plasma membrane; these tubules branch and send extensions into the filamentous matter (69). Studies on isolated smooth muscle membranes have shown that microsomes, which are presumably derived from the sarcoplasmic reticulum, are able to capture Ca^{2+} and that this is related to muscle relaxation. This suggests that the sarcoplasmic reticulum of smooth muscle cells may function as a regulator of actomyosin activity, as it does in striated muscle; however, other evidence indicates that the Ca^{2+} content of smooth muscle cells may be regulated from outside the cell through the plasma membrane or, at least partly, by mitochondria, which are able to accumulate considerable amounts of Ca^{2+} (174).

In striated muscle the external control of contraction occurs by changes in the electrical membrane potential, which is related to transient modifications in the permeability of specific pores of the plasma membrane for Na^+ and Ca^{2+}. This action potential extends deep into the cell along the transverse tubules (T tubules); the sarcoplasmic reticulum establishes close contact with the T tubules, and its permeability for Ca^{2+} becomes changed as an action potential arrives. It is likely, but not established, that a similar though not identical mechanism is involved in regulating smooth muscle activity (40, 193). The structure of the membrane system of smooth muscle cells is definitely less elaborate, as there is no equivalent to the T tubules; the large number of caveolae observed at the plasma membrane does not appear to be equivalent to the T tubules, although they seem related to Ca^{2+} transport. Physiologically the action potential of smooth muscle cells is largely due to Ca^{2+} flux rather than Na^+ flux; if this is true the contractile matter could be controlled, at least in part, directly from the plasma membrane by regulating the Ca^{2+} content of the cell.

Smooth muscle cells form bundles, similar to myocardial cells, that are electrically coupled so they can contract synchronously. Cell-to-cell coupling occurs through nexus or gap junctions, as they were described in *Epithelium of Conducting Airways*, p. 56, for epithelial cell coupling. Nexus have been found on smooth muscle cells (Figs. 20 and 23) but not consistently (35, 69); there is large variability in the size and frequency of such membrane connections.

Mitochondria are the most prominent cytoplasmic organelles in smooth muscle cells (except for filamentous matter), occupying 2%–5% of the cytoplasm (Figs. 20 and 23). Groups of mitochondria are found near poles of the elongated nuclei, but profiles of single mitochondria are found throughout the filamentous matter to the area beneath the plasma membrane; their role is to supply ATP for contraction and possibly for active Ca^{2+} uptake by the sarcoplasmic reticulum. It appears that there is only one type of smooth muscle cell (168), in contrast to skeletal muscle, where mitochondria-rich aerobic and mitochondria-poor glycolytic fibers can be distinguished.

MYOFIBROBLASTS AND PERICYTES. Recently it has been shown that many fibroblasts, if not all, are endowed with notable contractile properties. Such cells contain bundles of thin microfilaments (6–7 nm diam) that are anchored in dense patches beneath the plasma membrane (Fig. 24). Immunocytochemical methods have shown that these filaments consist of actin, which is able to bind to myosin (100–102). Although Kapanci et al. (101) have also demonstrated the presence of myosin with such techniques, it has not been possible to demonstrate thick filaments on electron micrographs; intermediate (10-μm) filaments and microtubules are found, however, and both are interpreted as elements of the cytoskeleton. Fibroblasts differ considerably in the amount of actomyosin bundles they contain. In some locations the filament bundles become so prominent that the cells have been called myofibroblasts (68); this is true, for instance, in granulation tissue of healing wounds, where contractile fibroblasts are believed to help approximate the wound edges (68). In the lung such prominent myofibroblasts are found in the strong connective tissue rings that circle the alveolar mouths, but here we may find all transitions toward actual smooth muscle cells. Myofibroblasts differ in two respects from smooth muscle cells: *1*) they contain an appreciable amount of nonfilamentous cytoplasm and organelles, so that the filaments occur in clearly separated bundles, and *2*) their plasma membrane is not enwrapped with a basement membrane. However, some myofibroblasts may eventually differentiate into smooth muscle cells.

The fibroblasts of alveolar septa appear to be a special kind of myofibroblast. As shown in Figure 22 they form multiple cytoplasmic branches that follow the septal fiber network and contain ER in a clear cytoplasm. However, short bundles of filaments occur randomly (Fig. 22), generally extending crosswise from cell membrane to cell membrane (more or less perpendicular to the main axis of the cytoplasmic branch or to the course of the fibers). As shown in Figure 24, such bundles span the entire width of the cell and the width of the interstitial space; the membrane of the fibroblasts is regularly attached to either the epithelial or the endothelial basement membrane in the places where it is connected to the filament bundles (204). Thus contraction of the filament bundle acts on these basement membranes and indirectly on the epithelium or endothelium. The function of these fibroblastic myofibrils is not yet known. They may regulate the width of the capillary sheet by shortening the height of the posts (100–102), or they may regulate the compliance of the interstitial space for fluid accumulation (204); their arrangement could serve both functions equally well. An intriguing observation is that strips of lung parenchyma—presumably a sequence of alveolar septa—shorten under appropriate pharmacological stimulation (62, 100). If this is an effect of contracting septal myofibroblasts, at least part of the actomyosin bundles must be parallel to the septal fiber system; this has not been observed. Alternatively, one suspects that a parenchymal strip has a sufficient amount of

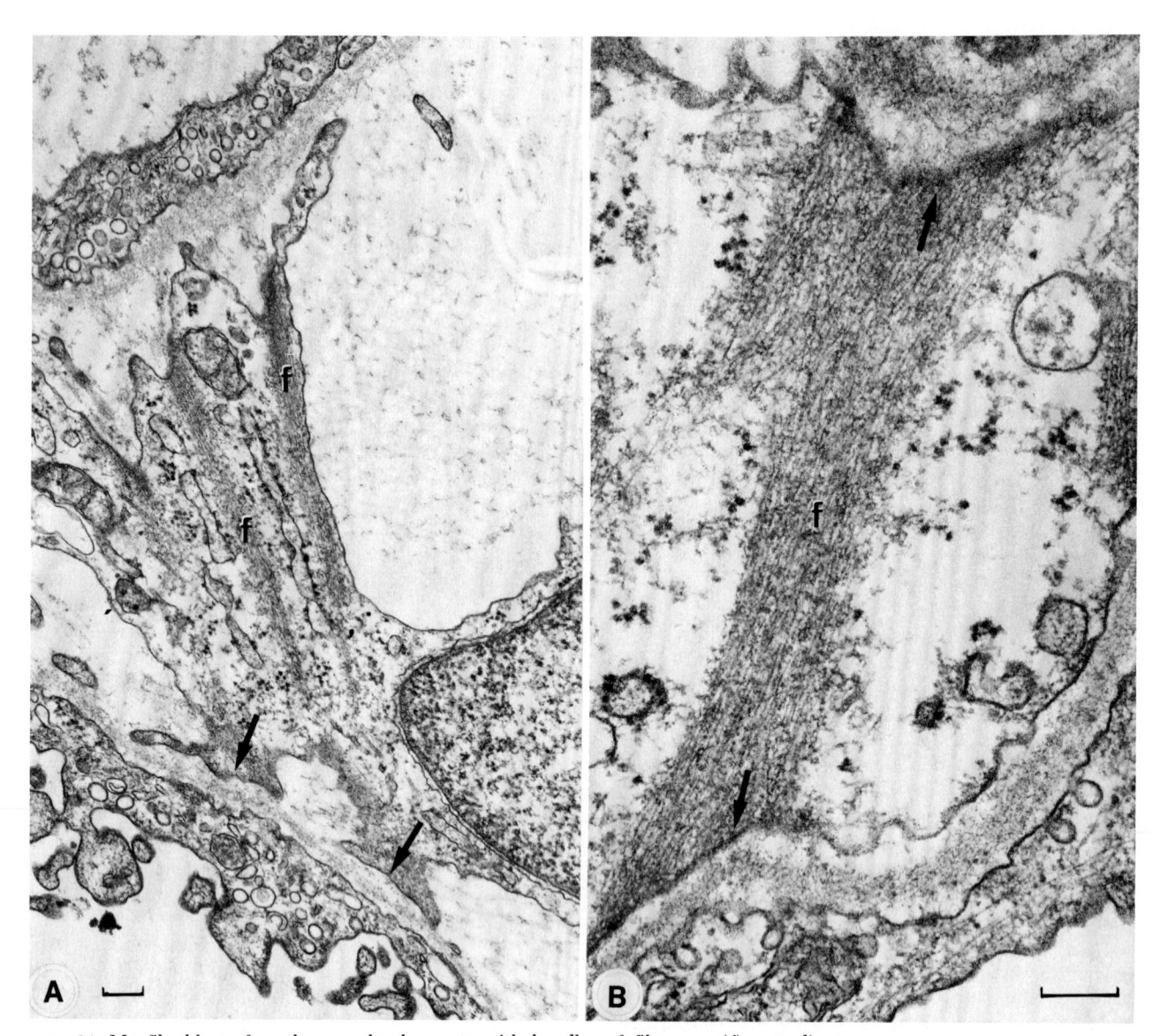

FIG. 24. Myofibroblasts from human alveolar septa with bundles of filaments (*f*) extending obliquely or crosswise between dense insertion spots on plasma membrane, which appears affixed to basement membrane (*arrows*). Bars, 0.2 μm.

alveolar duct walls (with their network of smooth muscle fibers) to account for this effect. Conclusive evidence on the role of the septal myofibroblasts can only be procured with better controlled preparations of septal tissue.

The alveolar wall contains a second set of interstitial cells with putative contractile properties: the capillary pericytes (200). These cells, which have long and branched extensions, are closely apposed to the capillary endothelial basement membrane; some of their processes penetrate beneath the basement membrane to directly contact the endothelial cells (Fig. 25). The outer surface of these cells, however, is partially covered by a basement membrane that is connected to that of the endothelium. Thus pericytes are "sandwiched" between leaflets of the capillary basement membrane. Pericytes may have contractile prop-

erties because they contain fine filaments like those of myofibroblasts; these filaments are usually arranged in a condensed layer closely apposed to the plasma membrane, which faces the endothelial basement membrane (Fig. 25). They resemble the smooth muscle cells of small venules, where the contractile filamentous matter is also concentrated on the luminal side of the cell; caveolae occur mostly, though not exclusively, on the side facing the interstitium in both venular smooth muscle and pericytes (200).

Pericytes have been assigned putative functions other than contractility, notably that of being part of the defense system, because phagosomes are sometimes observed in their cytoplasm, but there is no strong evidence for this. They seem to be quite labile cells, because one often observes swollen cytoplasmic processes (Fig. 25), particularly if there was a delay

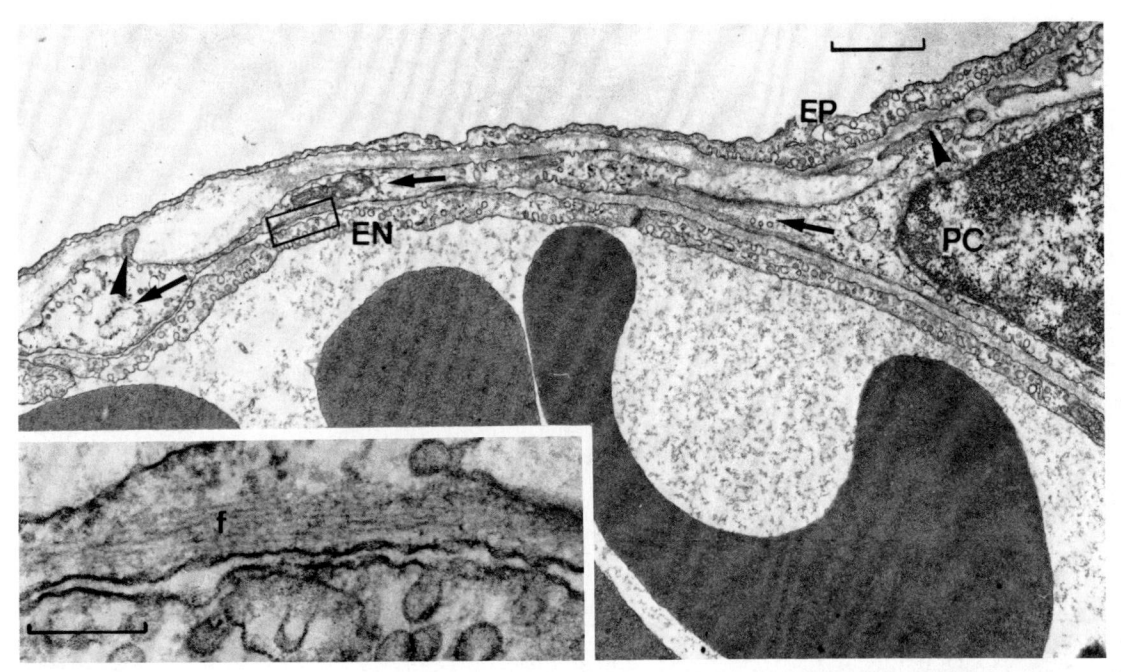

FIG. 25. Capillary pericyte (*PC*) with extension (*arrows*) that lies between the endothelial cell (*EN*) and its basement membrane in its peripheral part. Other processes of same cell make contact with epithelial (*EP*) basement membrane (*arrowheads*). Inset, pericyte filaments (*f*). Bars: 1 μm; 0.1 μm (inset).

between death and fixation or in pathological specimens (8).

The peculiar location of pericytes between endothelium and interstitium raises the question of their nature. They resemble fibroblasts in many respects, except that fibroblasts are never covered by a basement membrane. However, the pericyte is rarely completely enwrapped in a basement membrane; there are regions where it extends toward the epithelial basement membrane with a short process that contains fine filaments (Fig. 25). This is no different from the disposition of the myofibroblast processes described above (see Fig. 27). The question remains whether pericytes are a distinct differentiated cell type or merely partially specialized myofibroblasts.

Lymphatics and Free Cells

It is generally maintained that lymphatics occur only in a juxta-alveolar position in large perivascular connective tissue beds (112, 113, 116) and that the alveolar septa lack lymphatic capillaries. The endothelial cell of lymphatics differs distinctly from that of capillaries in that it does not have a basement membrane. Its cytoplasmic leaflets furthermore have a rather irregular surface texture, which is partly caused by large fluid-filled blebs; these blebs may be related to the active bulk transfer of fluid (lymph) into the vessel by large "gulps." In juxta-alveolar connective tissue beds one can often find cells that have all the characteristics of a fibroblast and whose broad extensions appear to enwrap large interstitial fluid pockets; such structures may be lymphatic capillaries being newly formed from fibroblasts.

Lymphatic capillaries are often associated with groups of free interstitial cells comprising lymphocytes, plasma cells, and histiocytes, in particular; for a discussion of these cells see CELLS OF PULMONARY DEFENSE SYSTEM, p. 82. Free interstitial cells are rarely encountered in the alveolar septa.

In the normal lung, mast cells are also found predominantly in perivascular and subpleural connective tissue, but they may occasionally be located in alveolar septa, often at the junction between three septa (Fig. 26). In fibrotic lungs, mast cells are most frequently found in the thickened septa (105). Mast cells produce and secrete heparin and histamine, products that are stored in granules whose structure shows considerable species differences. In the human mast cell the granules have a very characteristic substructure in the form of scrolls (Fig. 26), whereas in the rat the granules are more homogeneous or granular (105, 199, 202). Note that the granules of basophilic granulocytes, considered to be the blood mast cells, have a substructure different from that of tissue mast cells. The mast cell becomes "degranulated" on release of histamine and heparin; the granules do not completely disappear, but they lose their characteristic substructure (105).

Nerves

Nerve cells are rare in the lung; occasional small ganglia occur in the wall of larger bronchi. Nerve fibers are, however, found all along the airway tree, usually therefore maintain an elaborate defense system. This begins with the mechanical cleansing devices in the nasal cavity and larger airways in the form of a mucous stream and continues to the alveolar surface, which has a cell population that acts both through the immune system and by direct nonimmune defense.

Alveolar and Interstitial Macrophages

The nonimmune defense is essentially carried out by macrophages that can ingest noxious materials by phagocytosis, digest them partially in the lysosomal system, and, if necessary, store residues in intracellular compartments. Such phagocytic cells occur in several locations in the lung: in the surface lining layer of alveoli, in the mucous layer of conducting airways, and in the interstitial space (particularly in perivascular and peribronchial sheaths, subpleural tissues, and interlobular septa).

The alveolar macrophages constitute the actual cell population of the alveolar surface lining layers. They are loosely attached to the surface of the alveolar epithelium, particularly on type I cells, with which they establish a patchwise close contact; the nature and function of these contact zones are not yet understood, but they may explain why only a limited fraction of alveolar macrophages can be harvested through endobronchial lavage with saline (30). Although in conventional preparations alveolar macrophages sit on the surface of the epithelium (Figs. 27 and 28), they are not directly exposed to alveolar air; rather they are covered by a thin film of surface lining layer (Fig. 29). This is important in two respects: *1*) the macrophages do not intercept extraneous matter di-

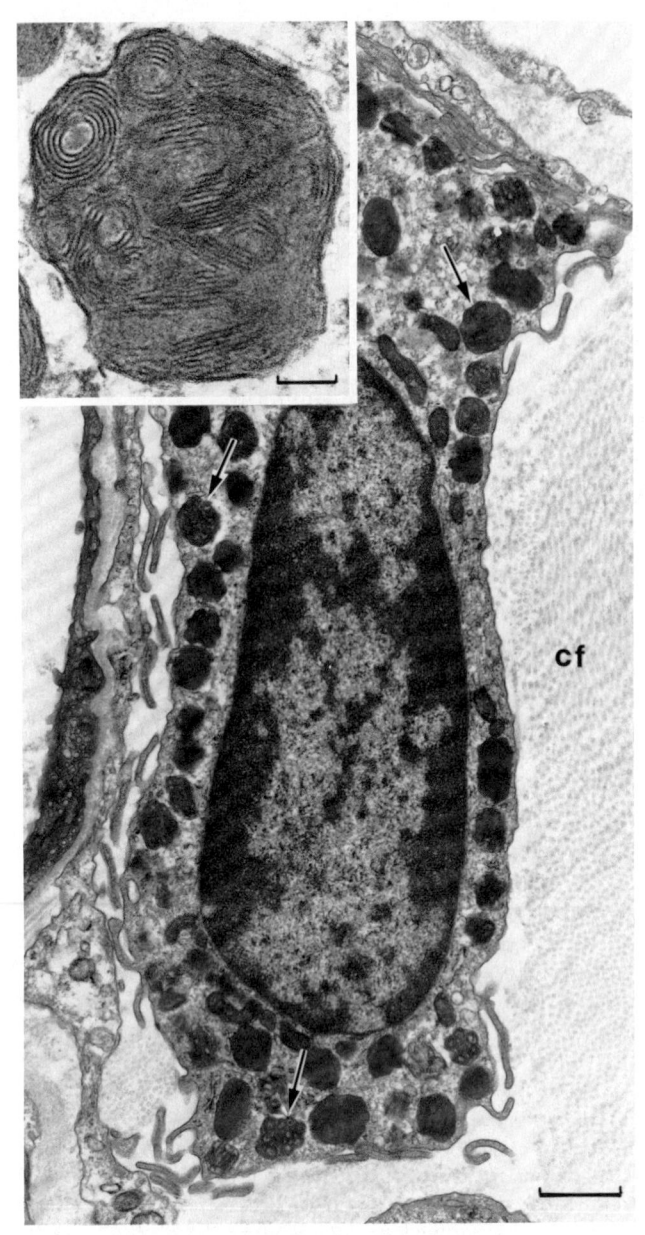

FIG. 26. Mast cell from human alveolar septum contains granules (*arrows*) with scroll-like substructure. Inset, scroll-like substructure of mast cell at higher magnification. *cf*, Collagen fibrils. Bars, 1 μm; 0.1 μm (*inset*).

enwrapped in small bundles by a typical perineural sheath. Most of these fibers are unmyelinated, but small myelinated axons are also observed. How far these nerve fibers penetrate into the lung parenchyma and with what density is not known. Although the occurrence of unmyelinated nerve fibers in alveolar septa has repeatedly been documented (69, 91, 131), they are rare.

CELLS OF PULMONARY DEFENSE SYSTEM

Because of its large surface open to outside air the lung is exposed to multiple potential hazards and must

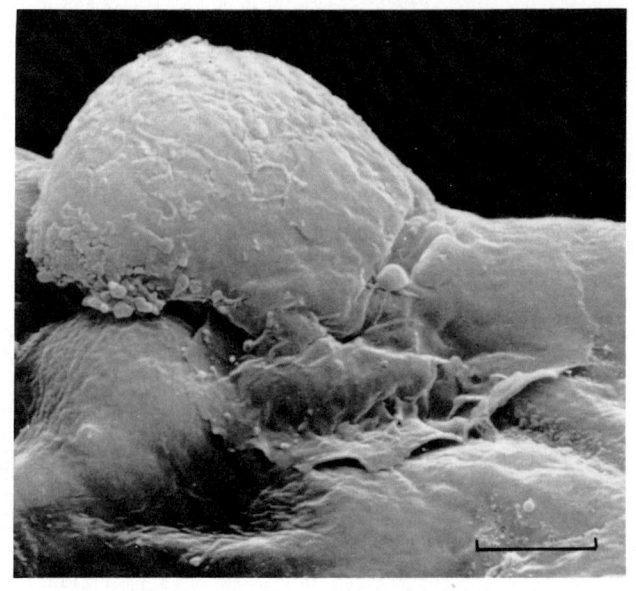

FIG. 27. Scanning electron micrograph of human alveolar macrophage on alveolar epithelial surface. Thin advancing cytoplasmic lamella appears partly attached to epithelium. Bar, 5 μm. [From Weibel (202).]

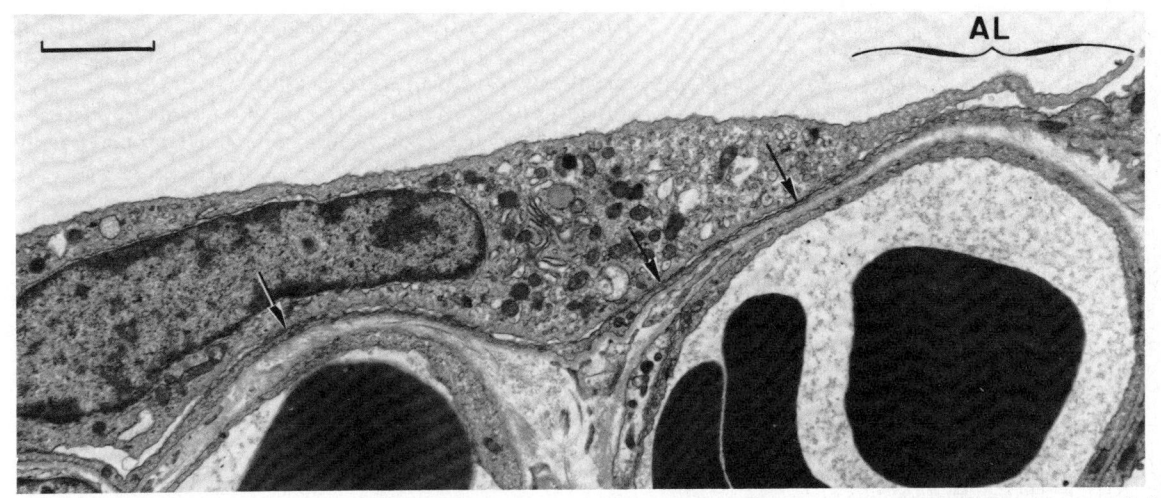

FIG. 28. Alveolar macrophage of human lung apposed to epithelium in several places (*arrows*). Advancing lamella (*AL*) is free of organelles that are rich in perinuclear cytoplasm. *Bar*, 2 μm.

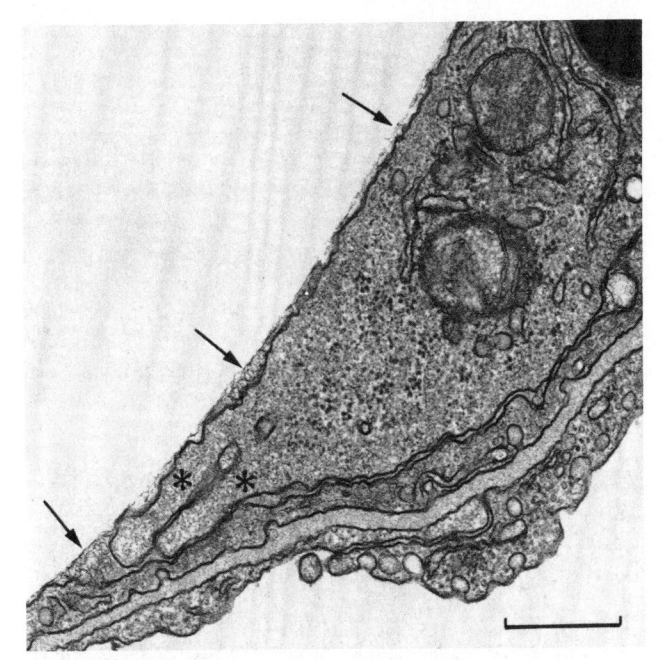

FIG. 29. Alveolar macrophage lies beneath thin film of surface lining layer (*arrows*). Exclusion of organelles from short peripheral cytoplasmic flaps (*asterisks*). *Bar*, 1 μm.

rectly but rather after its absorption to the lining layer; 2) the lining layer defines the space through which macrophages can move over the alveolar surface, and because the lining layer fills most alveolar pores, macrophages can move from one alveolus to the other through these pores. The latter pathway is significant because it appears that macrophages move throughout the acinus and tend to accumulate in the central acinar region (24, 80). From there they may move on to the bronchiolar surface and be removed up the bronchial escalator, finally ending in the pharynx with the mucus. Dust-laden cells or hemosiderin-containing heart failure cells that originate in alveoli may thus end up in the expectorate or in the digestive tract.

Macrophages that populate the mucous blanket of the bronchial surface (see Fig. 8A) are thus partially of alveolar origin, but evidence exists that there is a genuine population of bronchial macrophages that reach the mucous blanket through the bronchial epithelium (178).

The third group of macrophages resides in all major connective tissue beds, e.g., perivascular and peribronchial sheaths, interlobular septa, subpleural layers, and bronchial walls. Such cells are often grouped near small lymphatics with cells of the immune defense system (Fig. 30). They can also enter lymphatics and be removed to lymph nodes, where they are deposited in the lymphatic tissue (98).

One important functional property of macrophages is their ameboid mobility (70, 152, 178, 186). This is particularly marked in surface macrophages, which develop prominent cytoplasmic extensions in the form of leaflets that are free of organelles but rich in filamentous matter of the actomyosin type [Figs. 27-29; (185, 186)]. These leaflets are the advancing edge of the cells by which they move forward, dragging the main part of the cells behind. Interstitial macrophages also have such extensions by which they move through interstices of the connective tissue in much the same way. The movement of macrophages is directed by chemotaxins (52, 212).

The capacity to ingest fluid and particulate matter also seems related to motility of the cell periphery (185). The macrophage forms cytoplasmic flaps, which enwrap the extracellular material (Fig. 31A); the lips of the pocket thus generated close and the membranes fuse, releasing into the cytoplasm a phagosome bounded by a membrane. This particle is translocated into the interior of the cell, probably by the action of

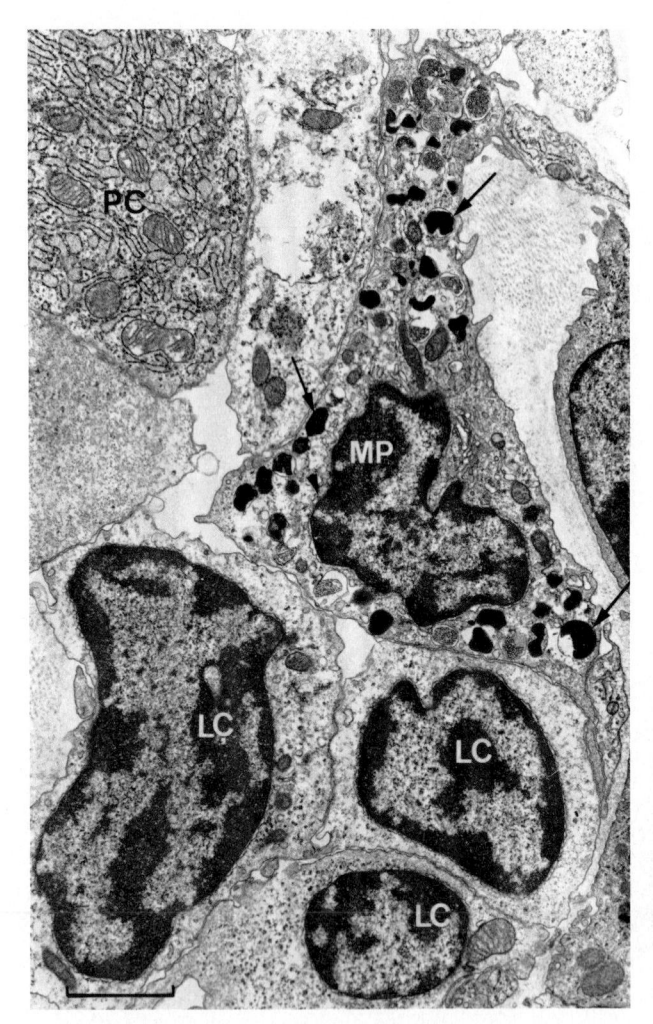

FIG. 30. Interstitial macrophage (*MP*) from human lung contains heterogeneous dark material in phagolysosomes or residual bodies (*arrows*). Macrophage is in group of free cells with lymphocytes (*LC*) and plasma cell (*PC*). *Bar*, 2 μm.

factant removal, but how important this is in quantitative terms is not clear. On the other hand, alveolar macrophages have some capability of synthesizing phospholipids, but this capability differs considerably from that of type II epithelial cells, both quantitatively and qualitatively (123, 171).

Not all materials ingested by macrophages are accessible to digestion by lysosomal enzymes. Macrophages sequester inorganic dust particles, carbon, asbestos, and silica but do not modify these materials. The dust particles are eliminated if the macrophage containing them leaves the lung via the airways. How-

contractile filaments; primary lysosomes originating in the GERL fuse with the phagosome and release their enzyme content into its interior, thus initiating intracellular digestion of the phagocytosed material. The fate of the phagolysosome depends on its content, which is very heterogeneous, including foreign bodies such as dust particles or bacteria and endogenous material. Organic material can be broken down to small molecular units that can partly be reutilized. For example, alveolar macrophages ingest large portions of the material of the surface lining layer; the phagosome then contains tubular myelin (Fig. 31*B*), which is disassembled by various hydrolytic enzymes common in lysosomes. Many intracellular granules of alveolar macrophages contain lamellar osmiophilic material, probably phospholipids resulting from surfactant resolution. The role of alveolar macrophages in surfactant metabolism is not completely understood. They seem to constitute one pathway for sur-

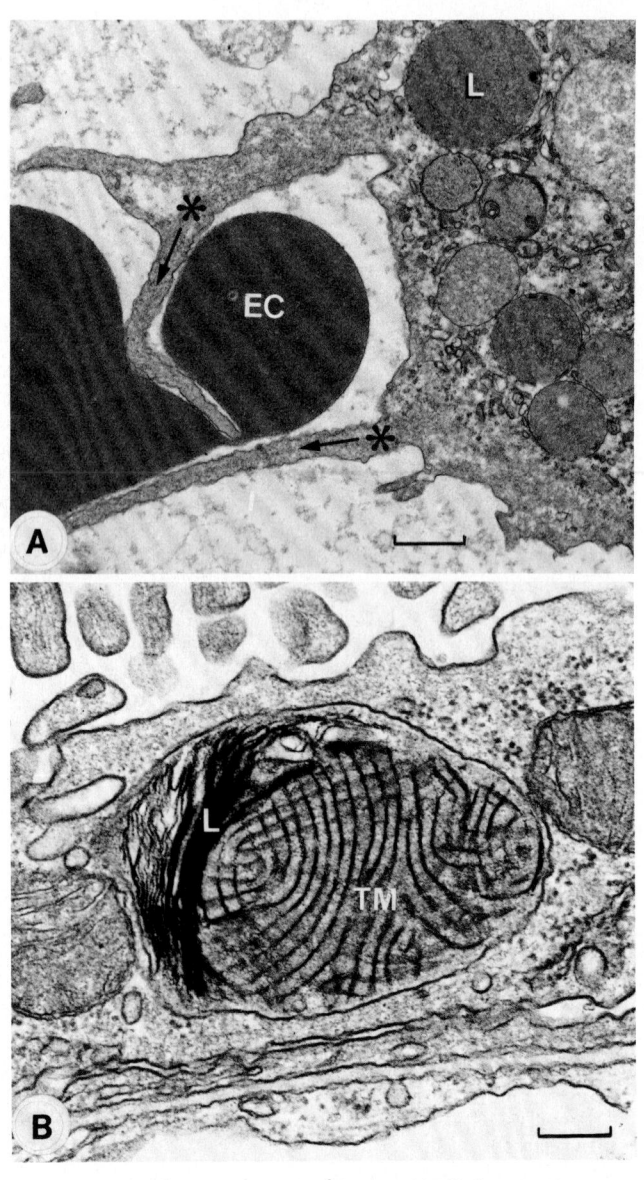

FIG. 31. *A*: phagocytosis of erythrocyte (*EC*) by alveolar macrophage. Ectoplasmic "lips" (*asterisks*) are pinching off fragment. *B*: phagolysosome may contain tubular myelin (*TM*) and lamellar (*L*) osmiophilic material, possibly the result of enzymatic disassembly of surface lining material. *Bars*: 1 μm (*A*); 0.2 μm (*B*).

ever, an unknown fraction of such foreign material is transferred to the interstitial space from where there are no routes for elimination; the particle is sequestered and stored in cytoplasmic vacuoles of histiocytes. The fate of these cells is varied, depending partly on the material contained: some cells are deposited in the connective tissue of peribronchial sheaths and interlobular septa; others enter the lymphatics and are sequestered in lymph nodes. Two points are uncertain in respect to this storage of inorganic particles. *1)* How do they get from the alveolar into the interstitial space? Alveolar macrophages are probably first to intercept them: do these cells traverse the epithelium and migrate into the interstitium, or do they transfer their indigestible material to other cells in the interstitium? *2)* What is the turnover rate of particle-laden histiocytes? Do they retain their particles indefinitely, or do they (perhaps because of cell damage) release them into the interstitial space to be taken up by new cells? The answers to these questions are important because of the tissue damage caused by such particles, which often results in pneumoconiosis.

The origin and the interrelation of alveolar and interstitial macrophages have long been debated. For some time it has been maintained that alveolar macrophages may be derived from type II epithelial cells; there is little strong evidence supporting this view; much data indicate instead that these cells are metabolically clearly different (123, 171), despite superficial resemblances, such as the content in lamellar phospholipid granules. On the other hand the evidence indicating that alveolar macrophages derive directly or indirectly from monocytes and thus originate in the bone marrow is increasingly convincing (30). A recent series of studies that used [³H]thymidine to estimate DNA synthesis and colchicine to arrest cells in mitosis showed that alveolar macrophages are probably renewed from blood monocytes by a two-stage process involving an intermediate stage in the interstitium (28). An increased demand for macrophages, induced by carbon loading of the airways, is first met by an accelerated egress of blood monocytes into the pulmonary interstitium and then onto the alveolar surface; in a second phase, interstitial cells go through the cell cycle and divide (3). Whether alveolar macrophages simply pass through the interstitium or whether a division of interstitial cells is required to prime them is not certain. From such convincing studies it appears that pulmonary macrophages are of hematopoietic origin and that the need for increased phagocytic activity requires a sequence of events: increased monocyte production in the bone marrow, accelerated egress of monocytes into the pulmonary interstitium, and finally an increased rate of interstitial cell division from where alveolar macrophages are recruited. There may also be some limited cell proliferation within the alveolar macrophage population.

Phagocytosis is not limited to specialized macrophages; other cells, such as neutrophil granulocytes, share this capacity (178). Under certain circumstances even type I epithelial cells can engage in phagocytosis of foreign material (178).

Cells of Immune Defense System

The pulmonary interstitium contains a variable amount of cells of the immune defense system, notably lymphocytes and plasma cells. The lymphocytes have a small compact nucleus surrounded by a narrow shell of cytoplasm, which has a few small mitochondria, a Golgi complex, and some free ribosomes but very little ER (Fig. 30). Based on their function, two classes of lymphocytes are differentiated (for review see refs. 80, 89): B cells generate immunoglobulins and thus are related to plasma cells and humoral defense through antibodies; T cells exert their defense function through their cell membrane, which carries receptors that allow the T lymphocyte to bind to cells bearing certain antigens. The T cells are the principal mediators of tissue incompatibility.

In plasma cells the cytoplasm is abundant and filled with cisternae of RER (Fig. 32). These cisternae are the site of immunoglobulin synthesis; it is well established that each plasma cell makes one specific antibody for which it has been programmed in germinal centers of lymphatic nodules, either in lymph nodes or in lymphoepithelial tissue (80).

Immune defense cells are commonly assembled at strategically favorable sites. Thus they are concentrated along the conducting air passages where the major part of noxious intruders (dust particles and airborne bacteria) are intercepted. This so-called bronchus-associated lymphoid tissue (BALT) serves a function similar to that of the lymphoid tissue of the gastrointestinal tract (18–20). Through this tissue a complete chain of the immune defense system is at the disposal of the lung, because germinal centers forming in the lymph nodules of BALT probably serve as programming centers for plasma cells against antigens that enter the body via the airways (18, 20, 95). Such local programming appears to provide a more effective defense against airborne infections than that through the general lymphatic system of the body; however, immunoglobulin A (IgA) cells can apparently distribute between the lymphoid tissues associated with gut and bronchi (20).

Immune defense cells decrease in density from the larger bronchi to the bronchioles, and lymphocytes and plasma cells are rarely encountered in lung parenchyma, except in juxta-alveolar connective tissue beds, which contain lymphatics and a variety of free interstitial cells. There, as in other places, lymphocytes are often associated with macrophages (Fig. 30); this may be related to the mediator function that macrophages may play in programming immunocompetent cells for synthesis of specific antibodies (165, 194).

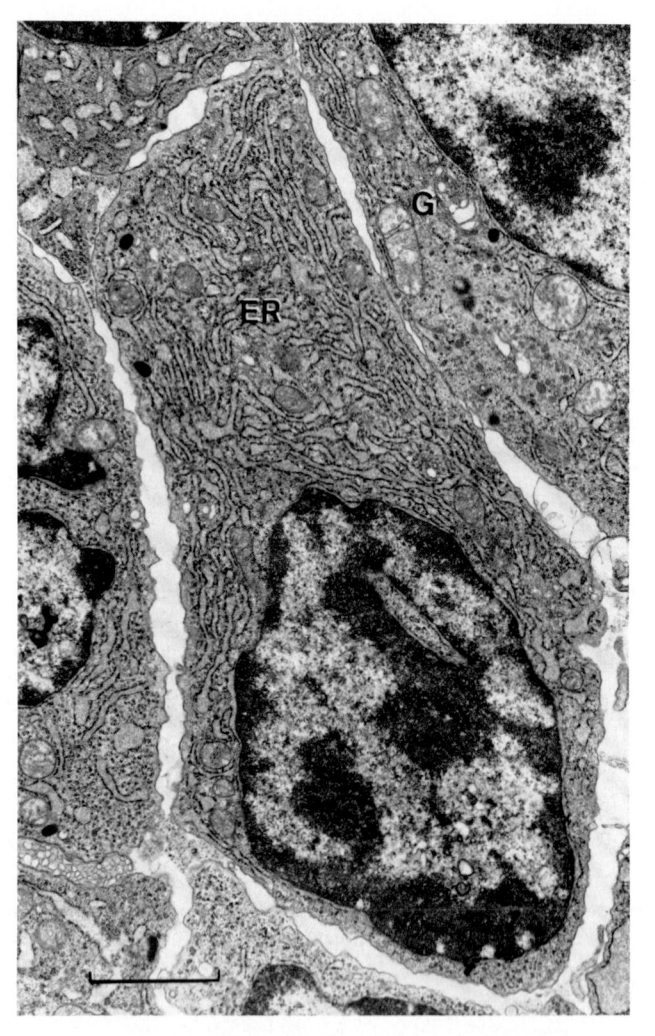

FIG. 32. Plasma cell from small rat lymph node contains massive rough endoplasmic reticulum (*ER*). Golgi complexes (*G*) are in adjacent plasma cell. *Bar*, 2 μm.

Besides the obvious abundance of such cells in lymph nodes one other location of immunocompetent cells is noteworthy. Groups of plasma cells are closely associated with the glandular acini and ducts in the small bronchial glands; probably these cells produce secretory antibodies similar to those made in salivary glands (78, 127, 132). The IgA made by these glandular plasma cells is transferred to the secretory cells, which link them to a polypeptide called secretory piece and prepare them for secretion onto the airway surface. Secretory plasma cells of salivary glands are programmed in germinal centers of Peyer's plaques, the major constituents of mucosal lymphoid tissue of the intestine, from where they leave by the bloodstream to "home" eventually in the salivary gland interstitium (127). Whether a similar mechanism is effective in the lung, i.e., whether plasma cells programmed in BALT can specifically "home" in bronchial mucous glands, is not known.

Granulocytes

In order to complete the list of cells of the defense system that may transiently settle in the lung, it should be mentioned that granulocytes, particularly eosinophils and neutrophils, are regularly found (though in small number) in places where other free cells also occur, particularly in the wall of bronchi. They very rarely occur in the alveolar septal interstitium, however.

Granulocytes are found on lung sections as constituents of the blood (see Fig. 13*B*) and often appear to be sticking to the vascular endothelium. Under the effect of chemotactic substances, partly secreted by macrophages or by lymphocytes, these cells may migrate into the tissue, traversing the endothelium; neutrophils are known to have ameboid mobility. Greater numbers of neutrophils in the tissue are a sign of inflammatory reaction, a great danger for the integrity of lung tissue because neutrophils are able to secrete into their environment a variety of hydrolytic enzymes, such as proteases and in particular elastase, which can damage the delicate supporting tissue. Eosinophils commonly are enriched in allergic diseases.

MESOTHELIAL CELLS OF PLEURA

The cells that form a squamous epithelial lining of both the visceral and parietal pleura and thus bound the pleural space have received little attention. These cells derive from the celomic epithelium of the embryo and thus are genetically identical to the cells bounding the peritoneal and pericardial cavities.

The mesothelium is a single layer of flattened polygonal cells that are joined by the usual junctional complexes of tight junctions and some desmosomes; the degree of tightness of these junctions is not well defined. At the apical surface the cells form numerous slender and long microvilli that show considerable regional variations (111, 118). The cytoplasm of mesothelial cells is rich in ER, which suggests a high level of synthetic activity, possibly related to the formation of pleural fluid. Little is known about the metabolic activity of these cells, which appear to have some capacity for phagocytosis, at least when stimulated with foreign material in tissue culture (95).

Mesothelial cells form a relatively small fraction of lung cells. They merit more attention, however, if only because such cells may be important contaminants of lung cell cultures, particularly those obtained from peripheral strips of lung parenchyma, which tend to enrich such cells merely by the process of tissue selection.

The author's work was supported by grants from the Swiss National Science Foundation.

The help of Gayle Kaufman, Gertrud Reber, Karl Babl, Fabienne Doffey, and Marianne Rüfenacht in preparing this review is gratefully acknowledged.

REFERENCES

1. ADAMSON, I. Y. R., AND D. H. BOWDEN. The intracellular site of surfactant synthesis: autoradiographic studies on murine and avian lung explants. *Exp. Mol. Pathol.* 18: 112–124, 1973.
2. ADAMSON, I. Y. R., AND D. H. BOWDEN. The type 2 cell as progenitor of alveolar epithelial regeneration. A cytodynamic study in mice after exposure to oxygen. *Lab. Invest.* 30: 35–42, 1974.
3. ADAMSON, I. Y. R., AND D. H. BOWDEN. Role of monocytes and interstitial cells in the generation of alveolar macrophages. II. Kinetic studies after carbon loading. *Lab. Invest.* 42: 518–524, 1980.
4. AFZELIUS, B. A. The immotile-cilia syndrome and other ciliary diseases. *Int. Rev. Exp. Pathol.* 19: 1–43, 1979.
5. ASHTON, F. T., A. V. SOMLYO, AND A. P. SOMLYO. The contractile apparatus of vascular smooth muscle: intermediate high voltage stereo electron microscopy. *J. Mol. Biol.* 98: 17–29, 1975.
6. ASKIN, F. B., AND C. KUHN. The cellular origin of pulmonary surfactant. *Lab. Invest.* 25: 260–268, 1971.
7. ATWAL, O. S., AND L. M. BROWN. Membrane-bound glycoprotein in the alveolar cells of the caprine lung. *Am. J. Anat.* 159: 275–283, 1980.
8. BACHOFEN, M., AND E. R. WEIBEL. Alterations of the gas exchange apparatus in adult respiratory insufficiency associated with septicemia. *Am. Rev. Respir. Dis.* 116: 589–615, 1977.
9. BAKHLE, Y. S., AND J. R. VANE (editors). *Lung Biology in Health and Disease. Metabolic Functions of the Lung.* New York: Dekker, 1977, vol. 4.
10. BARTELS, H. The air-blood barrier in the human lung. A freeze-fracture study. *Cell Tissue Res.* 198: 269–285, 1979.
11. BARTELS, H. Freeze-fracture demonstration of communicating junctions between interstitial cells of the pulmonary interalveolar septa. *Am. J. Anat.* 155: 125–129, 1979.
12. BARTELS, H., H. J. OESTERN, AND G. VOSS-WERMBTER. Communicating-occluding junction complexes in the alveolar epithelium. A freeze-fracture study. *Am. Rev. Respir. Dis.* 121: 1017–1024, 1980.
13. BASERGA, R. (editor). *Multiplication and Division in Mammalian Cells.* New York: Dekker, 1976, vol. 6. (Biochem. Dis. Ser.)
14. BATENBURG, J. J. Isolated type II cells from fetal lung as model in studies on the synthesis and secretion of pulmonary surfactant. *Lung* 158: 177–192, 1980.
15. BATENBURG, J. J., M. POST, V. OLDENBORG, AND L. M. G. VAN GOLDE. The perfused isolated lung as a possible model for the study of lipid synthesis by type II cells in their natural environment. *Exp. Lung Res.* 1: 57–65, 1980.
16. BELTON, J. C., D. BRANTON, H. V. THOMAS, AND P. K. MUELLER. Freeze-etch observations of rat lung. *Anat. Rec.* 170: 471–483, 1971.
17. BENSCH, K. G., G. B. GORDON, AND L. R. MILLER. Studies on the bronchial counterpart of the Kulchitzky (argentaffin) cell and innervation of bronchial glands. *J. Ultrastruct. Res.* 12: 668–686, 1965.
18. BIENENSTOCK, J., R. L. CLANCY, AND D. Y. E. PEREY. Bronchus associated lymphoid tissue (BALT): its relation to mucosal immunity. In: *Immunologic and Infectious Reactions in the Lung*, edited by C. H. Kirkpatrick and H. Y. Reynolds. New York: Dekker, 1976, p. 29–58.
19. BIENENSTOCK, J., N. JOHNSTON, AND D. Y. E. PEREY. Bronchial lymphoid tissue. I. Morphometric characteristics. *Lab. Invest.* 28: 686–691, 1973.
20. BIENENSTOCK, J., M. MCDERMOTT, D. BEFUS, AND M. O'NEILL. A common mucosal immunologic system involving the bronchus, breast and bowel. *Adv. Exp. Med. Biol.* 107: 53–59, 1978.
21. BLOBEL, G. Synthesis and segregation of secretory proteins: the signal hypothesis. In: *International Cell Biology, 1976–1977*, edited by B. R. Brinkley and K. R. Porter. New York: Rockefeller Univ. Press, 1977, p. 318–325.
22. BLOBEL, G. Intracellular protein topogenesis. *Proc. Natl. Acad. Sci. USA* 77: 1496–1500, 1980.
23. BOLENDER, R. P., D. PAUMGARTNER, G. LOSA, D. MUELLENER, AND E. R. WEIBEL. Integrated stereological and biochemical studies on hepatocytic membranes. I. Membrane recoveries in subcellular fractions. *J. Cell Biol.* 77: 565–583, 1978.
24. BOORMAN, G. A., L. W. SCHWARTZ, AND D. L. DUNGWORTH. Pulmonary effects of prolonged ozone insult in rats: morphometric evaluation of the central acinus. *Lab. Invest.* 43: 108–115, 1980.
25. BOREN, H. G., AND L. J. PARADISE. Cytokinetics of lung. In: *Lung Biology in Health and Disease. Pathogenesis and Therapy of Lung Cancer*, edited by C. C. Harris. New York: Dekker, 1978, vol. 10, chapt. 7, p. 369–418.
26. BOUHUYS, A. (editor). *Lung Cells in Disease.* Amsterdam: North-Holland, 1976.
27. BOUHUYS, A. Action and interaction of pharmacological agents on airway smooth muscle. In: *The Biochemistry of Smooth Muscle*, edited by N. L. Stephens. Baltimore, MD: University Park, 1977, p. 703–722.
28. BOWDEN, D. H., AND I. Y. ADAMSON. Role of monocytes and interstitial cells in the generation of alveolar macrophages. I. Kinetic studies in normal mice. *Lab. Invest.* 42: 511–517, 1980.
29. BRADLEY, K. H., O. KAWANAMI, V. J. FERRANS, AND R. G. CRYSTAL. The fibroblast of human lung alveolar structures: a differentiated cell with a major role in lung structure and function. *Methods Cell Biol.* 21A: 37–64, 1980.
30. BRAIN, J. D., J. J. GODLESKI, AND S. P. SOROKIN. Quantification, origin, and fate of pulmonary macrophages. In: *Lung Biology in Health and Disease. Respiratory Defense Mechanisms*, edited by J. D. Brain, D. F. Proctor, and L. M. Reid. New York: Dekker, 1977, vol. 5, pt. II, chapt. 20, p. 849–892.
31. BRINKLEY, B. R., AND K. R. PORTER (editors). *International Cell Biology, 1976–1977.* New York: Rockefeller Univ. Press, 1977.
32. BRUNS, R. R., AND G. E. PALADE. Studies on blood capillaries. II. Transport of ferritin molecules across the wall of muscle capillaries. *J. Cell Biol.* 37: 277–299, 1968.
33. BUCKINGHAM, S., H. O. HEINEMANN, S. C. SOMMERS, AND W. F. MCNARY. Phospholipid synthesis in the large pulmonary alveolar cells. *Am. J. Pathol.* 48: 1027–1041, 1966.
34. BÜLBRING, E., A. F. BRADING, A. W. JONES, AND T. TOMITA (editors). *Smooth Muscle: An Assessment of Current Knowledge.* Austin: Univ. of Texas Press, 1981.
35. BURNSTOCK, G. Development of smooth muscle and its innervation. In: *Smooth Muscle: An Assessment of Current Knowledge*, edited by E. Bülbring, A. F. Brading, A. W. Jones, and T. Tomita. Austin: Univ. of Texas Press, 1981, p. 431–457.
36. BURRI, P. H. The postnatal growth of the rat lung. III. Morphology. *Anat. Rec.* 180: 77–98, 1974.
38. BURRI, P. H., AND E. R. WEIBEL. The ultrastructure and morphometry of the developing lung. In: *Lung Biology in Health and Disease. Development of the Lung*, edited by W. A. Hodson. New York: Dekker, 1977, vol. 6, chapt. 5, p. 215–268.
39. CALDWELL, P. R. B., B. C. SEEGAL, K. C. HSU, M. DAS, AND R. L. SOFFER. Angiotensin converting enzyme: vascular endothelial localization. *Science* 191: 1050–1051, 1976.
40. CASTEELS, R. Membrane potential in smooth muscle cells. In: *Smooth Muscle: An Assessment of Current Knowledge*, edited by E. Bülbring, A. F. Brading, A. W. Jones, and T. Tomita. Austin: Univ. of Texas Press, 1981, p. 105–126.
41. CASTLE, J. D., J. D. JAMIESON, AND G. E. PALADE. Radioautographic analysis of the secretory process in the parotid acinar cell of the rabbit. *J. Cell Biol.* 53: 290–311, 1973.
42. CHEVALIER, G., AND A. J. COLLET. In vivo incorporation of choline-^{3}H, leucine-^{3}H, and galactose-^{3}H in alveolar type II pneumocytes in relation to surfactant synthesis. A quantitative radioautographic study in mouse by electron microscopy. *Anat. Rec.* 174: 289–310, 1972.
43. CLEMENTS, J. A., AND R. KING. Composition of surface active

material. In: *Lung Biology in Health and Disease. The Biochemical Basis of Pulmonary Function*, edited by R. G. Crystal. New York: Dekker, 1976, vol. 2, chapt. 10, p. 363–387.
44. COOKE, P. A filamentous cytoskeleton in vertebrate smooth muscle fibers. *J. Cell Biol.* 68: 539–556, 1976.
45. COUPLAND, R. E. *The Natural History of the Chromaffin Cell.* London: Longman, 1965.
46. COUPLAND, R. E., AND T. FUJITA (editors). *Chromaffin, Enterochromaffin and Related Cells.* Amsterdam: Elsevier, 1976. (NATO Found. Symp.)
47. CRAPO, J. D., B. E. BARRY, H. A. FOSCUE, AND J. SHELBURNE. Structural and biochemical changes in rat lung occurring during exposure to lethal and adaptive doses of oxygen. *Am. Rev. Respir. Dis.* 122: 123–143, 1980.
48. CRAPO, J. D., B. E. BARRY, P. GEHR, M. BACHOFEN, AND E. R. WEIBEL. Cell numbers and cell characteristics of the normal human lung. *Am. Rev. Respir. Dis.* 125: 332–337, 1982.
49. CRAPO, J. D., J. MARSH-SALIN, P. INGRAM, AND P. C. PRATT. Tolerance and cross-tolerance using NO_2 and O_2. II. Pulmonary morphology and morphometry. *J. Appl. Physiol.: Respirat. Environ. Exercise Physiol.* 44: 370–379, 1978.
50. CUTZ, E., W. CHAN, V. WONG, AND P. E. CONEN. Endocrine cells in rat fetal lungs. Ultrastructural and histochemical study. *Lab. Invest.* 30: 458–464, 1974.
51. DARRAH, H. K., AND J. HEDLEY-WHYTE. Rapid incorporation of palmitate into lung: site and metabolic fate. *J. Appl. Physiol.* 34: 205–213, 1973.
52. DAUBER, J. H., AND R. P. DANIELE. Secretion of chemotaxins by guinea pig lung macrophages. I. The spectrum of inflammatory cell responses. *Exp. Lung Res.* 1: 23–32, 1980.
53. DEVEREUX, T. R., AND J. R. FOUTS. Isolation and identification of Clara cells from rabbit lung. *In Vitro* 16: 958–968, 1980.
54. DEVEREUX, T. R., AND J. R. FOUTS. Xenobiotic metabolism by alveolar type II cells isolated from rabbit lung. *Biochem. Pharmacol.* 30: 1231–1237, 1981.
55. DEVEREUX, T. R., G. E. R. HOOK, AND J. R. FOUTS. Foreign compound metabolism by isolated cells from rabbit lung. *Drug Metab. Dispos.* 7: 70–75, 1979.
56. DEY, R. D., R. ECHT, AND R. J. DINERSTEIN. Morphology, histochemistry and distribution of serotonin-containing cells in tracheal epithelium of adult rabbit. *Anat. Rec.* 199: 23–31, 1981.
57. DIGLIO, C. A., AND Y. KIKKAWA. The type II epithelial cells of the lung. IV. Adaptation and behavior of type II cells in culture. *Lab. Invest.* 37: 622–631, 1977.
58. DOUGLAS, W. H., J. A. MCATEER, J. R. SMITH, AND W. R. BRAUNSCHWEIGER. Type II alveolar pneumonocytes in vitro. *Int. Rev. Cytol.* 10: 45–65, 1979.
59. DOUGLAS, W. H., R. L. SANDERS, AND K. R. HITCHCOCK. Maintenance of human and rat pulmonary type II cells in an organotypic culture system. *Methods Cell Biol.* 21A: 79–94, 1980.
60. EDMONDSON, N. A., AND D. J. LEWIS. Distribution and ultrastructural characteristics of Feyrter cells in the rat and hamster airway epithelium. *Thorax* 35: 371–374, 1980.
61. ETHERTON, J. E., AND D. M. CONNING. Enzyme histochemistry of the lung. In: *Lung Biology in Health and Disease. Metabolic Functions of the Lung*, edited by Y. S. Bakhle and J. R. Vane. New York: Dekker, 1977, vol. 4, chapt. 8, p. 233–258.
62. EVANS, J. N., AND K. B. ADLER. The lung strip: evaluation of a method to study contractility of pulmonary parenchyma. *Exp. Lung Res.* 2: 187–195, 1981.
63. EVANS, M. J., L. J. CABRAL, R. J. STEPHENS, AND G. FREEMAN. Transformation of alveolar type 2 cells to type 1 cells following exposure to NO_2. *Exp. Mol. Pathol.* 22: 142–150, 1975.
64. EVANS, M. J., L. J. CABRAL-ANDERSON, AND G. FREEMAN. Role of the Clara cell in renewal of the bronchiolar epithelium. *Lab. Invest.* 38: 648–655, 1978.
65. FISHER, A. B., AND G. G. PIETRA. Comparison of serotonin uptake from the alveolar and capillary spaces of isolated rat lungs. *Am. Rev. Respir. Dis.* 123: 74–78, 1981.
66. FOLIQUET, B., AND L. ROMANOVA. Le pneumocyte de type III de l'alvéole pulmonaire de rat. *Biol. Cell.* 38: 221–224, 1980.
67. FOX, B., T. B. BULL, AND A. GUZ. Innervation of alveolar walls in the human lung: an electron microscopic study. *J. Anat.* 131: 683–692, 1980.
68. GABBIANI, G., B. J. HIRSCHEL, G. B. RYAN, P. R. STATKOV, AND G. MAJNO. Granulation tissue as a contractile organ. A study of structure and function. *J. Exp. Med.* 135: 719–734, 1972.
69. GABELLA, G. Structure of smooth muscle cells. In: *Smooth Muscle: An Assessment of Current Knowledge*, edited by E. Bülbring, A. F. Brading, A. W. Jones, and T. Tomita. Austin: Univ. of Texas Press, 1981, p. 1–46.
70. GEE, J. B. L., AND A. S. KHANDWALA. Motility, transport, and endocytosis in lung defense cells. In: *Lung Biology in Health and Disease. Respiratory Defense Mechanisms*, edited by J. D. Brain, D. F. Proctor, and L. M. Reid. New York: Dekker, 1977, vol. 5, pt. II, chapt. 22, p. 927–981.
71. GIL, J., AND J. M. MCNIFF. Interstitial cells at the boundary between alveolar and extraalveolar connective tissue in the lung. *J. Ultrastruct. Res.* 76: 149–157, 1981.
72. GIL, J., AND O. K. REISS. Isolation and characterization of lamellar bodies and tubular myelin from rat lung homogenates. *J. Cell Biol.* 58: 152–171, 1973.
73. GIL, J., D. A. SILAGE, AND J. M. MCNIFF. Distribution of vesicles in cells of air-blood barrier in the rabbit. *J. Appl. Physiol.: Respirat. Environ. Exercise Physiol.* 50: 334–340, 1981.
74. GIL, J., AND E. R. WEIBEL. Extracellular lining of bronchioles after perfusion fixation of rat lungs for electron microscopy. *Anat. Rec.* 169: 185–199, 1971.
75. GILULA, N. B. Gap junctions and cell communication. In: *International Cell Biology, 1976–1977*, edited by B. R. Brinkley and K. R. Porter. New York: Rockefeller Univ. Press, 1977, p. 61–69.
76. GMELICH, J. T., K. G. BENSCH, AND A. A. LIEBOW. Cells of Kultschitzky type in bronchioles and their relation to the origin of peripheral carcinoid tumor. *Lab. Invest.* 17: 88–98, 1967.
77. GOLDFISCHER, S., Y. KIKKAWA, AND L. HOFFMAN. The demonstration of acid hydrolase activities in the inclusion bodies of type II alveolar cells and other lysosomes in the rabbit lung. *J. Histochem. Cytochem.* 16: 102–109, 1968.
78. GOODMAN, M. R., D. W. LINK, W. R. BROWN, AND P. K. NAKANE. Ultrastructural evidence of transport of secretory IgA across bronchial epithelium. *Am. Rev. Respir. Dis.* 123: 115–119, 1981.
79. GOULD, K. G. Dispersal of lung into individual viable cells. In: *Lung Biology in Health and Disease. The Biochemical Basis of Pulmonary Function*, edited by R. G. Crystal. New York: Dekker, 1976, vol. 2, chapt. 2, p. 49–71.
80. GREEN, G. M., G. J. JAKAB, R. B. LOW, AND G. S. DAVIS. Defense mechanisms of the respiratory membrane. *Am. Rev. Respir. Dis.* 115: 479–514, 1977.
81. HAGE, E. Light and electron microscopic characteristics of the various lung endocrine cell types. *Invest. Cell Pathol.* 3: 345–351, 1980.
82. HAIES, D. M., J. GIL, AND E. R. WEIBEL. Morphometric study of rat lung cells. I. Numerical and dimensional characteristics of parenchymal cell population. *Am. Rev. Respir. Dis.* 123: 533–541, 1981.
83. HALLMAN, M., AND L. GLUCK. Phosphatidylglycerol in lung surfactant. II. Subcellular distribution and mechanism of biosynthesis in vitro. *Biochim. Biophys. Acta* 409: 172–191, 1975.
84. HANCE, A. J., AND R. G. CRYSTAL. Collagen. In: *Lung Biology in Health and Disease. The Biochemical Basis of Pulmonary Function*, edited by R. G. Crystal. New York: Dekker, 1976, vol. 2, chapt. 7, p. 215–271.
85. HASSETT, R. J., W. ENGELMAN, AND C. KUHN. Extramem-

branous particles in tubular myelin from rat lung. *J. Ultrastruct. Res.* 71: 60–67, 1980.
86. HITCHCOCK, K. R. Lung development and the pulmonary surfactant system: hormonal influences. *Anat. Rec.* 198: 13–34, 1980.
87. HITCHCOCK-O'HARE, K. R., E. MEYMARIS, J. BONACCORSO, AND S. B. VANBUREN. Separation and partial characterization of surface-active fractions from mouse and rat lung homogenates. Identification of a possible marker system for pulmonary surfactant. *J. Histochem. Cytochem.* 24: 487–507, 1976.
88. HOGG, J. C., P. D. PARÉ, AND R. C. BOUCHER. Bronchial mucosal permeability. *Federation Proc.* 38: 197–201, 1979.
89. HOOD, L. E., J. H. WILSON, AND W. B. WOOD. *The Molecular Biology of Eukaryotic Cells.* Menlo Park, CA: Benjamin, 1975.
90. HORWITZ, A. L., N. A. ELSON, AND R. G. CRYSTAL. Proteoglycans and elastic fibers. In: *Lung Biology in Health and Disease. The Biochemical Basis of Pulmonary Function*, edited by R. G. Crystal. New York: Dekker, 1976, vol. 2, chapt. 8., p. 273–311.
91. HUNG, K. S. Innervation of rabbit fetal lungs. *Am. J. Anat.* 159: 73–83, 1980.
92. HUNG, K. S., A. L. CHAPMAN, AND M. A. MESTEMACHER. Scanning electron microscopy of bronchiolar neuroepithelial bodies in neonatal mouse lungs. *Anat. Rec.* 193: 913–926, 1979.
93. INOUÉ, S., R. P. MICHEL, AND J. HOGG. Zonulae occludentes in alveolar epithelium of dog lungs studied with the freeze-fracture technique. *J. Ultrastruct. Res.* 56: 215–225, 1976.
94. JAMIESON, J. D., AND G. E. PALADE. Production of secretory proteins in animal cells. In: *International Cell Biology, 1976–1977*, edited by B. R. Brinkley and K. R. Porter. New York: Rockefeller Univ. Press, 1977, p. 308–317.
95. JAURAND, M. C., H. KAPLAN, J. THIOLLET, M. C. PINCHON, J. F. BERNAUDIN, AND J. BIGNON. Phagocytosis of chrysotile fibers by pleural mesothelial cells in culture. *Am. J. Pathol.* 94: 529–538, 1979.
96. JEFFERY, P. K., AND L. M. REID. The respiratory mucous membrane. In: *Lung Biology in Health and Disease. Respiratory Defense Mechanisms*, edited by J. D. Brain, D. F. Proctor, and L. M. Reid. New York: Dekker, 1977, vol. 5, pt. I, chapt. 7, p. 193–245.
97. JOBE, A., E. KIRKPATRICK, AND L. GLUCK. Labeling of phospholipids in the surfactant and subcellular fractions of rabbit lung. *J. Biol. Chem.* 253: 3810–3816, 1978.
98. JOHANSSON, A., AND P. CAMNER. Are alveolar macrophages translocated to the lymph nodes? *Toxicology* 15: 157–162, 1980.
99. KALTREIDER, H. B., AND S. E. SALMON. Immunology of the lower respiratory tract. Functional properties of bronchioalveolar lymphocytes obtained from the normal canine lung. *J. Clin. Invest.* 52: 2211–2217, 1973.
100. KAPANCI, Y., A. ASSIMACOPOULOS, C. IRLE, A. ZWAHLEN, AND G. GABBIANI. "Contractile interstitial cells" in pulmonary alveolar septa. A possible regulator of ventilation/perfusion ratio? Ultrastructural immunofluorescence and in vitro studies. *J. Cell Biol.* 60: 375–392, 1974.
101. KAPANCI, Y., P. M. COSTABELLA, P. CERUTTI, AND A. ASSIMACOPOULOS. Distribution and function of cytoskeletal proteins in lung cells with particular reference to "contractile interstitial cells." *Methods Achiev. Exp. Pathol.* 9: 147–168, 1979.
102. KAPANCI, Y., P. M. COSTABELLA, AND G. GABBIANI. Location and function of contractile interstitial cells of the lungs. In: *Lung Cells in Disease*, edited by A. Bouhuys. Amsterdam: North-Holland, 1976, p. 69–82.
103. KAUFFMAN, S. L. Cell proliferation in the mammalian lung. *Int. Rev. Exp. Pathol.* 22: 131–191, 1980.
104. KAUFFMAN, S. L., P. H. BURRI, AND E. R. WEIBEL. The postnatal growth of the rat lung. II. Autoradiography. *Anat. Rec.* 180: 63–76, 1974.
105. KAWANAMI, O., V. J. FERRANS, J. D. FULMER, AND R. G. CRYSTAL. Ultrastructure of pulmonary mast cells in patients with fibrotic lung disorders. *Lab. Invest.* 40: 717–734, 1979.

106. KIKKAWA, Y., AND K. YONEDA. The type II epithelial cells of the lung. I. Method of isolation. *Lab. Invest.* 30: 76–84, 1974.
107. KIKKAWA, Y., K. YONEDA, F. SMITH, B. PACKARD, AND K. SUZUKI. The type II epithelial cells of the lung. II. Chemical composition and phospholipid synthesis. *Lab. Invest.* 32: 295–302, 1975.
108. KING, R. J. Utilization of alveolar epithelial type II cells for the study of pulmonary surfactant. *Federation Proc.* 38: 2637–2643, 1979.
109. KING, R. J., H. MARTIN, D. MITTS, AND F. M. HOLMSTROM. Metabolism of the apoproteins in pulmonary surfactant. *J. Appl. Physiol.: Respirat. Environ. Exercise Physiol.* 42: 483–491, 1977.
110. KÖHLER, G., AND C. MILSTEIN. Continuous culture of fused cells secreting antibody of predefined specificity. *Nature London* 256: 495–497, 1975.
111. KUHN, C. The cells of the lung and their organelles. In: *Lung Biology in Health and Disease. The Biochemical Basis of Pulmonary Function*, edited by R. G. Crystal. New York: Dekker, 1976, vol. 2, chapt. 1, p. 3–48.
112. LAUWERYNS, J. M. The juxta-alveolar lymphatics in the human adult lung. *Am. Rev. Respir. Dis.* 102: 877–885, 1970.
113. LAUWERYNS, J. M., AND J. H. BAERT. Alveolar clearance and the role of pulmonary lymphatics. *Am. Rev. Respir. Dis.* 115: 625–683, 1977.
114. LAUWERYNS, J. M., M. COKELAERE, AND P. THEUNYNCK. Neuro-epithelial bodies in the respiratory mucosa of various mammals. A light optical, histochemical and ultrastructure investigation. *Z. Zellforsch. Mikrosk. Anat.* 135: 569–592, 1972.
115. LAUWERYNS, J. M., M. COKELAERE, AND P. THEUNYNCK. Serotonin producing neuroepithelial bodies in rabbit respiratory mucosa. *Science* 180: 410–413, 1973.
116. LEAK, L. V. Pulmonary lymphatics and their role in the removal of interstitial fluids and particulate matter. In: *Lung Biology in Health and Disease. Respiratory Defense Mechanisms*, edited by J. D. Brain, D. F. Proctor, and L. M. Reid. New York: Dekker, 1977, vol. 5, pt. II, chapt. 17, p. 631–685.
117. LEBLOND, C. P., AND A. BENNETT. Role of the Golgi apparatus in terminal glycosylation. In: *International Cell Biology, 1976–1977*, edited by B. R. Brinkley and K. R. Porter. New York: Rockefeller Univ. Press, 1977, p. 326–340.
118. LEESON, T. S. Visceral pleura of the adult rat lung. *Folia Morphol. Prague* 25: 25–33, 1977.
119. LIEBER, M., B. SMITH, A. SZAKAL, W. NELSON-REES, AND G. TODARO. A continuous tumor-cell line from a human lung carcinoma with properties of type II epithelial cells. *Int. J. Cancer* 17: 62–70, 1976.
120. LOEWENSTEIN, W. R. Junctional intercellular communication: the cell-to-cell membrane channel. *Physiol. Rev.* 61: 829–913, 1981.
121. LOW, F. N. The pulmonary alveolar epithelium of laboratory animals. *Anat. Rec.* 117: 241–263, 1953.
122. LUCIANO, L., E. REALE, AND H. RUSKA. Ueber eine "chemorezeptive" Zelle in der Trachea der Ratte. *Z. Zellforsch. Mikrosk. Anat.* 85: 350–375, 1968.
123. MASON, R. J. Metabolism of alveolar macrophages. In: *Lung Biology in Health and Disease. Respiratory Defense Mechanisms*, edited by J. D. Brain, D. F. Proctor, and L. M. Reid. New York: Dekker, 1977, vol. 5, pt. II, chapt. 21, p. 893–926.
124. MASSARO, D., AND G. D. MASSARO. Synthesis, intracellular transport and secretion of macromolecules by the lung. In: *Lung Biology in Health and Disease. The Biochemical Basis of Pulmonary Function*, edited by R. G. Crystal. New York: Dekker, 1976, vol. 2, chapt. 11, p. 389–416.
125. MASSARO, G. D., AND D. MASSARO. Granular pneumocytes: electron microscopic radioautographic evidence of intracellular protein transport. *Am. Rev. Respir. Dis.* 105: 927–931, 1972.
126. MAVIS, R. D., J. N. FINKELSTEIN, AND B. P. HALL. Pulmonary surfactant synthesis. A highly active microsomal phosphatidate phosphohydrolase in the lung. *J. Lipid Res.* 19: 467–477, 1978.

127. McGhee, J. R., J. Mestecky, and J. L. Babb (editors). *Secretory Immunity and Infection.* New York: Plenum, 1978. (Adv. Exp. Med. Biol. Ser., vol. 107.)
128. Meban, C. The inclusion bodies in granular pneumonocytes of hamster lung: a combined cytochemical and ultrastructural study. *J. Anat.* 112: 195–206, 1972.
129. Meban, C. Localization of phosphatidic acid phosphatase activity in granular pneumonocytes. *J. Cell Biol.* 53: 249–252, 1972.
130. Meyrick, B., and L. Reid. The alveolar brush cell in rat lung—a third pneumocyte. *J. Ultrastruct. Res.* 23: 71–80, 1968.
131. Meyrick, B., and L. Reid. Nerves in rat intra-acinar alveoli: an electron microscopic study. *Respir. Physiol.* 11: 367–377, 1971.
132. Montgomery, P. C., K. M. Connelly, J. Cohn, and C. A. Skandera. Remote-site stimulation of secretory IgA antibodies following bronchial and gastric stimulation. *Adv. Exp. Med. Biol.* 107: 113–122, 1978.
133. Nardone, L. L., and S. B. Andrews. Cell line A549 as a model of the type II penumocyte: phospholipid synthesis from native and organometallic precursors. *Biochim. Biophys. Acta* 573: 276–295, 1979.
134. Neutra, M., and C. P. Leblond. Synthesis of the carbohydrate of mucus in the Golgi complex as shown by electron microscope autoradiography of goblet cells from rats injected with glucose-H^3. *J. Cell Biol.* 30: 119–136, 1966.
135. Novikoff, A. B. The endoplasmic reticulum: a cytochemist's view (a review). *Proc. Natl. Acad. Sci. USA* 73: 2781–2787, 1976.
136. O'Brien, T. W. Transcription and translation in mitochondria. In: *International Cell Biology, 1976–1977,* edited by B. R. Brinkley and K. R. Porter. New York: Rockefeller Univ. Press, 1977, p. 245–255.
137. Ody, C., and A. F. Junod. Converting enzyme in endothelial cells isolated from pig pulmonary artery and aorta. *Am. J. Physiol.* 232 (*Cell Physiol.* 1): C95–C98, 1977.
138. O'Hare, K. H., O. K. Reiss, and A. E. Vatter. Esterases in developing and adult rat lung. I. Biochemical and electron microscopic observations. *J. Histochem. Cytochem.* 19: 97–115, 1971.
139. O'Hare, K. H., and P. L. Townes. Morphogenesis of albino rat lung: an autoradiographic analysis of the embryological origin of the type I and II pulmonary epithelial cells. *J. Morphol.* 132: 69–88, 1970.
140. Pack, R. J., L. H. Al-Ugaily, G. Morris, and J. G. Widdicombe. The distribution and structure of cells in the tracheal epithelium of the mouse. *Cell Tissue Res.* 208: 65–84, 1980.
141. Palade, G. E. Intracellular aspect of the process of protein synthesis. *Science* 189: 347–358, 1975.
142. Palade, G. E., M. Simionescu, and N. Simionescu. Structural aspects of the permeability of the microvascular endothelium. *Acta Physiol. Scand. Suppl.* 463: 11–32, 1979.
143. Palisano, J. R., and J. Kleinerman. APUD cells and neuroepithelial bodies in hamster lung: methods, quantitation, and response to injury. *Thorax* 35: 363–370, 1980.
144. Palmer, K. C., G. L. Snider, and J. A. Hayes. Cellular proliferation induced in lung by cadmium aerosol. *Am. Rev. Respir. Dis.* 112: 173–179, 1975.
145. Pearse, A. G. E. The cytochemistry and ultrastructure of polypeptide hormone-producing cells of the APUD series and the embryologic, physiologic and pathologic implications of the concept. *J. Histochem. Cytochem.* 17: 303–313, 1969.
146. Pinkstaff, C. A. The cytology of salivary glands. *Int. Rev. Cytol.* 63: 141–263, 1980.
147. Plopper, C. G., L. H. Hill, and A. T. Mariassy. Ultrastructure of the nonciliated bronchiolar epithelial (Clara) cell of mammalian lung. I–III. *Exp. Lung Res.* 1: 139–180, 1980.
148. Porter, K. R., and J. B. Turner. The ground substance of the living cell. *Sci. Am.* 244: 56–67, 1981.
149. Prockop, D. J. Collagen, elastin, and proteoglycans: matrix for fluid accumulation in the lung. In: *Pulmonary Edema,* edited by A. P. Fishman and E. M. Renkin. Bethesda, MD: Am. Physiol. Soc., 1979, chapt. 9, p. 125–135.
150. Racker, E. *A New Look at Mechanisms in Bioenergetics.* New York: Academic, 1976.
151. Rambourg, A., and C. P. Leblond. Electron microscope observations on the carbohydrate-rich cell coat present at the surface of cells in the rat. *J. Cell Biol.* 32: 27–53, 1967.
152. Reaven, E. P., and S. G. Axline. Subplasmalemmal microfilaments and microtubules in resting and phagocytizing cultivated macrophages. *J. Cell Biol.* 59: 12–27, 1973.
153. Rooney, S. A., B. A. Page-Roberts, and E. K. Motoyama. Role of lamellar inclusions in surfactant production: studies on phospholipid composition and biosynthesis in rat and rabbit lung, subcellular fractions. *J. Lipid Res.* 16: 418–425, 1975.
154. Ross, R. R., and E. P. Benditt. Wound healing and collagen formation. V. Quantitative electron microscope radioautographic observations of proline-H^3 utilization by fibroblasts. *J. Cell Biol.* 27: 83–106, 1965.
155. Rossman, C. M., J. B. Forrest, R. E. Ruffin, and M. T. Newhouse. Immotile cilia syndrome in persons with and without Kartagener's syndrome. *Am. Rev. Respir. Dis.* 121: 1011–1016, 1980.
156. Roth, J., M. Bendayan, and L. Orci. Ultrastructural localization of intracellular antigens by the use of protein-A-gold complex. *J. Histochem. Cytochem.* 26: 1074–1081, 1978.
157. Roth, J., H. Winkelmann, and H. W. Meyer. Electron microscopic studies in mammalian lungs by freeze-etching. IV. Formation of the superficial layer of the surfactant system by lamellar bodies. *Exp. Pathol.* 8: 354–362, 1973.
158. Ryan, U. S., and J. W. Ryan. Correlations between the fine structure of the alveolar-capillary unit and its metabolic activities. In: *Lung Biology in Health and Disease. Metabolic Functions of the Lung,* edited by Y. S. Bakhle and J. R. Vane. New York: Dekker, 1977, vol. 4, chapt. 7, p. 197–232.
159. Ryan, U. S., J. W. Ryan, C. Whitaker, and A. Chiu. Localization of angiotensin converting enzyme (kininase II). II. Immunocytochemistry and immunofluorescence. *Tissue Cell* 8: 125–145, 1976.
161. Schneeberger, E. E. Barrier function of intercellular junctions in adult and fetal lungs. In: *Pulmonary Edema,* edited by A. P. Fishman and E. M. Renkin. Bethesda MD: Am. Physiol. Soc., 1979, chapt. 2, p. 21–37.
162. Schneeberger, E. E. Heterogeneity of tight junction morphology in extrapulmonary and intrapulmonary airways of the rat. *Anat. Rec.* 198: 193–208, 1980.
163. Schneeberger, E. E., and M. J. Karnovsky. The ultrastructural basis of alveolar-capillary membrane permeability to peroxidase used as a tracer. *J. Cell Biol.* 37: 781–793, 1968.
164. Schneeberger, E. E., and M. J. Karnovsky. Substructure of intercellular junctions in freeze-fractured alveolar-capillary membranes of mouse lung. *Circ. Res.* 38: 404–411, 1976.
165. Schwartz, S. L., and J. A. Bellanti. The relationship of the alveolar macrophage to the immunologic responses of the lung. In: *Lung Biology in Health and Disease. Respiratory Defense Mechanisms,* edited by J. D. Brain, D. F. Proctor, and L. M. Reid. New York: Dekker, 1977, vol. 5, pt. II, chapt. 25, p. 1053–1074.
166. Simionescu, N., M. Simionescu, and G. E. Palade. Permeability of muscle capillaries to small heme-peptides. Evidence for the existence of patent transendothelial channels. *J. Cell Biol.* 64: 586–607, 1975.
167. Sleigh, M. A. The nature and action of respiratory tract cilia. In: *Lung Biology in Health and Disease. Respiratory Defense Mechanisms,* edited by J. D. Brain, D. F. Proctor, and L. M. Reid. New York: Dekker, 1977, vol. 5, pt. I, chapt. 8, p. 247–288.
168. Small, J. V. The contractile apparatus of the smooth muscle cell: structure and composition. In: *The Biochemistry of Smooth Muscle,* edited by N. L. Stephens. Baltimore, MD: University Park, 1977, p. 379–411.

169. SMALL, J. V. Studies on isolated smooth muscle. *J. Cell Sci.* 24: 327–349, 1977.
170. SMITH, D. S., U. SMITH, AND J. W. RYAN. Freeze-fractured lamellar body membranes of the rat lung great alveolar cell. *Tissue Cell* 4: 457–468, 1972.
171. SMITH, F. B., AND Y. KIKKAWA. The type II epithelial cells of the lung. III. Lecithin synthesis: a comparison with pulmonary macrophages. *Lab. Invest.* 38: 45–51, 1978.
172. SMITH, F. B., Y. KIKKAWA, C. A. DIGLIO, AND R. C. DALEN. The type II epithelial cells of the lung. VI. Incorporation of ^{3}H-choline and ^{3}H-palmitate into lipids of cultured cells. *Lab. Invest.* 42: 296–301, 1980.
173. SMITH, M. N., S. D. GREENBERG, AND H. J. SPJUT. The Clara cell: a comparative ultrastructural study in mammals. *Am. J. Anat.* 155: 15–30, 1979.
174. SOMLYO, A. P., J. VALLIÉRES, R. E. GARFIELD, H. SHUMAN, A. SCARPA, AND A. V. SOMLYO. Calcium compartmentalization in vascular smooth muscle: electron probe analysis and studies on isolated mitochondria. In: *The Biochemistry of Smooth Muscle*, edited by N. L. Stephens. Baltimore, MD: University Park, 1977, p. 563–583.
175. SOMLYO, A. V., F. T. ASHTON, L. F. LEMANSKI, J. VALLIÉRES, AND A. P. SOMLYO. Filament organization and dense bodies in vertebrate smooth muscle. In: *The Biochemistry of Smooth Muscle*, edited by N. L. Stephens. Baltimore, MD: University Park, 1977, p. 445–471.
176. SOROKIN, S. Centrioles and the formation of rudimentary cilia by fibroblasts and smooth muscle cells. *J. Cell Biol.* 15: 363–377, 1962.
177. SOROKIN, S. P. A morphological and cytochemical study on the great alveolar cell. *J. Histochem. Cytochem.* 14: 884–897, 1966.
178. SOROKIN, S. P. Phagocytes in the lung. In: *Lung Biology in Health and Disease. Respiratory Defense Mechanisms*, edited by J. D. Brain, D. F. Proctor, and L. M. Reid. New York: Dekker, 1977, vol. 5, pt. II, chapt. 19, p. 711–848.
179. SPICER, S. S., I. MOCHIZUKI, M. E. SETSER, AND J. R. MARTINEZ. Complex carbohydrates of rat tracheobronchial surface epithelium visualized ultratructurally. *Am. J. Anat.* 158: 93–109, 1980.
180. SPITZER, H. L., J. M. RICE, P. C. MACDONALD, AND J. M. JOHNSTON. Phospholipid biosynthesis in lung lamellar bodies. *Biochem. Biophys. Res. Commun.* 66: 17–23, 1975.
181. STAUBLI, W., R. HESS, AND E. R. WEIBEL. Correlated morphometric and biochemical studies on the liver cell. II. Effects of phenobarbital on rat hepatocytes. *J. Cell Biol.* 42: 92–112, 1969.
182. STEPHENS, N. L. (editor). *The Biochemistry of Smooth Muscle*. Baltimore, MD: University Park, 1977.
183. STONER, G. D. Explant culture of human peripheral lung. *Methods Cell Biol.* 21A: 65–77, 1980.
184. STONER, G. D., Y. KIKKAWA, A. J. KNIAZEFF, K. MIYAI, AND R. M. WAGNER. Clonal isolation of epithelial cells from mouse lung adenoma. *Cancer Res.* 35: 2177–2185, 1975.
185. STOSSEL, T. P. The mechanism of phagocytosis. *J. Reticuloendothel. Soc.* 19: 237–245, 1976.
186. STOSSEL, T. P. The mechanism of leucocyte locomotion. In: *Leukocyte Chemotaxis: Methods, Physiology, and Clinical Implications*, edited by J. I. Gallin and P. G. Quie. New York: Raven, 1978, p. 143–157.
187. STURGESS, J. M. Mucous secretions in the respiratory tract. *Pediatr. Clin. North Am.* 26: 481–501, 1979.
188. STURGESS, J. M., J. CHAO, J. WONG, N. ASPIN, AND J. A. TURNER. Cilia with defective radial spokes: a cause of human respiratory disease. *N. Engl. J. Med.* 300: 53–56, 1979.
189. STURGESS, J. M., M. MOSCARELLO, AND H. SCHACHTER. The structure and biosynthesis of membrane glycoproteins. *Curr. Top. Membr. Transp.* 11: 15–105, 1978.
190. SUEISHI, K., K. TANAKA, AND T. ODA. Immunoultrastructural study of surfactant systems. Distribution of specific protein of surface active material in rabbit lung. *Lab. Invest.* 37: 136–142, 1977.
191. SUZUKI, Y. Fenestration of alveolar capillary endothelium in experimental pulmonary fibrosis. *Lab. Invest.* 21: 304–308, 1969.
192. TARTAKOFF, A. M. The Golgi complex: crossroads for vesicular traffic. *Int. Rev. Exp. Pathol.* 22: 227–251, 1980.
193. TOMITA, T. Electrical activity (spikes and slow waves) in gastrointestinal smooth muscles. In: *Smooth Muscle: An Assessment of Current Knowledge*, edited by E. Bülbring, A. F. Brading, A. W. Jones, and T. Tomita. Austin: Univ. of Texas Press, 1981, p. 127–156.
194. UNANUE, E. R. The regulation of lymphocyte function by the macrophage. *Immunol. Rev.* 40: 227–255, 1978.
195. WALDMAN, R. H., AND C. S. HENNEY. Cell-mediated immunity and antibody responses in the respiratory tract after local and systemic immunization. *J. Exp. Med.* 134: 482–494, 1971.
196. WANGENSTEEN, D., H. BACHOFEN, AND E. R. WEIBEL. Lung tissue volume changes induced by hypertonic NaCl: morphometric evaluation. *J. Appl. Physiol.: Respirat. Environ. Exercise Physiol.* 51: 1443–1450, 1981.
197. WEIBEL, E. R. *Morphometry of the Human Lung*. Heidelberg: Springer-Verlag, 1963.
198. WEIBEL, E. R. The mystery of "non-nucleated plates" in the alveolar epithelium of the lung explained. *Acta Anat.* 78: 425–443, 1971.
199. WEIBEL, E. R. Morphological basis of alveolar-capillary gas exchange. *Physiol. Rev.* 53: 419–495, 1973.
200. WEIBEL, E. R. On pericytes, particularly their existence on lung capillaries. *Microvasc. Res.* 8: 218–235, 1974.
201. WEIBEL, E. R. Oxygen demand and the size of respiratory structures in mammals. In: *Lung Biology in Health and Disease. Evolution of Respiratory Processes. A Comparative Approach*, edited by S. C. Wood and C. Lenfant. New York: Dekker, 1979, vol. 13, chapt. 7, p. 289–346.
202. WEIBEL, E. R. Design and structure of the human lung. In: *Pulmonary Diseases and Disorders*, edited by A. P. Fishman. New York: McGraw-Hill, 1980, p. 224–271.
203. WEIBEL, E. R. Functional morphology of lung parenchyma. In: *Handbook of Physiology. The Respiratory System. Mechanics of Breathing*, edited by P. T. Macklem and J. Mead. Bethesda, MD: Am. Physiol. Soc., in press.
204. WEIBEL, E. R., AND H. BACHOFEN. Structural design of the alveolar septum and fluid exchange. In: *Pulmonary Edema*, edited by A. P. Fishman and E. M. Renkin. Bethesda, MD: Am. Physiol. Soc., 1979, chapt. 1, p. 1–20.
205. WEIBEL, E. R., G. S. KISTLER, AND G. TÖNDURY. A stereologic electron microscope study of "tubular myelin figures" in alveolar fluids of rat lungs. *Z. Zellforsch. Mikrosk. Anat.* 69: 418–427, 1966.
206. WEIBEL, E. R., AND G. E. PALADE. New cytoplasmic components in arterial endothelia. *J. Cell Biol.* 23: 101–112, 1964.
207. WEIBULL, C., E. CARLEMALM, W. VILLIGER, E. KELLENBERGER, J. FAKAN, A. GAUTIER, AND C. LARSSON. Low-temperature embedding procedures applied to chloroplasts. *J. Ultrastruct. Res.* 73: 233–244, 1980.
208. WEISSMANN, G., AND R. CLAIBORNE (editors). *Cell Membranes: Biochemistry, Cell Biology and Pathology*. New York: Hospital Practice, 1975.
209. WELLS, A. B. The kinetics of cell proliferation in the tracheobronchial epithelia of rats with and without chronic respiratory disease. *Cell Tissue Kinet.* 3: 185–206, 1970.
210. WILLIAMS, M. C. Freeze-fracture studies of tubular myelin and lamellar bodies in fetal and adult rat lungs. *J. Ultrastruct. Res.* 64: 352–361, 1978.
211. WILSON, M., K. R. HITCHCOCK, W. H. J. DOUGLAS, AND R. A. DELELLIS. Hormones and the lung. II. Immunohistochemical localization of thryoid hormone binding in type II pulmonary epithelial cells clonally-derived from adult rat lung. *Anat. Rec.* 195: 611–619, 1979.
212. ZIGMOND, S. H. Chemotaxis by polymorphonuclear leucocytes. *J. Cell Biol.* 77: 269–287, 1978.

CHAPTER 3

Pulmonary circulation

ALFRED P. FISHMAN | *Cardiovascular-Pulmonary Division, Department of Medicine, University of Pennsylvania School of Medicine, Philadelphia, Pennsylvania*

CHAPTER CONTENTS

Pulmonary Hemodynamics
  Pulmonary blood flow: general aspects
    Rest
    Exercise
    Posture
    Respiration
    Aging
    Distribution
  Pulmonary blood flow and pressure waves
    Propagation of flow and pressure waves
    Changes in patterns of propagation
  Mechanical influences on pulmonary blood flow
    Vascular waterfall
    Zones of the lungs
    Distension and recruitment
    Alveolar, corner, and extra-alveolar vessels
    Inflation
  Pulmonary vascular pressures
    Pulmonary artery
    Pulmonary microcirculation
    Pulmonary veins and left atrium
    Pulmonary arteriovenous pressure differences
    Pulmonary wedge pressure
    Influence of intrathoracic pressure on pulmonary vascular pressures
    Transmural versus luminal pressures
    Mechanical ventilation
    Exercise
  Pulmonary blood volume
    Measurement
    Changes
    Normal values
    Partition
  Pressure-volume, pressure-flow relationships
    Distensibility
    Pulmonary vascular resistance
    Pulmonary vascular impedance
Vasomotor Regulation
  Level of initial tone
  Detection of a vasomotor response
  Sites of pulmonary vasoconstriction
  Vasomotor mechanisms
    Nervous control
    Chemical control
Bronchial Circulation
  Determination of bronchial blood flow
  Normal levels of bronchial blood flow
  Bronchial circulation in the normal lung
  Bronchial circulation in disease

Fetal and Neonatal Pulmonary Circulation
  Morphologic changes
  Regulation of fetal pulmonary circulation
  Postnatal pulmonary vasodilation
Pulmonary Hypertension
  Pathogenesis
  Experimental chronic pulmonary hypertension
    Hypoxic model
    Dietary model
    Sepsis model
    Blood component model
    Other models
  Pulmonary vasodilators
  Endothelium-dependent pulmonary vasodilation

THE PULMONARY CIRCULATION is a low-resistance, highly compliant vascular bed that is markedly influenced by pressures generated by the heart and the thorax. Normally it appears to be maximally dilated, uninfluenced by maneuvers to decrease its initial tone (28, 140, 300, 420, 440). Because of its intrinsic properties and its meager endowment for vasomotor control, modest external forces can exert relatively large hemodynamic effects, complicating attempts to distinguish between active and passive changes in vascular calibers. Indeed detection of pulmonary vasomotor activity requires unflagging attention to perivascular pressures generated during respiration and to the effects of cardiac performance on blood pressures at the two ends of the pulmonary circulation, pulmonary blood flow, and pulmonary blood volume (99, 138, 231).

The passive influences can exert their effects quite subtly. For example, during a single heartbeat, as the right ventricle empties, part of the ejectate is retained within the pulmonary arterial tree and distends its walls, while the remainder courses through the pulmonary microcirculation en route to the left side of the heart (332, 443). The partition of the stroke output between the amount retained in the arterial tree and the amount exiting from the pulmonary capillary bed is determined by the interplay among the intrinsic properties of the pulmonary arterial tree, the pressure drop along the length of the pulmonary arterial tree, the transmural pressures, and the resistance to outflow at the distal end of the arterial tree. A dramatic change in breathing pattern or cardiac performance, or a shift from rest to exercise, can passively affect the partition between the stored and pass-through components of the stroke volume as well as modify the peripheral transmission of the pressure and flow pulses.

A second example of the difficulty in distinguishing between passive and active influences is moderate exercise, which is often used in the intact, unanesthetized human subject to construct passive pressure-flow curves (138). This device for defining the passive behavior of pulmonary arterial pressures in response to increments in blood flow assumes that if proper precautions are taken pulmonary vasomotor tone will not increase during the exercise and the concentration of circulating catecholamines will remain unchanged. This assumption may not be entirely valid (415). A third instance is illustrated by the detection and quantification of vasomotor activity in response to hypoxia: one set of problems arises from attempts to interpret measurements made during an unsteady state, i.e., when both breathing patterns and cardiac dynamics are changing; a second set is encountered when the steady state of respiration, circulation, and metabolism is achieved (144). This chapter considers approaches for dealing with these diverse problems.

Until about 15 years ago interest in the pulmonary circulation focused almost entirely on hemodynamics and gas exchange. Since then the span has widened to include the nonrespiratory and water-exchanging functions of the lungs (215). Some of the nonrespiratory functions of the pulmonary circulation (e.g., the sieving of particulate matter) are simply mechanical. Others are metabolic and essential not only for the integrity of pulmonary structure and function (e.g., the generation of surfactant) but also as components of the neurohumoral and metabolic machinery of the body (e.g., the renin-angiotensin system) (Fig. 1). The nonrespiratory functions of the lungs are extraordinarily diverse and stem from their architecture, organization, location within the thorax between the two ventricles, cellular composition, and enormous air-blood interface (513).

The pulmonary circulation is not the sole blood supply to the lungs; systemic arterial branches (the "bronchial circulation") ensure the vitality of the conducting airways of the lungs and of the structures that support the gas-exchanging apparatus (99). Ordinarily this blood supply is exceedingly small. However, it is capable of remarkable proliferation when the pulmonary blood is compromised or when the lungs are the seat of certain chronic inflammatory processes (136).

A final word sets the stage for considering the behavior of the pulmonary circulation. Both structure and function often differ not only between species

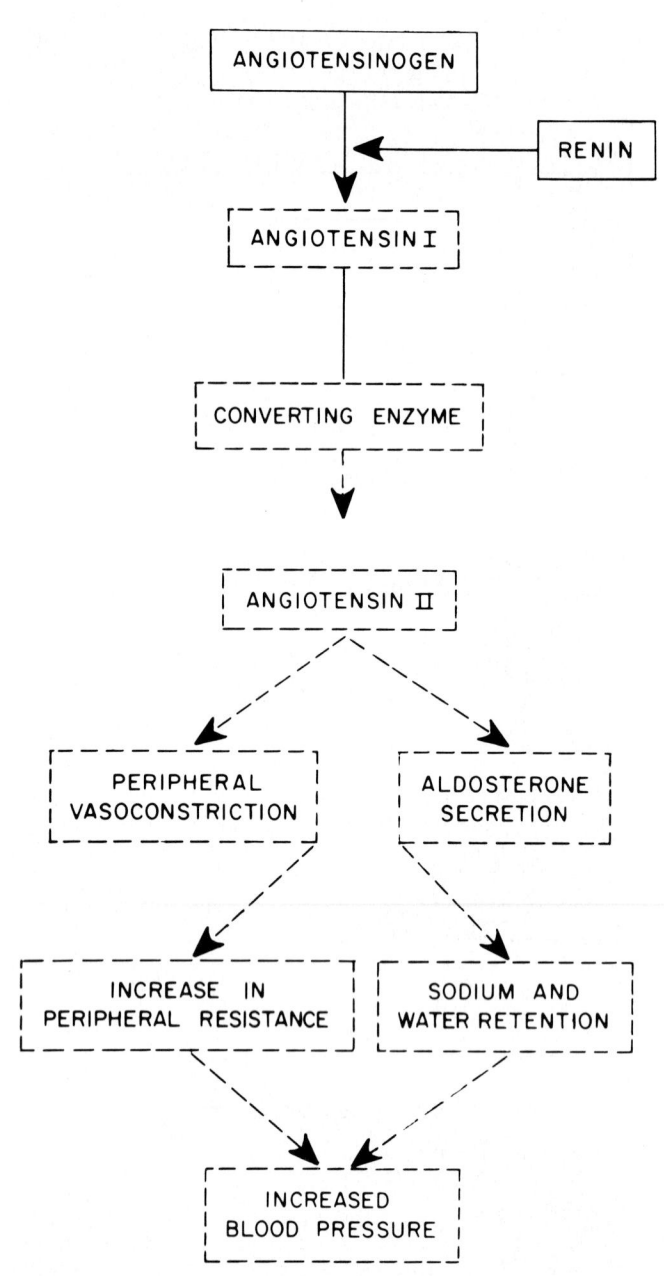

FIG. 1. Renin-angiotensin system. The lungs play a central role in control of systemic blood pressure because of the converting enzyme on the luminal aspect of pulmonary capillary endothelium. Strategic disposition of the enzyme and huge expanse of pulmonary capillary endothelium enable rapid and efficient conversion of angiotensin I to angiotensin II as blood courses through the lungs.

(Fig. 2) but sometimes within species. For example, the pulmonary resistance vessels (small arteries and veins) of native residents at high altitude are more muscular than those of sea-level natives, apparently an adaptation to chronic hypoxia. Also responsiveness to the same acute hypoxic stimulus often differs strikingly not only between native residents at sea level and at high altitude but also among individuals and

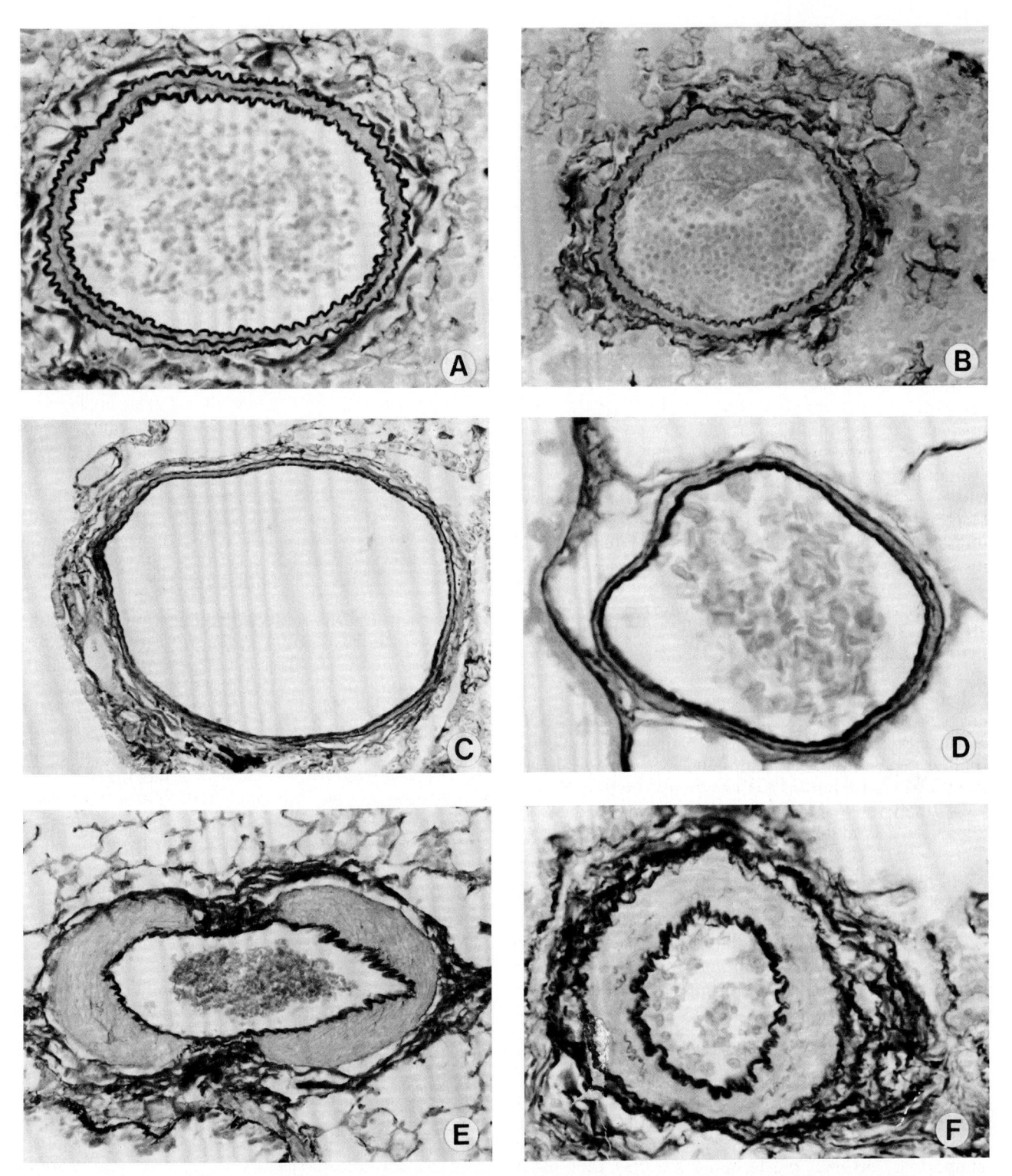

FIG. 2. Muscular pulmonary arteries (resistance vessels) in pulmonary circulation of various animal species. Elastic Van Gieson's stain. *A*: dog; × 500. *B*: cat; × 500. *C*: human; × 200. *D*: rat; × 800. *A–D*: tunica media is relatively thin. *E*: guinea pig; × 200. Tunica media consists of crescentic masses of circular smooth muscle disposed in discontinuous segments resembling sphincters. In areas between sphincterlike masses of smooth muscle the wall consists only of an elastic lamina. *F*: cow; × 500. Tunica media is thick. (Micrographs courtesy of J. M. Kay.)

species born and raised at the same altitude. Fetal pulmonary blood vessels differ distinctively from those of the adult not only in structure but also in responsiveness. Finally, when disease afflicts either the pulmonary vessels or the surrounding parenchyma, not only is the structure altered but the behavior of the vessels may be seriously modified by the vascular or perivascular localization of the injury and by the components of the inflammatory process.

In this chapter, unless otherwise stipulated, the designation "normal pulmonary circulation" signifies the pulmonary circulation of the normal adult dweller at sea level.

PULMONARY HEMODYNAMICS

Pulmonary Blood Flow: General Aspects

Reynolds numbers (peak 5,000–9,000) in the main pulmonary artery suggest that the pattern of flow there borders on turbulence. The mean velocity of blood flow in the pulmonary artery is ~18 cm/s in the human and dog. This value is about the same as that in the large pulmonary veins and aorta (332).

During a single heartbeat the outputs of the two ventricles need not be the same because of differential effects of breathing on pulmonary and systemic venous return. However, averaged over several respiratory cycles the outputs of the two ventricles are well matched except that the output of the left ventricle is consistently higher than that of the right ventricle because the bronchial (systemic) veins drain into the pulmonary veins. This anatomical venous admixture is ~1%–2% of the total left ventricular output (93).

For men and women the cardiac output is generally expressed per square meter of body surface area (cardiac index). Although this practice has been widely adopted for human studies, it is more reliable when applied to consecutive measurements in the same individual than to subjects of different age, sex, and body build. Whether it is a reliable basis for comparing cardiac outputs of different mammalian species or whether body weight is a more meaningful standard of reference within a given species is unsettled (218, 474, 475).

In the intact animal or human, cardiac output is generally determined by some application of the indicator-dilution or Fick principles. For both, reliable determinations require the achievement of a steady state (144). Of the two, the indicator-dilution approach has become increasingly popular because a briefer period of stability in the respiration and circulation is needed to obtain accurate and reproducible results. Body plethysmography has been used in special experimental circumstances but is impractical for general use. Pulmonary capillary blood flow has also been determined in humans by breath-holding and rebreathing methods on the basis of the relative disappearance rates of a soluble and a poorly soluble gas. Improvements in analytic techniques promise new practical applications of this approach (379, 460).

In normal unanesthetized dogs and humans the cardiac output is matched to the metabolic rate (187, 396). Thus an increase in O_2 uptake ($\Delta \dot{V}_{O_2}$) of 100 ml generally elicits an increase in cardiac output ($\Delta \dot{Q}_T$) of 600–800 ml/min. The reproducibility in individual test subjects is greatly enhanced by measures designed to promote relaxation, comfort, and a near-normal state in the control periods (138, 415). Not infrequently, control values for $\dot{V}_{O_2}$ are lower after exercise than before, i.e., when anxiety about an unfamiliar procedure has been relieved by successful withstanding of the test. Heart failure is associated with subnormal values for $\Delta \dot{Q}_T / \dot{V}_{O_2}$.

In contrast to the roughly linear relation between O_2 uptake and cardiac output during exercise, the relation between O_2 uptake and the arteriovenous O_2 difference is hyperbolic. The relative contribution of an increase in cardiac output and a widening of the arteriovenous O_2 difference to satisfying the tissue requirements for O_2 varies with the situation (e.g., type of exercise and temperature), but training does not seem to affect the relationship (151).

REST. In normal, supine human adults in the postprandial state, the cardiac index averages ~3.12 liters· $min^{-1} \cdot m^{-2}$ (SD ± 0.40); the corresponding O_2 uptake is 138 ml· $min^{-1} \cdot m^{-2}$ (SD ± 14) (138). In the resting, unanesthetized dog the cardiac output is ~150 ml/kg.

Blood spends little time in gas exchange in the pulmonary capillaries, i.e., ~0.80 s at rest (138). During exercise the transit time is abbreviated. Direct observation of red cell movement in the subpleural capillaries of the open-chest dog suggests that the transit time is not as rapid as previously described for the intact animal (509). However, part of the discrepancy may arise from nonuniform transit times in the lungs and the possibility that blood flow in subpleural vessels is slower than in the substance of the lungs (536).

EXERCISE. Depending on its type and severity, exercise evokes a series of adaptive responses in the respiration, circulation, and metabolism. Part of this integrated response is an increase in the pulmonary blood flow (Fig. 3). Pulmonary blood flow may increase up to 20-fold during exercise; the increase is accommodated by a combination of recruitment of vessels that are ordinarily closed at rest and by distension of open vessels; it is accompanied by an increase in pulmonary arterial pressure. In unanesthetized human subjects the treadmill and bicycle ergometer are the conventional devices for achieving calibrated and reproducible levels of exercise. Anxiety caused by unfamiliarity with the procedure may dominate the response not only at rest but also as maximum tolerable levels are approached. Quantification of the level of

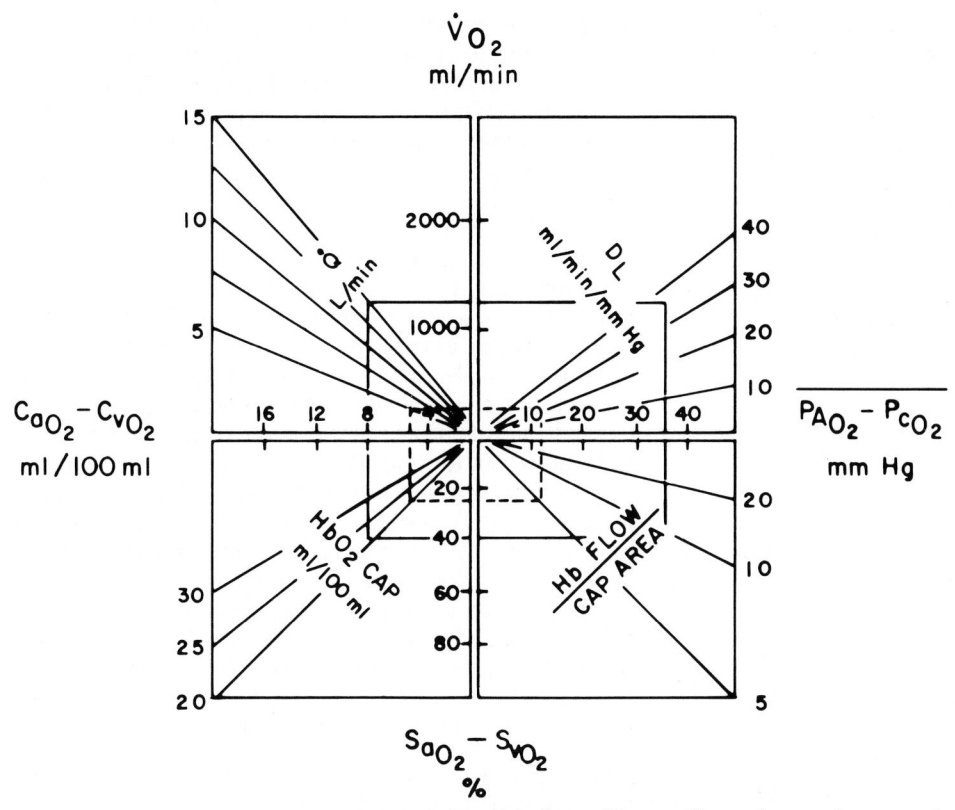

FIG. 3. Four-quadrant diagram illustrating respiratory and circulatory adaptation by which O_2 requirement ($\dot{V}_{O_2}$) is satisfied at rest (*inner rectangle*) and during exercise (*outer rectangle*). Ca_{O_2}, concentration of O_2 in arterial blood; Cv_{O_2}, concentration of O_2 in venous blood; CAP area, capillary area; D_L, diffusing capacity of the lungs; Hb, hemoglobin; Hb_{O_2}, O_2 capacity of hemoglobin; $\bar{P}A_{O_2}$, mean alveolar O_2 tension; $\bar{P}c_{O_2}$, mean capillary O_2 tension; Sa_{O_2}, arterial O_2 saturation; Sv_{O_2}, venous O_2 saturation. [Adapted from Barcroft (21a).]

exercise is accomplished either by determining O_2 uptake or by assessing the work load (138).

In normal human subjects lying supine, in whom pulmonary blood flow is increased to both lungs by moderate exercise or to one lung by occlusion of the opposite pulmonary artery, calculated resistance does not change appreciably or consistently. This observation and the experimental evidence that pulmonary blood volume undergoes little if any change under these conditions suggest that the full pulmonary vascular bed is fully open while the subject is supine (291). The situation is quite different in the vertical lung. Thus, as the cardiac output and pulmonary arterial pressure increase during moderate exercise in the sitting position (subject on a bicycle), blood flow to the upper zones increases preferentially (231, 523). Accordingly, calculated resistance decreases during exercise in the upright position.

POSTURE. Under the influence of gravity a change in posture automatically redirects blood flow to the dependent parts of the lungs (148, 466). Thus apical blood flow increases in the supine position, whereas basal blood flow undergoes little change (523). In this position, although blood flow at the apices and bases tends to equalize, the uppermost (anterior) parts of the lungs receive less of the cardiac output than the lowermost (posterior). Similarly, redistribution of blood flow, again favoring the dependent parts of the lungs, occurs when the lateral or prone position is assumed (246). In the individual standing on his head, blood flow at the apex exceeds that at the base (114, 278). Predictable rearrangement of pulmonary blood flow also occurs when the body is exposed to centrifugal forces (170).

RESPIRATION. Respiration affects the pulmonary circulation via venous return, pleural pressure, and the degree of inflation of the lungs. During breathing, matched changes in the filling pressures of the right ventricle, effected by phasic changes in venous return, induce corresponding changes in pulmonary arterial inflow (386). In artificial circumstances the ventilatory pressures and patterns can dissociate blood flow in the consecutive segments of the pulmonary vascular bed (412).

At the start of a normal breath the lungs increase in vertical height, largely through expansion below the hilum. The main pulmonary artery distends as its intravascular pressure increases with respect to the mediastinal pressure that surrounds it. Pulmonary arterial pressures remain unchanged with respect to alveolar pressure but increase with respect to pleural pressure. Pulmonary venous and left atrial pressures decrease as the surrounding pressures fall. Within one heartbeat after the start of inspiration, right ventricular stroke output generally increases; in those instances in which inspiration has little effect on right ventricular stroke output, heart rate generally speeds up to increase pulmonary blood flow. The net effect of inspiration is a slight decrease in pulmonary vascular resistance (386). Pulmonary capillary blood flow increases at the start of inspiration but gradually tapers as inspiration continues (499). Outflow from the lungs follows the increase in right ventricular output within 0.1–0.2 s, i.e., after sufficient time for the pulse wave to be transmitted (342); the time lag between the output of the two ventricles depends on the rate and depth of inspiration.

A large, deep breath may collapse both the systemic veins at their entry to the thorax and the pulmonary veins as they exit from the lungs (waterfall effect) (444).

During expiration the opposite effects occur, beginning with slowing of systemic venous return as pleural pressure increases. As explained elsewhere in this chapter, not only the magnitude but even the direction of the mechanical effects on the pulmonary vessels varies from site to site along the pulmonary vascular tree, e.g., collapse of alveolar vessels as extra-alveolar vessels dilate. Also, as expiration continues, extra-alveolar vessels from the top of the lungs downward tend to close. These effects are exaggerated during obstructive airways disease in which swings in pleural pressure are quite marked.

AGING. In standing humans 65–75 yr old the distribution of pulmonary blood flow is more uniform than in young normals. However, the bases continue to be better perfused. The improved uniformity may be due to the higher pulmonary arterial pressures in the elderly (377).

DISTRIBUTION. Matching of blood flow to alveolar ventilation is a prime concern for efficiency in gas exchange. Some of the stimuli for local rearrangement of blood flow (e.g., hypoxia) are considered in great detail in the volume on gas exchange in preparation for this *Handbook* section on the respiratory system.

Pulmonary Blood Flow and Pressure Waves

PROPAGATION OF FLOW AND PRESSURE WAVES. Propagation of the flow (and pressure) waves is a function of the architecture of the vascular tree, the viscoelastic properties of the vascular wall, the distensibility of the vasculature, other physical attributes of the vascular tree, and the motion of the blood (89, 332). In the pulmonary circulation, flow is pulsatile from the beginning to the end of the pulmonary vascular tree (Fig. 4), but the amplitude of the flow (and pressure) pulsations decreases along the length of the pulmonary arterial tree, remaining distinctly pulsatile in the capillaries and even in the large pulmonary veins. Pulsatility is more marked in pulmonary capillaries than in systemic capillaries (342). About 50% of the pulmonary arterial pressure pulse reaches precapillary vessels (~100 μm), and ~35% penetrates the midcapillary region. The pressure waves are then greatly attenuated in the pulmonary venous bed, the degree of damping depending on the frequency (495). Although the origins of pulmonary venous pulsatility have been debated, it seems clear that in the normal pulmonary circulation more of the pulsatility in the pulmonary veins is attributable to orthograde transmission via the pulmonary artery than to retrograde transmission from the left atrium (138, 332).

Although attenuation of the pressure and flow pulses provides some insight into the mechanical properties of the intervening vascular bed, little is known about the physiological significance of wave velocities in the circulation. One possibility for the pulmonary circulation is that the transmission time for the flow pulse through the normal lungs operates to deliver blood into the left atrium just at the onset of rapid ventricular filling, thereby maintaining a balance between the outputs of the two ventricles (238).

Wiener et al. (527) used direct recordings of flow and pressure pulses at consecutive segments of the pulmonary circulation in the dog and Womersley's equations for a tethered elastic tube to reconstruct the patterns of wave propagation in the pulmonary circulation (arteries, microcirculation, and veins) (Fig. 5). In their model, ~50% of the arterial pressure pulse reached the precapillary region in accord with direct experimental observations (332, 527). Also both pressure and flow pulses decreased markedly at the entry to the microcirculation. In the microcirculation (diam ≤ 120 μm) the pressure pulse became severely damped, whereas the flow purse was little affected. This approach is useful in examining the hemodynamic properties of an entire vascular bed and provides realistic models that can be tested experimentally.

CHANGES IN PATTERNS OF PROPAGATION. Simultaneous registration of peak flows in the pulmonary artery and capillaries—a formidable technical undertaking—has encouraged the idea that an inverse relation exists between pulmonary arterial compliance and vascular resistance under a variety of experimental conditions in the dog and human (238, 405, 471). According to this concept the time constant (resistance times capacitance) of the pulmonary arterial tree tends to be self-adjusting, because agents that decrease the caliber of the resistance vessels (small arteries and arterioles) in the lungs simultaneously stiffen the larger pulmonary arteries (capacitance vessels). Thus, in response to interventions or pathologic processes, automatic counterbalancing adjustments occur in the tension of the large elastic arteries and in the calibers of the precapillary vessels that contribute the bulk of

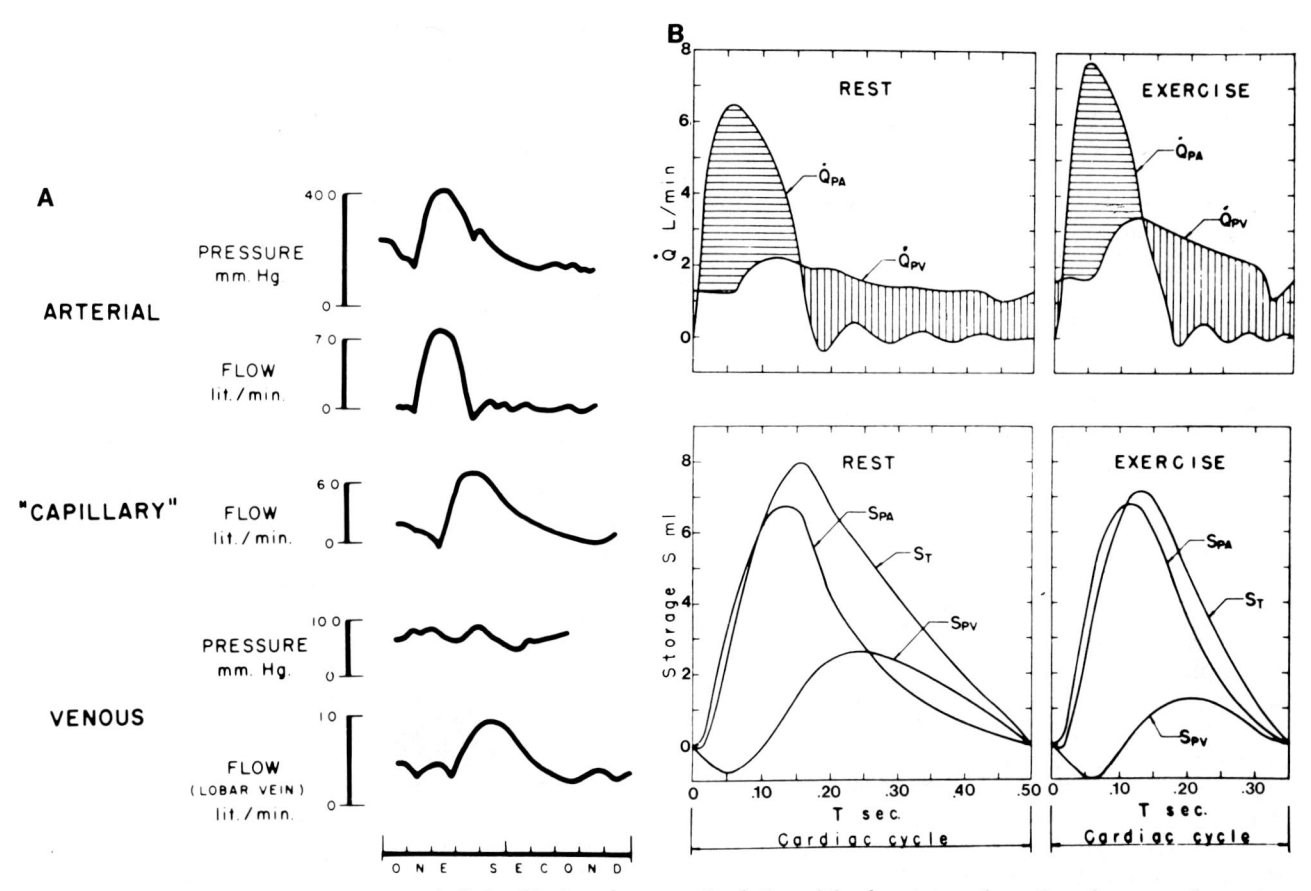

FIG. 4. Pulsatility in pulmonary circulation of the dog. *A*: transformation of pressure-flow pulses along length of pulmonary circulation. Transmission time for pressure pulse from pulmonary artery to capillaries ~0.09 s; from capillaries to veins, transmission time ~0.03 s. *B: top*, changes in pulmonary blood volume of the dog at rest and exercise during a single cardiac cycle. Rate of change in pulmonary blood volume (*striped area*) equals difference between flows in main pulmonary artery (Qpa) and in pulmonary veins (Qpv). *Bottom*, storage as calculated from discharge curves at consecutive sections of pulmonary vascular tree during a cardiac cycle. Spa, storage in pulmonary arteries; Spv, storage in pulmonary veins; S_T, total storage. Most storage occurs within the pulmonary arterial tree. [*A* from Wiener, Fishman, et al. (527), by permission of the American Heart Association, Inc. *B* from Skalak, Fishman, et al. (443).]

the pulmonary vascular resistance (407, 472). For example, in response to acute hypoxia the resistance vessels appeared to constrict and the larger arteries to stiffen, so that transmission of flow to the capillaries remained virtually unchanged (404).

An attempt has also been made in the dog to use the pattern of transmission of the pulmonary flow pulse to predict the predominant site of pulmonary vasoconstriction during hypoxia (343). The results have suggested precapillary vasoconstriction but are not conclusive because of the technical difficulty of simultaneously recording blood flow in the pulmonary capillaries and pulmonary artery.

Mechanical Influences on Pulmonary Blood Flow

As noted at the outset, the major purpose of the lung is to arterialize the venous blood. Because regional inhomogeneities exist in structure, mechanical forces, ventilation, and gas exchange, the design of the cardiorespiratory apparatus provides for regional differences in blood flow and automatic mechanisms for rearrangement that match blood flow to alveolar ventilation when appropriate.

A variety of techniques have been used to determine the topographical distribution of blood delivered to the lungs. Mention of three techniques illustrates the approaches that have been used and the problems in interpretation. *1*) A poorly soluble gas (e.g., xenon) is dissolved in saline and intravenously injected; the gas escapes into the alveolar gas and external counters record the intrapulmonary distribution of radioactivity (69). *2*) A very soluble gas (e.g., CO_2) is inhaled; the rate of its disappearance from a particular region of the lung is recorded (522). *3*) Macroaggregated albumin is intravenously injected; the distribution of radioactivity is then determined from a radiograph.

Comparison of results obtained with these different techniques is complicated on several accounts. *1*) Spontaneous variations in pulmonary arterial blood

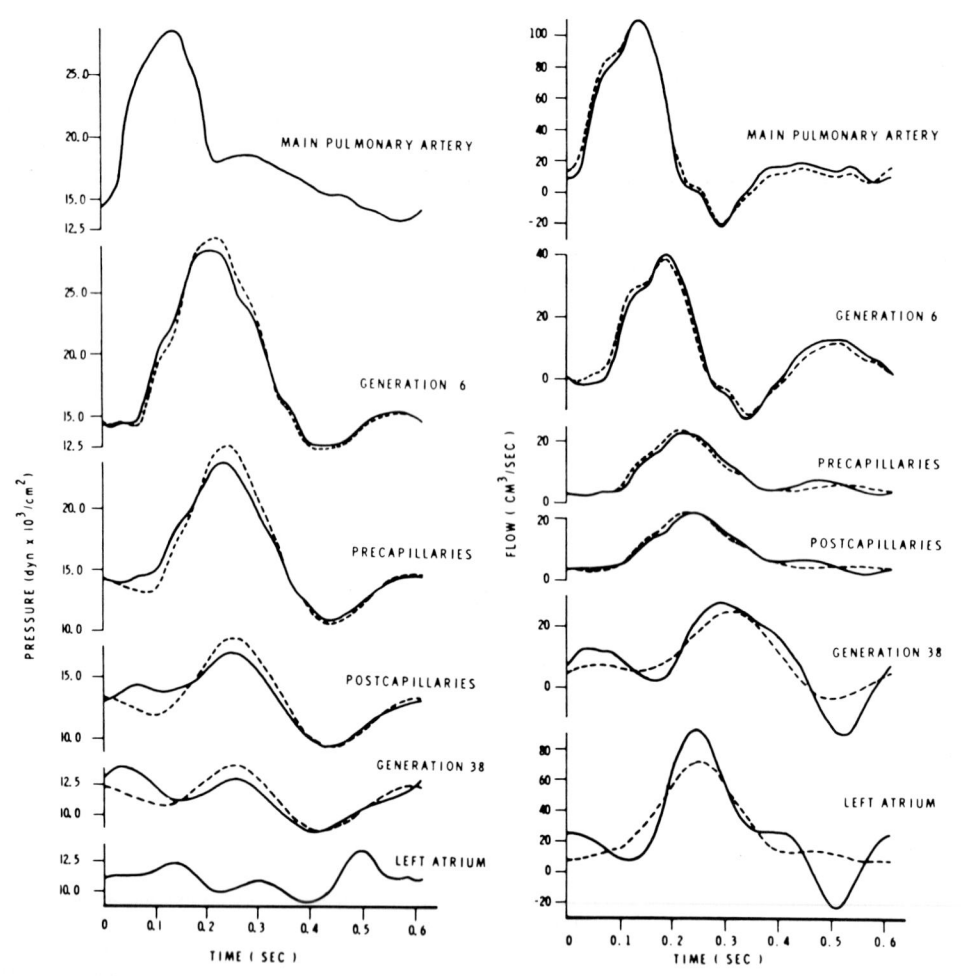

FIG. 5. Propagation of pressure pulses (*left*) and flow pulses (*right*) through pulmonary circulation. *Left*: *top* and *bottom* curves, measured boundary pressures from which all other pressures and flows in the model were calculated. *Dashed curves*, sum of the mean pressure plus pressure oscillations propagated from right ventricle (arterial pulse). *Solid curves* include contribution of oscillatory part of left atrial pressure (venous pulse) and represent total (mean + arterial pulse + venous pulse) pressure at each location. *Right*: corresponding curves for flow. In contrast to *left panel*, for which *top* and *bottom* curves were determined experimentally, all *curves* in *right panel* were computed. *Tracings*, from *top* to *bottom*: main pulmonary artery, segmental pulmonary artery (generation 6), precapillaries, postcapillaries, segmental pulmonary vein (generation 38), and left atrium. [From Wiener, Fishman, et al. (527), by permission of the American Heart Association, Inc.]

pressure in the course of sequential testing may modify distribution of pulmonary blood flow. *2*) The tests are designed to compare, rather than to measure in absolute terms, the blood flow in different regions. *3*) The different tests do not provide the same kind of information about regional blood flow: in one laboratory, regional blood flow is expressed per unit of alveolar gas volume (69); in another, regional blood flow is per alveolus (13); and, in a third, regional blood flow is per unit of lung volume (air and tissue).

Nonetheless the results of all techniques agree that in the upright lungs the blood flow decreases steadily from the bottom to the top, that gravity is the compelling force, and that an interplay among pulmonary arterial, alveolar, and pulmonary venous pressures is involved. As a consequence of these influences, the apices of the lungs in a relaxed, seated subject—particularly in one with an elongated thorax—may be unperfused, especially in states of pulmonary hypotension or increased alveolar pressure (13, 69).

VASCULAR WATERFALL. In 1960 Banister and Torrance (21) demonstrated that the level of alveolar pressure could influence pressure-flow relationships in the pulmonary circulation and drew an analogy between the behavior of the pulmonary arterial, pulmonary venous, and alveolar pressures and that of a Starling resistor. The crucial point of their demonstration was that when alveolar pressure (chamber pressure) exceeded venous (downstream) pressure, the driving pressure became arterial minus alveolar pressure and not arterial minus venous pressure (21).

Permutt et al. (373) compared this behavior to that of a waterfall where height does not influence the flow of water over its brink (Fig. 6).

ZONES OF THE LUNGS. Recognition of the effects of alveolar pressure on pressure-flow relationships in the pulmonary circulation and the formulation of the behavior of pulmonary microvessels in terms of the Starling resistor [Fig. 6; (21, 373)] paved the way for a model of the topographic distribution of blood flow in the lungs under the influence of gravity (524). As a result it is now commonplace to use "zones" of blood flow in the lungs to specify the interplay between pulmonary arterial, alveolar, and pulmonary venous pressures (Fig. 7).

In the normal, upright lung [estimated height 25 cm at functional residual capacity (FRC)], ~15 cm is above the left atrium and ~10 cm is below (Fig. 8). If it is assumed that the mean pulmonary arterial pressure measured at the level of the left atrium is ~15 cmH$_2$O and that left atrial pressure is ~7 cmH$_2$O, the top few centimeters of the lung will be hypoperfused during most of the cardiac cycle except for flushes of blood during the peak ejection phase of systole. This zone has been designated zone 1. Below zone 1, flow increases regularly with distance down the lung (zone

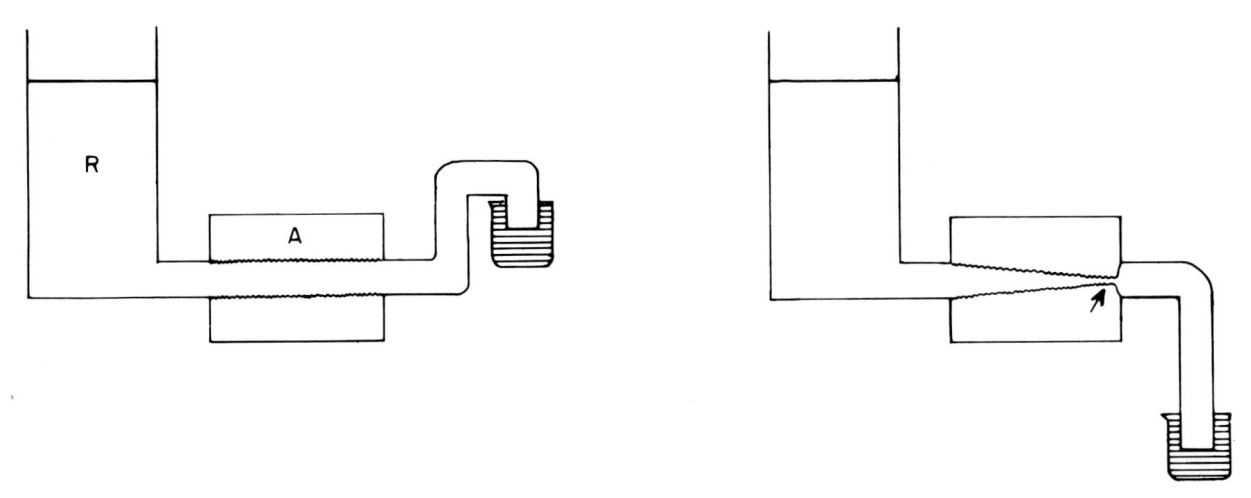

FIG. 6. Principle of a Starling resistor. Thin-walled collapsible tube traverses a closed chamber (A) in which pressure can be varied at will. Fluid flows from reservoir (R) into collecting vessel (striped area), traversing collapsible tube en route. When outflow pressure exceeds chamber pressure (left), flow is determined by difference between inflow and outflow pressure. However, when chamber pressure exceeds outflow pressure, so that collapsible tube closes (arrow), flow is determined by difference between inflow and chamber pressure. [Adapted from West et al. (524).]

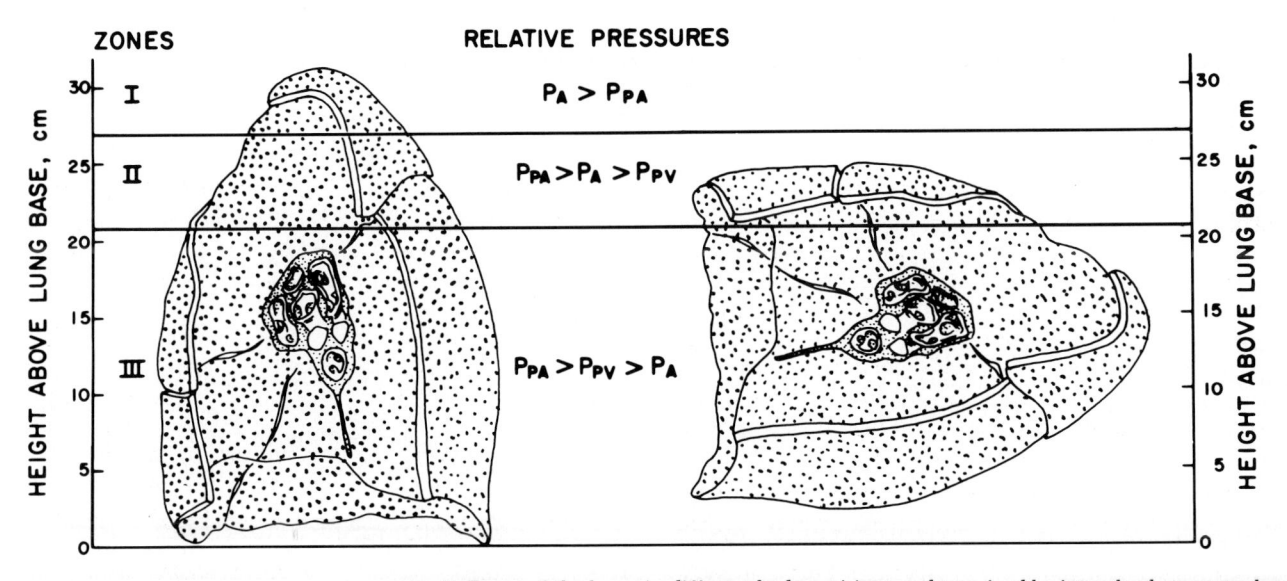

FIG. 7. Zones of the lungs in different body positions as determined by interplay between pulmonary vascular (Ppv) and alveolar pressures (PA). For simplicity, only zones 1, 2, and 3 are shown. Ppa, pulmonary arterial pressure. [Adapted from Hughes (231).]

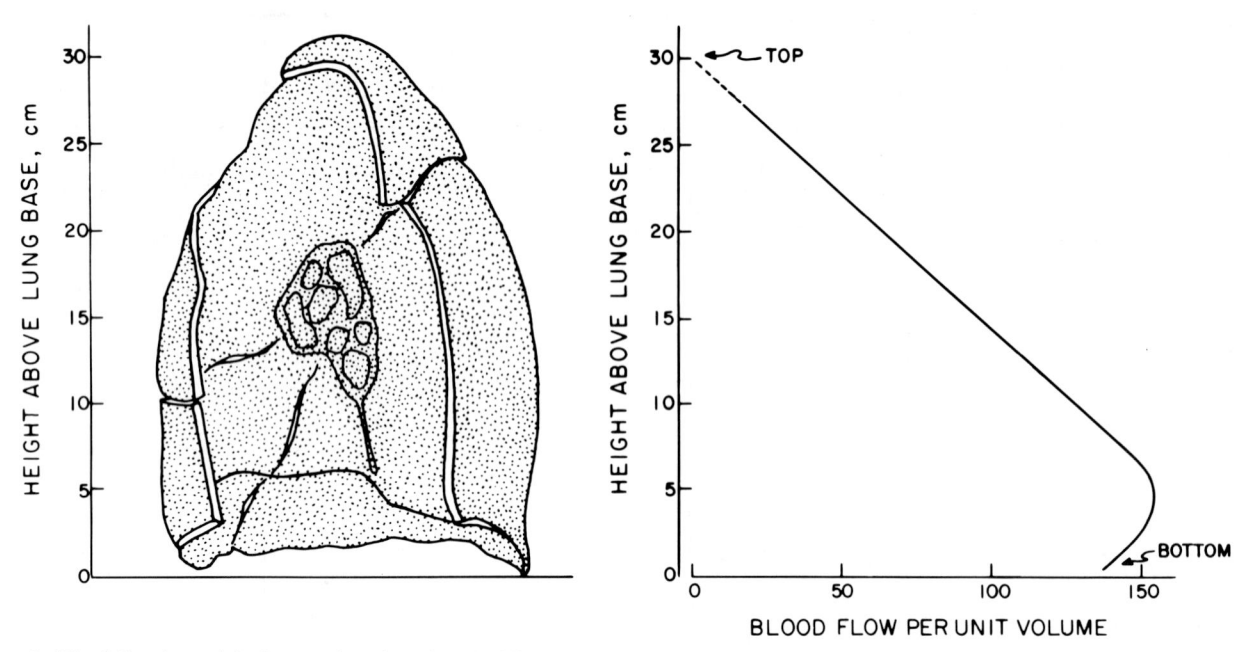

FIG. 8. Blood flow in upright lung as function of vertical height. [Adapted from Glazier et al. (172).]

2). Below zone 2 is another zone of increasing blood flow (zone 3) that may be interrupted by a zone of decreasing flow near the base (zone 4). The mechanisms responsible for blood flow in the different zones differ considerably and are dealt with next.

Zone 1. Blood flow in zone 1 of the vertical lung is minimal, as determined by both physiological testing and histologic examination. In zone 1, alveolar pressure exceeds pulmonary arterial pressure (PA > Ppa) (Fig. 9). Note that in this zone, although most alveolar capillaries appear on histologic examination to be attenuated or collapsed—causing their resistance to blood flow to approach infinity—extra-alveolar vessels in the corners of the alveoli often remain open, emphasizing that the extra-alveolar vessels are exposed to different forces than are the alveolar vessels. Moreover, although the model illustrated in Figure 9 deals with alveolar pressures, the pericapillary pressure is somewhat less than the alveolar pressure because of the surface tension of the alveolar lining layer (163, 256). In principle, persistence of blood flow through parts of zone 1, even though alveolar pressure exceeds pulmonary arterial pressure, could be due to the lowering effect of surface tension on pericapillary pressure. However, a more likely explanation is that much of the persistent flow in zone 1 is through extra-alveolar vessels (corner vessels) that expand during inspiration (410, 416).

Clearly the apices of the lungs cannot be continuously deprived of pulmonary blood flow. The expedient for flushing apical pulmonary capillaries is the pulsatility of pulmonary arterial blood flow, which enables the apices to be perfused, although mean pulmonary arterial pressure is too low to sustain blood flow to the apices (522).

Zone 2. In zone 2, pulmonary arterial pressure exceeds alveolar pressure, which in turn exceeds pulmonary venous pressure (Ppa > PA > Ppv) (Fig. 9). As with the Starling resistor, blood flow is determined by the pulmonary arterial-alveolar pressure difference rather than by the pulmonary arterial-pulmonary venous pressure difference. This hemodynamic situation in which flow is independent of downstream pressure has been likened to a vascular waterfall (373). Under the influence of gravity the pulmonary arterial pressure increases by ~1 cmH$_2$O per centimeter of distance down the lung, whereas alveolar pressure remains unchanged; the driving pressure, and therefore the blood flow, increases down this zone. According to this model the capillaries of zone 2 operate as a "sluice gate" (21), opening and closing in response to imbalance in luminal and pericapillary pressures. Whether the collapse points shown in Figure 9 actually do develop is debatable (155). Moreover it has been suggested that under zone 2 conditions alveolar pressure compresses microvessels other than capillaries, particularly pulmonary venules.

Zone 3. In this part of the lungs, pulmonary venous pressure is greater than alveolar pressure (Ppa > Ppv > PA) and flow is determined by the arteriovenous difference in pressure (because both exceed PA) (Fig. 9). Resistance to blood flow in zone 3 is less than in zone 2. The driving pressure here remains fixed down to the bottom of the lung because the effect of gravity causes arterial and venous pressures to increase equally per centimeter of distance. Despite the con-

PRESSURES IN ZONES		ALVEOLAR CAPILLARY FLOW	FLOW DEPENDS ON:
I $P_A > P_{pa} > P_{pv}$	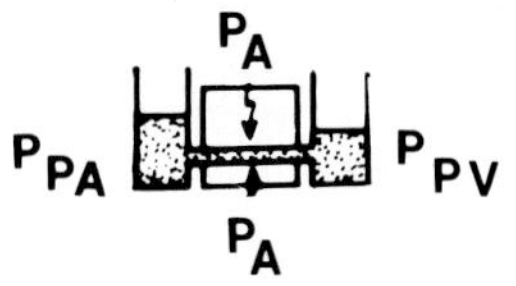 P_A, P_{pa}, P_{pv}, P_A	NONE TO LOW	PULSATILITY (FLOW CONTINUES THROUGH CORNER VESSELS)
II $P_{pa} > P_A > P_{pv}$	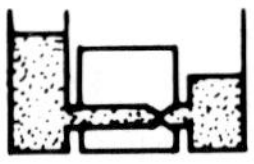	INTERMEDIATE	$P_{pa} - P_A$ (STARLING RESISTOR)
III $P_{pa} > P_{pv} > P_A$	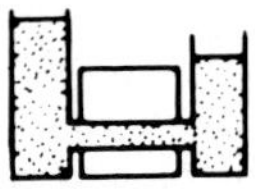	HIGH	$P_{pa} - P_{pv}$
IV $P_{pa} > P_{pv} > P_A$ $P_{INTERSTITIAL}$	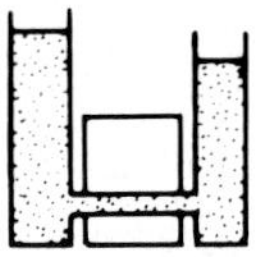	INTERMEDIATE	RESISTANCE IN EXTRA-ALVEOLAR VESSELS

FIG. 9. Topographical distribution of pulmonary blood flow according to relationship among pulmonary arterial pressure (Ppa), pulmonary venous pressure (Ppv), and alveolar pressure (PA). Because of effect of surface tension, PA is more accurately pericapillary pressure. Zone 1 (apex): PA > Ppa > Ppv. No flow (except through corner vessels) because collapsible vessels close when pericapillary pressure exceeds the pressure inside the vessels. Vessels that close are capillaries and other alveolar vessels up to ~30 μm diam. Zone 2: Ppa > PA > Ppv. Driving pressure is Ppa − PA. This difference increases down lung and so does flow. Zone 3: Ppa > Ppv > PA. Driving pressure is Ppa − Ppv. Although Ppa − Ppv does not change down lung, Ppa and Ppv continue to increase from top to bottom. Flow down zone 3 is less than zone 2. Zone 4 (appears at residual volume): this region of decreased flow appears during forced exhalation and has been attributed to either an increase in interstitial pressure at lung bases or to closure of small airways at low lung volumes as the increase in PA creates either zone 1 or zone 2 conditions. [Adapted from West et al. (524) and Anthonisen and Milic-Emili (13).]

stant driving pressure, flow increases toward the bottom of the lungs as resistance decreases. In contrast to zone 2, where the increase in blood flow from top to bottom of the zone is predominantly due to recruitment of vessels that were previously closed, in zone 3 a comparable increase in blood flow is effected largely by distension of patent capillaries (157).

Zone 4. In the isolated vertical lung and in normal upright humans, the most dependent part—where vascular pressures are highest—includes an area of decreased blood flow [Figs. 8 and 9; (231, 330)]. The zone of reduced flow (zone 4) disappears on deep inflation. This paradox of high vascular pressures and low blood flow is not explicable in terms of the three-zone model in which pulmonary arterial and pulmonary venous pressures are related to alveolar pressures in predicting distribution of blood flow. The mechanism is believed to reside in the extra-alveolar rather than in the alveolar vessels. Indeed, at residual volume, because of the increase in perivascular pressure and mechanical distortion of extra-alveolar vessels, the distribution of blood flow throughout the lung is attributable to extra-alveolar vessels (13, 231).

Note that "zones" are a functional rather than an anatomical concept; instead of being fixed topographically, they vary in vertical height according to shifts in the relationships between pulmonary arterial, pulmonary venous, and alveolar pressures. For example, positive-pressure breathing enlarges zone 2 at the expense of zone 3, and zone 1 at the expense of zone 2 (523). Awareness of the function of these relationships affects the interpretation of changes in calculated pulmonary vascular resistance: for vessels in zone 2 the conventional calculation of pulmonary vascular resistance is meaningless, because alveolar pressure rather than pulmonary venous pressure is the outlet pressure; oppositely, for vessels in zone 3 the calculation is meaningful, because pulmonary venous pressure—rather than alveolar pressure—determines the quantity of blood flow.

DISTENSION AND RECRUITMENT. It is now generally accepted that the extent of the alveolar capillary network is quite variable and that the number, size, and shape of the open capillaries depend on the method of fixation for histologic examination as well as on the experimental circumstances. Some uncertainty still persists, however, about the relative roles played by recruitment (opening of new capillaries) or distension (increase in the caliber of patent capillaries) in enlarging the capillary network.

Not very long ago pulmonary capillary distension was discounted largely on the basis of extrapolation from the behavior of systemic capillaries. However, attempts to draw an analogy between the distensibility of systemic and pulmonary capillaries appear predestined to fail because pulmonary capillaries are suspended in a sea of air and not embedded in tissue. Indeed it has now been amply shown that pulmonary vascular calibers do increase appreciably as transmural pressures are raised (516). It has also become evident, however, that the relationship between vascular calibers and transmural pressure is far from simple (525). Moreover there is no consensus about the extent to which the alveolar capillary bed is distensible (155, 525).

How recruitment is effected remains unsettled. When blood flow is minimal (as in zone 1) (Figs. 8 and 9) only few capillaries are open; these are predominantly corner vessels lodged within septal pleats (164). As transmural pressures increase, the extent of the open capillary bed enlarges, primarily by recruitment in zone 2 and by dilation in zone 3 (164, 512). Some believe that as pulmonary arterial pressure increases, critical opening pressures of different arterioles are successively overcome to open new arteriolar domains to blood flow (231, 374). Others favor the view that capillaries control their own destinies, i.e., that capillaries per se, rather than arterioles, are responsible for opening new portions of the capillary bed and that both distensibility and recruitment occur at the capillary level (172, 512, 525).

Despite lingering doubts about the mechanisms involved in the operation of recruitment and distensibility under different conditions, three generalizations can be made. *1*) Pulmonary capillaries are more distensible than systemic capillaries, presumably because of the lack of supporting connective tissue in the lung (155, 172). *2*) Both recruitment and distensibility are more affected by changes in pulmonary arterial than in pulmonary venous pressure. *3*) Recruitment is the predominant mechanism for enlarging the capillary bed in the apices of the lungs in response to pulsatile flow, whereas recruitment and distensibility probably both contribute—although to different degrees, depending on the circumstances—in the more dependent parts of the lungs.

The concepts about recruitment and distensibility outlined above, based on detailed morphologic observations and tube flow, differ from those provided by the sheet-flow model, which relies heavily on fluid mechanics and in which capillary recruitment is completely discounted (157). Whether a middle ground exists between these opposite views remains to be seen (17, 164).

ALVEOLAR, CORNER, AND EXTRA-ALVEOLAR VESSELS. As the pulmonary vessels branch their way to the capillaries and then regroup to form venous trunks leading to the left atrium, the consecutive segments are subjected to different surrounding pressures (Fig. 10). These perivascular pressures strongly influence vascular calibers, because intravascular pressures in the pulmonary circulation are low and vessel diameters depend heavily on transmural pressures (intravascular minus perivascular pressure) (323). Appreciation of the importance of the different perivascular pressures has encouraged useful distinctions between extra- and intrapulmonary vessels and among three types of intrapulmonary vessels.

Extrapulmonary vessels. Vessels outside of the lungs and within the mediastinum are subjected to subcostal pleural pressure modified by local mechanical distortions. Because of the local effects the pressures surrounding the hilar vessels during inflation are somewhat less negative than subcostal pleural pressures (455). Extrapulmonary veins are thin walled and collapsible. Blood flow through them is pulsatile. Their cross section changes shape as left atrial pressure increases, and the waveform of pulmonary venous blood flow is related inversely to left atrial pressure (395).

Intrapulmonary vessels. When the lungs are inflated under conditions designed to simulate the natural state, intrapulmonary arteries and veins lengthen without appreciable narrowing (264). However, the effect of lung inflation on the calibers of intrapulmonary vessels is not uniform because of the regional differences in pleural pressure, the nonuniform transmission of pleural pressures to the walls of consecutive vascular segments, the original vascular dimensions and degree of distension, the physical characteristics of the vascular walls, the anatomical incorporation of the vessel into the surrounding lung, and the level of vascular tone. Depending on the perivascular pressures to which they are exposed, three types of intrapulmonary vessels have been distinguished: alveolar, corner, and extravascular (Fig. 10).

Alveolar vessels. Alveolar vessels are capillaries that are contained within the walls that separate adjacent alveoli. They are surrounded by interstitium that varies in thickness and in the nature and content of cells, collagen, and elastic fibers [Fig. 11; (139, 309, 515)]. The appearance of the alveolar capillaries depends heavily on the route of fixation. Thus fixation via the airways (which removes the surfactant lining) causes

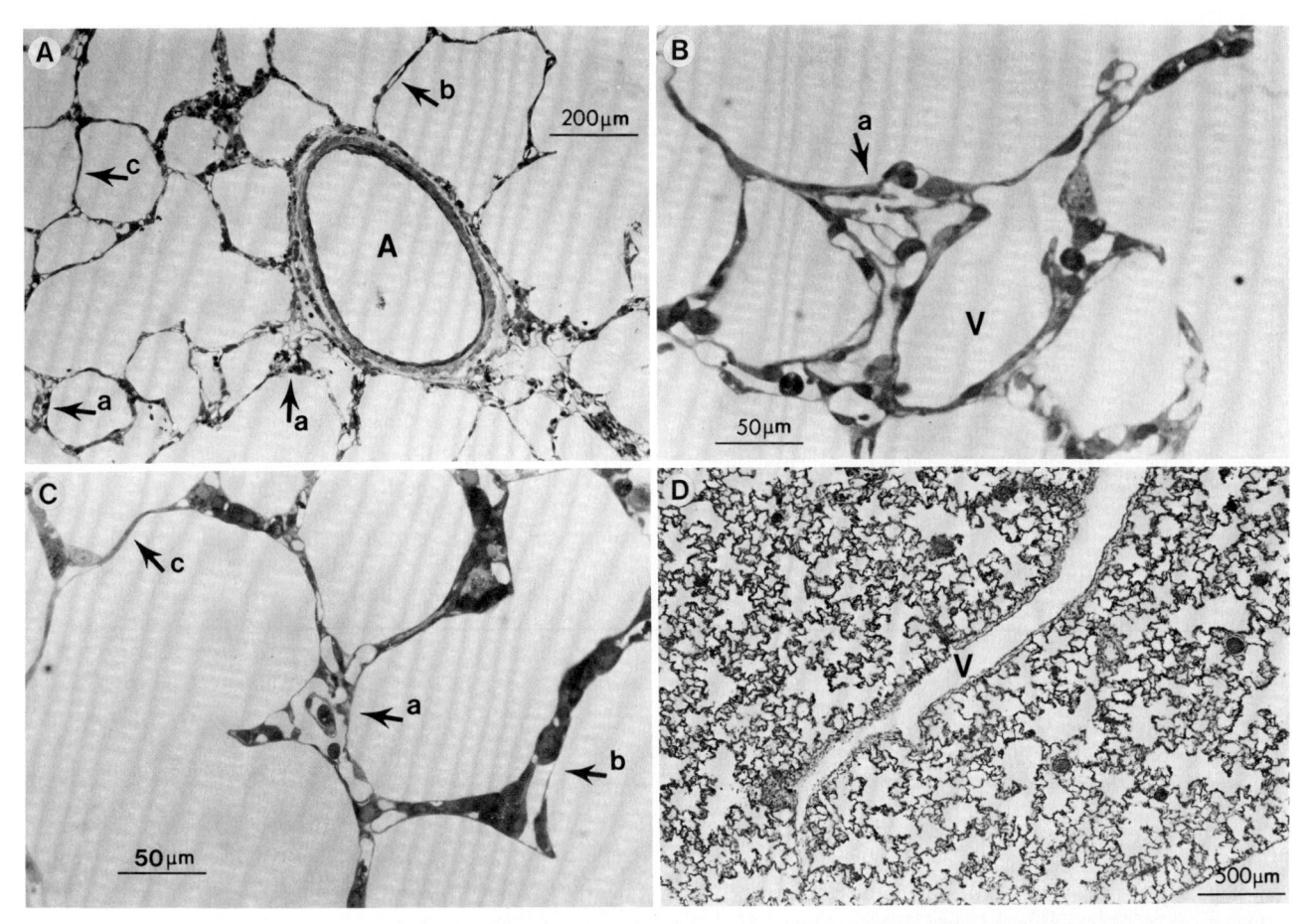

FIG. 10. Alveolar, corner, and extra-alveolar vessels. *A*: large extra-alveolar artery (*A*) showing its muscle layer surrounded by a loose connective tissue sheath. Alveolar septa, inserted radially, presumably exert a radial outward pull that is responsible for dilation of these vessels as the lung is inflated. Lung parenchyma is characteristic of zone 2. *a*, Bundles of capillaries (corner vessels); *b*, flat septa containing open but smoothened, slitlike capillaries; *c*, septa containing completely closed (derecruited) capillaries. Normal rabbit lung fixed under zone 2 conditions by vascular perfusion of OsO_4 into the pulmonary artery. After 2 full inflations, peak arterial pressure = 11–12 mmHg, alveolar pressure = 10 mmHg. Thin epoxy section. *B*: bundle of wide-open capillaries (*a*) within reversible folds of alveolar walls in a corner area. Bundles communicate with vessels (*V*) larger than capillaries, here probably a small nonmuscular artery that is part of the corner arrangement. Although this vessel cannot expand with inflation, it is also protected against collapse. In other locations, small veins are also visible in this arrangement. Normal rabbit lung fixed under zone 2 conditions by vascular perfusion of OsO_4 into the pulmonary artery. Thin epoxy section. *C*: capillaries inside a bundle of capillaries (*a*) in corner presumably connect small arteries with small veins (cf. *B*) and are protected against excess alveolar pressure. Arrangement is due to reversible pleating of alveolar walls. Some septal capillaries (*b*) are open but flattened, whereas others (*c*) are derecruited. Normal rabbit lung fixed under zone 2 conditions by vascular perfusion of OsO_4 into the pulmonary artery. Thin epoxy section. *D*: large extra-alveolar vein (*V*) is surrounded by a loose connective tissue sheath. *Bottom right*, pleural surface. Normal rat lung fixed by instillation of fixatives into trachea after lung collapse. Relatively thick paraffin section, hematoxylin and eosin stain. (Micrographs courtesy of J. Gil.)

the capillaries to bulge into the alveoli, whereas fixation by perfusion (so that the lung remains air-filled) eliminates these deformations, widens capillaries unnaturally, and does away with alveolar pleats and folds (164). As the lung expands, alveolar walls unfold and the connective tissue elements surrounding them are rearranged. The calibers of the alveolar capillaries depend on the level of lung inflation; the capillaries undergo compression (without change in wall thickness) (310) when alveolar pressures increase. Clearly impressions of alveolar morphology are meaningful only when full account is taken not only of the route of fixation but also of the way in which the lung was handled during fixation.

As the lungs expand, the alveolar pericapillary pressure is less than the alveolar pressure (largely because of the surfactant lining of the alveoli) but higher than the pressure surrounding extra-alveolar vessels. This

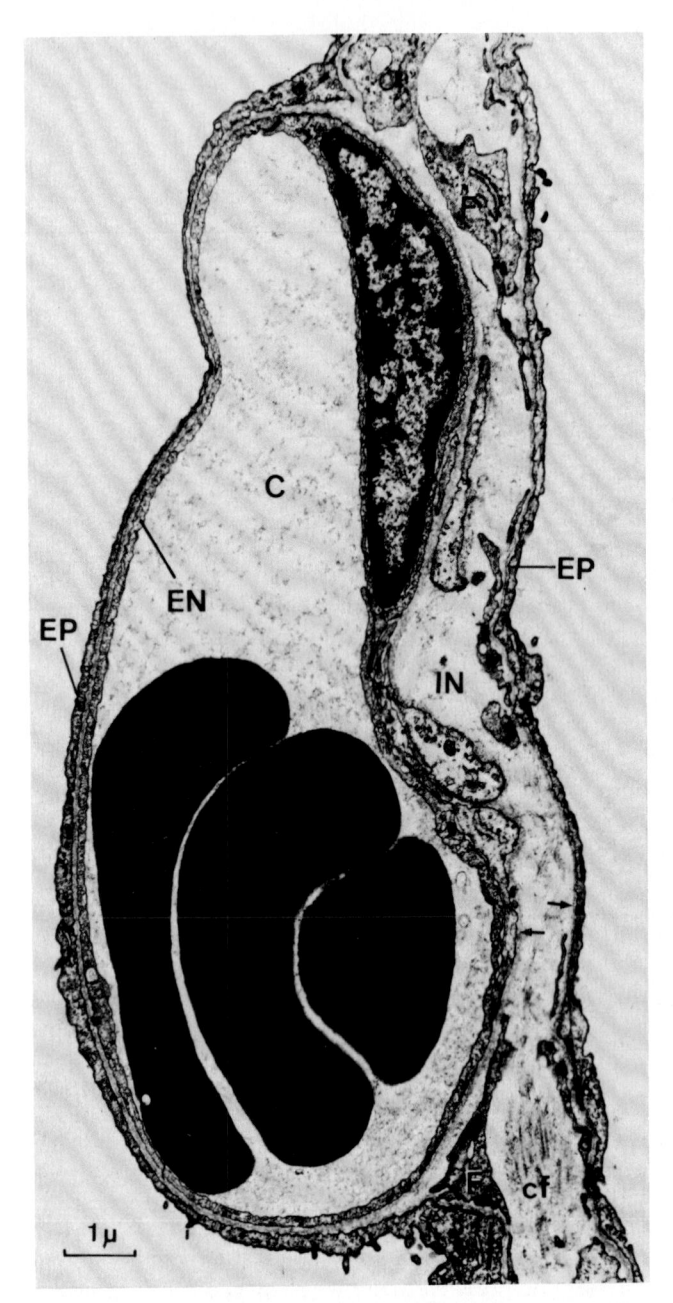

FIG. 11. Cross section of alveolar capillary from human lung lined by endothelium (*EN*). Endothelial nucleus is striking. Alveolar-capillary barrier is organized into thick (*right*) and thin (*left*) portions. Thick side includes considerable interstitial space (*IN*), containing connective tissue elements, e.g., fibers (*cf*). In contrast, interstitial space on thin side is obliterated by fusion of basement membranes, which forms a minimal air-blood barrier. C, capillary containing 3 red corpuscles in its lumen; *EP*, alveolar epithelium; *F*, fibroblast. [From Weibel (515).]

difference between the interstitial pressures to which alveolar and extra-alveolar vessels are exposed is exaggerated at high levels of lung inflation.

To simplify the hemodynamic analysis of blood flow in the alveolar walls Fung and Sobin (155, 156, 449) pictured the alveolar capillary bed as a "sheet" between two membranes separated at regular intervals by "posts." From this point of departure they constructed a sheet-flow model, which pictures the architecture of the pulmonary capillary bed as though it were an underground garage in which posts of septal tissue separate the two layers of endothelium that constitute the roof and floor (157). This model provides a distinct anatomical alternative to that of Weibel (513), who regards the capillary bed as a meshwork of wedged, short cylinders. However, despite striking dissimilarities in appearance the two models do not have markedly different implications for the behavior of pulmonary capillary blood flow: elastic deformation occurs in both models in response to a change in distending pressure, and neither model invokes Poiseuille-type flow in the capillary bed (157). However, the sheet-flow model is deceptively simple in design until full account is taken of *1*) the conceptual and experimental infrastructure of the morphometry, the geometry, and, the elasticity of the capillary network, *2*) the interplay between red blood cells and the vascular wall, *3*) the structure of alveoli, and *4*) the topology of the arteries, capillaries, and venules in the lung.

The most recent application of the sheet-flow model has been to the quantitative analysis of the pulmonary circulation of the cat under steady-state conditions, with particular reference to pressure-flow relationships in the whole lung, the longitudinal distribution of pressures, and the transit time for red blood cells (536). Unfortunately the results of this impressive analysis are not entirely consistent with the observations of others (357). As Zhuang et al. (536) recognize, part of the discrepancy exists because their data base (although extensive) is still incomplete, some of the morphological and mechanical properties assumed for the model can be challenged, and their physiological-anatomical correlations are handicapped by the sparsity of relevant physiological data for the cat. Nonetheless, this analysis challenges prevailing concepts concerning the distensibility of pulmonary capillaries and the role of the capillaries in critical closure; the reconciliation of this analysis with conclusions about the pulmonary circulation drawn from other experimental approaches and theoretical frameworks is needed (66, 159).

Corner vessels. These vessels (Fig. 10) are located at sites where three alveoli abut (172, 416); there they are contained within pleats in the alveolar walls beneath sharp curvatures in the overlying alveolar film of surfactant (163, 166). They are neither extra-alveolar vessels (see next section)—in that they lack a surrounding sleeve of connective tissue—nor conventional components of the pulmonary microcirculation. Their location and anatomical arrangement within pleats seem to offer considerable protection against fluctuations in alveolar pressure. Indeed blood flow persists in these vessels when alveolar pressure exceeds pulmonary arterial pressure by 10 cmH$_2$O (416). Originally pictured as arteriovenous anastomoses, they are now viewed as preferential channels through which blood flow continues despite wide swings in alveolar pressure (164).

Extra-alveolar vessels. By definition extra-alveolar vessels are small vessels that are not affected by changes in alveolar pressure but do enlarge during lung inflation [Fig. 10; (230, 295, 522)]. The definition is far more precise for physiologists than for anatomists, because the designation "extra-alveolar vessel" appears to include diverse components of the pulmonary microcirculation, notably veins, venules, arteries, and precapillaries (164).

Despite this morphologic diversity, the key to the physiological behavior of the extra-alveolar vessels appears to be the connective tissue sheath that they share (95, 164). Surrounding the extra-alveolar vessels is an interstitial space that is bounded by extensions of the fascial sheaths that envelop the trachea and esophagus. Within the perivascular interstitial space lie loose areolar tissue, collagenous fibers, and lymph vessels that drain lymph from the lung parenchyma; in pulmonary edema, excess fluid (and protein) accumulates within this space. The sheaths extend further peripherally along the pulmonary arteries than the bronchi [Fig. 12; (207)]; for pulmonary arteries and probably for pulmonary veins the perivascular sheaths continue peripherally to vessels ~100 μm in diameter. Dilatation of extra-alveolar vessels during inflation is a consequence of a drop in the surrounding interstitial pressure (231).

The degree to which extra-alveolar vessels widen during inflation depends on their initial calibers, which in turn vary with lung volume (34, 263). During deflation to levels below FRC, small arteries and veins tend to close, possibly because of inherent vascular tone (263) abetted by alveolar hypoxia in the poorly expanded regions (95). At this time the site of maximum resistance to blood flow shifts proximally in the arterial tree (106).

It has proved difficult to sort out the effect of a change in lung volume from that of a change in transpulmonary pressure on the resistance of either alveolar or extra-alveolar vessels. As a rule the isolated lung has been used in attempts to make this distinction. Depending on the experimental circumstances, the influence of one or the other may predominate, or the two may act in concert (95).

The alveolar and extra-alveolar interstitial spaces are generally pictured as a continuous pathway for the movement toward the lymphatics of fluid and protein that enter the alveolar-pericapillary space. However, Gil (165) recently suggested that the alveolar and extra-alveolar spaces may be discontinuous. This suggestion implies that pulmonary lymph collected from large lymphatic vessels is derived solely from extra-alveolar vessels without any contribution from alveolar vessels (165). This revolutionary concept needs testing.

INFLATION. Some aspects of the effect of inflation on consecutive pulmonary vascular segments are dealt with in ALVEOLAR, CORNER, AND EXTRA-ALVEOLAR VESSELS, p. 104. Only a few general aspects are reviewed here.

Pulmonary vascular resistance approaches its nadir during normal breathing. At either very high or low levels of lung inflation—no matter how accomplished—pulmonary vascular resistance increases. Inflation of the collapsed, isolated lung with negative pressure first decreases resistance and then increases resistance as high levels of inflation are reached. These observations can be reconciled by attributing *1)* the high resistance at high levels of inflation (P$_A$ held constant) to narrowing of alveolar capillaries, *2)* the high resistance during lung collapse to closure, narrowing, and kinking of the bulk of alveolar capillaries of both kinds, and *3)* the transient drop in resistance as the collapsed lung is inflated to a gradual opening of corner vessels and then usual alveolar vessels followed by narrowing of the usual alveolar vessels at high levels of inflation (95).

Pulmonary Vascular Pressures

For pressure measured within an intrathoracic vessel to be quantifiable, the recording system must be adequate and the reference level must be specified. Conventional measurements are related to atmospheric pressure by taking into account the hydrostatic pressure difference between the intrathoracic site from which pressure is being recorded and the externally placed sensing element of the manometer. For this purpose the plane of the sensing element is set in relationship to both the heart and some thoracic landmark. In human subjects, different hydrostatic zero

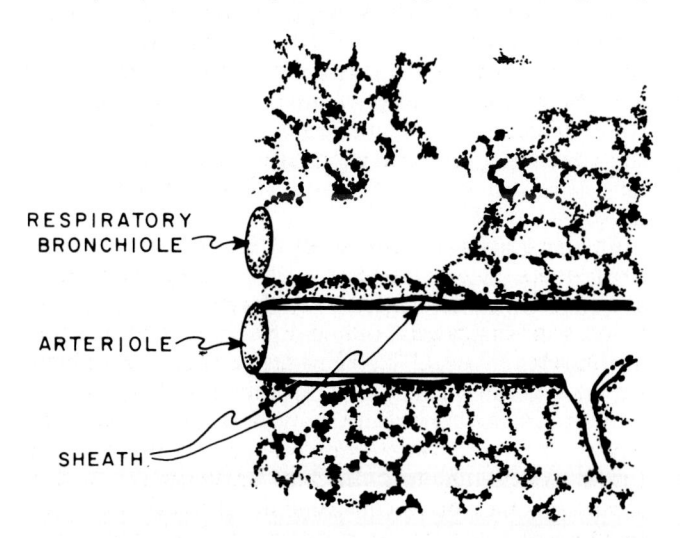

FIG. 12. Schematic representation of fascial sheath extending down wall of pulmonary arteriole. [Adapted from Hayek (207).]

levels have been used as a preference level for pulmonary arterial pressures: the most popular levels are 5 cm below the angle of Louis and 10–12 cm above the tabletop. Although different reference levels do complicate comparison of data from different laboratories, each is a reliable standard for consecutive measurements in the same individual (138). The implications for the measurement of pulmonary wedge pressure of impacting a cardiac catheter in other than zone 3 of the lung are considered next.

PULMONARY ARTERY. With each breath, as the lungs fill with air, pressures in the pulmonary artery fall by a few millimeters of mercury, reflecting a combination of changes in systemic venous return, intrathoracic pressure, and mechanical deformation of the pulmonary vascular tree. The rate and depth of breathing modifies the time lag between blood flow into and out of the lungs: left ventricular pressure falls steadily during a deep breath in human subjects and increases after a lag of 2–3 s following the start of expiration. Pulmonary vascular resistance increases during inspiration (138).

With minor differences the contour of the pulmonary arterial pressure pulse mirrors that at the root of the aorta: as may be seen in Figure 4, the pulmonary arterial pressure pulse is small in amplitude as compared to the aortic pulse and characteristically displays a rapid rise to a rounded peak during systole, a brisk small incisura, and a gradual decrease in pressure during diastole (60). Classic pulmonary arterial curves are more apt to be recorded in pulmonary hypertensive states than in pulmonary normotensive states; at the lower levels of pulmonary arterial pressure, distorting artifacts are exceedingly common. In contrast to pressure-velocity relationships in the aorta, the pulmonary arterial pressure and velocity curves are quite similar: the velocity of blood flow in the pulmonary artery lags slightly behind the pulmonary arterial pressure (332).

In all species studied, pressure pulses, like flow pulses, diminish as they travel peripherally in the pulmonary vascular tree (332). Although reflections do occur in the transmission of the pressure pulses, in the normal pulmonary circulation they are insufficient to amplify the pulmonary arterial pressure pulse appreciably.

Ordinarily the pulmonary arterial mean pressure in the human, dog, cat, and rabbit averages one-fifth to one-sixth that in the systemic circulation (Fig. 13). In the human the level of the pulmonary arterial pressure seems to increase slightly with age (377). There is no fixed relationship between the pressures in the two circuits. At the end of diastole the pulmonary arterial pressure in human subjects is ~7–12 mmHg; during systole it rises abruptly to 20–30 mmHg; the corresponding mean pressure is ~12–15 mmHg. In the dog, pulmonary arterial pressures tend to be somewhat higher, so that a mean pressure of 20 mmHg is not unusual (138).

PULMONARY MICROCIRCULATION. The pulmonary arterial and venous trees are connected by a complicated microcirculation in which distinctions between capillaries and contiguous arterioles and venules tend to be indistinct and consecutive segments are often exposed to perivascular pressures that differ not only in degree but also in direction (see Fig. 10). Consequently many physiologists have forsaken the designation "capillary" for terms in which anatomical precision is sacrificed for the sake of physiological description and analysis. Among these are the designations "alveolar vessels," "microvessels," and "extraalveolar vessels."

One important implication of this incorporation of anatomical terms in interpreting physiological measurements is that the terms impart to them more of an operational than a structural reality; the methods used have considerable implications for identifying the particular segment(s) of the microcirculation that is involved. For example, direct measurement of pressures in subpleural vessels by micropuncture indicates that most of the arteriovenous pressure drop occurs in the pulmonary capillaries (49, 357). Somewhat different results were obtained on the basis of morphometry of the pulmonary arterial tree, which indicated that more than half of the pressure drop from pulmonary artery to pulmonary vein occurs proximal to the pulmonary capillaries, particularly in vessels smaller than 0.8 mm in diameter (96).

Gas-exchanging techniques, which presumably operate by way of precapillaries and capillaries, generally attribute most of the pressure drop to precapillary vessels (110, 511). A second experimental approach that depends on inflation of the lungs to distinguish between alveolar and extra-alveolar vessels casts doubt on this conclusion: the results from one laboratory implicated arterial extra-alveolar, alveolar, and venous extra-alveolar vessels about equally in the pulmonary arteriovenous pressure drop (312); the results from another laboratory attributed most of the pressure drop to alveolar vessels (149). A third experimental approach that depends on determinations of water exchange in the pulmonary microcirculation has the additional ambiguity that not only alveolar capillaries but also extra-alveolar vessels appear to be involved.

The inconsistent results with different techniques underscore uncertainties about the anatomical equivalents of physiologically designated "capillaries," "alveolar vessels," "gas-exchanging vessels," and "fluid-exchanging vessels." Certainly they need not refer to the same anatomical structures under different experimental conditions. For example, experiments designed to apply water-exchanging techniques sometimes ignore changes in lung volumes that may strongly influence the outcome. Even direct measurements can be misleading: accurate measurements of subpleural pressures may fail to provide values that are meaningful for vessels buried within the substance

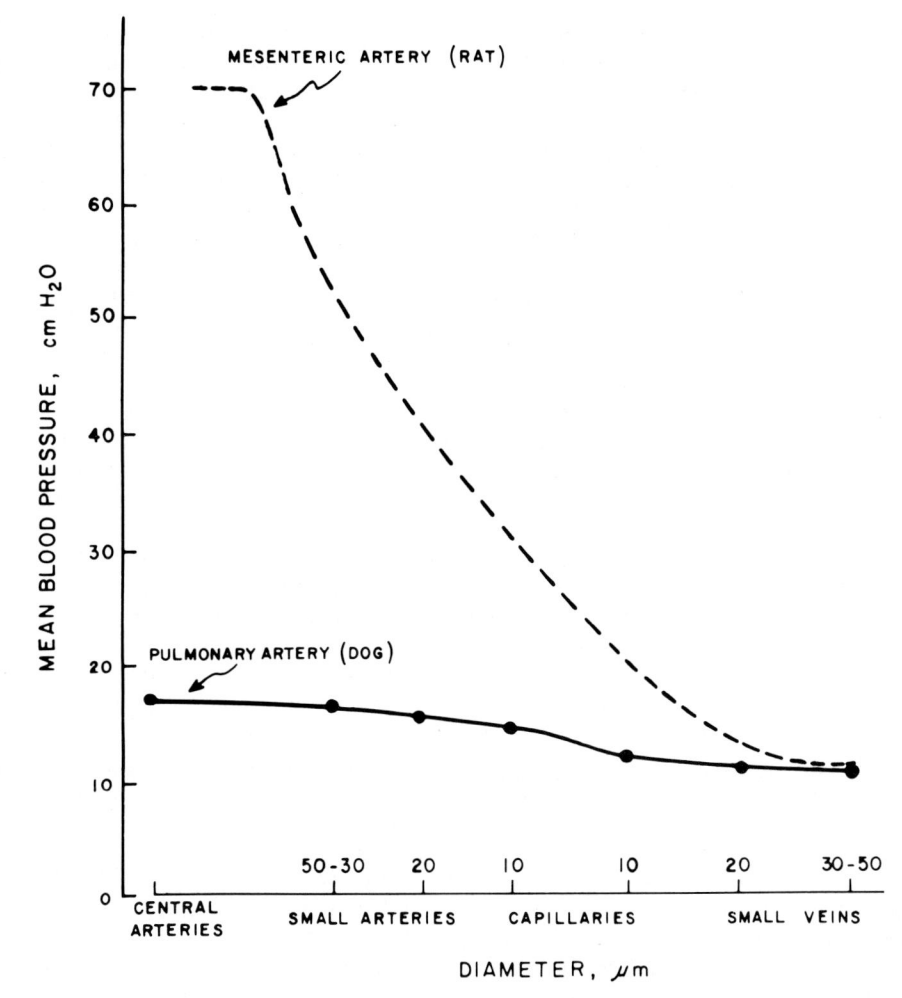

FIG. 13. Pulmonary vascular pressures in consecutive segments of the pulmonary vascular tree and in comparable segments of a systemic artery. Measurements were made by direct puncture of arterial and venous segments of the subpleural microcirculation. [Adapted from Bhattacharya et al. (49, 50).]

of the lungs. Certainly the isolated perfused lung exposed to atmospheric pressures operates under different transmural pressures and microcirculatory dimensions than those of the normal lung, which is subjected to rhythmic changes in pleural pressure within the confines of the intact thorax.

Of great interest to those concerned with water exchange and Starling forces in the lungs is the average pressure and the average intravascular pressure drop between the beginnings and ends of the fluid-exchanging components of the pulmonary microcirculation (358). Unfortunately none of the available techniques provide a reliable measure of these important hemodynamic parameters (50).

PULMONARY VEINS AND LEFT ATRIUM. Blood pressures have been recorded directly from the left atrium and pulmonary veins in dogs and humans (Figs. 4, 5, and 14). Because pulmonary venous pressure pulse appears to be a record only of left atrial events, the pulmonary arterial pressure pulse seems to be damped out as it traverses small pulmonary vessels. As in the systemic veins and right atrium, the A, C, and V waves are clearly defined, but in contrast to the right heart the summit of the V wave is usually the highest part of the pressure pulse and pressure variations during the cardiac cycle are greater in the left atrium and pulmonary veins. Thus, in both the unanesthetized and anesthetized dog, pulmonary venous pressures during a single cardiac cycle range between 3 and 12 mmHg. In intact unanesthetized humans the mean left atrial pressure is ~5–10 mmHg (482). Although physiological and anatomical observations have raised the possibility that the pulmonary venous–left atrial junctions can act as sphincters, proof, in the form of suitably recorded pulmonary venous–left atrial pressure gradients or differences between the contours of the pulmonary venous and left atrial pressure pulses, has yet to be published.

PULMONARY ARTERIOVENOUS PRESSURE DIFFERENCES. In the human, cat, and dog the pressure drop across the pulmonary vascular bed is ~10% of the pressure drop across the systemic circulation (Fig. 13). The pulmonary arterial–left atrial pressure gradient is maximal early in systole; it decreases late in systole and may even approach zero if diastole is sufficiently prolonged. Unfortunately because both the pulmonary

FIG. 14. Simultaneous tracings in the dog of pulmonary arterial and venous flow and pulmonary arterial and venous pressure. Variations in pulmonary arterial and venous flow are nearly simultaneous; maxima and minima in venous flow lag from corresponding points in arterial flow record only by the 0.09 s necessary for flow pulse to be propagated across pulmonary circulation. [From Morkin, Fishman, et al. (342).]

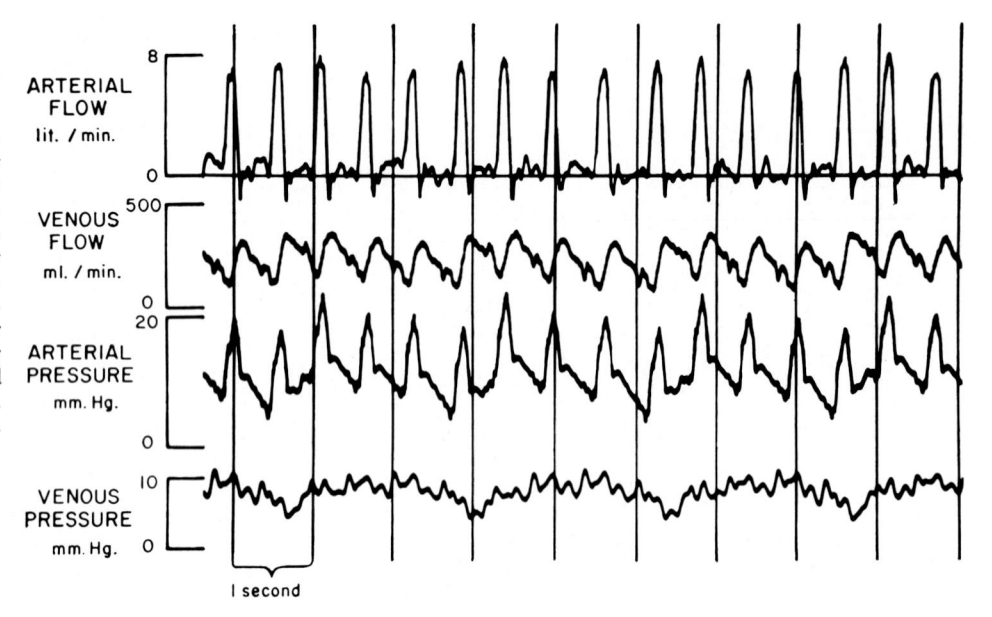

arterial and pulmonary venous pressure pulses have different origins (right and left sides of the heart, respectively) it is not possible to predict the shape of the pressure pulses of the intervening vascular bed from the pulmonary arterial–pulmonary venous pressure gradient.

PULMONARY WEDGE PRESSURE. The pulmonary arterial wedge pressure is recorded by introducing a cardiac catheter into a systemic vein and advancing it through the right side of the heart into the pulmonary arterial tree until it impacts in a small precapillary vessel (Fig. 15). In this way a continuous channel is formed, consisting of the catheter in series with the wedged vessel (usually an artery ~1,500–3,000 mm), the intervening segment of the pulmonary capillary bed, and the pulmonary veins that drain into the left atrium. If the vessels between the wedged catheter and left atrium are open (as under zone 3 conditions) the mean wedge pressure equals that in the left atrium. Because the catheter is easy to place and because clinical interest in left atrial pressure is high on several accounts—not the least of which is the opportunity it provides for the calculation of pulmonary vascular resistance—reliance on the wedge pressure is widespread in human studies.

In the normal pulmonary circulation of the dog and human the wedge pressure is usually ~5–10 mmHg, but it reflects mean left atrial pressure reliably only when the catheter tip is properly wedged below the level of the left atrium (zone 3) (481, 482). In this circumstance the wedge pressure mirrors left atrial pressure both during an acute increase in left atrial pressure, as is produced by transfusion, and in chronic left atrial hypertension, as in chronic mitral stenosis. However, the wedge pressure cannot be counted on to mirror left atrial pressures during states of left atrial

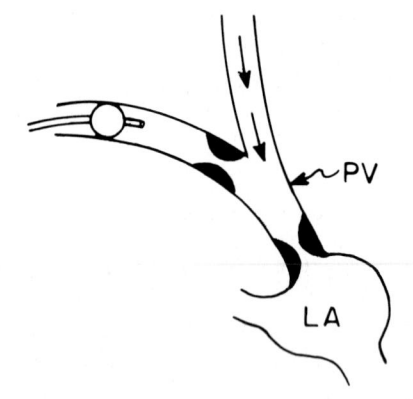

FIG. 15. Principle of determination of pulmonary wedge pressure. Pressure sensed by wedged catheter (*left*, balloon inflated) is same as that at conjunction of flowing (*2 arrows*) and static streams (distal to wedged catheter). Nonocclusive constriction distal to occlusive catheter does not affect determination of pulmonary wedge pressure. However, constriction distal to confluence, as in pulmonary venule (PV), may cause pulmonary wedge pressure to exceed left atrial (LA) pressure. [Adapted from Marini (304).]

hypotension, as in systemic arterial hypotension (Fig. 16).

Another practical approach that is used to estimate left atrial pressure is inflating a balloon in one pulmonary artery and recording distally to the occlusive balloon. The tracing obtained in this way resembles that of the pulmonary arterial wedge pressure (138).

Various criteria have been advanced to ensure that a wedge pressure value is a reliable measure of mean left atrial pressure: *1*) checking to be sure that wedge pressure is less than mean pulmonary arterial and diastolic pressures, *2*) the withdrawal of fully oxygenated blood from the impacted catheter, *3*) the characteristic snap of the catheter as it is withdrawn from the wedge position, and *4*) the distinctive configura-

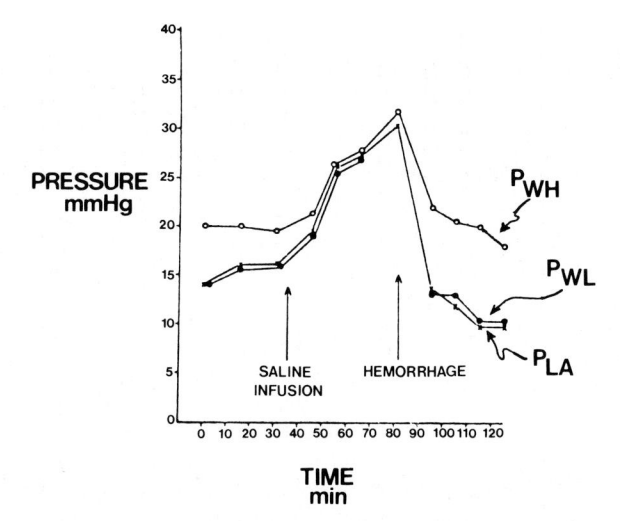

FIG. 16. Effect of location of tip of wedged catheter on validity as measure of left atrial pressure (Pla); one catheter was wedged high (Pwh) and the other low (Pwl) in the lung. Initially the upper catheter was located in zone 2 of the lung and did not reflect left atrial pressure. Saline infusion increased left atrial pressure and converted lung containing upper wedged catheter to zone 3 conditions; both catheters then reflected left atrial pressures. Subsequent hemorrhage restored zone 2 conditions and original discrepancy between pulmonary wedge and left atrial pressures. Catheter that was wedged low operated throughout under zone 3 conditions. [From Todd et al. (481).]

tion of the wedge tracing. Unfortunately, even when all criteria are met the wedge pressure may fail to provide a measure of mean left atrial pressure if the catheter fails for anatomical reasons to be wedged properly, if the tip is wedged in zone 1 or 2 of the lung instead of zone 3, if vessels between the catheter tip and the left atrium are the seat of occlusive disease (392), or if the parenchyma of the intervening lung is structurally deranged, e.g., by fibrosis or emphysema (138).

When the catheter wedges in zones 1 or 2 rather than in zone 3 the pressure that is recorded relates more closely to alveolar than to atrial pressure. This situation is more apt to occur during blind passage of a Swan-Ganz catheter under hemodynamic guidance than during placement with fluoroscopic control. Hemorrhagic shock (481) and positive-pressure breathing favor this occurrence because these states are characterized by an increase in the extent of zones 1 and 2 at the expense of zone 3; wedge pressure then exceeds mean left atrial pressure (481, 482).

The use of pulmonary arterial wedge pressure to measure mean left atrial pressure is on sounder footing than is its use for registering the fleeting components of the left atrial pressure pulse. Except in states of pulmonary venous congestion, i.e., left ventricular failure or mitral regurgitation, the wedge catheter cannot be expected to reliably reproduce cyclic events in the left atrium; the likelihood of artifacts is compounded by exercise and deep breathing.

In brief, when used critically the pulmonary arterial wedge pressure can usually provide a measure of the mean left atrial pressure. It provides no measure of pulmonary capillary pressure, i.e., the average hydrostatic pressure in the alveolar capillaries.

INFLUENCE OF INTRATHORACIC PRESSURE ON PULMONARY VASCULAR PRESSURES. If the manometer that records the pressure is balanced against atmospheric pressure, all pressure changes within the thorax arising from ventilation (e.g., a cough) will be immediately propagated across the walls of the pulmonary vessels and heart to the incompressible blood that they contain; the intrathoracic pressure changes will therefore be registered as an integral part of the pressure pulse. However, pressures recorded in this way (luminal pressures) provide no measure of the pressure that distends the vessels (transmural pressures): during a cough, while the pressure recorded by a manometer balanced against atmospheric pressure rises precipitously, a manometer balanced against pleural pressure shows that the transmural pressure has remained virtually unchanged (138).

Values for the pleural pressures have been obtained in various ways, including direct measurements from gas pockets and balloons within the pleural or mediastinal space and indirect estimates from the esophagus. Unfortunately the introduction of a catheter, balloon, or transducer invariably distorts the local molecular, cohesive, and adhesive forces between the pleural surfaces. Resorting to the determination of liquid pleural pressures (by widely separating the pleural surfaces so as to minimize intermolecular forces) provides no clue about the surface pleural pressures in the intact animal or human, although it does furnish a reproducible artifact that can be measured with great accuracy. New initiatives at indirect determinations of local pleural pressures still have to be reconciled with more direct observations (223).

These measurement difficulties underscore the problem in obtaining precise measurements of the pleural pressures that are operating at the surface of particular pulmonary vascular segments: not only is it likely that topographical differences in pleural pressure do exist but the possibility is strong that extramural pressures differ from segment to segment. The use of indirect measures, such as the esophageal balloon, is practical if care is exerted in interpretation. Current teaching estimates a vertical gradient of pleural pressure in the normal lung of ~0.2–0.5 cmH$_2$O/cm.

TRANSMURAL VERSUS LUMINAL PRESSURES. During each respiratory cycle the changing pleural pressures affect all intrathoracic vessels except those apposed to alveoli (223, 315). Consequently the pressure that determines the caliber of the alveolar capillaries, i.e., transmural pressure, is customarily calculated as the difference between estimated intracapillary pressure and alveolar pressure; the transmural pressure of all other vessels is calculated as the difference between the luminal and the pleural pressure. The practical difficulties in estimating perivascular pressure from pleural pressure have been mentioned above; pericapillary pressures also have an element of uncertainty because of the prospect that tissue forces (e.g., alveolar surface tension) may decrease pericapillary pressure to subatmospheric levels.

It has also been noted above that, depending on the purpose of the observation, pulmonary vascular pressures are referred either to atmospheric or to pleural pressure. Considerable confusion has arisen from the indiscriminate use of transmural pressures for luminal pressures in the calculation of pulmonary vascular resistance. As long as left atrial pressure exceeds alveolar pressure the measurement of the driving pressure across the lung requires only the simultaneous measurements of luminal pulmonary arterial and venous pressures—no matter what the intrathoracic pressure may be.

MECHANICAL VENTILATION. Although mechanical ventilation is now commonplace both in the experimental laboratory and in the clinical setting, and even though a consensus exists about many of its general effects on the respiration and circulation, considerable uncertainty exists about details. One source of ambiguity is the various patterns in which the different machines inflate the lungs; another that relates to the determination of the transmural pressures affecting key intrathoracic vessels, cardiac chambers, and potential spaces is the difficulty in obtaining accurate estimates of local intrathoracic pressures.

Among the more thoroughly analyzed types of mechanical ventilation from the hemodynamic point of view are positive-pressure ventilation and positive end-expiratory pressure (PEEP) (391). In normal humans and animals, PEEP at a level of 5 cmH$_2$O decreases stroke volume, cardiac output, and central blood volume, leaving heart rate unaffected; pulmonary arterial pressures also increase and blood flow through the lungs is redistributed—presumably favoring alveolar corner vessels in the uppermost, hypoperfused areas—resulting in high ventilation-perfusion ratios ($\dot{V}_A/\dot{Q}$) (213); these effects are exaggerated as the PEEP level is raised. In those respiratory and cardiac disorders characterized by pulmonary edema (e.g., the adult respiratory distress syndrome) the same phenomena occur but at higher levels of PEEP, ranging from 15 to 40 cmH$_2$O (533). How the reduction in cardiac output is effected is enigmatic. At least three mechanisms are currently advocated: 1) a decrease in venous return (preload) to the right ventricle (the most traditional mechanism) (91), 2) a decrease in left ventricular preload (240), and 3) impairment of both right and left ventricular performance (411). To complicate the situation further the prospects have been raised that an increase in PEEP inhibits cardiovascular regulatory mechanisms in the brain (78) and that prostaglandins contribute to a negative inotropic effect of PEEP (127). Presently it is not possible to quantify the roles played by each of these influences in the various experimental or clinical settings in which PEEP has been assessed. Information along these lines is even more fragmentary for other forms and modifications of mechanical ventilation, e.g., continuous positive-pressure ventilation (506).

EXERCISE. Before considering changes in pulmonary artery pressure during exercise, it should be noted that 1) pulmonary vascular pressures are difficult to measure accurately during exercise because respiratory swings are marked and the records are apt to be distorted by artifacts, 2) especially during severe exercise, shifts in midposition of the lung and changes in compliance confuse the recognition of the mechanisms involved in a change of pressure, and 3) the increase in mean pulmonary arterial pressure and the concomitant increase in pulsatility (Fig. 17) improve perfusion of the apices of the lungs (522).

The behavior of the pulmonary arterial pressure during light exercise is quite predictable: at the start of the exercise the (luminal) pulmonary arterial mean pressure increases abruptly by 3–5 mmHg. As exercise is continued a plateau is reached, generally at 1–2 mmHg less than peak values; the increase in systolic pressure exceeds the increase in diastolic pressure. In

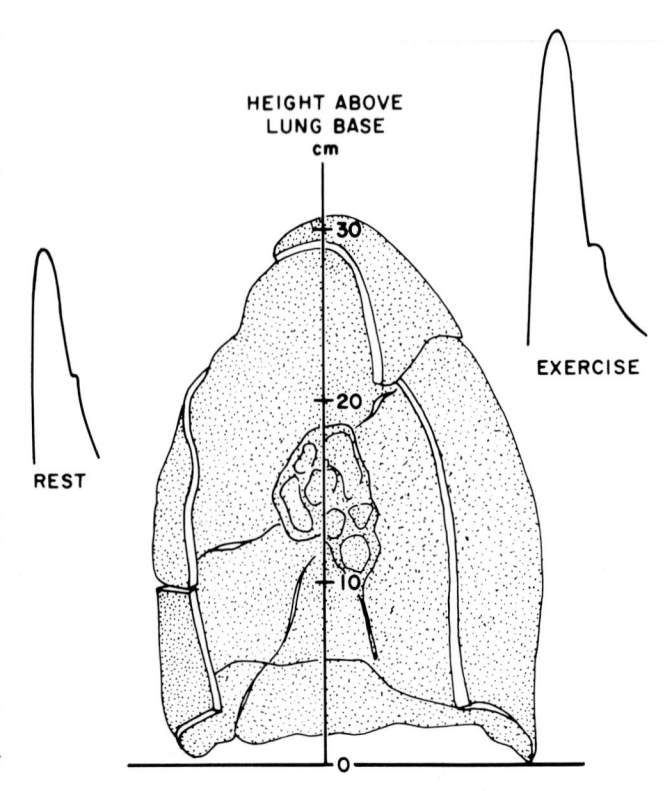

FIG. 17. Effect of exercise on upright lung. Increase in mean pulmonary arterial pressure, coupled with increase in pulsatility, favors apical perfusion. [Adapted from West (522).]

upright, normal human lungs the modest increment in the level of the mean pulmonary arterial pressure, coupled with the increase in pulsatility, suffices to improve perfusion of the apices (522). As a rule, the higher the preexercise level of the pulmonary arterial pressures, the higher the values reached during exercise. Immediately after the exercise the pulmonary arterial pressure often falls below control resting values (138).

Figure 18 shows pulmonary hemodynamics in normal young men and women during supine exercise. The exercise involved two different work loads on a bicycle ergometer; particular care was exerted to achieve a steady state. Not shown is that the studies confirmed a positive linear correlation between the level of physical activity and the O_2 uptake at the low and medium work rates; at higher work rates the curve for O_2 uptake approached an asymptote. Although the patterns of hemodynamic change in the young men and women were qualitatively similar, the work loads were not the same and the patterns of response are not identical (187).

Direct measurements of the left atrial pressure during exercise in intact humans or dogs have not been reported. However, in dogs exercised by electrical stimulation of the extremities the left atrial pressure remains unchanged (132); unfortunately the level of exercise in these experiments is unknown. In humans the slight increments of the pulmonary arterial pressure during mild exercise suggest that if the left atrial pressure does increase, the increase cannot exceed a few millimeters of mercury. The pulmonary wedge pressure is unaffected by mild exercise but may increase slightly as the intensity of the exercise increases (120).

Pulmonary Blood Volume

The volume of blood contained in the lungs of intact animals or humans has been of interest along at least five different lines: *1)* as a determinant of the mechanical behavior of the lungs, *2)* as an important element in external gas exchange, *3)* as a prime factor in ensuring an adequate preload for the left ventricle, *4)* as a contributor in the pathogenesis of hemodynamic pulmonary edema, and *5)* as a stimulus to the sensation of dyspnea. In large measure the quantity of blood contained in the lungs at any instant is

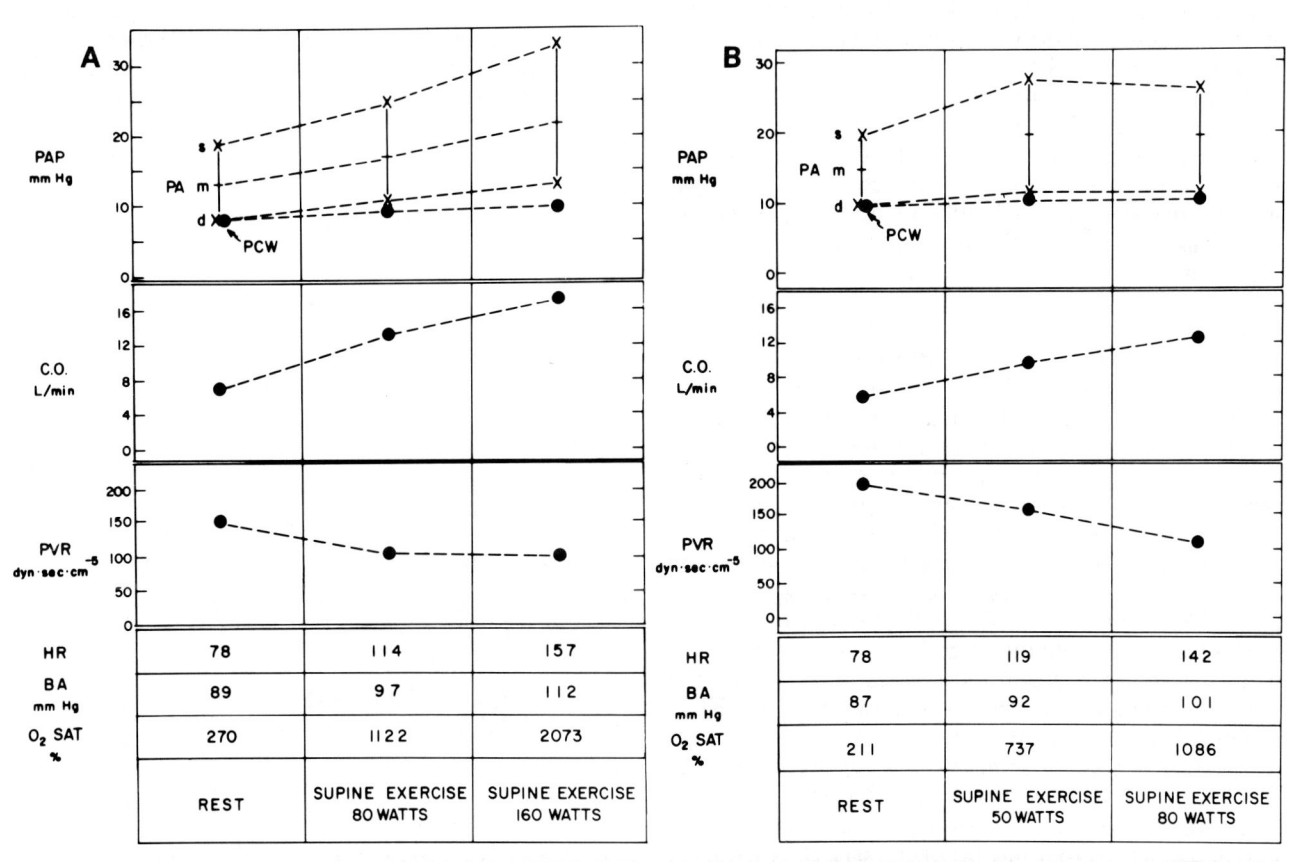

FIG. 18. Pulmonary hemodynamics at rest and during steady-state supine exercise in humans. *A*: normal males, avg age 23.6 ± 2.1 SD. *B*: normal females, avg age 23.8 ± 3.9 SD. BA, brachial arterial pressure; C.O., cardiac output; d, diastolic pressure; HR, heart rate; m, mean pressure; PAP, pulmonary arterial pressure; PCW, pulmonary capillary wedge pressure; PVR, pulmonary vascular resistance; s, systolic pressure. [Adapted from Gurtner et al. (187).]

determined passively by the balance between pulmonary inflow and outflow, i.e., between the outputs of the two ventricles (see Fig. 4); it is also influenced considerably by the ventilation. Whether an element of self-control is also provided by pulmonary vasomotor activity, particularly on the part of the veins or of hypothetical venous sinuses, is conjectural.

MEASUREMENT. Most methods for determining the pulmonary blood volume are designed to provide a measure of the total volume of blood in the lungs; a few are designed to partition this volume (see Fig. 4; Table 1). In intact animals and humans, indicator-dilution techniques are generally used. As a rule the indicator-dilution volume depends on the sites of injection and sampling. Few methods are designed to detect a change in pulmonary blood volume per se.

In the isolated lung or in thoracotomized animals the pulmonary blood volume is available for direct mensuration, but because of the surgical manipulations and the drastic experimental conditions the measured volume may differ considerably from the volume that prevails under more natural conditions.

The traditional Stewart-Hamilton method entails the introduction of a test substance into the venous side of the circulation and the registration, from a systemic artery, of its changing concentration with time. This technique defines only a "central blood volume" that includes not merely the blood volume between the needles but also the volume of blood contained in the other branches of the venous and arterial trees having equivalent circulation times. It is meaningless to use the central blood volume—with its vague boundaries and its potential for internal rearrangement—to estimate the pulmonary blood volume as long as the test substance is injected into a peripheral vein. The first step to narrow the boundaries of the central blood volume was the pulmonary arterial injection of the test substance coupled with peripheral arterial sampling; this central blood volume approximates 20%–25% of the total circulating blood volume (265). The second step was to couple the pulmonary arterial injection either with sampling from the left atrium or with the injection of a second tracer into the left atrium. With this technique the pulmonary blood volume has proved to be ~10% of the total circulating blood volume.

It is surprising how closely the indicator-dilution value of ~10% in the intact human corresponds to the more direct measurements of pulmonary blood volume in the dog, rabbit, and rat. The indicator-dilution value of 10% also coincides with estimates based on pulmonary vascular dimensions in the dog (332).

CHANGES. The pulmonary blood volume has been reported to increase under the following circumstances: *1)* the increase in pulmonary blood flow caused by acute infusion of plasma expanders, *2)* inflation of an antigravity suit, *3)* negative-pressure (pleural) breathing, *4)* assumption of the supine position, *5)* systemic

TABLE 1. *Partition of Pulmonary Microvascular Resistances in Dogs*

Preparation	Condition by Zone	Method	Ra/RT	Rv/RT	Ref.
Spontaneous partition					
Intact	III	Fluid absorption	0.40	0.60	6
			0.60	0.40	362
		Starling resistor	0.71	0.29	168
		Segmental pressures	0.62	0.38	262
		Isofiltration	0.52	0.48	106, 160
		Swan-Ganz transients	0.60	0.40	226
Isolated	III	Isogravimetric	0.56	0.44	159
			0.53	0.47	366
			0.67	0.33	428
		Low-viscosity bolus	0.63	0.37	66
			0.69	0.31	109, 189
		Occlusion	0.60	0.40	363
			0.67	0.33	189
		Micropuncture	0.61	0.39	49
Intact	II, low	Fluid absorption	0.60	0.40	364
	II, high	Fluid absorption	0.40	0.60	364
Effects of vasomotor agents					
Intact	III	Arachidonic acid, bisenoic prostaglandins, PGH$_2$; segmental pressures		Increased	244
Isolated	III	Serotonin; occlusion and viscous bolus	0.79	0.21	64, 189, 225
		Histamine; occlusion and viscous bolus	0.30	0.70	62, 64, 189, 244
		Alveolar hypoxia; isogravimetric	0.81	0.19	365
		Alveolar hypoxia; occlusion and viscous bolus	0.67	0.33	189, 235

Ra, arterial (precapillary) resistance; RT, total pulmonary vascular bed resistance; Rv, venous (postcapillary) resistance. Data from A. E. Taylor and J. C. Parker, unpublished observations.

vasoconstriction from a variety of causes, *6*) immersion in water, *7*) clamping the pulmonary veins, and *8*) left ventricular failure and mitral stenosis (133, 138).

Conversely a decrease in pulmonary blood volume results from other types of interventions: *1*) after venesection and the consequent reduction in cardiac output, *2*) during positive-pressure breathing or the Valsalva maneuver, *3*) during systemic vasodilation (as from warming), *4*) on assumption of the upright posture, and *5*) on exposure to acute hypoxia (2). Expansion of the pulmonary blood volume while the lung is upright—as by infusion, exercise, heart disease (mitral stenosis), or limitation in the extent of the pulmonary vascular bed—tends to make the blood flow through the lungs more uniform and to diminish the likelihood of redistribution when posture is changed.

Many different approaches have been used to estimate changes in pulmonary blood volume, including *1*) lung volumes, *2*) mechanics of breathing, *3*) radioactive tracers, and *4*) other methods, such as the teeterboard.

Lung volumes. In normal subjects the vital capacity is less in the supine than in the upright position. Although part of this decrease may reflect a change in the position and tone of the diaphragm, an increase in the pulmonary blood volume also seems to be involved, because measures that interfere with systemic venous return to the lungs minimize or prevent the decrease in vital capacity. Clinically a low vital capacity is found in pulmonary congestion. However, in such patients, particularly if pulmonary venous hypertension has been prolonged and severe, the lung volumes may be more limited by pulmonary edema and fibrosis than by an expanded pulmonary blood volume (138).

Mechanics of breathing. Pathologists have long been aware that the chronically congested lung is a stiff lung. In 1934 Christie and Meakins showed by measuring pleural pressure in vivo that the chronically congested lung requires a greater distending force than the normal lung. Since then more elaborate ways of measuring and expressing pulmonary distensibility, such as "compliance" (change in lung volume per unit change in pleural pressure), have come into general use for the study of both acute and chronic pulmonary congestion; for the sake of safety and expediency, and at some risk of uncertainty and inaccuracy, esophageal pressures have been substituted for pleural pressures (322).

The effects of acute pulmonary engorgement on pulmonary distensibility have been examined in animals and in humans (179). Such studies have shown that pulmonary venous hypertension has a considerably greater effect in reducing pulmonary compliance than does either pulmonary arterial hypertension or an increase in pulmonary blood flow; moreover a decrease in vital capacity parallels a decrease in pulmonary compliance. However, these studies have also clarified some of the problems with the use of a change in compliance as a qualitative measure of the state of the pulmonary blood volume: *1*) an increase in pulmonary interstitial fluid during acute pulmonary venous hypertension may be indistinguishable from an associated increase in pulmonary blood volume; *2*) the discrepancies between esophageal pressure and pleural pressure are exaggerated in the supine position because mediastinal contents compress the esophagus to yield artificially high values for pleural pressures; and *3*) changes in the lung volume may, per se, affect apparent pulmonary distensibility. Nonetheless, despite the inherent limitations of available methods and prevailing uncertainties in interpretation, exploration of pulmonary mechanics in pulmonary congestion continues to be illuminating. For example, the mechanical work and energy cost of moving congested lungs has proved to be abnormally high; even more impressive is the repeated demonstration that stiff lungs are associated with a distinctive breathing pattern (rapid frequency, small tidal volume).

Radioactive tracers. Radioactive tracers administered intravenously in conjunction with external counting devices have been used to uncover changes in regional pulmonary blood volume after a variety of experimental manipulations (352). The validity of this approach rests heavily on the assumption that the external detector continues to survey an unchanged geometry throughout the control and test periods. It is difficult to prove that this assumption is valid in experiments that involve either respiratory maneuvers or changes in body position.

Other methods. Some experiments require only the recognition that a change has occurred in thoracic (instead of pulmonary) blood volume. One noninvasive approach along this line has been the use of the critically balanced teeterboard to detect a shift in the center of gravity of the body as blood is displaced from one end of the body to the other. Another is the "cardiopneumogram," which provides an index of the changes in thoracic blood volume during each cardiac cycle (198).

NORMAL VALUES. In the normal lungs of a 75-kg man the pulmonary blood volume is generally estimated to be ~500 ml, i.e., ~10%–12% of the total blood volume (532). In a 20-kg dog the corresponding value is ~200 ml, i.e., ~8%–10% of the total blood volume (332).

PARTITION. The distribution of the pulmonary blood volume within the pulmonary vascular tree is strongly influenced by the experimental circumstance and the preparation under study (110, 135, 385). In both the human and dog, arteries, capillaries, and veins share about equally in the partition of the blood volume. Thus in a 20-kg dog the volume of blood in arteries, capillaries, and veins is ~56, 68, and 76 ml, respectively. The partition is somewhat less equal for the human lung, i.e., ~120, 250, and 150 ml, respectively (96, 442). The value of ~250 ml for the normal human lung agrees well with the morphometric estimate of 213 ml (161). However, values for the partition of pulmonary blood volume should be regarded as estimates and are more apt to be characteristic of a particular preparation and experimental circumstance than of the unmolested natural state (138).

For those concerned with alveolar-capillary gas exchange, the size of the capillary blood volume is of considerable interest (504, 505). In the model of the human lung proposed by Cumming et al. (96), the pulmonary capillary blood volume is ~150 ml. This value is larger than that usually obtained by measuring the diffusing capacity for CO, possibly because of recruitment and distension of capillaries incident to fixing the autopsy specimen (96). An even larger value has been obtained by morphometry (213 ml), attributable in part to the method of fixation (161); the corresponding endothelial surface area was 126 m^2. Other approaches estimate that the pulmonary capillary blood volume at rest constitutes about one-third of the total pulmonary blood volume (32, 532).

The pulmonary capillary blood volume falls when the sitting position is assumed (148, 532). During exercise, as the cardiac output increases, the pulmonary capillary volume increases; during strenuous exertion it can virtually double (532). This increase has been attributed more to the recruitment of additional areas of the capillary bed than to widening of capillaries already open.

Pressure-Volume, Pressure-Flow Relationships

DISTENSIBILITY. A key feature of the pulmonary vasculature is the combination of high distensibility and low resistance to blood flow (167, 184, 406). Compared to the systemic vascular bed, the pulmonary vascular compliance is ~1:6 or 1:7 (438). In the isolated dog lung and in the intact human the values for compliance and resistance (obtained by different methods) are quite similar. Also, at normal levels of blood pressure the pressure-volume curve is approximately linear (as in the case of the pressure-flow curve) but becomes nonlinear at very low driving pressures (Ppa − Ppv). As do other vascular beds, the pulmonary circulation displays pressure-volume behavior that depends on its stress history; i.e., it exhibits hysteresis (33).

Attempts to partition total pulmonary vascular compliance have yielded inconsistent values, differing not only from species to species (374) but also within species (374, 438). Nor does a consensus exist about the major determinants of pulmonary vascular distensibility: one view is that most of the compliance is in the larger pulmonary vessels (416, 438); another is that most of the compliance resides in the microcirculation (110, 504). It has also proved difficult to isolate pulmonary vascular segments for assessments of distensibility. For example, pulmonary venous compliance is difficult to estimate reliably because of uncertainty about the contribution of the left atrium. Indeed different techniques have resulted in opposite interpretations. One type of experiment suggests that the pulmonary venous bed should be regarded as a vasculature that is virtually rigid; i.e., a change in venous pressure exerts no influence on pulmonary blood volume. Another suggests that it is highly distensible and that the compliance of the pulmonary venous bed is ~0.1236 ml·mmHg^{-1}·kg^{-1} in the dog (438).

PULMONARY VASCULAR RESISTANCE. This term is generally used as a measure of the hindrance offered by a vascular bed to the flow of blood through it. In the normal pulmonary circulation an increase in cardiac output or in pulmonary artery pressure decreases vascular resistance. The decrease is not linear, depends on the level of initial tone, and becomes less marked at the higher levels of pressure and flow. In addition to displaying pressure-volume hysteresis, the pulmonary circulation also displays pressure-flow hysteresis (33).

Although vascular resistance is sometimes expressed without reference to control or standard values, more often vascular resistances are compared before and after an intervention has been applied. Usually two questions are being entertained. *1*) Has a change occurred in the calibers of the resistance vessels, as manifested by a change in the value of calculated resistance? *2*) If a change in calculated resistance has followed the intervention, was this change mediated passively or by vasomotor activity?

Anatomical basis. Morphometric analysis indicates that the major site of pulmonary vascular resistance is in the small muscular arteries (100–1,000 μm) and arterioles (<100 μm) [Fig. 2; (96, 228, 442)]. In contrast to the trumpetlike pattern of expansion by which the cross-sectional area of the bronchial tree branches from trachea to terminal bronchioles, the cross-sectional area of the vascular tree expands suddenly, resembling a thumbtack at the precapillary level. The frequent branching pattern probably interferes with laminar flow, although the Reynolds numbers for all but the central pulmonary arteries are too low for turbulence. In infants, where vessels are quite narrow and angulations more acute than in the adult, larger vessels probably also contribute to pulmonary vascular resistance. A similar situation occurs in chronic hypoxia, which is associated with medial hypertrophy of the small pulmonary arteries and peripheral extension of vascular smooth muscle toward the capillary bed (402).

Calculation. A variety of approaches have been used to detect changes in pulmonary vascular resistance (138, 266). These include pressure-flow curves and the pressure gradient across the pulmonary vascular bed at the end of diastole. However, traditionally pulmonary vascular resistance is calculated as the drop in pressure across any segment of the circulation divided by the rate of flow across it. The calculation for the pulmonary circulation, with mean values of pressure and flow, is

$$R = \frac{Ppa - Ppv}{\dot{Q}}$$

where R is pulmonary vascular resistance [either in R (resistance) units, as here, or in $dyn \cdot s^{-1} \cdot cm^{-5}$], Ppa − Ppv is the pressure drop across the pulmonary circuit, and $\dot{Q}$ is pulmonary blood flow in milliliters per second. Pulmonary wedge pressure is generally substituted for pulmonary venous pressure; on rare occasions left atrial pressure is used instead. For the normal pulmonary circulation the value for R is ∼0.1. To express pulmonary vascular resistance in $dyn \cdot s^{-1} \cdot cm^{-5}$, the numerator of the equation is multiplied by 1,332; the normal value is then ∼100.

Worthy of emphasis is the pressure difference in the numerator of the equation. Occasionally attempts are made to short-cut the calculation by omitting the outflow pressure and to interpret the result in terms of "total pulmonary vascular resistance." Unfortunately the value obtained in this way is bereft of either physiological or physical meaning, although it may be useful empirically, especially in states of pulmonary hypertension (292).

The analogy of the above hydrodynamic formulation with Ohm's law is evident. Unfortunately the nature of biological systems imposes serious restraints on the interpretation of calculated values for resistance: blood flow under natural conditions is neither constant nor laminar, vascular walls are not rigid, and blood is not a homogeneous fluid (138, 351). These limitations are evident in certain features of the pulmonary circulation: the marked distensibility of the pulmonary vascular tree, the pulsatility of blood flow not only in the large arteries but also in the minute vessels of the lungs, the anomalous viscosity of blood, the pulse-wave velocity, the inertia of components of the vascular walls, and reflected waves. Accordingly, instead of calculated pulmonary vascular resistance measuring a fixed attribute of the vascular tree, it is an operational ratio that depends strongly on the levels of pressures, volume, and flow within the pulmonary circulation.

In the supine human subject the relationship between pressure drop and flow appears to be approximately linear when pulmonary blood flow is doubled (292); i.e., the entire bed is opened and does not distend appreciably at modest increments in blood flow. However, in the upright position, linearity is not preserved when cardiac output is increased experimentally, presumably because of the recruitment of additional vessels at the top of the lungs (522).

Interpretation of a change. Although the concept of pulmonary vascular resistance has been used extensively to detect a change in the overall caliber of pulmonary resistance vessels and to infer that the mechanism responsible for the change is either active or passive, confidence in the interpretation rests heavily on the degree to which the assumptions underlying the assumptions have been respected. Two categories of assumptions are involved. *1)* Laminar flow, a rigid system of pipes and a homogeneous perfusate, is obviously suspect in the normal low-pressure, high-flow, vigorously pulsatile circulation of the lungs. *2)* A vascular system in which the vessels are all open is even more dubious, because not only caliber but also recruitment can affect the cross-sectional area of the pulmonary vascular bed—the major variable on which the value for calculated resistance is presumed to depend.

Given these physical attributes it is evident that other influences can affect the values used to calculate pulmonary vascular resistance. For example, the pulmonary circulation is encased within lungs and thorax, i.e., in a box within a box and juxtaposed to the beating heart. As a result opportunities for mechanical interplay are great and vary with the experimental situation. These influences certainly differ in the isolated lung from those in the intact animal. Moreover because pressures in the pulmonary circulation are low and elongate catheters are used to determine them in the intact animal and human, prospects for artifacts and error are ever present, notably in clinical studies when pulmonary wedge pressures are recorded in patients with lung disease.

One familiar source of difficulty in interpreting a change in calculated pulmonary vascular resistance occurs when pulmonary blood pressures, or blood flow, or both, change concurrently (Fig. 19). In this situation, insight into the passive characteristics of the system can be exceedingly helpful in deciding how much of the change in resistance is a passive consequence of the change in pressure or flow, per se. Most helpful in this regard is the passive pressure-flow relationship, e.g., the change in pressure drops across the pulmonary circulation (Ppa − Pw; Pw, wedge pressure) evoked by simply increasing pulmonary blood flow ($\dot{Q}$). As indicated above, in the upright position the pressure-flow relationship in the normal pulmonary circulation is not linear; nor does it traverse the origin. In contrast, both in the supine position and in the hypertensive pulmonary circulation, linearity is apt to be more marked but the position of the curve is less certain. One useful strategy for delineating the passive pressure-flow curve is to exercise the subject in the supine position and assume that no change in vasomotor activity is evoked by this procedure. It then becomes possible to compare the position of the pressure-flow curve before and after applying a test stimulus. Indeed once the control pressure-flow curve is known a single test point (Fig. 20) may suffice to uncover vasomotor activity.

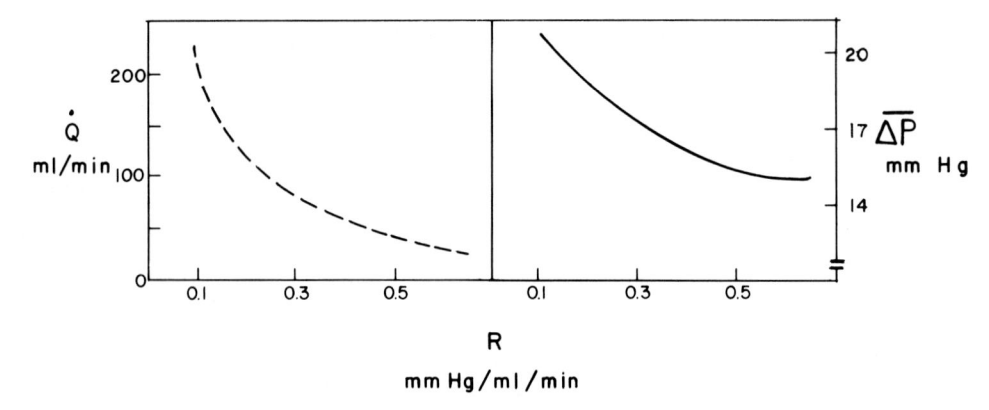

FIG. 19. Passive changes in pulmonary vascular resistance (R) at different levels of driving pressure ($\Delta \overline{P}$) and pulmonary blood flow ($\dot{Q}$). Pulmonary venous pressure is assumed to remain constant. Pulmonary vascular resistance decreases as either blood flow or pressure drop increases.

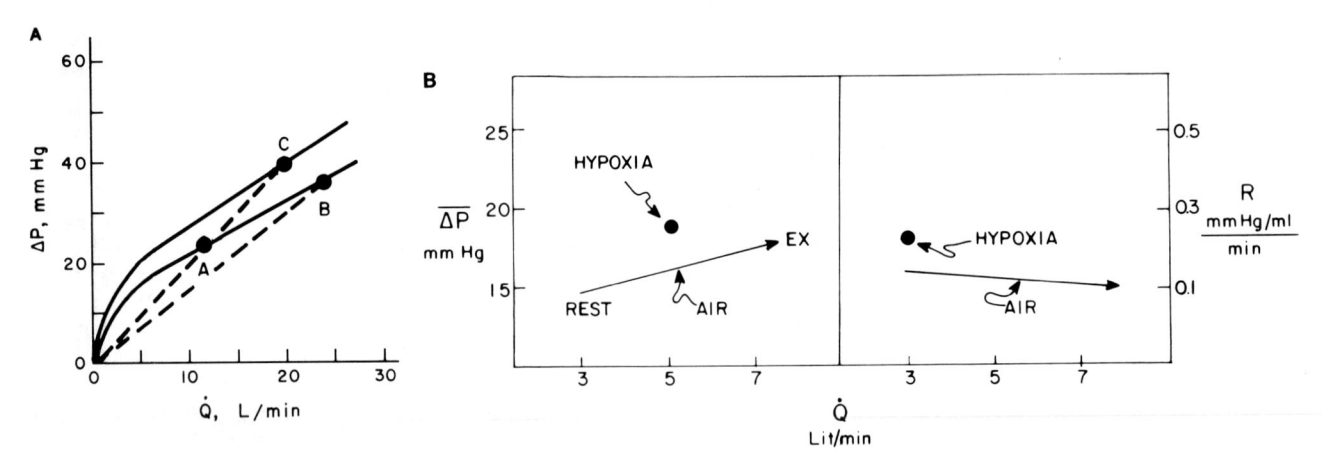

FIG. 20. Pulmonary vascular pressure-flow curves for detection of pulmonary vasomotor activity. A: theoretical basis for detecting pulmonary vasomotor activity with respect to passive pressure-flow curves in the same individual. *Solid line*, passive pressure-flow curve for the individual. *Points A and B*, linear incremental changes in pressure and flow along passive pressure-flow curve. *Point C*, active change in pulmonary vascular resistance. B: practical application of passive pressure-flow curves to detect vasomotor activity. *Left*: passive pressure-flow curve has been established for the individual by measurements at 2 levels of blood flow, i.e., at rest and during exercise (EX). During a single trial of acute hypoxia, point falls above passive pressure-flow curve, i.e., on a new curve that lies above the passive curve, suggesting that pulmonary vasoconstriction has occurred. *Right*: similar plot with calculated pulmonary vascular resistance instead of pressure drop as ordinate. (A courtesy of D. Silage.)

These considerations pertain to the current intense interest in using vasodilator agents for treating pulmonary hypertension. Unfortunately care has to be taken before attributing a decrease in calculated resistance to vasodilation unless pulmonary arterial pressure or blood flow remains unchanged. Moreover without some indication that the left atrial pressure has remained unchanged between the control and test periods the consequences of passive changes in outflow pressure are not easily taken into account. As indicated above, to discount left atrial pressure renders the calculation of pulmonary vascular resistance meaningless.

Although the pulmonary circulation of native residents at high altitude retains these general features (Fig. 21), it differs in certain particulars, i.e., thicker muscular media in the small arteries and arterioles and peripheral extension of precapillary smooth muscle. As a result, pulmonary vascular resistance is ordinarily higher at high altitude than at sea level. In either case—at sea level or at high altitude—the advent of diffuse pulmonary disease is apt to increase pulmonary vascular resistance and to decrease pulmonary vascular compliance by inducing vascular occlusive disease, by increasing the stiffness of the parenchyma surrounding the resistance vessels, and by evoking severe hypoxia (occasionally with acidosis), which evokes pulmonary vasoconstriction (293).

Modifiers. Because of the architecture of the lungs and the way in which they are accommodated in the thorax, changes in vascular calibers (and in their resistance to blood flow) may be accomplished in a

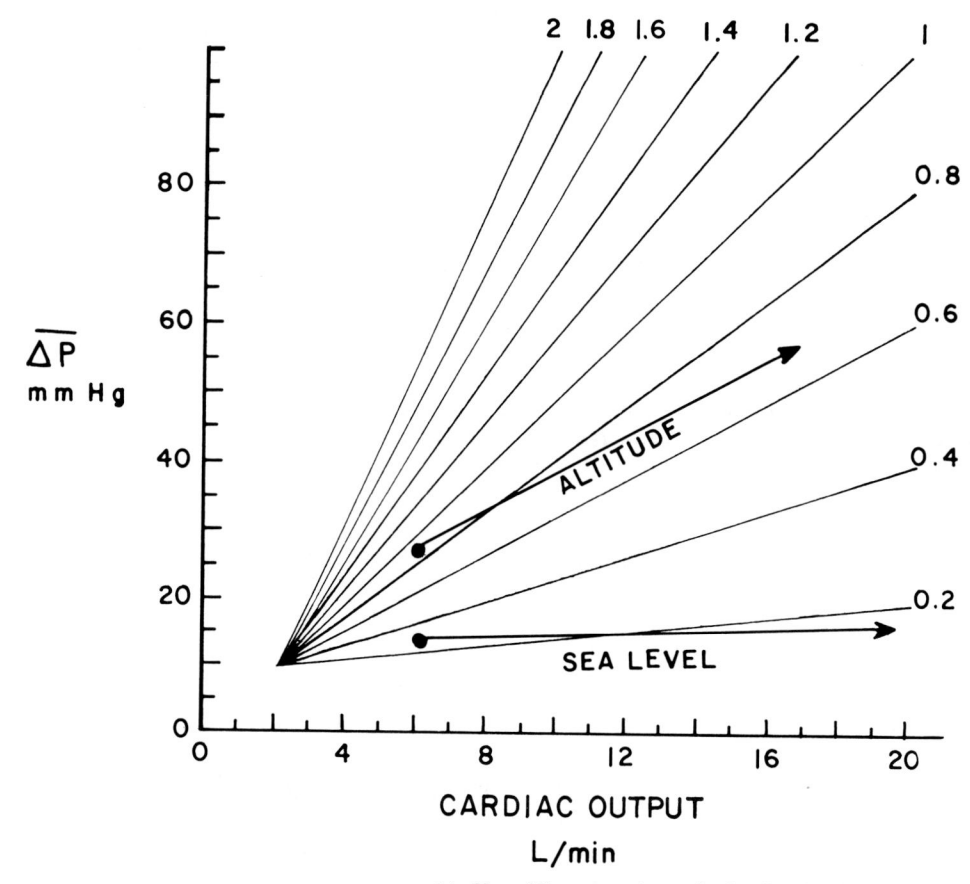

FIG. 21. Use of linear portions of a family of pulmonary vascular resistance curves as isopleths to display effect of test procedure on pulmonary vascular resistance. *Right*, resistance values (R units). At rest (●), pulmonary vascular resistance is higher at sea level than at altitude. During exercise (→), resistance values decrease in both instances, moving in each case to a lower resistance isopleth.

variety of passive ways—some of which are arcane—rather than by a change in vasomotor tone. The following merit special notice.

1. An increase in pulmonary arterial or pulmonary venous pressure automatically causes resistance to fall either by opening segments of the pulmonary microcirculation (recruitment) or by distending minute vessels that are already open (Fig. 19). The process of recruitment and derecruitment may be a function of random differences in the geometry of the complex microcirculatory network of the lungs or operate via critical opening and closing pressures; e.g., a specific opening pressure has to be exceeded in a particular arteriole before it will conduct blood to its capillary bed.

2. Lung volumes passively affect vascular resistance. Thus extra-alveolar vessels are pulled open and their resistance decreases as the lungs expand; conversely, alveolar capillaries are compressed at high lung volumes, which stretch alveolar walls. This opposite behavior also applies at low lung volumes: extra-alveolar vessels increase, and alveolar vessels decrease, their resistance. The tone of smooth muscle in the walls of the extra-alveolar vessels (small arteries and veins) introduces a separate variable in determining the resistance of these vessels. For example, this tone is susceptible to change under the influence of vasoactive drugs.

Zones of lungs and calculated resistance. In the normal pulmonary circulation, vascular resistance is so low that in the human subject at rest a driving pressure (Ppa − Pla; Pla, left atrial pressure) of only 6–7 cmH$_2$O elicits a blood flow of ~6 liters/min. Resistance is normally lowest at FRC and increases both at higher and lower lung volumes and transpulmonary pressures (71). Exercise sufficient to triple the blood flow is associated only with a doubling of the pressure gradient.

Interpreting a change in calculated resistance [(Ppa − Pla)/Q] can be troublesome in a vertical lung unless it is clear that the portion of the vascular bed under consideration is operating under zone 3 conditions so that the driving pressure is the pressure difference between the pulmonary arterial pressure and left atrial (or pulmonary venous) pressure. Otherwise the outlet pressure is the alveolar rather than the left atrial pressure (47).

In the vertical lung, resistance automatically decreases on several accounts as flow increases: *1)* an increase in flow causes the ratio to decrease as it increases zone 3 at the expense of zone 2, *2)* an increase in pressure causes distension of open vessels as well as recruitment of vessels previously closed, and *3)* stress relaxation becomes manifest in the pulmonary vessels if flow is increased abruptly (95).

Critical closure. Critical closure is discussed in the section devoted to pulmonary vasomotor activity in the chapter by Fishman in volume II of the *Handbook* section on circulation (138). This was a carry-over from the systemic circulation for which critical closure was originally advocated as a measure of vasomotor tone. Presently this concept seems more relevant to understanding recruitment of vessels in the pulmonary circulation than as a measure of vascular tone.

In both the pulmonary and systemic circulations this value is determined by observing the transmural pressure at which flow stops as the driving pressure is decreased (Fig. 21). Because of the need for tight control of blood pressures, airway pressure, and the degree of lung inflation, observations on critical closure are generally made on isolated perfused lungs or lobes. One handicap of these preparations is that they deteriorate with time and tend to become edematous, undergoing spontaneous changes in compliance and resistance. Moreover the pulmonary circulation is inherently difficult to examine for critical closure because neither extraluminal nor interstitial forces are constant, changes in lung inflation impose large and often divergent stresses on consecutive pulmonary vascular segments (230, 375), and distinctions between the behavior of alveolar and extra-alveolar vessels can only be inferred (178). Because of the artificial circumstances, the difficulty in separating and quantifying forces that are being applied to consecutive vascular segments, and the prospect of gradual, undetected loss in viability of the preparations under study, observations on critical closure generally leave unsettled the extent to which the results are applicable to more intact preparations, which, except in clinical disorders, operate under less stressful conditions.

With these caveats in mind, under zone 2 conditions the isolated lobe does display critical closure; i.e., a positive driving pressure (Ppa − PA) is accompanied by zero flow. Where and how this critical closure occurs is debatable (Fig. 21); although alveolar vessels lack smooth muscle in their walls, the possibility exists that pericapillary myofibroblasts or other interstitial cells could constrict alveolar capillary lumens to the point of closure (178, 231, 247, 335). Alternatively, extra-alveolar vessels—which do contain smooth muscle in their walls—have also been invoked to account for critical closure (178, 294).

These observations are relevant to the possibility that control of blood flow to the gas-exchanging surfaces of the lungs may be at the alveolar level (508, 512). They also suggest that in addition to the usual control of distribution of blood exerted by pulmonary precapillary vessels, under special conditions closure of alveolar vessels by pericapillary forces and even congregated blood constituents within capillary lumens (508) may deflect blood flow from one pulmonary capillary area to another. Finally, they reinforce the notion of preferential channels in the gas-exchanging areas—possibly corner vessels—which could be the last to close as driving pressure decreases (and the first to open as driving pressure is increased), thereby setting the critical closing pressure.

Sites of vascular resistance. The longitudinal distribution of pulmonary vascular resistance (106, 108, 190) is of interest on several accounts: *1)* for the understanding of the hemodynamics of the pulmonary circulation, *2)* for the determination of the capillary pressure responsible for transudation of fluid from the microcirculation into the pulmonary interstitium (see the chapter by Taylor and Parker in this *Handbook*), and *3)* for the identification of the vascular segments that undergo a change in caliber after a particular intervention, such as exposure to acute hypoxia or the administration of a pharmacologic agent (107).

Until the recent advent of micropuncture studies in the lung (49), attempts to partition the pulmonary microvascular resistances were indirect, involving a wide variety of experimental designs and manipulations. Consequently the possibility was strong that the outcome would depend heavily on the nature of the experiment. Somewhat surprisingly the results have been quite consistent, suggesting that in the normal lung, pre- and postcapillary resistances are about equal, favoring a slightly higher precapillary resistance, i.e., 60:40 (see Table 1). Nevertheless some of the differences in outcome and experimental design warrant mention. For example, in experiments on the isolated lung in which Starling's law of transcapillary exchange was applied to the pleura, precapillary resistance proved to be ∼40% of the total pulmonary vascular resistance (5). Somewhat higher values were obtained when the isogravimetric technique was applied to the isolated lung of the dog, i.e., precapillary resistance was generally ∼60% of the total (363), or even higher (109, 168, 189). In the open-chest dog, application of the isogravimetric method indicated that pre- and postcapillary resistances in the pulmonary microcirculation are about equal (160).

Among the influences that can strongly affect the longitudinal distribution of pulmonary vascular resistance in the different preparations is the degree of inflation of the lungs. As pointed out above, lung inflation influences not only total pulmonary vascular resistance (106), the partition of blood volume within the consecutive vascular segments (230), and vascular calibers (172) but also affects alveolar and extra-alveolar vessels oppositely. During inflation, alveolar capillaries are stretched and narrowed and resistance to blood flow through them increases (172). At the same time the calibers and the volumes of the extraalveolar vessels (small arteries and veins) increase and their resistance to blood flow decreases (34). A second important influence is the way in which the lungs are suspended: in the upright lung, vertical topographic zones are created by the effects of gravity, thereby creating the complicated interplay among alveolar, arterial, and venous pressures that has been described in ZONES OF THE LUNGS, p. 101. For example, under zone 3 conditions, precapillary resistance predominates, whereas further up the lung where zone 2 conditions prevail the balance shifts in favor of postcapillary resistances as zone 1 is approached (106, 189, 364).

Recent direct determinations by microvascular puncture in the isolated dog lung are in line with most of the previous indirect observations on the isolated lung preparation in indicating that the ratio of pre- to postcapillary resistances is 60:40. However, the direct determinations also suggest that the pulmonary capillaries have not received their full due in previous attempts to partition pulmonary vascular resistance, because they do contribute importantly to the overall hindrance to blood flow in the lungs (49).

As may be seen in Table 1 (data from A. E. Taylor and J. C. Parker, unpublished observations), different experimental interventions influence the partition of pulmonary vascular resistances in different ways. Acute hypoxia consistently increases precapillary resistance (52, 107, 189, 235, 366). In contrast, histamine exerts its predominant effect on postcapillary vessels (62, 63) via an H_1-receptor system. The effects of serotonin on the partition of resistances remain problematic (50, 64, 189).

PULMONARY VASCULAR IMPEDANCE. Traditionally, hemodynamic studies of the pulmonary circulation are based on the Poiseuille relationship, which deals with vascular resistance in terms of mean pressure and flow. This approach tacitly assumes a model of the vascular system in which pressure-volume relations are static, flow is constant, and recruitable pathways are at hand. Values for resistance calculated in this way have proved useful in detecting changes in the cross-sectional area of the pulmonary vascular bed that is being perfused.

The concept of vascular impedance extends that of resistance with the use of the relationship between pulsatile pressure and pulsatile flow to provide information about the viscoelastic properties of the vessels, their dimensions, and wave reflections. Vascular impedance is calculated as the ratio of corresponding frequency components in the arterial pressure and flow waves; by means of frequency analysis, sinusoidal signals derived from pulse waves under natural conditions are used to solve the appropriate impedance equations. Among the different types of vascular impedance that can be calculated, input impedance (the ratio of pressure to flow at a particular vascular cross section) is commonly used to define the pressure-flow relationships of the vascular bed beyond the site under consideration. Another useful category is that of characteristic impedance, which discounts the contribution to the pulse contour of reflected waves, thereby affording a measure of the dimensions and elastic properties of the vascular walls (311, 381, 382, 443).

Although the determination of pulmonary vascular impedance is considerably more complicated than that of vascular resistance and also more vulnerable to misinterpretation (355), it does afford the opportunity for additional insights into 1) the geometry and viscoelastic properties of the system (368, 381), 2) the matching of the mechanical performance and energetics of the right ventricle with that of the pulmonary vascular bed (332, 368, 389, 404, 443), 3) the quantitative relationships between mean and pulsatile pressure and pulsatile pressure and flow (332), and 4) pulmonary vasomotor activity (343, 380).

In general, pulmonary vascular impedance is similar to impedance in the ascending aorta except for differences arising from the lower resistance and greater distensibility of the pulmonary vascular tree [Fig. 22; (355)]. Also, in contrast to the systemic circulation, the normal pulmonary circulation acts as though there were only a single reflecting site (~17 cm from the main pulmonary artery) (38), and the characteristic impedance is about half of that in the ascending aorta because its elastic modulus and phase velocity are

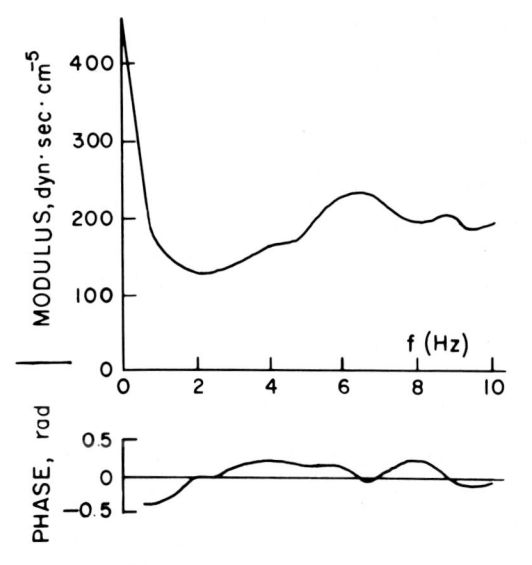

FIG. 22. *Top*: input impedance spectrum in main pulmonary artery of normal anesthetized dog. Pattern is similar to that of the ascending aorta but lower in amplitude. Minimal value of impedance modulus and crossover of impedance phase occurs at ~6-8 Hz. Pulmonary hypertension secondary to valvular heart disease is associated with an increase in pulmonary arterial input impedance and a shift of minimal impedance modulus to right. *Bottom*: impedance phase. Flow in normal lung leads pressure at lower frequencies (negative phase); situation is reversed at higher frequencies. [Adapted from Milnor (332).]

lower. Experimental pulmonary hypertension, such as that produced either acutely by infusing serotonin (38) or chronically by embolization of the lungs with acrylic beads, increases the elastic modulus and pulse-wave velocity (311). The concept of impedance has also been applied to the recognition of alterations in the physical attributes and energetics of the pulmonary vascular system in experimental pulmonary hypertension produced in the dog by a chronic increase in pulmonary blood flow (227). However, interpretation of results along these lines may be troublesome (355).

Because of the information that is provided about the physical properties and behavior of the pulmonary vascular bed, analysis of pulsatile flows and application of the concept of impedance have enabled the construction of more realistic models of the pulmonary (and systemic) circulation (332). For example, the model of Wiener, Fishman, et al. (527) in the dog, which is based on extensive anatomical and hemodynamic measurements (see Fig. 5), is quite consistent with values obtained experimentally for wave transmission in the pulmonary circulation and for the partition of pulmonary vascular resistances (5).

Another instructive consequence of the impedance concept has been the determination of how energy delivered to the pulmonary vascular bed by the right ventricle is partitioned: the oscillatory components, which comprise about one-third of the total energy delivered by the right ventricle per unit, are dissipated primarily in the large arteries, whereas the steady-flow components are spent primarily in the microcirculation, i.e., where resistance to blood flow is high (333). Most of the energy delivered by the right ventricle is spent in overcoming the frictional resistance to blood flow and only a small fraction is used to distend the arteries during right ventricular ejection. Little kinetic energy is delivered into the large pulmonary veins (443).

VASOMOTOR REGULATION

Contractile elements in the substance of the lungs are not confined to vascular media. Some, such as contractile interstitial cells in the alveolar wall (247, 308, 514) and myofibroblasts in the walls of the small pulmonary arteries (325), could change vascular calibers independent of the smooth muscle in the media of the small pulmonary arteries and arterioles. Indeed active contraction of alveolar interstitial cells has been proposed on morphologic grounds to account for the increase in pulmonary vascular resistance during hypoxia (247). Moreover the arrangement within the pulmonary parenchyma of the supporting structures of the lungs is such as to alter pulmonary vascular calibers passively as well as actively. For example, a decrease in lung volume or in transpulmonary pressure could increase pulmonary vascular resistance by deforming alveolar-capillary walls.

One intriguing aspect of vasomotor control that has not yet been fully explored for the pulmonary circulation is the role of endothelium in mediating the pressor response to biologically active molecules within the vascular lumen [see *Endothelium-Dependent Pulmonary Vasodilation*, p. 152; (158)]. In the systemic circulation, agents such as acetylcholine are endothelium dependent for their relaxing effects on large blood vessels; the same is true of the vasoconstricting action of norepinephrine. The extent to which endothelium-dependent behavior of vascular smooth muscle occurs in the pulmonary circulation is unknown. Clearly this prospect has great implications not only for normal pulmonary vasomotor tone and regulation but also for vascular diseases that affect the intima of the blood vessels and for the effective use of vasodilator agents.

Another caution with respect to interpreting tests for pulmonary vasomotor activity is the concern that any experimental deviation from natural conditions entails the risk of modifying the pulmonary vasoconstrictive response (154). The pulmonary pressor response to acute hypoxia is an example. As a rule the more prolonged and elaborate the manipulations before hypoxic testing and the deeper the anesthesia the more apt is the pulmonary circulation to show a high threshold for stimulation, a blunted vasoconstrictor response, and distortions in the time course of the pressor response. Also after an hour or so the hypoxic pressor response of the isolated perfused lobe of the dog tends to decrease and then disappear, even though vasoactive drugs can still elicit vasoconstriction (177, 202).

High on the list of causes for blunting of reactivity are abnormal perfusates. Substitution of platelet-free plasma for blood hastens the process, and a decrease in temperature from 38°C to 27.5°C also abolishes the response (202). Acid-base disturbances, electrolyte imbalances, protein abnormalities, blood substitutes (see Acute acidosis, p. 142), and even kinins from glass connections in the perfusing system can diminish the pressor response (77). Covert abnormalities in the perfusate may also be operative. The discordant results obtained by different investigators who seemingly have applied the same hypoxic stimulus to apparently identical preparations may be utterly incomprehensible without an appreciation of the variability in the pattern of the pulmonary pressor response with time under natural conditions: manipulations induce modifications, artifacts arise from the experimental circumstances, and lungs removed from their natural situation suffer inexorable deterioration.

Four topics of special interest concerning vasomotor regulation can be identified: *1*) the level of initial tone, *2*) detection of a vasomotor response (an active change in vascular caliber in response to an applied stimulus, e.g., the vasomotor effects of acute hypoxia), *3*) identification of the site or sites of pulmonary vasoconstriction [the particular vascular segment(s) involved in the vasomotor response], and *4*) clarification of the vasomotor mechanisms underlying an active change in pulmonary vascular tone.

Level of Initial Tone

One important element in determining whether a pulmonary vessel constricts or dilates on stimulation is its initial tone. In the normal adult at sea level, initial tone in the pulmonary circulation is low even though mixed venous blood is hypoxic (see 4. Intrinsic chemical mediators, p. 132). As a result the normal adult pulmonary circulation at sea level is in a state of near-maximal dilation (300, 420). Initial tone is higher in the fetus (104) and in the native resident at high altitude (371). Whether tone increases further during exercise as mixed venous partial pressure of O_2 (Pv_{O_2}) decreases is not known. One prevalent notion is that vasodilator prostaglandins contribute importantly to the low initial tone of the pulmonary circulation under natural or near-natural states (10, 270, 517).

Daly and Hebb (99) wondered if the vasoconstrictor effect of hypoxia depended on "the pre-existing state of tonus in the same (responding) vessels, or in the vessels belonging to some other part of the circuit." Others subsequently voiced concern about initial tone and its importance (138, 229, 283). Clearly, experimental manipulations and stress can modify initial tone.

A variety of influences could reset initial tone in the experimental setting: in some circumstances, catecholamines might predominate (28); in others, angiotensin (46), serotonin (99), vasoconstrictor prostaglandins (162, 193), or mysterious plasma factors (56). When initial tone is high, as during combined hypoxia and acidosis, stimulators of the β-receptor adrenergic mechanisms and the infusion of acetylcholine (200) elicit an impressive vasodilation, whereas neither does much to the normal pulmonary circulation. Nowhere is a high level of initial pulmonary vascular tone better illustrated than in the fetus. Before birth the pulmonary circulation responds vigorously to certain vasodilator agents (e.g., bradykinin) that the adult pulmonary circulation virtually ignores (77).

As a rule pulmonary resistance vessels that manifest high initial tone show a blunted response to pulmonary vasoconstrictors, as though vascular tone operated over a range and increased tone brought the vessels closer to their contractile ceiling. Conversely, when initial tone is high in the pulmonary circulation the effects of vasodilators are more impressive (25, 37, 290). In the fetus, high initial tone of the pulmonary resistance vessels is associated with a brisk reactive hyperemia, a vasomotor response that has not been elicitable in the adult pulmonary circulation (M. G. Magno and A. P. Fishman, unpublished observations). Initial tone is also high in the pulmonary circulation of high-altitude dwellers (320). However, although the considerations above do serve as bases for useful generalizations about initial tone—particularly for experiments done on a single species under controlled experimental conditions—exceptions do occur, especially when results from different species and experimental conditions are compared. Indeed, even within a single species, genetic variability can cause differences in initial tone and responsiveness (182).

Detection of a Vasomotor Response

As indicated above (see PULMONARY VASCULAR RESISTANCE, p. 116, and Fig. 20), most experiments designed to detect a vasomotor response rely heavily on a comparison of calculated values for resistance before and after applying a stimulus. In some instances the results of this comparison are easy to explain, as vasodilation is the combination of a decrease in pulmonary arterial pressure while cardiac output increases and left atrial pressure remains unchanged. Equally convincing for pulmonary vasoconstriction are the experiments involving tolerable levels of acute hypoxia; in these experiments pulmonary arterial pressure increases while pulmonary blood flow and left atrial pressure remain virtually unchanged. Indeed, in the latter circumstance, when other hemodynamic parameters remain unchanged, calculations are unnecessary because an increase in pulmonary arterial pressure suffices as evidence of pulmonary vasoconstriction.

However, interpretation tends to become much more complicated when an increase in pulmonary arterial pressure or unchanged pulmonary vascular pressure is accompanied by an increase in pulmonary blood flow. This is now commonplace in trials of pharmacologic agents that are administered to pulmonary hypertensive patients in the attempt to elicit pulmonary vasodilation. Many of these agents increase pulmonary blood flow by a positive inotropic effect on the heart. In this circumstance, prior determination of the individual's passive pressure-flow ($\Delta P/\dot{Q}$) curve—as by exercise—is often useful in sorting out the contribution of passive effects evoked by the increase in pulmonary blood flow per se (Fig. 22).

Sites of Pulmonary Vasoconstriction

Different physiological approaches have been used to identify the segment(s) of the pulmonary vascular tree involved in vasoconstriction after applying a stimulus, such as acute hypoxia. However, some have dealt with alveolar vessels, extra-alveolar vessels, or both. Because these segments of the pulmonary circulation are not readily available for testing, ingenious experiments that vary greatly in concept and design have been applied. One protocol takes advantage of the reasonable proposition that predominant constriction of either pre- or postcapillary pulmonary vessels should affect water exchange in the lungs in a predictable and measurable way. Others resort to special preparations to obtain data for mathematical modeling.

Not surprisingly the results differ considerably. For example, one model suggests that certain stimuli—notably acute hypoxia, stimulation of sympathetic nerves, and the administration of serotonin or PGF$_{2\alpha}$—exert their maximal vasoconstrictive effects toward the arterial end of the pulmonary circulation, whereas histamine, norepinephrine, epinephrine, or an increase in cerebrospinal fluid pressure exert their predominant effects toward the venous end of the pulmonary circulation (283). Other experimental preparations have yielded conflicting results: serotonin, which elicits primarily precapillary vasoconstriction in one experimental preparation (189), affects predominantly the postcapillary vessels in another (64, 65). A similar discrepancy has occurred for arachidonic acid (57, 235). The discrepancies underscore the importance of taking into account the nature of the test procedures and the experimental preparations. For example, testing the effects of prostaglandins by administering arachidonic acid (a biological precursor that can be processed by alternate pathways that involve the generation of diverse vasoactive materials) is apt to yield different results when different preparations are used.

Vasomotor Mechanisms

As noted in PULMONARY VASCULAR RESISTANCE, p. 116, analysis of vasomotor mechanisms in the pulmonary circulation is complicated in two ways: *1*) passive influences acting on highly distensible, low-resistance vessels play a predominant role under natural conditions, and *2*) the contribution of local hormones—released and destroyed within the lungs—to the setting of pulmonary vascular tone is difficult to uncover. For example, vasoactive prostaglandins, released in the vicinity of blood vessels, may have too short a half-life for detection in systemic arterial or even in pulmonary venous blood. Also, as in the case of certain catecholamines, distinguishing between the effects of locally released transmitters and those brought to pulmonary vessels from afar may not be possible (356).

Nerves, chemical mediators, or both may alter vasomotor tone in the pulmonary circulation. Which effect is predominant depends on the experimental conditions. Clearly any intervention that inordinately tilts the balance in favor of one or the other of these mechanisms will distort the natural situation. Among the more overt deranging influences in common use are anesthesia, denervation, mechanical ventilation, surgical manipulation, and artificial perfusates. Additional distortions are sometimes produced by pulmonary inflammatory processes, such as infection of the rat lung by *Pneumocystis carinii*, which are capable of generating biologically active materials that can modify vascular tone.

NERVOUS CONTROL. *Nerves and receptors.* Except for the possibility of a modest contribution to the initial tone (which is low) of the pulmonary arterial tree, there is no evidence to suggest involvement of the autonomic nervous system of the lungs in the regulation of the pulmonary circulation as long as the individual is unstressed (415). In contrast, as is considered in *Vasomotor reflexes*, p. 125, during stress the sympathetic component of pulmonary vascular innervation is very evident. Mapping of the autonomic nerves to the pulmonary circulation—particularly of the parasympathetic components to the minute vessels—is still incomplete (212). Nonetheless, despite considerable variation in the number, distribution, and concentration of nerve endings from species to species and between fetal and adult life, adrenergic and cholinergic nerves have been identified in the pulmonary vasomotor nerves of all species in which they have been sought (212, 334). Also, vagal stimulation dilates the pulmonary vasculature (347), whereas sympathetic nervous stimulation elicits pulmonary vasoconstriction (99). The cholinergic nerves exert their vasodilatory effect by releasing acetylcholine, which acts on muscarinic receptors in the pulmonary vessels (347).

With respect to the sympathetic nervous supply, both α- and β-adrenergic receptors are present and may be stimulated simultaneously (290). However, α-receptors predominate both numerically and functionally under normal conditions at rest (212, 229, 388). During states of increased vascular tone—as elicited by acute hypoxia in the fetal lamb—the converse is true (290). However, generalization from the fetal to the adult pulmonary circulation is complicated not only by the higher initial tone of the fetus but also by its inherent exaggerated responsiveness to all sorts of stimuli (123, 278). In contrast to ample evidence for the functional importance of the adrenergic mechanism, no particular role has yet been demonstrated for the cholinergic mechanism in the control of the pulmonary circulation.

Except for sporadic attempts to identify the role played by the parasympathetic nervous system in the regulation of the pulmonary circulation (347), attention has focused on the adrenergic nerves (90, 99, 128, 473). Still cloudy is the contribution of local and circulating hormones—including the catecholamines—to the setting of the initial tone of the pulmonary vessels. Another uncertainty is the contribution made by the endothelium to pulmonary vascular tone, because the endothelium not only processes circulating catecholamines as they traverse the lungs (356) but also interacts with the smooth muscle cells in the media in some mysterious way to shape the vasomotor response to certain biologically active substances, e.g., acetylcholine (158).

Nonetheless, certain features of the adrenergic innervation are now quite distinct. *1)* The innervation of the pulmonary vascular tree is more modest than that of the systemic arterial tree (including the bronchial arteries) (99). *2)* The concentration of fibers is greatest in large vessels and decreases peripherally, becoming exceedingly sparse in the vicinity of the arterioles (<30 μm) (99). *3)* The fibers are both myelinated and nonmyelinated on the one hand and sympathetic and parasympathetic on the other (454). *4)* Functional connections have been shown to exist between the adrenergic nerves to the pulmonary circulation and the central nervous system (12, 122, 288, 297, 472). *5)* Afferent pathways link the carotid and aortic chemoreceptors and the systemic baroreceptors to sympathetic efferent nerves to the pulmonary blood vessels (471).

The sympathetic innervation to the pulmonary circulation includes α- and β-adrenergic receptors on pulmonary vascular smooth muscle. The α-adrenergic receptors constrict, whereas the β-adrenergics dilate (421). The α-adrenergic receptors appear to predominate. Norepinephrine, a potent α-agonist, evokes pulmonary vasoconstriction. In contrast, isoproterenol, a β-adrenergic agonist, causes pulmonary vasodilation (440, 441). Epinephrine, which is both an α- and β-agonist, sometimes elicits pulmonary vasoconstriction and at other times pulmonary vasodilation, depending on the degree to which experimental circumstances have influenced the relative availability of the adrenergic binding sites (40).

Many reports dating to the first studies of the pulmonary circulation attest to the responsiveness of the pulmonary vasculature to stimulation of components of the autonomic nervous system (98). For example, under controlled mechanical conditions in the isolated lung, electrical stimulation of the stellate ganglion evokes pulmonary vasoconstriction (99); both the capacitance and resistance vessels seem to be affected (237, 360); depending on experimental conditions, the effect on the resistance vessels or capacitance vessels predominates. Unfortunately, because of the complexity of the experimental preparations used in these studies, it is difficult to assess the implications of these observations for the behavior of the pulmonary circulation under natural conditions. For example, in the days of extensive surgical sympathectomy for essential hypertension, the pulmonary pressor response of unanesthetized humans to hypoxia seemed unaffected (137). Nor did reserpine, given to animals in doses sufficient to block the release of norepinephrine from sympathetic nerve endings, appreciably modify the pressor response (176). Finally, α-adrenergic blockade with phenoxybenzamine has failed to block the pressor response in intact animals (440). These observations suggest that under natural conditions the sympathetic nervous system contributes little to pulmonary vascular tone but that its influence may be greatly increased under stressful conditions. Indeed the demonstration that the walls of the pulmonary arterial tree stiffen during sympathetic nervous stimulation, thereby increasing pulsatility in the pulmonary circulation, suggests that intense sympathetic nervous stimulation improves perfusion of underperfused or nonperfused portions of the lungs (238, 258).

The central connections of the adrenergic nerves to the pulmonary circulation provide a mechanism by which the pulmonary circulation can quickly engage in the circulatory adjustments that accompany a sudden fright, rage, or fight-or-flight reaction. In the fight-or-flight reaction, catecholamines are poured into the bloodstream, reinforcing the effects of adrenergic nerve stimulation (238, 258).

Attempts have also been made to sort out the relative contributions of these remote sensors: ordinarily the aortic chemoreceptors appear to be more effective than the carotid chemoreceptors in evoking pulmonary vasoconstriction (459); however, if the experimental conditions are right, opposite responses can be obtained (97). Although these observations do establish the existence of reflex extrapulmonary pathways, they provide no insight into the extent to which they are operative under natural conditions.

In the normal resting adult at sea level, in whom autonomic tone in the pulmonary circulation is slight and the level of circulating catecholamines is low, it can be shown with reasonable assurance (although often with some difficulty) that adrenergic influences are active and that α-adrenergic influences predominate (41, 290).

Vasomotor reflexes. With each heartbeat, baroreceptors, located primarily in the main pulmonary arteries near the bifurcation, send impulses via afferent vagal fibers synchronously with the fluctuations in pulmonary arterial pressure (88). However, these receptors do not seem to exert an appreciable hemodynamic effect within the lungs. In particular, no evidence exists that baroreceptors are involved in the pulmonary redistribution of blood, e.g., as during a change in posture. Nor is there much evidence behind other proposed mechano- or chemoreflexes that could operate locally (138).

Remote reflexes appear to be functionally much more important than local reflexes. Among the remote reflexes that have been studied are *1)* a systemic depressor reflex, in which a considerable and abrupt increase in pulmonary arterial or venous pressure elicits modest (and inconsistent) bradycardia and systemic hypotension; sectioning the vagi abolishes this reflex (138, 276); *2)* a complicated chain reflex that originates deep within the substance of the lung but that also engages the central nervous system (243); one example of this phenomenon is the J reflex, in which stimulation of juxtacapillary receptors in the alveolar walls is followed not only by tachypnea and bronchoconstriction but also by sagging at the knees (139); *3*) effects of stimulating systemic baro- and chemoreceptors on pulmonary vasomotor tone (98); *4*) the Bainbridge reflex, in which distension of the pulmonary venoatrial junction elicits reflex tachycardia (138); and *5*) stimulation of the ventilation by an increase in pulmonary blood flow, possibly due to stimulation of CO_2-sensitive receptors within the lungs (180). Because of the elaborate techniques generally required to uncover these reflex pathways, the extent to which they operate under natural conditions remains speculative.

Rhythmic swings in pulmonary arterial blood pressure—independent of the respiration or events in the heart or systemic circulation—have occasionally been noted, especially in deteriorating experimental preparations. A similar phenomenon has also been reported in an occasional patient with pulmonary hypertension of unknown cause (primary pulmonary hypertension) (138, 397). Although these vascular rhythms are reminiscent of Traube-Hering-Mayer waves and strongly suggest a central vasomotor mechanism as their basis, their genesis remains unsettled.

Much remains to be learned about the functional implications of the generous adrenergic innervation of the pulmonary blood vessels. The uncertainties encourage speculation. One notion is that this innervation promotes the efficiency of external gas exchange by helping to match alveolar blood flow to alveolar ventilation (92, 471). Another is that the pulmonary nerves contribute to the proper adjustment of the resistance and compliance characteristics of the pulmonary circulation (407, 471) and to balance between the ouputs of the two ventricles.

CHEMICAL CONTROL. Important insight into the complexity of the control of the pulmonary circulation was provided by the demonstration that vasomotor agents, such as angiotensin I, serotonin, and bradykinin, were also processed by pulmonary vascular endothelium en route through the lungs. It could then be reasoned that the location of the pulmonary endothelial apparatus between the venous and arterial segments of the systemic circulation was strategically disposed not only for protecting the vital organs of the body against potentially noxious humoral substances and particulate matter but also for generating substances that were essential for the proper functioning of the rest of the body (215). Subsequent chapters in this volume deal extensively with the metabolic handling of vasoactive materials by the lungs. However, a new understanding of the regulation of the pulmonary circulation by biologically active materials materialized when it was shown that endothelial-media interplay in the isolated systemic artery was involved in effecting a vasomotor response to certain agents. For example, in a large systemic artery the vasodilator effect of acetylcholine can be eliminated by damaging the intimal lining of the vessel (158).

Biologically active agents. How vasoactive substances exert their effects on the pulmonary circulation is currently under active investigation, with particular reference to the use of vasodilator agents to relieve pulmonary hypertension (see *Pulmonary Vasodilators*, p. 151). Some of the mechanisms of action appear to operate directly on the membrane of smooth muscle cells of the media, e.g., nifedipine; others operate via endothelial smooth muscle interactions, e.g., acetylcholine; a third group seems to involve intermediary substances that are biologically active, e.g., the release of prostaglandins. Three categories of agents have been extensively tested: vasoactive amines, polypeptides, and the prostaglandins. Some of these agents evoke pulmonary vasoconstriction; others evoke pulmonary vasodilation.

Vasoconstrictors. Norepinephrine and phenylephrine, potent stimulators of the α-adrenergic system in the pulmonary circulation, consistently elicit pulmonary vasoconstriction, whereas epinephrine, which possesses α- and β-adrenergic effects, not only evokes less vasoconstriction on a weight-for-weight basis but can also, depending on the preparation, cause vasodilation (40).

1. Angiotensin II. This octapeptide, formed in the lungs by the action of converting enzyme from angiotensin I, a decapeptide, generally but not invariably (22) elicits pulmonary vasoconstriction (18, 39). Small doses (~ 0.03 $\mu g \cdot kg^{-1} \cdot min^{-1}$) administered intravenously suffice to increase pulmonary arterial pressure without discernible effect on the systemic circulation (200).

2. Histamine. In doses of $\sim 10^{-5}$ g (given intravenously over a 2-min period) histamine elicits more variable responses. Although species difference and the type of experimental preparation seem to influence the outcome (435), most reports conclude that histamine (like hypoxia) is a powerful pulmonary vasoconstrictor and a systemic vasodilator (18). The combination of a pulmonary pressor effect and the location of histamine in pulmonary mast cells adjacent to muscular pulmonary arteries raised suspicion that histamine acts as an important local mediator in the regulation of pulmonary circulation (203). However, close experimental scrutiny has failed to support this notion (141).

A possible explanation of the apparent discrepancies in the effects of histamine on the pulmonary circulation has been provided by the identification of H_1 and H_2 receptors and the use of blocking agents to distinguish between their effects: chlorpheniramine has been used to block H_1 receptors selectively; metiamide has been used to block H_2 receptors (25, 41, 224, 359, 486, 530). The use of these agents suggests that pulmonary vasoconstriction is mediated by H_1 receptors and vasodilation by H_2 receptors. Chlorpheniramine not only prevents histamine-induced vasoconstriction but elicits vasodilation; oppositely, metiamide enhances the pulmonary vasoconstrictor effect of histamine. In contrast to the systemic circulation, H_1 receptors appear to be more plentiful than H_2 receptors in the pulmonary circulation. Moreover, differences in the disposition and concentration of the two receptors seem to account for the divergent responses of the pulmonary arterial and venous segments to histamine (41). See 4b. Histamine, p. 133, for further discussion.

3. Serotonin. In doses of ~10^{-5} g (given intravenously in a few min) serotonin is another vasoconstrictive amine that occurs in the mast cells of some species (169) but not others. It is synthesized from dietary tryptophan in the enterochromaffin cells of the gut. The overflow from these cells is largely removed by the liver; the remainder is almost completely removed and deaminated in the endothelial cells of the pulmonary circulation. Serotonin, escaping the metabolic machinery of the liver and lungs, is stored as dense granules in circulating platelets and released during platelet aggregation (480, 537). In addition to its direct effects on vessels, airways, and platelets, serotonin enhances vasoconstriction and platelet aggregation produced by other vasoactive agents, such as norepinephrine and angiotensin II.

In recent years, serotonergic receptors have been postulated, but it now seems clear that different receptors were being investigated (498). However, in vitro studies seem to have sorted out two distinct binding sites for serotonin: S_1-receptor binding sites that are labeled by serotonin and S_2-receptor binding sites that are labeled by serotonin antagonists, e.g., spiperone and ketanserin (279, 376, 498). The physiological and pharmacologic effects of serotonin (vasomotor activity, bronchoconstriction platelet aggregation) appear to be related to the binding of serotonin to the S_2 receptor; no such effects have been attributed to binding to the S_1 receptor.

The distinction between S_1 receptors and S_2 receptors holds great promise for reexamining the role of serotonin in the bronchoconstriction and pulmonary vasoconstriction evoked by pulmonary embolism (234, 408, 409). In contrast to histamine, which seems to affect both pulmonary arterial and venous components (66, 173), serotonin seems to exert its vasoconstrictor effect largely on vessels proximal to the pulmonary microcirculation (50, 283).

Vasodilators. Much of the response to vasodilators appears to depend on the initial tone of the pulmonary resistance vessels.

1. Isoproterenol. In the normal pulmonary circulation, isoproterenol usually evokes a barely detectable drop in pressure; this modest response has been attributed either to the paucity of β-receptors or to the low level of their activity in the normal state. However, the vasodilator response is much more impressive in animal preparations in which initial tone is high (28, 421) and in some patients with pulmonary hypertension (437). Rubin and Lazar (421) suggest that the pulmonary vasodilator effect of isoproterenol when pulmonary vascular tone is high does not depend entirely on pulmonary vascular adrenergic receptors but also on vasodilator prostaglandins.

2. Acetylcholine. The influence of initial tone is even more dramatically illustrated by acetylcholine: this agent elicits virtually no vasodilator response in the normal pulmonary circulation. Conversely, when administered intravenously (in doses of ~0.1 mg·kg^{-1}·min^{-1}) it elicits brisk vasodilation if the pulmonary circulation is in a state of heightened tone, as in the fetus (277) or in adults during exposure to alveolar hypoxia (153).

3. Bradykinin. This pulmonary vasodilator, a member of a family of vasoactive polypeptides, is inactivated by the same converting enzyme(s) in the lungs that converts angiotensin I to II. Although it is consistently a powerful systemic vasodilator, it is not as predictable as a pulmonary vasodilator, usually evoking pulmonary vasodilation (367). The pulmonary vasodilator effect is much more consistent and striking in the lungs of the fetus and newborn than in the adult (77). The biological role of bradykinin in regulating the pulmonary circulation is unclear. The possibility has been raised that the origin of bradykinin in the pulmonary vascular endothelium constitutes a source of vasodilator agent for the systemic circulation (457). Although angiotensin II and bradykinin share a dependency on converting enzyme for their genesis, they act differently on vascular smooth muscle: angiotensin acts without intermediaries, whereas vasoactive prostaglandins are involved in the effects of the kallidins (367). Indeed, at least in some of the species, the variability in the vasoactive effects of bradykinin and the kallidins has been attributed to variations in the extent to which different prostaglandins are engaged as mediators of the vasodilator response.

Vasoactive prostaglandins and their precursors. In the search for chemical mediators of pulmonary vasomotor activity, arachidonic acid has almost achieved the status of the philosophers' stone because of the multitude of biologically active products that it generates (Fig. 23).

Arachidonic acid (eicosatrienoic acid, a 20-carbon polyunsaturated fatty acid) is the precursor of the prostaglandins. It is released from tissues by deacylation of cellular phospholipids. On release it is metabolized by either the cyclooxygenase or lipoxygenase enzyme systems (430). Because the arachidonic acid metabolites released from membrane lipids are organ and cell specific, and because experimental conditions strongly influence the metabolism of arachidonic acid (236, 453), either the cyclooxygenase or lipoxygenase pathway may predominate (Fig. 23). Administered arachidonic acid need not have the same metabolic consequences as that generated in response to endogenous stimuli. Nor are physiological and pharmacologic doses and patterns of release apt to be identical. Therefore it is difficult to predict which pathway will dominate or how experimental circumstances are in-

FIG. 23. Arachidonic acid cascade, illustrating 2 pathways and some metabolic products able to change pulmonary vasomotor tone. Metabolic pathways of arachidonic acid initiated by cyclooxygenase and lipoxygenase catalyzed reactions. By stimulating a phospholipase the leukotrienes may in turn cause release of products of cyclooxygenase pathway.

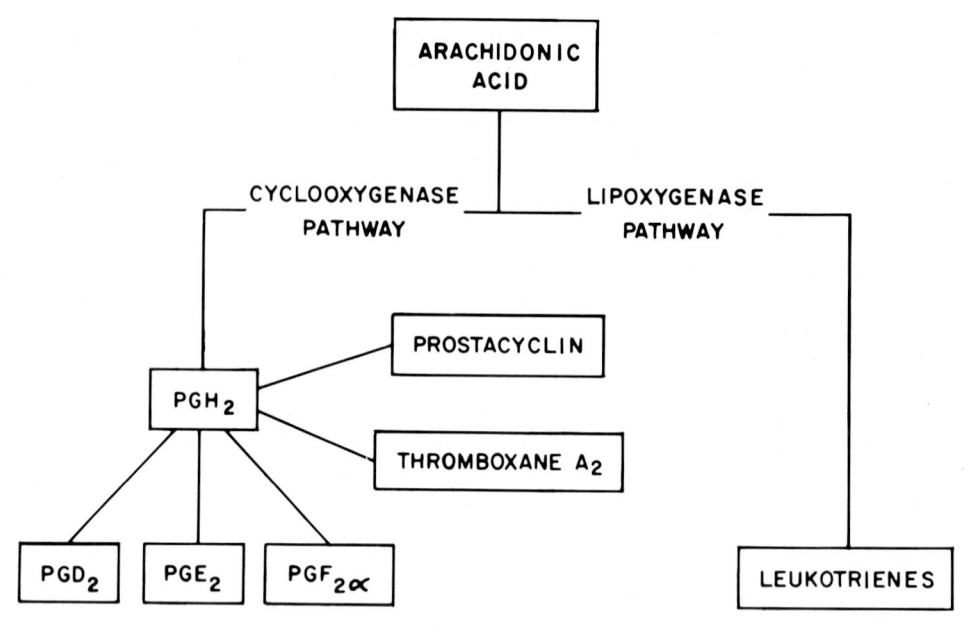

fluencing the biological effects. As a rule, arachidonic acid injected intravenously elicits pulmonary vasoconstriction (500), largely because of the predominant effect of thromboxane A_2, even though prostacyclin (PGI_2), a potent vasodilator, is also released (162); leukotrienes do not appear to operate in this circumstance.

Pharmacologic interruption of one pathway has been used to uncover the effect of metabolites produced by the other. For example, indomethacin, which inhibits prostaglandin synthetase, is a popular agent for blocking the cyclooxygenase pathway to disclose the actions exerted by metabolites of the lipoxygenase pathway. Diethylcarbamazine, which interferes with the lipoxygenase pathway, serves the same purpose for the cyclooxygenase pathway. However, specificity of these and other inhibitors for particular sites in the arachidonic acid cascade is rarely complete. Moreover alternate pathways in the metabolism of arachidonate provide opportunity for subtle experimental quirks to channel the cascade into one pathway or another, thereby covertly shaping the vasomotor response of the pulmonary circulation, not only to prostaglandins (exogenous as well as endogenous) but also to inapparent neurohumoral influences and to biologically active molecules. Finally, considerable species variation exists in the intensity of the vasomotor response to particular products of arachidonic acid metabolism. According to these considerations, results from one organ or tissue are not readily extrapolated to another; each experimental circumstance is destined to imprint its own distinctive mark on arachidonic acid metabolism.

The various products of arachidonate metabolism are described elsewhere in this chapter and volume. A few remarks here illustrate the diversity of biological effects that these ubiquitous substances can elicit.

1) Certain metabolic products of the cyclooxygenase pathway are pulmonary vasoconstrictors, e.g., $PGF_{2\alpha}$, PGE_2, and thromboxane A_2, whereas others are pulmonary vasodilators, e.g., PGE_1 and PGI_2 (245, 447); PGE_2, which constricts the adult pulmonary vascular bed, dilates the neonatal pulmonary vascular bed (289). *2)* Leukotrienes, generated by the lipoxygenase pathway, include potent pulmonary vasoconstrictors. *3)* Suspicion is high that the prostaglandins are involved as intermediaries in pulmonary vasomotor responses to other agents, e.g., the kallidins, histamine, and isoproterenol (183, 421). *4)* It is also suspected that a balance between prostaglandin vasodilator activity and the constrictor effect of thromboxane A_2 is importantly involved in setting the low initial tone of the normal pulmonary circulation (162, 193, 245). *5)* Hemodynamic (and other mechanical) factors influence both the release of vasoactive prostaglandins, e.g., PGI_2, and the endothelial metabolism of prostaglandins (128, 456).

Of all the prostaglandins, PGI_2 is currently attracting most attention as a potent pulmonary (and systemic) vasodilator and antithrombogenic agent (496). This agent is formed by the action of prostacyclin synthase on the prostaglandin endoperoxide PGH_2. Sheer stress of the endothelium is a potent stimulus to the release of PGI_2 from endothelium. The endothelium appears to have higher concentrations of prostacyclin synthase than do the other layers of the vessel wall, a preferential distribution that may relate to the role of PGI_2 as an inhibitor of platelet-platelet interaction and possibly to the communication links between endothelium and the subadjacent vascular smooth muscle (119). Bradykinin releases PGI_2 in cell culture and stimulates endothelial cells (from large pulmonary arteries) to produce more PGI_2 than $PGF_{2\alpha}$. Because bradykinin is plentiful in the lungs, its effects on endothelium suggest a mechanism to account for predominant release of PGI_2 in the pulmonary circulation.

Another major line of experimental interest involving the prostaglandins has been the ductus arteriosus and its mechanism of closure. One intriguing aspect of the ductus arteriosus is that despite its embryologic origin (as the distal segment of the left 6th aortic arch) and its location as a bridge between the pulmonary artery and the descending aorta, it leads a vasomotor life of its own with respect to the two circulations that it bridges. For example, immediately postpartum, i.e., on switching from the hypoxic environment in utero to the air-breathing, O_2-rich environment of independent neonatal life, the ductus arteriosus contracts vigorously to the point of self-obliteration of its lumen; at the same time the pulmonary circulation vasodilates (219, 423).

Closure of the ductus arteriosus immediately after birth depends heavily on prostaglandins in its walls; conversely, premature closure of the ductus arteriosus before birth, as by the placental transfer of indomethacin from mother to fetus, may cause fetal pulmonary arterial hypertension or interfere with the morphologic development of the pulmonary vascular bed (273). The responses of the ductus arteriosus to prostaglandins and to inhibitors of the cyclooxygenase pathway have been turned to clinical advantage: PGE_2 or PGE_1 has been used to maintain patency of the ductus arteriosus in newborns with congenital heart disease who would benefit from this continued communication between the pulmonary and systemic circulations; conversely, indomethacin, an inhibitor of the prostaglandin synthetase element of the cyclooxygenase pathway, has been used to promote closure of a persistent ductus arteriosus in premature infants (353, 423).

Interest is high in the role of arachidonic metabolites in the consequences of lung injury. After the infusion of *Escherichia coli* endotoxin or ethchlorvynol, a two-phased response occurs (61, 171). The first phase, characterized by marked pulmonary hypertension and leukopenia, involves the cyclooxygenase pathway and is associated with the release of thromboxane A_2 (and PGI_2) into lymph and blood. In the subsequent phase, in which the composition of pulmonary lymph signifies that a striking increase in pulmonary microvascular permeability has occurred, the lipoxygenase pathway is primarily involved (344). Thus, although pulmonary hypertension can be alleviated by administering either indomethacin or imidazole, the subsequent permeability phase is unaffected by cyclooxygenase inhibition, suggesting that the lipoxygenase-derived products are involved in the increase in microvascular permeability (344). In the adult respiratory distress syndrome the types of arachidonic acid metabolites have been found to vary greatly and often unpredictably; gravely ill patients with sepsis generally manifest high levels of thromboxane and PGI_2.

Another line of potential clinical interest is pulmonary embolism. The literature dealing with experimental replicas of the human disorder is extensive and has been summarized recently (299). The role of prostaglandins in producing the clinical syndrome is being explored. Prostaglandins seem to be more involved in the genesis of increased pulmonary microvascular permeability than in the genesis of pulmonary hypertension or metabolism. For example, after infusion of glass beads to produce modest pulmonary hypertension, the pulmonary removal of PGE_1 (and serotonin) was only slightly reduced, whereas that of norepinephrine was unaffected. However, after vascular occlusion in the lungs the combination of pulmonary leukostasis and the release of thromboxane A_2 seems to play an important role in increasing pulmonary microvascular permeability. The pulmonary hypertension produced by administering autologous zymosan-activated plasma as a bolus to sheep has been related partly to thromboxane A_2 release. Attempts to implicate arachidonic acid metabolites in the increased vascular permeability that follows air embolization have been unsuccessful.

Respiratory gases and pH. Acute hypoxia. More than 40 years have elapsed since the hypothesis was advanced that acute hypoxia elicits pulmonary vasoconstriction (48) and, as a corollary, that the vasoconstrictive response to hypoxia automatically adjusts pulmonary capillary blood flow to alveolar ventilation (132). This hypothesis has withstood intense scrutiny since then, and the pressor response has been elicited in virtually all species tested. However, depending on species (369) and experimental conditions, acute hypoxia has evoked pulmonary vasoconstriction (118, 147, 287, 452, 469), vasodilation (286), neither (529), or both (117, 467).

Not all the species that do vasoconstrict in response to acute hypoxia, do so with the same vigor. Indeed, Beyne (48) and Euler and Liljestrand (132), the early proponents, were fortunate in their choice of the cat rather than the dog or guinea pig as the test animal, because the feline pulmonary circulation responds well. Even more impressive responses to acute hypoxia have since been obtained in certain cattle (182) and in the newborn of several different species (104). Ingenious attempts to reconcile the diversity in the hypoxic pressor response among different species (305) have encountered difficulty in predicting the magnitude of the vasoconstrictor response in a given animal (534).

The route by which hypoxia exerts its pressor effect on the pulmonary circulation pertains both to its mechanism and site of action. The major focus has been on hypoxia by airways, i.e., by decreasing inspired P_{O_2} (141); this general strategy for reducing alveolar P_{O_2} (PA_{O_2}) has been supplemented by sporadic observations on the effects of experimentally manipulating ambient barometric pressure (370). Since the 1950s, however, doubt has arisen about the airways as the sine qua non for eliciting the pressor response. Indeed, evidence has been adduced that the pulmonary pressor response can also be evoked by decreasing the P_{O_2} of mixed venous blood (Pv_{O_2}), a natural occurrence during exercise. The two routes, alveolar and blood, by which the smooth muscle of the small pulmonary arteries (and venules) could be affected by hypoxia are shown schematically in Figure 24. This consideration raises the possibility that alveolar hypoxia has been overemphasized in the search for mechanisms underlying the pressor response and that the inordinate stress on the induction of hypoxia by airways is more a function of experimental design than of intrinsic biological design (268).

Most studies of the vasomotor effects of acute hypoxia have relied on determinations of the pulmonary vascular pressure drop and blood flow and/or the calculation of pulmonary vascular resistance. The pros and cons of this approach have been discussed in PULMONARY VASCULAR RESISTANCE, p. 116. Another approach has depended on unilateral hypoxia, with diversion of blood flow from one part of the lung to another as the end point. Just as secondary influences (e.g., acidosis, lung volumes, and temperature) introduced by the experimental circumstances can shape the intensity of the pulmonary vascular response to acute hypoxia in pressure-flow experiments, so can subtle factors, particularly the relative volume and elastic properties of the hypoxic area, affect the outcome of the diversion experiments (305).

Nonetheless the results obtained by the two approaches provide a coherent and consistent picture of the effects of hypoxia on the pulmonary circulation. *1*) In human subjects and in conventional laboratory animals, acute hypoxia (generally induced by lowering the concentration of O_2 in inspired air) causes pulmonary arterial pressure to increase (132) while leaving left atrial pressure—and usually the cardiac output—unaffected (260, 321, 341). *2*) The hypoxic pressor response can be elicited in the isolated perfused lung devoid of all nervous connections as well as in the intact animal or human (141, 195, 354). *3*) In contrast to the vasoconstriction that acute hypoxia elicits in the pulmonary circulation, it evokes vasodilation in the systemic circulation (137, 319, 470). *4*) The gain of the hypoxic pressor response (under sea-level conditions) is maximum at PA_{O_2} values of ~60–70 mmHg. *5*) The intensity of the hypoxic vasoconstriction varies from subject to subject, among species, and in different parts of the same lung (14, 143, 182, 369, 478, 484, 485, 491). *6*) On exposure to acute hypoxia the pressor response starts within a few breaths, generally reaching its peak by 3 min (301) and, depending on the preparation and the concentration of inspired O_2, it may persist for hours (420) or days (491); generally the response attenuates within hours toward control levels (302), but instances of enhanced responsiveness with time have also been reported (10). *7*) The mechanism(s) responsible for the gradual subsidence of pulmonary vasoconstriction during severe hypoxia [partial pressure of O_2 in arterial blood (Pa_{O_2}) = 30–37 mmHg] is not understood (302). *8*) The hypoxic pressor response may be enhanced in different ways: concurrent acidosis (45, 131); repeated exposure to intermittent hypoxia (491), ethyl alcohol (121), cyclooxygenase inhibitors (193), and vanadate [a trace metal essential for life (502)]; and certain metabolic inhibitors, e.g., sodium cyanide and dinitrophenol (284) and iodoacetate and 2-deoxyglucose (458). *9*) More ways (ranging from chemical to mechanical) have been described for blunting than for enhancing the hypoxic pressor response: hypocapnia and alkalosis (37, 300, 301), Ca^{2+} antagonists

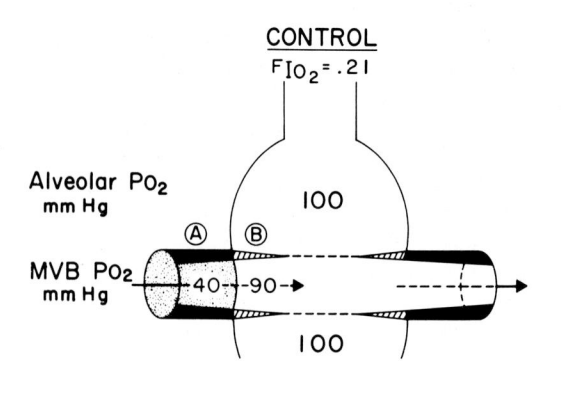

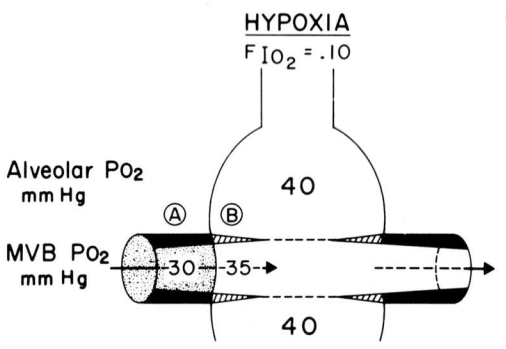

FIG. 24. Putative sites of action of acute hypoxia. Pulmonary microvessel (artery, capillary, and vein) is shown traversing alveolar portion of the lung. Precapillary vessel is subdivided into proximal conducting segment (*A*), in which mixed venous blood P_{O_2} (MVB P_{O_2}) affects some critical element of the vascular smooth muscle, and terminal segment (*B*), in which alveolar P_{O_2} ordinarily is the major influence (*striped area*). *Top*: air breathing. Low mixed venous P_{O_2} is responsible for normal tone of proximal pulmonary vascular segments; high alveolar P_{O_2} is responsible for tone of distal segments. *Bottom*: hypoxia (breathing 10% O_2 mixture). During hypoxia the mixed venous P_{O_2} in proximal segment (*A*) undergoes little change, whereas alveolar P_{O_2} decreases to a level that is not appreciably different from blood P_{O_2} in distal segment (*B*); to the high tone of proximal segment is added the increase in tone of distal segment. Main component of pressor response to hypoxia is due to smooth muscle contraction in distal segment. FI_{O_2}, fraction of O_2 in inspired gas. [From Fishman (141), by permission of the American Heart Association, Inc.]

(316), lung inflation (390), an increase in pulmonary artery pressure or cardiac output, anesthesia, pregnancy, circulating vasoactive substances (338), endotoxin (431, 493), curious interplays between Pa_{O_2} and Pv_{O_2} on the one hand (370) and Pa_{O_2} and systemic Pa_{O_2} on the other (275), genetic predisposition (520), aging (277, 446), and female sex hormones (339, 446, 526). 10) Certain characteristic features of the pulmonary pressor response to acute hypoxia—notably the increase in pulmonary arterial pressure, the unchanged left atrial pressure, and the freedom from pulmonary edema—favor (even though they do not clinch) the idea that the pulmonary precapillary vessels (small pulmonary muscular arteries and arterioles) are the predominant site of vasoconstriction. 11) The vasoconstriction produced by acute hypoxia can be relieved by vasodilators (35). 12) The degree of hypoxic pulmonary vasoconstriction may be modulated by the production of one or more vasodilator prostaglandins (501, 520). 13) Diversion of blood flow during local hypoxia favors improvement in oxygenation of systemic arterial blood by readjusting pulmonary blood flow to alveolar ventilation (27, 124, 138). 14) The degree of diversion during local hypoxia is strongly affected (and may be strikingly reduced) by opposing mechanical influences (305, 390).

No consensus exists about many of the items on this list. For example, not all investigators have been able to demonstrate differences between the pressor responses of male and female rats to acute hypoxia (450). Nor have observations based on the use of metabolic inhibitors been consistent (126, 458). However, the list does illustrate the many approaches that have been used to explore the pulmonary pressor response evoked by acute hypoxia. Earlier in this chapter (see CHEMICAL CONTROL, p. 126) it was shown that chronic hypoxia, like acute hypoxia, also entails an increase in pulmonary vasomotor tone, i.e., pulmonary vasoconstriction (341).

1. Extrinsic nerves and reflexes. Almost 25 years ago two separate groups of investigators used exceedingly elegant preparations to show that hypoxic stimulation of the carotid and aortic chemoreceptors was able to reflexly elicit pulmonary vasoconstriction (19, 97). About 10 years later, operation of this reflex pathway was demonstrated under somewhat less artificial conditions in immature fetal lambs (75). However, these experiments left unsettled the role of these reflex pathways under more natural conditions (275). The focus of the experiments cited above was on the resistance vessels. A new turn was taken with the demonstration that hypoxic stimulation of the carotid and aortic chemoreceptors reflexly decreased the distensibility of the large pulmonary arteries (471). Indeed, if resistance to blood flow did increase through the small vessels, the effect was completely overshadowed by the decrease in compliance of the large vessels.

Although the sympathetic motor innervation may contribute under special circumstances (notably during stress) to the pulmonary pressor response of the adult lung to hypoxia, under most experimental conditions its role is negligible. This conclusion is based on the ability to elicit the hypoxic pressor response in the isolated lung (125, 126, 388) in sympathectomized humans and animals (140) and in animals after adrenergic depletion and the administration of adrenergic blocking agents (28, 136, 440, 441).

However, a contribution of the sympathetic nervous system to the pulmonary pressor response to hypoxia cannot be automatically discounted. For example, in the fetal lamb studied near term the pulmonary pressor response to asphyxia depends heavily on the adrenergic nervous system; this nervous component attenuates gradually during the neonatal period (76). Moreover a contribution of the adrenergic nervous system to the hypoxic pressor response has been detected not only in the awake dog (476) but also in the perfused lung lobe (28, 388) and in the sympathectomized dog exposed to unilateral hypoxia (255). Finally, it has been shown that systemic hypoxia also contributes reflexly to the pulmonary pressor response by a pathway involving peripheral chemoreceptors and pulmonary sympathetic fibers (473).

These observations leave the distinct impression that the extent to which adrenergic vasomotor innervation affects the pulmonary resistance vessels during hypoxia depends on the experimental circumstance, species, and level of maturity. In the manipulated, intact fetus (75, 76) the role of adrenergic nerves is more readily discernible than in the normal adult or in the isolated denervated lung.

2. Intrinsic pulmonary mechanisms (local effects). Acute hypoxia has repeatedly been shown to elicit pulmonary vasoconstriction in the isolated perfused lung (126, 138, 285). This ability to elicit pulmonary vasoconstriction in the denervated lung that is entirely devoid of extrinsic neurohumoral influences or bronchial circulation is persuasive evidence that at least a large component of the hypoxic pressor effect begins and ends within the lungs.

This is not to imply that external influences play no role in the intact animal or human. For example, clearly the initial tone of the vessels before the hypoxic stimulus is applied can contribute to the vigor of the response (141). Extrapulmonary influences, operating via the autonomic nervous system and bloodstream, can also shape the response. Finally, different animals appear to have different inherent capabilities (susceptibility) for responding (138, 211). Altogether, although there is no question that pulmonary vasoconstriction can begin and end within the lungs (i.e., locally), there is little doubt that this pressor response can be strongly influenced by extrapulmonary stimuli.

Mechanisms proposed to account for the intrinsic (intrapulmonary) effects of hypoxia seem to fall into four categories: 1) local reflexes (i.e., confined to the lungs), 2) vasoactive substances (including H^+) in the perfusate, 3) chemical mediators that originate within the lungs, and 4) cellular events in the pulmonary vascular smooth muscle. The last two of these are currently the focus of attention.

3. *Local reflexes.* Evidence favoring intrapulmonary chemoreceptors is meager. However, Lauweryns and Van Lommel (268) continue to adduce evidence to support the idea that neuroepithelial bodies in the intrapulmonary airways are hypoxia-sensitive chemoreceptors that are stimulated by a change in the O_2 composition of inspired air both to local secretory activity and to participation in a reflex arc modulated by the central nervous system (268). To date, this hypothesis rests heavily on morphologic observations with few physiological data to support it.

4. *Intrinsic chemical mediators.* Recent insights into the interplay among biologically active molecules have heightened awareness that the isolation of a unique chemical mediator in the pulmonary pressor response to acute hypoxia is a formidable undertaking. The six criteria are based on those enunciated by Burnstock for chemical transmitters released by vasomotor nerves during stimulation. *1*) The mediator or its precursors must exist in the lungs. *2*) The source of mediator must be strategically disposed with respect to the resistance vessels so as to gain ready access to their media during acute hypoxia. *3*) The effect of the mediator must be mimicked by the application of the proposed mediator to the pulmonary blood vessels. *4*) A mechanism must be present to turn on and to inactivate the mediator. *5*) Agents that modify the pressor response elicited by the mediator should have similar effects on responses to the exogenously administered mediator. *6*) Inhibition or depletion of the mediator, as by pharmacologic agents, should depress the hypoxic response.

Four experimental observations have encouraged the search for a unique chemical intermediate that is released or generated within the lungs during hypoxia: *1*) the proximity of mast cells to pulmonary muscular arteries (188); *2*) the diametrically opposite responses of pulmonary and systemic arteries to hypoxia, i.e., vasoconstriction and vasodilation, respectively (137); *3*) the ability of a strip of pulmonary artery to constrict during hypoxia only if it retains a collar of parenchyma (287); and *4*) the abolition of the hypoxic pressor response in the isolated perfused lung by antihistamines (203).

Exceptions have been taken to each of these lines of evidence. Particularly noteworthy are the following: *1*) the idea of a primary role for the mast cell in the pulmonary pressor response has not withstood experimental scrutiny (141, 191), *2*) stripping the pulmonary artery of the rabbit (287) entails the risk of deranging electrolyte composition (and reactivity) of the vascular wall in a species that is poorly responsive to the pressor effects of acute hypoxia (451), and *3*) the abolition of the pressor response by antihistamines (203) may be nonspecific (451). Despite these reservations the search for a unique chemical mediator has received new impetus in recent years because of the surge of interest in vasoactive substances that are generated in or processed by the lungs.

For the prospector in search of chemical mediators the cells of the lung offer a treasure trove of biologically active substances. In most species, pulmonary mast cells contain histamine, serotonin, ATP, and slow-reacting substance; in some a great deal of dopamine is present (212). Other pulmonary parenchymal cells also contain serotonin, histamine, and ATP. The autonomic nerve endings constitute a ready source of neurotransmitter substances, and the endothelium constitutes a metabolic machine that is deeply involved in processing blood constituents that are brought to it from elsewhere in the body (145, 145a). For a while serotonin was a serious candidate for the role of the unique chemical mediator (23, 68, 348). This possibility has been discounted, but four chemicals remain viable candidates for this role: catecholamines, histamine, prostaglandins, and angiotensin.

4a. *Catecholamines.* The rich innervation of the pulmonary circulation by the autonomic nervous system (98, 123, 462) and the ample supply of α-receptors (constrictor) and β-receptors (dilator) in pulmonary vascular smooth muscle (41, 231) have nurtured the idea that the adrenergic system may not only help to set the initial tone of the pulmonary vasculature (141) but may also make an important contribution to the pulmonary vasomotor response to acute hypoxia. The adrenergic nerves could conceivably contribute to the hypoxic pressor response by *1*) a hypoxic effect on the synthesis, uptake, storage, and handling of norepinephrine at nerve endings (414), *2*) interference with the handling and disposition of circulating catecholamines, and *3*) other more subtle effects on the adrenergic system for vasomotor control of the pulmonary circulation (39). The evidence that the hypoxic pressor is blunted or abolished by α-adrenergic blockade with phenoxybenzamine and enhanced by β-adrenergic blockade with propranolol supports the important involvement of the adrenergic nervous system (23, 28, 67, 388).

Unfortunately, although the metabolism and release of norepinephrine are distinctly affected by acute hypoxia (414), the results may be more meaningful for the pharmacology of pulmonary vascular nerve endings and receptors than for the integrated pulmonary vascular response to acute hypoxia. Misgivings about the physiological significance of studies with blocking agents heighten the uncertainties about the role played by norepinephrine and the adrenergic nervous system in mediating the hypoxic pulmonary pressor response. Moreover, despite successful α-adrenergic blockade, both in animal preparations (98, 285) and in intact animals (100, 176, 300, 440) the pulmonary pressor response to acute hypoxia has persisted. Thus, although norepinephrine and the adrenergic nervous system may contribute to the hypoxic response under certain experimental conditions, norepinephrine cannot be implicated as the unique chemical mediator that operates under natural or near-natural conditions.

4b. *Histamine.* For a while enthusiasm was high for histamine as the unique chemical mediator of the pulmonary pressor response to hypoxia: histamine appeared in pulmonary veins during acute hypoxia, presumably from strategically dispersed perivascular mast cells (188); the pulmonary pressor response to hypoxia was blunted by antihistamines and histamine depleters (203) and was enhanced by a histamine inhibitor (semicarbazide) (205, 206, 463). Also chronic hypoxia was shown to be associated with both pulmonary hypertension and hyperplasia of mast cells in the lungs of rats, calves, and pigs (250, 254).

However, time has not been kind to the notion of histamine as the unique chemical mediator (28, 191, 250, 254). Histamine can cause pulmonary vasodilation as well as vasoconstriction (25), and agents effective in blocking the pressor response in some species (e.g., the rat and ferret) (25) have proved ineffective in others (e.g., the cat or dog) (191, 487). Mast cell depletion is not a regular feature of the pressor response to acute hypoxia (254), and mast cell stabilizers or depleters are without effect on hypoxic vasoconstriction in the cat (25). Nor has it been possible consistently to show increased concentrations of histamine in the effluent from hypoxically vasoconstricted lungs (59). Finally, the histamine content of the lungs does not decrease during acute hypoxia (254). These observations challenge the notion that release of histamine from perivascular mast cells is involved in the hypoxic pressor response.

The experience with pulmonary mast cells has proved too inconsistent and inconclusive to designate them the seat of the unique chemical mediator in the hypoxic pressor response. The evidence against histamine from mast cells is summarized above. In addition, large species differences exist in the number and pulmonary perivascular disposition of mast cells and in their contents of biologically active material (25, 28, 188, 212, 484). For example, one inconsistency is the high density of pulmonary perivascular mast cells in the dog and guinea pig, which react rather poorly to the pulmonary pressor effects of acute hypoxia (484). Another is the sluggish degranulation of mast cells (254) in the face of abrupt vasoconstriction produced by acute hypoxia. Finally, the hypoxic pressor response can be elicited in the mast cell–deficient cat (306) and mouse (535), suggesting that if histamine is involved it must originate from intrapulmonary sources other than the mast cell (350, 535).

From this tangle of contradictory evidence and uncertainty it is not possible to implicate histamine as the unique mediator of the pressor response to acute hypoxia, especially because histamine is a potent releaser of prostaglandins and products of the lipoxygenase pathway, primarily prostacyclins from endothelial cells. It shares this property with thrombin, mellitin, and bradykinin. By the same token, as in the case for the catecholamines (487), the evidence does not exclude a subsidiary role for histamine (229), either in setting initial tone or in modulating the pressor response.

Nonetheless interest in the role of histamine in the pulmonary pressor response to acute hypoxia has not waned completely, because of the demonstration of two types of histamine receptors by the use of blocking agents: chlorpheniramine to block the H_1 (vasoconstrictor) actions and metiamide to block the H_2 (vasodilator) actions. Under ordinary (nonhypoxic) conditions, depending on the species and experimental circumstances, either pulmonary vasoconstriction or vasodilation may predominate after histamine release, presumably depending on the balance of interactions between H_1 and H_2 receptors (25, 486). Usually, however, pulmonary vasodilation results, particularly if initial tone is high, as during acute hypoxia (105, 435). Chronic hypoxia affords a different prospect, i.e., a shift in balance from predominant H_1 (vasoconstrictor) actions to H_2 (vasodilator) actions.

These considerations suggest that at least part of the variability in the pulmonary pressor response may reflect differences in initial tone, stimulation of β-adrenergic receptors in the pulmonary circulation by release of epinephrine from the adrenal glands (86, 229), or relative distributions of H_1 and H_2 receptors in different species. The predominant site of pulmonary vasomotor effects is generally held to be the small pulmonary veins (173). The same is true for the effects of histamine on pulmonary vascular permeability (384). However, histamine receptors have been identified in large pulmonary arteries (479).

The overall experience with histamine is a useful reminder of at least three axioms in the use of pharmacologic agents to uncover mechanisms involved in vasomotor activity. *1*) Few drugs are sufficiently specific in their actions to settle the receptors or pathways that are affected. *2*) Rarely can subtle concomitant influences, such as the release of interfering biologically active substances—locally or afar, be excluded. *3*) Alternate vasomotor mechanisms may predominate at different times because of a complex interplay between different receptor sites and mechanisms for a single pharmacologic agent or because of shared receptors for different pharmacologic agents (141, 316).

4c. *Angiotensin.* Angiotensin II began to attract serious attention as a potential chemical mediator of the pulmonary pressor response to hypoxia when it was shown that the addition of subpressor quantities of angiotensin I to the perfusate of a lung unresponsive to hypoxia would restore the pressor response for 30–60 min (46). However, important misgivings soon developed about the validity of this hypothesis. *1*) The experiments did not exclude the possibility that restoration of responsiveness by angiotensin may have been a nonspecific effect operating in exceedingly artificial circumstances. *2*) Because angiotensin I is converted to angiotensin II at the endothelial surface, some form of endothelial-medial interaction had to be invoked. *3)* The administration of saralasin—a competitive inhibitor of angiotensin II—did not prevent the pressor response to acute hypoxia (192, 316).

Presently it seems likely that angiotensin does little more than contribute to initial tone, a property that different vasoactive substances may share to different degrees, depending on the species and experimental conditions.

4d. Prostaglandins. Because the intravenous administration of arachidonate elicits vasoconstriction (500) and because of the prospect that a balance between PGI_2 and thromboxane A_2 may be important in setting initial tone during ambient air breathing, it was natural for investigators to probe the cyclooxygenase pathway in search of a chemical mediator responsible for the pulmonary pressor response to acute hypoxia (see Fig. 23). However, with meclofenamate, an inhibitor of prostaglandin synthesis, no evidence could be adduced for a prostaglandin role in eliciting hypoxic pulmonary vasoconstriction either in the awake calf, anesthetized dog, or isolated perfused rat lung (413); nor could $PGF_{2\alpha}$ be implicated (40). Indeed, instead of serving in a pulmonary pressor role the cyclooxygenase pathway seemed to dampen the pulmonary vasoconstriction evoked by acute hypoxia. Several lines of evidence favor this view. *1)* Inhibition of cyclooxygenase increased the strength of pulmonary hypoxic vasoconstriction (492, 517). *2)* Differences in cyclooxygenase activity appear to be responsible for individual differences in the pressor response (193). *3)* Prostacyclin has the potential for serving as an intrinsic agent that automatically blunts the pulmonary pressor response to acute hypoxia (162, 197, 490, 500). *4)* In sheep that hyporespond to acute hypoxia, inhibitory prostaglandins seem to be involved in the blunted response (7). *5)* The pulmonary arterial pressor response to acute hypoxia can be abolished by administering minute doses of endotoxin (15 μm/kg) intravenously, presumably because of the production of a dilator prostaglandin (518). Thus, even though products of the cyclooxygenase pathway may modulate tone and the pressor response, they do not appear to be involved via the cyclooxygenase pathway in the genesis of the pulmonary pressor response to acute hypoxia (162).

With the discovery of the lipoxygenase pathway and the availability (in small quantities) of the leukotrienes, attention has shifted to components of this pathway. The leukotrienes, notably leukotriene C_4, have been shown to be pulmonary vasoconstrictors (199, 531), and the suggestion has been made that the leukotrienes may be involved in the pulmonary pressor response to acute hypoxia (7, 8). The evidence rests heavily on the use of inhibitors (e.g., diethylcarbamazine) that are not entirely specific, and not all of the complexities of the lipoxygenase pathway are unraveled. Whether the leukotrienes are the elusive chemical mediator or simply another biological agent that can, under proper conditions, affect pulmonary vascular tone remains to be clarified.

4e. Nonadrenergic, noncholinergic polypeptides. The physiological effects of these substances (including vasoactive intestinal polypeptide, two other vasoactive polypeptides, and substance P) on the pulmonary circulation are uncertain (429).

5. *Cellular events in vascular smooth muscle (direct effect).* Those who do not advocate a chemical mediator in the pulmonary pressor response to acute hypoxia espouse a direct effect, but if a direct effect on pulmonary vascular smooth muscle is responsible, how it is responsible is still speculative (141, 483). One attractive prospect is that acute hypoxia may elicit contraction of pulmonary arteries and arterioles by a direct effect on pulmonary vascular smooth muscle (55). Somewhat troublesome to proponents of this view is the fact that (depending on the species, experimental preparation, and test procedure) the response of isolated large pulmonary arteries to acute hypoxia has been inconsistent, i.e., constriction, dilation, or a combination of the two. However, advocates of a direct effect continue to gain strength with each failure to identify a unique chemical mediator and with the conceptual difficulty of reconciling the synergistic effects of acidosis and hypoxia on the pulmonary pressor response with the intervention of a special chemical agent.

Before considering how hypoxia might exert a direct vasoconstrictor effect on pulmonary vascular smooth muscle, it is necessary to note three important experimental realities. *1)* Isolating and handling vascular smooth muscle without modifying its reactivity or extinguishing its viability is difficult (451). *2)* The sparseness of muscle in the small pulmonary vessels and the difficulty in handling these vessels experimentally compel the experimenter to resort to large vessels, which need not behave the same as small pulmonary arteries and arterioles (44). *3)* Adaptation of precapillary vessels to chronic hypoxia may modify their response pattern, because they are chronically exposed to O_2-poor mixed venous blood, whereas blood in postcapillary vessels (venules and veins) is constantly perfused by O_2-rich blood (Fig. 24).

Acute hypoxia could act on pulmonary arterial smooth muscle by affecting either mechanisms that control membrane excitation, or excitation-contraction coupling, or chemomechanical transduction (116, 118, 134). These three options are currently the subject of intense investigations. In contrast, no evidence has been adduced to support the notion that hypoxia acts directly on the contractile process. Nor is there much compelling evidence in favor of an intracellular sensor and transduction mechanism even though, by analogy with the effects of hypoxia on the carotid body, the idea remains intuitively attractive (241, 483). Paramount among the likely candidates for an intracellular sensing and transduction agent are the metalloporphyrins (126, 331, 468). For example, cytochrome P-450 might induce pulmonary vasoconstriction when its heme-binding site is unoccupied and relax when either O_2 or CO occupies the binding site (257). Unfortunately, the involvement of hemoglobin, myoglobin, cytochrome oxidase, or cytochrome P-450 has not been convincingly demonstrated (468).

The attention of those who espouse a direct hypoxic effect as the mechanism for the hypoxic pressor response is focused presently on one or both of the two universal requirements for contraction: the energy source (ATP) and the regulator ion (Ca^{2+}) (Fig. 25). This approach presupposes that the rate of contraction may be limited by constraints on either the fuel (ATP) or the activator (Ca^{2+}) (242). Because hypoxia is apt to affect ATP production, the direct effects of hypoxia on the rate of contraction of pulmonary vascular smooth muscle may be limited by the ATP concentration. Another possibility involving ATP is its critical role in making activator Ca^{2+} available to the contractile machinery.

Presently these suggestions only can be regarded as intriguing hypotheses, but (aside from indicating directions for future research) they do have at least two important implications. *1*) The divergent responses to hypoxia of systemic and pulmonary vascular smooth muscle (470) may entail different biochemical mechanisms involving either ATP or Ca^{2+} or an interplay of the two (115, 378). *2*) The disparate contractile behavior of vascular smooth muscle from different

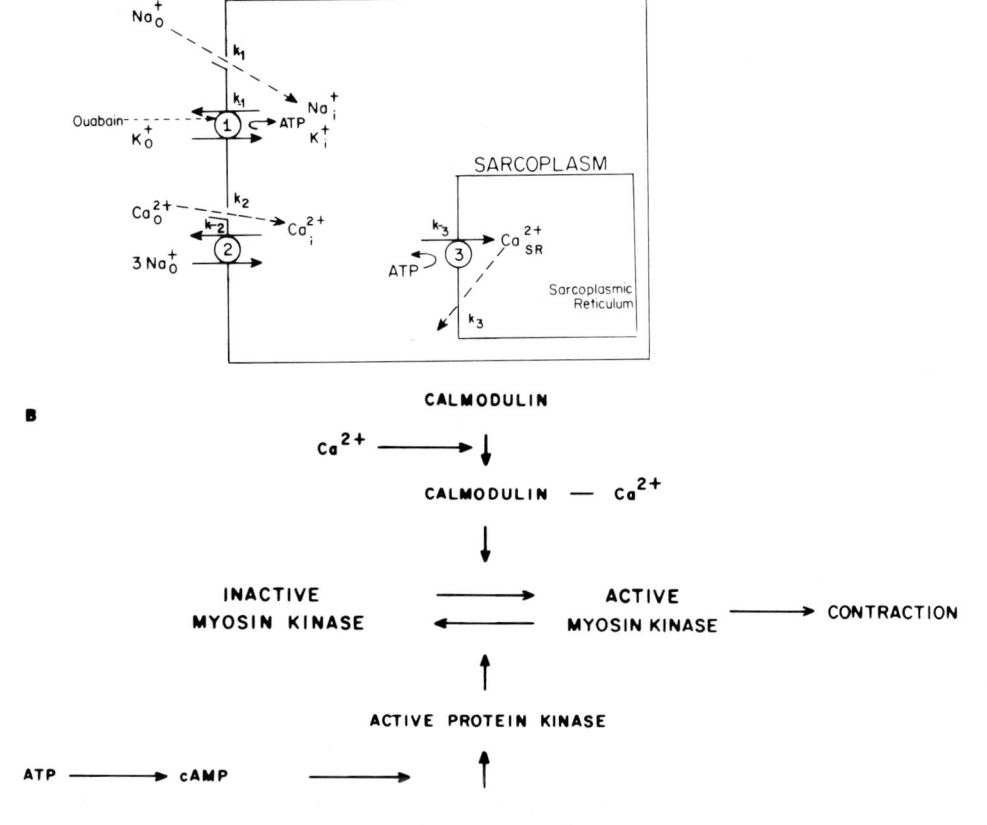

FIG. 25. Calcium and smooth muscle contraction. *A*: block diagram of compartmentalization of Ca^{2+} in muscle fibers. Also shown are main pathways and transport systems for Na^+ and Ca^{2+}: *1*) ATP-dependent, ouabain-sensitive Na^+-K^+ exchange pump; *2*) sarcolemmal Na^+-Ca^{2+} exchange mechanism (shown operating in forward or Ca^{2+} extrusion mode); *3*) sarcoplasmic reticulum (SR) ATP-dependent Ca^{2+} pump. Most of entering Na^+ and Ca^{2+} is assumed to come through voltage-sensitive conductance channels associated with action potential. k, Rate coefficient for fluxes of Na^+ and Ca^{2+} across sarcolemma and sarcoplasmic reticulum membranes in directions indicated. *B*: contraction of vascular smooth muscle. When intracellular Ca^{2+} levels exceed a critical level (10^{-6} M), Ca^{2+} binds to calmodulin, a Ca^{2+}-binding protein; Ca^{2+}-calmodulin complex binds in turn to myosin kinase, thereby activating the enzyme. Active kinase then catalyzes phosphorylation of myosin, which can interact with actin to produce contraction. Cyclic AMP plays an important role in activating a cAMP-dependent protein kinase that can transfer phosphate from ATP to proteins directly involved in regulation of intracellular Ca^{2+} levels and in interaction of actin with myosin. [*A* adapted from Blaustein (53).]

sources suggests that the requirements for contraction may differ from site to site: rate limitation by ATP may be more critical in pulmonary vascular smooth muscle, whereas rate limitation by Ca^{2+} may be more critical in systemic vascular smooth muscle (118). To what extent these generalizations, based largely on experiments with large vessels, apply to resistance vessels in the pulmonary circulation is enigmatic, but they do underscore the biochemical credibility of a direct effect of hypoxia on pulmonary vascular smooth muscle.

5a. *Metabolic effects.* A key question is whether a decrease in the rate of oxidative phosphorylation in pulmonary vascular smooth muscle elicits the hypoxic pressor response (418). Liljestrand (281) interpreted the experimental evidence then on hand [evidence largely based on the previous experiments of others (126) and his own experience with the effects of iodoacetate on the pressor response to acute hypoxia] and proposed that hypoxia elicited pulmonary vasoconstriction by increasing glycolysis, thereby liberating lactic acid within the pulmonary vascular smooth muscle. However, recent observations with 2-deoxyglucose or iodoacetate (competitive inhibitors of glucose metabolism) (317) and low levels of glucose in the perfusate (419) undermined the earlier evidence (126) by demonstrating an increase (rather than a decrease) in the hypoxic pressor response. These observations challenged the possibility that hypoxic pulmonary vasoconstriction is attributable to an increase in the rate of anaerobic glycolysis (418, 419) and left unclear why a decrease in the rate of glucose metabolism increases the pulmonary pressor response. Further exploration of this question in the isolated rat lung reaffirmed that inhibition of glucose metabolism enhances hypoxic pulmonary vasoconstriction and negated the possibility that hypoxic pulmonary vasoconstriction is due to an increase in the rate of anaerobic glycolysis (281). The link between the metabolic change and the hemodynamic response is still uncertain. However, it has been reasoned that this relationship is attributable to a decrease in the production of pyruvate rather than to a decrease in the glycolytic generation of ATP. As Rounds and co-workers (418, 419) recognize, neither the experiments nor the reasoning have excluded the possibility of either limitation of mitochondrial oxidative phosphorylation in an O_2-sensing cell (as yet unidentified) or of a change in either the concentration or activity of some intracellular or intercellular constituent (peptide, fatty acid, or lipid).

5b. *Electrical activity and electrical-mechanical coupling.* Few observations have been made on the smooth muscle cells of the pulmonary vascular tree, and most of these have been confined to the main or large pulmonary vessels (81, 82). One possible way by which acute hypoxia might elicit its pulmonary pressor response is by depolarizing the cell membrane of pulmonary vascular smooth muscle. By changing the activity of the Na^+-K^+ pump or the distribution of ions across the cell membrane, hypoxia could decrease the transmembrane potential, thereby bringing the cell closer to its threshold potential for activation (44, 53). The difficulties inherent in testing this proposal are great but not insurmountable (451). In the isolated main pulmonary artery of the rat, resting membrane potentials recorded intracellularly during acute hypoxia proved to be less negative than during normoxic control periods. One major article of faith is that observations made on the large pulmonary artery and vein—which can be tested with microelectrodes or the sucrose gap technique—are pertinent to the behavior of the small arteries and arterioles that constitute the pulmonary resistance vessels. Direct measurements of membrane potentials have been made with isolated pulmonary vessels from rats rendered chronically (464, 465) and acutely hypoxic.

In current studies of the hypoxic pulmonary pressor response, Ca^{2+} is featured prominently [Fig. 25; (55, 316, 501)]; along related lines Mg^+ has received some, but much less, attention (488). Acute hypoxia is pictured as increasing the Ca^{2+} concentration in the vascular smooth muscle cell either by increasing the permeability of the cell membrane, promoting intracellular shifts, or both (55). The tone of the vascular smooth muscle could then be set by an interplay between Ca^{2+} and the supply of ATP. Support for a major role of Ca^{2+} in the hypoxic pressor response has been obtained in a variety of ways: Ca^{2+} antagonists in an isolated blood-perfused rat lung preparation indicate that hypoxia can act directly to depolarize pulmonary vascular smooth muscle and to initiate the transmembrane flow of Ca^{2+} into the cell where it can activate the contractile machinery; autoradiographs of the pulmonary artery of chronically hypoxic rats are consistent with an increase in intracellular Ca^{2+}; Ca^{2+} antagonists block the hypoxic pressor response (316, 487).

How Ca^{2+} operates in the hypoxic pressor response remains a fruitful area for exploration. A strong case has been made for its role as a mediator in excitation-contraction coupling (316), but only glimpses are available of how the disposition and flux of Ca^{2+} within the myoplasm relates to the contractile proteins (451). Nor are the actions of Ca^{2+} channel blockers entirely clear (345). The observations on membrane potentials during chronic and acute hypoxia (464), the influence of ions and electrogenic pumps on resting membrane potentials during hypoxia, the role of Ca^{2+} in the hypoxic pulmonary pressor response, and the differences in the patterns of depolarization with time during hypoxia also require clarification. Indeed the possibility has not been excluded that Ca^{2+} operates by way of local chemical mediators or the release of transmitter substances from the parenchyma around the vessels (287). Those who believe in a direct effect of acute hypoxia can find support in the observations cited above and conclude that a Ca^{2+}-

dependent mechanism is involved in hypoxic pulmonary hypertension. However, nonbelievers continue to regard this evidence as unconvincing and have not been deflected from their search for a unique chemical mediator in the pulmonary hypoxic pressor response.

Although the evidence favoring a unique chemical mediator and that for a direct effect have been presented separately, the possibility has not even been excluded that an interplay between both mechanisms may be involved. Recent demonstrations of interplay between endothelium and vascular smooth muscle (158) raise questions about whether the reason for the uncertainty is in the complexity of the mechanism or in a biological reaction or substance that has not yet been identified. It may well be that once again scientists are looking "where the light is" and that the answer is still in the unexplored darkness.

6. Sites of pulmonary vasoconstriction. The extensive literature on this subject allows considerable latitude in interpretation. Indeed it can be interpreted to mean that, depending on the experimental circumstances and the preparation, acute hypoxia can increase tone of the whole pulmonary vascular tree or constrict any or all of its segments, i.e., arterial, capillary, alveolar and extra-alveolar, or venous [Fig. 24; (141)]. Among the influences that determine the pulmonary vascular site(s) affected by acute hypoxia are the nature of the preparation or model, the species, and the age of the animal under study. The bulk of the experimental evidence assigns a predominant role to the muscular precapillary vessels, i.e., the small arteries and arterioles (1, 11, 107, 141, 181). However, as is indicated next, no consensus exists about this point.

The evidence favoring the pulmonary arteries and arterioles is both direct and indirect. *1)* The media is thicker and better organized for vasoconstriction in the pre- than in the postcapillary vessels of the lungs; this difference is heightened by chronic hypoxia (201, 410). *2)* In principle, alveolar-capillary water exchange would be in jeopardy if the predominant site of vasoconstriction were postcapillary (138). *3)* The pressor response to hypoxia is virtually instantaneous when PA_{O_2} is dropped (239). *4)* In cross-circulated fetal lambs, selective decrease in mixed Pv_{O_2} produced by asphyxia of the donor causes pulmonary vasoconstriction in the unasphyxiated recipient (76). *5)* In the isolated perfused lung a decrease in the mixed Pv_{O_2} during ventilatory arrest elicits pulmonary vasoconstriction (204). *6)* The increase in pulmonary artery pressure during hypoxia can be blunted by perfusing the pulmonary artery with well-oxygenated blood (54, 204). *7)* The synergistic effect of acidosis on the pulmonary pressor response to hypoxia (131) is in keeping with the imputation that pulmonary arterial smooth muscle is involved in the vasoconstriction. *8)* Carbon monoxide and 2,4-dinitrophenol, which selectively decrease the mixed Pv_{O_2}, concomitantly evoke the pulmonary pressor response (42).

Although the evidence that the small muscular arteries and arterioles are the predominant sites of the increase in pulmonary vascular resistance during acute hypoxia is strong, it is not conclusive. Much of the evidence for this view rests on the assumption that vessels devoid of vascular media cannot undergo an active change in caliber. Whether this generalization applies to the pulmonary capillaries is currently under investigation (336). About 30 years ago pulmonary capillary vasoconstriction was proffered as an explanation for the responses to acute hypoxia obtained during forward and retrograde perfusion of the isolated lung of the cat (125). This proposition subsequently lay dormant until observations on alveolar-capillary morphology rekindled interest in the possibility (248, 249, 308, 309). These observations suggested that during acute hypoxia, alveolar septa were deformed and able to interfere with the passage of formed elements (309, 504). Clearly these morphologic observations cannot determine the mechanism or distinguish cause from effect.

One way capillaries might change their calibers actively is by increased tone of the contractile interstitial cells in the alveolar wall (248). Although this idea is consistent with the larger concept that smooth muscle everywhere in the lungs constricts on exposure to acute hypoxia (141), no decrease in pulmonary compliance during acute hypoxia has been reported.

Physiological observations during acute hypoxia (51, 335, 521) have suggested that not only capillaries (alveolar vessels) but also extra-alveolar vessels constrict during acute hypoxia. However, these experiments do little more in anatomical terms than suggest that minute pre- and postcapillary vessels that contain smooth muscle in their walls, as well as capillaries, can participate in the pressor response to acute hypoxia. Consequently it is difficult to relate the physiological to the morphologic observations or to do more than recognize that these results are probably more characteristic of special experimental circumstances than of the intact animal or human under natural conditions.

Evidence also exists that under the proper set of experimental conditions pulmonary postcapillary venules may be the predominant site of pulmonary vasoconstriction. As a rule, these experiments have relied on the fluid-exchanging function of the lungs to distinguish between pre- and postcapillary vasoconstriction. However, the results have been inconsistent, varying from preparation to preparation and from species to species (335).

Presently it seems reasonable to underscore that many different contractile elements in the lungs seem to be able to contribute to the pressor response to acute hypoxia. Under natural conditions precapillary vasoconstriction appears to predominate. This view has indirect support from the muscular hypertrophy and peripheral extension of muscle in the pulmonary precapillary vessels in chronic hypoxia. Under special experimental conditions, however, other sites and mechanisms may predominate. Often these special conditions blur distinctions between active and passive changes.

7. *Overview of pressor response to acute hypoxia.* In the last few decades hypoxia has emerged as the most effective, straightforward, and reproducible stimulus for eliciting pulmonary vasoconstriction. When hypoxia is confined to part of the lung—as by bronchospirometry or as a result of lung disease—blood flow is diverted to the nonhypoxic parts of the lungs. However, when hypoxia affects all parts of the lungs, the result is pulmonary hypertension. Because of its effectiveness at tolerable levels in the laboratory, as well as its spontaneous occurrence at high altitude and in patients with cardiopulmonary disorders, a large research effort has been directed at uncovering the pattern of the pulmonary vasoconstrictor response and the mechanisms by which it is effected. As a result the phenomenon has been approached in many ways, ranging from local to widespread pulmonary hypoxia and from physiological and biochemical studies of the interplay between the hypoxic and H^+ stimuli on the one hand to genetics on the other. The surfeit of experimental observations has made it clear that both intrapulmonary (local) and extrapulmonary influences are engaged in the response, that generally the local influences predominate, but that the vigor of the response may be strongly modified both by initial tone of the resistance vessels and by stimuli converging on the reactive smooth muscle. Striking differences in the magnitude of the response occur not only between one experimental preparation and another but also between species and between fetus and adult.

Because of the inaccessibility of the pulmonary circulation, artificial conditions that depress responsiveness of pulmonary vascular smooth muscle are often part of the study. Nonetheless the results have directed attention to the pulmonary vascular smooth muscle and framed the question, Does hypoxia exert its effects indirectly, via a mediator released within the lung, or does it act directly on pulmonary vascular smooth muscle? Efforts to uncover a unique chemical mediator have failed, and attempts to uncover a direct mechanism by which hypoxia could elicit pulmonary vasoconstriction have not settled the issue.

8. *Hypoxia in atelectasis.* It cannot be assumed that an apparently atelectatic lung is an airless lung unless special precautions have been taken to ensure complete alveolar collapse, i.e., an adequate period of prior O_2 breathing to eliminate N_2. Thus the rate of collapse depends on the prior history of the experimental lobe or lung, and interpretation in terms of mechanical effects generally have to take into account a low cardiac output and arterial hypoxemia. After induction of unilateral atelectasis, ipsilateral blood flow decreases progressively as the lung shrinks: within 15 min ipsilateral flow falls to ~50% of control values and a considerable retrograde flow occurs during diastole from the pulmonary artery on the affected side (349). Not only mechanical influences but also hypoxia and hypercapnia contribute to the increase in ipsilateral pulmonary vascular resistance (26, 28).

Of these three influences, hypoxic pulmonary vasoconstriction, acting locally, is generally the most powerful (28, 35, 36, 387). However, systemic hypoxemia has been reported to increase blood flow through the atelectatic lung (35, 36, 349), an effect that is presumably reflexly mediated via the systemic arterial chemoreceptors (275). This reflex pulmonary vasodilation evoked in the atelectatic lung by systemic hypoxemia is difficult to reconcile with observations made in another context that systemic hypoxemia elicits pulmonary vasoconstriction via the systemic arterial chemoreceptors (238). Shock, acidosis, and the ipsilateral administration of sodium nitroprusside increase blood flow through the atelectatic lung.

Chronic hypoxia. For more than 20 years it has been known that life at high altitude is associated with chronic hypoxia, arterial hypoxemia, and pulmonary hypertension [Fig. 26; (210, 318, 340, 341, 417)]. It has also long been appreciated that chronic hypoxia affects the pulmonary and systemic circulations oppositely, relaxing systemic vascular smooth muscle while eliciting pulmonary vasoconstriction (141, 210). Chronic hypoxia produced experimentally at sea level—either by decreasing the O_2 content of inspired air or by dropping ambient pressure—also evokes pulmonary hypertension (232, 393). The degree of pulmonary hypertension depends heavily but not exclusively on the level of chronic hypoxia [Fig. 27; (210, 371)]. At Morococha, Peru (4,540 m), where the ambient P_{O_2} is ~80 mmHg (Table 2), mean pulmonary arterial pressure in adults is ~28 mmHg, compared to an average value of 12 mmHg in sea-level residents (Lima, Peru). Cardiac output and pulmonary wedge pressures do not differ appreciably at sea level and at high altitude. Until the age of 5 yr, children have uniformly higher pulmonary arterial pressure than adults at the same alitutde (Fig. 28). During moderate exercise, mean pulmonary arterial pressure increases considerably [Fig. 27; (372)]. In individuals suffering from chronic mountain sickness, in which severe arterial hypoxemia and hypercapnia are secondary to alveolar hypoventilation, the corresponding pressures are much higher [Fig. 29; (210, 371)]. Striking species differences in reactivity have been observed in humans and animals that are native to high altitude (182, 399).

A variety of influences—hemodynamic, morphologic, and genetic—influence the degree of vasomotor responsiveness during chronic hypoxia (394). As a rule the more muscle in the pulmonary muscular arteries and arterioles, the greater is the vasomotor response. Thus certain cattle (mostly calves) at high altitude not only have thick muscle in their small pulmonary arteries but also develop extraordinarily high pulmonary arterial pressures when exposed to hypoxia. As a result they develop a syndrome of right ventricular

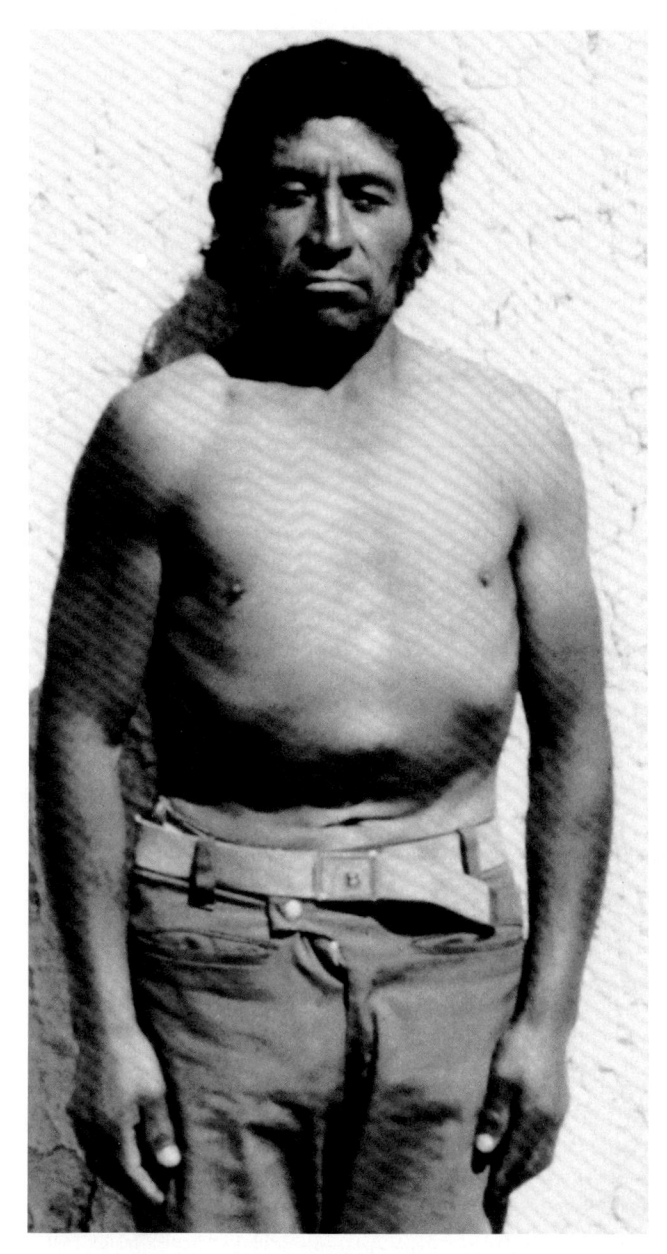

FIG. 26. Native resident of Lake Titicaca (Peruvian Andes, ~4,500 m). Barrel chest is generally held to be one of several adaptations to life in rarified atmosphere. (Courtesy of R. B. Eckhardt.)

failure, which includes edema of the brisket (the dependent portions between the forelegs and neck) (261).

Genetic predisposition features prominently in determining pulmonary vascular hyperresponders and the development of brisket disease. Indeed it has been possible to sort these calves into genetic hypo- and hyperresponders (427, 519). Cold, which often accompanies hypoxia at high altitude, appears to enhance the pulmonary pressor response in the hyperresponders, leaving the hyporesponders unaffected (528). Genetic factors also seem to influence human suscep-

tibility to pulmonary hypertension at high altitude (503).

It is suspected but not proved that the pulmonary vascular responses to acute and chronic hypoxia involve related mechanisms. However, it also seems likely that subtle adaptive mechanisms may be operative in the chronically hypoxic individual. For example, the chronic hypoxia consequent to lung disease need not involve the same adjustments as the normal chronic hypoxia at high altitude where the fetus, neonate, and adult live unremittingly in an O_2-poor environment. The mechanisms operating in the hypoxic native resident at high altitude or in the sea-level dweller who acquires lung disease late in life also need not be the same as those in the individual with congenital cyanotic heart disease.

In contrast to the prompt reversal of the pressor response when acute hypoxia is discontinued, pulmonary arterial pressure and pulmonary vascular resistance remain high when chronically hypoxic animals or humans are exposed to normoxia, as when native residents of high altitude move to sea level. In large measure the persistent increase in pulmonary vascular

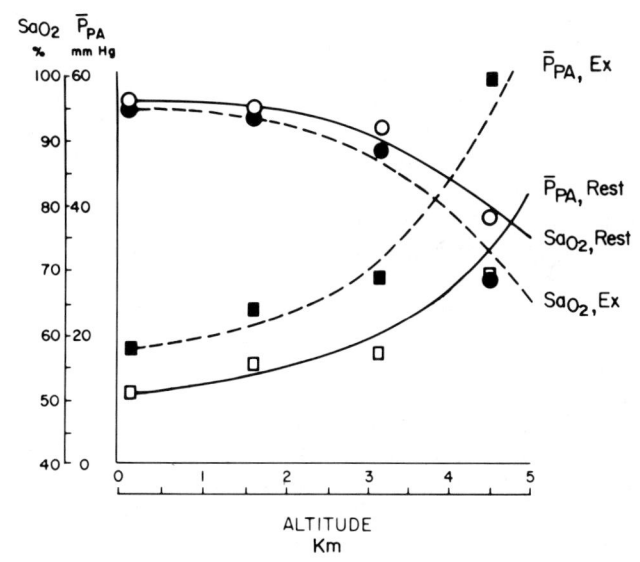

FIG. 27. Relation in Peruvian Andes between altitude, arterial O_2 saturation (Sa_{O_2}), and mean pulmonary arterial pressure ($\bar{P}pa$). Appreciable levels of arterial hypoxemia and of pulmonary hypertension occur at ~3,000 m. During exercise (EX) arterial hypoxemia and pulmonary arterial pressure increase. [From Penaloza and Gamboa (371).]

TABLE 2. *Representative Normal Values for Native Residents at High Altitude*

Altitude, m	4,540
Ambient P_{O_2}, mmHg	80
Arterial O_2 saturation, %	78
Pulmonary artery pressures, mmHg*	40/15, 28
Pulmonary wedge pressure, mmHg	5
Cardiac output, liters·min⁻¹·m⁻²	3.70

Values are for residents of Morococha, Peru. * Systolic/diastolic, mean.

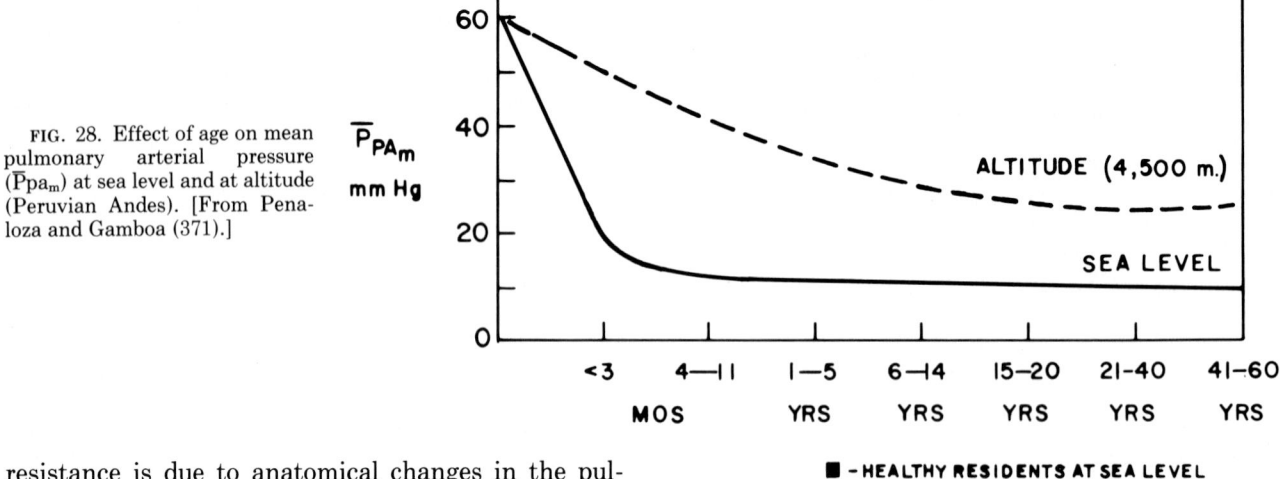

FIG. 28. Effect of age on mean pulmonary arterial pressure ($\overline{P}pa_m$) at sea level and at altitude (Peruvian Andes). [From Penaloza and Gamboa (371).]

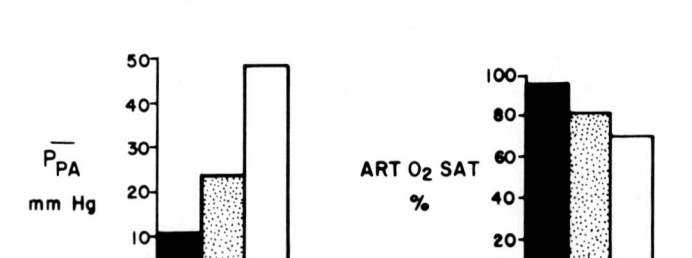

FIG. 29. Mean pulmonary arterial pressure ($\overline{P}pa$) and arterial O_2 saturation (ART O_2 SAT) in 3 groups of individuals. In healthy highlanders, arterial oxygenation is lower than in healthy sea-level residents. This discrepancy is greatly widened in chronic alveolar hypoventilators (Monge's disease) at high altitude. Level of pulmonary arterial pressure is inversely related to degree of arterial hypoxemia. [Adapted from Heath and Williams (210).]

resistance is due to anatomical changes in the pulmonary arterial tree elicited by the chronic hypoxia (129, 152, 208) abetted by polycythemia (152). Age and possibly sex influence the degree of muscularization of the terminal branches of the pulmonary arterial tree (446).

The anatomical lesions of hypoxic pulmonary hypertension are reversible (261). On withdrawal of the hypoxic stimulus, as by relocating native residents from high altitude to sea level, the pulmonary arterial pressure falls (210, 293). However, complete return to levels of pulmonary arterial pressure that are normal for sea-level dwellers is not usually achieved for a number of years. Even as long as 2 yr after moving to sea level, the native resident of high altitude responds to exercise with an inordinate increase in pulmonary arterial pressure for the level of cardiac output, presumably due to residual muscularization of the small pulmonary arteries. On return to normoxic conditions the pulmonary circulation of altitude dwellers responds to acute hypoxia by vasoconstricting. However, the vigor of the response has varied from laboratory to laboratory, apparently depending on the preparation and the time chosen for testing after return to normoxic conditions (129, 152, 317).

Interest remains high in the morphologic changes that occur on exposure to chronic hypoxia. In sea-level dwellers the small muscular arteries at the acinar level (15–30 μm diam) are thin tubes of endothelium resting on a sparse collagen framework and containing only traces of muscle in their walls (445, 450). These "arterioles" are part of the "resistance vessels." Shortly after the start of exposure to hypoxia, morphologic changes begin in the walls of these vessels (450). As hypoxia is prolonged, the media of the pulmonary arterioles hypertrophies and undergoes hyperplasia while extending peripherally into precapillary vessels that are ordinarily nonmuscular (15, 222); whether the number of patent resistance vessels also decreases is unsettled (222, 252). Despite this precapillary restructuring, the pulmonary capillaries and veins remain unchanged (450). Similar changes occur spontaneously in humans and most animals native to high altitude (15). Calves susceptible to pulmonary hypertension during hypoxia have more smooth muscle in the small pulmonary arteries than do calves that are poorly reactive (520). Certain species native to high altitude, notably the llama, alpaca, and the vizcacha in South America, do not develop medial hypertrophy (210, 211).

Polycythemia contributes to the pulmonary hypertension associated with chronic hypoxia (24, 450). This effect depends on an increase in blood viscosity (152). Pulmonary arterial pressure tends to remain high when the hypoxic stimulus is acutely removed and the pulmonary pressor response to acute hypoxia is preserved, at least for a day or two (152). The morphologic changes, the polycythemia, and the level of pulmonary hypertension tend to regress after removal from the hypoxic environment (4, 208, 450), but the return toward normal pulmonary arterial pressure is gradual (217). Mast cell depletion (in the mouse) does not interfere with the pulmonary hypertensive or morphologic response to chronic hypoxia (535).

Several issues remain to be clarified: *1*) the nature of the precursor cell for the new smooth muscle cells in the media, i.e., pericyte (328, 329) or fibroblast (450); *2*) whether peripheral pulmonary arteries do decrease in number during chronic hypoxia (129, 222, 232, 401); and *3*) the effect of sex on the muscularization of the pulmonary arterioles (392, 446, 450). Finally, it is extremely difficult to compare observations in the isolated lung (318) with those made in intact animals (152). Discrepancies often appear to be a function of experimental manipulation rather than an innate characteristic of the intact animal operating under natural conditions.

As at sea level, supine exercise increases pulmonary arterial pressure: at 4,540 m in the Peruvian Andes, exercise sufficient to quadruple the O_2 uptake is associated with intensification of the arterial hypoxemia, a doubling of the cardiac output (from 3.65 to 7.49 liters·min^{-1}·m^{-2}), and a doubling of the pulmonary arterial pressure [from 41/15, 29 mmHg (systolic/diastolic, mean) to 77/40, 60 mmHg] (417).

After birth at high altitude, involution of pulmonary arterial pressures is delayed: young children (1–5 yr) raised at high altitude have higher pulmonary arterial pressures (~58/32, 44 mmHg) than do older children (~41/18, 28 mmHg).

1. *Site of increased pulmonary vascular resistance.* The distal ramifications of the pulmonary arterial tree, i.e., the small muscular arteries and arterioles, are generally held to be responsible for the increase in pulmonary vascular resistance in chronic hypoxia (15). This conclusion is based primarily on anatomical evidence: *1*) in chronic hypoxia the media of the small pulmonary arteries undergoes hypertrophy and the vascular smooth muscle extends peripherally into minute precapillary vessels that are ordinarily devoid of smooth muscle (222, 393, 520); *2*) the number of peripheral arteries is reduced morphologically (222), even though the pulmonary blood volume remains within normal limits (129); and *3*) in some species the intimal lining also undergoes proliferation, thereby contributing to pulmonary vascular obstruction (9).

The pulmonary pressor response to chronic hypoxia consists of vasoconstrictive and morphologic components (129, 293, 318, 327). The morphologic changes have been attributed to a combination of hypoxia and the persistent pulmonary hypertension that it elicits. These combined stimuli affect large and small pulmonary arteries differently (365). The muscular hypertrophy of the small pulmonary vessels induced by chronic hypoxia gradually reverses on restoration of sea-level O_2 tensions in the ambient air (217, 269, 327). An intriguing exception to the effects of chronic hypoxia is the llama, a mammal indigenous to the Peruvian Andes (4,720 m). In contrast to the Quechua Indians who also live at this altitude, the llama develops neither muscularization of the terminal portion of the pulmonary arterial tree, nor (presumably) pulmonary hypertension, nor right ventricular hypertrophy (209).

What purpose is served by the pulmonary hypertension of high altitude? With respect to gas exchange, pulmonary hypertension could ensure better blood flow to the apices of the lungs, thereby improving oxygenation. More subtle benefits for gas exchange or for hemodynamics are conceivable. However, the possibility also exists that the pressor response lingers as an evolutionary throwback in the adult but serves a useful purpose in ensuring a small pulmonary blood flow in the fetus.

2. *Functional component of increased pulmonary vascular resistance.* It has been tacitly assumed that the vasomotor mechanisms underlying the sustained increase in pulmonary vascular tone during chronic hypoxia are directly related to, if not the same as, those that operate during acute hypoxia. This need not be so. Although the circumstance of lifelong hypoxia is difficult to reproduce in the laboratory, it is conceivable that in pulmonary vascular smooth muscle (118), as in systemic vascular smooth muscle, chronic hypoxia may introduce major detours in the metabolic pathways of pulmonary vascular smooth muscle (117). To what extent the changes in energetics modify pulmonary vascular tone and reactivity is unexplored.

With respect to a unique chemical mediator as the basis for the sustained pulmonary hypertension during chronic hypoxia, it is difficult to picture either histamine, or the catecholamines, or angiotensin II (141) in this role. Much simpler to imagine than a unique chemical mediator is a direct effect of chronic hypoxia on vascular smooth muscle. For example, the adaptation to the lack of O_2 might favor anaerobic over aerobic metabolism in the vascular smooth muscle, or reset the flow of ions across the smooth muscle membrane, or readjust electromechanical coupling (117). With respect to the latter, chronic hypoxia was recently shown to change membrane potentials recorded from isolated pulmonary vessels of pulmonary hypertensive rats (465); whereas the resting membrane potential of smooth muscle in the main pulmonary artery was depolarized, that of the small pulmonary arteries (resistance vessels) was hyperpolarized. Increased chloride conductance of the membrane was proposed to account for the membrane potentials in the main pulmonary artery; for the small pulmonary arteries a different mechanism, i.e., an increase in the Na^+-K^+, was suggested. Of necessity the observations were made under highly artificial conditions. Nonetheless they are of great interest not only in suggesting an avenue for further exploration of direct mechanisms involved in hypoxic pulmonary vasoconstriction but also as a reminder that different vessels in the pulmonary vascular tree need not respond the same way to the same stimulus (327). In essence, with respect to mechanisms responsible for the pulmonary pressor effect, the same alternatives seem to apply as for acute hypoxia. However, for direct observation and manipulation, chronic hypoxia seems more attractive because of the possibility that hypertrophied media in chronically hypoxic animals are apt to be more manageable experimentally.

3. *Teleological considerations.* Inevitably questions are raised about the advantages gained from pulmonary hypertension. In the fetus, pulmonary hypertension is necessary because the lung is not a gas-exchanging organ and the high pulmonary vascular resistance directs blood flow through the ductus arteriosus toward the gas-exchanging apparatus, the placenta. Other advantages are less certain: with respect to gas exchange, pulmonary hypertension could improve oxygenation by increasing blood flow to the apices of the lungs. Conversely the possibility remains that pulmonary hypertension exhausts its benign function in the fetus and is a vestigial mechanism that serves no useful purpose in the adult.

Acute hyperoxia. The resistance vessels of the normal pulmonary circulation at sea level manifest little vasomotor "tone," so an increase in $P_{A_{O_2}}$ above normoxic levels can only be expected to cause minimal vasodilation (27). The degree of atony is somewhat surprising, because systemic venous blood reaching the pulmonary microcirculation is hypoxemic, i.e., it should elicit vasoconstriction unless there is a special adaptation of precapillary vessels to unremitting hypoxemia from birth.

In contrast to the lack of effect of acute hyperoxia on the normal pulmonary circulation, hypoxic pulmonary hypertension in experimental animals and human subjects usually responds to improved oxygenation. Pulmonary vasodilation is more marked after relief of acute than of chronic hypoxia (138, 175). Pulmonary hypertension, unassociated with arterial hypoxemia, rarely responds to acute hyperoxia.

Acute hypercapnia. Testing the effects of inhaled CO_2 with respect to the chemical control of the pulmonary circulation was part of the first experiments on the regulation of the pulmonary circulation (132). Since then this subject has been much less studied than the effects of acute hypoxia. As in the case of acute hypoxia, exposure to acute hypercapnia does not always elicit the same pulmonary vascular response (130). However, with conventional laboratory animals and conditions, the usual response is pulmonary vasoconstriction (along with bronchodilation). Moreover acute hypercapnia, e.g., breathing a 5% CO_2 mixture, almost invariably elicits a weaker response than does acute hypoxia, e.g., breathing a 10% O_2 mixture.

The magnitude of the pulmonary pressor response to acute hypercapnia depends not only on the experimental circumstance but also on the species and age. Thus acute hypercapnia elicits more marked pulmonary vasoconstriction in the fetus than in the adult (104). Even more impressive is its role as an enhancer of the pressor response to acute hypoxia (45, 130, 131). The constrictor effect is presumably by way of the formation of carbonic acid and the resultant decrease in the local concentration of H^+ (30, 45). Attempts to assess the role of β-adrenergic receptors in this response have been inconclusive (130). Whether the vascular site affected by acute hypercapnia is the same as that for acute hypoxia is also unsettled (43, 259).

Acute acidosis. Acute acidosis elicits pulmonary vasoconstriction. How the acidosis is produced appears to be irrelevant, because hypercapnia or mineral acids can produce the same pressor effect by equivalent changes in the concentration of H^+; neither the anions nor molecular CO_2 seem to count. Acidosis must be moderately severe (blood pH ~7.2) to be effective. Alkalemia generally causes pulmonary vasodilation (426).

Not only does the acid-base balance of the perfusate contribute to the tone of the pulmonary vessels but acidosis also acts, in some unknown way, to potentiate the hypoxic pressor response (29, 30, 202, 441). Indeed hypoxia and acidosis seem to interact, each facilitating the effect of the other (131, 301, 477); the effect of alkalosis in depressing the hypoxic pressor response has not been as consistent (441). This interplay may be of considerable importance in lung disease in which local acidosis in a region of alveolar hypoventilation can enhance the effect of local hypoxia in diverting blood flow to better-ventilated parts of the lungs (132, 202). The interaction between these two stimuli—hypoxia imposed on the pulmonary circulation predominantly via the alveoli and acidosis via the bloodstream—has important implications for the site at which this interaction is occurring (39).

In areas of alveolar hypoventilation the effects of local hypoxia and acidosis (due to formation of carbonic acid) are believed to operate synergistically to divert pulmonary capillary blood flow to the better-ventilated areas of the lungs (141). In hemorrhagic shock, metabolic acidosis contributes to the characteristic increase in pulmonary vascular resistance, but its effects are apt to be overshadowed by other complicated features of this condition, e.g., atelectasis, edema, heightened sympathetic tone, and intravascular coagulation (298).

BRONCHIAL CIRCULATION

Bronchial circulation (or pulmonary collateral circulation) refers to the systemic blood supply to the lungs (Fig. 30). Although usage has firmly entrenched the designation "bronchial," the term is inadequate on two accounts: *1*) the systemic blood supply to the lungs originates not only from bronchial arteries but

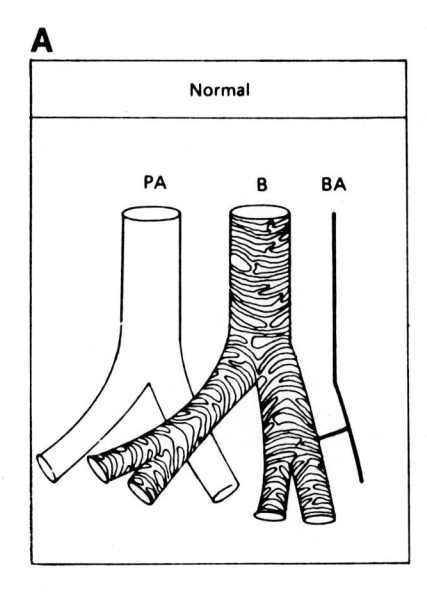

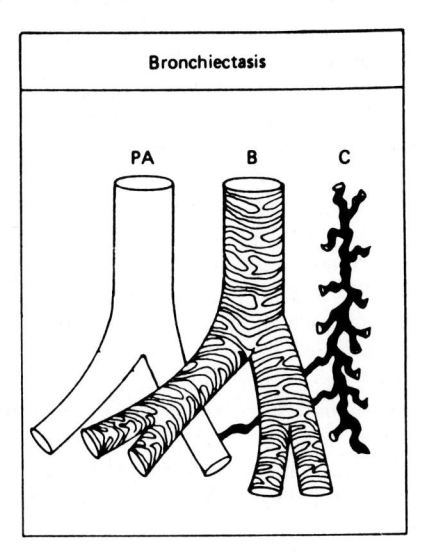

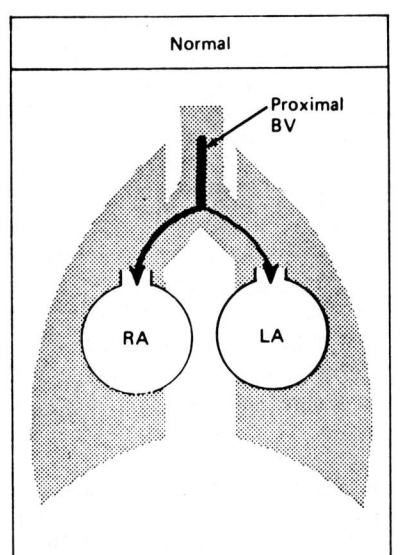

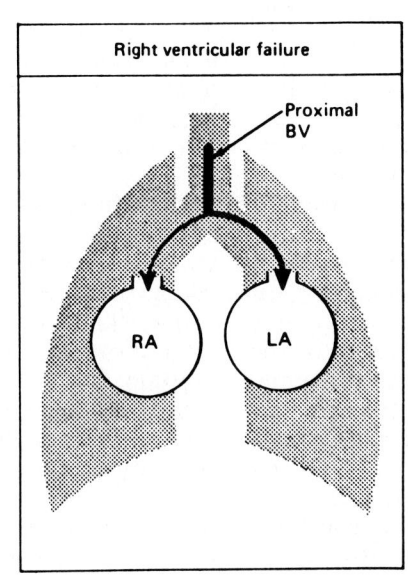

FIG. 30. *A*: schematic representations of bronchial circulation in different disorders. *Top*: bronchial arteries (BA). In chronic suppurative diseases of the lungs, bronchial arteries undergo considerable proliferation. *Bottom*: bronchial veins (BV). Proximal bronchial veins drain either into right atrium (RA) or left atrium (LA), depending on pressure levels in these 2 cardiac chambers. Normally most bronchial venous outflow from the lungs enters right atrium (*thicker curved arrow*). However, in right ventricular failure, bronchial venous drainage to left atrium increases. B, bronchus; C, expanded bronchial arterial circulation; PA, pulmonary artery. *B*: indicator-dilution curves from pulmonary artery and brachial artery (BA) in a normal individual (*left*) and in a patient with bronchiectasis (*right*). Curves from the patient are identical in appearance, time, and height, indicating that catheter tip in pulmonary artery (in vicinity of bronchiectatic area) had sampled systemic arterial blood. [*A* from Fishman (136), by permission of the American Heart Association, Inc. *B* from Cudkowicz (93).]

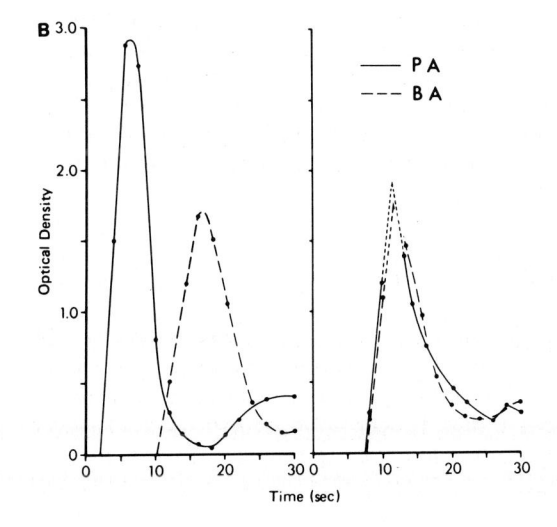

also from the aorta and other intrathoracic arteries, and *2)* the systemic arterial blood is delivered not only to the walls of the bronchi but also to the adventitia of large vessels and structures of the lungs (93, 99, 138).

The size, pattern of origin, and distribution of the systemic arteries to the lungs vary from species to species. In the dog, human, and pig, the arteries are small, arise from multiple sites, and reach the lungs as small twigs (74, 99); in the sheep, horse, and seal, a single, large vessel conveys most of the systemic arterial blood supply to the lungs [Fig. 30; (296)]. In birds, information about the bronchial circulation is incomplete and contradictory (3).

In the normal lung the bronchial circulation has the features of a nutrient circulation: it is modest in size, carries arterialized blood, and is distributed primarily to the airways, blood vessels, and supporting structures of the lungs. At the level of the respiratory bronchioles the bronchial arteries give rise to capillaries that communicate with pulmonary capillaries (136, 296).

Venous return from the bronchial circulation is via either bronchial or pulmonary veins. From the hilar structures and large bronchi, bronchial venous blood is returned to the right atrium via systemic veins. From more peripheral airways and the substance of the lung, bronchial venous blood is returned to the left atrium by two routes: via bronchial-pulmonary capillary anastamoses and via "bronchopulmonary veins" that connect bronchial capillaries to small pulmonary veins. The direction taken by bronchial venous outflow is determined by the relative pressures at the outlet of the two systems. For example, an increase in left atrial pressure detours bronchial venous drainage toward the right, rather than the left, atrium (291, 433). In some animals, functioning communications exist not only between the bronchial and pulmonary capillary circulations but also between the bronchial arteries and other systemic arteries (296).

Certain features of the bronchial circulation merit special attention. *1)* Although difficult to demonstrate and of doubtful functional significance, microscopic anastomoses between bronchial and pulmonary arteries do appear to exist at the precapillary level in the normal lung (433). *2)* The bronchial arteries proliferate remarkably in certain lung, liver, and congenital heart diseases, which are often associated with clubbing of the digits (136). *3)* The mechanisms responsible for the proliferation of the bronchial circulation are unclear, but certain influences (e.g., cortisone) retard its expansion, whereas growth hormone stimulates it (280). *4)* Pharmacologic agents, injected via the bronchial arteries as well as via the pulmonary arteries, reach end organs within the lungs (16). *5)* Cardiothoracic surgery stimulates proliferation of the bronchial circulation (439). *6)* The bronchial veins are organized in the submucosa of the airways into a large plexus that runs the entire length of the tracheobronchial tree (383). *7)* Bronchial venules respond like the systemic venules to certain vasoactive agents, notably histamine and bradykinin (383). *8)* The bronchial venous circulation is involved in the pathogenesis of experimental pulmonary edema produced in the dog and sheep by histamine, endotoxin, and bradykinin (383).

Determination of Bronchial Blood Flow

Because the bronchial arteries of most conventional laboratory animals are small and difficult to handle, elaborate experimental preparations have been adopted over the years for measuring bronchial blood flow and for determining its responses to vasoactive agents and manipulations (20, 136, 303, 433). In the intact human and dog, however, the traditional approaches have been the indicator-dilution principle and some modification of the Fick principle (138). These are intended to measure total bronchial blood flow. In recent years radioactive microsphere techniques have been tried in experimental animals. These techniques offer the prospect not only of quantifying total bronchial blood flow but also of partitioning it with respect to airways and parenchyma (337). One haunting problem in this approach is the prospect of recirculation if the tracer is injected into the left atrium, a step that is usually required to ensure proper mixing of the tracer, especially in species with minute bronchial arteries.

Because bronchial blood flow in the normal lung is so small, it is difficult to measure by techniques that depend on indicator-dilution or Fick principles. This task becomes easier when the bronchial circulation increases, as after ligation of a major pulmonary artery (136). The one caveat to this generalization is that the airways and lungs be free of widespread disease, such as chronic obstructive airways disease, which may complicate the application of the indicator-dilution or Fick principles because of early recirculation (291).

It was noted above that in some species a single large bronchial artery is responsible for carrying the bulk of the systemic arterial blood supply to the lungs (308). This fortunate anatomical arrangement has recently been exploited in the sheep, in which one large bronchial artery (the carinal artery) supplies 88% of the lungs (all but the fraction served by the bronchi to the right apical lobe). By placing an electromagnetic flow probe around this artery at thoracotomy, resting bronchial blood flow has been measured directly and the responses of the bronchial circulation to various manipulations (e.g., reactive hyperemia, airway pressures, vasoactive agents) have been tested (296). In the open-chest sheep, carinal artery flow averaged 0.46 ml·min^{-1}·kg^{-1} body wt. Clearly the availability of this large vessel affords the prospect not only for acute manipulations in the open-chest animal but also for chronic implantation of flow probes for observations under more natural conditions.

Normal Levels of Bronchial Blood Flow

Although different values for bronchial blood flow have been found in different species and preparations (296), the consensus is that in the normal human and dog lung, bronchial blood flow constitutes 1%–2% of the cardiac output (153, 296). Some of the recorded discrepancies are the result of the procedures and manipulations. In the thoracotomized sheep the level of bronchial arterial flow varies with the cardiac output (296). In other experimental preparations, other influences, particularly the systemic arterial blood pressure, the airway pressures, and the occurrence of arterial hypoxemia, play primary roles in setting the level of bronchial blood flow (296).

Bronchial Circulation in the Normal Lung

As indicated above, the bronchial circulation has as its major functions the circulation of nutrients for the conducting airways and blood vessels and the support of the framework of the lungs proximal to the sites of gas exchange. Beyond the respiratory bronchioles the pulmonary circulation becomes the nutrient circulation for the supporting structures of the lungs (93, 291). The conditioning of the temperature and water content of the inspired air is another presumed function of the bronchial circulation (111, 314, 384).

Bronchial Circulation in Disease

In the normal lung the bronchial circulation operates covertly, as long as the pulmonary circulation is intact. However, should the pulmonary circulation to an area be compromised or lost—as by ligation or an embolus—viability and function of the affected area depend on the integrity and adequacy of the bronchial blood supply (136, 282). The full potential of the bronchial circulation for expanding and assuming the function of a collateral circulation is strikingly disclosed after occlusion of a main pulmonary artery has persisted for years. The stimulus for this proliferation is unclear.

Expansion of the bronchial circulation occurs clinically in two major categories of disease: those involving *1*) severe curtailment of pulmonary blood flow, as in congenital pulmonary atresia (136), and *2*) a chronic inflammatory bronchopulmonary process, such as bronchiectasis or chronic lung abscess (199). Because clubbing of the digits (occasionally accompanied by hypertrophic osteoarthropathy) is also common in these disorders, the relationship between clubbing of the digits and expansion of the collateral circulation to the lungs is often questioned (94).

Another clinically important aspect of the expanded bronchial circulation is bronchial arterial bleeding as the source of hemoptysis in chronic lung disease, a condition that was portrayed by Leonardo da Vinci. The usual disorders associated with this type of hemoptysis are bronchiectasis, lung abscess, old inflammatory cavities, and lung cancer (403). In contrast, in chronic mitral stenosis, hemoptysis usually originates from bronchial veins underlying the tracheal mucosa. At one time, failure of the nutrient circulation to the lungs was considered to be a likely mechanism for certain types of emphysema (461). However, this concept now has few advocates.

Because primary carcinoma of the lungs often receives much of its blood supply from systemic arteries, particularly if the neoplasm obstructs blood flow to the pulmonary artery (93), attempts have been made to deliver chemotherapeutic agents to the cancerous site via a bronchial artery. This approach has proved ineffective. Also, in some patients in whom life-threatening hemoptysis complicates a carcinoma of the lungs, particulate matter has been injected as bronchial arterial emboli in the hope of occluding the feeder bronchial artery. Unfortunately the effect of selective embolization is transient (403).

A different consequence of the expanded collateral circulation, as in bronchiectasis, is its potential role as a hemodynamic burden (136), but rarely does the large left-to-right shunt constituted by the expanded circulation cause cardiac embarrassment even though the shunt may become quite large (136, 291). Note also that when the collateral circulation is enlarged in the vicinity of a wedged pulmonary arterial catheter, the pulmonary wedge pressure is apt to be misleading if the catheter tip is lodged in the vicinity of bronchial-pulmonary arterial anastomoses (138).

As noted above, bronchial venous blood that drains into the left atrium contributes to the anatomical venous admixture. Another source of the anatomical venous admixture occurs in some patients with cirrhosis of the liver in whom abnormal anatomical connections allow the passage of portal venous blood into the pulmonary venous system. In an occasional patient with hepatic cirrhosis, the portal-pulmonary blood flow becomes quite large, i.e., ~5%–15% of the cardiac output (84, 346). Occasionally these anastomatic channels enlarge sufficiently to be demonstrable during life with indicators or angiography (324). More often the quantity of blood shunted from the portal to pulmonary venous system is too small to be measured reliably.

FETAL AND NEONATAL PULMONARY CIRCULATION

Before birth the lungs play no role in gas exchange; this function is carried on by the placenta. Instead the lungs serve as a metabolic organ, and for this purpose they are provided with a modest blood flow: most of the blood returning to the right side of the heart is diverted toward the systemic circulation by way of the foramen ovale and ductus arteriosus (Fig. 31). As a result of this diversion the lungs before birth receive ~10%–15% of the right ventricular output (423). After birth, as the lungs assume gas-exchanging functions and the fetal connections close, the entire output of the right ventricle perfuses the lungs.

Considerable ingenuity and manipulation are required to gain access to the remote fetal pulmonary circulation. In the 1950s and 1960s pulmonary hemodynamic measurements were confined to exceedingly artificial and stressful conditions (103, 104). Because the fetal pulmonary circulation is highly reactive, the experimental circumstances and the interventions strongly influenced hemodynamic behavior, generally by provoking inordinate sympathetic nervous activity. Oppositely, prolonged surgery under deep anesthesia often depressed the cardiopulmonary apparatus. However, in recent years increasing reliance on chronically implanted recording and sampling devices in fetal animals, particularly the lamb, has provided opportunities for observing the fetal pulmonary circulation under more natural conditions (277).

In the fetal lamb approaching term, pulmonary arterial and aortic pressure levels are virtually identical; during gestation, blood pressures in both circuits increase in parallel, from a mean of 30 mmHg in the 60-day lamb to 50 mmHg at term, i.e., ~140 days [Fig. 32; (422)]. During the same period, pulmonary blood

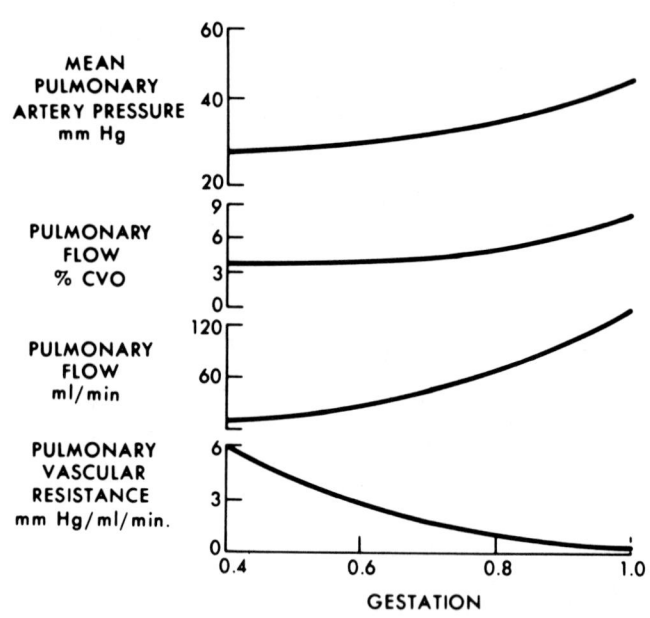

FIG. 32. Schematic representation of changes in mean pulmonary arterial pressure, proportion of combined ventricular output (CVO) distributed to the lungs, actual pulmonary blood flow, and calculated pulmonary vascular resistance in fetal lambs during gestational development from 0.4 to 1.0 gestation. Progressive decrease in resistance is attributable to an increase in cross-sectional area of pulmonary vascular bed, in large measure due to growth of new vessels. [From Rudolph (423). Reproduced, with permission, from the Annual Review of Physiology, vol. 41, © 1979 by Annual Reviews, Inc.]

flow increases dramatically, i.e., ~40-fold (422). At the same time, pulmonary vascular resistance decreases from 6 mmHg·ml^{-1}·min^{-1} to 0.3 mmHg·ml^{-1}·min^{-1} at term. The principal mechanism responsible for this dramatic decrease in resistance is an increase in the number of minute vessels as gestation proceeds; mechanical increase in vascular calibers associated with breathing and a decrease in vasomotor tone exert appreciable but much smaller influences (423).

The patterns of blood flow have been examined in the pulmonary trunk and in pulmonary arterial branches: in the pulmonary trunk the velocity profile before birth is about the same as after birth; distally in a branch pulmonary artery the pattern before birth is different, not only with respect to contour during early systole but also because of backflow in late systole. These different patterns (Fig. 33) can be explained by the relative resistances of the pulmonary and systemic circulation and the magnitude of blood flow through the ductus arteriosus (277). As may be seen in Figure 33, flow in the pulmonary trunk, which receives the entire right ventricular output, is forward continuously throughout systole, whereas in the main pulmonary artery, flow is forward only early in systole, followed by a pronounced reversal of flow in late systole. In accord with this explanation, patterns of pulmonary blood flow can be greatly modified by interventions that either affect the caliber of the ductus arteriosus or the balance of resistances in the pulmonary and systemic circulations.

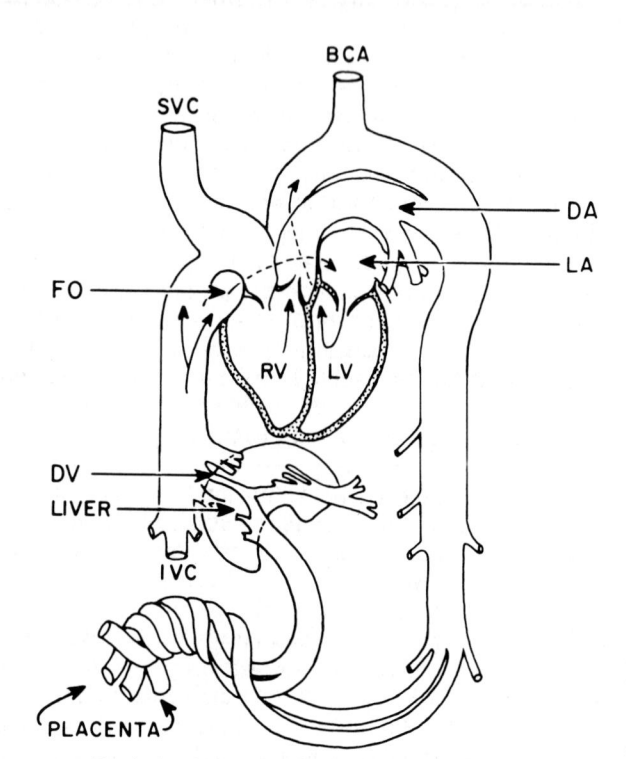

FIG. 31. Fetal circulation in the lamb. BCA, brachiocephalic artery; DA, ductus arteriosus; DV, ductus venosus; FO, foramen ovale; IVC, inferior vena cava; LA, left atrium; LV, left ventricle; RV, right ventricle; SVC, superior vena cava. [From Dawes (103).]

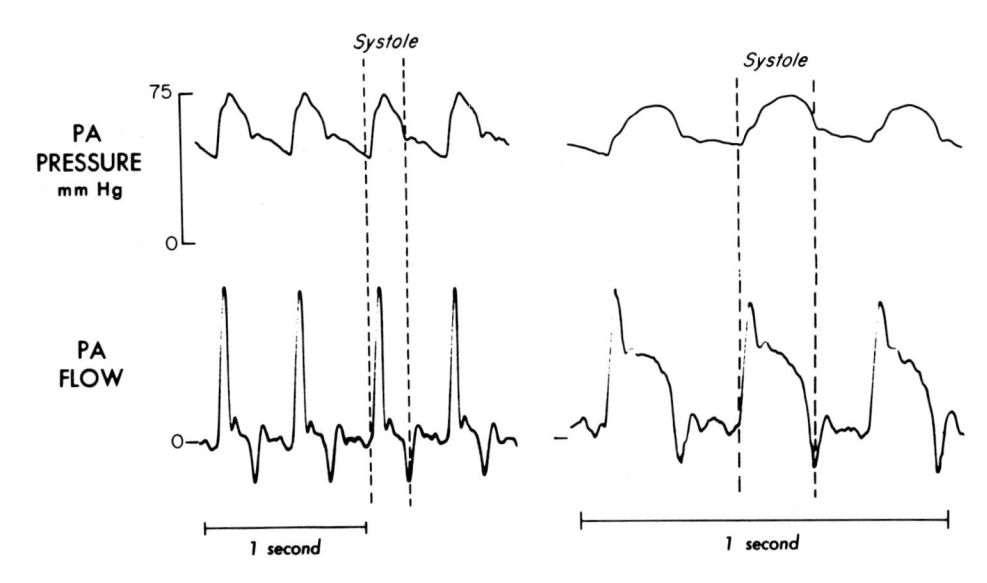

FIG. 33. Changes in patterns of pulmonary arterial (PA) pressure and flow after birth. *Left*: in the fetus. *Right*: after birth. [From Rudolph (423). Reproduced, with permission, from the Annual Review of Physiology, vol. 41, © 1979 by Annual Reviews, Inc.]

Morphologic Changes

In the lung of the lamb near term, the small muscular arteries, which constitute the resistance vessels, are well endowed with smooth muscle. Until ~80 days of gestation (term ~140 days) the small muscular arteries undergo medial hypertrophy, particularly in the 5th and 6th generations (274). Various interventions before birth can augment the thickness of this vascular smooth muscle: maternal hypoxia (174), systemic and/or pulmonary arterial hypertension in the fetus (273), and maternal ingestion of prostaglandin synthetase inhibitors (causing constriction of the ductus arteriosus, pulmonary vasoconstriction, or both) (220).

The media of the small muscular arteries regresses rapidly after birth (102). However, prolonging hypoxia, as by exposing the newborn to a continued decrease in inspired P_{O_2} for 2 wk, not only retards the normal involution of pulmonary vascular smooth muscle but also leads to the development of new muscle in peripheral precapillary vessels that would otherwise be expected to be devoid of muscle (222).

Regulation of Fetal Pulmonary Circulation

Compared to the adult pulmonary circulation, the fetal circulation affords much more vascular resistance, a higher initial tone, and (as has been noted above) a greater vascular reactivity; this reactivity increases with gestational age (277). Thus an infusion of bradykinin (77) or acetylcholine (105)—which is virtually without effect in the adult pulmonary circulation—evokes in the fetus (and newborn) a prompt and dramatic drop in pulmonary arterial pressure and an impressive increase in pulmonary blood flow (77). The response to acetylcholine also increases as the fetus grows older. Finally, the characteristic reactive hyperemia, a hallmark of the autonomic control of the adult systemic circulation, is also vigorous and easily demonstrable in the fetus at term, even though it cannot be elicited in the adult pulmonary circulation (296). In the fetus as in the adult, initial vasomotor tone is important in determining the vigor of the vasomotor response to pharmacologic agents; as in the adult, initial tone determines not only the magnitude but also the direction of the fetal pulmonary vascular response to acetylcholine (424).

Fetal hypoxia, induced in a variety of ways, consistently elicits pulmonary vasoconstriction (75–77). The increase in resistance is considerable and the increment in pressure is large, often associated with a decrease in pulmonary blood flow. The pulmonary pressor response of the fetus to maternal hypoxia increases curvilinearly with the decrease in fetal Pa_{O_2}; the magnitude of the response increases as gestation advances, consistent with the idea that pulmonary vascular smooth muscle grows increasingly responsive to hypoxia as gestation advances (277).

In the adult, neither vagotomy nor thoracic sympathectomy affects the pressor response to acute hypoxia (138). Nor is the response impaired by α- or β-adrenergic or parasympathetic blockade in the newborn lamb (277) or calf (440). On the other hand, after the elaborate interventions inherent in cross-perfusing fetal lambs, the sympathetic nervous system contributes importantly to the pressor response to acute hypoxia, the extent varying with the gestational age (75, 76).

In the fetus, electrical stimulation of the cut end of the vagus or of the thoracic sympathetic chain (87) evokes a dramatic change in pulmonary vasomotor tone, i.e., vasodilation or vasoconstriction, respectively. The fetal pulmonary circulation also responds briskly to cholinergic stimulation by acetylcholine (105), to stimulation of α-receptors by methoxamine and norepinephrine (31, 79, 80), and to stimulation of β-receptors (79, 80). These results were obtained after considerable experimental manipulation. In contrast the fetal circulation studied under more natural conditions is unaffected by the administration of propranolol (a β-adrenergic blocking agent) or phentolamine (an α-adrenergic blocking agent) (277). The injection of atropine or bilateral cervical vagotomy does not appreciably modify pulmonary vascular tone in the fetus (87). These observations illustrate that sympathetic activity plays an important role in setting initial vasomotor tone in the fetal pulmonary circulation and that in the undisturbed fetus, initial vasomotor tone is low.

As in the adult, acidosis elicits pulmonary vasoconstriction and greatly enhances the pulmonary pressor response to acute hypoxia (426); the more severe the acidosis, the greater the pressor and enhancing effects.

Postnatal Pulmonary Vasodilation

Ventilation of the lungs with air causes a marked drop in pulmonary vascular resistance. Two factors are involved: predominant is the increase in P_{O_2}; a much lesser role is played by physical expansion of the lungs (104, 425). Attempts to uncover the mechanism by which relief of hypoxia exerts its vasodilator effect in the fetus have been drawn to the possibility that a local mediator may be involved, bradykinin in particular because of its powerful vasodilator effect in the fetus (221). However, although the kinins may play some role in the immediate vasodilation after birth, their effects seem to be too fleeting to account for the persistent lowering of pulmonary vascular resistance once the fetus is born.

The prostaglandins are more viable candidates (85). This prospect stems from two observations: 1) distension of the lungs of adult animals results in the release of prostaglandins, particularly those of the E series, and 2) indomethacin blunts the continued drop in pulmonary vascular resistance that otherwise would be expected to occur during the 10–20 min after the initial fall (271). In contrast, the renin-angiotensin system, which develops early in gestation, does not appear to be involved in either the high initial pulmonary vasomotor tone of the fetus or the vasoconstrictor response to hypoxia (423). Moreover, in the fetus, prostaglandin synthetase inhibitors enhance the pulmonary pressor response to acute hypoxia (490). In essence, in the fetus, as in the adult, it is still *sub judice* whether O_2 exerts its vasodilator effect by a direct effect on pulmonary vascular smooth muscle, or by the release of a mediator, or both.

Attention has been called repeatedly in this section to the marked reactivity of the fetal pulmonary circulation. The purposes served by the marked pulmonary vasoreactivity are not certain, but an increase in fetal pulmonary vascular tone causes redistribution of the pulmonary blood flow (only 8%–10% of the output of both ventricles late in gestation), favoring blood flow to vital organs (brain, myocardium, and placenta). Conversely, pulmonary vasodilation could be importantly involved in the circulatory rearrangements after birth.

PULMONARY HYPERTENSION

Pathogenesis

The designation "pulmonary hypertension" (pulmonary arterial hypertension) depends on the altitude: at sea level, where mean pressures in the pulmonary artery rarely exceed 15–18 mmHg, pulmonary hypertension is generally said to exist at mean pressures of 25–30 mmHg; at high altitude, where normal pulmonary arterial pressures are higher than at sea level, an increase in mean pressure of 10–15 mmHg above normal is generally accepted as evidence of pulmonary hypertension (185).

It is not easy to raise the pulmonary arterial pressure experimentally by more than a few millimeters of mercury. Removal of an entire lung generally elicits an increment in pulmonary arterial pressure of ~5 mmHg if the remaining lung is normal (Fig. 34). Indeed to achieve pulmonary hypertension by amputating portions of the pulmonary vascular tree requires the ablation of at least one entire lung plus a lobe of the remaining lung. Another remarkable aspect of this low-resistance, capacious, and highly expansile circulation is that embolization of the lung is rarely successful in causing sustained pulmonary hypertension unless the process is repeated often enough to accomplish an enduring obliteration of extensive areas of the pulmonary arterial tree.

Table 3 lists the six categories of mechanisms that may cause (or contribute to the pathogenesis of) pulmonary hypertension. Distinction is made between the first two (primary) that set the stage for an increase in pulmonary arterial pressure and the contributory mechanisms that aggravate the process (142).

Note that external influences rarely cause pulmonary hypertension unless accompanied by alveolar hypoxia, i.e., by alveolar hypoventilation. In contrast is the preeminent role played by anatomical restriction in one form or another, i.e., extensive parenchymal disease that somehow affects the resistance and distensibility of the pulmonary arterial tree or obliterative pulmonary vascular disease where vascular lumens are encroached on from within; often the anatomical changes are associated with pulmonary vasoconstriction. Hypoxia, often abetted in clinical situations by acidosis, has proved to be the most effective stimulus of vasoconstriction. Although the collateral (bronchial) circulation to the lungs may undergo considerable expansion in certain lung diseases, rarely is the increase sufficient to contribute appreciably to the pathogenesis of pulmonary hypertension.

Experimental Chronic Pulmonary Hypertension

Experimental pulmonary hypertension has been produced in a variety of different ways (216). Each is important, because it is difficult to raise pressures in the pulmonary circulation to hypertensive levels and

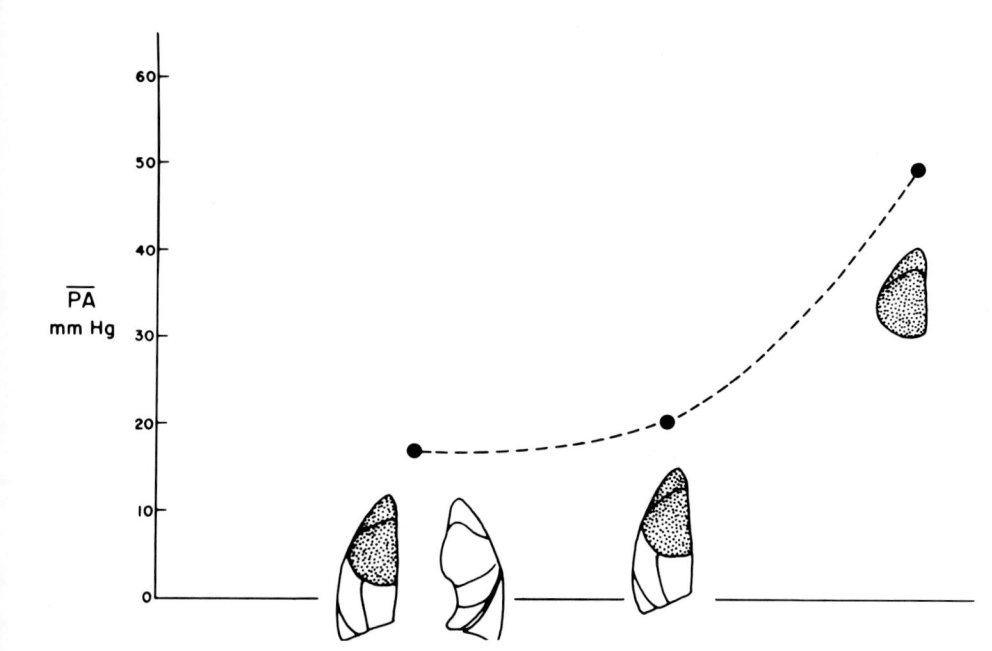

FIG. 34. Schematic representation of effects of progressive restriction of pulmonary vascular bed by successive amputation of lobes of the lungs on mean pulmonary arterial (PA) pressure (assuming that pulmonary blood flow remains unchanged). Pneumonectomy (*middle*) evokes only a modest increase in pulmonary arterial pressure (to 22 mmHg). Subsequent removal of right lower and middle lobes leads to considerable pulmonary arterial hypertension (to 55 mmHg). [Data from Lategola (267).]

TABLE 3. *Potential Pathogenic Mechanisms Leading to Pulmonary Arterial Hypertension and Cor Pulmonale*

Mechanism	Example
Primary	
Anatomical decrease in cross-sectional area distensibility of pulmonary resistance vessels	Interstitial fibrosis and granuloma
Vasoconstriction of pulmonary resistance vessels	Hypoxia and acidosis
Contributory	
Large increments in pulmonary blood flow	Exercise
Increased pressures of left heart and pulmonary veins	Left ventricular failure or pulmonary venous-occlusive disease
Increased viscosity of blood	Secondary polycythemia of chronic hypoxia
Unproved	
Compression of pulmonary resistance vessels by raised alveolar pressures in their vicinity	Asthmatic bronchitis
Bronchial arterial–pulmonary arterial anatomoses	Expanded bronchial circulation

to sustain these levels. Four of the currently popular experimental models have broad implications for understanding the behavior of the pulmonary circulation: the hypoxic, dietary, sepsis, and blood component models.

HYPOXIC MODEL. This model takes advantage of the fact that hypoxia—acute and chronic—is the most direct, effective, and reproducible way to elicit pulmonary hypertension. Indeed a natural reservoir of this type of pulmonary hypertension exists in native dwellers at high altitude. Pulmonary hypertension at tolerable altitudes (up to ~4,570 m) is generally modest in degree, but the development of alveolar hypoventilation in this population elicits striking increments in the level of pulmonary arterial pressure.

DIETARY MODEL. Interest in a laboratory model of dietary pulmonary hypertension was sparked in two ways: *1*) experimental pulmonary hypertension produced by ingestion of the seed of a leguminous plant, *Crotalaria spectabilis*, and *2*) the spontaneous outbreak of pulmonary hypertension in normal individuals that occurred in Switzerland, Austria, and Germany between 1966 and 1968, almost exclusively in those who had ingested Aminorex (5-amino-5-phenylooxazoline), an appetite depressant (140).

Crotalaria spectabilis. This is an annual shrub indigenous to the tropics and subtropics (140, 251, 489). *Crotalaria* is poisonous to humans and animals because of the pyrrolizidine alkaloids that it contains. The major offending pyrrolizidine alkaloid in *Crotalaria spectabilis* is monocrotaline. Other species of the shrub, such as *Crotalaria fulva*, contain their own distinctive alkaloids, e.g., fulvine. Ingestion of *Crotalaria* by domestic animals (and humans) leads to incapacitating damage of the liver, lungs, and central nervous system (83). In the West Indies, where poisoning by *Crotalaria spectabilis* is endemic in the native population, hepatotoxicity predominates. However, in the rat (70, 251, 489) and the nonhuman primate (*Macaca*) (83) the sequelae of pulmonary arterial hypertension, i.e., right heart failure and death, are characteristic features.

The pyrrolizidine alkaloid, monocrotaline, does not act directly on the pulmonary circulation of the rat (251). Instead, monocrotaline is converted by the liver to dehydromonocrotaline (72, 307), as a prerequisite for pulmonary vascular toxicity. At autopsy the pulmonary vascular lesions resemble those produced by severe, long-standing mitral stenosis in the human: medial hypertrophy, necrotizing arteriolitis, and proliferation of mast cells. Moreover the lesions appear to be morphologically distinct from those of primary pulmonary hypertension, because neither intimal fibrosis nor plexiform lesions are regular features (326, 507, 510).

These experiments have demonstrated that substances taken by mouth can cause obliterative vascular lesions in the pulmonary circulation. Attempts have failed to implicate intrinsic lung damage or release of vasoactive substances from the pulmonary mast cells in the pathogenesis of the pulmonary hypertension. More likely is the prospect that interplay between damaged pulmonary capillary endothelium and platelet aggregation may be pathogenetically involved (72).

Aminorex. Another type of pulmonary hypertension that may have involved the gut-liver-lung axis (Fig. 35) occurred in Europeans between 1966 and 1968 (186). In Switzerland, Austria, and Germany the incidence of unexplained pulmonary hypertension suddenly increased 20-fold. In contrast to the pulmonary vascular lesions produced by pyrrolizidine alkaloids in the rat, the pathology in humans was typical of primary pulmonary hypertension, including plexiform lesions and intimal fibrosis; the liver was spared. By coincidence or as a consequence the epidemic followed the introduction in November 1965 of the appetite depressant Aminorex, which resembles epinephrine and amphetamine in chemical structure; both of these agents release endogenous stores of catecholamines. As yet, however, the clinical entity of "catecholamine pulmonary hypertension" does not exist; nor could amphetamine or epinephrine be implicated in the outbreak. The epidemic subsided in 1968 when Aminorex could no longer be bought over the counter.

Note that relatively few of those who ingested Aminorex developed pulmonary hypertension. To explain the peculiar pulmonary pressor effect of Aminorex in some individuals, some type of predisposition, possibly genetic, had to be assumed as prerequisite for the development of obliterative pulmonary vascular lesions. In this regard, Aminorex pulmonary hypertension—if it is a true entity—resembles the inordinate pulmonary hypertension of some breeds of cattle at high altitude (182).

Attempts to reproduce pulmonary hypertension by administering Aminorex to animals have been uniformly unsuccessful. Not only did large oral doses to rats (for up to 43 wk) and to dogs (20 wk) fail to elicit the vascular lesions of pulmonary hypertrophy (253) but also prior hypersensitization by chronic exposure to the hypoxia of high altitude proved to be of no avail (73). Quite different clinically, but possibly related pathogenetically, is the pulmonary venous occlusion that sometimes occurs after medicinal use of "bush tea" prepared from *Crotalaria retusa* (58).

Gut-liver-lung axis. The experience with *Crotalaria*

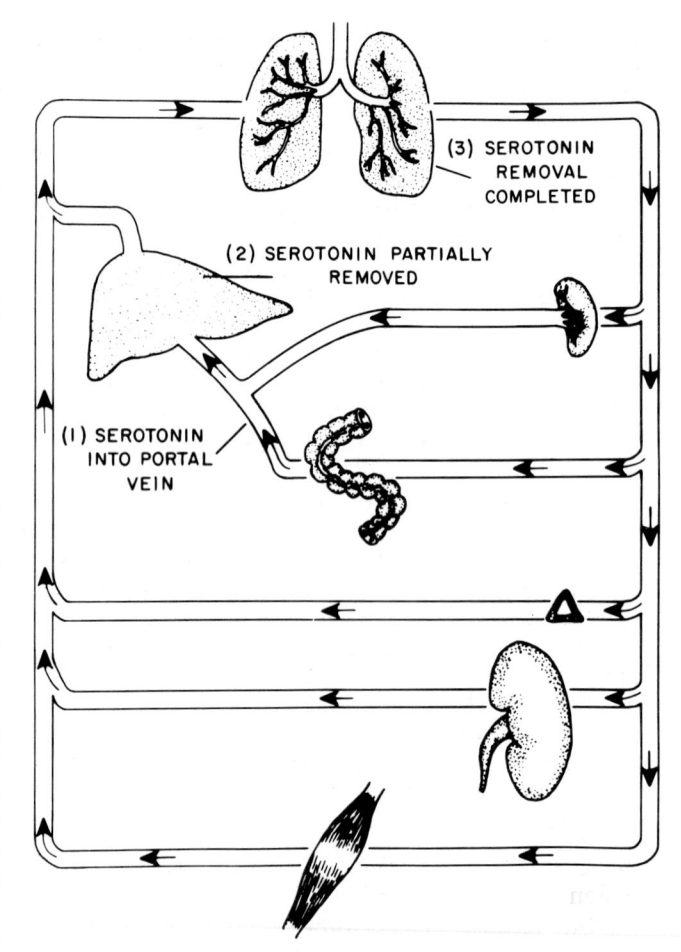

FIG. 35. Gut-liver-lung axis. Serotonin, brought to the liver via the portal vein, is partially removed by the liver. Removal is completed in the lungs.

suggests that metabolites of ingested foods may induce pulmonary hypertension if they gain access to the pulmonary circulation or block a metabolic pathway that ordinarily exerts a pulmonary antihypertensive effect. Alternatively, by damaging the liver, vasoactive substances such as histamine, serotonin, and catecholamines might escape metabolic pathways to reach and injure the pulmonary vessels. Indeed nucleotides that gain access to the pulmonary circulation have been shown to increase pulmonary arterial blood pressure by producing extensive pulmonary vascular obstruction (398). Thus it is possible to imagine a wide variety of gut-liver-pulmonary interplays that might evoke pulmonary hypertension. Nonetheless it must be kept in mind that no product of digestion has yet been identified that is able to elicit pulmonary hypertension. The one intestinal hormone that has been identified has potent vasodilator properties (428). Also patients with hepatic cirrhosis seem to blunt their pulmonary pressor response to hypoxia (101). Finally, if entry of intestinal hormones and the products of digestion into the pulmonary circulation were as damaging as the foregoing considerations imply, portacaval shunts would be an inevitable disaster. However, they are not.

If it is assumed that dietary pulmonary hypertension is a distinct entity, the nature of the initiating lesion merits consideration. One possible common denominator is endothelial damage, which increases capillary permeability in the lungs and is followed by the sequelae and consequences of injury: platelet aggregation, local release of vasoactive substances, endothelial dehiscence, naked basement membranes, and obstruction of the minute pulmonary vessels (494).

Because of the outpouring of new drugs, nostrums, and natural foods, dietary pulmonary hypertension is apt to be a consequence of more agents than monocrotaline, fulvine, Aminorex, and phenformin. Inevitably attempts will be made to link primary pulmonary hypertension to ingested materials, and many questions await solution. Why does vulnerability vary from individual to individual and from species to species? Is genetic failure of a single hepatic enzyme sufficient for some forms of dietary pulmonary hypertension? What are the respective roles of the liver and the pulmonary capillary endothelium in coping with vasoactive substances that enter by way of the gut? Is pulmonary vasoconstriction, mechanical obstruction by platelet aggregates, or a combination of the two the initiating event?

SEPSIS MODEL. Transient pulmonary arterial hypertension, succeeded in 2–3 h by a phase of increased alveolar-capillary permeability, has been produced acutely in several different species by the intravenous infusion of endotoxin derived from *E. coli* (194, 201, 367). This is a complicated model involving an interplay among blood constituents, O_2 radicals, and the vessel wall. Among the potential players in this reaction are leukocytes, platelets, complement, reactive O_2 radicals, proteolytic enzymes, histamine, kinins, serotonin, endorphins, and arachidonic acid metabolites (194). The initial pulmonary vasoconstriction is greatly reduced or prevented by the administration of cyclooxygenase inhibitors (e.g., indomethacin) before the infusion of endotoxin (367), suggesting that cyclooxygenate products of arachidonate metabolism (eicosanoids) are involved in the pulmonary vasoconstriction; thromboxane A_2 has been identified as the primary vasoconstrictor in mediating this pressor response (233); as indicated in a prior section, the leukotrienes are involved in the subsequent phase of increased permeability.

BLOOD COMPONENT MODEL. Interactions between blood constituents and endothelium have proved to be able to elicit pulmonary hypertension (214). For example, infusion into sheep of plasma containing zymosan-activated complement produces leukopenia and leukostasis in pulmonary circulation; thromboxane A_2 has been implicated in this response: leukocytes, on exposure to activated complement, damage pulmonary vascular endothelial cells and stimulate the synthesis of thromboxane A_2, which evokes pulmonary vasoconstriction (313).

Another mechanism for generating pulmonary hypertension is via the leukotrienes, products (along with thromboxanes and prostaglandins) of arachidonic acid metabolism. The leukotrienes were first discovered in leukocytes (434). These substances, notably leukotriene C_4, have proved to be able to cause edema followed by pulmonary vasoconstriction. However, much remains to be learned about their release and mechanisms of action, because they are constituents of a general biological control system that begins with arachidonic acid and entails not only alternate pathways (prostaglandins, thromboxanes, and leukotrienes) but also the prospect of complicated interplay among the various products.

OTHER MODELS. Among the various models (216), two others may have particular clinical relevance: *1)* systemic arterial—pulmonary lobar arterial anastomoses to produce a severe and accelerated pulmonary hypertension (432) and *2)* multiple pulmonary emboli to curtail the pulmonary vascular bed (267) while creating a facsimile of the human disorder (436).

Pulmonary Vasodilators

The therapeutic need for relieving pulmonary hypertension has recently given great impetus to the search for pulmonary vasodilators. A national registry has been set up in the attempt to standardize the use of vasodilator agents and collate the results.

Trials of vasodilator therapy and pulmonary hypertension traditionally begin with the administration of enriched O_2 mixtures. The rationale for this approach is the demonstrated ability of improved oxygenation to relieve the pulmonary pressor response elicited by hypoxia. However, unless systemic hypoxemia is present the use of enriched O_2 mixtures for pulmonary vasodilation is generally disappointing (146).

Acetylcholine, bradykinin, and PGI_2 administered intravenously have been used to achieve maximal vasodilation in a single circulation. The use of acetylcholine is encumbered by the need to prepare the solution immediately before injection; supplies of PGI_2 are still too limited for widespread use. Both appear to be powerful vasodilators that exert their effects by different mechanisms (497). No comparison of the pulmonary vascular responses to these two potent vasodilators is available. One reason for this omission is that vasodilation by these agents is exceedingly difficult to demonstrate in the normotensive pulmonary circulation where initial tone is low. Because of their ephemeral effects, these agents are more valuable diagnostically than therapeutically. The vasoactive intestinal polypeptide exerts a vasodilator effect on isolated pulmonary arterial strips. This effect is unrelated to cholinergic and adrenergic receptors. The practical use of this agent as a pulmonary vasodilator remains to be explored (196).

All pulmonary vasodilators also cause systemic vasodilation if allowed to enter the systemic circulation. Because of their ability to act within a single pulmonary circulation, the effects of acetylcholine, PGI_2, and bradykinin are more easily attributed to direct effects on the pulmonary circulation than are those of other agents that are infused for longer periods and can elicit systemic vasodilation that is covert because of the systemic baroregulatory apparatus.

The other agents that have been tried can be sorted into four categories: 1) directly acting drugs, 2) drugs that act on adrenergic receptors, 3) drugs that block Ca^{2+} transport, and 4) agents that influence components of the renin-angiotensin system (394). Interpretation of the clinical use of these agents is often complicated by heavy reliance on the use of calculated pulmonary vascular resistance in situations where pulmonary vascular pressure, volume, and flow are changing simultaneously.

Paramount among the directly acting drugs are nitroprusside, hydralazine, and diazoxide. Their effects have been inconsistent from patient to patient and often attended by untoward reactions attributable to the extrapulmonary circulatory actions of these agents. For example, hydralazine elicits an increase in cardiac output and tachycardia as well as a direct vasodilator effect on pulmonary vascular smooth muscle. On the other hand, diazoxide promotes salt and water retention, often to a marked degree. All of these agents entail the risk of evoking systemic hypotension.

Of the drugs in the second category that act on adrenergic receptors, isoproterenol and phentolamine are the most popular. Isoproterenol is a powerful sympathomimetic amine that acts on β-receptors everywhere, leaving α-receptors virtually unaffected. Its use as a pulmonary vasodilator is accompanied by chronotropic and inotropic effects on the heart, coupled with peripheral vasodilation. Phentolamine dilates pulmonary vascular smooth muscle directly, by interfering slightly with sympathetic nervous activity and by antagonizing circulating catecholamines.

The drugs that block Ca^{2+} transport include verapamil, nifedipine, and, more recently, diltiazem. They illustrate Ca^{2+} blockers in general, which constitute an exceedingly heterogeneous group of agents that differ considerably in structure, pharmacologic activity, and electrophysiological effects (345).

The fourth group consists of agents that block the effects of angiotensin II (saralasin acetate) or inhibit the converting enzyme for angiotensin (and bradykinin). Their efficacy as pulmonary vasodilators is open to serious question (272).

Endothelium-Dependent Pulmonary Vasodilation

A fresh look at the mechanisms involved in pulmonary vasodilation has been prompted by the demonstration that in the isolated aortic preparation, vasodilation in response to cholinergic agents requires the presence of an intact endothelial layer [Fig. 36; (113, 158)]. Subsequently the same requirement was found to apply to the pulmonary (and systemic) vasodilator response to acetylcholine, bradykinin, histamine, Ca ionophores, thrombin, and adenosine nucleotides (112, 150, 400). Not all vasodilator agents seem to use this pathway. For example, nitrovasodilators are not affected by removing endothelium. The mechanisms involved in the endothelium-dependent vascular relaxation are currently under investigation. In the pulmonary vessels the dilation seems to be nonneuronal in character (150). Nor does a vasodilating product of arachidonic acid seem to be involved. Instead the possibility has been raised that stimulation of the endothelium elicits pulmonary vasodilation by the release of one or more agents that diffuse into the smooth muscle to cause relaxation of vascular tone (150).

Presently it is not known if endothelial–smooth muscle interactions in the pulmonary and systemic vascular beds operate in the same way to produce pulmonary vasodilation. The nature of the bridge between endothelium and smooth muscle is unclear. The postulated release of a vasodilator substance awaits proof, and the possibility of anatomical connections has not been excluded. Finally, the respective roles played by endothelium-dependent mechanisms, neuronal mechanisms, and other mechanisms in effecting vasodilation await elucidation.

It seems likely that roles of each of these mechanisms vary considerably depending on the vasodilator agent, the experimental conditions, and the vascular bed under consideration. Moreover now that acetyl-

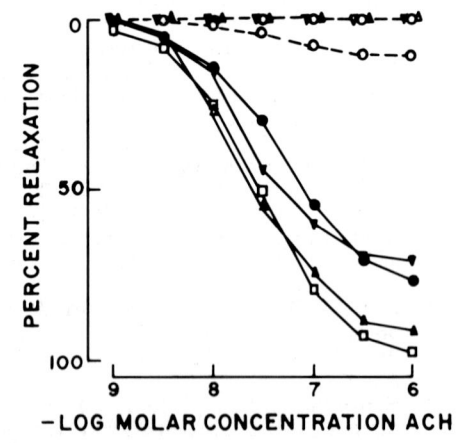

FIG. 36. Influence of endothelium on responses of different vessels to acetylcholine (ACH). Increasing concentrations of acetylcholine were applied to rings of femoral, saphenous, splenic, and pulmonary arteries (*circles*) that had previously been contracted with norepinephrine. Those vessels in which endothelium was intact (*solid curves*) responded with increasing vasodilation. In vessels without endothelium (*dashed curves*), virtually no vasodilation occurred. [Adapted from De Mey and Vanhoutte (113).]

choline receptor genes have been cloned, the full complexity of vasodilator (and vasoconstrictor) mechanisms is destined to be reexamined at the levels of molecular and cell biology. It does not seem farfetched to speculate that at these levels different agents engage the vasodilator system in different ways—possibly by a final common pathway—to accomplish relaxation (or constriction) of vascular smooth muscle.

The original work referred to in this chapter was supported by grants from the National Institutes of Health, primarily HL-08805.

REFERENCES

1. AARSETH, P., L. BJERTNAES, AND J. KARLSEN. Changes in blood volume and extravascular water content in isolated perfused rat lungs during ventilation hypoxemia. *Acta Physiol. Scand.* 109: 61–67, 1980.
2. AARSETH, P., AND J. KARLSEN. Blood volume and extravascular water content in the rat lung during acute alveolar hypoxia. *Acta Physiol. Scand.* 100: 236–245, 1977.
3. ABDALLA, M. A., AND A. S. KING. The functional anatomy of the bronchial circulation of the domestic fowl. *J. Anat.* 121: 537–550, 1976.
4. ABRAHAM, A. S., J. M. KAY, R. B. COLE, AND A. C. PINCOCK. Hemodynamic and pathological study of the effect of chronic hypoxia and subsequent recovery of the heart and pulmonary vasculature of the rat. *Cardiovasc. Res.* 5: 95–102, 1971.
5. AGOSTONI, E., AND J. PIIPER. Capillary pressure and distribution of vascular resistance in isolated lung. *Am. J. Physiol.* 202: 1033–1036, 1962.
6. AGOSTONI, E., A. TAGLIETTI, AND I. SETNIKAR. Absorption force of the capillaries of the visceral pleura in determination of the intrapleural pressure. *Am. J. Physiol.* 191: 277–282, 1957.
7. AHMED, T., AND W. OLIVER, JR. Does slow-reacting substance of anaphylaxis mediate hypoxic pulmonary vasoconstriction? *Am. Rev. Respir. Dis.* 127: 566–571, 1983.
8. AHMED, T., W. OLIVER, JR., AND A. WANNER. Variability of hypoxic pulmonary vasoconstriction in sheep. Role of prostaglandins. *Am. Rev. Respir. Dis.* 127: 59–62, 1983.
9. ALEXANDER, A. F. The bovine lung: normal vascular histology and vascular lesions in high mountain disease. *Med. Thorac.* 19: 528–542, 1962.
10. ALEXANDER, J. M., M. D. NYBY, AND K. A. JASBERG. Prostaglandin synthesis inhibition restores hypoxic pulmonary vasoconstriction. *J. Appl. Physiol.: Respirat. Environ. Exercise Physiol.* 42: 903–908, 1977.
11. ALLISON, D. J., AND H. S. STANBROOK. A radiologic and physiologic investigation into hypoxic pulmonary vasoconstriction in the dog. *Invest. Radiol.* 15: 178–190, 1980.
12. ANDERSON, F. L., AND A. M. BROWN. Pulmonary vasoconstriction elicited by stimulation of the hypothalamic integrative area for the defense reaction. *Circ. Res.* 21: 747–756, 1967.
13. ANTHONISEN, N. R., AND J. MILIC-EMILI. Distribution of pulmonary perfusion in erect man. *J. Appl. Physiol.* 21: 760–766, 1966.
14. ARBORELIUS, M., JR. Influence of moderate hypoxia in one lung on the distribution of the pulmonary circulation and ventilation. *Scand. J. Clin. Lab. Invest.* 17: 257–259, 1965.
15. ARIAS-STELLA, J., AND M. SALDANA. The terminal portion of the pulmonary arterial tree in people native to high altitudes. *Circulation* 28: 915–925, 1963.
16. ARMSTRONG, D. J., AND J. C. LUCK. Accessibility of pulmonary stretch receptors from the pulmonary and bronchial circulations. *J. Appl. Physiol.* 36: 706–710, 1974.
17. ASSIMACOPOULOS, A., R. GUGGENHEIM, AND Y. KAPANCI. Changes in alveolar capillary configuration at different levels of lung inflation in the rat: an ultrastructural and morphometric study. *Lab. Invest.* 34: 10–22, 1976.
18. AVIADO, D. M. Anoxia and the pulmonary circulation: systemic mechanisms. In: *The Lung Circulation.* Oxford, UK: Pergamon, 1965, vol. 1, p. 3–83.
19. AVIADO, D. M., JR., J. S. LING, AND C. F. SCHMIDT. Effects of anoxia on pulmonary circulation: reflex pulmonary vasoconstriction. *Am. J. Physiol.* 189: 253–262, 1957.
20. BAILE, E. M., J. M. B. NELEMS, M. SCHULZER, AND P. D. PARÉ. Measurement of regional bronchial arterial blood flow and bronchovascular resistance in dogs. *J. Appl. Physiol.: Respirat. Environ. Exercise Physiol.* 53: 1044–1049, 1982.
21. BANISTER, J., AND R. W. TORRANCE. The effects of tracheal pressure upon flow-pressure relations in the vascular bed of isolated lungs. *Q. J. Exp. Physiol.* 45: 352–367, 1960.
21a. BARCROFT, J. *The Respiratory Function of the Lung. Lessons From High Altitudes.* Cambridge, UK: Cambridge Univ. Press, pt. I, 1913.
22. BARER, G. R. A comparison of the circulatory effects of angiotensin, vasopressin, and adrenaline in the anesthetized cat. *J. Physiol. London* 156: 49–66, 1961.
23. BARER, G. R. Reactivity of the vessels of collapsed and ventilated lungs to drugs and hypoxia. *Circ. Res.* 18: 366–378, 1966.
24. BARER, G. R., D. BEE, AND R. A. WACH. Contribution of polycythaemia to pulmonary hypertension in simulated high altitude in rats. *J. Physiol. London* 336: 27–38, 1983.
25. BARER, G. R., C. J. EMERY, F. H. MOHAMMED, AND I. P. MUNGALL. H_1 and H_2 histamine actions on lung vessels: their relevance to hypoxic vasoconstriction. *Q. J. Exp. Physiol.* 63: 157–169, 1978.
26. BARER, G. R., P. HOWARD, J. R. MCCURRIE, AND J. W. SHAW. Changes in the pulmonary circulation after bronchial occlusion in anesthetized dogs and cats. *Circ. Res.* 25: 747–764, 1969.
27. BARER, G. R., P. HOWARD, AND J. W. SHAW. Stimulus-response curves for the pulmonary vascular bed to hypoxia and hypercapnia. *J. Physiol. London* 211: 139–155, 1970.
28. BARER, G. R., AND J. R. MCCURRIE. Pulmonary vasomotor responses in the cat: the effects and interrelationships of drugs, hypoxia and hypercapnia. *Q. J. Exp. Physiol.* 54: 156–172, 1969.
29. BARER, G. R., J. R. MCCURRIE, AND J. W. SHAW. Effect of changes in blood pH on the vascular resistance in the normal and hypoxic cat lung. *Cardiovasc. Res.* 5: 490–497, 1971.
30. BARER, G. R., AND J. W. SHAW. Pulmonary vasodilator and vasoconstrictor actions of carbon dioxide. *J. Physiol. London* 213: 633–645, 1971.
31. BARRETT, C. T., M. A. HEYMANN, AND A. M. RUDOLPH. Alpha and beta adrenergic receptor activity in fetal sheep. *Am. J. Obstet. Gynecol.* 112: 1114–1121, 1972.
32. BATES, D. V., C. J. VARVIS, R. E. DOWEVAN, AND R. V. CHRISTIE. Variations in the pulmonary capillary blood volume and membrane diffusion component in health and disease. *J. Clin. Invest.* 39: 1401–1412, 1960.
33. BECK, K. C., AND J. HILDEBRANDT. Adaptation of vascular pressure-flow-volume hysteresis in isolated rabbit lungs. *J. Appl. Physiol.: Respirat. Environ. Exercise Physiol.* 54: 671–679, 1983.
34. BENJAMIN, J. J., P. S. MURTAGH, D. F. PROCTOR, H. A. MENKES, AND S. PERMUTT. Pulmonary vascular interdependence in excised dog lobes. *J. Appl. Physiol.* 37: 887–894, 1974.
35. BENUMOF, J. L. Hypoxic pulmonary vasoconstriction and infusion of sodium nitroprusside. *Anesthesiology* 50: 481–483, 1979.
36. BENUMOF, J. L. Mechanism of decreased blood flow to atelectatic lung. *J. Appl. Physiol.: Respirat. Environ. Exercise Physiol.* 46: 1047–1048, 1979.
37. BENUMOF, J. L., J. M. MATHERS, AND E. A. WAHRENBROCK.

Cyclic hypoxic pulmonary vasoconstriction induced by concomitant carbon dioxide changes. *J. Appl. Physiol.* 41: 466–469, 1976.
38. BERGEL, D. H., AND W. R. MILNOR. Pulmonary vascular impedance in the dog. *Circ. Res.* 16: 401–415, 1965.
39. BERGOFSKY, E. H. Mechanisms underlying vasomotor regulation or regional pulmonary blood flow in normal and disease states. *Am. J. Med.* 57: 378–397, 1974.
40. BERGOFSKY, E. H. Active control of the normal pulmonary circulation. In: *Lung Biology in Health and Disease. Pulmonary Vascular Diseases*, edited by K. M. Moser, New York: Dekker, 1979, vol. 14, chapt. 3, p. 233–277.
41. BERGOFSKY, E. H. Humoral control of the pulmonary circulation. *Annu. Rev. Physiol.* 42: 221–233, 1980.
42. BERGOFSKY, E. H., B. G. BASS, R. FERRETTI, AND A. P. FISHMAN. Pulmonary vasoconstriction in response to precapillary hypoxemia. *J. Clin. Invest.* 42: 1201–1215, 1963.
43. BERGOFSKY, E. H., F. HAAS, AND R. PORCELLI. Determination of the sensitive vascular sites from which hypoxia and hypercapnia elicit rises in pulmonary arterial pressure. *Federation Proc.* 27: 1420–1425, 1968.
44. BERGOFSKY, E. H., AND S. HOLTZMAN. A study of the mechanism involved in the pulmonary arterial pressor response to hypoxia. *Circ. Res.* 20: 506–519, 1967.
45. BERGOFSKY, E. H., D. E. LEHR, AND A. P. FISHMAN. The effect of changes in hydrogen ion concentration on the pulmonary circulation. *J. Clin. Invest.* 14: 1492–1502, 1962.
46. BERKOV, S. Hypoxic pulmonary vasoconstriction in the rat: the necessary role of angiotensin II. *Circ. Res.* 35: 257–261, 1974.
47. BERRYHILL, R. E., AND J. L. BENUMOF. PEEP-induced discrepancy between pulmonary arterial wedge pressure and left atrial pressure: the effects of controlled vs. spontaneous ventilation and compliant vs. noncompliant lungs in the dog. *Anesthesiology* 31: 303–308, 1979.
48. BEYNE, J. Influence de l'anoxemie sur la grande circulation et sur la circulation pulmonaire. *C. R. Soc. Biol. Paris* 136: 399–400, 1942.
49. BHATTACHARYA, J., S. NANJO, AND N. C. STAUB. Factors affecting lung microvascular pressure. *Ann. NY Acad. Sci.* 384: 107–114, 1982.
50. BHATTACHARYA, J., S. NANJO, AND N. C. STAUB. Micropuncture measurement of lung microvascular pressure during 5-HT infusion. *J. Appl. Physiol.: Respirat. Environ. Exercise Physiol.* 52: 634–637, 1982.
51. BJERTNAES, L. J., A. HAUGE, AND T. TORGRIMSEN. The pulmonary vasoconstrictor response to hypoxia. The hypoxia-sensitive site studied with a volatile inhibitor. *Acta Physiol. Scand.* 109: 447–462, 1980.
52. BLAND, R. D., R. DEMLING, S. SELINGER, AND N. C. STAUB. Effects of alveolar hypoxia on lung fluid and protein transport in unanesthetized sheep. *Circ. Res.* 40: 269–274, 1977.
53. BLAUSTEIN, M. P. Sodium ions, calcium ions, blood pressure regulation, and hypertension: a reassessment and a hypothesis. *Am. J. Physiol.* 232 (*Cell Physiol.* 1): C165–C173, 1977.
54. BOAKE, W. C., R. DALEY, AND I. K. R. McMILLAN. Observations on hypoxic pulmonary hypertension. *Br. Heart J.* 21: 31–39, 1959.
55. BOHR, D. F. The pulmonary hypoxic response. State of the field. *Chest* 71, Suppl. 2: 244–246, 1977.
56. BOHR, D. F., AND B. JOHANSSON. Contraction of vascular smooth muscle in response to plasma. *Circ. Res.* 19: 593–601, 1966.
57. BOWERS, R. E., K. BRIGHAM, AND P. J. OWEN. Salicylate pulmonary edema. Mechanism in sheep and review of the clinical literature. *Am. Rev. Respir. Dis.* 115: 261–268, 1977.
58. BRAS, G., D. M. BERRY, AND P. GYORGY. Plants as etiological factors in veno-occlusive disease of the liver. *Lancet* 1: 960–962, 1957.
59. BRASHEAR, R. E., R. R. MARTIN, AND J. C. ROSS. In vivo histamine levels with hypoxia and compound 48/80. *Am. J. Med. Sci.* 260: 21–28, 1970.
60. BRAUNWALD, E., A. P. FISHMAN, AND A. COURNAND. Time relationship of dynamic events in the cardiac chambers, pulmonary artery and aorta in man. *Circ. Res.* 4: 100–107, 1956.
61. BRIGHAM, K. L., R. BOWERS, AND J. HAYNES. Increased sheep lung vascular permeability caused by *Escherichia coli* endotoxin. *Circ. Res.* 45: 292–297, 1979.
62. BRIGHAM, K. L., R. E. BOWERS, AND P. J. OWEN. Effects of antihistamines on the lung vascular response to histamine in unanesthetized sheep. Diphenhydramine prevention of pulmonary edema and increased permeability. *J. Clin. Invest.* 58: 391–398, 1976.
63. BRIGHAM, K. L., T. R. HARRIS, AND P. J. OWEN. [^{14}C]urea and [^{14}C]sucrose as permeability indicators in histamine pulmonary edema. *J. Appl. Physiol.: Respirat. Environ. Exercise Physiol.* 43: 99–101, 1977.
64. BRIGHAM, K. L., AND P. J. OWEN. Increased sheep lung vascular permeability caused by histamine. *Circ. Res.* 37: 647–657, 1975.
65. BRIGHAM, K. L., AND P. J. OWEN. Mechanism of the serotonin effect on lung transvascular fluid and protein movement in awake sheep. *Circ. Res.* 36: 761–770, 1975.
66. BRODY, J. S., E. J. STEMMLER, AND A. B. DUBOIS. Longitudinal distribution of vascular resistance in the pulmonary arteries, capillaries, and veins. *J. Clin. Invest.* 47: 783–799, 1968.
67. BRUTSAERT, D. Influence of reserpine and of adrenolytic agents on the pulmonary arterial pressor response to hypoxia and catecholamines. *Arch. Int. Physiol. Biochim.* 72: 395–412, 1964.
68. BRUTSAERT, D. The effects of reserpine and adrenolytic agents on the pulmonary arterial pressor response to serotonin. *Exp. Med. Surg.* 23: 13–27, 1965.
69. BRYAN, A. C., L. G. BENTIVOGLIO, F. BEEREL, H. MACLEISH, A. ZIDULKA, AND D. V. BATES. Factors affecting regional distribution of ventilation and perfusion in the lung. *J. Appl. Physiol.* 19: 395–402, 1964.
70. BURNS, J. Heart and pulmonary arteries in rats fed on *Senecio jacobaea. J. Pathol.* 106: 187–194, 1972.
71. BUTLER, J., AND H. W. PALEY. Lung volume and pulmonary circulation. *Med. Thorac.* 19: 261–267, 1962.
72. BUTLER, W. H., A. R. MATTOCKS, AND J. M. BARNES. Lesions in the liver and lungs in rats given pyrrole derivatives of pyrrolizidine alkaloids. *J. Pathol.* 100: 169–175, 1970.
73. BYRNE-QUINN, E., AND R. F. GROVER. Aminorex (Menocil) and amphetamine: acute and chronic effects on pulmonary and systemic haemodynamics in the calf. *Thorax* 27: 127–131, 1972.
74. CALKA, W. Vascular supply of the lungs through direct branches of the aorta in domestic pig. *Folia Morphol. Warsaw Engl. Transl.* 34: 135–142, 1975.
75. CAMPBELL, A. G. M., F. COCKBURN, G. S. DAWES, AND J. E. MILLIGAN. Pulmonary vasoconstriction in asphyxia during cross-circulation between twin foetal lambs. *J. Physiol. London* 192: 111–121, 1967.
76. CAMPBELL, A. G. M., G. S. DAWES, A. P. FISHMAN, AND A. I. HYMAN. Pulmonary vasoconstriction and changes in heart rate during asphyxia in immature fetal lambs. *J. Physiol. London* 192: 93–110, 1967.
77. CAMPBELL, A. G. M., G. S. DAWES, A. P. FISHMAN, A. I. HYMAN, AND A. M. PERKS. The release of a bradykinin-like pulmonary vasodilator substance in foetal and new-born lambs. *J. Physiol. London* 195: 83–96, 1968.
78. CASSIDY, S. S., F. A. GAFFNEY, AND R. L. JOHNSON, JR. A perspective on PEEP. *N. Engl. J. Med.* 304: 421–422, 1981.
79. CASSIN, S., G. S. DAWES, J. C. MOTT, B. B. ROSS, AND L. B. STRANG. The vascular resistance of the foetal and newly ventilated lung of the lamb. *J. Physiol. London* 171: 61–79, 1964.
80. CASSIN, S., G. S. DAWES, AND B. B. ROSS. Pulmonary blood flow and vascular resistance in immature foetal lambs. *J. Physiol. London* 171: 80–89, 1964.
81. CASTEELS, R., K. KITAMURA, H. KURIYAMA, AND H. SUZUKI.

The membrane properties of the smooth muscle cells of the rabbit main pulmonary artery. *J. Physiol. London* 271: 41–61, 1977.

82. CASTEELS, R., K. KITAMURA, H. KURIYAMA, AND H. SUZUKI. Excitation-contraction coupling in the smooth muscle cells of the rabbit main pulmonary artery. *J. Physiol. London* 271: 63–79, 1977.

83. CHESNEY, C. F., AND J. R. ALLEN. Endocardial fibrosis associated with monocrotaline-induced pulmonary hypertension in nonhuman primates (*Macaca arctoides*). *Am. J. Vet. Res.* 34: 1577–1581, 1973.

84. CHIESA, A., G. CIAPPI, L. BALBI, AND L. CHIANDUSSI. Role of various causes of arterial desaturation in liver cirrhosis. *Clin. Sci.* 37: 803–814, 1969.

85. COCEANI, F., I. BISHAI, E. WHITE, E. BODACH, AND P. M. OLLEY. Action of prostaglandins, endoperoxides, and thromboxanes on the lamb ductus arteriosus. *Am. J. Physiol.* 234 (*Heart Circ. Physiol.* 3): H117–H122, 1978.

86. COLEBATCH, H. J. H. Adrenergic mechanisms in the effects of histamine in the pulmonary circulation of the cat. *Circ. Res.* 26: 379–396, 1970.

87. COLEBATCH, H. J. H., G. S. DAWES, J. W. GOODWIN, AND R. A. NADEAU. The nervous control of the circulation in the foetal and newly expanded lungs of the lamb. *J. Physiol. London* 178: 544–562, 1965.

88. COLERIDGE, J. C. G., AND C. KIDD. Relationship between pulmonary arterial pressure and impulse activity in pulmonary arterial baroreceptor fibres. *J. Physiol. London* 158: 197–205, 1961.

89. COLLINS, R., AND J. A. MACCARIO. Blood flow in the lung. *J. Biomech.* 12: 373–395, 1979.

90. COURNAND, A. Air and blood. In: *Circulation of the Blood. Men and Ideas*, edited by A. P. Fishman and D. W. Richards. New York: Oxford Univ. Press, 1964, p. 3–70.

91. COURNAND, A., H. L. MOTLEY, L. WERKO, AND D. W. RICHARDS, JR. Physiological studies of the effects of intermittent positive pressure breathing on cardiac output in man. *Am. J. Physiol.* 152: 162–174, 1948.

92. CRANDALL, E. D., AND R. W. FLUMERFELT. Effects of time-varying blood flow on oxygen uptake in the pulmonary capillaries. *J. Appl. Physiol.* 23: 944–953, 1967.

93. CUDKOWICZ, L. Bronchial arterial circulation in man: normal anatomy and responses to disease. In: *Lung Biology in Health and Disease. Pulmonary Vascular Diseases*, edited by K. M. Moser. New York: Dekker, 1979, vol. 14, chapt. 2, p. 111–232.

94. CUDKOWICZ, L., AND D. G. WRAITH. A method of study of the pulmonary circulation in finger clubbing. *Thorax* 12: 313–321, 1957.

95. CULVER, B. H., AND J. BUTLER. Mechanical influences on the pulmonary microcirculation. *Annu. Rev. Physiol.* 42: 187–198, 1980.

96. CUMMING, G., R. HENDERSON, K. HORSFIELD, AND S. S. SINGHAL. The functional morphology of the pulmonary circulation. In: *Pulmonary Circulation and Interstitial Space*, edited by A. P. Fishman and H. H. Hecht. Chicago, IL: Univ. of Chicago Press, 1969, p. 327–340.

97. DALY, I. DE B., AND M. DE B. DALY. The effects of stimulation of the carotid body chemoreceptors on the pulmonary vascular bed in the dog: the vasosensory controlled perfused living animal preparation. *J. Physiol. London* 148: 201–219, 1959.

98. DALY, I. DE B., AND M. DE B. DALY. The nervous control of the pulmonary circulation. In: *Problems of Pulmonary Circulation*, edited by A. V. S. de Reuck and M. O'Connor. Boston, MA: Little, Brown, 1961, p. 44–60. (Ciba Found. Study Group 8.)

99. DALY, I. DE B., AND C. O. HEBB. *Pulmonary and Bronchial Vascular Systems*. London: Arnold, 1966.

100. DALY, I. DE B., C. C. MICHEL, D. J. RAMSAY, AND B. A. WAALER. Conditions governing the pulmonary vascular response to ventilation hypoxia and hypoxaemia in the dog. *J. Physiol. London* 196: 351–379, 1968.

101. DAOUD, F. S., J. T. REEVES, AND J. W. SCHAFFER. Failure of hypoxic pulmonary vasoconstriction in patients with liver cirrhosis. *J. Clin. Invest.* 51: 1076–1080, 1972.

102. DAVIES, G., AND L. REID. Growth of the alveoli and pulmonary arteries in childhood. *Thorax* 25: 669–681, 1970.

103. DAWES, G. S. Physiological changes in the circulation after birth. In: *Circulation of the Blood. Men and Ideas*, edited by A. P. Fishman and D. W. Richards. New York: Oxford Univ. Press, 1964, p. 743–816.

104. DAWES, G. S. *Fetal and Neonatal Physiology*. Chicago, IL: Year Book, 1968, p. 98.

105. DAWES, G. S., AND J. C. MOTT. The vascular tone of the foetal lung. *J. Physiol. London* 164: 465–477, 1962.

106. DAWSON, C. A., D. J. GRIMM, AND J. H. LINEHAM. Effects of lung inflation on longitudinal distribution of pulmonary vascular resistance. *J. Appl. Physiol.: Respirat. Environ. Exercise Physiol.* 43: 1089–1092, 1977.

107. DAWSON, C. A., D. J. GRIMM, AND J. H. LINEHAN. Influence of hypoxia on the longitudinal distribution of pulmonary vascular resistance. *J. Appl. Physiol.: Respirat. Environ. Exercise Physiol.* 44: 493–498, 1978.

108. DAWSON, C. A., D. J. GRIMM, AND J. H. LINEHAN. Lung inflation and longitudinal distribution of pulmonary vascular resistance during hypoxia. *J. Appl. Physiol.: Respirat. Environ. Exercise Physiol.* 47: 532–536, 1979.

109. DAWSON, C. A., R. L. JONES, AND L. H. HAMILTON. Hemodynamic responses of isolated cat lungs during forward and retrograde perfusion. *J. Appl. Physiol.* 35: 95–102, 1973.

110. DAWSON, C. A., J. H. LINEHAN, AND D. A. RICKABY. Pulmonary microcirculatory hemodynamics. *Ann. NY Acad. Sci.* 384: 90–105, 1982.

111. DEAL, E. C., JR., E. R. MCFADDEN, JR., R. H. INGRAM, JR., AND J. J. JAEGER. Esophageal temperature during exercise in asthmatic and nonasthmatic subjects. *J. Appl. Physiol.: Respirat. Environ. Exercise Physiol.* 46: 484–490, 1979.

112. DE MEY, J. G., AND P. M. VANHOUTTE. Role of the intima in cholinergic and purinergic relaxation of isolated canine femoral arteries. *J. Physiol. London* 316: 347–355, 1981.

113. DE MEY, J. G., AND P. M. VANHOUTTE. Heterogeneous behavior of the canine arterial and venous wall. Importance of the endothelium. *Circ. Res.* 51: 439–447, 1982.

114. DENISON, D., J. ERNSTING, AND D. I. FRYER. The effect of the inverted posture upon the distribution of blood flow in man. *J. Physiol. London* 172: 49–50, 1964.

115. DETAR, R. Mechanism of physiological hypoxia-induced depression of vascular smooth muscle contraction. *Am. J. Physiol.* 238 (*Heart Circ. Physiol.* 7): H761–H769, 1980.

116. DETAR, R., AND D. F. BOHR. Oxygen and vascular smooth muscle contraction. *Am. J. Physiol.* 214: 241–244, 1968.

117. DETAR, R., AND D. F. BOHR. Contractile responses of isolated vascular smooth muscle during prolonged exposure to anoxia. *Am. J. Physiol.* 222: 1269–1277, 1972.

118. DETAR, R., AND M. GELLAI. Oxygen and isolated vascular smooth muscle from the main pulmonary artery of the rabbit. *Am. J. Physiol.* 221: 1791–1794, 1971.

119. DEWITT, D. L., J. S. DAY, W. K. SONNENBURG, AND W. L. SMITH. Concentrations of prostaglandin endoperoxide synthase and prostaglandin I_2 synthase in the endothelium and smooth muscle of bovine aorta. *J. Clin. Invest.* 72: 1882–1888, 1983.

120. DEXTER, L., J. L. WHITTENBERGER, F. W. HAYNES, W. T. GOODALE, R. GORLIN, AND C. G. SAWYER. Effect of exercise on circulatory dynamics of normal individuals. *J. Appl. Physiol.* 3: 439–453, 1951.

121. DOEKEL, R. C., E. K. WEIR, R. LOOGA, R. F. GROVER, AND J. T. REEVES. Potentiation of hypoxic pulmonary vasoconstriction by ethyl alcohol in dogs. *J. Appl. Physiol.: Respirat. Environ. Exercise Physiol.* 44: 76–80, 1978.

122. DOWNING, S. E., AND T. H. GARDNER. Cephalic and carotid reflex influences on cardiac function. *Am. J. Physiol.* 215: 1192–1199, 1968.

123. DOWNING, S. E., AND J. C. LEE. Nervous control of the pulmonary circulation. *Annu. Rev. Physiol.* 42: 199–210, 1980.

124. DUGARD, A., AND A. NAIMARK. Effect of hypoxia on distribution of pulmonary blood flow. *J. Appl. Physiol.* 23: 663–671, 1967.
125. DUKE, H. N. The site of action of anoxia on the pulmonary blood vessels of the cat. *J. Physiol. London* 125: 373–382, 1954.
126. DUKE, H. N., AND E. M. KILLICK. Pulmonary vasomotor responses of isolated perfused cat lungs to anoxia. *J. Physiol. London* 117: 303–316, 1952.
127. DUNHAM, B. M., G. A. GRINDLINGER, T. UTSUNOMIYA, M. M. KRAUSZ, H. B. HECHTMAN, AND D. SHEPRO. Role of prostaglandins in positive end-expiratory pressure-induced negative inotropism. *Am. J. Physiol.* 241 (*Heart Circ. Physiol.* 10): H783–H788, 1981.
128. ELLSWORTH, M. L., T. J. GREGORY, AND J. C. NEWELL. Pulmonary prostacyclin production with increased flow and sympathetic stimulation. *J. Appl. Physiol.: Respirat. Environ. Exercise Physiol.* 55: 1225–1231, 1983.
129. EMERY, C. J., D. BEE, AND G. R. BARER. Mechanical properties and reactivity of vessels in isolated perfused lungs of chronically hypoxic rats. *Clin. Sci.* 61: 569–580, 1981.
130. EMERY, C. J., P. J. M. SLOAN, F. H. MOHAMMED, AND G. R. BARER. The action of hypercapnia during hypoxia on pulmonary vessels. *Bull. Eur. Physiopathol. Respir.* 13: 763–776, 1977.
131. ENSON, Y., C. GIUNTINI, M. L. LEWIS, T. Q. MORRIS, M. I. FERRER, AND R. M. HARVEY. The influence of hydrogen ion concentration and hypoxia on the pulmonary circulation. *J. Clin. Invest.* 43: 1146–1162, 1964.
132. EULER, U. S. VON, AND G. LILJESTRAND. Observations on the pulmonary arterial blood pressure in the cat. *Acta Physiol. Scand.* 12: 301–320, 1946.
133. FALCH, D. K., AND S. B. STROMME. Pulmonary blood volume and interventricular circulation time in physically trained and untrained subjects. *Eur. J. Appl. Physiol. Occup. Physiol.* 40: 211–218, 1979.
134. FAY, F. S. Guinea pig ductus arteriosus. I. Cellular and metabolic basis for oxygen sensitivity. *Am. J. Physiol.* 221: 470–479, 1971.
135. FEISAL, K., J. SONI, AND A. DUBOIS. Pulmonary circulation time, pulmonary arterial blood volume, and the ratio of gas to tissue volume in the lungs of dogs. *J. Clin. Invest.* 41: 390–400, 1962.
136. FISHMAN, A. P. The clinical significance of the pulmonary collateral circulation. *Circulation* 24: 677–690, 1961.
137. FISHMAN, A. P. Respiratory gases in the regulation of the pulmonary circulation. *Physiol. Rev.* 41: 214–280, 1961.
138. FISHMAN, A. P. Dynamics of the pulmonary circulation. In: *Handbook of Physiology. Circulation*, edited by W. F. Hamilton. Bethesda, MD: Am. Physiol. Soc., 1963, sect. 2, vol. II, chapt. 48, p. 1667–1743.
139. FISHMAN, A. P. Pulmonary edema. The water-exchanging function of the lung. *Circulation* 46: 390–408, 1972.
140. FISHMAN, A. P. Dietary pulmonary hypertension. *Circ. Res.* 35: 657–660, 1974.
141. FISHMAN, A. P. Hypoxia on the pulmonary circulation: how and where it acts. *Circ. Res.* 38: 221–231, 1976.
142. FISHMAN, A. P. (editor): *Pulmonary Diseases and Disorders*. New York: McGraw-Hill, 1980.
143. FISHMAN, A. P., H. W. FRITTS, JR., AND A. COURNAND. Effects of acute hypoxia and exercise on the pulmonary circulation. *Circulation* 22: 204–215, 1960.
144. FISHMAN, A. P., J. MCCLEMENT, A. HIMMELSTEIN, AND A. COURNAND. Effects of acute anoxia on the circulation and respiration in patients with chronic pulmonary disease studied during the steady state. *J. Clin. Invest.* 31: 770–781, 1952.
145. FISHMAN, A. P., AND G. G. PIETRA. Handling of bioactive materials by the lung. Pt. 1. *N. Engl. J. Med.* 291: 884–889, 1974.
145a. FISHMAN, A. P., AND G. G. PIETRA. Handling of bioactive materials by the lung. Pt. 2. *N. Engl. J. Med.* 291: 953–959, 1974.
146. FISHMAN, A. P., AND G. G. PIETRA. Vasodilator treatment of primary pulmonary hypertension. In: *Update: Pulmonary Diseases and Disorders*, edited by A. P. Fishman. New York: McGraw-Hill, 1982, p. 396–408.
147. FORREST, J. B., AND A. FARGAS-BABJAK. Variability of the pulmonary vascular response to hypoxia and relation to gas exchange in dogs. *Can. Anaesth. Soc. J.* 25: 479–487, 1978.
148. FOURNIER, P., J. MENSCH-DECHÈNE, B. RANSON-BITKER, W. VALLADARES, AND A. LOCKHART. Effects of sitting up on pulmonary blood pressure, flow, and volume in man. *J. Appl. Physiol.: Respirat. Environ. Exercise Physiol.* 46: 36–40, 1979.
149. FOWLER, K. T., J. B. WEST, AND M. C. F. PAIN. Pressure flow characteristics of horizontal lung preparations of minimal height. *Respir. Physiol.* 1: 88–98, 1966.
150. FRANK, G. W., AND J. A. BEVAN. Electrical stimulation causes endothelium-dependent relaxation in lung vessels. *Am. J. Physiol.* 244 (*Heart Circ. Physiol.* 13): H793–H798, 1983.
151. FREEDMAN, M. E., G. L. SNIDER, P. BROSTOFF, S. KIMELBLOT, AND L. N. KATZ. Effects of training on response of cardiac output to muscular exercise in athletes. *J. Appl. Physiol.* 8: 37–47, 1955.
152. FRIED, R., B. MEYRICK, M. RABINOVITCH, AND L. REID. Polycythemia and the acute hypoxic response in awake rats following chronic hypoxia. *J. Appl. Physiol.: Respirat. Environ. Exercise Physiol.* 55: 1167–1172, 1983.
153. FRITTS, H. W., JR., P. HARRIS, R. H. CLAUSS, J. E. ODELL, AND A. COURNAND. The effect of acetylcholine on the human pulmonary circulation under normal and hypoxic conditions. *J. Clin. Invest.* 37: 99–108, 1958.
154. FUCHS, K. I., L. G. MOORE, AND S. ROUNDS. Pulmonary vascular reactivity is blunted in pregnant rats. *J. Appl. Physiol.: Respirat. Environ. Exercise Physiol.* 53: 703–707, 1982.
155. FUNG, Y. C., AND S. S. SOBIN. Elasticity of the pulmonary alveolar sheet. *Circ. Res.* 30: 451–469, 1972.
156. FUNG, Y. C., AND S. S. SOBIN. Pulmonary alveolar blood flow. *Circ. Res.* 30: 470–490, 1972.
157. FUNG, Y.-C. B., AND S. S. SOBIN. Pulmonary alveolar blood flow. In: *Lung Biology in Health and Disease. Bioengineering Aspects of the Lung*, edited by J. B. West. New York: Dekker, 1977, vol. 3, chapt. 4, p. 267–359.
158. FURCHGOTT, R. F. Role of endothelium in responses of vascular smooth muscle. *Circ. Res.* 53: 557–573, 1983.
159. GAAR, K. A., JR., A. E. TAYLOR, L. J. OWENS, AND A. C. GUYTON. Effect of capillary pressure and plasma protein on development of pulmonary edema. *Am. J. Physiol.* 213: 79–82, 1967.
160. GABEL, J. C., AND R. E. DRAKE. Pulmonary capillary pressure in intact dog lungs. *Am. J. Physiol.* 235 (*Heart Circ. Physiol.* 4): H569–H573, 1978.
161. GEHR, P., M. BACHOFEN, AND E. R. WEIBEL. The normal human lung: ultrastructure and morphometric estimation of diffusion capacity. *Respir. Physiol.* 32: 121–140, 1978.
162. GERBER, J. G., N. VOELKEL, A. S. NIES, I. F. MCMURTRY, AND J. T. REEVES. Moderation of hypoxic vasoconstriction by infused arachidonic acid: role of PGI_2. *J. Appl. Physiol.: Respirat. Environ. Exercise Physiol.* 49: 107–112, 1980.
163. GIL, J. Influence of surface forces on pulmonary circulation. In: *Pulmonary Edema*, edited by A. P. Fishman and E. M. Renkin. Bethesda, MD: Am. Physiol. Soc., 1979, p. 53–64.
164. GIL, J. Organization of microcirculation in the lung. *Annu. Rev. Physiol.* 42: 177–186, 1980.
165. GIL, J. Alveolar and extraalveolar connective tissue compartments and origin of pulmonary lymph. *Microcirculation* 1: 407–420, 1981.
166. GIL, J. Alveolar wall relations. *Ann. NY Acad. Sci.* 384: 31–43, 1982.
167. GIL, J., AND E. R. WEIBEL. Morphological study of pressure-volume hysteresis in rat lungs fixed by vascular perfusion. *Respir. Physiol.* 15: 190–213, 1972.
168. GILBERT, R. D., J. R. HESSLER, D. V. EITZMAN, AND S. CASSIN. Site of pulmonary vascular resistance in fetal goats. *J. Appl. Physiol.* 32: 47–53, 1972.
169. GILLIS, C. N. Metabolism of vasoactive hormones by lung. *Anesthesiology* 39: 626–632, 1973.

170. GLAISTER, D. H. Effect of acceleration. In: *Regional Differences in the Lung*, edited by J. B. West. New York: Academic, 1977, p. 331–346.
171. GLAUSER, F. L., R. P. FAIRMAN, J. E. MILLEN, AND R. K. FALLS. Indomethacin blunts ethchlorvynol-induced pulmonary hypertension but not pulmonary edema. *J. Appl. Physiol.: Respirat. Environ. Exercise Physiol.* 53: 563–566, 1982.
172. GLAZIER, J. B., J. M. B. HUGHES, J. E. MALONEY, AND J. B. WEST. Measurements of capillary dimensions and blood volume in rapidly frozen lungs. *J. Appl. Physiol.* 26: 65–76, 1969.
173. GLAZIER, J. B., AND J. F. MURRAY. Site of pulmonary vasomotor reactivity in the dog during alveolar hypoxia and serotonin and histamine infusion. *J. Clin. Invest.* 50: 2550–2558, 1971.
174. GOLDBERG, S. J., R. A. LEVY, B. SIASSI, AND J. BETTEN. Effects of maternal hypoxia and hyperoxia upon the neonatal pulmonary vasculature. *Pediatrics* 48: 528–533, 1971.
175. GOLDRING, R. M., G. M. TURINO, D. H. ANDERSEN, AND A. P. FISHMAN. Cor pulmonale in cystic fibrosis of the pancreas (Abstract). *Circulation* 24: 942, 1961.
176. GOLDRING, R. M., G. M. TURINO, G. COHEN, A. G. JAMESON, B. G. BASS, AND A. P. FISHMAN. The catecholamines in the pulmonary arterial pressor response to acute hypoxia. *J. Clin. Invest.* 41: 1211–1221, 1962.
177. GORSKY, B. H., AND T. C. LLOYD, JR. Effects of perfusate composition on hypoxic vasoconstriction in isolated lung lobes. *J. Appl. Physiol.* 23: 683–686, 1967.
178. GRAHAM, R., C. SKOOG, L. OPPENHEIMER, J. RABSON, AND H. S. GOLDBERG. Critical closure in the canine pulmonary vasculature. *Circ. Res.* 50: 566–572, 1982.
179. GRAY, B. A., D. R. MCCAFFREE, E. D. SIVAK, AND H. T. MCCURDY. Effect of pulmonary vascular engorgement on respiratory mechanics in the dog. *J. Appl. Physiol.: Respirat. Environ. Exercise Physiol.* 45: 119–127, 1978.
180. GREEN, J. F., AND N. D. SCHMIDT. Mechanism of hyperpnea induced by changes in pulmonary blood flow. *J. Appl. Physiol.: Respirat. Environ. Exercise Physiol.* 56: 1418–1422, 1984.
181. GRIMM, D. J., C. A. DAWSON, T. S. HAKIM, AND J. H. LINEHAN. Pulmonary vasomotion and the distribution of vascular resistance in a dog lung lobe. *J. Appl. Physiol.: Respirat. Environ. Exercise Physiol.* 45: 545–550, 1978.
182. GROVER, R. F., J. H. K. VOGEL, K. H. AVERILL, AND S. G. BLOUNT, JR. Pulmonary hypertension: individual and species variability relative to vascular reactivity (Editorial). *Am. Heart J.* 66: 1–3, 1963.
183. GRUETTER, C. A., D. B. MCNAMARA, A. L. HYMAN, AND P. J. KADOWITZ. Contractile responses of intrapulmonary vessels from three species to arachidonic acid and an epoxymethano analog of PGH2. *Can. J. Physiol. Pharmacol.* 56: 206–215, 1978.
184. GUINTINI, C., A. MASERI, AND R. BIANCHI. Pulmonary vascular distensibility and lung compliance as modified by dextran infusion and subsequent atropine injection in normal subjects. *J. Clin. Invest.* 45: 1770–1789, 1966.
185. GURTNER, H. P. Hypertensive pulmonary vascular disease: some remarks on its incidence and aetiology. In: *Proc. Meet. Eur. Soc. Study Drug Toxic., 12th, Uppsala, 1970*, edited by S. B. Baker. Amsterdam: Excerpta Med., 1971, p. 81–88.
186. GURTNER, H. P. L'hypertension pulmonaire apres absorption d'un anorexigene, le fumarate d'aminorex. *Rev. Med. Paris* 14: 911–920, 1974.
187. GURTNER, H. P., P. WALSER, AND B. FASSLER. Normal values for pulmonary hemodynamics at rest and during exercise in man. *Prog. Respir. Res.* 9: 295–315, 1975.
188. HAAS, F., AND E. H. BERGOFSKY. Role of the mast cell in the pulmonary pressor response to hypoxia. *J. Clin. Invest.* 51: 3154–3162, 1972.
189. HAKIM, T. S., C. A. DAWSON, AND J. H. LINEHAN. Hemodynamic responses of dog lung lobe to lobar venous occlusion. *J. Appl. Physiol.: Respirat. Environ. Exercise Physiol.* 47: 145–152, 1979.
190. HAKIM, T. S., R. P. MICHEL, AND H. K. CHANG. Partitioning of pulmonary vascular resistance in dogs by arterial and venous occlusion. *J. Appl. Physiol.: Respirat. Environ. Exercise Physiol.* 52: 710–715, 1982.
191. HALES, C. A., AND H. KAZEMI. Role of histamine in the hypoxic vascular response of the lung. *Respir. Physiol.* 24: 81–88, 1975.
192. HALES, C. A., E. T. ROUSE, AND H. KAZEMI. Failure of saralasin acetate, a competitive inhibitor of angiotensin II, to diminish alveolar hypoxic vasoconstriction in the dog. *Cardiovasc. Res.* 11: 541–546, 1977.
193. HALES, C. A., E. T. ROUSE, AND J. L. SLATE. Influence of aspirin and indomethacin on variability of alveolar hypoxic vasoconstriction. *J. Appl. Physiol.: Respirat. Environ. Exercise Physiol.* 45: 33–39, 1978.
194. HALES, C. A., L. SONNE, M. PETERSON, D. KONG, M. MILLER, AND W. D. WATKINS. Role of thromboxane and prostacyclin in pulmonary vasomotor changes after endotoxin in dogs. *J. Clin. Invest.* 68: 497–505, 1981.
195. HALES, C. A., AND D. M. WESTPHAL. Pulmonary hypoxic vasoconstriction: not affected by chemical sympathectomy. *J. Appl. Physiol.: Respirat. Environ. Exercise Physiol.* 46: 529–533, 1979.
196. HAMASAKI, Y., M. MOJARAD, AND S. I. SAID. Relaxant action of VIP on cat pulmonary artery: comparison with acetylcholine, isoproterenol, and PGE_1. *J. Appl. Physiol.: Respirat. Environ. Exercise Physiol.* 54: 1607–1611, 1983.
197. HAMASAKI, Y., H.-H. TAI, AND S. I. SAID. Hypoxia stimulates prostacyclin generation by dog lung in vitro. *Prostaglandins Leukotrienes Med.* 8: 311–316, 1982.
198. HAMILTON, W. F., AND E. A. LOMBARD. Intrathoracic volume changes in relation to the cardiopneumogram. *Circ. Res.* 1: 76–82, 1953.
199. HANNA, C. J., M. K. BACH, P. D. PARE, AND R. R. SCHELLENBERG. Slow-reacting substances (leukotrienes) contract human airway and pulmonary vascular smooth muscle in vitro. *Nature London* 290: 343–344, 1981.
200. HARRIS, P., AND D. HEATH. The effect of drugs. In: *The Human Pulmonary Circulation*. Baltimore, MD: Williams & Wilkins, 1977, p. 113–126.
201. HARRIS, R. H., M. ZMUDKA, Y. MADDOX, P. W. RAMWELL, AND J. R. FLETCHER. Relationships of TXB_2 and 6-keto-$PGF_{1\alpha}$ to the hemodynamic changes during baboon endotoxic shock. *Adv. Prostaglandin Thromboxane Res.* 7: 843–849, 1980.
202. HARVEY, R. M., Y. ENSON, R. BETTI, M. L. LEWIS, D. F. ROCHESTER, AND M. I. FERRER. Further observations on the effect of hydrogen ion on the pulmonary circulation. *Circulation* 35: 1019–1027, 1967.
203. HAUGE, A. Conditions governing the pressor response to ventilation hypoxia in isolated perfused rat lungs. *Acta Physiol. Scand.* 72: 33–44, 1968.
204. HAUGE, A. Hypoxia and pulmonary vascular resistance: the relative effects of pulmonary arterial and alveolar PO_2. *Acta Physiol. Scand.* 76: 121–130, 1969.
205. HAUGE, A., AND K. L. MELMON. Role of histamine in hypoxic pulmonary hypertension in the rat. II. Depletion of histamine, serotonin, and catecholamines. *Circ. Res.* 22: 385–392, 1968.
206. HAUGE, A., AND N. C. STAUB. Prevention of hypoxic vasoconstriction in cat lung by histamine-releasing agent 48/80. *J. Appl. Physiol.* 26: 693–699, 1969.
207. HAYEK, H. VON. *The Human Lung*. New York: Hafner, 1960.
208. HEATH, D., C. EDWARDS, M. WINSON, AND P. SMITH. Effects on the right ventricle, pulmonary vasculature, and carotid bodies of the rat of exposure to, and recovery from, simulated high altitude. *Thorax* 28: 24–28, 1973.
209. HEATH, D., P. SMITH, D. WILLIAMS, P. HARRIS, J. ARIAS-STELLA, AND H. KRUGER. The heart and pulmonary vasculature of the llama (*Lama glama*). *Thorax* 29: 463–471, 1974.
210. HEATH, D., AND D. R. WILLIAMS. *Man at High Altitude. The Pathophysiology of Acclimatization and Adaptation* (2nd ed.). New York: Churchill Livingstone, 1981.
211. HEATH, D., D. WILLIAMS, P. HARRIS, P. SMITH, H. KRÜGER, AND A. RAMIREZ. The pulmonary vasculature of the mountain-

viscacha (*Lagidium peruanum*). The concept of adapted and acclimatized vascular smooth muscle. *J. Comp. Pathol.* 91: 293–301, 1981.
212. HEBB, C. Motor innervation of the pulmonary blood vessels of mammals. In: *Pulmonary Circulation and Interstitial Space*, edited by A. P. Fishman and H. H. Hecht. Chicago, IL: Univ. of Chicago Press, 1969, p. 195–222.
213. HEDENSTIERNA, G., F. C. WHITE, R. MAZZONE, AND P. D. WAGNER. Redistribution of pulmonary blood flow in the dog with PEEP ventilation. *J. Appl. Physiol.: Respirat. Environ. Exercise Physiol.* 46: 278–287, 1979.
214. HEFFNER, J. E., S. A. SHOEMAKER, E. M. CANHAM, M. PATEL, I. F. MCMURTRY, H.G. MORRIS, AND J. E. REPINE. Acetyl glyceryl ether phosphorylcholine-stimulated human platelets cause pulmonary hypertension and edema in isolated rabbit lungs. Role of thromboxane A$_2$. *J. Clin. Invest.* 71: 351–357, 1983.
215. HEINEMANN, H. O., AND A. P. FISHMAN. Nonrespiratory functions of mammalian lung. *Physiol. Rev.* 49: 1–47, 1969.
216. HERGET, J., AND F. PALEČEK. Experimental chronic pulmonary hyertension. In: *International Review of Experimental Pathology*, edited by G. W. Richter and M. A. Epstein. New York: Academic, 1978, vol. 18, p. 347–406.
217. HERGET, J., A. J. SUGGETT, E. LEACH, AND G. R. BARER. Resolution of pulmonary hypertension and other features induced by chronic hypoxia in rats during complete and intermittent normoxia. *Thorax* 33: 468–473, 1978.
218. HEUSNER, A. A. Body size, energy metabolism, and the lungs. *J. Appl. Physiol.: Respirat. Environ. Exercise Physiol.* 54: 867–873, 1983.
219. HEYMANN, M. A., AND A. M. RUDOLPH. Control of the ductus arteriosus. *Physiol. Rev.* 55: 62–78, 1975.
220. HEYMANN, M. A., AND A. M. RUDOLPH. Effects of acetylsalicylic acid on the ductus arteriosus and circulation in fetal lambs in utero. *Circ. Res.* 38: 418–422, 1976.
221. HEYMANN, M. A., A. M. RUDOLPH, A. S. NIES, AND K. L. MELMON. Bradykinin production associated with oxygenation of the fetal lamb. *Circ. Res.* 25: 521–534, 1969.
222. HISLOP, A., AND L. REID. New findings in pulmonary arteries of rats with hypoxia-induced pulmonary hypertension. *Br. J. Exp. Pathol.* 57: 542–554, 1976.
223. HOFFMAN, E. A., S. J. LAI-FOOK, J. WEI, AND E. H. WOOD. Regional pleural surface expansile forces in intact dogs by wick catheters. *J. Appl. Physiol.: Respirat. Environ. Exercise Physiol.* 55: 1523–1529, 1983.
224. HOFFMAN, E. A., M. L. MUNROE, A. TUCKER, AND J. T. REEVES. Histamine H$_1$- and H$_2$-receptors in the cat and their roles during alveolar hypoxia. *Respir. Physiol.* 29: 255–264, 1977.
225. HOLCROFT, J. W., D. D. TRUNKEY, AND M. A. CARPENTER. Sepsis in the baboon: factors affecting resuscitation and pulmonary edema in animals resuscitated with Ringer's lactate versus Plasmanate. *J. Trauma* 17: 600–610, 1977.
226. HOLLOWAY, H., M. PERRY, J. DOWNEY, J. PARKER, AND A. TAYLOR. Estimation of effective pulmonary capillary pressure in intact lungs. *J. Appl. Physiol.: Respirat. Environ. Exercise Physiol.* 54: 846–851, 1983.
227. HOPKINS, R. A., J. W. HAMMON, JR., P. A. MCHALE, P. K. SMITH, AND R. W. ANDERSON. Pulmonary vascular impedance analysis of adaptation to chronically elevated blood flow in the awake dog. *Circ. Res.* 45: 267–274, 1979.
228. HORSFIELD, K. Morphometry of the small pulmonary arteries in man. *Circ. Res.* 42: 593–597, 1978.
229. HOWARD, P., G. R. BARER, B. THOMPSON, P. M. WARREN, C. J. ABBOTT, AND I. P. F. MUNGALL. Factors causing and reversing vasoconstriction in unventilated lung. *Respir. Physiol.* 24: 325–345, 1975.
230. HOWELL, J. B. L., S. PERMUTT, D. F. PROCTOR, AND R. L. RILEY. Effect of inflation of the lung on different parts of pulmonary vascular bed. *J. Appl. Physiol.* 16: 71–76, 1961.
231. HUGHES, J. M. B. Pulmonary circulation and fluid balance. In: *Respiratory Physiology II*, edited by J. G. Widdicombe. Baltimore, MD: University Park, 1977, vol. 14, p. 135–183. (Int. Rev. Physiol. Ser.)
232. HUNTER, C., G. R. BARER, J. W. SHAW, AND E. J. CLEGG. Growth of the heart and lungs in hypoxic rodents. A model of human hypoxic diseases. *Clin. Sci. Mol. Med.* 46: 375–391, 1974.
233. HÜTTEMEIER, P. C., W. D. WATKINS, M. B. PETERSON, AND W. M. ZAPOL. Acute pulmonary hypertension and lung thromboxane release after endotoxin infusion in normal and leukopenic sheep. *Circ. Res.* 50: 688–694, 1982.
234. HUVAL, W. V., M. A. MATHIESON, L. I. STEMP, B. M. DUNPAM, A. G. JONES, D. SHEPRO, AND H. D. HECHTMAN. Therapeutic benefits of 5-hydroxytryptamine inhibition following pulmonary embolism. *Ann. Surg.* 197: 220–225, 1983.
235. HYMAN, A. L., AND P. S. KADOWITZ. Effects of alveolar and perfusion hypoxia and hypercapnia on pulmonary vascular resistance in the lamb. *Am. J. Physiol.* 228: 397–403, 1975.
236. HYMAN, A. L., E. W. SPANNHAKE, AND P. J. KADOWITZ. Divergent responses to arachidonic acid in the feline pulmonary vascular bed. *Am. J. Physiol.* 239 (*Heart Circ. Physiol.* 8): H40–H46, 1980.
237. INGRAM, R. H., J. P. SZIDON, AND A. P. FISHMAN. Response of the main pulmonary artery of dogs to neuronally released versus blood-borne norepinephrine. *Circ. Res.* 26: 249–269, 1970.
238. INGRAM, R. H., J. P. SZIDON, R. SKALAK, AND A. P. FISHMAN. Effects of sympathetic nerve stimulation on the pulmonary arterial tree of the isolated lobe perfused in situ. *Circ. Res.* 22: 801–815, 1968.
239. JAMESON, A. G. Gaseous diffusion from alveoli into pulmonary arteries. *J. Appl. Physiol.* 19: 448–456, 1964.
240. JARDIN, F., J. FARCOT, L. BOISANTE, N. CURIEN, A. MARGAIRAZ, AND J. BOURDARIAS. Influence of positive end-expiratory pressure on left ventricular performance. *N. Engl. J. Med.* 304: 387–392, 1981.
241. JOBSIS, F. F. What is a molecular oxygen sensor? What is a transduction process? *Adv. Exp. Med. Biol.* 78: 3–18, 1977.
242. JOHANSSON, B. Determinants of vascular reactivity. *Federation Proc.* 33: 121–126, 1974.
243. KABINS, S. A., J. FRIDMAN, J. NEUSTADT, G. ESPINOSA, AND L. N. KATZ. Mechanisms leading to lung edema in pulmonary embolization. *Am. J. Physiol.* 198: 543–546, 1960.
244. KADOWITZ, P. J., C. A. GRUETTER, F. W. SPANNHAKE, AND A. C. HYMAN. Pulmonary vascular responses to prostaglandins. *Federation Proc.* 40: 1991–1996, 1981.
245. KADOWITZ, P. J., P. D. JOINER, AND A. L. HYMAN. Effect of prostaglandin E$_2$ on pulmonary vascular resistance in intact dog, swine and lamb. *Eur. J. Pharmacol.* 31: 72–80, 1975.
246. KANEKO, K., J. MILIC-EMILI, M. B. DOLOVICH, A. DAWSON, AND D. V. BATES. Regional distribution of ventilation and perfusion as a function of body position. *J. Appl. Physiol.* 21: 767–777, 1966.
247. KAPANCI, Y., A. ASSIMACOPOULOS, C. IRLE, A. ZWAHLEN, AND G. GABBIANI. "Contractile interstitial cells" in pulmonary alveolar septa: a possible regulator of ventilation/perfusion ratio? *J. Cell Biol.* 60: 375–392, 1974.
248. KAPANCI, Y., AND P. M. COSTABELLA. Studies on structure and function of contractile interstitial cells (CIC) in pulmonary alveolar septa (Abstract). *Federation Proc.* 38: 964, 1979.
249. KAPANCI, Y., P. M. COSTABELLA, P. CERUTTI, AND A. ASSIMACOPOULOS. Distribution and function of cytoskeletal proteins in lung cells with particular reference to "contractile interstitial cells." *Methods Achiev. Exp. Pathol.* 9: 147–168, 1979.
250. KAY, J. M., AND R. F. GROVER. Lung mast cells and hypoxic pulmonary hypertension. *Prog. Respir. Res.* 9: 157–164, 1975.
251. KAY, J. M., AND D. HEATH. *Crotalaria Spectabilis. The Pulmonary Hypertension Plant.* Springfield, IL: Thomas, 1969, 136 p.
252. KAY, J. M., P. M. KEANE, K. L. SUYAMA, AND D. GAUTHIER. Angiotensin converting enzyme activity and evolution of pulmonary vascular disease in rats with monocrotaline pulmonary

hypertension. *Thorax* 37: 88–96, 1982.
253. KAY, J. M., P. SMITH, AND D. HEATH. Aminorex and the pulmonary circulation. *Thorax* 26: 262–270, 1971.
254. KAY, J. M., J. C. WAYMIRE, AND R. F. GROVER. Lung mast cell hyperplasia and pulmonary histamine-forming capacity in hypoxic rats. *Am. J. Physiol.* 226: 178–184, 1974.
255. KAZEMI, H., P. E. BRUECKE, AND E. F. PARSONS. Role of autonomic nervous system in the hypoxic response of the pulmonary vascular bed. *Respir. Physiol.* 15: 245–254, 1972.
256. KING, R. J. Pulmonary surfactant. *J. Appl. Physiol.: Respirat. Environ. Exercise Physiol.* 53: 1–8, 1982.
257. KNOBLAUCH, A., A. SYBERT, N. J. BRENNAN, J. T. SYLVESTER, AND G. H. GURTNER. Effect of hypoxia and CO on a cytochrome P-450-mediated reaction in rabbit lungs. *J. Appl. Physiol.: Respirat. Environ. Exercise Physiol.* 51: 1635–1642, 1981.
258. KORNER, P. I., AND S. W. WHITE. Circulatory control in hypoxia by sympathetic nerves and adrenal medulla. *J. Physiol. London* 184: 272–290, 1966.
259. KOYAMA, T., AND M. HORIMOTO. Pulmonary microcirculatory response to localized hypercapnia. *J. Appl. Physiol.: Respirat. Environ. Exercise Physiol.* 53: 1556–1564, 1982.
260. KOYAMA, T., S. NAKAJIMA, AND Y. KAKIUCHI. Quick increase of pulmonary blood flow in response to an acute alveolar hypoxia in human subjects. *Jpn. J. Physiol.* 27: 1–11, 1977.
261. KUIDA, H., H. H. HECHT, R. L. LANGE, A. M. BROWN, T. J. TSAGARIS, AND J. L. THORNE. Brisket disease. III. Spontaneous remission of pulmonary hypertension and recovery from heart failure. *J. Clin. Invest.* 42: 589–596, 1964.
262. KURAMOTO, K., AND S. RODBARD. Effects of blood flow and left atrial pressure on pulmonary venous resistance. *Circ. Res.* 11: 240–246, 1962.
263. LAI-FOOK, S. J. A continuum mechanics analysis of pulmonary vascular interdependence in isolated dog lobes. *J. Appl. Physiol.: Respirat. Environ. Exercise Physiol.* 46: 419–429, 1979.
264. LAI-FOOK, S. J., AND R. E. HYATT. Effect of parenchyma and length changes on vessel pressure-diameter behavior in pig lungs. *J. Appl. Physiol.: Respirat. Environ. Exercise Physiol.* 47: 666–669, 1979.
265. LAMMERANT, J. *Le volume sanguin des poumons.* Brussels: Arscia, 1957.
266. LANDIS, E. M., AND J. R. PAPPENHEIMER. Exchange of substances through the capillary walls. In: *Handbook of Physiology. Circulation*, edited by W. F. Hamilton. Bethesda, MD: Am. Physiol. Soc., 1963, sect. 2, vol. II, chapt. 29, p. 961–1034.
267. LATEGOLA, M. T. Pressure-flow relationships in the dog lung during acute, subtotal pulmonary vascular occlusion. *Am. J. Physiol.* 192: 613–619, 1958.
268. LAUWERYNS, J. M., AND A. VAN LOMMEL. Morphometric analysis of hypoxia-induced synaptic activity in intrapulmonary neuroepithelial bodies. *Cell Tissue Res.* 226: 201–214, 1982.
269. LEACH, E., P. HOWARD, AND G. R. BARER. Resolution of hypoxic changes in the heart and pulmonary arterioles during intermittent correction of hypoxia. *Clin. Sci. Mol. Med.* 52: 153–162, 1977.
270. LEFFLER, C. W., AND J. R. HESSLER. Pulmonary and systemic effects of exogenous prostaglandin I$_2$ in fetal lambs. *Eur. J. Pharmacol.* 54: 37–42, 1979.
271. LEFFLER, C. W., T. L. TYLER, AND S. CASSIN. Effect of indomethacin on pulmonary vascular response to ventilation of fetal goats. *Am. J. Physiol.* 234 (*Heart Circ. Physiol.* 3): H346–H351, 1978.
272. LEIER, C. V., D. BAMBACH, S. NELSON, J. B. HERMILLER, P. HUSS, R. MAGORIEN, AND D. V. UNVERFERTH. Captopril in primary pulmonary hypertension. *Circulation* 67: 155–161, 1983.
273. LEVIN, D. L., L. J. MILLS, M. PARKEY, J. GARRIOTT, AND W. CAMPBELL. Constriction of the fetal ductus arteriosus after administration of indomethacin to the pregnant ewe. *J. Pediatr.* 94: 647–650, 1979.
274. LEVIN, D. L., A. M. RUDOLPH, M. A. HEYMANN, AND R. H. PHIBBS. Morphological development of the pulmonary vascular bed in fetal lambs. *Circulation* 53: 144–151, 1976.
275. LEVITZKY, M. G. Chemoreceptor stimulation and hypoxic pulmonary vasoconstriction in conscious dogs. *Respir. Physiol.* 37: 151–160, 1979.
276. LEWIN, R. J., C. E. CROSS, P. RIEBEN, AND P. F. SALISBURY. Stretch reflexes from the main pulmonary artery to the systemic circulation. *Circ. Res.* 9: 585–588, 1961.
277. LEWIS, A. B., M. A. HEYMANN, AND A. M. RUDOLPH. Gestational changes in pulmonary vascular responses in fetal lambs in utero. *Circ. Res.* 39: 536–541, 1976.
278. LEWIS, M. L., AND L. C. CHRISTIANSON. Behavior of the human pulmonary circulation during head-up tilt. *J. Appl. Physiol.: Respirat. Environ. Exercise Physiol.* 45: 249–254, 1978.
279. LEYSEN, J. E. Serotonergic receptors in brain tissue: properties and identification of various ^{3}H-ligand binding sites in vitro. *J. Physiol. Paris* 77: 351–362, 1981.
280. LIEBOW, A. A. Recent observations on pulmonary collateral circulation. *Med. Thorac.* 19: 609–622, 1962.
281. LILJESTRAND, G. Chemical control of distribution of pulmonary blood flow. *Acta Physiol. Scand.* 44: 216–240, 1958.
282. LILKER, E. S., AND E. J. NAGY. Gas exchange in the pulmonary collateral circulation of dogs. *Am. Rev. Respir. Dis.* 112: 615–620, 1975.
283. LINEHAN, J. H., AND C. A. DAWSON. A three-compartment model of the pulmonary vasculature: effects of vasoconstriction. *J. Appl. Physiol.: Respirat. Environ. Exercise Physiol.* 55: 923–928, 1983.
284. LLOYD, T. C., JR. Effect of alveolar hypoxia on pulmonary vascular resistance. *J. Appl. Physiol.* 19: 1086–1094, 1964.
285. LLOYD, T. C., JR. Role of nerve pathways in the hypoxic vasoconstriction of the lung. *J. Appl. Physiol.* 21: 1351–1355, 1966.
286. LLOYD, T. C., JR. Influences of P_{O_2} and pH on resting and active tensions of pulmonary arterial strips. *J. Appl. Physiol.* 22: 1101–1109, 1967.
287. LLOYD, T. C., JR. Hypoxic pulmonary vasoconstriction: role of perivascular tissue. *J. Appl. Physiol.* 25: 560–565, 1968.
288. LLOYD, T. C., JR. Effect of increased intracranial pressure on pulmonary vascular resistance. *J. Appl. Physiol.* 35: 332–335, 1973.
289. LOCK, J. E., P. M. OLLEY, AND F. COCEANI. Direct pulmonary vascular responses to prostaglandins in the conscious newborn lamb. *Am. J. Physiol.* 238 (*Heart Circ. Physiol.* 7): H631–H638, 1980.
290. LOCK, J. E., P. M. OLLEY, AND F. COCEANI. Enhanced β-adrenergic-receptor responsiveness in hypoxic neonatal pulmonary circulation. *Am. J. Physiol.* 240 (*Heart Circ. Physiol.* 9): H697–H703, 1981.
291. LOCKHART, A. Functional aspects of the pulmonary collateral circulation. In: *Pulmonary Circulation in Health and Disease*, edited by G. Cumming and G. Bonsignore. New York: Plenum, 1980, p. 43–65.
292. LOCKHART, A. Pressure-flow-volume relationships in the normal human pulmonary circulation at sea-level and at altitude. In: *Pulmonary Circulation in Health and Disease*, edited by G. Cumming and G. Bonsignore. New York: Plenum, 1980, p. 337–355.
293. LOCKHART, A., M. ZELTER, J. MENSCH-DECHENE, G. ANTEZANA, M. PAZ-ZAMORA, E. VARGAS, AND J. COUDERT. Pressure-flow-volume relationships in pulmonary circulation of normal highlanders. *J. Appl. Physiol.* 41: 449–456, 1976.
294. LOPEZ-MUNIZ, R., N. L. STEPHENS, B. BROMBERGER-BARNEA, S. PERMUTT, AND R. RILEY. Critical closure of pulmonary vessels analyzed in terms of Starling resistor model. *J. Appl. Physiol.* 24: 625–635, 1968.
295. MACKLIN, C. C. Evidence of increase in the capacity of the pulmonary arteries and veins of dogs, cats and rabbits during inflation of the freshly excised lung. *Rev. Can. Biol.* 5: 199–232, 1946.
296. MAGNO, M. G., AND A. P. FISHMAN. Origin, distribution, and

blood flow of bronchial circulation in anesthetized sheep. *J. Appl. Physiol.: Respirat. Environ. Exercise Physiol.* 53: 272–279, 1982.
297. MALIK, A. B. Pulmonary vascular response to increase in intracranial pressure: role of sympathetic mechanisms. *J. Appl. Physiol.: Respirat. Environ. Exercise Physiol.* 42: 335–343, 1977.
298. MALIK, A. B. The role of metabolic acidosis in the pulmonary vascular response to hemorrhage and shock. *J. Trauma* 18: 108–114, 1978.
299. MALIK, A. B. Pulmonary microembolism. *Physiol. Rev.* 63: 1114–1207, 1983.
300. MALIK, A. B., AND B. S. L. KIDD. Adrenergic blockade on the pulmonary vascular response to hypoxia. *Respir. Physiol.* 19: 96–106, 1973.
301. MALIK, A. B., AND B. S. L. KIDD. Independent effects of changes in H^+ and CO_2 concentrations on hypoxic pulmonary vasoconstriction. *J. Appl. Physiol.* 34: 318–323, 1973.
302. MALIK, A. B., AND B. S. L. KIDD. Time course of pulmonary vascular response to hypoxia in dogs. *Am. J. Physiol.* 224: 1–6, 1973.
303. MALIK, A. B., AND S. E. TRACY. Bronchovascular adjustments after pulmonary embolism. *J. Appl. Physiol.: Respirat. Environ. Exercise Physiol.* 49: 476–481, 1980.
304. MARINI, J. J. *Respiratory Medicine and Intensive Care.* Baltimore, MD: Williams & Wilkins, 1981.
305. MARSHALL, B. E., AND C. MARSHALL. Continuity of response to hypoxic pulmonary vasoconstriction. *J. Appl. Physiol.: Respirat. Environ. Exercise Physiol.* 49: 189–196, 1980.
306. MARTIN, L. F., A. TUCKER, M. L. MUNROE, AND J. T. REEVES. Lung mast cells and hypoxic pulmonary vasoconstriction in cats. *Respiration* 35: 73–77, 1978.
307. MATTOCKS, A. R. Toxicity of pyrrolizidine alkaloids. *Nature London* 217: 723–728, 1968.
308. MAY, N. D. S. *Anatomy of the Sheep* (3rd ed.). St. Lucia, Australia: Univ. of Queensland Press, 1970.
309. MAZZONE, R. W. Influence of vascular and transpulmonary pressures on the functional morphology of the pulmonary microcirculation. *Microvasc. Res.* 20: 295–306, 1980.
310. MAZZONE, R. W., C. M. DURAND, AND J. B. WEST. Electron microscopy of lung rapidly frozen under controlled physiological conditions. *J. Appl. Physiol.: Respirat. Environ. Exercise Physiol.* 45: 325–333, 1978.
311. MCDONALD, D. A. *Blood Flow in Arteries.* London: Arnold, 1974.
312. MCDONALD, I. G., AND J. BUTLER. Distribution of vascular resistance in the isolated perfused dog lung. *J. Appl. Physiol.* 23: 463–474, 1967.
313. MCDONALD, J. W. D., M. ALI, E. MORGAN, E. R. TOWNSEND, AND J. D. COOPER. Thomboxane synthesis by sources other than platelets in association with complement-induced pulmonary leukostasis and pulmonary hypertension in sheep (Abstract). *Circ. Res.* 52: 1–6, 1983.
314. MCFADDEN, E. R., JR. Respiratory heat and water exchange: physiological and clinical implications. *J. Appl. Physiol.: Respirat. Environ. Exercise Physiol.* 54: 331–336, 1983.
315. MCMAHON, S. M., D. F. PROCTOR, AND S. PERMUTT. Pleural surface pressure in dogs. *J. Appl. Physiol.* 27: 881–885, 1969.
316. MCMURTRY, I. F., A. B. DAVIDSON, J. T. REEVES, AND R. F. GROVER. Inhibition of hypoxic pulmonary vasoconstriction by calcium antagonists in isolated rat lungs. *Circ. Res.* 38: 99–104, 1976.
317. MCMURTRY, I. F., K. G. MORRIS, AND M. D. PETRUN. Blunted hypoxic vasoconstriction in lungs from short-term high-altitude rats. *Am. J. Physiol.* 238 (*Heart Circ. Physiol.* 7): H849–H857, 1980.
318. MCMURTRY, I. F., M. D. PETRUN, AND J. T. REEVES. Lungs from chronically hypoxic rats have decreased pressor response to acute hypoxia. *Am. J. Physiol.* 235 (*Heart Circ. Physiol.* 4): H104–H109, 1978.
319. MCMURTRY, I. F., M. D. PETRUN, A. TUCKER, AND J. T. REEVES. Pulmonary vascular reactivity in the spontaneously hypertensive rat. *Blood Vessels* 16: 61–70, 1979.
320. MCMURTRY, I. F., J. T. REEVES, D. H. WILL, AND R. F. GROVER. Reduction of bovine pulmonary hypertension by normoxia, verapamil and hexaprenaline. *Experientia* 33: 1192–1194, 1977.
321. MCMURTRY, I. F., S. ROUNDS, AND H. S. STANBROOK. Studies of the mechanism of hypoxic pulmonary vasoconstriction. *Adv. Shock. Res.* 8: 21–33, 1982.
322. MEAD, J. Mechanical properties of lungs. *Physiol. Rev.* 41: 281–330, 1961.
323. MEAD, J., T. TAKISHIMA, AND D. LEITH. Stress distribution in lungs: a model of pulmonary elasticity. *J. Appl. Physiol.* 28: 596–608, 1970.
324. MELLEMGAARD, K., K. WINKLER, N. TYGSTRUP, AND J. GEORG. Sources of venoarterial admixture in portal hypertension. *J. Clin. Invest.* 42: 1399–1405, 1963.
325. MEYRICK, B., K. FUJIWARA, AND L. REID. Smooth muscle myosin in precursor and mature smooth muscle cells in normal pulmonary arteries and the effect of hypoxia. *Exp. Lung Res.* 2: 303–313, 1981.
326. MEYRICK, B., W. GAMBLE, AND L. REID. Development of *Crotalaria* pulmonary hypertension: hemodynamic and structural study. *Am. J. Physiol.* 239 (*Heart Circ. Physiol.* 8): H692–H702, 1980.
327. MEYRICK, B., AND L. REID. The effect of continued hypoxia on rat pulmonary arterial circulation. An ultrastructural study. *Lab. Invest.* 38: 188–200, 1978.
328. MEYRICK, B., AND L. REID. Hypoxia and incorporation of ^{3}H-thymidine by cells of the rat pulmonary arteries and alveolar wall. *Am. J. Pathol.* 96: 51–70, 1979.
329. MEYRICK, B., AND L. REID. Ultrastructural features of the distended pulmonary arteries of the normal rat. *Anat. Rec.* 193: 71–98, 1979.
330. MILIC-EMILI, J., AND N. M. SIAFAKAS. The nature of zone 4 in regional distribution of pulmonary blood flow. In: *Pulmonary Circulation in Health and Disease*, edited by G. Cumming and G. Bonsignore. New York: Plenum, 1980, p. 211–224.
331. MILLER, M. A., AND C. A. HALES. Role of cytochrome P-450 in alveolar hypoxic pulmonary vasoconstriction in dogs. *J. Clin. Invest.* 64: 666–673, 1979.
332. MILNOR, W. R. *Hemodynamics.* Baltimore, MD: Williams & Wilkins, 1982.
333. MILNOR, W. R., D. H. BERGEL, AND J. D. BARGAINER. Hydraulic power associated with pulmonary blood flow and its relation to heart rate. *Circ. Res.* 19: 467–480, 1966.
334. MILSOM, W. K., B. L. LANGILLE, AND D. R. JONES. Vagal control of pulmonary vascular resistance in the turtle *Chrysemys scripta*. *Can. J. Zool.* 55: 359–367, 1977.
335. MITZNER, W., AND J. T. SYLVESTER. Hypoxic vasoconstriction and fluid filtration in pig lungs. *J. Appl. Physiol.: Respirat. Environ. Exercise Physiol.* 51: 1065–1071, 1981.
336. MITZNER, W., J. T. SYLVESTER, AND Y. K. NGEOW. Evidence for hypoxic constriction of alveolar vessels (Abstract). *Physiologist* 23: 154, 1980.
337. MODELL, H. I., K. BECK, AND J. BUTLER. Functional aspects of canine bronchial-pulmonary vascular communications. *J. Appl. Physiol.: Respirat. Environ. Exercise Physiol.* 50: 1045–1051, 1981.
338. MOORE, L. G., I. F. MCMURTRY, AND J. T. REEVES. Effects of sex hormones on cardiovascular and hematologic responses to chronic hypoxia in rats. *Proc. Soc. Exp. Biol. Med.* 158: 658–662, 1978.
339. MOORE, L. G., AND J. T. REEVES. Pregnancy blunts pulmonary vascular reactivity in dogs. *Am. J. Physiol.* 239 (*Heart Circ. Physiol.* 8): H297–H301, 1980.
340. MORET, P. R. Coronary blood flow and myocardial metabolism in man at high altitude. In: *High Altitude Physiology. Cardiac and Respiratory Aspects*, edited by R. Porter and J. Knight. London: Churchill Livingstone, 1971, p. 131–148. (Ciba Found. Symp.)
341. MORET, P., E. COVARRUBIAS, J. COUDERT, AND F. DUCHOSAL. Cardiocirculatory adaptation to chronic hypoxia: comparative study of coronary flow, myocardial oxygen consumption and efficiency between sea level and high altitude residents. *Acta*

Cardiol. 27: 283-305, 1972.
342. MORKIN, E., J. A. COLLINS, H. S. GOLDMAN, AND A. P. FISHMAN. Pattern of blood flow in the pulmonary veins of the dog. *J. Appl. Physiol.* 20: 1118-1128, 1965.
343. MORKIN, E., O. R. LEVINE, AND A. P. FISHMAN. Pulmonary capillary flow pulse and the site of pulmonary vasoconstriction in the dog. *Circ. Res.* 15: 146-160, 1964.
344. MORRIS, H. R., P. J. PIPER, G. W. TAYLOR, AMD J. R. TIPPINS. The role of arachidonate lipoxygenase in the release of SRS-A from guinea-pig chopped lung. *Prostaglandins* 19: 371-383, 1980.
345. MOTULSKY, J. H., M. D. SNAVELY, R. J. HUGHES, AND P. A. INSEL. Interaction of verapamil and other calcium channel blockers with α_1- and α_2-adrenergic receptors. *Circ. Res.* 52: 226-231, 1983.
346. NAKAMURA, T., S. NAKAMURA, T. TAZAWA, S. ABE, T. AIKAWA, AND K. TOKITA. Measurement of blood flow through portopulmonary anastomosis in portal hypertension. *J. Lab. Clin. Med.* 65: 114-121, 1965.
347. NANDIWADA, P. A., A. L. HYMAN, AND P. J. KADOWITZ. Pulmonary vasodilator responses to vagal stimulation and acetylcholine in the cat. *Circ. Res.* 53: 86-95, 1983.
348. NAYAR, H. S., R. M. MATHUR, AND V. V. RANADE. The role of serotonin (5-hydroxytryptamine) in the pulmonary arterial pressor response during acute hypoxia. *Indian J. Med. Res.* 60: 1665-1673, 1972.
349. NEWELL, J. C., M. G. LEVITZKY, J. A. KRASNEY, AND R. E. DUTTON. Phasic reflux of pulmonary blood flow in atelectasis: influence of systemic Po_2. *J. Appl. Physiol.* 40: 883-888, 1976.
350. NEWMAN, J. H., N. F. VOELKEL, C. M. ARROYAVE, AND J. T. REEVES. Distribution of mast cells and histamine in canine pulmonary arteries. *Respir. Physiol.* 40: 191-198, 1980.
351. NIHILL, M. R., D. G. MCNAMARA, AND R. L. VICK. The effects of increased blood viscosity on pulmonary vascular resistance. *Am. Heart J.* 92: 65-72, 1976.
352. OKADA, R. D., G. M. POHOST, H. D. KIRSHENBAUM, F. G. KUSHNER, C. A. BOUCHER, P. C. BLOCK, AND H. W. STRAUSS. Radionuclide-determined change in pulmonary blood volume with exercise. Improved sensitivity of multigated blood-pool scanning in detecting coronary-artery disease. *N. Engl. J. Med.* 301: 569-576, 1979.
353. OLLEY, P. M., AND F. COCEANI. Prostaglandins and the ductus arteriosus. *Annu. Rev. Med.* 32: 375-385, 1981.
354. ORCHARD, C. H., R. S. DE LEON, AND M. K. SYKES. The relationship between hypoxic pulmonary vasoconstriction and arterial oxygen tension in the intact dog. *J. Physiol. London* 338: 64-74, 1983.
355. O'ROURKE, M. F. Vascular impedance in studies of arterial and cardiac function. *Physiol. Rev.* 62: 570-623, 1982.
356. OSSWALD, W., AND S. GUIMARAES. Adrenergic mechanisms in blood vessels: morphological and pharmacological aspects. *Rev. Physiol. Biochem. Pharmacol.* 96: 54-122, 1983.
357. OVERHOLSER, K. A., J. BHATTACHARYA, AND N. C. STAUB. Microvascular pressures in the isolated, perfused dog lung: comparison between theory and measurement. *Microvasc. Res.* 23: 67-76, 1982.
358. OVERLAND, E. S., R. N. GUPTA, G. J. HUCHON, AND J. F. MURRAY. Measurement of pulmonary tissue volume and blood flow in persons with normal and edematous lungs. *J. Appl. Physiol.: Respirat. Environ. Exercise Physiol.* 51: 1375-1383, 1981.
359. OWEN, D. A. A. Histamine receptors in the cardiovascular system. *Gen. Pharmacol.* 8: 141-156, 1977.
360. PACE, J. B., R. H. COX, F. ALVAREZ-VARA, AND G. KARREMAN. Influence of sympathetic nerve stimulation on pulmonary hydraulic input power. *Am. J. Physiol.* 222: 196-201, 1972.
361. PARKER, J. C., A. C. GUYTON, AND A. E. TAYLOR. Pulmonary interstitial and capillary pressures estimated from intra-alveolar fluid pressures. *J. Appl. Physiol.: Respirat. Environ. Exercise Physiol.* 44: 267-276, 1978.
363. PARKER, J. C., P. R. KVIETYS, K. P. RYAN, AND A. E. TAYLOR. Comparison of isogravimetric and venous occlusion capillary pressures in isolated dog lungs. *J. Appl. Physiol.: Respirat. Environ. Exercise Physiol.* 55: 964-968, 1983.
364. PARKER, J. C., R. E. PARKER, D. N. GRANGER, AND A. E. TAYLOR. Vertical gradient in regional vascular resistance and pre to postcapillary resistance ratios in the dog lung. *Lymphology* 12: 191-200, 1979.
365. PARKER, R. E., D. N. GRANGER, B. H. COOK, H. J. GRANGER, AND A. E. TAYLOR. A histochemical analysis of vascular and nonvascular smooth muscles in the canine lung. *Microvasc. Res.* 18: 167-174, 1979.
366. PARKER, R. E., D. N. GRANGER, AND A. E. TAYLOR. Estimates of isogravimetric capillary pressures during alveolar hypoxia. *Am. J. Physiol.* 241 (*Heart Circ. Physiol.* 10): H732-H739, 1981.
367. PARRATT, J. R., AND R. M. STURGESS. Evidence that prostaglandin release mediates pulmonary vasoconstriction induced by *E. coli* endotoxin (Abstract). *J. Physiol. London* 246: 79P-80P, 1975.
368. PATEL, D. J., D. P. SCHILDER, AND A. J. MALLOS. Mechanical properties and dimensions of the major pulmonary arteries. *J. Appl. Physiol.* 15: 92-96, 1960.
369. PEAKE, M. D., A. L. HARABIN, N. J. BRENNAN, AND J. T. SYLVESTER. Steady-state vascular responses to graded hypoxia in isolated lungs of five species. *J. Appl. Physiol.: Respirat. Environ. Exercise Physiol.* 51: 1214-1219, 1981.
370. PEASE, R. D., J. L. BENUMOF, AND F. R. TROUSDALE. Pa_{O_2} and $P\bar{v}_{O_2}$ interaction on hypoxic pulmonary vasoconstriction. *J. Appl. Physiol.: Respirat. Environ. Exercise Physiol.* 53: 134-139, 1982.
371. PEÑALOZA, D., AND R. GAMBOA. Hipertension pulmonar. In: *Cardiología Pediátrica*. Madrid: Salvat, in press.
372. PEÑALOZA, D., I. SIME, N. BANCHERO, AND R. GAMBOA. Pulmonary hypertension in healthy men born and living at high altitude. *Am. J. Cardiol.* 11: 150-157, 1963.
373. PERMUTT, S., B. BROMBERGER-BARNEA, AND H. N. BANE. Alveolar pressure, pulmonary venous pressure and the vascular waterfall. *Med. Thorac.* 19: 239-260, 1962.
374. PERMUTT, S., P. CALDINI, A. MASERI, W. H. PALMER, T. SASAMORI, AND K. ZIERLER. Recruitment versus distensibility in the pulmonary vascular bed. In: *Pulmonary Circulation and Interstitial Space*, edited by A. P. Fishman and H. H. Hecht. Chicago, IL: Univ. of Chicago Press, 1969, p. 375-387.
375. PERMUTT, S., J. B. L. HOWELL, D. F. PROCTOR, AND R. L. RILEY. Effect of lung inflation on static pressure-volume characteristics of pulmonary vessels. *J. Appl. Physiol.* 16: 64-70, 1961.
376. PEROUTKA, S. J., AND S. H. SNYDER. Multiple serotonin receptors: differential binding of [^{3}H]5-hydroxytryptamine, [^{3}H]lysergic acid diethylamide and [^{3}H]spiroperidol. *Mol. Pharmacol.* 16: 687-699, 1979.
377. PERRAULT, J. L., J. MORINET, F. A. NADER, AND A. LOCKHART. Influence de l'age et de l'exercice physique sur les pressions dans la circulation pulmonaire de sujects normaux ages de plus de quarante ans. *Bull. Physio-Pathol. Respir.* 5: 505-522, 1969.
378. PETERSON, J. W., AND R. J. PAUL. Aerobic glycolysis in vascular smooth muscle: relation to isometric tension. *Biochim. Biophys. Acta* 357: 167-176, 1974.
379. PETRINI, M. F., B. T. PETERSON, AND R. W. HYDE. Lung tissue volume and blood flow by rebreathing: theory. *J. Appl. Physiol.: Respirat. Environ. Exercise Physiol.* 44: 795-802, 1978.
380. PIENE, H. The influence of pulmonary blood flow rate on vascular input impedance and hydraulic power in the sympathetically and noradrenaline stimulated cat lung. *Acta Physiol. Scand.* 98: 44-53, 1976.
381. PIENE, H. Influence of vessel distension and myogenic tone on pulmonary arterial input impedance. A study using a computer model of rabbit lung. *Acta Physiol. Scand.* 98: 54-66, 1976.
382. PIENE, H., AND T. SUND. Flow and power output of right ventricle facing load with variable input impedance. *J. Appl. Physiol.* 237 (*Heart Circ. Physiol.* 6): H125-H130, 1979.

383. PIETRA, G. G., M. MAGNO, L. JOHNS, AND A. P. FISHMAN. Bronchial veins and pulmonary edema. In: *Pulmonary Edema*, edited by A. P. Fishman and E. M. Renkin. Bethesda, MD: Am. Physiol. Soc., 1979, p. 195–206.
384. PIETRA, G. G., J. P. SZIDON, M. M. LEVENTHAL, AND A. P. FISHMAN. Histamine and interstitial pulmonary edema in the dog. *Circ. Res.* 29: 323–337, 1971.
385. PIIPER, J. Grosse des Arterien-, des Capillar- und des Venenvolumens in der isolierten Hundelunge. *Pfluegers Arch. Gesamite Physiol. Menschen Tiere* 269: 182–193, 1959.
386. PINSKY, M. R., W. R. SUMMER, R. A. WISE, S. PERMUTT, AND B. BROMBERGER-BARNEA. Augmentation of cardiac function by elevation of intrathoracic pressure. *J. Appl. Physiol.: Respirat. Environ. Exercise Physiol.* 54: 950–955, 1983.
387. PIRLO, A. F., J. L. BENUMOF, AND F. R. TROUSDALE. Atelectatic lobe blood flow: open vs. closed chest, positive pressure vs. spontaneous ventilation. *J. Appl. Physiol.: Respirat. Environ. Exercise Physiol.* 50: 1022–1026, 1981.
388. PORCELLI, R. J., AND E. H. BERGOFSKY. Adrenergic receptors in pulmonary vasoconstrictor responses to gaseous and humoral agents. *J. Appl. Physiol.* 34: 483–488, 1973.
389. POULEUR, H., J. LEFEVRE, C. VAN EYLL, P. M. JAUMIN, AND A. A. CHARLIER. Significance of pulmonary input impedance in right ventricular performance. *Cardiovasc. Res.* 12: 617–629, 1978.
390. QUEBBEMAN, E. J., AND C. A. DAWSON. Influence of inflation and atelectasis on the hypoxic pressor response in isolated dog lung lobes. *Cardiovasc. Res.* 10: 672–677, 1976.
391. QVIST, J., H. PONTOPPIDAN, R. S. WILSON, E. LOWENSTEIN, AND M. B. LAVER. Hemodynamic responses to mechanical ventilation with PEEP. *Anesthesiology* 42: 45–55, 1975.
392. RABINOVITCH, M., W. J. GAMBLE, O. S. MIETTINEN, AND L. REID. Age and sex influence on pulmonary hypertension of chronic hypoxia and on recovery. *Am. J. Physiol.* 240 (*Heart Circ. Physiol.* 9): H62–H72, 1981.
393. RABINOVITCH, M., W. GAMBLE, A. S. NADAS, O. S. MIETTINEN, AND L. REID. Rat pulmonary circulation after chronic hypoxia: hemodynamic and structural features. *Am. J. Physiol.* 236 (*Heart Circ. Physiol.* 5): H818–H827, 1979.
394. RABINOVITCH, M., M. A. KONSTAM, W. J. GAMBLE, N. PAPANICOLAU, S. TREVES, AND L. REID. Changes in pulmonary blood flow affect vascular response to chronic hypoxia in rat. *Circ. Res.* 52: 432–441, 1983.
395. RAJAGOPALAN, B., C. D. BERTRAM, T. STALLARD, AND G. DE J. LEE. Blood flow in pulmonary veins. III. Simultaneous measurements of their dimensions, intravascular pressure and flow. *Cardiovasc. Res.* 13: 684–692, 1979.
396. REEVES, J. T., R. F. GROVER, G. F. FILLEY, AND S. G. BLOUNT, JR. Circulatory changes in man during mild supine exercise. *J. Appl. Physiol.* 16: 279–282, 1961.
397. REEVES, J. T., AND B. M. GROVES. Approach to the patient with pulmonary hypertension. In: *Pulmonary Hypertension*, edited by E. K. Weir and J. T. Reeves. Mount Kisco, NY: Futura, 1984, p. 1–44.
398. REEVES, J. T., P. JOKL, J. MERIDA, AND J. E. LEATHERS. Pulmonary vascular obstruction following administration of high-energy nucleotides. *J. Appl. Physiol.* 22: 475–479, 1967.
399. REEVES, J. T., W. W. WAGNER, JR., I. F. MCMURTRY, AND R. F. GROVER. Physiological effects of high altitude on the pulmonary circulation. In: *Environmental Physiology III*, edited by D. Robertshaw. Baltimore, MD: University Park, 1979, vol. 20, p. 289–310. (Int. Rev. Physiol. Ser.)
400. REGOLI, D., J. MIZRAHI, P. D'ORLEANS-JUSTE, AND S. CARANIKAS. Effects of kinins on isolated blood vessels. Role of endothelium. *Can. J. Physiol. Pharmacol.* 60: 1580–1583, 1982.
401. REID, L. M. The pulmonary circulation remodeling in growth and disease. *Am. Rev. Respir. Dis.* 119: 531–546, 1979.
402. REID, L., AND B. MEYRICK. Hypoxia and pulmonary vascular endothelium. In: *Metabolic Activities of the Lung*. Amsterdam: Excerpta Med., 1980, p. 37–60. (Ciba Found. Symp. 78.)
403. REMY, J., A. ARNAUD, H. FARDOU, R. GIRAUD, AND C. VOISIN. Treatment of hemoptysis by embolization of bronchial arteries. *Radiology* 122: 33–37, 1977.
404. REUBEN, S. R. Wave transmission in the pulmonary arterial system in disease in man. *Circ. Res.* 27: 523–529, 1970.
405. REUBEN, S. R. Compliance of the human pulmonary arterial system in disease. *Circ. Res.* 29: 40–50, 1971.
406. REUBEN, S. R., B. J. GERSH, J. P. SWADLING, AND G. DE J. LEE. Measurement of pulmonary arterial distensibility. *Cardiovasc. Res.* 4: 473–481, 1970.
407. REUBEN, S. R., J. P. SWADLING, B. J. GERSH, AND G. DE J. LEE. Impedance and transmission properties of the pulmonary arterial system. *Cardiovasc. Res.* 5: 1–9, 1971.
408. RICKABY, D. A., C. A. DAWSON, AND M. B. MARON. Pulmonary inactivation of serotonin and site of serotonin pulmonary vasoconstriction. *J. Appl. Physiol.: Respirat. Environ. Exercise Physiol.* 48: 606–612, 1980.
409. RICKABY, D. A., J. H. LINEHAN, T. A. BRONIKOWSKI, AND C. A. DAWSON. Kinetics of serotonin uptake in the dog lung. *J. Appl. Physiol.: Respirat. Environ. Exercise Physiol.* 51: 405–414, 1981.
410. RILEY, R. L. Effect of lung inflation upon the pulmonary vascular bed. In: *Pulmonary Structure and Function*, edited by A. V. S. de Reuck and M. O'Connor. Boston, MA: Little, Brown, 1962, p. 261–272. (Ciba Found. Symp.)
411. ROBOTHAM, J. L., W. LIXFELD, L. HOLLAND, D. MACGREGOR, B. BROMBERGER-BARNEA, S. PERMUTT, AND J. L. RABSON. The effects of positive end-expiratory pressure on right and left ventricular performance. *Am. Rev. Respir. Dis.* 121: 677–683, 1980.
412. RODBARD, S., AND H. MURAO. Ventilatory effects on pulmonary vascular inflow and outflow patterns. *Cardiovasc. Res.* 11: 177–186, 1977.
413. ROOS, S. D., E. K. WEIR, AND J. T. REEVES. Meclofenamate does not reduce chronic hypoxic pulmonary vasoconstriction. *Experientia* 32: 195–196, 1976.
414. RORIE, D. K., AND G. M. TYCE. Effects of hypoxia on norepinephrine release and metabolism in dog pulmonary artery. *J. Appl. Physiol.: Respirat. Environ. Exercise Physiol.* 55: 750–758, 1983.
415. ROSE, C. E., JR., J. A. ALTHAUS, D. L. KAISER, E. D. MILLER, AND R. M. CAREY. Acute hypoxemia and hypercapnia: increase in plasma catecholamines in conscious dogs. *Am. J. Physiol.* 245 (*Heart Circ. Physiol.* 14): H924–H929, 1983.
416. ROSENZWEIG, D. Y., J. M. B. HUGHES, AND J. B. GLAZIER. Effects of transpulmonary and vascular pressures on pulmonary blood volume in isolated lung. *J. Appl. Physiol.* 28: 553–560, 1970.
417. ROTTA, A., A. CÁNEPA, A. HURTADO, T. VELÁSQUEZ, AND R. CHÁVEZ. Pulmonary circulation at sea level and at high altitudes. *J. Appl. Physiol.* 9: 328–336, 1956.
418. ROUNDS, S., AND I. F. MCMURTRY. Inhibitors of oxidative ATP production cause transient vasoconstriction and block subsequent pressor responses in rat lungs. *Circ. Res.* 48: 393–400, 1981.
419. ROUNDS, S., I. F. MCMURTRY, AND J. T. REEVES. Glucose metabolism accelerates the decline of hypoxic vasoconstriction in rat lungs. *Respir. Physiol.* 44: 239–249, 1981.
420. RUBIN, L. J., AND J. D. LAZAR. Influence of prostaglandin synthesis inhibitors on pulmonary vasodilatory effects of hydralazine in dogs with hypoxic pulmonary vasoconstriction. *J. Clin. Invest.* 67: 193–200, 1981.
421. RUBIN, L. J., AND J. D. LAZAR. Nonadrenergic effects of isoproterenol in dogs with hypoxic pulmonary vasoconstriction. Possible role of prostaglandins. *J. Clin. Invest.* 71: 1366–1374, 1983.
422. RUDOLPH, A. M. Fetal and neonatal pulmonary circulation. *Am. Rev. Respir. Dis.* 115: 11–18, 1977.
423. RUDOLPH, A. M. Fetal and neonatal pulmonary circulation. *Annu. Rev. Physiol.* 41: 383–395, 1979.
424. RUDOLPH, A. M., P. A. M. AULD, R. J. GOLINKO, AND M. H. PAUL. Pulmonary vascular adjustments in the neonatal period. *Pediatrics* 28: 28–34, 1961.
425. RUDOLPH, A. M., M. A. HEYMANN, AND A. B. LEWIS. Physi-

ology and pharmacology of the pulmonary circulation in the fetus and newborn. In: *Lung Biology in Health and Disease. Development of the Lung*, edited by W. A. Hodson. New York: Dekker, 1977, vol. 6, chapt. 14, p. 497–523.

426. RUDOLPH, A. M., AND S. YUAN. Response of the pulmonary vasculature to hypoxia and H+ ion concentration changes. *J. Clin. Invest.* 45: 399–411, 1966.

427. RUIZ, A. V., G. E. BISGARD, AND J. A. WILL. Hemodynamic responses to hypoxia and hyperoxia in calves at sea level and altitude. *Pfluegers Arch.* 344: 275–286, 1973.

428. RYAN, K., P. KVIETYS, J. C. PARKER, AND A. E. TAYLOR. Comparison of venous occlusion and isogravimetric capillary pressures in isolated dog lungs (Abstract). *Physiologist* 23: 76, 1980.

429. SAID, S. I. Pulmonary metabolism of prostaglandins and vasoactive peptides. *Annu. Rev. Physiol.* 44: 257–268, 1982.

430. SAID, S. I. Vasodilator action of VIP: introduction and general considerations. In: *Vasoactive Intestinal Peptide*, edited by S. I. Said. New York: Raven, 1982, p. 145–148.

431. SAID, S. I., T. YOSHIDA, S. KITAMURA, AND C. VREIM. Pulmonary alveolar hypoxia: release of prostaglandins and other humoral mediators. *Science* 185: 1181–1183, 1974.

432. SALDANA, M. E., R. A. HARLEY, A. A. LIEBOW, AND C. B. CARRINGTON. Experimental extreme pulmonary hypertension and vascular disease in relation to polycythemia. *Am. J. Pathol.* 52: 935–981, 1968.

433. SALISBURY, P. F., P. WEIL, AND D. STATE. Factors influencing collateral blood flow to the dog's lung. *Circ. Res.* 5: 303–309, 1957.

434. SAMUELSSON, B. Leukotrienes: mediators of immediate hypersensitivity reactions and inflammation. *Science* 220: 568–575, 1983.

435. SHAW, J. W. Pulmonary vasodilator and vasoconstrictor actions of histamine (Abstract). *J. Physiol. London* 215: 34P–35P, 1971.

436. SHELUB, I., A. VAN GRONDELLE, R. MCCULLOUGH, S. HOFMEISTER, AND J. T. REEVES. A model of embolic chronic pulmonary hypertension in the dog. *J. Appl. Physiol.: Respirat. Environ. Exercise Physiol.* 56: 810–815, 1984.

437. SHETTIGAR, U. R., H. N. HULTGREN, M. SPECTER, R. MARTIN, AND D. H. DAVIES. Primary pulmonary hypertension: favorable effect of isoproterenol. *N. Engl. J. Med.* 295: 1414–1415, 1976.

438. SHOUKAS, A. S. Pressure-flow and pressure-volume relations in the entire pulmonary vascular bed of the dog determined by two-part analysis. *Circ. Res.* 37: 809–818, 1975.

439. SIEGELMAN, S. S., J. W. C. HAGSTROM, S. K. KOERNER, AND F. J. VEITH. Restoration of bronchial artery circulation after canine lung allotransplantation. *J. Thorac. Cardiovasc. Surg.* 73: 792–795, 1977.

440. SILOVE, E. D., AND R. F. GROVER. Effects of alpha adrenergic blockade and tissue catecholamine depletion on pulmonary vascular responses to hypoxia. *J. Clin. Invest.* 47: 274–285, 1968.

441. SILOVE, E. D., T. INOUE, AND R. F. GROVER. Comparison of hypoxia, pH, and sympathomimetic drugs on bovine pulmonary vasculature. *J. Appl. Physiol.* 24: 355–365, 1968.

442. SINGHAL, S., R. HENDERSON, K. HORSFELD, K. HARDING, AND G. CUMMING. Morphometry of the human pulmonary arterial tree. *Circ. Res.* 33: 190–197, 1973.

443. SKALAK, R., F. WIENER, E. MORKIN, AND A. P. FISHMAN. The energy distribution in the pulmonary circulation. II. Experiments. *Phys. Med. Biol.* 11: 437–449, 1966.

444. SMITH, H. C., AND J. BUTLER. Pulmonary venous waterfall and perivenous pressure in the living dog. *J. Appl. Physiol.* 38: 304–308, 1975.

445. SMITH, P., AND D. HEATH. Ultrastructure of hypoxic hypertensive pulmonary vascular disease. *J. Pathol.* 121: 93–100, 1977.

446. SMITH, P., H. MOOSAVI, M. WINSON, AND D. HEATH. The influence of age and sex on the response of the right ventricle, pulmonary vasculature and carotid bodies to hypoxia in rats. *J. Pathol.* 112: 11–18, 1974.

447. SNAPPER, J. R., A. A. HUTCHISON, M. L. OGLETREE, AND K. L. BRIGHAM. Effects of cyclooxygenase inhibitors on the alterations in lung mechanics caused by endotoxemia in the unanesthetized sheep. *J. Clin. Invest.* 72: 63–76, 1983.

449. SOBIN, S. S., H. M. TREMER, AND Y. C. FUNG. Morphometric basis of the sheet-flow concept of the pulmonary alveolar microcirculation in the cat. *Circ. Res.* 26: 397–414, 1970.

450. SOBIN, S. S., H. M. TREMER, J. D. HARDY, AND H. P. CHIODI. Changes in arteriole in acute and chronic hypoxic pulmonary hypertension and recovery in rat. *J. Appl. Physiol.: Respirat. Environ. Exercise Physiol.* 55: 1445–1455, 1983.

451. SOMLYO, A. P., AND A. V. SOMLYO. Vascular smooth muscle. II. Pharmacology of normal and hypertensive vessels. *Pharmacol. Rev.* 22: 249–353, 1970.

452. SOUHRADA, J. F., D. W. DICKEY, AND R. A. SCHULTZ. The role of substrate in the hypoxic response of the pulmonary artery. *Chest* 71: 252–253, 1977.

453. SPANNHAKE, E. W., A. L. HYMAN, AND P. J. KADOWITZ. Dependence of the airway and pulmonary vascular effects of arachidonic acid upon route and rate of administration. *J. Pharmacol. Exp. Ther.* 212: 584–590, 1980.

454. SPENCER, H., AND D. LEOF. The innervation of the human lung. *J. Anat.* 98: 559–609, 1964.

455. SPIRO, S. G., B. H. CULVER, AND J. BUTLER. Pressure outside the extrapulmonary airway in dogs. *J. Appl. Physiol.: Respirat. Environ. Exercise Physiol.* 45: 437–441, 1978.

456. SPRAGUE, R. S., A. H. STEPHENSON, L. J. HEITMANN, AND A. J. LONIGRO. Differential response of the pulmonary circulation to PGE_2 and $PGF_{2-\alpha}$ in the presence of unilateral alveolar hypoxia (Abstract). *Clin. Res.* 30: A784, 1982.

457. STALCUP, S. A., P. J. LEUENBERGER, J. S. LIPSET, M. M. OSMAN, J. M. CERRETA, R. B. MELLINS, AND G. M. TURINO. Impaired angiotensin conversion and bradykinin clearance in experimental canine pulmonary emphysema. *J. Clin. Invest.* 67: 201–209, 1981.

458. STANBROOK, H. S., AND I. F. MCMURTRY. Inhibition of glycolysis potentiates hypoxic vasoconstriction in rat lungs. *J. Appl. Physiol.: Respirat. Environ. Exercise Physiol.* 55: 1467–1473, 1983.

459. STERN, S., R. E. FERGUSON, AND E. RAPAPORT. Reflex pulmonary vasoconstriction due to stimulation of the aortic body by nicotine. *Am. J. Physiol.* 206: 1189–1195, 1964.

460. STOCKS, J., K. COSTELOE, C. P. WINLOVE, AND S. GODFREY. Measurement of pulmonary capillary blood flow in infants by plethysmography. *J. Clin. Invest.* 59: 490–499, 1977.

461. STRAWBRIDGE, H. T. G. Chronic pulmonary emphysema. An experimental study. *Am. J. Pathol.* 37: 161–174, 1960.

462. SU, C., AND J. A. BEVAN. Pharmacology of pulmonary blood vessels. *Pharmacol. Ther. B* 2: 275–288, 1976.

463. SUSMANO, A., AND R. A. CARLETON. Prevention of hypoxic pulmonary hypertension by chlorpheniramine. *J. Appl. Physiol.* 31: 531–535, 1971.

464. SUZUKI, H., AND B. M. TWAROG. Membrane properties of smooth muscle cells in pulmonary arteries of the rat. *Am. J. Physiol.* 242 (*Heart Circ. Physiol.* 11): H900–H906, 1982.

465. SUZUKI, H., AND B. M. TWAROG. Membrane properties of smooth muscle cells in pulmonary hypertensive rats. *Am. J. Physiol.* 242 (*Heart Circ. Physiol.* 11): H907–H915, 1982.

466. SVANBERG, L. Influence of posture on the lung volumes, ventilation and circulation in normals. *Scand. J. Clin. Lab. Invest. Suppl.* 25: 1–95, 1957.

467. SYLVESTER, J. T., A. L. HARABIN, M. D. PEAKE, AND R. S. FRANK. Vasodilator and constrictor responses to hypoxia in isolated pig lungs. *J. Appl. Physiol.: Respirat. Environ. Exercise Physiol.* 49: 820–825, 1980.

468. SYLVESTER, J. T., AND C. MCGOWAN. The effects of agents that bind to cytochrome P-450 on hypoxic pulmonary vasoconstriction. *Circ. Res.* 43: 429–437, 1978.

469. SYLVESTER, J. T., W. MITZNER, Y. NGEOW, AND S. PERMUTT. Hypoxic constriction of alveolar and extra-alveolar vessels in isolated pig lungs. *J. Appl. Physiol.: Respirat. Environ. Exercise*

Physiol. 54: 1660–1666, 1983.
470. SYLVESTER, J. T., S. M. SCHARF, R. D. GILBERT, R. S. FITZGERALD, AND R. J. TRAYSTMAN. Hypoxic and CO hypoxia in dogs: hemodynamics, carotid reflexes, and catecholamines. *Am. J. Physiol.* 236 (*Heart Circ. Physiol.* 5): H22–H28, 1979.
471. SZIDON, J. P., AND A. P. FISHMAN. Autonomic control of the pulmonary circulation. In: *Pulmonary Circulation and Interstitial Space*, edited by A. P. Fishman and H. H. Hecht. Chicago, IL: Univ. of Chicago Press, 1969, p. 239–268.
472. SZIDON, J. P., AND A. P. FISHMAN. Participation of pulmonary circulation in the defense reaction. *Am. J. Physiol.* 220: 364–370, 1971.
473. SZIDON, J. P., AND J. F. FLINT. Significance of sympathetic innervation of pulmonary vessels in response to acute hypoxia. *J. Appl. Physiol.: Respirat. Environ. Exercise Physiol.* 43: 65–71, 1977.
474. TAYLOR, C. R., AND E. R. WEIBEL. Design of the mammalian respiratory system. I. Problems and strategy. *Respir. Physiol.* 44: 1–10, 1981.
475. TENNEY, S. M. A comparative survey of the design of respiratory systems for gas exchange. In: *Pulmonary Diseases and Disorders*, edited by A. P. Fishman. New York: McGraw-Hill, 1980, p. 282–297.
476. THILENIUS, O. G., B. M. CANDIOLO, AND J. L. BEUG. Effect of adrenergic blockade on hypoxia-induced pulmonary vasoconstriction in awake dogs. *Am. J. Physiol.* 213: 990–998, 1967.
477. THILENIUS, O. G., AND C. DERENZO. Effects of acutely induced changes in arterial pH on pulmonary vascular resistance during normoxia and hypoxia in awake dogs. *Clin. Sci.* 42: 277–287, 1972.
478. THOMAS, H. M., III, AND R. C. GARRETT. Strength of hypoxic vasoconstriction determines shunt fraction in dogs with atelectasis. *J. Appl. Physiol.: Respirat. Environ. Exercise Physiol.* 53: 44–51, 1982.
479. THOMPSON, B., G. R. BARER, AND J. W. SHAW. The action of histamine on pulmonary vessels of cats and rats. *Clin. Exp. Pharmacol. Physiol.* 3: 399–414, 1976.
480. THOMPSON, J. H. Serotonin and the alimentary tract. *Res. Commun. Chem. Pathol. Pharmacol.* 2: 687–781, 1981.
481. TODD, T. R., E. M. BAILE, AND J. C. HOGG. Pulmonary arterial wedge pressure in hemorrhagic shock. *Am. Rev. Respir. Dis.* 118: 613–616, 1978.
482. TOOKER, J., J. HUSEBY, AND J. BUTLER. The effect of Swan-Ganz catheter height on the wedge pressure-left atrial pressure relationships in edema during positive-pressure ventilation. *Am. Rev. Respir. Dis.* 117: 721–725, 1978.
483. TORRANCE, R. W. The idea of a chemoreceptor. In: *Pulmonary Circulation and Interstitial Space*, edited by A. P. Fishman and H. H. Hecht. Chicago, IL: Univ. of Chicago Press, 1969, p. 223–237.
484. TUCKER, A., I. F. MCMURTRY, A. F. ALEXANDER, J. T. REEVES, AND R. F. GROVER. Lung mast cell density and distribution in chronically hypoxic animals. *J. Appl. Physiol.: Respirat. Environ. Exercise Physiol.* 42: 174–178, 1977.
485. TUCKER, A., I. F. MCMURTRY, J. T. REEVES, A. F. ALEXANDER, D. H. WILL, AND R. F. GROVER. Lung vascular smooth muscle as a determinant of pulmonary hypertension at high altitude. *Am. J. Physiol.* 228: 762–767, 1975.
486. TUCKER, A., E. K. WEIR, J. T. REEVES, AND R. F. GROVER. Histamine H_1- and H_2-receptors in pulmonary and systemic vasculature of the dog. *Am. J. Physiol.* 229: 1008–1013, 1975.
487. TUCKER, A., E. K. WEIR, J. T. REEVES, AND R. F. GROVER. Failure of histamine antagonists to prevent hypoxic pulmonary vasoconstriction in dogs. *J. Appl. Physiol.* 40: 496–500, 1976.
488. TURLAPATY, P. D. M. V., AND B. M. ALTURA. Extracellular magnesium ions control calcium exchange and content of vascular smooth muscle. *Eur. J. Pharmacol.* 52: 421–423, 1978.
489. TURNER, J. H., AND J. J. LALICH. Experimental cor pulmonale in the rat. *Arch. Pathol.* 79: 409–418, 1965.
490. TYLER, T., R. WALLIS, C. LEFFLER, AND S. CASSIN. The effects of indomethacin on the pulmonary vascular response to hypoxia in the premature and mature newborn goat. *Proc. Soc. Exp. Biol. Med.* 150: 695–698, 1975.
491. UNGER, M., M. ATKINS, W. A. BRISCOE, AND T. K. C. KING. Potentiation of pulmonary vasoconstrictor response with repeated intermittent hypoxia. *J. Appl. Physiol.: Respirat. Environ. Exercise Physiol.* 43: 662–667, 1977.
492. VAAGE, J., L. BJETNAES, AND A. HAUGE. The pulmonary vasoconstrictor response to hypoxia: effects of inhibitors of prostaglandin biosynthesis. *Acta Physiol. Scand.* 95: 95–101, 1975.
493. VAAGE, J., AND A. HAUGE. Prostaglandins and the pulmonary vasoconstrictor response to alveolar hypoxia. *Science* 189: 899–900, 1975.
494. VALDIVIA, E., Y. HAYASHI, J. J. LALICH, AND J. SONNAD. Capillary obstruction in experimental cor pulmonale (Abstract). *Circulation Suppl.* 32: 211, 1965.
495. VAN DEN BOS, G. C., N. WESTERHOF, AND O. S. RANDALL. Pulse wave reflection: can it explain the differences between systemic and pulmonary pressure and flow waves? *Circ. Res.* 51: 479–485, 1982.
496. VANE, J. R. Clinical potential of prostacyclin. In: *Advances in Prostaglandin, Thromboxane and Leukotriene Research*, edited by B. Samuelsson, R. Paoletti, and P. Ramwell. New York: Raven, 1982, vol. 11, p. 449–461.
497. VANE, J. R. Prostacyclin (Editorial). *J. R. Soc. Med.* 76: 245–249, 1983.
498. VAN NEUTEN, J. H., J. E. LEYSEN, J. A. J. SOHUURKES, AND P. M. VANHOUTTE. Ketanserum, a selective antagonist of 5-HT2 serotonergic receptors. *Lancet* 1: 297–298, 1983.
499. VERMEIRE, P., AND J. BUTLER. Effect of respiration on pulmonary capillary blood flow in man. *Circ. Res.* 22: 299–303, 1968.
500. VOELKEL, N. F., J. G. GERBER, I. F. MCMURTRY, A. S. NIES, AND J. T. REEVES. Release of vasodilator prostaglandin, PGI_2, from isolated rat lung during vasoconstriction. *Circ. Res.* 48: 207–213, 1981.
501. VOELKEL, N. F., I. MCMURTRY, AND J. REEVES. High extracellular calcium causes pulmonary vasodilation by stimulating Na + K + ATPase. Symposium on the mechanism of vasodilation (Abstract). *Blood Vessels* 17: 168, 1980.
502. VOELKEL, N. F., R. D. OLSON, I. F. MCMURTRY, AND J. T. REEVES. Vanadate potentiates hypoxic pulmonary vasoconstriction (Abstract). *Federation Proc.* 39: 766, 1980.
503. VOGEL, J. H. K., W. F. WEAVER, R. L. ROSE, S. G. BLOUNT, AND R. F. GROVER. Pulmonary hypertension and exertion in normal man living at 10,150 feet. *Med. Thorac.* 19: 461–477, 1962.
504. VREIM, C. E., AND N. C. STAUB. Indirect and direct pulmonary capillary blood volume in anesthetized open-thorax cats. *J. Appl. Physiol.* 34: 452–459, 1973.
505. VREIM, C. E., AND N. C. STAUB. Pulmonary vascular pressures and capillary blood volume changes in anesthetized cats. *J. Appl. Physiol.* 36: 275–279, 1974.
506. VUORI, A. Central hemodynamics, oxygen transport and oxygen consumption during three methods for CPAP. *Acta Anaesthesiol. Scand.* 25: 376–380, 1981.
507. WAGENVOORT, C. A., AND N. WAGENVOORT. *Pathology of Pulmonary Hypertension*. New York: Wiley, 1977, 345 p.
508. WAGNER, W. W., JR., AND L. P. LATHAM. Vasomotion in the pulmonary microcirculation. In: *Small Vessel Angiography. Imaging, Morphology, Physiology, and Clinical Applications*, edited by B. K. Hilal and S. Baum. St. Louis, MO: Mosby, 1973, p. 301–306. (Symp. Radiological Res., 3rd, Glen Cove, NY, 1972.)
509. WAGNER, W. W., JR., L. P. LATHAM, M. N. GILLESPIE, AND J. P. GUENTHER. Direct measurement of pulmonary capillary transit times. *Science* 218: 379–381, 1982.
510. WALCOTT, G., H. B. BURCHELL, AND A. L. BROWN. Primary pulmonary hypertension. *Am. J. Med.* 49: 70–79, 1970.
511. WANNER, A., R. BEGIN, M. COHN, AND M. A. SACKNER.

Vascular volumes of the pulmonary circulation in intact dogs. *J. Appl. Physiol.: Respirat. Environ. Exercise Physiol.* 44: 956–963, 1978.

512. WARRELL, D. A., J. W. EVANS, R. O. CLARKE, G. P. KINGABY, AND J. B. WEST. Pattern of filling in the pulmonary capillary bed. *J. Appl. Physiol.* 32: 346–356, 1972.

513. WEIBEL, E. R. *Morphometry of the Human Lung.* Heidelberg: Springer-Verlag, 1963.

514. WEIBEL, E. R. On pericytes, particularly their existence on lung capillaries. *Microvasc. Res.* 8: 218–235, 1974.

515. WEIBEL, E. R. Design and structure of the human lung. In: *Pulmonary Diseases and Disorders*, edited by A. P. Fishman. New York: McGraw-Hill, 1980. p. 224–271.

516. WEIBEL, E. R., AND J. GIL. Structure-function relationships at the alveolar level. In: *Lung Biology in Health and Disease. Bioengineering Aspects of the Lung*, edited by J. B. West. New York: Dekker, 1977, vol. 3, chapt. 1, p. 1–81.

517. WEIR, E. K., I. F. MCMURTRY, A. TUCKER, J. T. REEVES, AND R. F. GROVER. Prostaglandin synthetase inhibitors do not decrease hypoxic pulmonary vasoconstriction. *J. Appl. Physiol.* 41: 714–718, 1976.

518. WEIR, E. K., J. T. REEVES, AND R. F. GROVER. Prostaglandin E_1 inhibits the pulmonary vascular pressor response to hypoxia and prostaglandin $F_{2-\alpha}$. *Prostaglandins* 10: 623–631, 1975.

519. WEIR, E. K., A. TUCKER, J. T. REEVES, D. H. WILL, AND R. F. GROVER. The genetic factor influencing pulmonary hypertension in cattle at high altitude. *Cardiovasc. Res.* 8: 745–749, 1974.

520. WEIR, E. K., D. H. WILL, A. F. ALEXANDER, I. F. MCMURTRY, R. LOOGA, J. T. REEVES, AND R. F. GROVER. Vascular hypertrophy in cattle susceptible to hypoxic pulmonary hypertension. *J. Appl. Physiol.: Respirat. Environ. Exercise Physiol.* 46: 517–521, 1979.

521. WEISKOPF, R. B., AND J. W. SEVERINGHAUS. Diffusing capacity of the lung for CO in man during acute acclimation to 14,246 ft. *J. Appl. Physiol.* 32: 285–289, 1972.

522. WEST, J. B. *Regional Differences in the Lung.* New York: Academic, 1977, p. 85–165.

523. WEST, J. B., AND C. T. DOLLERY. Distribution of blood flow and the pressure-flow relations of the whole lung. *J. Appl. Physiol.* 20: 175–183, 1965.

524. WEST, J. B., C. T. DOLLERY, AND A. NAIMARK. Distribution of blood flow in isolated lung: relation to vascular and alveolar pressures. *J. Appl. Physiol.* 19: 713–724, 1964.

525. WEST, J. B., A. M. SCHNEIDER, AND M. M. MITCHELL. Recruitment in networks of pulmonary capillaries. *J. Appl. Physiol.* 39: 976–984, 1975.

526. WETZEL, R. C., AND J. T. SYLVESTER. Gender differences in hypoxic vascular response of isolated sheep lungs. *J. Appl. Physiol.: Respirat. Environ. Exercise Physiol.* 55: 100–104, 1983.

527. WIENER, F., E. MORKIN, R. SKALAK, AND A. P. FISHMAN. Wave propagation in the pulmonary circulation. *Circ. Res.* 19: 834–850, 1966.

528. WILL, D. H., I. F. MCMURTRY, J. T. REEVES, AND R. F. GROVER. Cold-induced pulmonary hypertension in cattle. *J. Appl. Physiol.: Respirat. Environ. Exercise Physiol.* 45: 469–473, 1978.

529. WILLIAMS, A., D. HEATH, P. HARRIS, D. WILLIAMS, AND P. SMITH. Pulmonary mast cells in cattle and llamas at high altitude. *J. Pathol.* 134: 1–16, 1981.

530. WOODS, J. R., JR., C. R. BRINKMAN III, A. DANDAVINO, K. MURAYAMA, AND N. S. ASSALI. Action of histamine and H_1 and H_2 blockers on the cardiopulmonary circulation. *Am. J. Physiol.* 232 (*Heart Circ. Physiol.* 1): H73–H78, 1977.

531. YOKOCHI, K., P. M. OLLEY, E. SIDEIS, F. HAMILTON, D. HUHTANER, AND F. COCEANI. Leukotriene D_4: a potent vasoconstrictor of the pulmonary and systemic circulations in the newborn lamb. In: *Advances in Prostaglandin, Thromboxane and Leukotriene Research*, edited by B. Samuelsson and R. Paoletti. New York: Raven, 1981, vol. 11, p. 211–214.

532. YU, P. N. *Pulmonary Blood Volume in Health and Disease.* Philadelphia, PA: Lea & Febiger, 1969.

533. ZAPOL, W. M., AND M. T. SNIDER. Pulmonary hypertension in severe acute respiratory failure. *N. Engl. J. Med.* 296: 476–480, 1977.

534. ZASSLOW, M. A., J. L. BENUMOF, AND F. R. TROUSDALE. Hypoxic pulmonary vasoconstriction and the size of hypoxic compartment. *J. Appl. Physiol.: Respirat. Environ. Exercise Physiol.* 53: 626–630, 1982.

535. ZHU, Y. J., R. KRADIN, R. D. BRANDSTETTER, G. STATON, J. MOSS, AND C. A. HALES. Hypoxic pulmonary hypertension in the mast cell-deficient mouse. *J. Appl. Physiol.: Respirat. Environ. Exercise Physiol.* 54: 680–686, 1983.

536. ZHUANG, F. Y., Y. C. FUNG, AND R. T. YEN. Analysis of blood flow in cat's lung with detailed anatomical and elasticity data. *J. Appl. Physiol.: Respirat. Environ. Exercise Physiol.* 55: 1341–1348, 1983.

537. ZUCKER, M. B. The platelet release reactions. In: *Platelets, Drugs, and Thrombosis*, edited by J. Hirsch, J. F. Cade, A. S. Gallus, and E. Schonbaum. Basel: Karger, 1975, p. 27–34.

CHAPTER 4

Pulmonary interstitial spaces and lymphatics

AUBREY E. TAYLOR | *Department of Physiology, University of South Alabama*
JAMES C. PARKER | *School of Medicine, Mobile, Alabama*

CHAPTER CONTENTS

Structure and Composition of Pulmonary Interstitium
  Pulmonary interstitial connective tissues
  Physicochemical properties of interstitial matrix
  Vascular and extravascular fluid compartments in the lung
  Effect of increased hydration on tissue fluid compartments
Starling Forces and Lymph Flow
  Theoretical considerations
  Endothelial pathways
  Filtration coefficient
    Gravimetric procedures
    Estimation of capillary filtration coefficients with Starling equation
    Estimation of changes in plasma-bound dye concentrations
    Estimation of capillary filtration coefficients with maximal filtration rates
  Capillary pressure
  Tissue fluid pressure
    Measurement theories
    Measurement of average interstitial pressure
    Estimation of average interstitial fluid pressure by analysis of transcapillary forces
    Calculation of perivascular pressure with mechanical stress analyses
    Measurement of hilar perivascular fluid pressure
    Measurement of septal perivascular fluid pressure
    Estimation of intra-alveolar fluid pressure by analysis of structure
    Effect of interdependence on interstitial fluid pressure
  Interstitial compliance
  Interstitial fluid pressure gradients
  Colloid osmotic pressure gradient
    Measurement of capillary selectivity to plasma proteins
    Effect of increasing capillary pressure on the colloid osmotic gradient
    Equilibration times of proteins between plasma and lymph
  Lymph flow
    Formation of lymph
    Effect of increased capillary pressure on lymph flow
    Mechanisms of lymph propulsion
    Effect of lymphatic obstruction
    Effect of airway pressure on capillary filtration
  Analyses of force changes during formation of alveolar edema: edema safety factor
Abnormal Capillary Permeability to Plasma Proteins (Leaky Lung Syndromes)
  α-Naphthylthiourea
  Hydrochloric acid aspiration
  Hemorrhagic shock
  Septic shock
  Histamine
  High-altitude pulmonary edema
  Neurogenic pulmonary edema
  Microemboli vascular damage
  Oxygen toxicity
  Other compounds
  Possible mechanisms: superoxide system
Sequence and Pathways for Pulmonary Edema Formation
Conclusions

THE CHAPTER BY Greene (186) in the 1965 edition of the *Handbook* section on respiration indicated that the mechanisms leading to the formation of pulmonary edema were poorly understood and that future research should focus on four areas: *1*) how tissues swell, *2*) how solutes and water traverse capillary walls, *3*) how tissues respond to altered capillary forces, and *4*) how vertical and horizontal levels of the lung tissue differ with respect to forces responsible for fluid accumulation. During the ensuing years each of these topics has been extensively studied; the state of the art has progressed from simply weighing lungs postmortem to measuring capillary and tissue pressures with micropuncture techniques (65, 131, 138, 366, 431, 469, 471, 477, 500, 502, 516).

To present this large amount of information sequentially, we divided this review into five distinct but related sections. The first section deals with the composition and physicochemical makeup of the pulmonary interstitium in normal and edematous lungs (84, 211, 298, 424, 533). The second section deals with each force and flow in the Starling equation, i.e., tissue fluid pressure, capillary pressure, tissue colloid osmotic pressure, plasma colloid osmotic pressure, and lymph flow (11, 135, 137, 200, 201, 233, 238, 385, 479, 489, 495, 541). The theoretical considerations involved in measuring the coefficients in the Starling equation (the filtration and osmotic reflection coefficients) are discussed as they relate to lung fluid balance (477). The importance of tissue fluid pressure in preventing excessive accumulation of lung water is presented as it relates to different forces operating between the apical and basal portions of the lung and the septal and perivascular spaces (3, 41, 131, 195, 232). The lymphatic system is discussed as it relates to lung fluid dynamics (198, 288, 289, 363, 520, 555). The third section discusses the data for increased vascular permeability (31, 52, 139, 140, 257, 312, 431, 481, 501). At least 31 classes of compounds produce leaky capillaries (2, 78, 134, 136, 439, 440, 505, 549). The data concerning leaky lungs apparently differs from species to species and laboratory to laboratory, yet a model of the superoxide system (a major mediator of lung damage) provides a means of integrating the "leaky capillary syndrome" data. The fourth section deals with the sequence of pulmonary edema formation in the different portions of the lung interstitium (160). The fifth section summarizes the possible directions of future research.

STRUCTURE AND COMPOSITION OF PULMONARY INTERSTITIUM

The architecture of the lung is exquisitely designed to maximize gas exchange between air and blood. Likewise, tissue hydration is normally maintained at a minimum to assure short diffusion distances for O_2 at the alveolar-capillary barrier. Special arrangements of the parenchyma cause rapid movement of filtered fluid away from the alveolar septal region and prevent increases in blood-air barrier thickness. Although it has been postulated that the physicochemical nature of the interstitial matrix also affects the passage of fluid and proteins as they move from vascular filtration sites to enter the terminal lymphatics, only a few of these proposed mechanisms have been tested.

The composition and organization of the pulmonary interstitium and its connective tissue are closely related to its ability to regulate water and macromolecular exchange between the microvasculature and the parenchyma (84, 183, 211, 519). The lung is composed of a three-dimensional fibrous framework forming a continuum throughout the interstitial spaces of the lungs (211, 533). Weibel and Bachofen (533) consider this fibrous skeleton to be subdivided into three components: an axial, a peripheral, and a septal fiber system. The axial fiber system includes type I collagen, which forms the dense connective tissue sheaths surrounding bronchi and blood vessels. These collagen fibers are from large, strong units that course longitudinally and circumferentially down the airways and blood vessels into the parenchyma. Many of these fibers radiate into the parenchyma and support alveolar ducts and septa. Elastic fibers are not only interwoven throughout the sheaths accompanying large blood vessels and bronchi but are also present throughout the alveolar septa and pleura (270). The peripheral fiber system, which is primarily type I collagen located within the visceral pleura, surrounds the entire lung and penetrates into the parenchyma as fibrous septa between acini, lobules, and segments. The septal system is composed of collagen fibers forming a lattice or netlike structure interwoven with capillaries within the alveolar walls and connecting with the axial and peripheral fiber systems. Although the septal fibers have high tensile strength and low elasticity, their netlike arrangement allows the septal walls to stretch, much like a nylon stocking; i.e., the entire meshwork may stretch by reorientation without actually stretching the collagen fibers. Elastic fibers also contribute to the elastic characteristics of the lung because they return to their original length after deformation and restore the collagen fiber orientation (270, 424). This structural arrangement is important for fluid balance because the fibrous network is under tension at all lung volumes and the space surrounding each fiber is a potential conduit for fluid.

Resistance to fluid movement along these fibers and maintenance of different fluid pressures within different regions of the lung interstitium are functions of the physicochemical properties of the ground substance interspersed between the fibers. The ground substance is composed of proteoglycans (mucoproteins) and glycosaminoglycans (mucopolysaccharides), which are long-chained polysaccharides. There are no membranous barriers to fluid or protein transport within the interstitium, but the ground substances could behave as a molecular sieve similar to gel columns (182, 270).

Pulmonary Interstitial Connective Tissues

Table 1 shows the composition, location, and function of the lung's interstitial matrix. The major structural component of the fibrous skeleton in lung parenchyma is type I collagen (211, 424). The basic unit of this collagen consists of three polypeptide chains, which form a stable triple helix. These fibrils coalesce to form large fibers (20–200 nm diam) that are stabilized by covalent cross-bonding between the lysine residues. The fibers form branching helical arrays that surround blood vessels and airways, form pleural sheets, branch into interlobular septa, and radiate through the interstitial spaces of alveolar septa. Figure 1 shows the distribution of collagen and ground substance in a slightly edematous septal interstitium. Lung connective tissue is ~60% type I collagen or ~15% of the lung's total dry weight and over 40% of the airway dry weight (424). Type III collagen (differing only slightly in protein composition from type I) comprises ~30% of the lung's connective tissue and has the same distribution pattern as type I. The very fine type III fibers are thought to make up the reticulum, which is dispersed throughout the lung interstitium (270). These fibers are presumed to be an important component of the fluid-exchange system within the interstitium, because they form loose networks around alveolar capillaries and are closely associated with the glycosaminoglycans. Collagen types IV and V are ~10% of the total lung collagen and are primarily located in the basement membranes, which separate the capillary wall and epithelial cells from the interstitium proper.

The remaining components of connective tissues (elastic fibers and proteoglycans) are present in smaller amounts than collagen, but their properties are very important in maintaining lung tissue integrity. Elastic tissue is present as a relatively amorphous elastin or hollow microtubule (~12 nm diam). Approximately 4%–5% of the lung's dry weight is elastic fibers. These elastic fibers are cross-linked and intertwined with collagen in blood vessel sheaths, airways, pleura, interlobular septa, and alveolar septa (424).

The amorphous ground substance in the interstitial spaces between cells and fibers is composed of proteoglycans and glycosaminoglycans. Although the exact concentration of these compounds within the interstitial fluid is not known, they do comprise ~0.5% of the lung's dry weight (424). Proteoglycans are composed of 20% protein and 80% glycosaminoglycans. The polysaccharide portions are usually repeating disac-

TABLE 1. *Connective Tissues of Pulmonary Interstitium*

Macromolecule	Location	Function	Fraction of Total Connective Tissue	Fraction of Dry Weight
Collagen				
Type I	Alveolar interstitium, pleura, surrounding basement membrane of vessels and bronchi	Thick support fibers	0.50	0.10
Type II	Airway cartilage	Support fibrils	0.03	0.10
Type III	Alveolar interstitium, vessels, bronchi, pleura	Fine reticulum, support fibers	0.20	0.04
Type IV	Basement membrane	Support fibers	0.02	0.01
Type V	Basement membrane	Support fibers	0.02	0.01
Elastic fiber	Alveolar interstitium, vessel walls, airways, pleura	Elasticity and support fibers	0.21	0.05
Proteoglycans	Interstitial matrix, basement membrane, cartilage	Cell adhesion, cell spacing?	0.01	<0.01
Glycosaminoglycans	Interstitial matrix	Fluid immobilization	0.01	<0.01

Data from Rennard et al. (424) and Taylor, Parker, et al. (502).

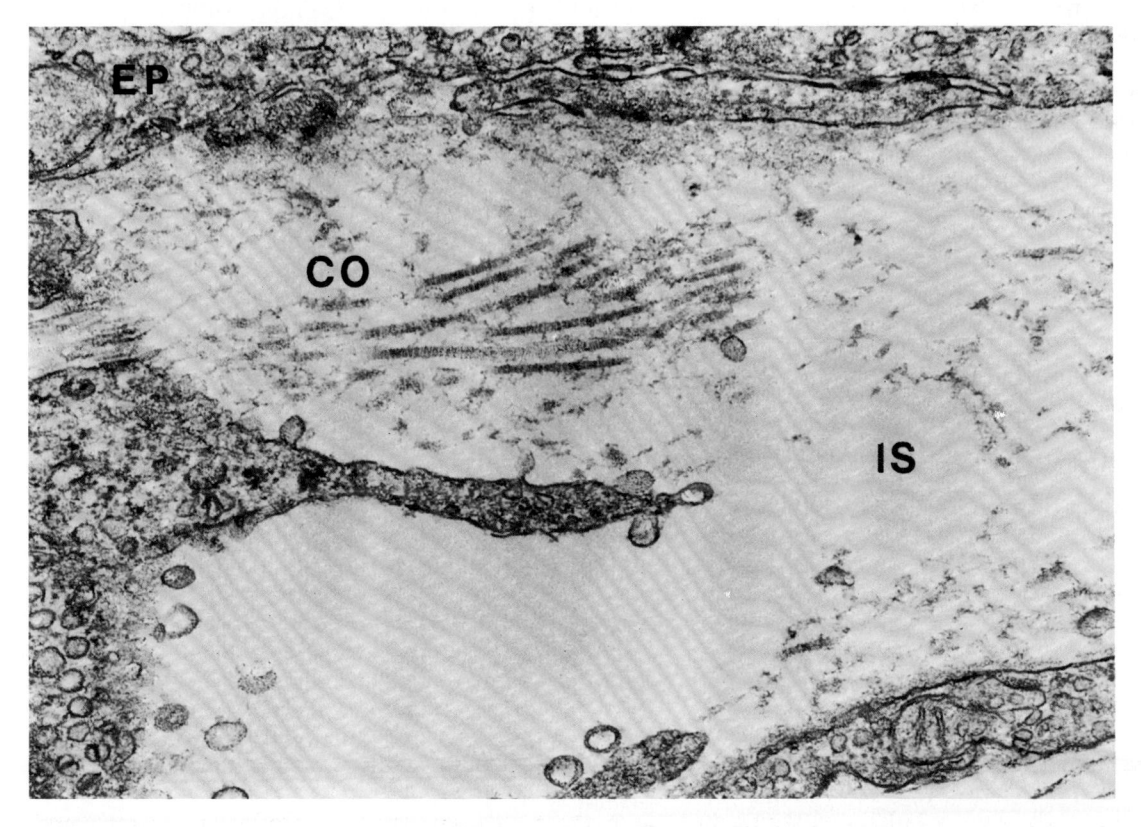

FIG. 1. Intra-alveolar interstitium (*IS*) showing filaments of proteoglycans throughout the slightly edematous interstitium. *CO*, bundle of collagen fibers; *EP*, epithelial barrier. × 6,100. (Micrograph courtesy of J. Gil.)

charides of an amino sugar (N-acetylglucosamine or N-acetylgalactosamine) and an acid sugar (glucuronic acid or iduronic acid). An exception is keratan sulfate, which incorporates galactose instead of a uronic acid. The distributions reported for the different glycosaminoglycans in lung tissue are 10%–38% hyaluronic acid, 30%–44% chondroitin and dermatan sulfates, and 26%–30% heparin and heparan sulfate (126, 229). The proteoglycans have molecular weights of 1–4 million and are anionic at body pH (416).

Physicochemical Properties of Interstitial Matrix

The anionic polysaccharides that fill the interstitial spaces of the lung are either unbound to other tissue components or combine with protein to form proteoglycans (84). The physicochemical properties of these compounds and their interactions with other connective tissue elements provide stability to the interstitial spaces and are responsible for the lung's ability to maintain a relatively dry state (182, 183). The proteoglycans are characterized by polysaccharide chains linked to a protein core in a brushlike configuration. Proteoglycans in cartilage are linked with hyaluronate to form aggregates, but hyaluronate does not bind strongly to other structural proteins. Hyaluronic acid is a linear polymer 10 Å wide and 2.5 μm long of N-acetylglycosamine and glucuronic acid units. It usually exists as a random coil and can swell in water to 10,000 times its original volume. In solutions of only a few tenths of a percent of hyaluronate and proteoglycans, the molecules become highly entangled and move as a single matrix unit during ultracentrifugation (84). Figure 2 is a diagram of a matrix of collagen fibers, hyaluronic acid, and proteoglycans. This matrix is stabilized by ionic, covalent, and hydrogen bonding between connective tissue elements, and water can be immobilized without direct chemical binding. However, physical compression can remove water from the matrix, much like wringing a sponge. Solutions of tissue polysaccharides and collagen also possess viscoelastic properties and can resist compression.

Because of the dense entanglement and cross-linked character of the interstitial matrix, small fluid areas are created between polysaccharide and collagen molecules into which water and small ions can gain access more easily than macromolecules (e.g., plasma proteins). This steric exclusion within the interstitial matrix fluid is directly related to solute size and polysaccharide concentration. Because of this property, filtered plasma proteins distribute into a smaller absolute volume of interstitial water than smaller molecules (e.g., Na^+ and K^+).

Generally the theoretical equations derived by Ogston (371) to describe the exclusion phenomenon are based on a model that incorporates rods and spherical molecules. Ogston's model predicts that excluded volumes for plasma proteins in hyaluronic acid solutions depend on both the protein's molecular radius and the hyaluronate concentration. However, exclusion of protein by collagen solutions is not greatly affected by the protein's size and is insignificant below collagen concentrations of ~5 g/100 ml (182). Laurent (287) found that albumin was excluded from 25% of the water volume of a 0.5 g/100 ml hyaluronate solution, whereas Wiederhielm et al. (542) reported an excluded volume of 30% for albumin (2 g/100 ml) in a 10% collagen solution. If the glycosaminoglycans were distributed evenly in the interstitial volumes of dog lungs (383), the total concentration of glycosaminoglycans in lung tissues (424) would be ~0.3 g/100 ml. However, this estimate does not incorporate the possibility of glycosaminoglycans combining with proteins in the interstitial tissues or of regional variations in the distribution of glycosaminoglycans.

In addition to restricting macromolecule entry into some fluid regions, the interstitial matrix also offers considerable steric hindrance to the diffusion of protein molecules. Diffusion of albumin in normally hydrated umbilical cord matrix was 25% of its diffusion rate in water, whereas that of γ-globulin was <20% (182). Albumin diffuses at half its free-diffusion rate in a 1% hyaluronate solution (372), which means that molecules will be selectively restricted when diffusing through the gel matrix and that the amount of restriction is directly related to molecular size for uncharged molecules. However, the transport of larger molecules through free-fluid channels surrounding the gel will be enhanced because of their smaller available volume in the matrix (182). Whether protein is transported primarily by diffusive flux or bulk flow in the interstitium of the normal lung is not known, but convective processes should predominate when volume flows

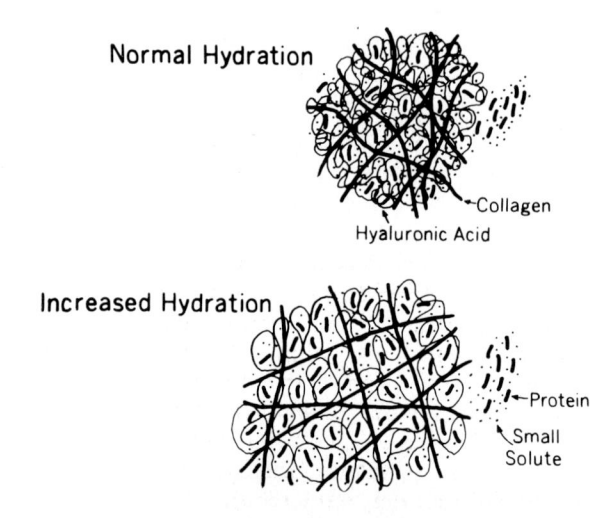

FIG. 2. Diagram of the extracellular matrix showing a collagen mesh with interspersed proteoglycans and glycosaminoglycans. Effect of increased hydration on matrix density and intragel dispersion of proteins and small solutes is also shown. [From Parker, Taylor, et al. (383), by permission of the American Heart Association, Inc.]

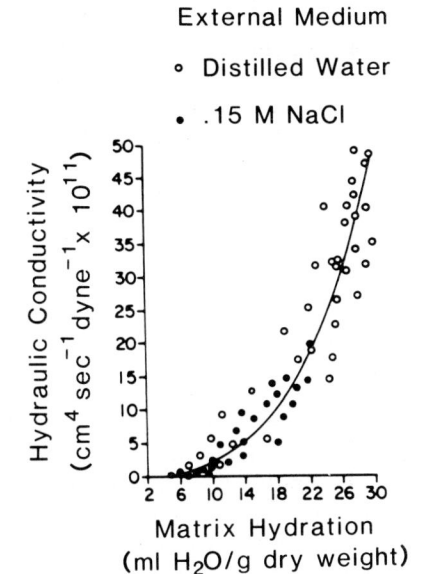

FIG. 3. Effect of increased hydration on hydraulic conductivity of umbilical interstitial matrix. Normal hydration, ~9 ml H$_2$O/g dry wt. [Adapted from Granger (182).]

through the tissues are large and diffusional fluxes would predominate when flows are normal.

The interstitial matrices of umbilical cord and subcutaneous tissues have low hydraulic conductivities when normally hydrated (182, 197), but the resistance to water movement within these tissues decreases dramatically as the tissues become increasingly hydrated. Figure 3 shows the effects of tissue hydration on the hydraulic conductivity of umbilical cord tissue. A 20-fold increase in hydraulic flow was associated with only a 3-fold increase in matrix volume (182). Presumably the interstitial matrix in lung tissue behaves similarly during edema formation, but no measurements of hydraulic conductivity in lung interstitium are available. However, because of the small septal spaces and the long distances between capillaries and lymphatics, the interstitium could offer considerable resistance to the formation of lymph at normal hydration states.

Another consequence of having hyaluronic acid and the proteoglycans in the interstitial matrix is that excised tissues swell when immersed in isotonic saline (182, 341). Meyer and Silberberg (341) observed that excised umbilical matrix increased to 1.5 and 1.7 times its original volume when immersed in protein-saline solutions equivalent to those found in lymph and plasma, respectively. Granger (182) reported a swelling (or imbibition) pressure of −12 mmHg for Wharton's jelly placed in Tyrode's solution. This value indicates that the interstitial matrix in this tissue (as in many other tissues) is maintained below its unstressed volume by some combination of osmotic, hydrostatic, or mechanical forces operating within the interstitium. The relative contributions of these factors to this swelling pressure remain controversial. Many investigators envision the interstitial gel in a dehydrated state as a result of tissue and lymphatic forces (183, 201). The electrostatic repulsion of polyanions results in the gel's tendency to swell in normal tissues, but the small water volume restrains the swelling of the polysaccharide matrix (181, 182, 192, 209, 446). Others have proposed an osmotic mechanism for the gel's imbibition pressure (341, 456, 540). The collagen fiber network restrains the proteoglycans and glycosaminoglycans; thus they exert an osmotic force that tends to pull water into the matrix without exerting any tensile effect on the intragel fluid.

Defining osmotic activity in a solution of macromolecules is a major problem. Certainly the ideal van't Hoff osmotic pressure of hyaluronate and proteoglycans in solution would be negligible at physiological concentrations because of their large size (84, 209). Therefore the nonideal osmotic pressure exerted by these macromolecules cannot be attributed to simple thermal activity of molecules in the conventional sense. A more recent, highly controversial theory has been advanced by Hammel and Scholander (209), who proposed that the absorptive (osmotic) pressure for a fluid is the result of macromolecule overcrowding. Granger and Shepherd (181–183) attempted to characterize the mechanical and osmotic stresses within the interstitial gel and found that Donnan factors accounted for only 15% of the imbibition pressure in the umbilical cord. One practical consequence of the restrained gel matrix is that significant pockets of free fluid and large fluid channels would not be present in tissues until the negative tension within the matrix is relieved and the polysaccharides expand to their unstressed volume states (182, 195, 201).

Vascular and Extravascular Fluid Compartments in the Lung

Figure 4 shows the subdivisions of tissue fluid spaces in the normal lung (69). Both the residual blood and tissue compartments are composed of ~79%–80% water and ~20%–21% dry weight. The blood water volume and blood dry weight are shown on the *left side* of the figure; the blood-free dry weight is shown on the *center* and *right side* of the figure. The extravascular lung water is about evenly divided into interstitial volume and cell volume. Within the interstitial volume, albumin can distribute in ~60% of the fluid volume. The albumin-excluded volume is not anatomically separate from the total interstitial volume but results from restriction imposed by the interstitial matrix within lung tissue (383).

Very reproducible values are obtained for gravimetric extravascular lung water when corrections are made for residual blood volume with either the amount of hemoglobin or ^{51}Cr-labeled red blood cells contained

FIG. 4. Schematic representation of lung fluid compartments. BDW, blood dry weight; BFDW, blood-free dry weight; Q_W, extravascular lung water; V_A, albumin interstitial volume; V_{BW}, blood water volume; V_{cell}, cell volume; V_E, albumin-excluded volume; V_I, interstitial volume.

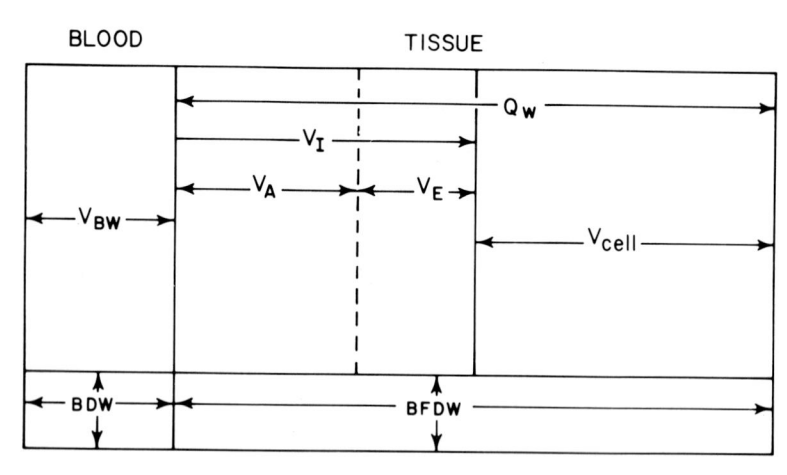

in the excised tissues (191, 291, 382, 383, 449, 474). A more accurate estimate of the vascular volume may be obtained with the distribution of a labeled protein when tissues are sampled rapidly after injecting protein into the plasma (14, 142, 339, 472). This method obviates any error due to differences between hematocrits of small and large blood vessels (59) but can cause an overestimation of plasma volume if significant amounts of labeled protein leak into the tissues prior to sampling. In most preparations the residual blood comprises 20%–30% of the total wet tissue weight (477).

Small ions (e.g., sodium and chloride) generally have greater extravascular distribution volumes than larger compounds [e.g., sucrose, ethylenediaminetetraacetic acid (EDTA), or diethylenetriamine pentaacetic acid (DTPA)] because small ions enter the parenchymal cells and larger molecules may be excluded from some tissue regions. Extravascular sodium spaces average 61% (40%–90%) of extravascular lung water, whereas chloride spaces average 52% (30%–69%) (449, 477). Simultaneous estimates of [^{14}C]sucrose and ^{36}Cl$^-$ indicate a sucrose space that is 64% of the chloride space (449). Sucrose spaces are good estimates of the lung's interstitial space because sucrose is inert, should not cross cell membranes, and is not significantly excluded by the interstitial matrix. The chelated complexes ^{51}Cr-labeled EDTA and ^{99m}Tc-labeled DTPA have permeability characteristics similar to those of sucrose but are easier to use because they contain γ-emitting isotopes (69, 382, 383). In several different species sucrose spaces in lung tissues measured during states of normal hydration have ranged from 33% to 60% of extravascular lung water (142, 339, 449, 474, 477).

At this time it is not possible to measure how the interstitial volume is compartmentalized within lung tissue; investigators must rely on the measurement of some blood-free total lung space to estimate the extravascular fluid volume in intact lungs. Obviously when measuring spaces the investigator must consider cell entry, size, and charge of the tracer molecule, especially in pathological states that may alter cell membrane characteristics.

Effect of Increased Hydration on Tissue Fluid Compartments

In most types of pulmonary edema the capillary filtrate enters the interstitial spaces and expands the extracellular matrix with little or no expansion of intracellular volume. Figure 5A shows the effect of three successive saline infusions (5% body wt) on the various fluid spaces within lung tissue (383). Extravascular lung water and the extravascular ^{99m}Tc-DTPA space increased in parallel as a function of increased extracellular expansion. The 34% increase in extravascular lung water that occurred after a volume load of 15% body weight is generally considered the maximum interstitial swelling that can occur before alveolar flooding (283).

Figure 5B shows the available volume for albumin and the excluded volume for albumin measured during interstitial edema formation produced by increased left atrial pressures (382). The calculation of the available volume was based on the albumin concentration measured in pulmonary lymph, because lymph was assumed to be at equilibrium with tissue fluid in these studies (361, 422). The sum of the two volumes equals the total interstitial fluid space. In Figure 5B the available volume and the excluded volume for albumin are shown as functions of pulmonary capillary pressures calculated with $P_c = P_{la} + 0.4(P_{pa} - P_{la})$, where P_c is capillary pressure, P_{la} is left atrial pressure, and P_{pa} is pulmonary arterial pressure. A small but significant decrease in the excluded volume occurred during edema formation as the available volume and the interstitial volume increased.

The excluded volume fraction (F_E) for albumin ($F_E = V_E/V_I$) is shown in Figure 5C as a function of the interstitial volume (V_I) for the same studies as shown in Figure 5B. The excluded volume fraction was calculated with

$$F_E = 1 - (V_{AV}/V_I) \quad (1)$$

where V_{AV} is the available volume of albumin, or

$$F_E = 1 - (Capp_A/C_{L,A}) \quad (2)$$

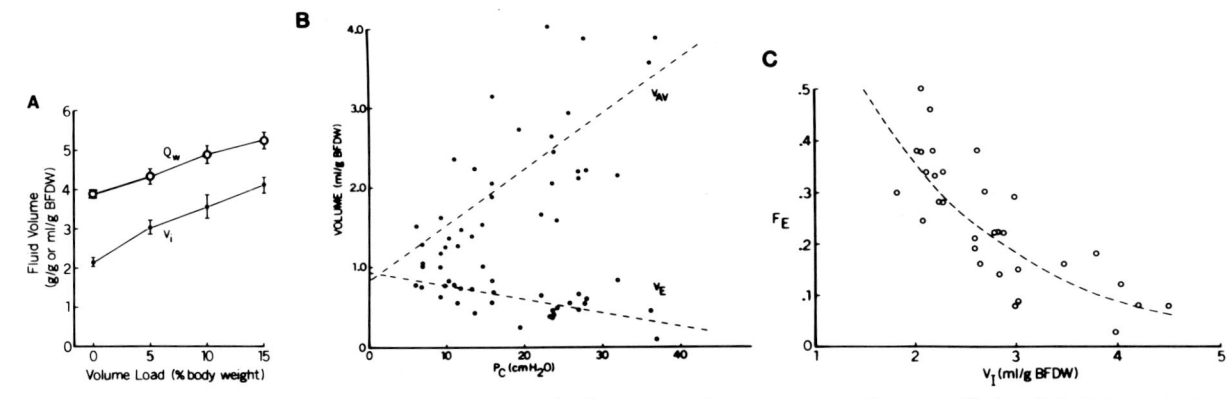

FIG. 5. *A*: effect of volume expansion on extravascular water (Q_W) and diethylenetriamine pentaacetic acid (DTPA) interstitial volume (V_I) in dog lung. BFDW, blood-free dry weight. *B*: effect of increased pulmonary capillary pressure (Pc) on interstitial volume (ordinate) available to albumin (V_{AV}) and excluded albumin volume (V_E) in dog lungs. *C*: effect of increasing extravascular ^{99m}Tc-DTPA V_I on albumin-excluded volume fraction (F_E). Increasing left atrial pressure produced interstitial pulmonary edema. [*A* from Parker, Taylor, et al. (383), by permission of the American Heart Association, Inc.; *B* and *C* from Parker, Taylor, et al. (382), by permission of the American Heart Association, Inc.]

where Capp$_A$ is the apparent tissue albumin concentration calculated by dividing the tissue albumin content by the interstitial volume and $C_{L,A}$ is the albumin concentration in pulmonary lymph. The excluded volume fraction decreased from 38% of interstitial volume in normal lungs to 10% when interstitial volume doubled. Apparently the relationship between volume and hydration of the interstitium depends on the behavior of the tissue matrix, because no significant differences were observed between curves generated with either volume loading or increased vascular pressures to produce edema (382, 383). The albumin-excluded volumes measured in lung interstitium are similar to those measured in 0.5% hyaluronic acid solutions (287). From Table 1 the concentration of glycosaminoglycans in lung interstitium can be computed to be 0.3%. However, the relative contributions of collagen and the different proteoglycans to the measured albumin exclusion are not known. Because the actual excluded volume decreased, half of the excluded volume could be attributed to the expandable glycosaminoglycan system, whereas the other half probably reflects the nonexpandable collagen interspaces (182, 542).

We have discussed the interstitium's effect on albumin exclusion as a function of the steric properties of the interstitial matrix. However, the components within the interstitium are highly charged; the glycosaminoglycans are negative and the collagen fibers positive. Therefore the exclusion of charged molecules such as plasma proteins by the interstitial matrix is a complex phenomenon resulting from both charge and steric factors. In fact the capillary wall appears to be a negative barrier, whereas the capillary wall–interstitium–lymphatics behaves as a positive barrier (496). Therefore the interstitial charge must greatly affect the distribution and movement of negatively charged plasma proteins within its confines.

STARLING FORCES AND LYMPH FLOW

Theoretical Considerations

The equations that describe solvent flow and the movement of neutral solutes across capillary walls have been explicitly defined by Kedem and Katchalsky (261) and Katchalsky and Curran (258) for an uncharged solute (S) and solvent (V) membrane system

$$J_V = L_P(\Delta P - \sigma_d \Delta \Pi) \qquad (3)$$

where J_V is the net volume flow occurring across the capillary wall (cm$^3 \cdot$s$^{-1} \cdot$cm^{-2} membrane), and

$$J_S = (1 - \sigma_f)\overline{C}_S J_V + \omega \Delta \Pi \qquad (4)$$

where J_S is the net solute flux occurring across the membrane (amount$\cdot$s$^{-1} \cdot$cm^{-2} membrane). The hydraulic conductivity (L_P) is in cm$^5 \cdot$dyn$^{-1} \cdot$s^{-1}. The hydrostatic pressure head acting across the capillary wall (ΔP) equals capillary pressure minus interstitial tissue fluid pressure (Pti,f; dyn/cm^2). The osmotic reflection coefficient (σ_d) equals 1 if the solute is impermeable and 0 if the solute is freely permeable. Equation 3 should contain a σ_d for all solutes in plasma, but for this review, only a σ_d for all plasma proteins is used. The osmotic pressure operating across the capillary wall ($\Delta \Pi$) equals the colloid osmotic pressure of the plasma (Π_P; dyn/cm^2) minus the colloid osmotic pressure of the tissues (Π_{ti}; dyn/cm^2). Whether the solvent-drag reflection coefficient (σ_f) equals σ_d in normally filtering capillaries is being debated (42, 43, 180, 392, 498, 499). In an ideal system $\sigma_d = \sigma_f$, but the pulmonary capillary system is far from ideal. The argument concerns the applicability of using Equation 4 to predict protein fluxes occurring across a heteroporous barrier with different ΔP and $\Delta \Pi$ values driving the solute and solvent fluxes (499, 501). At high J_V values, $\sigma_d = \sigma_f$ (49, 180). The average solute concentration ($\bar{C}_S$, amount/cm^3) is assumed to be equal to the average concentration between plasma (C_P) and tissue (C_{ti}); i.e., $\bar{C}_S = (C_P + C_{ti})/2$. The choice of $\bar{C}_S$ in Equation 4 may cause problems with estimating σ_d in Equation 3. The solute mobility (ω) is in amount·dyn^{-1}·s^{-1}. Kedem and Katchalsky's equations describe completely a membrane-solvent-solute system when σ_d, ω, and L_P are known and J_V is very close to zero; i.e., the system is close to equilibrium ($C_P \cong C_{ti}$) and the molecules are uncharged.

Equations 3 and 4 have been cast in more familiar terms by replacing $\omega\Delta\Pi$ with the permeability-surface area product (PS) times the concentration gradient ($\Delta C = C_P - C_{ti}$) and replacing L_P times the membrane area with the capillary filtration coefficient ($K_{f,c}$)

$$\dot{Q}_V = K_{f,c}[(Pc - Pti,f) - \sigma_d(\Pi_P - \Pi_{ti})] \quad (5)$$

and

$$\dot{Q}_S = (1 - \sigma_f)\dot{Q}_V \bar{C}_S + PS(C_P - C_{ti}) \quad (6)$$

Equations 5 and 6 now contain surface areas, and $\dot{Q}_V$ and $\dot{Q}_S$ (net volume and solute flows) are measured in terms of per 100 g of organ tissue rather than per square centimeter of membrane. Equation 5 is the Starling equation; Pc, Pti, and $\sigma_d(\Pi_P - \Pi_{ti})$ are Starling forces (475, 476). Because of the lung's complex architecture an equation should be written at each lung height; i.e., the lung should be divided into n vertical slices. However, this is impractical, and we must use weighted averages to discuss each force and its relationship to capillary filtration (75).

Attempts to apply Equation 6 to protein fluxes occurring across capillary walls have been made with data for protein concentrations in lymph (C_L). Unfortunately Equation 6 cannot be applied to this data because it is collected far from equilibrium, i.e., $C_L \ll C_P$. To remedy this, Bresler and Groome (49) derived an equation that predicts how solutes should move across membranes that are exchanging both solute and solvent in the same pathway (536). The equation is an algebraic manipulation of one derived earlier by Patlak et al. (392)

$$\dot{Q}_S = (1 - \sigma_d)\dot{Q}_V C_P + \frac{(1 - \sigma_d)\dot{Q}_V(C_P - C_L)}{e^x - 1} \quad (7)$$

where

$$x = (1 - \sigma_d)\dot{Q}_V/PS \quad (8)$$

The exponent in Equation 7 is called the Peclet number and provides a means of predicting the behavior of solute flux. As $\dot{Q}_V$ increases, x increases and $e^x - 1$ becomes so large that

$$\dot{Q}_S = (1 - \sigma_d)\dot{Q}_V C_P$$

or

$$\dot{Q}_V C_{ti} = (1 - \sigma_d)\dot{Q}_V C_P \quad (9)$$

or

$$C_{ti}/C_P = 1 - \sigma_d$$

Equation 7 can be rearranged to yield

$$C_{ti}/C_P = \frac{1 - \sigma_d}{1 - \sigma_d e^{-x}} \quad (10)$$

Equation 10 can be applied to the capillary-tissue-lymphatic system if one assumes that $C_L = C_{ti}$. When lymph is collected at different steady states after increasing capillary pressure then C_{ti}/C_P should approach $1 - \sigma_d$, i.e., become constant at high lymph flows. Granger and Taylor (180) introduced this approach for analyzing lymph protein fluxes in intestinal tissue. Not only did these investigators estimate σ_d for several endogenous proteins but they also described the selectivity of the intestinal capillaries to macromolecules in terms of a two-pore model. Because plasma proteins are charged, their permeability properties are not totally described by Equation 10. A recent review (496) of the effect of charge on macromolecular permeability indicates that the following equation describes the kinetics of charged protein fluxes

$$C_L/C_P = \frac{1 - \beta}{1 - \beta e^{-x}} \quad (11)$$

where $\beta = \sigma_d + KZ\Delta\psi(PS)/\dot{Q}_V$ and $x = (1 - \beta)\dot{Q}_V/PS$ (K is a constant that equals 0.03 at body temperature, Z refers to molecular charge, and $\Delta\psi$ is the diffusive potential in millivolts). The behavior of charged macromolecules has been studied in pulmonary tissue. Unlike the negatively charged glomerular membrane, the pulmonary blood-lymph barrier behaves as a positive barrier (99, 496, 497). The effect of charge on protein fluxes is an important area that is being intensely investigated in several different laboratories [see Fig. 22; (297)].

The applications of the different equations for analyzing the movement of molecules in various experimental models are discussed in *Colloid Osmotic Pressure Gradient*, p. 194. Mathematical and experimental models are now available to study the selectivity of the pulmonary capillary walls for different proteins present in plasma. Unfortunately most data collected with either tracer fluxes or lymphatic models do not lend themselves to rigorous mathematical treatment and provide at best only qualitative estimates of the selectivity characteristics of the pulmonary capillary wall.

Endothelial Pathways

Lung interstitial fluid contains all the proteins present in plasma, and the total protein concentration in lymph draining normal lungs is ~75% of that found in plasma. The lung tissue contains two anatomically different capillaries: *1*) pulmonary capillaries with a continuous endothelial lining at the inner surfaces and *2*) bronchial capillaries with fenestrated walls. Pulmonary capillaries have a far greater surface area than bronchial capillaries and comprise the major pulmonary blood vessels involved in fluid exchange between plasma and lung interstitium. However, the bronchial circulation must provide nutrient flow to the bronchial structures and visceral pleura and can leak large amounts of fluid into these areas when challenged by vasoactive compounds such as histamine (404, 408).

Volume flow at the endothelial barrier of the pulmonary circulation is thought to occur at the junctions between endothelial cells; the volume flow of the bronchial circulation occurs at the fenestrae. Endothelial vesicles are not thought to be involved in producing net volume movement across capillary walls unless they fuse to form open channels (533).

Investigators have used physiological studies to predict that pulmonary capillaries possess leakage sites, which can be described in terms of small pores (radius <45 Å) and large pores (radius 200–1,000 Å). Figure 6 depicts schematically the pathways by which molecules can cross capillary walls. In continuous capillaries solutes can move across the endothelial barrier in pinocytotic vesicles, through intercellular junctions located between endothelial cells, or through transendothelial channels formed by fused vesicles (1, 2, and 3, respectively, in Fig. 6). A large volume of the pulmonary endothelial cell is occupied by vesicles with radii of 250 Å. Tracer studies indicate that molecules up to 150 Å in radius may be ferried across the endothelial cells by the random motion of these vesicles between plasma and interstitium. Usually a greater density of vesicles is present at the venular ends of capillary walls, and different capillary beds have different populations of vesicles, i.e., muscle > lung > brain (63, 375, 376, 420, 457, 460, 543). However, studies indicate that vesicles are of minor significance in the movement of proteins across the endothelial barrier (150, 430). Therefore their function(s) is presently unclear.

Intercellular junctions of alveolar septal capillaries are relatively tight with respect to the passage of macromolecules, such as horseradish peroxidase and hemoglobin, at normal hydrostatic pressures (244, 407, 445). The tracers have been detected in minute amounts in pulmonary lymph, which is consistent with a slow but measurable turnover rate (343). In most capillary beds intercellular junctions have widths of 20–60 Å; however, the junctional dimensions in normal lungs are not known. Venular ends of septal capillaries have less well-organized junctional complexes (442, 443), which may be similar to the large junctions seen in other tissues (244, 376, 442–445, 459, 543). Transendothelial channels, the third pathway existing across endothelial cells (Fig. 6, 3), are the result of the fusion of two or more vesicles so that blood plasma communicates with the interstitium through "pores" with maximal diameters of 500 Å. Strictures reduce the internal diameter of these channels to 100–400 Å (Fig. 6, inset). In some instances the opening is covered by a diaphragm with a radius of 25–60 Å. Although transendothelial channels have not been demonstrated in lung tissue—presumably because there are so few—they could be the structural correlate of the large-pore system (63, 150, 375, 376). Interendothelial cell junctions may be the anatomical counterpart of the small-pore system (radius 50–80 Å), and the counterpart of the large-pore system (radius 200–250 Å) may be either transendothelial channels or venular intercellular junctions.

In addition to these pathways, the bronchial circulation has fenestrae (Fig. 6, bottom panel). Fenestrae are openings with radii of 200–300 Å within endo-

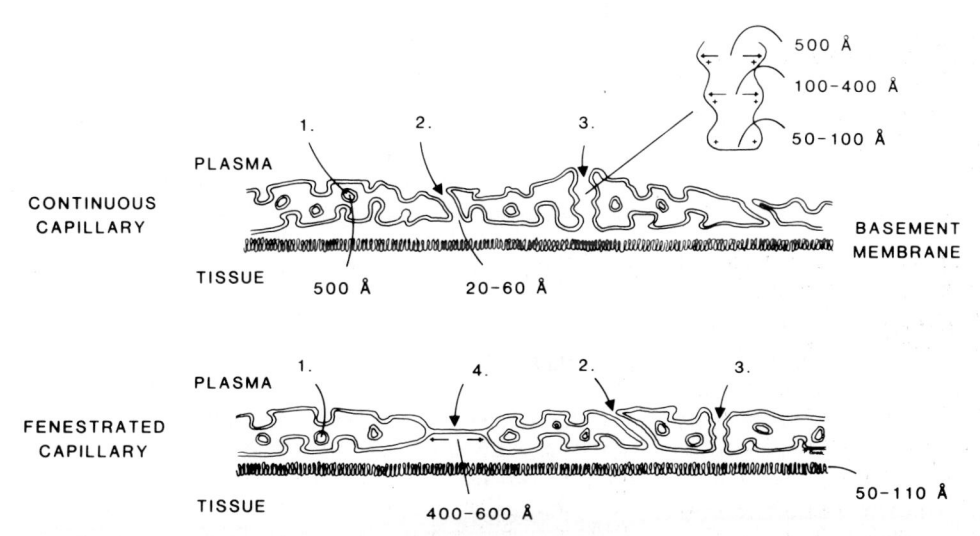

FIG. 6. Schematic representation of continuous and fenestrated capillary walls. 1, Plasmalemmal vesicles; 2, endothelial junctions; 3, transendothelial channels; 4, fenestrations. Diameters of structures are given. Top right, schematic of a transendothelial channel with its related structure and dimensions. [Adapted from Taylor and Granger (496).]

thelial cells (Fig. 6, 4). The fenestrae are covered by a diaphragm with an estimated radius of 50 Å (20, 71, 79, 80, 257, 376, 458, 459). Some fenestrae are open, and molecules with radii of <150 Å can easily penetrate these openings. The frequency of open fenestrae in the bronchial circulation is not known, but it is doubtful that it exceeds 40% of the total population of fenestrae (71).

After molecules cross the pulmonary endothelium they must cross the dense basement membrane to gain access to the interstitium. The basement membrane contains fine fibrillar material composed of type IV and V collagen and proteoglycans. The porosity of these structures is not known for lung endothelial basement membranes. In other capillary beds, however, tracer molecules with radii of 25–50 Å are not retained by basement membranes, whereas larger molecules with radii of 62–150 Å transiently accumulate in the spaces between vascular leak sites and the basement membrane (63, 458).

After passing through the basement membrane the molecules must percolate through the tissues to enter the lymphatic system. The permeability properties of the lung's interstitial matrix are not known. However, in normally hydrated tissues the matrix could provide considerable resistance to the movement of macromolecules and water.

From the interstitial compartments the molecules either cross the very leaky terminal lymphatic walls and leave the lung via lymph or pass into the alveolar spaces under certain conditions. Normally the epithelial membrane has a very tight junctional system between cells; molecules the size of plasma proteins do not cross this barrier in significant amounts (122, 123, 490, 527).

Filtration Coefficient

The amount of fluid that filters across any membrane per unit membrane area (J_V) is a function of the volume conductivity (L_P) of the membrane times the imbalance in hydrostatic (P) and osmotic (Π) forces acting across the barrier (258)

$$J_V = L_P(\Delta P - \Delta \Pi) \quad (12)$$

In organ systems the exact area through which the filtration is occurring is not known and what is actually measured is some transcapillary volume flow ($\dot{Q}_{V,c}$) that is a function of the membrane area A (378, 379): $\dot{Q}_{V,c} = L_P A(\Delta P - \Delta \Pi)$.

The coefficient relating the forces to the flow, $L_P A$, has been defined as the capillary filtration coefficient ($K_{f,c}$) (284, 285): $\dot{Q}_{V,c} = K_{f,c}(\Delta P - \Delta \Pi)$, where $K_{f,c}$ is directly related to A, radius to the fourth power, inversely related to membrane thickness and viscosity of the filtering fluid, and has the dimensions of milliliter per minute per mmHg per 100 g tissue. Because $K_{f,c}$ values are functions of the membrane area, their measurement has been used as an indicator of changes in capillary density (144, 183); however, because of this area dependency, comparison of $K_{f,c}$ values obtained in different organs is difficult. Obviously the lung has a tremendous surface area, and, although the hydraulic conductivity may be small, the filtration coefficient will be large (533).

The first $K_{f,c}$ was estimated for lung tissue by Guyton and Lindsey (196) in their classic study. These investigators determined the wet/dry weight ratios of lungs exposed to different left atrial pressures (Fig. 7). At left atrial pressures lower than ~25 mmHg the lungs gained no appreciable weight. When left atrial pressures exceeded this value the lungs gained weight rapidly. The $K_{f,c}$ was defined as the slope of the weight gain curve occurring at high vascular pressures.

The biphasic nature of the lung weight gain as a function of left atrial pressure is discussed in several sections of this chapter (*Lymph Flow*, p. 200; *Analyses of Force Changes During Formation of Alveolar Edema: Edema Safety Factor*, p. 206; and SEQUENCE AND PATHWAYS FOR PULMONARY EDEMA FORMATION, p. 214) relative to changes in Starling forces. When left atrial pressure is increased in the lower ranges, lymph flow increases, tissue pressure increases, the difference in colloid osmotic pressure across the capillary walls increases, and the increased capillary filtration gradient is reduced. When the ability of these forces and flows to change is exhausted the lungs gain weight continuously and intra-alveolar edema develops. It may not be possible to determine $K_{f,c}$ from Guyton and Lindsey's work (196), because fluid may be flowing across *both* the capillary and alveolar membranes during the rapid weight gain portion of the curve and the Starling forces are changing during the slow weight gain phase. Because the capillary and alveolar membranes are in series the total membrane filtration coefficient ($K_{f,T}$) is

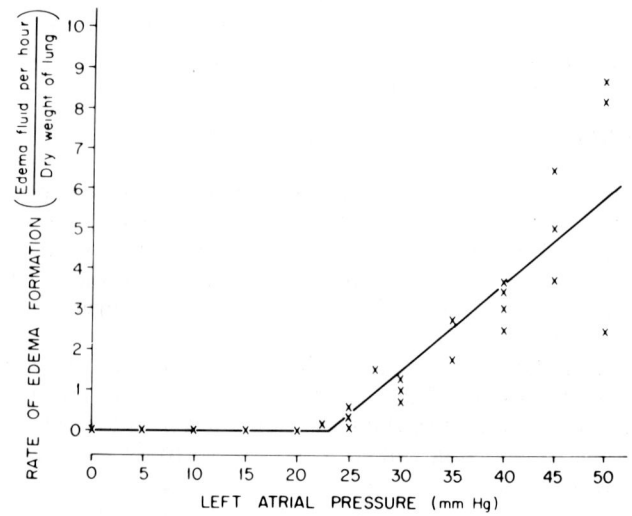

FIG. 7. Rate of pulmonary edema formation as a function of left atrial pressure. [From Guyton and Lindsey (196), by permission of the American Heart Association, Inc.]

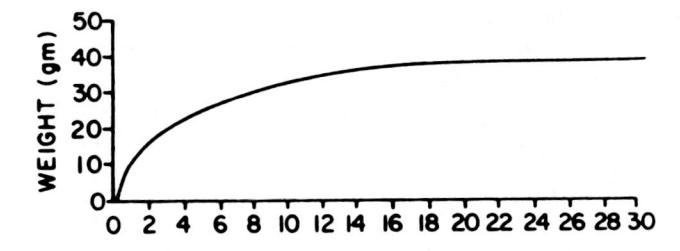

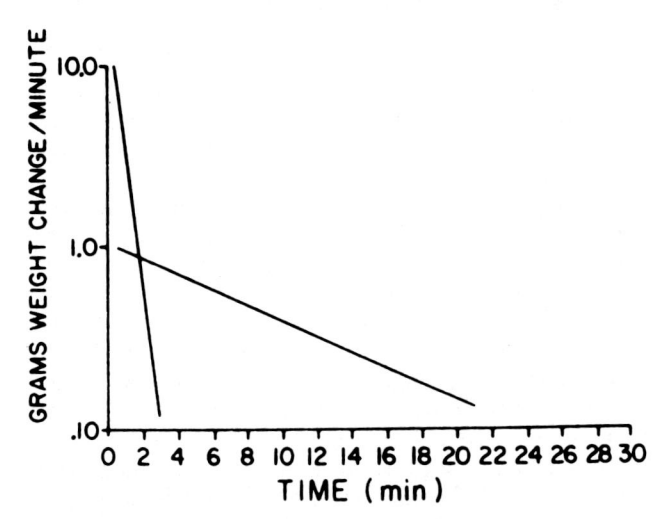

FIG. 8. Lung weight gain curve after elevation of capillary pressure in isolated dog lung (*top panel*). Slopes were plotted as functions of time with a semilogarithmic plot (*bottom panel*). Two distinct components are always observed: a rapid blood volume component and a slower capillary filtration component. [From Drake (112).]

$$K_{f,T} = \frac{K_f A K_{f,c}}{K_f A + K_{f,c}} \quad (13)$$

where $K_f A$ is the filtration coefficient of the alveolar membrane (93, 112, 115, 392, 491). When fluid is entering the alveoli, $K_{f,T}$ is measured; when fluid is entering only the interstitium, $K_{f,c}$ is measured. Because of the complexity associated with estimating $K_{f,c}$ in a double-membrane system when tissue forces are changing, three different techniques have been developed to evaluate $K_{f,c}$.

GRAVIMETRIC PROCEDURES. Several investigators (115, 154, 390, 492, 493) have measured $K_{f,c}$ with isolated dog lungs, which were perfused until they attained an isogravimetric state. Then both pulmonary arterial and venous pressures were increased by the same amount and the weight gain curve recorded as a function of time. The lung weight gain curve (Fig. 8) contains two components: *1*) a rapid phase as additional blood enters the lung and *2*) a slower phase that represents fluid filtration into the interstitium. As fluid filters into the tissue, changes in the Starling forces and lymph flow cause the lung to stop gaining weight. When the slopes of the weight gain curve are plotted as a function of time on semilogarithmic paper, the curves are analyzed as shown in the *bottom panel* of Figure 8. The curves are best fit by assuming that the slower component is a single exponential function. The zero time extrapolated value for the slow component [weight change/time change ($\Delta wt/\Delta t$)] divided by the imposed change in capillary pressure is used to calculate $K_{f,c}$. This estimate of $K_{f,c}$ is not complicated by the double-membrane system, because an isolated lung does not attain an isogravimetric state during the development of intra-alveolar edema. Also, because $\Delta wt/\Delta t$ is determined at zero time, any change in tissue forces would only minimally affect the estimate. However, $K_{f,c}$ could be underestimated because a portion of the pressure change could increase tissue pressure due to vascular distension and oppose filtration.

Several investigators have used a modification of this technique to estimate $K_{f,c}$. The estimates of $K_{f,c}$ in Table 2 have been converted to hydraulic conductivities to facilitate comparison. The table, which includes data for hydraulic conductivities for the capillary walls and the total alveolar-capillary membrane, presents quite variable results. The $K_{f,c}$ values estimated with some variation of the extrapolation technique are ~4 times greater than those determined with the analysis of Guyton and Lindsey (196), which measured $K_{f,T}$ (total alveolar-capillary membrane filtration coefficient). The alveolar membrane appears to have a conductivity ~10% of that of red blood cell membranes (455), and the capillary endothelium has

TABLE 2. *Filtration Coefficients and Hydraulic Conductivities for Pulmonary Membranes*

Membrane	Filtration Coefficient, ml·min⁻¹·100 g⁻¹·mmHg⁻¹	Hydraulic Conductivity, × 10¹¹ cm³· dyn⁻¹·s⁻¹	Ref.
Capillary			
Dog*	0.21	0.56	115
	0.15	0.40	115
	0.21	0.57	535
	0.26	0.70	492, 493
	0.13	0.35	395
	0.02–0.04	0.05–0.10	240
	0.96	2.60	348
	3.3	8.80	373
	0.11–0.38	0.31–1.03	350
	1.00	2.7	173
	33.3	90.1	373
Rabbit†	0.14	0.23	300
	0.67	1.10	324
	0.98	1.60	527
	2.15	3.50	262
	2.76	4.50	358, 402
Sheep*	0.009–0.014	0.025–0.038	129
Alveolar (maximum)			
Dog*	0.032	0.1	115, 153, 154
Alveolar-capillary			
Dog*	0.05–0.09	0.13–0.25	294
	0.09	0.25	115, 117, 156, 350
	0.06	0.16	115
	0.07	0.19	115

* Hydraulic conductivity calculated assuming surface area of 3,800 cm²/g.   † Hydraulic conductivity calculated assuming surface area of 6,300 cm²/g.

a volume conductivity 25%–50% of that found in skeletal muscle (378).

ESTIMATION OF CAPILLARY FILTRATION COEFFICIENTS WITH STARLING EQUATION. Erdmann et al. (129) and Staub (477) estimated $K_{f,c}$ for sheep lungs by measuring lymph flow and either measuring or assuming values for all Starling forces. The Starling equation (Eq. 4) was then solved for $K_{f,c}$

$$K_{f,c} = \frac{\dot{Q}_{L,T}}{(P_c - P_{ti}) - \sigma_d(\Pi_P - \Pi_{ti})} \quad (14)$$

The same approach yields similar estimates of $K_{f,c}$ for dog (388) and goat (547) lungs. The $K_{f,c}$ values determined by this procedure are 10–20 times smaller than $K_{f,c}$ values estimated with weight gain curves in isolated lungs. The reason for this large difference between $K_{f,c}$ values estimated with the two different approaches is not clear. However, $K_{f,c}$ values measured with a Starling force analysis reflect the volume conductance of the capillary wall and the tissue. The $K_{f,c}$ measured between plasma and lymph with a Starling force analysis is smaller than the smallest $K_{f,c}$ value in the fluid pathway, which leads to a gross underestimation of $K_{f,c}$ for lung capillaries because the tissues have a high resistance to volume flow (159, 199, 489, 495).

ESTIMATION OF CHANGES IN PLASMA-BOUND DYE CONCENTRATIONS. Oppenheimer et al. (373) determined $K_{f,c}$ by analyzing the venous outflow concentrations of a dye (confined to the vascular bed by protein binding) after increases in capillary pressure. They found that the pulmonary $K_{f,c}$ determined in this way may be 100 times greater than $K_{f,c}$ determinations made with the use of curves of lung weight gain. These studies indicate that the capillaries in the septal regions may have very high $K_{f,c}$ values, but when fluid filters into the small tissue spaces surrounding these blood vessels, tissue pressure increases and opposes further volume movement out of the capillaries. Then fluid begins to move from the filtering sites to more remote tissue areas in the lung, such as peribronchial and perivascular spaces. The lung continues to gain weight but at a much reduced rate. The extremely rapid filtration occurring between septal capillaries and their immediate tissue spaces is totally hidden in the early phase of the lung weight gain curve when large blood volume shifts are also occurring. The fluid movement between septal capillaries and more remote tissue sites may be associated with that portion of the lung weight gain that is more frequently used to estimate $K_{f,c}$. If these observations with plasma-bound dyes are correct, a $K_{f,c}$ estimated on the basis of extrapolated weighing techniques reflects tissue volume conductances rather than capillary wall conductances. However, Oppenheimer's studies were conducted with very small changes in capillary pressures and may reflect an experimental artifact. Future studies should repeat the procedure with higher filtration pressures.

ESTIMATION OF CAPILLARY FILTRATION COEFFICIENTS WITH MAXIMAL FILTRATION RATES. Gabel, Drake, Taylor, et al. (117, 156, 350) estimated $K_{f,c}$ by weighing the intact lung in an open-chest dog preparation, which is a modification of the Guyton-Lindsey technique (196). The lungs are forced to gain weight until a constant rate of weight gain is attained. The slope of the constant weight gain is then used to estimate $K_{f,c}$. Filtration coefficients determined with this technique are smaller than those in isolated lung (0.1 vs. 0.3 ml · min^{-1} · mmHg^{-1} · 100 g^{-1}). They have been useful for detecting alterations in capillary permeability (116, 156). The estimation of $K_{f,T}$, however, is complicated by the double-membrane system, and the values are very similar to those determined by Guyton and Lindsey (196).

Estimates of the hydraulic conductivity of capillaries with lung-weighing procedures yield values that are smaller than those for skeletal muscle, intestinal tissues, or subcutaneous tissues. Nonetheless, when the filtration forces in lung are changed, a large filtration is expected because of the large surface area. The importance of $K_{f,c}$ in the regulation of lung fluid balance is related to 1) the rapidity with which fluid can move in or out of the interstitium (198, 199, 478, 500, 502), 2) whether pores in different pathological conditions become larger (140, 362, 407), and 3) the ability of the lymphatics to cope with excess fluid arising from an increased capillary pressure (363). The amount of fluid that enters lung tissue when capillary pressure is increased is a function of how efficiently the Starling forces can change to slow transcapillary filtration. The magnitude of $K_{f,c}$ simply indicates how rapidly the process can occur but not how much the tissue volume will change for a given change in capillary pressure. The tissue volume is determined by the interstitial compliance, Starling forces, and lymph flow! After the tissue forces have adapted maximally and can change no further, $K_{f,c}$ determines how rapidly the lung's air spaces will fill with fluid. At this point, if the lung has an abnormally high $K_{f,c}$, alveolar fluid will accumulate more rapidly. Many investigators think that the filtration pathways (pores) across the pulmonary endothelium are altered when capillary pressure is increased (stretched-pore phenomena) or during different pathological conditions (139, 140, 362, 407, 452). If this occurs then greater accumulation of water is possible when the Starling forces and lymph flow can no longer change to buffer the increased filtration pressures.

Although the relationship of $K_{f,c}$ to lymph flow is discussed in detail later (see FORMATION OF LYMPH, p. 200), knowledge of $K_{f,c}$—at least its order of magnitude—is necessary to assess the lymphatic's ability to remove fluid from the pulmonary interstitium. This ability is not just a function of total lung lymph flow but is inversely proportional to $K_{f,c}$. Because estimates of $K_{f,c}$ differ by two orders of magnitude it is not possible to say how effectively the lymphatic system removes filtered fluid from the lung's interstitium, but the lymphatics easily remove proteins that have escaped the circulation (373).

Capillary Pressure

Pulmonary capillary pressure, the primary filtration force in the Starling equation, is responsible for fluid filtering out of the capillaries into the interstitium and finally forming lymph (198, 477). Physiologically, capillary pressure (which may have no real anatomical counterpart) is defined as a filtration midpoint. In this chapter the term *capillary* is used in the broadest sense because it is well known that fluid can filter from arterial and venous extra-alveolar and alveolar microvessels and that vascular pressures change at different lung heights because of hydrostatic factors (6, 34, 240, 537). In the Starling equation Pc is a functional capillary pressure, which is a weighted mean of all pressures in both a horizontal and vertical direction in the total lung tissue (199, 477, 489, 502).

Pappenheimer and Soto-Rivera (379) defined capillary pressure in two equations relating pulmonary arterial and left atrial pressures to the blood flow ($\dot{Q}_B$) occurring through precapillary (Ra) and postcapillary (Rv) resistances

$$Pc = Ppa - Ra\dot{Q}_B \qquad (15)$$

and

$$Pc = Pla + Rv\dot{Q}_B \qquad (16)$$

The equations have been cast in several forms; the most applicable form (477) is

$$Pc = Pla + \frac{Rv}{Ra + Rv}(Ppa - Pla) \qquad (17)$$

Hellems et al. (220) in 1948 were first to attempt to measure capillary pressure with small catheters placed into both the arterial and venous sides of the pulmonary circulation. Although the measured pressures were not the capillary pressures in the Starling equation, the technique led to the development of Swan-Ganz catheters for indirect estimates of left atrial pressures (428, 534).

Agostoni and Piiper (4) and Agostoni et al. (5) were the first to use a balance of Starling forces to estimate capillary pressure; they based their estimate on the determination of a pleural absorptive pressure and plasma colloid osmotic pressure. The difference between the pleural absorptive pressure for a colloid-free solution and the plasma colloid osmotic pressure was assumed to equal capillary pressure. From the calculated pulmonary capillary pressure they concluded that precapillary resistance was 40% of the total pulmonary vascular resistance. Subsequently Gaar, Taylor, and associates (153, 154) used Pappenheimer's isogravimetric techniques in an isolated dog lung preparation to estimate capillary pressures. They found that ~60% of the total vascular resistance was located in the precapillary segment of the pulmonary circulation. Isogravimetric studies by many investigators yielded similar results, indicating an approximately even division of resistance upstream and downstream from the filtration midpoint (98, 115, 204).

Because isogravimetric techniques are difficult to use in intact lungs, other approaches for assessing some effective capillary pressures have been developed. Dawson and co-workers (95, 97) measured the time course of the pressure drop when a low-viscosity bolus of saline passed through the pulmonary circulation in an isolated dog lung and used Poiseuille's equation to identify the major sites of vascular resistances in the pulmonary circulation. The low-viscosity bolus technique indicated that 60%-70% of the vascular resistance was located upstream from the vascular volume midpoint. Similar estimates of upstream resistances were also calculated by Gilbert et al. (167), who used the concept of a Starling resistor model and assumed that all zone II resistance (when alveolar pressure exceeds pulmonary venous pressure) was postcapillary. Kuramoto and Rodbard (273) placed nonobstructing small catheters into the venous side of the lung's circulation and measured a small drop in venous pressure. The small drop in pressure indicated that most of the resistance in the pulmonary circulation was located upstream from the small venous catheter sites. Gabel and Drake (155) used still another means of estimating vascular resistances. These investigators measured the weight of an in situ lung lobe in an open-chest dog preparation and estimated a postcapillary resistance by converging arterial and venous pressures in steps while maintaining a constant rate of lung weight gain (isofiltration). This technique yielded equal pre- and postcapillary resistances.

All techniques employing isolated lungs or open-chest preparations yielded very similar estimates of pre- and postcapillary resistances, but the measurements were made at normal pulmonary vascular pressures. For normal pulmonary arterial and left atrial pressures the average capillary pressure is 7-9 mmHg with precapillary resistance being slightly higher than postcapillary resistance.

A new approach for estimating capillary pressures has been developed based on studies of arterial and venous pressure transients after venous occlusion in the isolated dog lung (203). This technique measures a capacitance midpoint pressure, because the data were analyzed assuming that most of the vascular capacitance is located at the microcirculation. Values for upstream and downstream resistances demonstrated with this technique are surprisingly similar to capillary pressures estimated with the variety of experimental approaches discussed above.

Venous occlusion midpoint pressures ($P_{v,o}$) have

been compared with isogravimetric estimates (Pc,i) in the same isolated lung. The two estimates of capillary pressure were highly correlated over a Pc,i range of 5–16 mmHg (Pv,o = 1.1Pc,i − 2.1; r = 0.99). This indicates that most pulmonary vascular capacitance normally is located at or near the same region at which most capillary filtration occurs (226, 385a). Therefore occlusive techniques can be used in the unweighed lung to estimate capillary pressures (98, 226, 295).

The occlusion technique has since been modified for use in intact lungs (226, 295). Swan-Ganz catheters were placed into the pulmonary arteries and veins of intact dog lungs and the pressure transients were analyzed after occlusion of either venous or arterial cannulation sites. Because most vascular capacitance appears to be located at or near the capillary filtration midpoint, when an arterial catheter is wedged the pressure should immediately decrease to the pressure at the major capacitance region of the vasculature. Inverse transients should result when venous catheters are wedged (98, 203, 204, 226, 295). The occlusion technique can be used to estimate capillary pressure if the major capacitance site of the pulmonary circulation is at the same location as the filtration midpoint.

Holloway, Parker, Taylor, et al. (226) compared capillary pressures estimated with pulmonary arterial catheter transients (Pc,a) to calculated isogravimetric pressures [Pc,i = Pla + 0.4(Ppa − Pla)]. The correlation was excellent over a range of capillary pressures between 6 and 25 mmHg (Pc,i = 0.64 + 0.99 Pc,a; r = 0.97). The measurement is simple and can be made repeatedly in the same preparation. Apparently arterial pressure tracings can be used to yield reasonable capillary pressure values over a wide range of vascular pressures as compared with predicted values. However, to establish the validity of this measurement in other conditions the technique must be evaluated at different lung heights and when capillary pressure has been changed by various vasoactive compounds. A preliminary study in our laboratory with arterial Swan-Ganz catheter transients recorded during alveolar hypoxia indicates that the pulmonary resistance change is localized at the precapillary segment, which agrees with other published findings (96, 295, 390).

Another method for estimating isogravimetric capillary pressure has been introduced (384, 387). Capillary pressure was determined by measuring an absorptive pressure in small fluid-filled lung segments at different lung heights. Plasma colloid osmotic pressure and regional blood flows (with microspheres) were also measured in these studies. An equation similar to that used previously by Agostoni and Piiper (4) was derived that uses alveolar absorptive pressures to calculate capillary pressure at each lung height (387).

Figure 9A shows capillary pressure as a function of lung height. Note that for zone III conditions [Ppa > Pla > alveolar gas pressure (PA)] capillary pressure was approximately midway between the pulmonary arterial and venous pressures with pre- and postcapillary resistances being 60% and 40%, respectively.

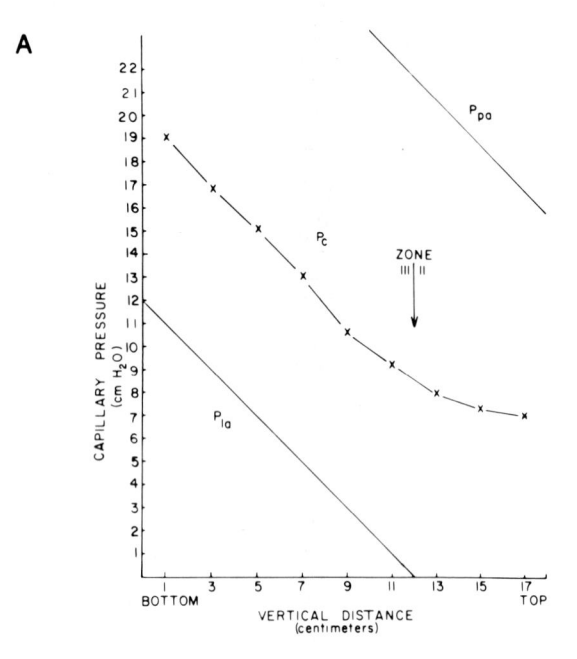

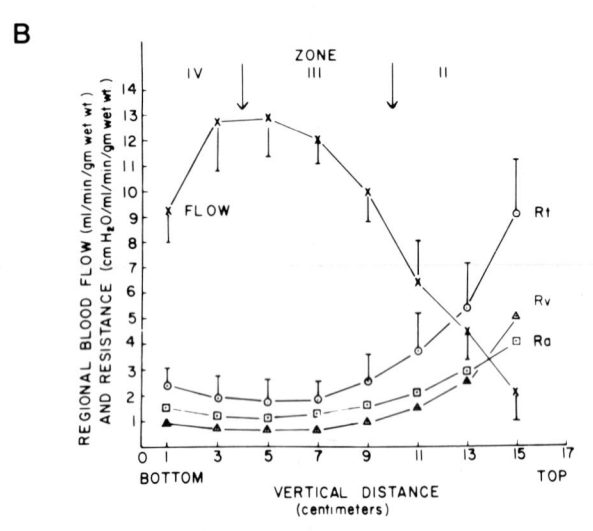

FIG. 9. A: estimation of capillary pressures (Pc) with alveolar absorptive measurements. Capillary pressure is shown as a function of vertical height. Distance between pulmonary arterial pressure (Ppa) and Pc represents precapillary resistance. Distance between left atrial pressure (Pla) and Pc represents postcapillary resistance. Arrow, transition from zone III to zone II perfusing conditions. Zone III, regions of the lung in which venous pressures exceed alveolar pressures. Zone II, areas in which alveolar pressures exceed venous pressures but not pulmonary arterial pressures. B: regional blood flow and resistances as a function of vertical height. Ra, precapillary resistance; Rt, total vascular resistance; Rv, postcapillary resistance. IV, III, and II: zonal conditions within the lung. Arrows, distance from bottom of the lung at which zonal conditions change. Zone IV, height at which vascular resistance increases after zone III condition. [From Parker, Taylor, et al. (387).]

However, as the lung becomes zone II (Ppa > PA > Pla) the resistance abruptly changes. Figure 9B, which shows regional lung blood flow as a function of lung height, indicates that both pre- and postcapillary resistances change in zone II conditions, but postcapillary resistance becomes the dominant resistance as the lung approaches a zone I condition, i.e., PA = Ppa. These findings indicate that alveolar pressures cause either a collapse of lung vascular segments downstream from the filtration sites or a narrowing of their vascular lumens. Hakim et al. (203) and Dawson et al. (95) used very different techniques for estimating pre- and postcapillary resistances and also observed that postcapillary resistances increase as lungs approach zone I conditions.

Parker, Taylor, et al. (387) empirically obtained the following equation, which is useful for estimating capillary pressure in zone II conditions

$$Pc = Ppa - [0.54 + 0.42 (Pa,tr - Pp,a)/Pa,tr](Pp,a - P_A) \quad (18)$$

where Pp,a is the pulmonary arterial pressure at the vertical height and Pa,tr is the pulmonary arterial pressure at which PA = Pla, i.e., the transition point between zone III and zone II conditions. Staub (477) derived a similar equation based on theoretical estimates of the two coefficients appearing in Equation 18.

Although capillaries have been punctured in many capillary beds, only recently have direct microvascular pressures been measured in lungs. Bhattacharya and Staub (27) measured a horizontal pulmonary vascular pressure profile in isolated dog lungs. The micropuncture study provides two very interesting observations: 1) the pre- and postcapillary resistances are ~60/40 when measured from the microvessel anatomical midpoint, and 2) the anatomical pulmonary capillaries provide considerable vascular resistance, which does not agree with more indirect estimates of capillary resistances (204).

Because of the complexities associated with measuring capillary pressure, only a few estimates have been reported for lungs challenged by various insults. However, the changes in pulmonary vascular resistance associated with alveolar hypoxia are well documented. Parker, Granger, and Taylor (390) used isogravimetric procedures to measure pre- and postcapillary resistance and found that precapillary resistance increased to 80% of the total lung resistance during alveolar hypoxia. Venous occlusion (203), low-viscosity bolus techniques (96), and measurement of small-vein resistances (239) yielded similar changes in vascular resistances with hypoxia. When lymph flow was used as an indicator of increased capillary filtration (i.e., an increased Pc), the results also suggested no change in postcapillary resistances during alveolar hypoxia (33).

Hakim et al. (203) reported the effects of several vasoactive substances on upstream and downstream resistances. They indicate that the upstream and downstream resistances measured by venous occlusion techniques in isolated dog lungs may be similar to pre- and postcapillary resistances determined with isogravimetric techniques. The upstream and downstream resistances are determined by the major capacitance portion of the pulmonary circulation. If this is identical to the filtration midpoint, then upstream and downstream resistances are the same as pre- and postcapillary resistances. The results indicate that serotonin increases precapillary resistance, whereas histamine increases postcapillary resistance. The finding that histamine primarily affects postcapillary resistance through an H_1 system has also been demonstrated by Brigham et al. (55, 56) and more indirectly by Kadowitz et al. (255). However, the effects of serotonin on pre- and postcapillary resistances are unsettled: some studies conclude that serotonin primarily affects precapillary resistance (203); others (26, 57) indicate that capillary pressure increases during serotonin infusions. This controversy points out the inadequacy of using upstream and downstream resistances to predict changes in filtration pressures without knowing the relationship between filtration and capacitance sites within the lung's microcirculation. In addition, Rippe, Allison, Parker, and Taylor (429a) recently demonstrated that the effects of histamine, serotonin, and norepinephrine on capillary pressure are different when constant flow through the lung is maintained after introducing these compounds. During constant-flow conditions all compounds increased both pre- and postcapillary resistance and capillary pressure, but only histamine increased capillary pressure in the constant-pressure condition. Therefore, capillary pressure should be measured when possible, because extrapolated values from different experimental models may lead to serious errors in estimating this important determinant of fluid balance.

Hyman, Kadowitz, and colleagues (239, 255) demonstrated that arachidonic acid and its products affect both pre- and postcapillary resistance as determined with small- and large-vein pressure measurements, which agrees with the prostaglandin data obtained by Hakim et al. (203) and Dawson et al. (98). The effects of arachidonic acid on lymph flow and lymph protein concentrations indicate that these compounds affect postcapillary resistances (38). In fact recent studies (M. Townsley, unpublished observations) indicate that arachidonate primarily increases postcapillary resistance and indomethacin totally blocks the effect.

Very little information exists concerning the effects of different physiological and pathological interventions on pulmonary capillary pressure. For the most part very indirect estimates have been used; only recently have methods been developed that may allow measurement of this important determinant of lung fluid balance in closed-chest animals. Future research should evaluate the effects of various pathological conditions on pulmonary microvascular pressures. Interestingly the filtration, resistance, capacitance, and anatomical midpoints appear to be located at the same sites within the pulmonary vasculature in normal lungs.

Tissue Fluid Pressure

MEASUREMENT THEORIES. Several investigators have reviewed the physical and physiological factors that determine tissue fluid pressure in the lung (131, 195, 199, 200, 232, 477). The disagreement surrounding measurements of tissue pressure in subcutaneous tissue has been extended to measurements of tissue fluid pressure conducted in the lung. The major uncertainty is whether micropipettes and cotton wicks inserted into tissues and chronically implanted plastic capsules actually measure the hydrostatic pressure of the interstitial fluid (40, 41, 44, 45, 192, 195, 200, 209, 412, 446, 470). Previous reservations concerning these techniques focused on two possible problems: *1*) colloid osmotic pressure acts across the limiting membrane that forms around implanted devices and affects the measured pressure (11, 540), and *2*) either the osmotic pressure of interstitial mucopolysaccharides (456, 468, 473, 555) or the Donnan effect of small ions within the gel matrix affects wick measurements (182). Because capsular lining membranes are highly permeable to plasma proteins, the first problem is not a great one (184). In addition the intragel Donnan effect contributes only a small portion of the matrix absorptive pressure; thus its effect on wick pressures will be minimal (181, 182, 212). The debate over the osmotic pressure effect of tissue collagens and polysaccharides on wick pressure measurements continues because the nature of interstitial matrix swelling is difficult to define (209, 468, 541).

Another serious problem with describing interstitial fluid pressure is the exact definition of the pressure measured by different techniques. Agostoni (3) studied pressures in the pleural spaces and proposed definitions for interstitial spaces similar to those of Guyton, Taylor, and associates (194, 195). The interstitial tissue fluid pressure (Pti,f) is the hydrostatic pressure that exists within the interstitial fluid. This pressure is responsible for fluid movement within the tissue interstitial gel and across the capillary wall. Agostoni defined the pleural fluid pressure (Ppl,f) as pressure that is in equilibrium with the tissue forces acting across the parietal and visceral pleural surfaces. Many solid components within interstitial spaces touch one another, and pressure will be transmitted between these contact points. Guyton called this pressure solid tissue pressure (Pti,s), whereas Agostoni called the equivalent pleural pressure the deformation pressure ($Pdef$). The other pressure that exists in all tissues is the total tissue pressure (Pti,T). For interstitial spaces, Pti,T is the pressure tending to collapse blood vessels. In the pleural spaces it is the pleural (or surface-averaged) pressure (Ppl). If no solid pressure acts in the tissue spaces, then $Pti,f = Pti,T$; if no deformation pressure acts in the pleural spaces, then $Ppl = Ppl,f$. Agostoni (3) found that pleural fluid pressure decreased (became more subatmospheric) by 1 cmH_2O/cm of height from lung base to apex. Yet when the tendency of the lungs to collapse (surface-averaged pressure) was measured the pressure changed by only 0.3 cmH_2O/cm of height from lung base to apex. Because pleural fluid pressure pulls the lungs outward (expansion), whereas surface-averaged pressure equals the lung's tendency to pull away from the pleural space, another force acting in an opposite direction to pleural fluid pressure must be present if pleural fluid pressure is more negative than pleural pressure. This would be the deformation pressure as described in the following relationship

$$Ppl = Ppl,f + Pdef \qquad (19)$$

and similarly for tissue spaces

$$Pti,T = Pti,f + Pti,s \qquad (20)$$

Permutt, Caldini, et al. (398, 399) applied these concepts to the lung and esophagus and demonstrated that the surface or total tissue pressure and fluid pressures need not be identical if a mechanical pressure is also acting on the tissue space. Lai-Fook (276) used a continuum mechanics analysis to describe the stresses and pressures that surround extra-alveolar vessels and concluded that perivascular fluid and surface-averaged pressures were the same. However, regional differences in fluid pressure within the perivascular sheath can only exist if there is a high resistance to fluid movement within the sheath and between interstitial and pleural spaces (282).

MEASUREMENT OF AVERAGE INTERSTITIAL PRESSURE. Early attempts to determine interstitial fluid pressures in lungs were estimates of the average perimicrovascular pressure surrounding filtration vessels (112, 335, 338, 384). More recent studies show the existence of fluid pressure gradients between different interstitial compartments within lung tissue (222). These interstitial pressure gradients prevent excess accumulation of edema fluid within the gas-exchanging regions of the lung. When excess fluid is filtered by the alveolar septal vessels the interstitial pressure gradient favors the flow of fluid away from the septal gas-exchanging regions into perivascular and peribronchial spaces (cuff fluid formation) (484).

All direct measurements of interstitial fluid pressures in lung tissue have been subatmospheric (279, 338, 380, 384, 389). For more meaningful comparisons of these measured pressures, all tissue pressures should be referenced to both alveolar gas and pleural or surface-averaged pressures. Pressures determined by several different techniques are summarized in Table 3 and referenced to both alveolar gas pressure and pleural or surface-averaged pressure. In spontaneously breathing animals, average alveolar gas pressure and pleural or surface-averaged pressure were assumed to be 0 and −5 cmH$_2$O, respectively, at functional residual capacity (3).

Meyer et al. (338) obtained the first direct measurements of lung tissue fluid pressures with chronically implanted perforated plastic capsules. Mean values for interstitial fluid pressures were −7.9 and −9.9 cmH$_2$O relative to alveolar gas pressures or −3 and −5 cmH$_2$O relative to pleural or surface-averaged pressures in spontaneously breathing dogs. Pressures as low as −21.8 cmH$_2$O were sometimes measured. Mean interstitial fluid pressures increased in response to Tyrode's infusion, increased left atrial pressures, and positive end-expiratory pressures (PEEP). Also transiently negative inspiratory decrements in fluid pressures of 8-10 cmH$_2$O occurred during lung expansion, and greater negative fluid pressures were obtained when the capsules were in a more superior location with respect to the heart. However, pressures at different vertical lung heights were not compared systematically. Parker and Taylor (389) used implanted capsules to measure interstitial fluid pressures in the lungs of spontaneously breathing dogs. A mean interstitial fluid pressure of −7.8 cmH$_2$O was measured at heart level, but these pressures became more negative when capsules were located in more superior regions. The dependency of fluid pressure on vertical lung height explains the variability of interstitial fluid pressures measured in earlier studies (338).

Agostoni and Piiper (4) and Agostoni et al. (5) determined that the mean absorptive pressures for Tyrode's solution at the visceral pleura were −11.8 and −21.3 cmH$_2$O relative to alveolar gas pressure. These absorptive pressure measurements indicate that a negative interstitial fluid pressure surrounds these subpleural lung capillaries. Any contribution of tissue colloid osmotic pressure to the measured absorptive pressures must be small, because the visceral pleura is highly permeable to plasma proteins (263).

Parker, Guyton, and Taylor (384) estimated interstitial fluid pressure by introducing fluid into small airway segments of dog lung. An equilibration pressure was measured in degassed, intralobar lung segments that were filled with fluid after the airways were occluded with a balloon catheter. Average pressures were −14.4 cmH$_2$O relative to alveolar gas pressure for segments filled with Tyrode's solution and −8.2 cmH$_2$O for segments filled with plasma. An interstitial fluid pressure of −10.5 cmH$_2$O was consistent with these measurements. The segment fluid pressures responded to volume loading and increased left atrial pressure changes, as predicted by the Starling equation. In a recent study (380), dogs were ventilated with positive pressure and a mean fluid pressure of −4.8 cmH$_2$O was measured in lung segments filled with Tyrode's solution; this mean fluid pressure increased to −1.1 cmH$_2$O during lung edema. Dynamic decreases in segmental fluid pressures occurred in response to lung inflation, but the average integrated segmental fluid pressure increased in response to increased pulmonary vascular pressure and increased tissue hydration. These studies confirmed that interstitial fluid pressure in the lung was negative and extremely sensitive to interstitial fluid volume changes.

Although quantitative differences exist between steady-state interstitial fluid pressures estimated by either capsules or alveolar absorptive pressures, the dynamic responses of both methods are qualitatively similar (338, 380, 384, 389). For example, both fluid pressure measurements decrease during lung inflation, and both pressures become less negative when either pulmonary vascular pressures or lung interstitial volumes are increased. Generally a sudden elevation of left atrial pressure rapidly increases tissue fluid pressure measurements because the vascular volume expands. This rapid phase is followed by a slower change in fluid pressure as fluid filters into the interstitium. In some instances the fluid pressure plateaus as filtration becomes equal to lymph flow.

The similar dynamic behavior of the two tissue fluid pressure measurements may be due to similar parenchymal stresses acting on the capsules and fluid-filled airways. Both methods use a relatively noncompliant structure embedded within a more compliant homogenous parenchyma. A limiting membrane of connective tissue surrounds the implanted capsules (184). Alveolar wall attachments to this membrane transmit radial stresses during lung expansion because of the low capsule compliance. Because septal fluid communicates with capsular fluid through a length of septal interstitium and through alveolar attachments at the capsular membrane, the capsular fluid pressure should have the same approximate relationship to septal interstitial fluid pressures as that in the sheaths that surround small blood vessels.

If epithelial permeability in the small airways is greater than that in the septa, fluid can move out of the filled airways into the more negative interstitial regions within the perivascular sheaths (160, 161, 479). This should cause the measured absorptive pressures to be weighted toward the interstitial pressures surrounding extra-alveolar or junctional blood vessels, which are not the same as septal pressures. In fact fluid placed into alveoli may directly communicate with perivascular spaces at alveolar ducts without having to traverse the alveolar membranes (160). Regional lobar distortions surrounding these fluid-filled segments may also influence the airway absorptive pressures (94, 127, 554).

ESTIMATION OF AVERAGE INTERSTITIAL FLUID PRESSURE BY ANALYSIS OF TRANSCAPILLARY FORCES. Interstitial fluid pressures have been estimated by measuring or assuming values for the Starling forces and solving the resulting equation for tissue fluid pressure. Levine et al. (293) and Mellins et al. (335) estimated

TABLE 3. *Pulmonary Interstitial Pressures in Dog*

Method	Reference Pressure — Alveolar pressure*	Reference Pressure — Pleural surface pressure	Transpulmonary Pressure	Vascular Pressure	Ref.
Average perimicrovascular fluid pressures					
Fluid absorption by subpleural capillaries					
Open chest, positive airway pressure	−9.8	−21.3	8.5	7.5† (10.2)	5
Isolated lung, negative pressure	−7.9	−11.8	6	8.8†	4
Calculated from Starling force balance					
Intact	−12.2	−8.2	8	14.3†	293
Isolated blood-perfused lobe	−7.4	−4.7	2.7	9†	112
Isolated perfused lobe, alloxan pretreatment	3.6	8.6	5	8.7†	473
Chronically implanted capsules					
Intact	−7.8	−2.8	5‡	14.0†	389
	−9.9 to −7.9	−4.9 to −3.9	5‡	5§	338
Intact, increased left atrial pressure	3.4	8.4	5‡	41§	338
Intact, increased airway pressure	−11	4	16	5§	338
Alveolar fluid absorptive pressures					
Intact, base line	−11	−6	5‡	10*	384
	−9.4	−4.4	5‡	17.7†	268
Intact, 40% lung weight gain	4	9	15†		384
Intact, oleic acid, edema	8.9	13.9	5‡	16.3†	268
Intact, positive airway pressure	−13	−4	8	10.9†	380
Intact, 18% increase in extravascular lung water	−9	0	8	12.0†	380
Perivascular extra-alveolar pressures					
Isolated lobe, wick-catheter hilar peribronchial-perivascular pressures with unperfused plasma-filled vessels, base-line tissue hydration	−6	0.5	6	10	283
	−39	−14	25	10	283
	−14	−9	5	30	222
	−62	−32	30	30	222
Edema, 20%–50% weight gain	−1	4	6	20	283
	−25	0	25	20	283
Edema, 103% weight gain	−6	−1	5	−5	222
	−38	−8	30	−5	222
Negative-pressure inflation	−13	−8	5	10	243
	−27	−2	25	30	243
	−45	−20	25	10	243
	−55	−30	25	−15	243
Negative-pressure inflation, edema, 145% weight gain	−5	−5	0	−15	243
	−38	−13	25	−15	243
Air-filled vessels, positive-pressure inflation	−7	−2	5	25	177
	−34	−9	25	25	177
	−8	−3	5	10	177
	−36	−11	25	10	177
Isolated lobe, hilar extraparenchymal vessels, wick-catheter pressure					
Unperfused plasma-filled vessels	−4.8	−4.8	0	0	242
	−4.8	−4.8	30	0	242
Isolated lobe, intraparenchymal vessels, wick-catheter fluid pressure					
Unperfused plasma-filled vessels	−4.8	−4.8	0	0	242
	−60	−30	30	0	242
Isolated lobe, perivascular pressure calculated from pressure-diameter behavior					
Medium-size extra-alveolar vessels					
Arteries	−6	−1	5	5	465
	−41	−11	30	5	465
	−4.5	0.5	5	20	465
	−25	5	30	20	465
Veins	−5.1	0	5	5	465
	−36.2	−6.2	30	5	465
	−4	1	5	12.5	465
	−33	−3	30	12.5	465
Air-filled vessels, >2 mm diam					
Arteries	−7	−3	4	10	276
	−43	−18	25	10	276
Veins	−4	0	3	10	276
	−33	−8	25	10	276

TABLE 3—Continued

Method	Reference Pressure		Transpul-monary Pressure	Vascular Pressure	Ref.
	Alveolar pressure*	Pleural surface pressure			
Perivascular alveolar pressures					
Isolated lobe, micropuncture of subpleural intra-alveolar fluid, plasma-filled vessels, edema					
60% Weight gain	−2.4	2.6	5		279
	−17.5	7.5	25		279
280% Weight gain	2	3	5		279
	−13.7	11.3	25		279
Isolated lobe, micropuncture of subpleural junctional interstitium, air-filled vessels, edema	−3.6	1.4	5		25
	−2	3	5		25
Isolated lobe, hilar wick pressure, transition point between interstitial filling and alveolar flooding, 20%–50% weight gain	−2	3	5	20	283
	−25	0	25	20	283

All pressures in cmH₂O.   * Assumed equal to atmospheric pressure during tidal breathing in intact animals.   † Capillary pressure at filtration midpoint in perfused vessels based on Pc = 0.4 (Ppa − Pla) + Pla, where Pc is capillary pressure, Ppa is pulmonary arterial pressure, and Pla is left atrial pressure (154).   ‡ Estimated transpulmonary pressure in intact closed-chest animal during tidal breathing.   § Left atrial pressure.

tissue fluid pressure by measuring the net transcapillary pressure needed to produce continuous edema formation during either volume loading or left atrial pressure elevation. An interstitial pressure of −12 cmH₂O (relative to PA) was calculated from these studies. Although the lung interstitial colloid osmotic pressure was not measured in these experiments, the estimated value of 3 mmHg was similar to lymph values reported for dogs with similar degrees of hemodilution (383). This estimate was based on the assumption that the interstitial fluid pressure required to produce alveolar flooding was approximately equal to alveolar gas pressure.

Drake (112) and Drake and Taylor (118) measured capillary pressure, plasma and lymph colloid osmotic pressures, lymph flow, and the capillary filtration coefficient in isolated, blood-perfused dog lungs. They placed these values into the Starling equation and calculated interstitial fluid pressure. In these unique experiments, all parameters were measured in a given experiment except tissue pressure and σ_d. Also the lymph was not contaminated by nonpulmonary sources. Initial estimates of Pti,f − PA ranged from −5.3 to 1.0 mmHg for seven lobes at an average airway pressure of 2 mmHg, and the calculated interstitial pressures increased after each increase in lobe weight.

In similar studies Snashall et al. (473) estimated tissue fluid pressure in unventilated, blood-perfused dog lung lobes at 5 cmH₂O airway pressure. By assuming small values for the lymphatic safety factor and oncotic pressure gradient in the volume flow equation, they equated perivascular interstitial pressure to isogravimetric capillary pressure. Alloxan increased vascular permeability, which was thought to decrease the osmotic pressure gradient in the fluid flux equation because σ_d was smaller and the tissue fluid colloid osmotic pressure (Π_{ti}) was higher. As expected, the calculated tissue pressures were positive relative to alveolar gas pressure (3.7 and 4.4 cmH₂O) when other parameters in the flux equation were considered unimportant. Drake and Taylor (118) identified two sets of isolated lungs in their studies. The first set of lungs had negative tissue fluid pressures in the range of isogravimetric capillary pressures between 4 and 11 mmHg. Tissue fluid pressure increased in direct proportion to capillary pressure with a slope of 1 as the tissues became edematous, i.e., tissue fluid pressure changed by the same amount as capillary pressure. A second set of lungs had positive tissue fluid pressures over the entire range of capillary pressures, and the tissue pressure changed by only 35% of the imposed change in capillary pressure.

Thus a large range of tissue fluid pressures can be calculated with a Starling force analysis. This emphasizes that a solution of the Starling equation may be misleading if all forces are not known. The assumption that the colloid osmotic gradient is unimportant in "leaky lungs" may be incorrect, because σ_d approaches 0.4 for total protein in very leaky lung capillaries and $\Delta\Pi$ is not 0 mmHg but 4–6 mmHg in these studies (473). In addition, alloxan does not always alter lung vascular permeability.

CALCULATION OF PERIVASCULAR PRESSURE WITH MECHANICAL STRESS ANALYSES. The interstitial fluid pressures that surround extra-alveolar blood vessels and bronchi are also important determinants of fluid movement within the interstitium. The mechanical features of these structures are such that negative pressures should exist in these spaces, especially during lung inflation (334, 336, 398). The loss of this negative fluid pressure surrounding extra-alveolar vessels and the favorable gradient for fluid movement from the gas-exchange regions in the septum occur concomitantly with alveolar flooding (279, 283).

Several investigators have calculated peribronchial and perivascular interstitial pressures based on a purely mechanical stress analysis of lung tissue (19,

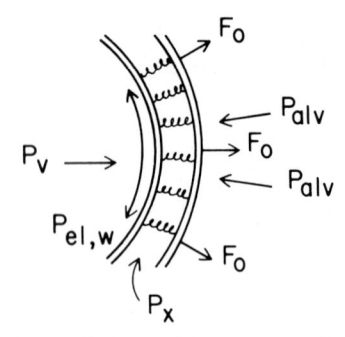

FIG. 10. Schematic representation of balance of forces surrounding an extra-alveolar vessel. F_O, outward acting stress exerted by alveolar wall attachments; P_{alv}, alveolar gas pressure; P_v, vascular pressure; Pel,w, elastic vessel wall tension; Px, interstitial pressure.

27, 334, 465). However, these are actually surface-averaged or total tissue pressures and may be different from the matrix fluid pressure operating in the tissues surrounding extra-alveolar vessels.

Figure 10 is a diagram of the forces acting on the interstitial spaces surrounding an extra-alveolar vessel. The interstitium is bordered by the vessel wall on one side and the vessel sheath on the other. Transmural pressure across the vessel is the difference between vascular pressure (Pvas) and interstitial pressure (Px, which is the same as Pti,T in Eq. 20) and equals the elastic tension on the vessel wall (Pel,w)

$$\text{Pvas} - \text{Px} = \text{Pel,w} \quad (21)$$

Forces across the sheath are represented by

$$\text{Px} = \text{P}_A - \frac{\Sigma F_O}{\text{area}} \quad (22)$$

where ΣF_O/area is the surface-averaged stress of alveolar wall attachments. Thus the forces tending to produce more negative interstitial pressures are the elastic wall tension of the vessel and radial traction exerted by alveolar attachments during lung inflation. Increased vascular and alveolar gas pressures tend to cause less-negative interstitial pressures at a given lung volume. However, the resultant total pressure may differ from the interstitial fluid pressure by the contribution of solid elements (shown as springs in Fig. 10) to the total interstitial pressure (Eqs. 19 and 20).

Lai-Fook and associates (276, 280–282) calculated perivascular and peribronchial surface pressures by relating the stresses that act on these structures to the elastic properties of the lung parenchyma. Vessels and bronchi were treated as thin-walled tubes and lung parenchyma as a homogenous isotropic continuum. Interstitial pressures [referenced to the pleural pressure (Px − Ppl)] decreased linearly with increased transpulmonary pressure from −1 cmH$_2$O to −15 cmH$_2$O around arteries and by a smaller amount around veins. The perivascular pressures were less negative when vascular pressures were increased at any given transpulmonary pressure. Peribronchial pressures were less affected than perivascular pressure with increased lung inflation and were only −1 cmH$_2$O below pleural pressures over a wide range of transpulmonary pressures. Smith and Mitzner (465) obtained similar results in an extensive analysis of lung vascular interdependence. Figure 11 shows the perivascular pressures calculated for arteries and veins. These perivascular pressures were less negative for comparable intravascular pressures and transpulmonary pressures than those reported by others (177, 222, 276, 278), but the vascular compliances in these studies may have been biased toward the more compliant smaller vessels.

MEASUREMENT OF HILAR PERIVASCULAR FLUID PRESSURE. Direct measurements of fluid pressures surrounding large and medium parenchymal vessels and bronchi at the hilum of the lung generally agree with measurements calculated with stress analyses in the lung. To obtain these pressure measurements, either fluid-filled wick catheters or micropipettes are placed into the interstitial spaces between the large intraparenchymal artery and bronchus near the hilum. Wick fluid pressures around these vessels are slightly lower than pleural surface pressures at functional residual capacity (FRC) but decrease linearly relative to pleural pressure as transpulmonary pressures are increased. Fluid pressures become less negative for any given transpulmonary pressure when vascular pressures or tissue hydration increases (177, 222, 243, 283). When blood vessels in isolated lobes were filled with air at 10 cmH$_2$O, the perivascular-peribronchial fluid pressure measured with respect to pleural pressure (Px − Ppl) was −3 cmH$_2$O at a transpulmonary pressure of 5 cmH$_2$O; this pressure decreased to −11 cmH$_2$O at a transpulmonary pressure of 25 cmH$_2$O. Pressure measurements in isolated lobes with plasma-filled blood vessels resulted in similar Px − Ppl values (177). When vessels were completely collapsed with an intravascular pressure of −15 cmH$_2$O, Px − Ppl decreased from −10 to −35 cmH$_2$O as transpulmonary pressure was increased from 5 to 30 cmH$_2$O (222). These studies indicate that the fluid pressures surrounding hilar vessels and bronchi transiently become less negative with vascular distension and more negative with lung inflation. This reflects the balance of tensional forces acting on the interstitial space between the vessel wall on one side and the limiting membrane on the other, as depicted schematically in Figure 10.

The consensus is that perivascular surface pressure is lower than both pleural surface pressure and alveolar gas pressure at FRC and that the tissue fluid pressure becomes considerably lower when transpulmonary pressure is increased. Although some investigators consider perivascular fluid pressures surrounding extra-alveolar vessels and total surface pressure to be equal (276, 278), others have demonstrated a pressure differential of a few cmH$_2$O existing between

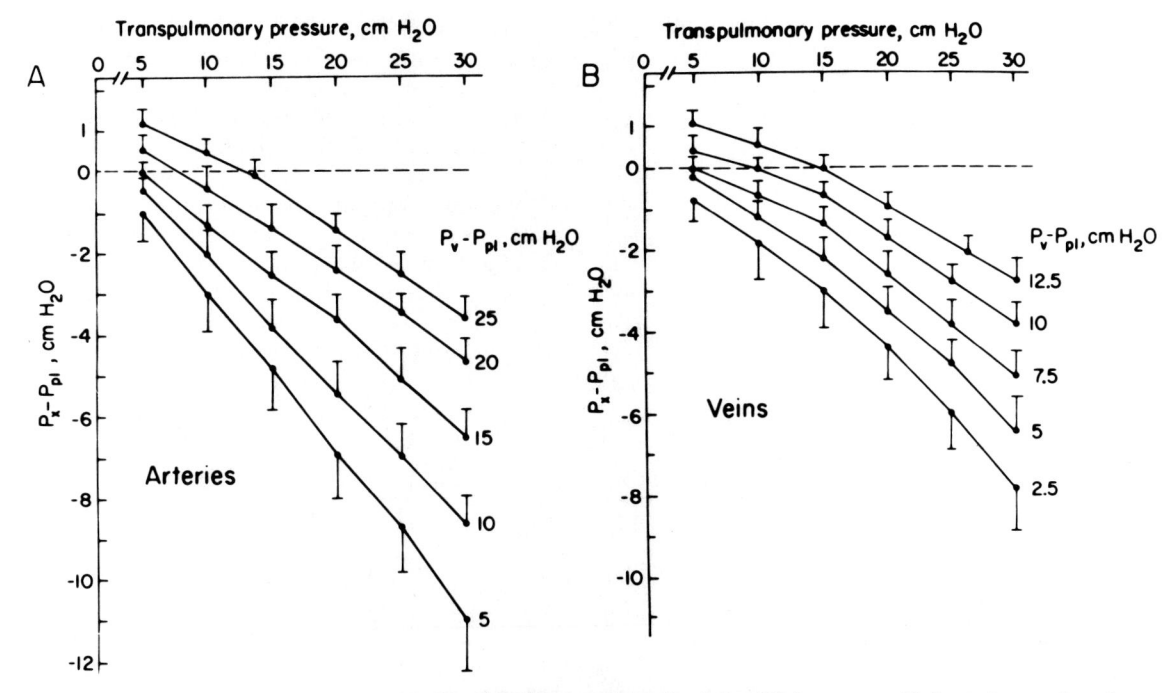

FIG. 11. Calculated perivascular interstitial pressures (Px) relative to pleural pressure (Ppl) as a function of transpulmonary pressure at different vascular pressures (P$_v$). [From Smith and Mitzner (465).]

perivascular surface-averaged and fluid pressures in normally hydrated pulmonary interstitium (222, 242, 243). At physiological pulmonary artery pressures the interstitial fluid pressures relative to alveolar gas pressures surrounding extra-alveolar vessels during a quiet breathing cycle must range between about −5 and −12 cmH$_2$O.

The greater compliance of successively smaller generations of bronchi and blood vessels can result in an interstitial fluid pressure gradient within the interstitium. Small vessels that are more compliant would offer less opposition to the distending forces acting on the limiting membrane. This would cause the tissue fluid pressure surrounding the smaller structures to be less negative than those pressures measured in the spaces surrounding the larger and less compliant blood vessels and bronchi (334, 465). The fluid pressure gradient would increase during inspiration because of the increased radial tension (279). In addition the movement of free fluid in the tissue spaces would always be toward the region surrounding the least compliant structure and away from the important gas-exchange portions of the lung.

MEASUREMENT OF SEPTAL PERIVASCULAR FLUID PRESSURE. Most studies of interstitial fluid pressures in the lung have been attempts to determine the average interstitial fluid pressure surrounding the septal capillaries and small extra-alveolar vessels. These pressures are of major importance in fluid balance because most fluid filtration is thought to occur from these small vessels (232, 240, 477). Although most studies indicate that pericapillary fluid pressure is 3 to 14 cmH$_2$O below alveolar gas pressure (4, 5, 112, 338, 380, 384, 389), some indirect measurements suggest that the average septal interstitial fluid pressure (Psf) may be either equal to or higher than alveolar gas pressure (108, 473, 477).

Pressures in the intra-alveolar fluid and interstitium of subpleural alveoli have recently been directly measured with micropipettes. Figure 12 summarizes these results. Pressures in these studies referenced to alveolar gas pressure were −3.6 cmH$_2$O at the septal junctions in control lungs and increased to −2 cmH$_2$O in edematous lungs (25, 279). In plasma-perfused lobes that had gained 60% of their initial weight, Psf − P$_A$ determined from alveolar liquid pressure measurements averaged −2.4, −11.8, and −17.5 cmH$_2$O at transpulmonary pressures of 5, 15, and 25 cmH$_2$O, respectively. These pressures increased to −2, −7, and −13.7 cmH$_2$O at the same transpulmonary pressures when the lobe was grossly edematous. Alveolar liquid pressures were estimated indirectly by Lai-Fook and Toporoff (283), who measured the transition point in the increasing hilar perivascular pressure during interstitial filling. This transition pressure was approximately −2 cmH$_2$O at a transpulmonary pressure of 6 cmH$_2$O but was reduced to −24 cmH$_2$O at a transpulmonary pressure of 24 cmH$_2$O.

These studies clearly indicate that pressures in the alveolar lining and septal interstitial fluids are subatmospheric in normally hydrated and edematous lungs. These fluid pressures are only 1–2 cmH$_2$O below airway pressure at FRC, but both become more negative

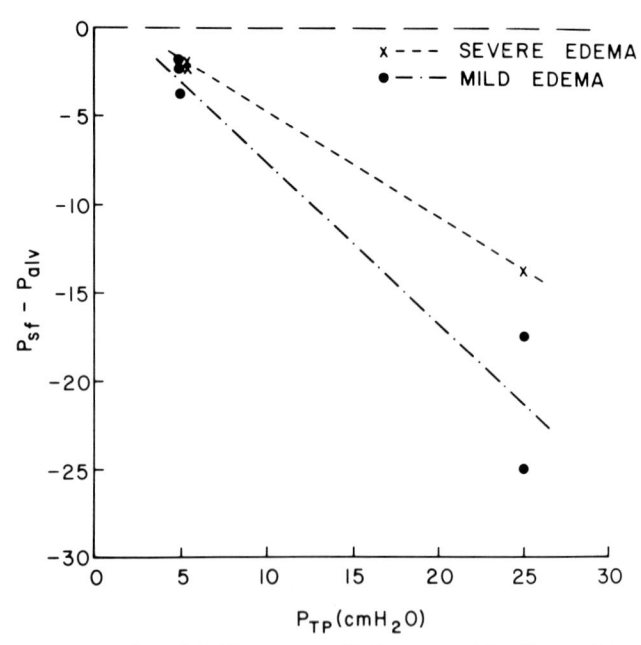

FIG. 12. Septal fluid pressures (Psf) measured by direct micropuncture and calculated from critical pressures for alveolar flooding. P$_{alv}$, alveolar pressure; Ptp, transpulmonary pressure. [Replotted data from Bhattacharya et al. (25), Lai-Fook and Beck (279), and Lai-Fook and Toporoff (283).]

when the lung is inflated. This can be attributed to the increased surface tension acting on the alveolar lining fluid during inflation. Fluid pressure in the alveolar lining layer probably does not become positive in air-filled alveoli, because alveolar flooding occurs before alveolar liquid pressure equals alveolar gas pressure (279).

ESTIMATION OF INTRA-ALVEOLAR FLUID PRESSURE BY ANALYSIS OF STRUCTURE. The forces that act on perivascular fluid surrounding alveolar vessels have been further investigated with ultrastructural techniques that allow the alveoli to be fixed with an intact fluid lining layer (163). The profound influence of surface tension forces on alveolar wall shape is evident when the lungs are preserved by rapid vascular fixation. The surface tension of the alveolar fluid lining layer tends to both minimize the intra-alveolar surface area and flatten any surface distortion of the alveolar wall (165). Therefore the surface geometry of the septal wall is regulated by interfacial surface tensions rather than tissue geometry. This leads to a smoothing of the septal walls in air-filled lungs and filling of intercapillary cusps with fluid, as shown in Figure 13. The smoothing effects of surface tension are particularly pronounced at high lung volumes because the surface tension of the lining layer is estimated to increase during inflation, i.e., from 2 dyn/cm in the collapsed lung to 50 dyn/cm at total lung capacity (12, 82, 165). This surface layer determines alveolar shape even during lengthening of alveolar walls as the septal wall pleats and unpleats within the confines of the fluid layer (166).

The intra-alveolar fluid in the cusps surrounding the septal capillaries is physically stable, whereas fluid pools on the large, concave alveolar surface are inherently unstable (545). The geometry of the cusp fluid pools and a surface tension of 1 dyn/cm have been used to calculate cusp fluid pressures of −9 cmH$_2$O below alveolar gas pressures. Using a similar approach, others have calculated fluid pressures of −20 cmH$_2$O below alveolar gas pressures at the alveolar corners because of their smaller radius of curvature (199).

A major determinant of such calculations is the surface tension assumed for the air-liquid interface. Recent estimates of alveolar surface tension range from 5 to 15 dyn/cm at FRC, but there is mounting evidence that surfactant may not be uniformly distributed over the alveolar surface (393, 394, 421, 447, 546). In particular, surfactant may accumulate in the cusp regions and at the alveolar corners because of the large number of type II pneumocytes in these regions (533, 546). The cusp fluid interface is believed to move in or out of the cusp to balance the fluctuations occurring in the subatmospheric interstitial fluid pressure. This surfactant accumulation may partly compensate for the very small radius of curvature at these cusp fluid interfaces. A critical fluid pressure of −0.4 cmH$_2$O for alveolar flooding has been calculated from the physical features of these cusps (545), indicating again that positive interstitial fluid pressure is not possible in air-filled lungs.

EFFECT OF INTERDEPENDENCE ON INTERSTITIAL FLUID PRESSURE. The interstitial pressures surrounding extra-alveolar vessels are influenced largely by the radial traction exerted on the outer limiting membrane of their interstitial spaces by alveolar wall attachments. These stresses (diagramed in Fig. 10) are responsible for a portion of the negative pressures surrounding extra-alveolar vessels when the lung is inflated. Mead et al. (334) described the mechanical basis for transmission of pleural pressure to all radial planes within the uniformly expanding lung. This interdependence of lung units leads to stability of the alveoli, vessels, and bronchi during changes in lung volume and helps create a pressure gradient for collateral ventilation when bronchi are occluded. The dynamic effects of interdependence may indirectly affect lung fluid balance by establishing a septal-to-hilar interstitial pressure gradient or by acutely decreasing pressure surrounding filtration vessels.

Investigators have observed that blood volume increases in extra-alveolar vessels when lung lobes are inflated (231, 400). This suggests that a distending force surrounds these blood vessels during lung inflation. Permutt et al. (400) proposed that a net force, Px − Ppl, decreases linearly from −20 to −30 cmH$_2$O when lungs are inflated to a transpulmonary pressure of 30 cmH$_2$O. This has been validated by direct perivascular pressure measurements. An index of interdependence (K'), which was derived from the pres-

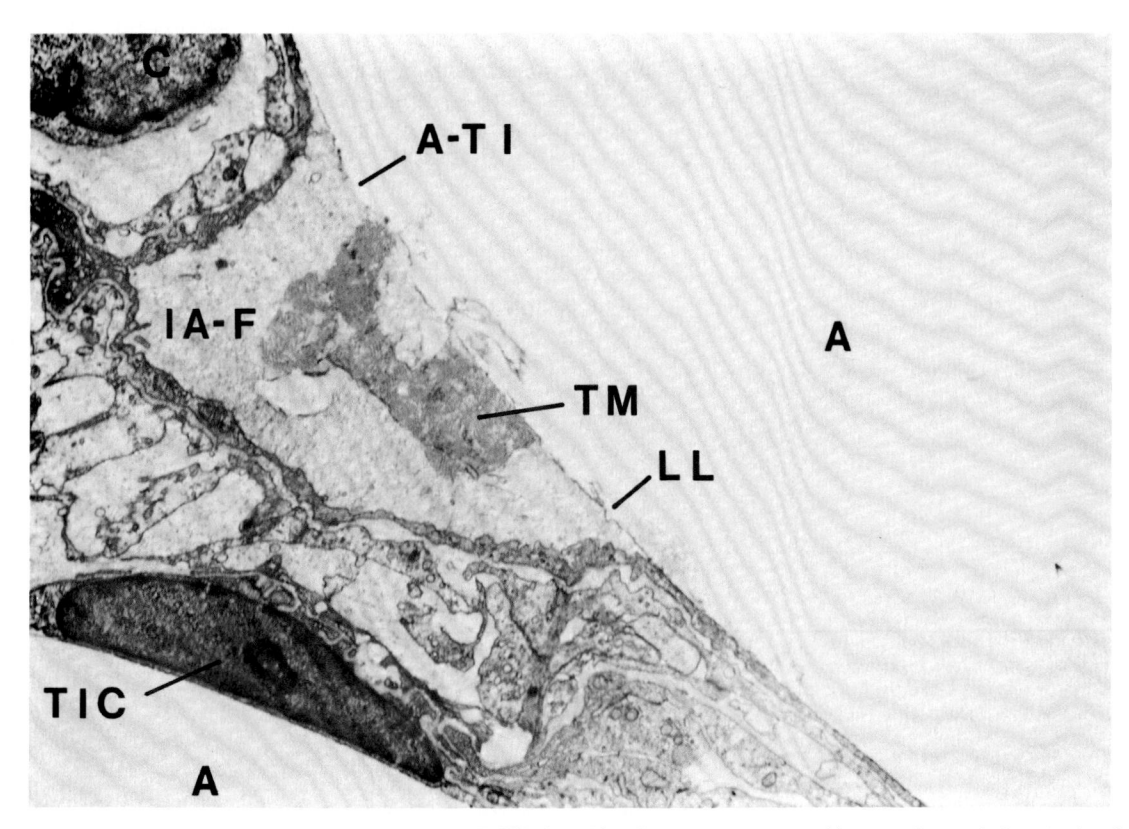

FIG. 13. Rabbit lung alveolar septum preserved by vascular perfusion. A, alveolar space; A-TI, air-tissue interface, which appears very smooth; C, capillary; IA-F, intra-alveolar cusp fluid; LL, lipid lining layer; TIC, type I alveolar cell; TM, tubular myelin (surfactant). × 6,100. (Micrograph courtesy of J. Gil.)

sure-diameter behavior of tantalum-insufflated blood vessels during lung inflation (19), is

$$K' = -\Delta(Px - Ppl)/\Delta Ptp \quad (23)$$

where Ptp is transpulmonary pressure. The K' is a measurement of the differences in distending pressures between the blood vessel and the surrounding lung parenchyma. Values for K' of 1.9 and 2.2 were calculated for extra-alveolar arteries and veins, respectively. These positive values indicate that the net distending force during lung inflation creates a negative pressure in the spaces surrounding the vessel walls (297, 401).

Values for K' can also be calculated with the slopes of the lines that relate perivascular pressure to transpulmonary pressure in the data from the study of Smith and Mitzner [see Fig. 10; (465)]. The K' for arteries decreased from 0.32 to 0.10 as arterial pressure increased from 10 to 25 cmH$_2$O, and K' for veins decreased from 0.25 to 0.17 as venous pressure increased from 5 to 10 cmH$_2$O. Values for K' calculated from the data of Goshy et al. (177) are 0.40 and 0.33 for arterial pressures of 10 and 25 cmH$_2$O, respectively.

The radial traction on such a blood vessel is related to the vessel volume (V$_0$) relative to the surrounding parenchymal volume (V) and the outward pressure that acts on the lung as it expands. The radial traction acting on the perivascular sheath is a function of the ratio of these volumes (V/V$_0$)$^{1/2}$. Interstitial edema increases the sheath volume and has the same effect on the net distending force as an increase in vascular volume. Figure 14 shows that K' values decreased from 0.92 to 0.28 as the lobe weight increased in isolated lung (243). Perivascular wick pressure measurements from the study of Hida et al. (222) yield K' values that decrease from 0.80 to 0.28 as the lung weight increases to similar values. These studies indicate a reduction in radial traction on the interstitial spaces as edema fluid collects, which results in a perivascular interstitial fluid pressure that is less negative. Either increased vascular distension or accumulation of perivascular edema can increase the perivascular interstitial fluid pressure and reduce the fluid pressure gradient that normally exists between septal and perivascular interstitial spaces (199, 279).

Interstitial Compliance

The pressure-volume relationship of the interstitium is a major determinant of lung fluid balance, because the slope of the relationship of $\Delta V/\Delta P$ (the interstitial compliance) indicates how the tissue fluid pressure responds to an increased tissue volume and

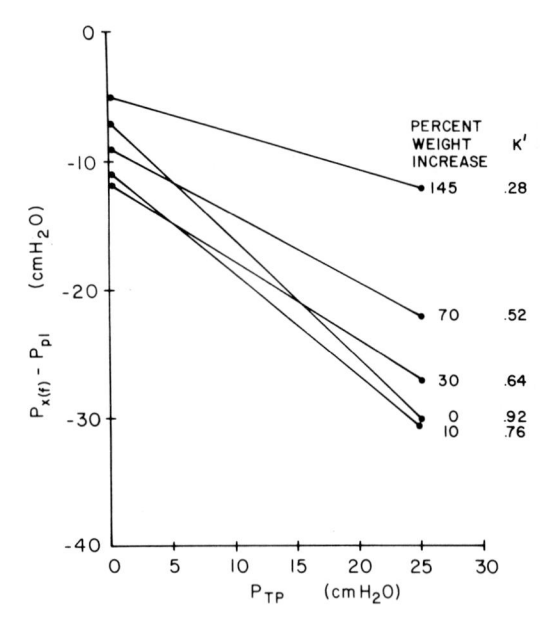

FIG. 14. Hilar perivascular pressure [Px(f) − Ppl] as a function of transpulmonary pressure (Ptp). Decreased values of K′ indicate a decreased radial traction exerted on the perivascular interstitial space as edema forms in the lung. [Data from Inoue et al. (243).]

limits filtration (201). Guyton et al. (193, 194) developed the general concept of interstitial compliance for subcutaneous tissue. These investigators established that the compliance of subcutaneous tissue is nonlinear. At low-hydration states, tissue pressure changes greatly for only small changes in volume (low tissue compliance), but as tissue elements begin to expand, tissue pressure changes very little for large changes in interstitial volume (high interstitial compliance).

Early experiments indicated a small change in interstitial fluid volume at low left atrial pressure, but at left atrial pressures above 25 mmHg edema fluid rapidly accumulated (196, 293, 335). Many investigators (112, 129, 173, 283, 384) have confirmed this nonlinear relationship between edema fluid and left atrial pressure. A typical relationship is shown in Figure 15. Tissue pressure changes markedly with only minimal changes in tissue volume (low compliance) until interstitial fluid pressure approaches alveolar gas pressure. Then tissue fluid volume accumulates at a rapid rate with only small changes in interstitial pressure. The high-compliance portion of the curve may be the transition point at which alveolar flooding occurs. However, the rapid phase of edema formation may also indicate an increased interstitial compliance. In fact interstitial volume has been reported to increase even during alveolar flooding. Moreover some alveolar flooding has been reported during the low-compliance phase of edema formation (340).

Experimental measurements of lung tissue compliance are summarized in Table 4. Most studies in this table are average perimicrovascular compliances constructed with weight gain curves of isolated lungs and estimated changes in interstitial pressure. The change in interstitial fluid pressure was either assumed to equal the change in imposed capillary pressure or was calculated with assumed values for the other forces in the volume flow equation. Drake (112) measured all Starling forces in isolated dog lobes and found that lymph oncotic pressure did not change significantly until capillary pressure exceeded 11 mmHg, but tissue pressure changed identically with capillary pressure over this range. However, if changes in $\Delta\Pi$ are not considered when calculating tissue pressure at higher capillary pressures, the tissue compliance will be overestimated. Average compliances obtained in isolated lobes are ~ 2 ml·cmH$_2$O^{-1}·100 g^{-1} wet wt at low tissue hydration states, increasing 6–10 times when interstitial volume is expanded by 20% to 50%.

Interstitial compliances have also been calculated for in vivo dog lungs with alveolar absorptive pressures as an indicator of tissue fluid pressure (293, 384). These in vivo compliances were computed with postmortem lung water and were $\sim 50\%$ of those values calculated in isolated lungs (112, 304, 348). In two instances the in vivo and in vitro compliances were identical (173, 262).

Direct measurements obtained by inserting wicks into peribronchial spaces have provided compliance curves for the hilar interstitial spaces (222, 243, 283). The compliance of the hilar spaces is 6–10 times the normal interstitial compliance for whole lung. This highly compliant compartment would cause large amounts of fluid to accumulate in these potential spaces during the early stages of edema formation.

The transition point at which the low-compliance phase of interstitial fluid filling abruptly changes to the higher compliance phase of interstitial fluid filling has been measured in isolated lungs with wicks (283). Figure 16 shows hilar wick pressure measurements made during interstitial swelling. The pressure inflection point may be the maximal interstitial volume prior to alveolar flooding, because it occurs at a weight gain of $\sim 35\%$. This transition pressure occurred at 2 cmH$_2$O below PA (Ptp = 6 cmH$_2$O) and at −25 cmH$_2$O below PA (Ptp = 25 cmH$_2$O). Although the total change in perivascular fluid pressure during intersti-

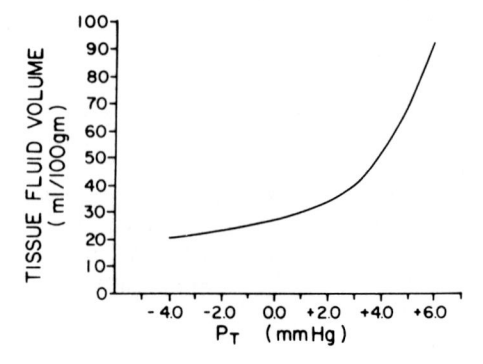

FIG. 15. Lung interstitial volume as a function of calculated interstitial fluid pressure (P$_T$). Slope of *curve* represents total interstitial compliance. [From Drake (112).]

TABLE 4. *Pulmonary Interstitial Compliance*

Method	Compliance Phases, g·cmH$_2$O^{-1}·100 g wet wt^{-1} Low	Compliance Phases, g·cmH$_2$O^{-1}·100 g wet wt^{-1} High	Transition Pressure,* cmH$_2$O	Transition Weight,* × Control	Transpulmonary Pressure, cmH$_2$O	Vascular Pressure, cmH$_2$O	Ref.
Average perimicrovascular compliance							
Dog, intact							
Absorptive pressure of alveolar fluid, gravimetric lung water	0.7	9.0	−1	1.21	5†		384
Starling force balance, safety factor for alveolar flooding	0.5	6.0	0	1.56	5†		293
Dog, isolated lobe							
Calculated tissue pressure change between isogravimetric states	0.7	10		1.07	5		173
	0.9	10		1.07	15		173
	2.2	13	0	1.20	2		112, 118
Vascular pressure change required to maintain isogravimetric state after filtration‡	1.8			>1.16	4		348
	0.9			>1.07	30		348
Rabbit, isolated lobe							
Calculated from Starling force balance	1.4				5.4		304
Calculated from fluid filtration between isogravimetric states	1.0						262
Hilar peribronchial-perivascular compliance							
Dog, isolated lobe							
Wick-catheter fluid pressures and lobe weight gain	10	60	−2	1.33	6	10–25	283
	4	60	−25	1.30	25	10–25	283
	30			2.5	0	−15	243
	8.8			2.5	25	−15	243
	12.9		−5	2.4	5	−15	222
	6.5		−20	2.1	20	−15	222
Calculated perivascular pressure from stress analysis	5.9						465

* Transition pressures are referenced to alveolar gas pressure. † Estimated for intact closed-chest dog at functional residual capacity. ‡ Assumes no transcapillary colloid osmotic pressure gradient.

tial filling was directly related to transpulmonary pressure, the fluid volume at which the transition occurred was independent of transpulmonary pressure. However, increasing the interstitial filling volume approximately twofold by decreasing vascular pressure to −15 cmH$_2$O is possible (222, 243). Apparently when the blood vessels are collapsed the displaced vascular volume is replaced by an equivalent volume of perivascular interstitial fluid prior to alveolar flooding. In general an increased transpulmonary pressure is associated with a decreased perivascular interstitial compliance, because measured interstitial compliances at a transpulmonary pressure of 25 cmH$_2$O were ~50% of those observed at a transpulmonary pressure of 5–6 cmH$_2$O (222, 243, 283).

In conclusion the total interstitial compliance of lung tissue has two distinct phases: *1*) a low-compliance phase at low interstitial fluid volumes and *2*) a high-compliance phase during advanced interstitial edema or alveolar flooding. The interstitial spaces surrounding larger blood vessels and bronchi have a much higher compliance than the interstitium as a whole, which may be weighted toward the less compliant interstitium located in the septal regions. At high lung volumes the tissues are stiffer and the interstitial spaces less compliant; the capacity for interstitial filling also appears to be inversely related to vascular filling. However, once the perivascular

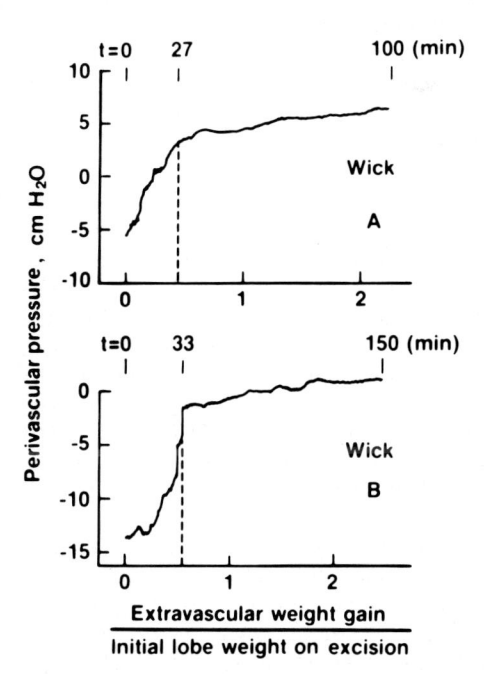

FIG. 16. Wick-catheter measurements of hilar perivascular fluid pressures as a function of lobe weight gain. Lobe A: vascular pressure, 25 cmH$_2$O; transpulmonary pressure, 20 cmH$_2$O. Lobe B: vascular pressure, 20 cmH$_2$O; transpulmonary pressure, 25 cmH$_2$O. Larger changes occur in perivascular fluid pressure during interstitial filling than alveolar flooding. [From Lai-Fook and Toporoff (283).]

spaces surrounding extra-alveolar vessels and bronchi are maximally filled with fluid, interstitial pressures equilibrate throughout all interstitial spaces. Further fluid filtration would then increase tissue fluid pressures to a critical level and intra-alveolar edema rapidly ensues.

Interstitial Fluid Pressure Gradients

The transvascular filtration occurring in the lung involves mostly alveolar vessels and small extra-alveolar vessels because of their large surface areas (233, 240, 477). The exact pathways for fluid movement through the interstitium have not been experimentally determined. However, it is generally believed that fluid filtered from the septal region moves along fluid pressure gradients to the terminal lymphatics, which are located in the tissue spaces surrounding the terminal bronchioles. Direct measurements of intra-alveolar fluid and septal fluid indicate a pressure below alveolar gas pressure but above the pressures that surround extra-alveolar vessels and bronchi (25, 279, 283, 465). Both intra-alveolar and extra-alveolar interstitial fluid pressures decrease markedly with lung inflation. At a transpulmonary pressure of 5 cmH$_2$O, an overall gradient between intra-alveolar or septal fluid and periarterial fluid pressure of 3–4 cmH$_2$O can be calculated. This gradient increases to 14 cmH$_2$O at a transpulmonary pressure of 25 cmH$_2$O (222, 242, 243, 277, 283). However, longitudinal gradients within the pulmonary tissues may differ in each vertical region because of the vertical gradients that exist in vascular and transpulmonary pressures.

Three major forces act on septal tissue fluid to move it toward the terminal lymphatics: *1*) interfacial surface tension forces, which act on the intra-alveolar lining fluid, *2*) tensional stresses, which act on the collagen support fibers that are interwoven with the septal capillaries (12, 164, 533, 546), and *3*) negative fluid pressures, which surround the extra-alveolar blood vessels and airways. Because surface tension tends to minimize the surface area of the lining fluid, a pressure is created over the alveolar surface that tends to compress protruding portions of septal capillaries and pull fluid from the intercapillary cusps between capillaries (Fig. 17, arrows). The solid arrows in Figure 17 indicate the force vectors created by the surface pressures. Vascular distending pressures force fluid from the compressed interstitial spaces toward the intercapillary cusp regions. Figure 17*A* shows these routes for fluid movement as dashed arrows (533). In addition an overall pressure gradient for fluid flow toward the alveolar corners is established by the negative pressures generated by their small radius of curvature (82, 199, 544). Preferential pathways or "drip channels" along the collagen support fibers within the thick portion of the interstitium provide routes for this fluid movement (85, 135, 533). An increased transpulmonary pressure and lung volume will increase the intra-alveolar surface tension and the pressure gradient for fluid movement toward septal junctions (82). In addition, as the elastic fibers are stretched and collagen fibers repositioned, they may compress the more deformable interstitial matrix and express interstitial fluid from its interior (182). Fluid can then preferentially migrate along the interstitial spaces at the junctions of the alveolar septal walls (544); this effect has been demonstrated by the migration of ink through a froth of soap bubbles (477). Migrating fluid next enters juxta-alveolar lymphatics or lymphatics surrounding terminal airways and within vascular sheaths (288, 289). The efficiency of such a system for fluid transport is evident by the absence of a marked increase in septal width until the late stages of edema formation (85, 100, 101), but cyclic lung inflation apparently facilitates fluid movement from the vascular filtration sites to the more remote perivascular and peribronchial tissue spaces (172).

Mechanical forces in the lung create the pressure gradients for fluid to move along the larger vessels and bronchi (Fig. 17*B*, dashed arrows). The decreasing interstitial compliance at successive generations of smaller extra-alveolar vessels and bronchi favors the creation of an interstitial pressure gradient between these smaller structures and lung hilum (279, 465). Hida et al. (222) failed to detect a difference between perivascular wick pressures measured around large and medium arteries in isolated lobes. However, the lower interstitial fluid pressure and higher interstitial compliance enhance the accumulation of excess tissue fluid in the perivascular interstitium (484). Appar-

FIG. 17. *A*: schematic representation of fluid pathways (– – →) and pressure vectors (——→) in septa and septal corner regions. *B*: fluid pathways in whole lung.

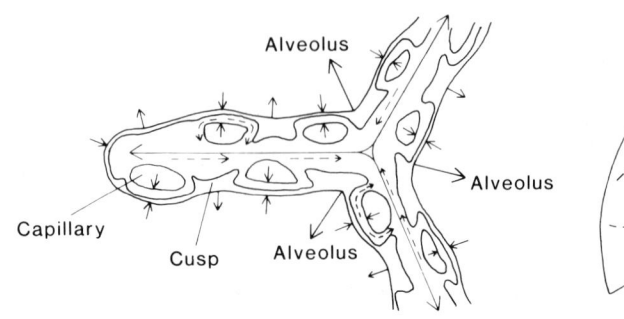

ently septal fluid pressures do not change greatly until the perivascular interstitial spaces are filled. Once these spaces are filled the perivascular pressure around septal vessels begins to increase and abolishes the fluid pressure gradient from alveolar-to-perivascular tissue (199, 279). This means that the tissue pressure gradient from septa to hilum acts as a "safety factor" against the formation of alveolar edema (200, 201). This gradient has been estimated to increase by 56% of the imposed increase in transpulmonary pressure (279, 283).

In addition to the longitudinal gradient in interstitial fluid pressure from alveolar septa to perivascular sheaths, vertical interstitial pressure gradients may exist between lung heights. Two factors could contribute to the establishment of the proposed gradients at different lung levels: 1) a vertical gradient in hydrostatic pressures within the blood vessels and 2) vertical gradients in pleural surface pressures and regional lung volumes (3, 169, 225, 477, 538). Theoretical estimates of the vertical pressure gradient of the interstitial fluid range from 1.0 cmH$_2$O/cm vertical distance to 0 cmH$_2$O/cm vertical distance (232, 477). An intermediate vertical gradient in tissue fluid pressure of 0.63 cmH$_2$O/cm vertical distance was calculated from the mathematical model of Guyton, Taylor, Drake, and Parker (199). Direct measurements of interstitial pressure have been reported at different heights in the lung. Vertical gradients of 0.60 cmH$_2$O/cm vertical distance for capsular fluid pressures and 0.78 cmH$_2$O/cm vertical distance for alveolar absorptive pressures were measured in intact spontaneously breathing dogs (389). However, no significant vertical gradient was obtained in the micropuncture studies of subpleural alveolar fluid pressures in excised lungs (25, 279). The absence of any vertical transpulmonary pressure gradient in excised lung lobes may account for this apparent difference in interstitial fluid pressure gradients between intact animals and excised lungs.

Table 5 summarizes the predicted perivascular pressures surrounding alveolar and extra-alveolar vessels at three vertical levels 7 cm apart in an intact lung. The distribution of these interstitial pressures is based on the measured relationship of the various interstitial pressures to transpulmonary and vascular pressures and the observed vertical gradients in in situ lungs. During spontaneous respiration, alveolar gas pressure equals atmospheric pressure; midlung pleural pressure was assumed to equal −5 cmH$_2$O with a vertical gradient of 0.3 cmH$_2$O/cm vertical distance (3). Alveolar septal fluid pressures were obtained at comparable transpulmonary pressures from Figure 12. Pulmonary arterial and left atrial pressures at the midlung level were 20 and 7 cmH$_2$O, respectively, with vertical gradients of 1 cmH$_2$O/cm vertical distance.

Capillary pressures were calculated with Pc = 0.4(Ppa − Pla) + Pla (154), and the arterial perivascular pressures were obtained from Lai-Fook's studies

TABLE 5. *Vertical Pressure Gradients in Zone III Lungs*

Pressures	Apex	Mid-lung	Base	Ref.
Alveolar gas pressure*	0	0	0	
Pleural surface pressure†	−7	−5	−3	3
Intra-alveolar and septal interstitial fluid pressure	−4.8	−2.9	−1	25, 279
Pulmonary arterial pressure	14	20	28	
Left atrial pressure	0	7	14	
Capillary pressure‡	5.6	12.2	19.6	154
Capillary transmural gradient	10.4	15.1	20.6	
Arterial minus pleural pressure	21	25	31	
Extra-alveolar perivascular minus pleural pressure	−5	−3.5	−2	276
Extra-alveolar perivascular minus alveolar gas pressure	−12	−8.5	−5	
Fluid pressure gradient from septal to periarterial interstitium§	7.2	5.6	4	

All pressures in cmH$_2$O. * Atmospheric pressure in spontaneously breathing animals. † Vertical gradient of 0.3 cmH$_2$O/cm vertical distance. ‡ Pc = 0.4 (Pa − Pla) + Pla, where Pc is capillary pressure, Pa is arterial pressure, and Pla is left atrial pressure. § Longitudinal pressure gradient.

(276, 278) for comparable vascular and transpulmonary pressures. Vertical gradients were calculated by dividing the pressure differences by the vertical distance. The vertical gradient in capillary transmural pressure (Pc − Psf) was 0.73 cmH$_2$O/cm vertical distance, and the vertical gradient in pulmonary arterial transmural pressure (Ppa − Ppl) was 0.71 cmH$_2$O/cm vertical distance. The vertical gradient in arterial perivascular pressure (Px − Ppl) was 0.21 cmH$_2$O/cm vertical distance, and the vertical gradient in the net driving pressure for fluid from the septal to perivascular interstitium (Psf − Px) was 0.23 cmH$_2$O/cm vertical distance. This indicates a reduced pressure gradient between septal and perivascular spaces at the base of the lung relative to the apex. However, static pressure gradients may be misleading when applied to the living lung, because the changes in regional gas volumes during tidal or forced inspirations are greater toward the base than the apex (169, 537). The increases in surface tension and interdependence could transiently produce a greater decrease in both alveolar fluid and perivascular fluid pressures (relative to PA) at the base of the lung than the apex. Menkes et al. (336) reported a greater interdependence in lung segments that were more dependent. A greater vascular interdependence at the base of the lung could theoretically produce a larger septal-to-perivascular pressure gradient at the base than at the apex. This could explain why no vertical gradient has been found for either extravascular water or the morphometric dimensions of interstitial spaces in the lung (12, 14, 142, 207, 472). Hales et al. (207) have proposed the possibility of a vertical perivascular interstitial pressure gradient to explain why early edema forms uniformly at all vertical levels when it has long been thought that fluid accumulates more readily in the more dependent areas of the lung. In addition the preferential appearance of edema in the basal lung lobes of dogs placed in either the head-up or head-down position may relate to the effects of parenchymal interdependence affecting fluid pressure gradients (292).

Although mechanical and surface forces undoubtedly influence interstitial fluid pressures, the interstitial matrix also has an important regulatory role in fluid movement. In a continuous interstitium such as that in the lung, fluid would move easily between interstitial regions if not impeded by the resistance of the interstitial gel. The hydraulic conductivity of the normally hydrated gel is extremely low but increases by orders of magnitude when gel hydration is increased (182, 197).

An equivalent pore can be calculated for the lung interstitium based on exclusion data obtained in normal and edematous dog lungs. The pore size required to predict albumin exclusion increased from 250 to 600 Å as the lung weights increased by 40% (383). The marked increase in interstitial pore size estimated during edema formation implies an increased hydraulic conductivity in the interstitial spaces. This could explain why the initial phase of edema formation is not gravity dependent, although edema fluid readily accumulates in the more dependent areas when the interstitial resistance decreases and fluid simply moves from the top to the bottom of the lung (207).

The arrangement of the gel matrix can also influence the transport of protein molecules. The presence of open free-fluid channels would facilitate the transport of large molecules in tissues, similar to the transport that occurs in gel columns (182). However, equilibration rates of albumin and fibrinogen between plasma and right duct lymph suggest a more rapid equilibration of the smaller macromolecules (339, 340) and indicate that free-fluid channels do not exist in normally hydrated lungs (149).

A mathematical model of fluid transport indicates that a low hydraulic conductance of the septal interstitium could cause a fluid filtration coefficient for lung tissue that is very low overall, even though the filtration coefficient of the fluid-exchanging blood vessels is large. As the pulmonary capillary pressure increases, both the hydration of the septal interstitial pathway and the hydraulic conductivity increase (Fig. 18). Fluid then will move more easily between the filtering capillaries and the perivascular interstitium, resulting in a progressive decrease in the septal-to-perivascular fluid pressure gradient (Fig. 18, *lower panel*) as perivascular fluid accumulates. However, the edema safety factors prevent excessive septal swelling and alveolar flooding until the septal-to-perivascular fluid pressure gradient no longer exists, which occurs

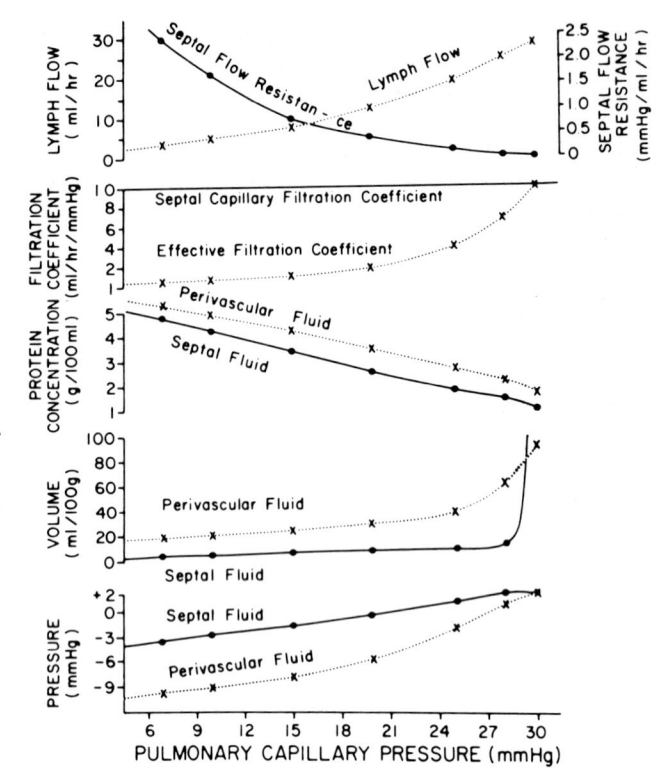

FIG. 18. Effect of steady-state increases in capillary pressure on pressure gradients between septal and extra-alveolar interstitial fluid, hydraulic conductivity of the septal interstitium, lymph flow, lymph protein concentration, and edema fluid accumulation in both the septal and perivascular interstitium. [From Guyton, Taylor, Drake, and Parker (199).]

in this model at a capillary pressure of 28 mmHg (199).

Colloid Osmotic Pressure Gradient

Since the early studies of Starling (476) and the more recent studies of Guyton and Lindsey (196) and Garr, Taylor, et al. (153, 154), physiologists and clinicians have recognized the importance of the colloid osmotic pressure as a primary regulator of fluid balance (23, 129, 195, 201, 477, 491, 516, 534). However, a complete analysis of this important force requires three different parameters. *1)* The osmotic reflection coefficient (σ_d), which is related to the selectivity of the pulmonary capillary membrane, must be measured. The $\sigma_d = 1$ for molecules that are impermeable at the capillary wall. If the capillary membrane is freely permeable to the plasma proteins then $\sigma_d = 0$ (258, 261). For pulmonary capillary membranes, $\sigma_d < 1$. Attempts to estimate this important parameter constitute one of the most active areas of research in pulmonary physiology (501). *2)* The colloid osmotic pressure of the plasma (Π_P) can now be measured with a simple membrane osmometer (413); however, in many instances, Π_P has been calculated from plasma protein concentrations and published equations (285,

354). *3*) The colloid osmotic pressure of the tissue (Π_{ti}) has never been directly measured in normal lung tissue. Most published information has used pulmonary lymph as an indicator of tissue fluids. A rigorous definition of a steady state between tissue volume, lymph flow, and capillary protein leakage is required before Π_{ti} and the colloid osmotic pressure of the lymph (Π_L) can be assumed equal. Although lymph may not reflect tissue fluids in a non–steady state, no evidence argues convincingly against equating Π_L with Π_{ti} (360, 361, 422, 483, 494, 522–524). Some investigators think that the bronchial circulation may contribute to lung lymph (85, 405, 406), and the concentration of protein can be altered in lymph during its passage through nodes (1, 422). Furthermore some pulmonary lymph preparations may be contaminated by nonpulmonary sources (113, 323). At this time lymph is the best choice for tissue fluid samples. However, serious problems do exist with equating Π_L to Π_{ti} in some experimental models.

MEASUREMENT OF CAPILLARY SELECTIVITY TO PLASMA PROTEINS. Drinker (119) and Warren and Drinker (528) developed the dog right duct lymph model that many investigators have used (36, 159, 339, 340, 367, 368, 521). However, studies indicate that right duct lymph is contaminated by extrapulmonary sources and may not accurately represent changes in capillary filtration or lung tissue fluids, unless the experimental maneuver affects only the lung (322, 323, 551). For example, when saline loading decreases plasma protein concentrations, a carefully cannulated right duct preparation will produce lymph flow increases of 120-fold, whereas lymph flow measured directly from a lung lymphatic that is cannulated before passing through nodes increases only 20-fold (159, 323, 383).

Parker, Taylor, and associates (190, 382, 383, 387, 437) developed a lung lymphatic model in which a small prenodal lymphatic is cannulated at the hilum of the lower left lobe in dogs. This preparation is useful for acute studies and is not contaminated by extrapulmonary sources. It does, however, require that the chest remain open during the experimental procedures.

The most widely used technique for studying pulmonary fluid balance has been the sheep lymphatic model (129, 347, 482). A caudal mediastinal efferent lymphatic is cannulated in the sheep and the animal allowed to recover from the surgery. The sheep can then be studied in an unanesthetized state, and lymph flow, left atrial pressure, and lymphatic protein concentrations can easily be monitored. Drake et al. (113) have challenged this experimental model. They contend that the lymph is contaminated from nonpulmonary sources (especially diaphragmatic and esophageal), which may lead to erroneous conclusions about pulmonary capillary selectivity to macromolecules, especially with substances such as histamine and endotoxin, which affect the systemic circulation. In addition the node appears to exchange proteins and fluid freely with plasma (1); studies indicate that histamine (320) and endotoxin (T. Adair, unpublished observations) greatly affect protein exchange within the node. The problem of contamination and nodal alteration of lymph is serious when this model is used to assess capillary permeability to plasma proteins.

Another interesting approach for evaluating selectivity of pulmonary capillaries to macromolecules has been used by Kern (262), who measured the accumulation of a radioactive macromolecule (^{131}I-labeled albumin) in lung tissue as a function of time in isolated, isogravimetric rabbit lungs. From this measurement an estimate of the permeability–surface area product can be determined, assuming only diffusion is occurring (29, 262). Then capillary pressure is increased and while the lung is gaining weight another isotopically labeled albumin (^{125}I) is injected into the perfusate and the contents of the tissues are analyzed. With these measurements and the following equation, σ_d can be estimated

$$J_S = (1 - \sigma_d)\overline{C}J_V + PS\Delta C \qquad (24)$$

where J_S is the solute flux, $\overline{C}$ is the average concentration, J_V is the volume flow, PS is the permeability–surface area product calculated in the isogravimetric state, and ΔC is the concentration gradient acting across the capillary wall. This technique can only be used in isolated and weighed lungs. A modification has been developed by Horovitz and Carrico (228), who measured isotopic flux of albumin into lung tissue over a given period. Although changes in capillary wall selectivity will certainly alter protein flux, the technique is limited because area changes and/or increased capillary filtration will also increase protein extraction. Nonetheless this approach allows qualitative estimates of changes in pulmonary capillary permeability after different experimental interventions and does not require lymphatic cannulation or total lung isolation to estimate a change in lung vascular permeability, at least in a qualitative sense.

Attempts have been made to use small molecules to assess pulmonary vascular selectivity (395, 493, 527). To accomplish this, osmotic transients were measured in isolated lungs for small molecules and the results were extrapolated to larger molecules. Although the agreement between most values extrapolated from small molecular osmotic transient data and lymphatic determinations of σ_d for albumin are good, direct osmotic estimates of σ_d by Wangensteen et al. (527) yielded much smaller σ_d values, which may reflect some experimental artifact rather than unselective pulmonary capillaries in rabbit lungs.

Other very promising techniques for evaluating pulmonary capillary permeability in intact lungs have been introduced by Gorin and Stewart (175), Gorin et al. (176), Prichard and Lee (414), and Prichard et al. (415). These methods involve external counting of radioisotopes over the lung fields to obtain a qualitative estimate of changes in lung vascular permeability in intact lungs of humans and animals. Other approaches use labeled albumin clearances into alveolar edema fluid (454) or analyses of the concentrations of plasma proteins in alveolar fluid to evaluate different types of clinical pulmonary edema (133). Both techniques are apparently easy to apply to the clinical setting and separate permeability edemas from hydrostatic-induced edema, because the concentration of proteins in edema fluid approaches plasma values in permeability edema.

Figure 19 shows the lymph-to-plasma concentration ratios for several protein fractions and povidone [polyvinylpyrrolidone (PVP)] as a function of the molecular radius of the probing molecules. As the molecular radius of the probing molecules increases, C_L/C_P decreases. Over the last several years many investigators have attempted to define both physical and physiological approaches for measuring σ_d (32, 42, 43, 180, 214, 332, 333, 388, 402, 497, 499, 501). One useful approach, which depends on the behavior of C_L/C_P at different lymph flows (180, 501), is described by the following equation developed by Granger and Taylor (180) from Patlak's (392) and Bresler's (49) equations

$$C_L/C_P = \frac{1 - \sigma_d}{1 - \sigma_d e^{-x}} \quad (25)$$

where $x = (1 - \sigma_d)\dot{Q}_L/PS$ (PS is the permeability-surface area product and $\dot{Q}_L$ is the lymph flow).

Figure 20 plots C_L/C_P for different-sized molecules and different PS values for a simple membrane system. As the volume flow increases across the membrane, C_L/C_P decreases; at high volume flows, C_L/C_P approaches a constant value, i.e., $C_L/C_P \rightarrow 1 - \sigma_d$. This occurs when the diffusional term is zero in the flux equation and $x \cong 2-4$ (388, 496, 497). When $\dot{Q}_L$ is large, C_L/C_P becomes filtration rate independent and does not change at higher $\dot{Q}_L$ values. For a given $\dot{Q}_L$, C_L/C_P is larger when the membrane is more permeable to the solute (Fig. 20A). To analyze the permeability characteristics of the pulmonary capillary membrane, the different proteins in lymph are measured by electrophoresis at normal lymph flows. Then venous pressure is increased in steps and steady-state C_L/C_P values are obtained. Once each protein becomes filtration rate independent, $\sigma_d = 1 - C_L/C_P$, and the appropriate pore theory can be applied to the results.

Figure 20B illustrates the problem associated with evaluating C_L/C_P at various lymph flow states. *Line 1* is for a σ_d of 0.9 and a surface area of 1; *line 2* is for a σ_d of 0.7 and a surface area of 1; *line 3* is for a σ_d of 0.9 and a surface area of 3. The same C_L/C_P (Fig. 20B, *points A, B, C*) can be obtained at different lymph flow states. For *point B* this represents an increased permeability (i.e., $\sigma_d = 0.7$), but for *point C* this results if only surface area (and not vascular permeability) is higher. Many investigators measure C_L/C_P at normal lymph flows and then challenge the lung with a compound such as histamine. If C_L/C_P was unchanged but lymph flow increased without any observable change in capillary filtration pressure, these investigators assumed that the particular challenge increased vascular permeability. Obviously this need not be the case. Figure 20B also depicts the relationship between C_L/C_P at the same lymph flow (Fig. 20B, points A', B', C'). Increased permeability increases C_L/C_P at the same lymph flow, but surface area changes give the same results. Therefore it is impossible to discuss vascular permeability by looking only at small changes in lymph flow and protein content. The only sure way of measuring a permeability factor (σ_d) is to force the system by elevating filtration forces until C_L/C_P for the solute(s) under study becomes constant. Then $C_L/C_P = 1 - \sigma_d$ for each protein in lymph.

The C_L/C_P values in the lung have been determined with several experimental models, but only a few studies have data for several protein fractions at high rates of volume flows; in these studies C_L/C_P approached a constant value (388, 391). Figure 21A shows a plot of $1 - \sigma_d$ versus the molecular radius for various proteins in dog lung lymph. The data for the large molecule were fitted by an equation developed by Drake and Davis (114)

$$\sigma_d = {}^{16}/_3(a/R)^2 - {}^{20}/_3(a/R)^3 + {}^7/_3(a/R)^4 \quad (26)$$

where a and R refer to the solute and pore radius, respectively.

The values of $1 - \sigma_d$ that fail to fit the curve of the large-pore distribution were then subtracted. The resulting points are then fit with another single pore line (423, 496, 497). These studies indicate that the pulmonary capillaries can be represented as two sets

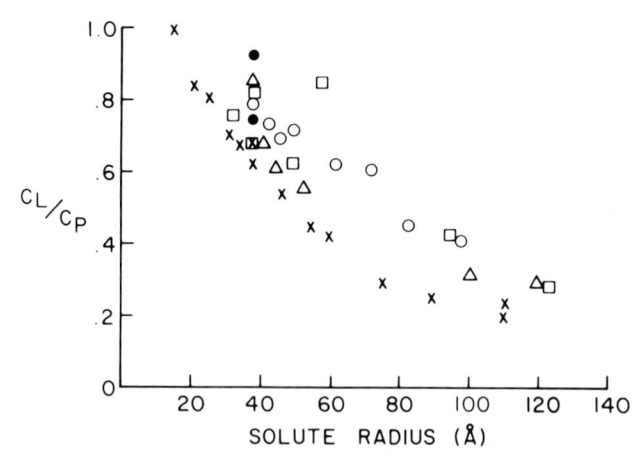

FIG. 19. Plot of lymph-to-plasma concentration ratios (C_L/C_P) for plasma protein fractions (○, ●, □, △) and povidone (×). ○, □, ×: C_L/C_P values obtained from sheep lymphatics by Brigham et al. (55), Parker et al. (391), and Boyd et al. (39), respectively. △, C_L/C_P values obtained from dog lung lymphatics by Parker, Taylor, et al. (387). [From Taylor and Granger (497).]

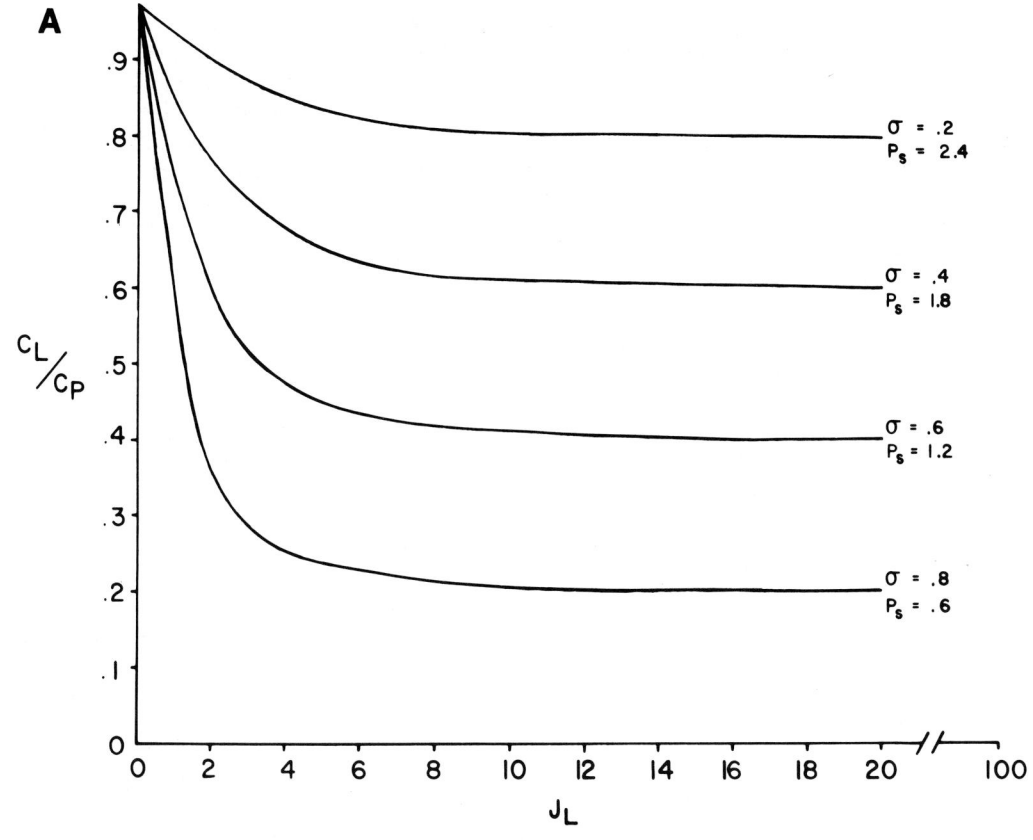

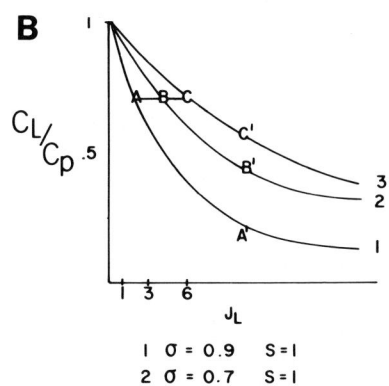

FIG. 20. *A*: lymph-to-plasma concentration ratios (C_L/C_P) as a function of lymph flow (J_L) for 4 different osmotic reflection coefficient (σ) values. P_S, calculated permeability coefficient–surface area product. *B*: C_L/C_P as a function of J_L for 2 different osmotic reflection coefficient values (σ) and surface areas (S). [From Taylor, Parker, et al. (501).]

of equivalent pores with radii of 80 and 200 Å in which 81% and 16% of the volume conductance reside, respectively. This interpretation agrees with the data obtained by Boyd et al. (39) and McNamee and Staub (333) with sheep models but not with the models that incorporate pores of 20, 125, and 1,000 Å radii developed by Brigham et al. (53) and Blake and Staub (32) with non-filtration-independent C_L/C_P values.

Any attempt to explain these discrepancies must note that dog lung data may not represent σ_d for the normal capillary membrane because *1*) raising left atrial pressures to high levels may cause the membrane to become leaky, *2*) a true capillary filtrate may not be obtainable for lung lymph because of the tremendous surface area for exchange, and *3*) not all solutes may have attained filtration rate independence. Recent data obtained in the sheep preparation (391) are shown in Figure 21*B*. Lymph obtained from the sheep model apparently provides a filtration-independent estimate of C_L/C_P for total protein. The σ_d for total protein is 0.75 for the sheep lung and ~0.70 for dog lung (388, 391). However, albumin was not at a filtration-independent state in either study, indicating that condition *1*, *2*, or *3* may be present in these studies. The large molecules (100 and 120 Å) provide filtration-independent estimates for σ_d in the dog lymph preparation of 0.94 and 0.98, respectively, but studies are needed to quantify the porosity of the

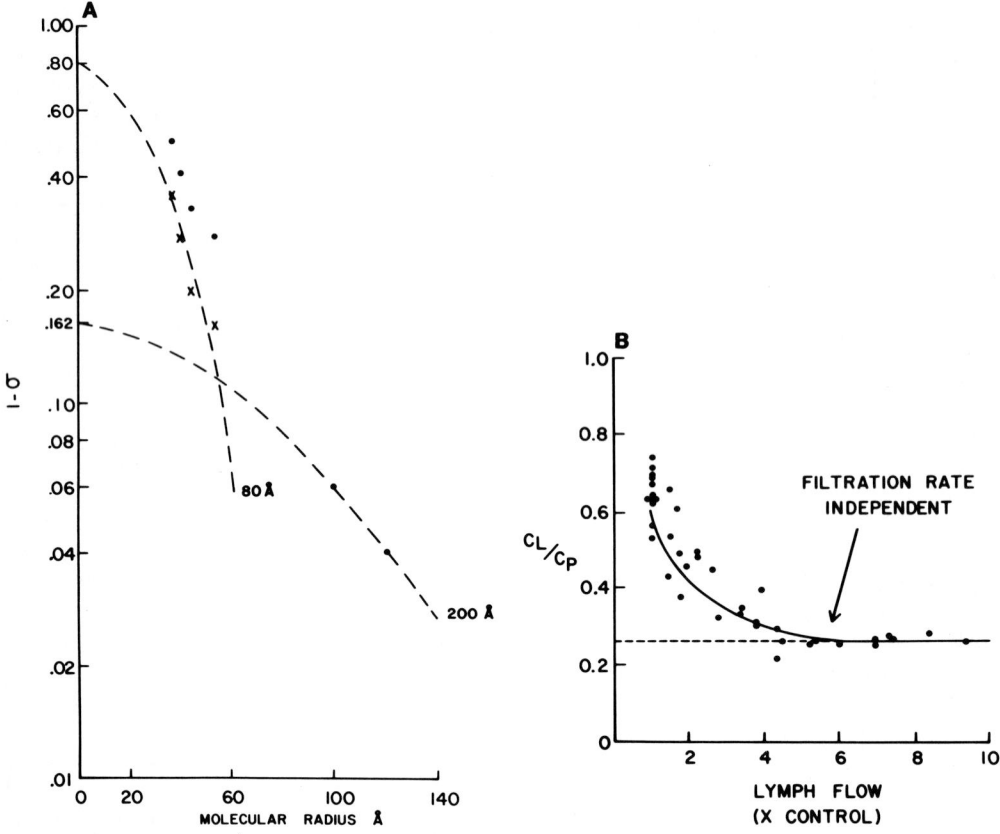

FIG. 21. *A*: $1 - \sigma$ as a function of molecular radii for 6 protein fractions. Renkin's method (423) was used to fit points to pore distributions. ●, Data points. ×, Differences between data points not falling on 200-Å curve and the predicted 200-Å curve; these points (×) were best fitted with an 80-Å curve. *B*: lymph-to-plasma concentration ratios (C_L/C_P) as a function of lymph flow from data obtained in sheep lymph by Parker (391). [*A* from Parker, Taylor, et al. (388), by permission of the American Heart Association, Inc.; *B* from Taylor and Granger (497).]

pulmonary capillary walls by obtaining filtration-independent states for all molecules studied. In addition to molecular size, solute charge also affects how molecules cross capillary walls. Figure 22 shows the effect of charge on C_L/C_P of lactate dehydrogenase isomers as a function of their isoelectric points. In Figure 22 the points to the *left* are more negatively charged isoenzymes. Positive molecules are more restricted than negative ones. To emphasize the importance of charge in macromolecular transport, an equivalent pore would apparently change from 105 Å to 70 Å radius to explain the difference observed between the negative and positive lactate dehydrogenase isozyme C_L/C_P values, respectively.

EFFECT OF INCREASING CAPILLARY PRESSURE ON THE COLLOID OSMOTIC GRADIENT. Figure 23 shows estimates of $\Pi_P - \Pi_L$ from two different animal models when capillary pressure was increased. In both studies the total protein concentrations in plasma and lymph were measured; in some instances albumin and globulin concentrations were also determined. The protein

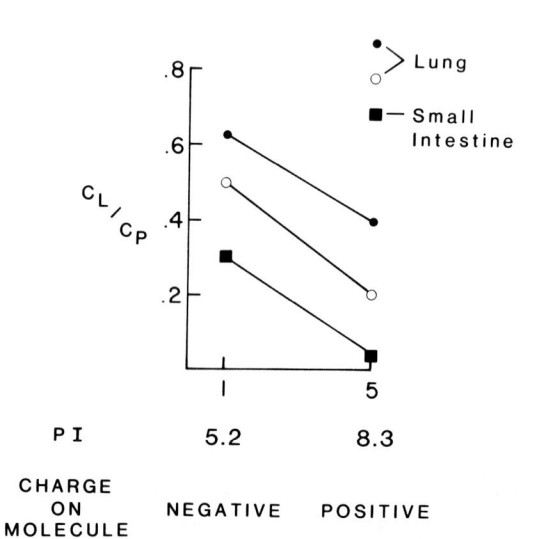

FIG. 22. Concentration ratios of lactate dehydrogenase in lymph and plasma (C_L/C_P) as a function of the isoelectric point (P_I) of the particular isoenzyme of lactate dehydrogenase. The more positive lactate dehydrogenase is more restricted than its more negative isomer. [Adapted from Taylor and Granger (496).]

concentrations (C) were then substituted into the following formulas to obtain either Π_P or Π_L [Eq. 27, dog, (354); Eqs. 28–30, human, (285)].

For total protein (T)

$$\Pi_T = 1.4C^2 + 0.22C^2 + 0.005C^3 \qquad (27)$$

or

$$\Pi_T = 2.1C^2 + 0.16C^2 + 0.009C^3 \qquad (28)$$

For albumin (A)

$$\Pi_A = 2.8C^2 + 0.18C^2 + 0.012C^3 \qquad (29)$$

For globulin (G)

$$\Pi_G = 1.6C^2 + 0.15C^2 + 0.006C^3 \qquad (30)$$

Figure 23 shows the change in $\Delta\Pi$ associated with increased capillary pressure based on lymph collected from isolated dog lungs (Fig. 23A) and the chronic sheep model (Fig. 23B). Based on these results and because σ_d for total protein is not known with any certainty for the lung, a change in $\Delta\Pi$ is estimated to be 30%–50% of the imposed change in capillary pressure if $\sigma_d = 0.75$.

Figure 24 shows data collected from sheep lungs when it was assumed that infusions of *Pseudomonas aeruginosa*, histamine, or endotoxin into the pulmonary circulation made capillaries leaky (53, 55, 58). The normal $\Delta\Pi$ for sheep lungs is ~10 mmHg. When left atrial pressure is increased to 30 mmHg, $\Delta\Pi$ increased to ~15 mmHg. After *P. aeruginosa*, histamine, and especially endotoxin challenge, $\Delta\Pi$ changed by lesser amounts when left atrial pressures were elevated. Because $\Delta\Pi$ must be multiplied by σ_d to obtain the effective osmotic pressure, the total osmotic force acting across the capillary wall will be even smaller when the capillary walls are more permeable to plasma proteins.

For several reasons $\Delta\Pi$ increases across capillary walls when capillary filtration increases: *1*) because the pulmonary capillaries are selective to plasma proteins, the protein concentrations in tissue fluids approach $C_P(1 - \sigma_d)$ as the limiting value, *2*) lymph removes proteins as a bulk phase unmixed with capillary filtrate from the interstitium (protein washout), *3*) the capillary filtrate mixes with and dilutes the interstitial proteins (198, 201, 495), and *4*) the plasma proteins are normally excluded from a large portion of interstitial water that is within the interstitial matrix. When the matrix expands, protein can enter its interior more easily and the protein's concentration in tissues decreases [Fig. 25; (181, 182)]. When interstitial volume doubled, a 25% greater decrease in interstitial colloid osmotic pressure occurred when exclusion decreased, as compared with dilution alone at the same tissue volume. These mechanisms determine the change in Π_T as capillary filtration and consequently tissue volume are elevated in steps. However, the minimal steady-state value for Π_T is only a function of $C_P(1 - \sigma_d)$.

In a recent study lymph was sampled at different lung heights (349, 502). Although the data vary, there apparently is a small difference in the lymph protein concentration at different lung levels. The difference

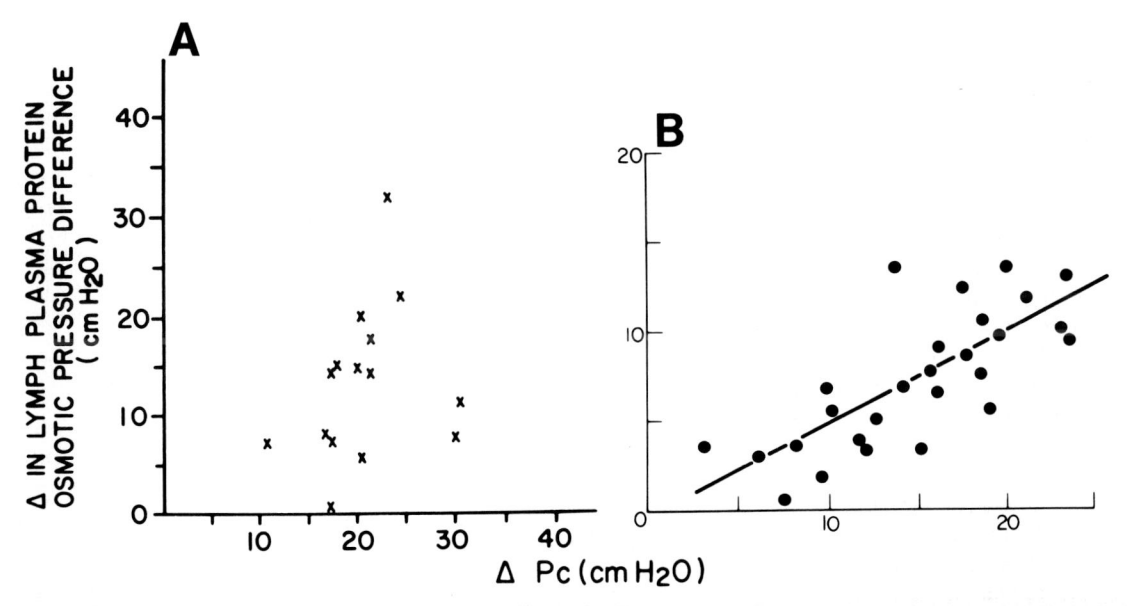

FIG. 23. *A*: change in plasma-lymph colloid osmotic pressure gradient in isolated dog lung lymph as a function of change in capillary pressure (ΔPc). *B*: change in plasma-lymph colloid osmotic pressure gradient in sheep lungs as a function of change in capillary pressure. [*A* adapted from Drake (112); *B* from Erdmann et al. (129), by permission of the American Heart Association, Inc.]

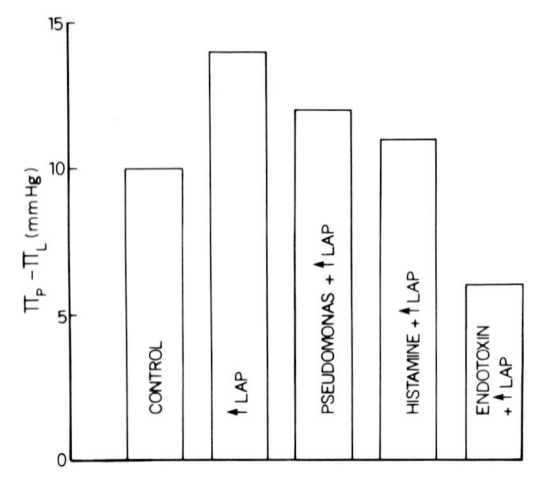

FIG. 24. Difference in colloid osmotic pressure gradient between plasma and lymph ($\Pi_P - \Pi_L$) when only left atrial pressures were elevated (↑LAP) and when the lung circulation of the sheep was exposed to *Pseudomonas aeruginosa*, histamine, and endotoxin in the studies of Brigham et al. (54, 55, 58). [From Taylor, Parker, et al. (500).]

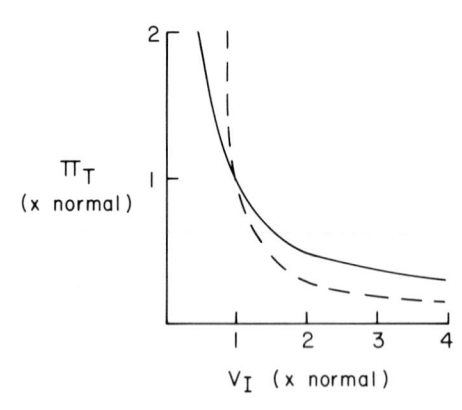

FIG. 25. Effect of protein exclusion on tissue colloid osmotic pressure (Π_T) when interstitial volume (V_I) is expanded. ———, Decrease in Π_T if no exclusion is present; – – – –, Π_T when protein is excluded from a portion of the interstitial space. Note that for the same interstitial value, Π_T is lower when exclusion is present. [From Taylor, Parker, et al. (502).]

in $\Pi_{ti} \cong 0.15$ cmH$_2$O change per centimeter of height from bottom to top of the lungs; Π_L is higher at the top of the lung. The $\Delta\Pi$ estimated with lung lymph is an average value that is a mixture of protein and fluid leaking from different lung heights. In addition, because the small blood vessels of the lung appear to be more porous toward their venous ends, this phenomenon also influences the average tissue protein concentrations.

EQUILIBRATION TIMES OF PROTEINS BETWEEN PLASMA AND LYMPH. The equilibration rate of a protein such as albumin between plasma and pulmonary lymph has been used to evaluate various characteristics of the blood-lymph barrier. Table 6 summarizes the reported equilibration rates for various proteins in lymph from sheep and dog lung. Half times for the equilibration of albumin range from 2.1 to 5.6 h for normal lung. Generally a bolus of isotope-labeled albumin is injected and first-order kinetics is assumed when the equilibration rate constant is estimated. In another study (339) a constant plasma infusion of labeled albumin was used to maintain the plasma tracer at a constant value. However, the equilibration rate constants can be calculated with a single injection of tracer and the assumption that a triple exponential relationship describes the biphasic decay of plasma tracer levels and the plasma-lymph rate constants (381, 436).

The plasma-lymph equilibration rate constant for albumin is directly proportional to the diffusive and convective fluxes and inversely proportional to the interstitial volume of distribution (249, 436). The transcapillary protein flux is a function of the permeability–surface area product of the endothelial barrier, the capillary filtration rate, and the blood-interstitium concentration gradient. Infusion of *P. aeruginosa* in sheep, which is thought to increase pulmonary vascular permeability, decreased the half times for albumin and transferrin equilibration to approximately one-third of their base-line values (176, 514). Increased left atrial pressures produced a modest decrease in equilibration half times because of increased convective transport of the tracer. Thus the equilibration times are a function of the protein transport gradients and permeability (see Eq. 25) as well as the interstitial fluid volumes. Although membrane coefficients and tissue distribution volumes have generally been derived with the linear flux equation (see Eq. 4), a kinetic analysis that incorporates the nonlinear flux equation provides a more accurate estimate of distribution volumes [see Eq. 10; (381)].

An interesting consequence of the increased turnover of albumin at high capillary pressures or in leaky capillary states is that albumin placed into the circulation in either of the two states equilibrates with lung tissue in <12 h. Therefore albumin will not remove fluid from the interstitium after a few hours and could increase lung fluid accumulation if capillary pressure increases with albumin therapy, which is usually the case (190).

Lymph Flow

FORMATION OF LYMPH. The sites at which fluid exchanges at the arterial and venous ends of the pulmonary circulation are not known, but fluid can leak out of alveolar and arterial and venous extra-alveolar vessels, depending on the pressure profile along the pulmonary vascular bed. Although the venous extra-alveolar vessel walls have the highest volume conductances, the blood pressure in arterial vessels is higher; therefore the arterial vessels could filter as much or more fluid than venous vessels. Because capillary pressure is higher at the bottom than the top

TABLE 6. *Plasma-Lymph Equilibration Times in Intact Animals*

Species, Condition, Tracer	Capillary Pressure*	Lymph Flow, μl/min	Lymph/ Plasma	Half Time, h	Rate Constant, h	Ref.
Dog, anesthetized						
RLD, ^{131}I-labeled albumin, control		21.1	0.80	5.6	0.124	339
TBN, ^{125}I-labeled albumin, Tyrode's infusion, edema	14.1	103.3	0.58	2.12	0.327	381
Sheep, anesthetized, CMN						
[125]I-albumin						
Control		81.5	0.86	4.00	0.173	175
Control, hemorrhage	11.6	190		2.9	0.239	106
Posthemorrhage	7.4	195		3.3	0.210	106
[113]In-labeled transferrin						
Control				2.4	0.289	176
Pseudomonas aeruginosa infusion				0.95	0.729	176
↑LAP				1.27	0.547	176
Sheep, unanesthetized, CMN, ^{125}I-albumin						
Control	10.7	88.3	0.87	2.9	0.239	514
↑LAP	25.4	268	0.63	2.2	0.315	514
P. aeruginosa infusion	12.9	620	0.77	0.7	0.990	514

CMN, caudal mediastinal node; ↑LAP, increased left atrial pressure; RLD, right lymph duct; TBN, tracheobronchial node lymphatic. * Calculated with Pc = 0.4 (Ppa − Pla) + Pla in cmH$_2$O, where Pc is capillary pressure, Ppa is pulmonary arterial pressure, and Pla is left atrial pressure.

of the lung, one would expect a larger amount of fluid to filter into the more dependent regions of the lungs (34, 240, 538). Recent studies have shown, however, that more fluid does not initially accumulate in the dependent portions of the lung (compared with upper areas) during the formation of hydrostatic edema (207). This indicates that other forces tending to move fluid out of the capillaries into the tissues must be higher at the top than the bottom of the lung; i.e., tissue pressure decreases, and/or tissue colloid osmotic pressure increases, and/or lymph flow decreases from lung base to apex (477, 478, 489, 502).

Therefore filtration gradients may differ within the pulmonary circulation in a longitudinal direction down the length of the small blood vessels and at each vertical height within the tissues. When lung weight or lymph flow is used as an index of capillary filtration the whole microvascular system is involved, which results in an average value that reflects cumulative filtration occurring across many microvessel walls at different regions of the pulmonary circulation. Most pulmonary physiologists believe that fluid normally leaks out of capillaries located in the alveolar walls, moves out of the very small septal interstitial spaces toward the corners, and then moves into the larger tissue spaces surrounding terminal airways (533). The fluid finally enters lymphatic capillaries in this vicinity. Therefore a pressure gradient must exist between the alveolar septal interstitial spaces and the more distant tissue areas containing the initial lymphatics (199, 277). The final product of capillary filtrate in normal lungs is lymph; the mechanisms involved in its formation represent a complex filtration process driven by a myriad of pressure gradients existing across several series and parallel barriers.

The rate at which filtered macromolecules and water enter the lymph in a steady state equals the rate at which they cross the capillary wall. When interstitial edema develops and the lung tissue cannot further expand, fluid containing large amounts of plasma protein begins to fill the alveoli. The mechanisms by which alveoli fill remain unsettled: alveolar epithelial junctions may open or epithelial cells may separate more easily at the junction of small airways and alveoli when sufficient forces act at these barriers (85, 124, 406, 479). Because the alveolar epithelial cells migrate toward alveolar ducts as they mature, they may be more easily displaced at the junction of the alveolar ducts and alveoli proper (160, 479). Of course the larger airways could also be the locus of edema fluid entry into the airways.

Once solutes and water enter the initial lymphatics they move by convection until they reach the funnel-shaped valves in the larger lymphatics. Then they move almost as a single bolus unit between valves, propelled either by tissue movement or the intrinsic contraction of the lymphatic walls. The collecting lymphatics coalesce in the hilar region of the lungs and join with the pleural lymphatics to enter the primary node (288, 289). The lymphatic drainage of the lungs in different animals has a variable number of communications with extrapulmonary lymphatic systems. The contribution from different portions of the lung to large collecting lymphatics not only varies from species to species but can differ between members of the same species (see *Interstitial Fluid Pressure Gradients*, p. 192). The initial lymphatics have large openings between endothelial cells and do not limit the entry of any plasma proteins into their lumen. Initial lymphatics also appear to be confined to larger tissue spaces surrounding terminal airways and have not been found in septal areas. Once lymph passes through nodes it may be altered in protein composition (1, 320, 422). Many experimental preparations used to study pulmonary microvascular permeability and capillary filtration use lymph that has passed through nodes and may drain different areas of the lung in different animals. In addition extrapulmonary lymphatics may join the large lymphatics at nodes or other junctional sites. Consequently lymph collected at the exit of large lymphatic channels may not have the same composition as lymph formed at the microcirculation level, and equating lymph to tissue fluids may be misleading.

EFFECT OF INCREASED CAPILLARY PRESSURE ON LYMPH FLOW. Lymph flow is ~0.062 ml·min^{-1}·100 g^{-1} wet wt (381) and increases ~20% for each 1-mmHg change in capillary pressure in several different lung lymphatic preparations (129, 346, 388). Figure 26 shows the effect of increasing capillary pressure on lymph flow when the lungs have been challenged with *P. aeruginosa* and endotoxin (52); lymph flow changes greatly for similar elevations in capillary pressure with the increased permeability of the capillary walls.

The importance of lymph flow as a means of removing excess capillary filtrate is difficult to assess, but one approach is to assume that lymph flow allows a certain imbalance to exist in forces operating across the capillary walls (11, 198, 363, 489, 491, 495). If total lymph flow ($\dot{Q}_{L,T}$) and the filtration characteristics of the pulmonary capillary walls ($K_{f,c}$) are known, the filtration pressure drop (ΔP_L) associated with forming lymph can be estimated as

$$\Delta P_L = \dot{Q}_{L,T}/K_{f,c} \quad (31)$$

Figure 27 is a schematic graph that predicts the importance of ΔP_L in removing filtrate associated with

FIG. 27. Lymphatic safety factor as a function of the filtration coefficient ($K_{f,c}$). *Shaded area*, range of $K_{f,c}$ values determined with weight analyses. [Adapted from Taylor and Drake (491).]

increased capillary pressure (491, 495). The *shaded area* represents the values associated with all estimates of $K_{f,c}$ determined in lung tissue. For normal lymph flows, ΔP_L will be small, buffering only a 5-mmHg change in capillary pressures, even when lymph flow increases to 5 times normal. However, if the lung interstitium is more resistant to the movement of fluid between filtering capillaries and lymph collection sites than the capillary walls, then estimates of $K_{f,c}$ made with Equation 14 will not predict the importance of the lymphatic system as a volume overload system. The ΔP_L for this case (199, 502) is described by

$$\Delta P_L = \dot{Q}_{L,T}/[K_{f,c}K_{f,ti}/(K_{f,c} + K_{f,ti})] \quad (32)$$

where $K_{f,ti}$ is the filtration coefficient of the tissues and the denominator is the total volume conductance of the microvascular wall, interstitial draining pathways, and lymphatic system. The lymphatics' apparent ability to remove filtered volume is significant at low tissue hydration states when the tissue conductance is small, because the denominator will be smaller than the smallest conductance. When the tissues expand during edema formation, the tissue resistance decreases and the lymphatic factor appears to become smaller (199, 271, 489). However, this calculation of the lymphatic safety factor has nothing to do with the difference in the Starling force balance at the capillary wall. For instance, if $K_{f,T}$ is calculated with the denominator in Equation 32 when $K_{f,c} = 0.3$ and $K_{f,ti} = 0.01$, then $K_{f,T} = 0.01$ and $\Delta P_L = 100\dot{Q}_L$. During tissue

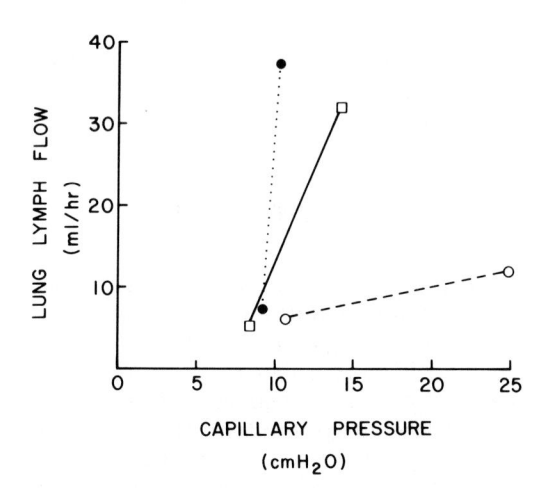

FIG. 26. Lung lymph flow as a function of capillary pressure for controls (o - - o) and lungs challenged with *Pseudomonas aeruginosa* (□——□) and endotoxin (●- -●). [Adapted from Brigham (52).]

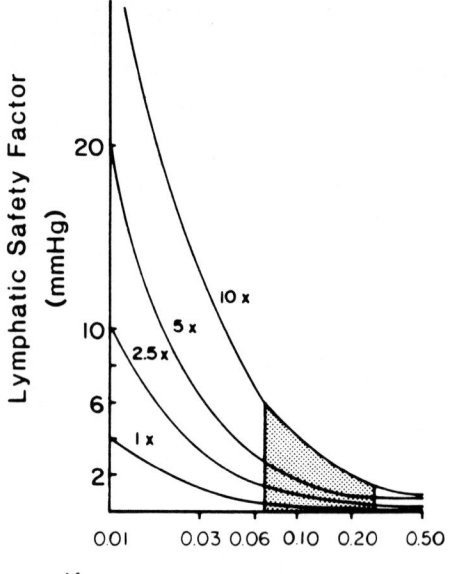

hydration, $K_{f,ti}$ increases 30-fold to 0.3, $K_{f,T} = 0.15$ and is still smaller than $K_{f,c}$, and $\Delta P_L = 6\dot{Q}_L$. Therefore $K_{f,c}$ cannot be estimated with Equation 14 because this calculates $K_{f,T}$. Inserting $K_{f,T}$ into Equation 31 produces a gross overestimation of the lymphatics' ability to remove interstitial volume, because in both examples ΔP_L should be $3.3\dot{Q}_L$.

Zarins et al. (553) have published a very interesting study concerning the effects of $\Delta \Pi$ on edema formation; Π_P was depleted and the lungs did not gain weight. The interpretation of this study was that tissue pressure and lymph flow increased sufficiently to balance the normal capillary pressure even when $\Delta \Pi \cong 0$. The study should be repeated and the capillary pressure increased to determine the total ability of tissue pressure and lymph flow to buffer changes in capillary pressures in the absence of $\Delta \Pi$.

Uhley et al. (511) demonstrated that chronic elevations in left atrial pressures induced a proliferation of lung lymphatics, which resulted in a much greater change in lymph flow than was observed in acute animals with similar left atrial pressures. This may explain how patients with chronic elevations of left atrial pressures can tolerate pressures exceeding 30–35 mmHg without developing intra-alveolar edema. The pulmonary lymph flow may provide a substantial safety factor in chronic edema, but other changes, e.g., decreased tissue compliance or capillary permeability, may also occur with chronic elevations of left atrial pressures.

At this time the lymphatic system's ability to remove fluid from the lung's interstitium is difficult to assess. Lymph flow is necessary to remove plasma proteins from the interstitium, but its ability to buffer changes in capillary filtration forces cannot be adequately assessed until the sites of vascular leakage and tissue fluid resistances are estimated under different experimental conditions. Because the lungs gain considerable water despite a great increase in lymph flow under some experimental conditions, a clear picture of the lymphatic system's contribution to the prevention of pulmonary edema is not available.

MECHANISMS OF LYMPH PROPULSION. The mechanisms responsible for lymph propulsion in lung tissue are poorly understood. Several mechanisms can propel lymph. *1*) Ventilation can alternately collapse and dilate larger lymphatic vessels to cause lymph to flow out of the lungs. Although lymph will not flow from unventilated isolated lungs, the role of ventilation in intact lungs is not established (112, 529). *2*) An increase in tissue pressure will provide better lymphatic filling at the lymphatic capillary because the pressure head for lymphatic filling is tissue pressure minus lymphatic hydrostatic pressure (70, 363, 494). *3*) Larger lymphatics contain smooth muscle and demonstrate phasic contractions that propel lymph in the valved system. Perhaps the endothelial cells in collecting lymphatics can also contract. Whether small lung lymphatics can actively contract has not been clearly established, but large pulmonary lymphatics do appear to contract, which would provide the force for lymph propulsion (68, 551). The relationship between tissue pressure and lymph flow (178, 494) needs to be clarified. *1*) Lymph flow can increase, decrease, or plateau when the tissues become grossly edematous. These responses may be explained by an increased tissue compliance accompanied by a decrease in tissue pressure or by sequestration of fluid into a space that is not well drained by the lymphatics (158, 159, 178). *2*) An increased venous pressure does not produce the same increase in lymph flow as does an equivalent decrease in $\Delta \Pi$ (170, 489, 494, 495). This discrepancy may be related to venous pressures acting on lymphatics to increase their outflow resistance or to a difference in the rapidity at which tissue pressure changes after either an elevation of capillary pressure or a reduction in $\Delta \Pi$. Interestingly, Chen, Granger, and Taylor (73) have postulated that the increased lymph flow in peripheral tissues after elevations in capillary pressure is a function of the rate of change of tissue pressure, not the absolute value. *3*) Saline infusions may decrease tissue resistance to fluid movement and promote greater lymphatic filling than occurs with vascular pressure elevations. This effect may be due to vascular distension with pressure elevations, which oppose lymphatic filling by causing tissue resistance to be higher. With saline infusions the tissue resistance is lower, and consequently more lymph flows. Increased lymph flows do not necessarily mean an increased ability of the lymphatic system to oppose edema formation. For instance, increased vascular permeability increases lymph flow to 20 times normal (437), yet the lungs are grossly edematous. One must be extremely cautious when lymph flow changes are used as indices of vascular permeability changes (Fig. 26) because they are determined both by the capillary filtrate (which is a function of the Starling force imbalance and vascular wall permeability) and by the ease with which volume moves away from the filtering portions of the microcirculation to the remote initial lymphatic, i.e., tissue resistance to fluid movement. In view of these uncertainties, the determination of tissue pressure in relation to lymph flow in lung tissue is clearly important, especially in the vicinity of terminal lymphatics.

EFFECT OF LYMPHATIC OBSTRUCTION. Because lymph removes fluid and protein from the interstitium, lymphatic vessel ligation would be expected to produce edema. Without removal of tissue proteins the lungs would gain water unless Pti = Pc. Lungs develop slight interstitial edema and tend to accumulate fluid when capillary pressure is elevated after ligation of the pulmonary lymphatics (305, 377). The maximum increase in tissue water after ligation occurs in 3 days, thereafter subsiding to reach normal levels within 5 days (353). The observation that lymphatics regenerate within the 1st wk after autologous lung transplantation explains why lung transplants do not develop intra-alveolar edema (87, 128). In these transplant studies the lung water also reached its maximum value 3 days after transplantation and returned to normal by the end of 6 wk.

Because lung lymphatics drain into veins, Bolton and Starling (35) and Starling (475) postulated that a rise in central venous pressure would cause a drop in lymph flow and consequently an accumulation of lung water and protein in heart failure. Several investigators proposed similar mechanisms to explain the formation of edema in right heart failure (121, 418, 487, 530, 532). Increases in venous pressure to 10 or 25 mmHg failed to influence the accumulation of lung edema fluid in the dog (353). It is unlikely that venous pressures in the range compatible with life interfere with lymph flow from the lungs, because lymphatics can pump against pressures as great as 25 mmHg (551).

EFFECT OF AIRWAY PRESSURE ON CAPILLARY FILTRATION. For many years the use of PEEP in treating pulmonary edema was based on the belief that an increased pressure on the surface of alveolar fluid would force fluid back into the capillaries. It is now known that much of the beneficial effect of PEEP on pulmonary gas exchange is the result of the opening of previously collapsed alveoli and the spreading of alveolar fluid over a larger surface area (477). A decrease in venous return and cardiac output also contributes to the improved pulmonary function by lowering pulmonary vascular pressures (135).

There are two major difficulties in predicting the net effect of PEEP on lung fluid balance: *1*) the different filtration responses of alveolar and extra-alveolar vessels to increased airway pressures and *2*) the effect of PEEP on pulmonary blood flow. Because of these complex interactions an increased airway pressure can produce opposite effects on the net capillary filtration rate, depending on whether the experiments are conducted with constant blood flow or constant perfusion pressures (397). Because PEEP increases lung volume it tends to increase the radial traction on extra-alveolar vessels, reduce their resistance to blood flow, and increase the transmural filtration gradient in these vessels. Fluid moves easily across the extra-alveolar vessel walls, and as much as half of the total transvascular filtration may occur from these vessels (240, 348, 464, 539). Lung inflation also imposes a longitudinal stress on the alveolar septa and tends to decrease the transmural pressure gradient across these vessels and to increase their resistance to blood flow (170, 233). A combination of the filtration from these vessel types determines the overall filtration from the pulmonary circulation (64, 433).

When alveolar gas pressure is increased at constant perfusion pressure, lung volume increases and presumably the filtration gradient for extra-alveolar vessels increases. However, because alveolar gas pressures increase relative to vascular pressures, there will be a decrease in the transmural pressure gradient across the alveolar septal vessels and a reduction in blood flow. Figure 28A is a diagram of the pressure gradients for blood flow and fluid filtration in a lobe perfused at constant vascular pressures as alveolar gas pressure is increased. The gradient for blood flow is determined by $P_{pa} - P_A$ when $P_A > P_{la}$, and it is determined by $P_{pa} - P_{la}$ when $P_{la} > P_A$ (396, 397, 400, 401). The transmural gradient for filtration from septal capillaries can be approximated by $P_c - P_A$. As shown in Figure 28A, the pressure gradients for both blood flow and filtration from septal vessels decreased as alveolar gas pressure increased. Therefore increasing the transpulmonary pressure at a constant perfusion pressure will slow the rate of fluid accumulation and decrease pulmonary blood flow, presumably because of a decrease in filtration gradients and the derecruitment of capillary networks (174).

When an isolated lobe is perfused at constant blood flow or cardiac output is maintained constant in animals, the rate of fluid filtration tends to increase in response to increased airway pressures (34, 66, 335, 510). Figure 28B illustrates the effect of increased PEEP on perfusion pressures in an isolated lobe perfused with constant blood flow (510). Inflow pressures and the filtration rate increased as PEEP increased; this was attributed to an increased transmural pressure gradient surrounding extra-alveolar vessels (397). However, others found no significant changes in either lung lymph flow or water accumulation with a PEEP of 10 cmH$_2$O, although lymph flow decreased transiently at the onset of PEEP (66, 108, 227, 240, 525). Permutt (396, 397) has postulated that the transmural gradients of the extra-alveolar blood vessels increase when PEEP is applied at constant blood flows. The alveolar transmural gradient should be reduced when $P_{la} > P_A$. Thus a net decrease in filtration is more likely in response to PEEP when left atrial pressure is high.

Bø et al. (34) defined the relationship between filtration and airway pressures with perfused lobes at constant pulmonary arterial and left atrial pressures under zone III conditions ($P_{pa} > P_{la} > P_A$). Transpulmonary and alveolar gas pressures could be varied independently in this preparation. The transcapillary filtration rate decreased in the lobe when alveolar gas pressure was increased, both when transpulmonary pressure increased in proportion to alveolar gas pressure and when transpulmonary pressure was maintained constant by elevating pleural pressure. The reduced filtration from alveolar vessels would account for this overall reduction in filtration rate. Although the mechanical tension surrounding extra-alveolar vessels would tend to increase the transmural filtration gradient, positive alveolar gas pressure partially offsets the mechanical forces. This explains why the filtration rate increased in the lobes when transpul-

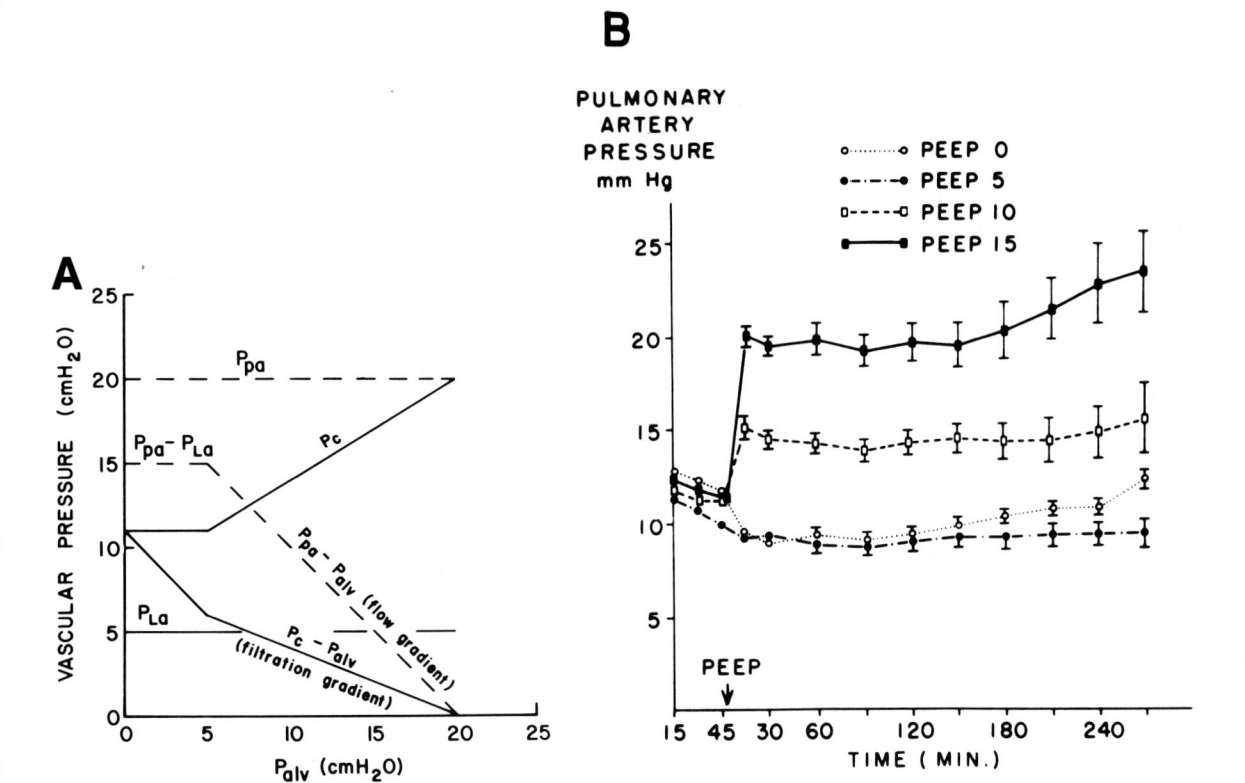

FIG. 28. *A*: pressure gradients for fluid filtration and blood flow as a function of alveolar gas pressure (P_{alv}) when pulmonary perfusing pressure is constant. Pc, capillary pressure; Ppa, pulmonary arterial pressure; Pla, left atrial pressure. Ppa − P_{alv} is considered to be the perfusing gradient; Pc − P_{alv} is the capillary filtration gradient. Flow would cease before pulmonary arterial pressure equaled alveolar gas pressure if all alveolar gas pressure was reflected to the capillary. *B*: pulmonary artery pressure as a function of time at 4 different levels of positive end-expiratory pressure (PEEP) in a dog lung perfused at constant blood flow (510). [*B* from Permutt (397).]

monary pressure was increased by negative pressure inflation at constant vascular pressures. Although these relationships are complex, the overall changes in the filtration rate are predictable from the transmural gradients acting across each set of blood vessels.

Several factors affect the filtration forces operating at the corner vessels of the septal junctions. Blood vessels located at these triple-line junctions (see Fig. 17) are exposed to *1*) radial traction exerted by the three septal walls as the lung expands, *2*) an outward force acting on the fluid lining layer, which is a function of surface tension and the radius of curvature at the corners, and *3*) alveolar gas pressure exerted on the fluid lining layer. Thus these vessels may behave similarly to either extra-alveolar vessels or septal capillaries. The equation describing the balance of forces at the corner vessels is

$$\mathrm{Pc} - \mathrm{PA} + f\left(\frac{3F_O}{L}\right) + K\left(\frac{ST}{r}\right) - \mathrm{Pel,w} = 0 \quad (33)$$

where $f(3F_O/L)$ is the stress exerted by the three septa at the junction, F_O is an outward-acting force, L is the length of the wall attached at the triple junction, ST is surface tension, r is the radius of curvature at the septal corner, and Pel,w is the capillary wall tension.

With $K = 0.0014$, equivalent pressures (mmHg) are given when surface tension is in dynes per centimeter and radius in centimeters (199). The two forces, $f(3F_O/L)$ and $K(ST/r)$, cause an increased transmural pressure in these blood vessels when lung volume increases, but an increased alveolar gas pressure results in a decreased transmural gradient. The special combination of these mechanical and interfacial forces acting on corner blood vessels has been implicated in blood flow studies to explain the persistent blood flow through the lungs even when alveolar gas pressure exceeds arterial pressure by 3–15 cmH$_2$O (62, 374, 434). Histological examination of lungs frozen when alveolar gas pressures exceed pulmonary arterial pressures by 24 cmH$_2$O reveals red blood cells in the corner vessels, but the septal walls are almost uniformly collapsed (170).

Nicolaysen and Hauge (359) recently demonstrated some of the filtration properties of these corner vessels with zone I lungs in which $P_A > \mathrm{Ppa} = \mathrm{Pla}$. When transpulmonary pressure was increased by increasing alveolar gas pressure at a constant pleural pressure, the filtration rate decreased; however, when transpulmonary pressure was increased by decreasing pleural pressure at a constant alveolar gas pressure, the filtration rate increased. In both maneuvers alveolar capillaries are collapsed and the extra-alveolar transmural gradient (i.e., Pvas − Pti) tends to increase because of increased radial traction acting on the vascular sheath. However, less of an increase in transmural pressure would be obtained when transpulmonary pressure is increased by alveolar gas pressure because alveolar gas pressure increases relative to vascular pressures. At the corner vessels the mechanical tension on the septal walls would be related only to transpulmonary pressure, but the outward force acting on the alveolar fluid layer would be diminished. The important role of these corner vessels in lung fluid balance is apparent from the examples given above; future anatomical and physiological studies should focus on the characteristics and behavior of these blood vessels with respect to fluid and protein exchange across the microvascular wall.

Analyses of Force Changes During Formation of Alveolar Edema: Edema Safety Factor

This chapter discusses many investigations that have evaluated one or more of the forces within the Starling equation

$$\bar{Q}_c = \bar{Q}_L = \bar{K}_{f,c}[(\bar{P}c - \bar{P}ti) - \bar{\sigma}_d(\bar{\Pi}_P - \bar{\Pi}_{ti})] \quad (34)$$

We emphasize that the Starling equation relates average capillary filtration ($\bar{Q}_c$) [or average lymph flow ($\bar{Q}_L$)] when the tissue volume is not changing to the average capillary filtration coefficient ($\bar{K}_{f,c}$) and average tissue forces: capillary ($\bar{P}c$), tissue fluid ($\bar{P}ti$), plasma colloid osmotic ($\bar{\Pi}_P$), and tissue fluid colloid osmotic ($\bar{\Pi}_{ti}$) pressures. In addition, a selectivity factor ($\bar{\sigma}_d$) is used to define the average selectivity of all pulmonary blood vessels that leak plasma proteins.

Guyton and Lindsey (196) presented the first study that clearly indicates an intrinsic edema-preventing mechanism in lung tissue that opposes the accumulation of lung water after elevations of capillary pressure. Only a slight amount of interstitial edema occurred in the lung when left atrial pressure was increased from normal to 25 mmHg. Lungs would also tolerate less elevation in left atrial pressure before excessive edema fluid accumulated when plasma colloid osmotic pressure was reduced to approximately half the normal values (12 mmHg instead of 25 mmHg). These authors surmised that there was not a sufficient change in tissue fluid pressure and tissue colloid osmotic pressure after the critical pressure was attained to oppose the tendency for fluid accumulation.

Levine et al. (293), in a similar study, postulated that tissue fluid pressure changed to oppose increased capillary pressure. These studies indicated that pulmonary interstitial fluid pressure was normally about −11 mmHg because left atrial pressures could be increased by this amount before the lungs began to rapidly form edema. Levine's study was the first Starling force analysis that considered changes in tissue pressure as important deterrents to fluid accumulation. In his classic study on plasma colloid osmotic pressure, Starling (476) also investigated the effect of tissue pressure in retarding capillary filtration; however, he rejected tissue pressure as an important regulator of tissue volume because positive tissue pressures increased both venous and capillary pressures. This would produce no net change in the hydrostatic pressure acting across the capillary walls. The definition by Guyton (192) and Guyton, Taylor, and Granger (195) of three types of tissue pressure explained Starling's study and provided both a conceptual and experimental basis for describing the behavior of interstitial fluid pressure during edema formation. Guyton, Taylor, and Granger (201) defined the ability of the Starling forces and lymph flow to change when filtration forces were altered as edema safety factors. When capillary pressure was increased, lymph flow, tissue pressure, and the osmotic pressure gradient across the capillary wall increased. These forces provided the tissues with an ability to maintain small interstitial volumes even when capillary pressure is elevated (or Π_P decreased).

Several studies of average Starling forces have been conducted in peripheral tissues (489), but only two have been conducted in lung tissue. Figure 29 shows two Starling force analyses conducted in lung tissue: 29A presents the results of a study by Erdmann et al. (129) in the awake sheep model; 29B depicts the results of a study by Drake (112) in isolated dog lungs. Erdmann et al. elevated left atrial pressures, measured lung lymph flow and lymph and plasma colloid osmotic pressure, and estimated capillary pressure with the equation of Garr, Taylor, et al. (154). Erdmann et al. assumed that interstitial fluid pressure equaled alveolar gas pressure. Their results indicated that ΔΠ changed by 50% of the imposed capillary pressure change. Because tissue pressure was assumed not to

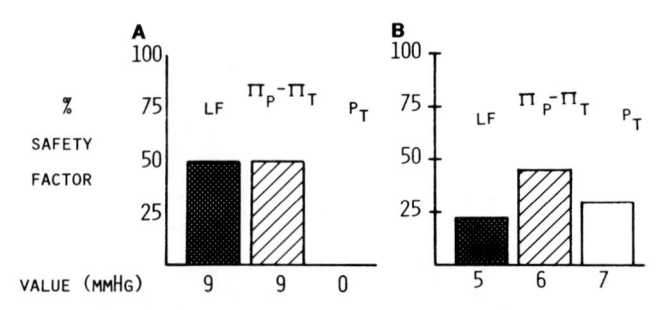

FIG. 29. Starling force analyses in sheep and dog lungs. Change (%) in lymph flow (LF), in colloid osmotic pressure gradient between plasma and tissues ($\Pi_P - \Pi_T$), and in tissue pressure (P_T) relative to change in capillary pressures. Numbers below each histogram are maximum change in each tissue force when capillary pressure was increased by 18 mmHg. [Adapted from Taylor (489).]

change, the remainder of the tissue's ability to buffer increases in capillary pressure was assigned to the lymph flow factor. Drake (112), Drake and Taylor (118), and Taylor et al. (495) measured the same parameters but calculated the ability of lymphatics to remove tissue fluid volume as equal to $\Delta P_L = \dot{Q}_L/K_{f,c}$. Their studies indicated that lymph flow, $\Delta\Pi$, and increased tissue pressures provided ~25%, ~50%, and ~25%, respectively, of the tissue's ability to buffer the changes in capillary pressure. Both studies have similar data, yet the interpretations are different. Each study required certain assumptions to calculate the Starling forces. *1)* The assumption that $P_{ti} = P_A$ is incorrect, as much of the information in this chapter indicates. *2)* The assumption that $\Pi_L = \Pi_{ti}$ appears to be correct (at least at high capillary pressures) because the change in $\Delta\Pi$ was similar in both studies and extrapulmonary sources cannot contaminate lymph-draining isolated lungs. *3)* The total lymph flow in the isolated lung study was assumed equal to right duct lymph flow. This appears to be a reasonable estimate for total lymph flow draining the lungs at elevated left atrial pressures (381). *4)* The assumption that the lymph flow factor is equal to $\bar{\dot{Q}}_L/K_{f,c}$ will be incorrect if the tissues offer more resistance than the capillary walls to the formation of lymph (502).

No Starling force analysis of leaky lung capillary conditions has been published. Obviously σ_d and the effective colloid osmotic gradient across the capillary wall decrease. The data obtained for α-naphthylthiourea (ANTU) challenge can help explain how increased capillary permeability alters the tissue's ability to oppose increased capillary pressures (437). After the ANTU damage, $\bar{\sigma}_d$ was 0.40 and the lymph-to-plasma protein concentration ratio was 0.6. The $\Delta\Pi$ was ~9.5 mmHg at normal capillary pressures. The $\Delta\Pi$ increased to 16.8 mmHg after elevations of capillary pressure. This difference in $\Delta\Pi$ is 7.3 mmHg and constitutes the colloid osmotic portion of the edema safety factor (Fig. 29). After ANTU challenge, $\Delta\Pi$ changed to only 12.1 mmHg and should be multiplied by 0.4 (σ_d) to obtain the effective $\Delta\Pi$ operating across the pulmonary capillary walls. The $\sigma_d\Delta\Pi$ for ANTU is ~5.0 mmHg. Therefore, after the lung has become leaky to plasma proteins, only a small osmotic pressure gradient is generated across capillary walls and changes in capillary pressure can only be opposed by alterations in tissue fluid pressure and lymph flow. Because the filtration pressure drop associated with forming lymph is inversely proportional to the filtration coefficient of the capillaries, which is directly proportional to capillary permeability, the lymphatic factor also decreases when permeability increases. In fact, if the lymphatic factor is a function of tissue resistance, it may decrease to zero after ANTU challenge.

Drake and Gabel (116) used a technique similar to that of Guyton and Lindsey (196) to evaluate a critical capillary pressure. This is the highest capillary pressure that can be attained prior to exhaustion of the tissue safety factors. At capillary pressures exceeding the critical capillary pressure, the tissue continuously gains edema fluid. When the lung is challenged with a compound such as alloxan, which increases vascular permeability, left atrial pressure is elevated until the lung gains weight at a continuous rate. The critical capillary pressure decreases when the capillaries are more leaky to plasma proteins. From such measurements the total edema safety factor can be calculated for many experimental conditions.

An average Starling force analysis simply does not describe how tissue fluid volume is regulated in different portions of lung tissue. However, until there are more studies of the vertical and horizontal force gradients and lymph flows within different sections of lung tissue we must rely on average Starling force analyses to explain studies of fluid balance in lungs.

ABNORMAL CAPILLARY PERMEABILITY TO PLASMA PROTEINS (LEAKY LUNG SYNDROMES)

Pulmonary edema most often results from increased left atrial pressure, but abnormal capillary permeability can also produce a rapid and fulminating pulmonary edema. Since development of the model for collection of lung lymph in chronic sheep, many investigators have measured lung lymph flow and the concentration of proteins in lymph and plasma to estimate capillary permeability. Several vasoactive substances and various experimental challenges thought to cause pulmonary capillaries to become abnormally leaky to plasma proteins have been studied with this model. In addition, models have been developed to collect lymph from small prenodal lymphatics in dog lungs.

α-Naphthylthiourea

Since the classic study of Drinker and Hardenbergh (120), investigators have shown that ANTU considerably damages both the lung capillary endothelium and alveolar epithelium (92, 157, 286, 302, 342, 429). However, only recently have lymphatic protein fluxes been analyzed in animals challenged by ANTU. Pine et al. (409) used right duct lymph to demonstrate an increased lymph flow and lung water after ANTU challenge. Figure 30 presents data from a more recent study. Rutili, Parker, Taylor, et al. (437) measured total protein content of lymph and plasma in a prenodal lymphatic model. Three hours after ANTU challenge they increased left atrial pressure and again determined C_L/C_P. Figure 30 demonstrates a filtration independent C_L/C_P state after ANTU challenge and left atrial pressure elevation. From these data a σ_d of 0.40 was calculated for dog lung capillaries after ANTU challenge as compared with a σ_d of 0.70 in

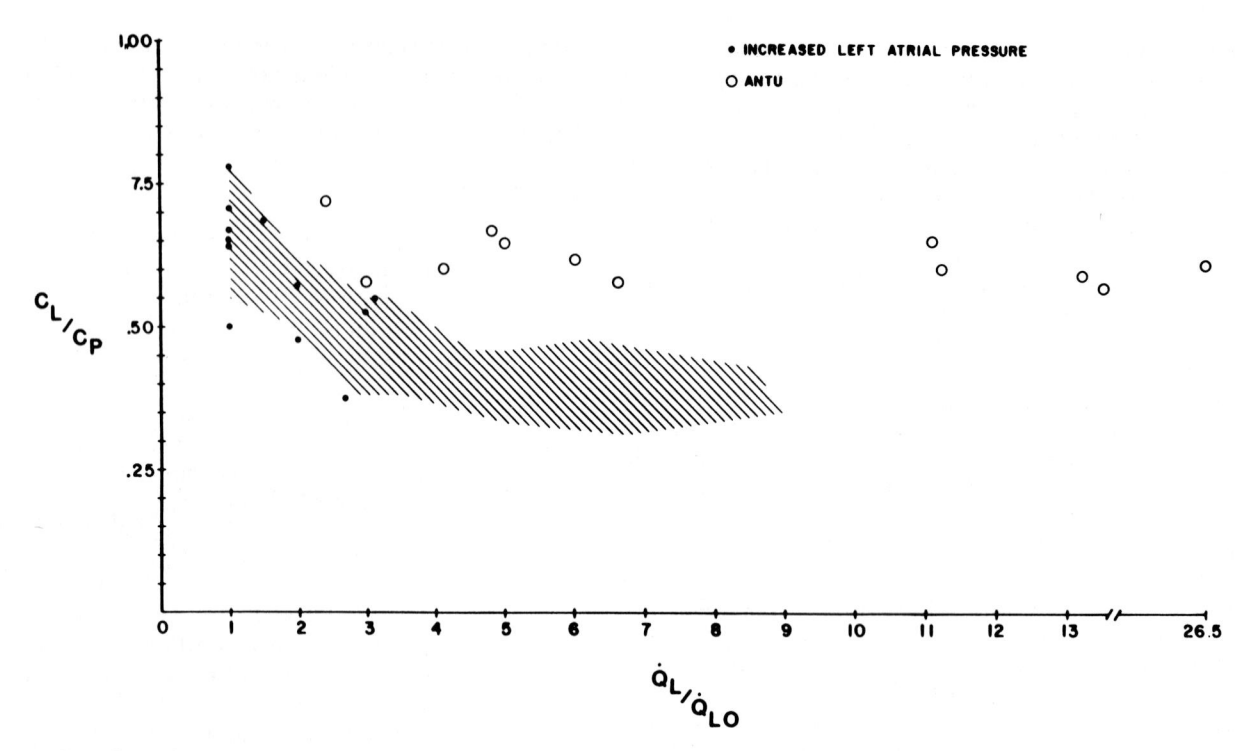

FIG. 30. Lymph-to-plasma concentration ratios (C_L/C_P) for total protein as a function of lymph flow ($\dot{Q}_L$) relative to control ($\dot{Q}_{L,0}$). [Adapted from Rutili, Parker, Taylor, et al. (437).]

control animals. In addition, when the pore analysis outlined in MEASUREMENT OF CAPILLARY SELECTIVITY TO PLASMA PROTEINS, p. 195, was used to fit the protein fractions, large pore radius increased from 200 to 280 Å and the volume conductance associated with the large pore system increased threefold. These data are from the only increased permeability study for which a plasma protein σ_d can be estimated with any degree of certainty in lung capillaries. The mechanism of ANTU edema formation is not known, but the damage appears to be confined to the lung endothelium (92, 409).

Hydrochloric Acid Aspiration

Acid aspiration results in severe lung damage and alveolar edema (187, 190, 251). Until recently the consensus was that acid simply damaged the lung tissue, thereby causing changes in the alveolar-capillary walls (251). However, this idea was challenged by the demonstration in the isolated dog lung that large doses of albumin tend to reverse the acid-related edema formation (67, 508, 509). Moreover corticosteroids appear to lessen the acid-induced damage (508).

Recently Grimbert, Parker, and Taylor (190) used prenodal lymph collection in the dog to study the effects of acid aspiration on pulmonary capillary permeability. Capillary permeability to plasma proteins increased markedly (Fig. 31), and albumin failed to reverse the lung damage. Indeed albumin resulted in a greater protein flux and a greater amount of lung water. Stothert et al. (485) used different techniques to confirm this finding. The differences observed in the protective effects of albumin may be related to the fact that flow was held constant in the studies of the isolated lung by Cameron et al. (67) and Toung et al. (508) and that the damage caused by aspiration is patchy. If blood flow is diverted from the damaged areas, fluid filtering from more normal areas of the lung may form lymph and mask a change in vascular permeability in an intact lung in which flow is more uniform.

Hemorrhagic Shock

The concept of a shock-lung syndrome has stimulated a great deal of research concerning whether lungs become overtly leaky to plasma proteins during the hypovolemic or reinfusion stages of hemorrhagic shock (136, 531). Fishman (136) designated shock lung a nonentity. As this section shows, lung damage associated with hypovolemic shock alone is minimal and probably not worthy of a syndrome status.

Structural changes and increased protein fluxes in right duct lymph have indicated that pulmonary capillaries become leaky to plasma proteins during hemorrhagic shock in the dog (321, 344, 368, 507). In contrast, other studies in both sheep and dog lung failed to demonstrate any effect on pulmonary capillary permeability during either the hemorrhagic or reinfusion states of shock (8, 104–106, 228, 265).

There is no doubt that lung water and protein fluxes

may increase after reinfusion of shed blood, but this is thought to be caused by increased vascular pressures (104, 106, 365). Changes (although small) may also occur in capillary permeability during the hemorrhagic phase of shock when studied in unanesthetized sheep (104, 106), although acute experiments in the same animal indicate no change in vascular permeability at this stage of shock (316).

Several factors may explain the divergent findings from many laboratories concerning alterations in capillary permeability in hemorrhagic shock. *1)* The effects of hypovolemic shock on lung vascular permeability are extremely variable from animal to animal in the same species (316). *2)* Dogs may respond differently than other species to hemorrhagic shock (46, 265). *3)* Many lymphatic studies do not appear to be in a steady state with respect to C_L/C_P, which seriously limits the use of lymph flux techniques to evaluate permeability in hemorrhagic shock (383, 501). *4)* Extrapulmonary sources contaminate lymphatics that are believed to drain primarily the lung interstitium, and lymph is definitely altered as its courses through nodes (1, 113, 319). Because hemorrhagic shock damages the viscera (179), any contamination of lung lymph by extrapulmonary sources would mask the true events occurring in pulmonary tissue, especially when right duct lymph is used as a lung lymph source in dogs (323, 367, 368). Some of the discrepancy may also stem from the type of hemorrhage used to induce shock, especially the duration and amount of hemorrhage. Heflin and Brigham (219) believe that ~6–8 h are required for neutrophils to be fully activated and affect lung capillary permeability. In most studies of severe hemorrhagic shock few animals survive more than 3–4 h. Although hemorrhagic shock alone does not apparently produce any great amount of damage to the lung vascular endothelium, the formation of emboli and the subsequent involvement of the neutrophil system may explain not only discrepant results but also why corticosteroids are sometimes helpful clinically in this disorder (54, 531).

Septic Shock

A controversy also exists over the effects of sepsis on lung vascular permeability and the subsequent development of pulmonary edema. Both the research and clinical communities have more or less accepted the notion that sepsis can cause lung vascular damage, which contributes to the adult respiratory distress syndrome (7, 76, 77, 151). However, the experimental evidence can be divided into two schools. *1)* In both dog and monkey no observable damage occurs to the lung endothelium after lethal doses of *Escherichia coli* endotoxin (156, 208, 215, 223, 265, 326). *2)* Other investigations, with conclusions that were based on collection of lymph in the chronically instrumented sheep, appear to demonstrate a substantial increase in pulmonary vascular permeability after infusions of either *E. coli* endotoxin or *P. aeruginosa*. Pulmonary vascular permeability appears to increase ~4–6 h after infusion of *P. aeruginosa* or endotoxin into the unanesthetized sheep (53, 54, 58). Methylprednisolone (given before or in the first 2–4 h after endotoxin challenge) blocks the permeability change (22, 54) and lessens the initial rise in pulmonary pressures (52). Indomethacin blocks the pressure rise associated with endotoxin challenge, indicating that some product of arachidonic acid increases the vascular resistance associated with septic shock (53, 369, 370). Finally granulocyte depletion partially prevents the increased vascular permeability associated with endotoxin (219), which agrees with the observations that O_2 radicals cause endothelial damage (438) and that endotoxin activates leukotaxic factors and complement (145, 221, 269, 410). Craddock et al. (88) invoked a similar mechanism to explain the pulmonary vascular damage associated with repeated hemodialysis in humans.

Physiologists and clinicians alike face the problem of explaining the two different findings concerning the effects of sepsis on vascular permeability. There are four possible explanations. *1)* A species difference may explain the different responses. *2)* Lymph collected with the sheep lung lymphatic model may be contaminated by nonpulmonary sources and altered by nodal effects, which could explain why the dog lung lymphatic model does not demonstrate the same response to sepsis as seen in the sheep model. In fact right duct lymph in the dog, which receives lymph from other thoracic and abdominal tissues and passes through numerous nodes, responds after endotoxin challenge in a manner similar to the sheep model (368). *3)* The bronchial circulation provides more lung lymph when affected by the toxin (406). However, lung lymph should be formed predominantly by the pulmonary blood vessels because they are so numerous

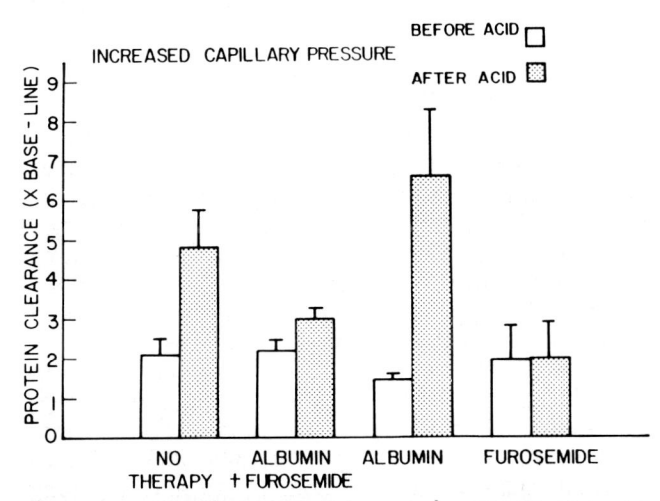

FIG. 31. Lymphatic protein clearances ($\dot{Q}_L \times C_L/C_P$) after acid aspiration in intact dog lungs. *Histograms*, protein clearance when capillary pressures were elevated in controls and after acid. Effects of albumin and furosemide on acid-induced clearance are also shown. [Data from Grimbert, Parker, and Taylor (190).]

relative to the bronchial vessels. *4)* The vascular damage in the dog model may require more time to develop than most experimental procedures have allowed.

Histamine

Histamine produces a transient increase in systemic vascular permeability to macromolecules (307, 308, 319). The effect appears to be mediated by contraction of endothelial cells, which produces large openings or gaps in the capillary wall (308). The effects of histamine on the permeability properties of lung capillaries appear to be different in sheep and dogs. In unanesthetized sheep, observations based on caudal mediastinal node lymph suggest a small increase in pulmonary vascular permeability after the administration of histamine; administration of an H_1 blocker abolished both the vascular constriction and the permeability effects (55, 56). Another study also supports the view that histamine causes pulmonary vessels to leak (417). Conversely several other laboratories used different preparations and failed to find a histamine effect on pulmonary vascular permeability (116, 171, 188, 319). Neither microscopic nor ultrastructural studies have demonstrated a histamine effect on vascular permeability in rabbit or dog lungs. Instead morphologic studies suggest that histamine causes bronchial venules to leak large molecules (404, 405, 408). More recent studies in the sheep show quite clearly that histamine changes surface area without any measurable change occurring in vascular permeability (K. L. Brigham, unpublished observations). It is interesting that histamine causes a greater leakage of plasma proteins into the lymph within a peripheral node and increases nodal lymph flow. The effect appears to be transient and may explain the histamine findings in the sheep preparation (320).

At this time a reasonable conclusion is that histamine may cause only minor changes in pulmonary vascular permeability. However, the question of how and where histamine acts in the lung circulation is intriguing for several reasons. For example, histamine dramatically increases lung vascular resistance, affecting primarily the postcapillary segments of the pulmonary circulation (98, 295, 429a). An increased capillary pressure then results, increasing lymph flow and protein flux without any change in vascular permeability. This increased fluid filtration may predispose the lung to intra-alveolar flooding. However, it is perplexing that the histamine damage, if it exists, is small. What protects the lung from histamine damage? Perhaps, in contrast to the systemic circulation, endothelial cells in the lung's vasculature do not contract in response to histamine. This may explain how the lung can be a tissue depot for mast cells, which constitute a defense mechanism for the airways, without running the added risk of pulmonary edema development each time histamine is released because of an airway challenge.

High-Altitude Pulmonary Edema

Decreasing alveolar partial pressure of O_2 ($P_{A_{O_2}}$) markedly increases pulmonary arterial pressures because of a large change in pulmonary vascular resistance (21, 96, 130, 310, 390, 526). Most investigators agree that vascular constriction occurs at the precapillary level of the circulation (33, 134, 259, 390), but others feel that postcapillary resistance changes may also occur during alveolar hypoxia (50, 310).

Why does ascent to high altitude sometimes produce pulmonary edema (236, 237, 267, 317, 517, 518)? Certainly the Indian troops involved in skirmishes with Chinese soldiers in the Himalayan Mountains were healthy individuals, "not sinful and gin-soaked old men" (317), yet ~500 of these well-trained individuals developed high-altitude pulmonary edema (337, 480)! Perhaps the high pulmonary arterial pressures actually rupture small arteries (539), or perhaps hyperperfusion occurs in focal regions of the lungs through short blood vessels that bypass the constricted arteries (an artery-to-capillary shunt) and cause the capillary pressure to rise in these focal areas. The latter idea is supported by the finding that individuals without a right pulmonary artery are prone to the development of high-altitude pulmonary edema (337). Individuals with a history of high-altitude pulmonary edema also have a larger rise in pulmonary arterial pressure during alveolar hypoxia than normal individuals (236). Hypoxia should increase cardiac output because of tissue demand and produce lung hyperperfusion. Courtice and Korner (86) showed that alveolar hypoxia caused a greater accumulation of lung water at high cardiac outputs, indicating that some edema may be caused by hyperperfusion. Because of the increased pulmonary blood flow, investigators have postulated that a diuretic (furosemide) may help prevent pulmonary edema during an ascent to higher altitudes (28, 480). However, the effectiveness of furosemide is questionable in both animal (274) and human (235) studies. It is interesting that furosemide partially reversed the damage associated with acid aspiration (190), which suggested that the diuretic caused either blood flow to bypass the damaged lung areas or the neutrophil system to be inactivated, because the involvement of neutrophil damage in alveolar hypoxia has also been postulated (448, 480, 486).

At this time the cause of high-altitude pulmonary edema is unclear. Indeed whether the excess fluid in the lungs is the consequence of local events or of neurogenic stimulation arising in the brain is not settled (346, 486, 513), but a few studies in dog lungs indicate that alveolar anoxia can produce an increased vascular permeability (119, 390, 529). The definitive observations have not been made because edema in subjects who rapidly ascended to high altitudes has been rare (0.1%–0.4%) (237).

Neurogenic Pulmonary Edema

Physiologists have recognized for many years that increasing cerebrospinal fluid (CSF) pressure by a Cushing maneuver, infusion of thrombin and fibrinogen into the cisterna magna, and intravenous or intrathecal infusion of massive amounts of catecholamines result in massive pulmonary edema. The associated pulmonary edema has been related to *1)* the increased blood volume and capillary pressure in the lungs associated with the transfer of blood from the vasoconstricted systemic vascular bed to the pulmonary circuit, *2)* an increased pulmonary capillary permeability to plasma proteins, and *3)* a direct neural effect on the pulmonary blood vessels mediated by the sympathetic system or an indirect neural effect mediated through circulating catecholamines.

Several investigations indicate that the edema is most likely due to the increased pulmonary blood volume with the subsequent increase in pulmonary capillary pressure (17, 72, 74, 299, 440, 461); it has even been argued that *neurogenic pulmonary edema* is a misnomer and that the disorder should be referred to as *neurohemodynamic pulmonary edema* (440). Theodore and Robin (505) described neurogenic edema as resulting from the increased pulmonary vascular pressure and the additional complication of leaky capillaries or stretched pores (140, 444, 452). The postulated increase in permeability of the vascular system would result in continued fluid filtration into the lung even when the pulmonary vascular pressures returned to normal. Raising intracranial pressure increases lung water, which can be blocked with a variety of agents (309, 513). However, Jones et al. (254) have shown that increasing CSF pressure does not produce leaky capillaries. These studies were evaluated by increasing left atrial pressures, which allowed a more rigorous evaluation of lung lymph protein fluxes.

Neurogenic pulmonary edema clearly results primarily from an increased pressure in the lung's microcirculation. In addition the permeability to macromolecules may increase because of stretched pores (185, 205, 206, 346, 462).

Microemboli Vascular Damage

The increased vascular permeability associated with microembolism has been the subject of much research over the last 20 years. Some investigators found that the endothelial damage associated with microembolism requires fibrin and some fibrin-degradation products (245, 247, 301, 311, 313–315, 318, 439, 512). Others dispute this view (30).

A substantial amount of information indicates that leukocytes are partially responsible for the microvascular damage associated with microemboli (15, 141, 246, 248, 329, 330). It is well known that leukocytes produce superoxides and may also release proteases, leading to extensive tissue damage; yet it is not clear whether fibrin, fibrin-degradation products, or complement acts as the messenger to signal the leukocyte attraction into lung tissues. Tissue damage alone will produce superoxides and leukotaxic substances such as leukotrienes. Thus the increased vascular pressures associated with microemboli may somehow cause sufficient pulmonary tissue damage to attract leukocytes (see the chapter by Fisher and Forman in this *Handbook*).

Oxygen Toxicity

High alveolar O_2 tensions cause severe endothelial damage (37, 89–91, 218, 266). The interstitial and perivascular edema associated with breathing high levels of O_2 indicates that vascular permeability probably increases in O_2 toxicity. In fact half of the pulmonary capillaries are destroyed in rats exposed to 99% O_2 for 72 h (18, 78, 549). High O_2 tension also appears to change postcapillary resistance and increase alveolar membrane permeability before any observable edema develops. In awake sheep breathing 100% O_2, capillary permeability to plasma proteins (as reflected by lung lymph) increased on the 4th day (51).

The excessive production of superoxide radicals is thought to cause O_2 toxicity (see the chapter by Fisher and Forman in this *Handbook*). The available amount of superoxide dismutase cannot buffer the increased superoxide production, and severe lung tissue damage results (328, 506). In addition the superoxide-dependent chemotactic factor is activated and neutrophils migrate into the lung tissue, which promotes further damage because of their release of more superoxides, the formation of hydroxyl radicals and peroxides, and the release of proteases. The result is lipid peroxidation or O_2 radical damage to the various membrane components within lung tissue. Paraquat is thought to also cause excessive O_2 radical production and produce lesions similar to those observed with O_2 toxicity, but the primary target apparently is the epithelial barrier rather than endothelial cells (111, 419, 427, 453, 466).

Recent startling results demonstrate that rats pretreated with small doses of ANTU (506), hypoxia (427), endotoxin (147, 148), and preadaptation with O_2 levels of ~80% (89–91, 256) tolerate 100% O_2 levels better than untreated animals. This is thought to be due to the increased production of tissue superoxide dismutase stimulated by the various mild challenges (148). The higher levels of superoxide dismutase will be more efficient in scavenging the superoxides formed either in response to the high partial pressure of O_2 (P_{O_2}) or by neutrophils that migrate to the exposed tissue in response to the chemotactic factor released by alveolar macrophages or other lung tissue cells (146, 466). In fact neutropenic animals survive hyperoxia much better than normal animals, indicating that neutrophils are also important in the promotion of the lung vascular injury associated with high levels of P_{O_2} (146, 451).

Other Compounds

Many compounds are thought to increase pulmonary capillary permeability. Iprindole, which is used to treat mental depression, causes considerable endothelial and epithelial damage (18). Salicylates also may increase vascular leakage of proteins and pulmonary edema in humans and sheep (38, 60), presumably by interfering with platelet function, which is important in maintaining normal capillary permeability (38, 439).

Oleic acid placed into the pulmonary circulation causes severe pulmonary edema, most likely by the damaging effects of free fatty acids on the endothelial membrane (10, 61, 109, 125, 189, 275).

Reexpansion of collapsed lungs sometimes results in intra-alveolar edema (48, 127, 306, 450, 465). The mechanism responsible for this capillary leak syndrome is not known, but it has been attributed to alterations in surfactant properties or to increased capillary pressure, which is related to the transpulmonary pressures required to reexpand the collapsed lungs (48).

Removal of Ca^{2+} from the perfusate with EDTA in isolated lungs increases capillary filtration (217, 230, 356, 357). The Ca^{2+} effect appears to be related to altered sieving characteristics of the endothelial basement membranes (80, 230).

Pulmonary edema is a common complication in acute hemorrhagic pancreatitis and is thought to be caused by the increased triglycerides and phospholipase released by the damaged pancreas (264). Microatelectasis and circulating pancreatic enzymes have also been implicated as the causative factors (290). In experimental pancreatitis a rise in pulmonary vascular resistance and a slight increase in lung protein flux have been observed. The data were interpreted as indicating an increased permeability caused either by *1*) histamine, *2*) pulmonary thrombosis, *3*) activation of the complement system, *4*) activation of the kallikrein system, or *5*) a direct effect of pancreatic lipases and proteases. A slight increase in protein flux and the increased pulmonary vascular resistance indicate that histamine may be responsible for the increased protein flux (290).

In some instances, certain compounds appear to increase or decrease permeability when lung weight change is used as an indicator of vascular permeability. For example, serotonin increases protein flux and vascular pressures in the intact sheep lung but does not appear to increase protein permeability at the capillary wall (57, 429a). Furosemide appears to decrease protein and fluid flux in acid-aspiration edema in dogs (190), but the results are thought to be due to decreases in vascular resistance and not necessarily a change in pulmonary vascular permeability (110).

On the basis of lymph flow and protein fluxes, prostaglandins have been implicated as causing permeability changes in endotoxemia (103). However, other mechanisms are only partially excluded. Indeed the prostaglandin studies indicate the difficulty in predicting permeability changes from only lymph flow and protein fluxes when the driving forces acting across the capillary wall are not measured simultaneously.

Coronary ligation (83), ketoacidosis (411), bradykinin (216), heroin overdose (260), cigarette smoke (253), etchlorvynol (132, 168, 345), ammonium chloride (364), alloxan (355, 524), and many other compounds have been reported to increase pulmonary vascular permeability.

Possible Mechanisms: Superoxide System

Several factors seem to increase capillary permeability to macromolecules. However, it is very clear that many factors (e.g., hemorrhage, shock, sepsis, alveolar hypoxia, and high $P_{A_{O_2}}$) do not always produce pulmonary edema. A simple physicochemical model may explain why edema develops in some experimental and clinical settings and not in other very similar conditions (500a). It is clear that neutrophils may be involved in the lung endothelial damage associated with different challenges because of free radical production [(9, 441); see also the chapter by Fisher and Forman in this *Handbook*]. Johnson et al. (250) demonstrated that instillation into alveoli of hypoxanthine plus xanthine oxidase results in lung damage that mimics the adult respiratory distress syndrome. The damage in these studies results from the production of superoxides, hydroxyl radicals, or hydrogen peroxide. Figure 32 is a model of the superoxide system in lung tissue that may explain how lung vascular damage is produced in many experimental forms of edema.

Breathing 100% O_2 for 4-5 days results in a large production of superoxides (78, 89, 250). Although pulmonary levels of superoxide dismutase also increase, they are insufficient to adequately buffer the high levels of superoxides formed. In addition a leukotaxin is released, stimulating the accumulation of neutrophils in lung tissues (327, 328). The neutrophils also produce superoxides and hydroxyl radicals that further damage the lung vascular tissue (425, 426). Another portion of the model (block 11) represents preconditioning: small amounts of endotoxin, hypoxia, ANTU, or preconditioning with 80% O_2 increases the tolerance of animals to 100% O_2 (89). This is due to two mechanisms: *1*) either the neutrophils stimulate superoxide scavenger production directly (210, 345) or *2*) the tissues respond with a greater production of

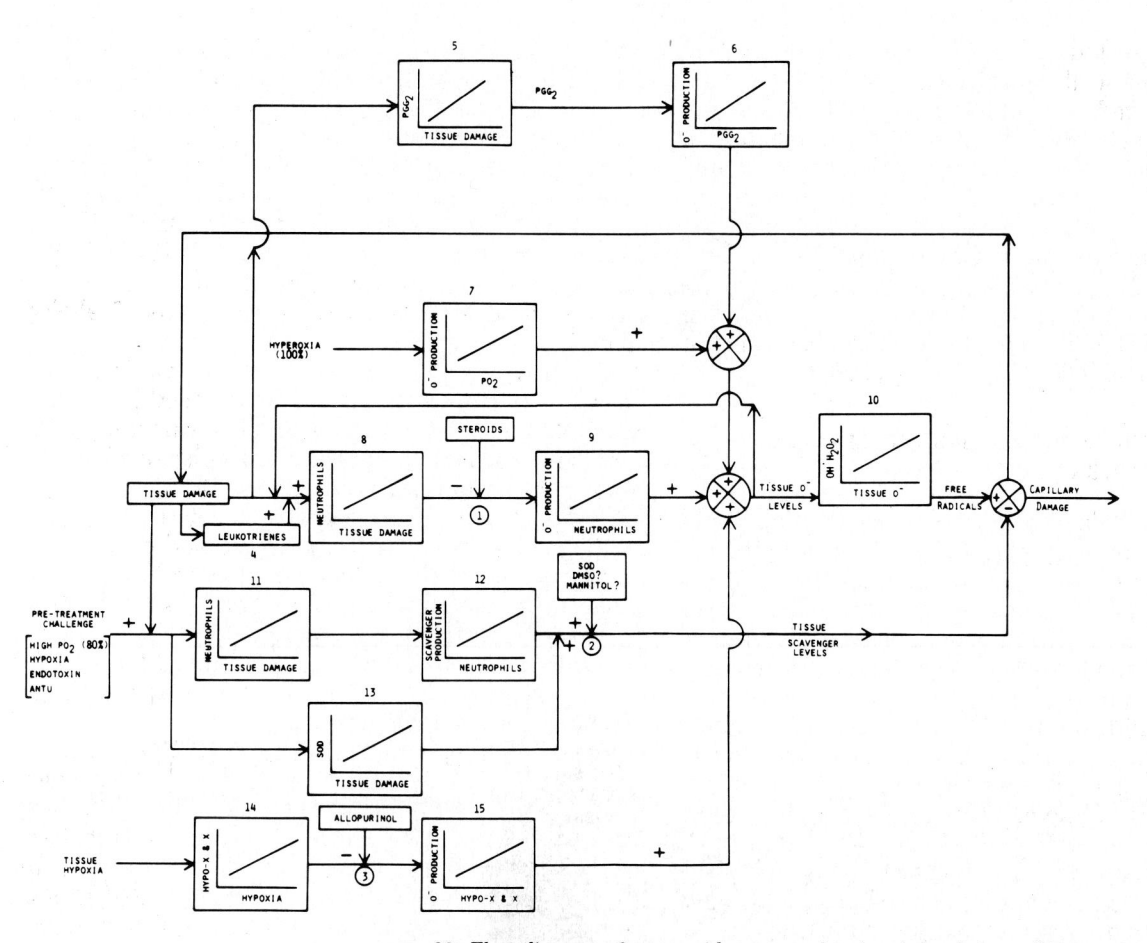

FIG. 32. Flow diagram of superoxide system showing tissue damage (*blocks 8–10*), pretreatments to increase free-radical scavengers (*blocks 11–13*), tissue hypoxic generation of superoxides (*blocks 14–15*), direct generation of O₂ radicals with hyperoxia (*block 7*), and generation of arachidonic acid metabolites and subsequent generation of superoxides (*blocks 5–6*). *Circled numbers*, proposed sites of actions of different compounds on the generation of superoxides, peroxides, and hydroxyl radicals. Ibuprofen would act at the entry to *block 5*. *Far right*, free radicals generated either by tissues or leukocytes are summed and ability of tissues to scavenge free radicals is subtracted. Interplay between generation and scavenging determines whether capillary damage results. [From Taylor and Martin (500a).]

superoxide scavenger (147, 148, 427, 506). This is especially true for the increased production of superoxide dismutase. When these lungs are then exposed to 100% O_2 the biochemical machinery is able to handle a greater load of superoxide formation and can buffer these tissue-destroying compounds to a greater degree.

The final portion of the model (block 14) shows how hypoxia may affect superoxide production through its effect on the xanthine and xanthine oxidase system. If free-radical generation exceeds the tissue's ability to inactivate this toxic compound, tissue damage will result. Block 5 shows how tissue damage produces prostaglandins and superoxide radicals. This may explain why indomethacin and ibuprofen are apparently beneficial in preventing some types of capillary damage (179).

It is quite likely that in many experimental conditions neutrophils are attracted to the tissues by leukotrienes released by platelet-activating factors (519).

In some instances the tissues make sufficient superoxide dismutase to buffer the increased superoxide production and no tissue damage results, especially if the particular animal model has a higher capacity to generate superoxide dismutase or other O_2 radical scavengers.

The proper intervention that may reverse each experimental condition is also shown in Figure 32. At step 1, methylprednisolone and depletion of neutrophils would act. At step 2, superoxide dismutase and perhaps dimethyl sulfoxide and mannitol would be beneficial as scavengers of the superoxides and hydroxyl radicals. Allopurinol, which competes with hypoxanthine for xanthine oxidase, can be used at step 3 to prevent the rise in superoxides associated with tissue hypoxia (179). A beneficial effect of corticosteroids has been demonstrated in endotoxin shock (54), and the beneficial effects of superoxide dismutase on the edema associated with microemboli and ANTU have also been demonstrated (141, 386). Allopurinol has not been tested in high-altitude exposure, where it may be beneficial, but furosemide may be a scavenger of free radicals, which accounts for its sometimes beneficial effect in high-altitude pulmonary edema and acid aspiration. Future research should provide much important information concerning the superoxide system's involvement in producing lung endothelial damage that results in pulmonary edema. Sufficient evidence exists to indicate that O_2 radicals are involved in pulmonary edema formation, and several papers have indicated that these compounds alter vascular permeability (179, 250, 386, 500a).

SEQUENCE AND PATHWAYS FOR PULMONARY EDEMA FORMATION

Although imbalances of the various Starling forces or increased capillary permeability can produce abnormally high capillary filtration rates, the progression of pulmonary edema follows a similar pattern regardless of etiology. In a comprehensive histological study, Staub et al. (484) described this sequence of events that occurs during the formation of pulmonary edema: *1)* filling of interstitial spaces surrounding extra-alveolar vessels and airways to form cuffs of edema fluid, *2)* thickening of the septal interstitial spaces, and *3)* alveolar flooding as an all-or-none phenomenon in individual alveoli. Note that fluid must leave the septal capillaries to move into the perivascular regions and that light microscopy cannot detect the slight volume changes occurring in the septal region.

The mechanical factors that favor accumulation of fluid around extra-alveolar vessels and airways are described in *Interstitial Fluid Pressure Gradients*, p. 192. Excess filtered fluid that cannot be cleared by the lymphatics moves into the connective tissue sheaths surrounding the smaller vessels and bronchioles. The fluid then migrates to the interstitial spaces surrounding successively larger vessels and bronchi at the hilum of the lung (464, 484). Edema fluid movement generally follows the interstitial pressure gradients shown in Figure 17. When an excess of fluid occurs (as in fluid-filled lobes) the edema cuff diameters are proportional to the transpulmonary pressure because of increased radial traction on the perivascular and peribronchial sheaths (161). Because the lymphatics course through the same connective tissue sheaths, these interstitial spaces constitute a parallel flow system for excess fluid that the lymphatics cannot accommodate. Evidence for movement of fluid down the longitudinal pressure gradient from smaller to larger perivascular-peribronchial sheaths includes the early swelling of the smaller peribronchial and perivascular interstitial spaces. Also both dye and radioactive labeled proteins equilibrate more rapidly with the fluid in small perivascular edema cuffs (<1 mm) (100, 158).

Fluid in the larger perivascular edema cuffs is functionally compartmentalized from the fluid continuously flowing through the interstitial spaces and cleared by the lymphatics. Gee and Havill (158) observed rapid movement of dye-labeled protein into the perivascular lymphatics during alloxan-induced pulmonary edema, but equilibration times for the dye with cuff edema fluid were in excess of 1 h. When lung interstitial fluid volume was increased by 78% with Tyrode's infusions in another study (381), half the interstitial edema was functionally sequestered and did not rapidly mix with an injected bolus of labeled albumin.

Although some investigators report an increased vascular resistance in vessels surrounded by edema cuffs (538), most studies indicate that vascular resistance is increased with significant alveolar flooding but is not affected by interstitial edema (24, 224, 241, 351, 352). The latter effect would be predicted from the mechanical properties of lung tissue and compliance measurements of the perivascular interstitium (276). Thus little compression of extra-alveolar vessels should occur until considerable fluid has accumulated in the lung. However, an elastic limit of the spaces within the vascular sheaths is reached at very high perivascular edema volumes (161).

An extravascular fluid gain of ~35% is generally considered the maximum interstitial volume change that can occur prior to alveolar flooding (112, 234, 240, 283, 382, 384, 474). However, a continued increase in interstitial volume (up to ~70%) during the alveolar flooding phase of edema has been demonstrated, which probably reflects patchy alveolar filling during intra-alveolar edema formation.

As the perivascular and peribronchial spaces fill with fluid, the septal interstitium also swells. Using morphometric techniques, DeFouw (100) and DeFouw and Berendsen (101) reported a 30%–56% increase in the mean width of the septal interstitial space for isolated lobe weight gains of 83%–88%. The edema is generally confined to the thick portion of the septal interstitium containing the collagen fibers (85, 488). The width of the endothelial and epithelial layers and of the fused basement membrane (thin) portion of the interstitial space increases minimally (13, 85, 100, 135, 140). In addition a vertical gradient in septal width was observed in severe hemodynamic and permeability edemas, with the septa in lower portions of the lung 30% wider than those in the upper zones (484). This gradient in septal width has not been observed in normally hydrated lungs (162). The temporal relationship of septal interstitial edema to the accumulation of extra-alveolar perivascular edema is not known, but septal swelling would be expected only after perivascular cuff formation.

Once the interstitium has reached its capacity to accommodate excess fluid, continued capillary filtration in excess of the lymphatic fluid transport will result in alveolar flooding. Estimates of alveolar fluid surface tension yield values of ~10–20 dyn/cm (393), but there is also evidence for an even lower surface tension (546). The negative pressure created by the surface tension tends to pull fluid into the alveoli. If the pressure gradient favors fluid movement into alveoli, they immediately fill with fluid (199, 200, 283). The patchy pattern of alveolar filling during edema (484) can be described by a system analysis of alveolar fluid balance (199). For these calculations a surface tension of 10 dyn/cm was assumed for an alveolus with a maximum 75 μm radius of curvature with a radius of 15 μm at the septal junctions. Intra-alveolar fluid pressure is determined by the smallest radius of curvature and is balanced by an identical interstitial fluid pressure (−10 mmHg). Figure 33 shows the effect on alveolar liquid volume as the fluid pressure became progressively less negative. Fluid pools that accumulate in the septal corners increased the radius of curvature at the air-liquid interface and reduced the inward acting force of surface tension. However, when the fluid pressure increased to −2 mmHg, the septal corners filled with fluid and the minimum radius of curvature decreased rather than increased. This effect is shown in the *upper panel* of Figure 33 for the radius of the fluid lining layer resulting from fluid pressures of −1.5, 0, and 2 mmHg. This increases the collapse pressure, and a stable alveolar liquid volume can only be maintained after the alveolus completely fills with fluid. This model predicts that alveoli of different radii would have different critical filling pressures; thus each alveolus (depending on its individual geometry and surface forces) would fill independently of other alveoli. Other calculations (545) indicate that fluid pools are maintained at a stable volume only in the region of intercapillary cusps, whereas fluid pools at the septal corners are inherently unstable (see Fig. 17). If these calculations are correct, only very small volumes of alveolar fluid can accumulate until a critical interstitial fluid pressure is attained. Once this occurs the alveolus immediately fills with interstitial fluid. Certainly this mechanism (especially the route by which fluid moves from the interstitium to the alveoli) requires further study.

The exact route by which fluid enters the alveoli from the interstitium remains controversial. There is general agreement that fluid enters by bulk flow through large channels that do not significantly sieve proteins (30, 160, 479, 522, 523). Staub (479) postulated that fluid moves through intercellular junctions of epithelium in small bronchioles during hemodynamic pulmonary edema and subsequently fills the alveoli. Evidence for this route of fluid entry includes the rapid movement of fluid and protein into peribronchiolar cuffs in fluid-filled lungs and the filling of intercellular junctions between bronchiolar epithelial cells with electron-dense tracers during edema formation (160, 479, 552). Hemoglobin and horseradish peroxidase filled intercellular clefts between epithelial cells, but the zonae occludens appeared to block passage of tracer into the airways. However, hemoglobin tracer appears to pass between alveolar epithelial cells

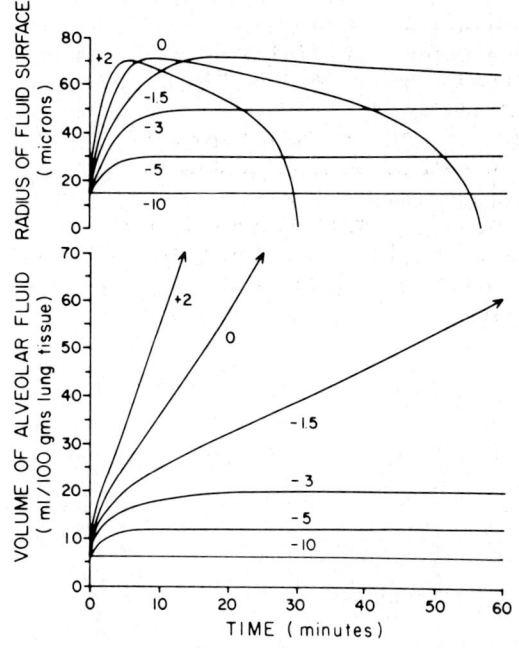

FIG. 33. Alveolar fluid volume and minimum radius of curvature at air-liquid interface at different steady-state interstitial fluid pressures. At a critical fluid pressure of −2 mmHg a stable fluid volume could not be maintained and the alveolus completely filled with fluid. [From Guyton, Taylor, Drake, and Parker (199).]

when pulmonary vascular pressures are increased to high levels (139, 552).

Interfacial tensions at the intra-alveolar fluid lining layer appear to favor fluid movement between the squamous epithelial cells lining the alveolar septa (81, 139, 164, 199). Certainly the widespread sloughing of septal epithelial cells observed in many clinical cases of respiratory distress leaves little doubt that considerable fluid moves directly from the uncovered interstitium into the alveolar spaces (13). Egan (122, 123) demonstrated the barrier function of the epithelial layer in preventing alveolar flooding. Disruption of the epithelial integrity by overinflation of the lung reduced the threshold left atrial pressure that was necessary to produce alveolar flooding in hydrostatic pulmonary edema.

CONCLUSIONS

This chapter has presented a comprehensive list of problems and possible solutions for evaluating the mechanisms responsible for the formation of pulmonary edema. The following summary is not intended to be as comprehensive. For a more complete discussion of a particular problem the reader is directed to the pertinent sections of the chapter and the references cited throughout the chapter.

1. *Tissue composition.* The swelling characteristics of the lung interstitium are a function of the makeup of the interstitium relative to collagen, proteoglycans, and other tissue constituents. Future work should

develop techniques for assessing the physicochemical makeup of different lung tissue components, such as basement membranes, septal interstitial spaces, and perivascular spaces.

2. *Theory of water and solute movement.* We feel that recent investigations have produced the correct physical and physiological approaches for assessing water and solute movement across pulmonary capillaries into the interstitium and finally into the lymphatics. However, many laboratories do not use the correct physical or experimental approaches when evaluating capillary permeability and should apply state-of-the-art techniques when assessing fluid and protein movement across the pulmonary microcirculation. In addition it is clear that the charge at the capillary wall, within the interstitium and possibly at the lymphatic vessel walls, affects the movement of the negatively charged plasma proteins. Studies with differently charged markers should enhance our understanding of the role of charge in transcapillary macromolecular exchange.

3. *Capillary pressure.* Because increases in capillary pressure are the most common cause of lung water accumulation, this parameter should be measured whenever possible. Most investigators have assumed a value for capillary pressure in intact animal studies. Techniques are now available that allow a direct determination of pulmonary pressures in intact animals.

4. *Tissue fluid pressure.* Pulmonary physiologists now readily accept the concept of a negative interstitial fluid pressure. The pressure is more negative surrounding extra-alveolar vessels (as compared with septal tissue spaces) and more negative at the top of the lung than at the bottom. Future studies should provide the necessary techniques to monitor the pressure gradients in lung tissue in both normal and pathological conditions.

5. *Colloid osmotic pressure.* This important regulator of capillary filtration can now be readily measured in terms of an average value, but techniques must be developed to either measure or evaluate tissue colloid osmotic pressure at different lung heights and at the same lung height in septal and perivascular fluids.

6. *Lymph flow.* Several excellent experimental models have been developed for estimating the lymph formation in an entire lung, but serious problems may be present in these models relative to contamination by extrapulmonary sources and changes occurring with lymph as it passes through nodes. These problems need to be resolved in the future and addressed when interpreting published data. It is important to know the difference in lymph formation rates at different horizontal and vertical sites within the lung tissue before average lymph flows can be interpreted relative to the mechanisms associated with capillary filtration.

7. *Abnormal capillary permeability.* As we reviewed the extensive literature in this area it became evident that most studies utilizing lymph did not assess pulmonary capillary permeability and that many models yield confusing data because of extrapulmonary sources contaminating lung lymph or because of lymph modification as it passes through nodes. For some lung pathological conditions, different laboratories obtained different results with the same experimental models. The problems associated with measuring pulmonary capillary permeability must be resolved before a complete theory describing mechanisms of formation and treatment of pulmonary edema can evolve. However, it is clear that many compounds cause pulmonary edema (31 in this chapter) by increasing capillary permeability and may have as a common denominator an overly active inflammatory response. The O_2 radicals or other compounds formed either by lung tissue or by activated neutrophils severely damage lung tissue. This research promises to provide important information relative to the mechanisms responsible for different forms of lung pathology.

8. *How does fluid enter and leave the alveoli?* This very basic question needs to be answered. Many investigators feel that interstitial fluid (when the pressure gradient is favorable) can enter the airways through epithelial junctions in the alveolar walls; others feel that fluid may enter the airways at bronchial-alveolar junctions. Research must settle this important issue before a complete model of lung edema formation can be developed. In addition the resolution of pulmonary edema is poorly understood. The fluid may be removed by active or passive mechanisms operating across the alveolar-epithelial membrane.

9. *Starling force analyses.* Past Starling force analyses have been based on average tissue and capillary forces and collection of lung lymph flow. Arguments have arisen as to the importance of various components of the Starling equation in opposing edema formation, because average Starling forces were used to interpret the data. It is now evident that *1)* tissue pressure becomes more negative from septal to perivascular spaces and in a vertical direction in the lung from base to apex, *2)* tissue fluid colloid osmotic pressure may differ in both a horizontal and a vertical direction within the lung tissues, *3)* vascular pressures decrease from arteries to veins and from base to apex in the lung, and *4)* the amount of lymph produced at different lung heights or the amount of capillary filtration that occurs in septal or perivascular tissue regions is not known.

The mechanisms responsible for capillary filtrate formation in lung tissue constitute a formidable and important area of research. Future studies need to develop appropriate physiological techniques for measuring the necessary forces and flows that describe the fluid and solute exchange occurring in different portions of lung tissue.

We thank Leigh Cosper, Sandy Worley, and Penny Cook for their diligent work on the preparation of this manuscript. In addition we thank Drs. N. Granger, P. Kvietys, M. Perry, and S. Lai-Fook for many helpful suggestions.

Research was supported by National Heart, Lung, and Blood Institute Grants HL-22549 and HL-24571 and the Parker B. Francis Pulmonary Fellows (now the Puritan-Bennet Foundation).

REFERENCES

1. ADAIR, T. H., D. S. MOFFATT, A. W. PAULSEN, AND A. C. GUYTON. Quantitation of changes in lymph protein concentration during lymph node transit. *Am. J. Physiol.* 243 (*Heart Circ. Physiol.* 12): H351–H359, 1982.
2. ADAMS, F. G., AND I. M. LEDINGHAM. The pulmonary manifestations of septic shock. *Clin. Radiol.* 28: 315–322, 1977.
3. AGOSTONI, E. Mechanics of the pleural space. *Physiol. Rev.* 52: 57–128, 1972.
4. AGOSTONI, E., AND J. PIIPER. Capillary pressure and distribution of vascular resistance in isolated lung. *Am. J. Physiol.* 202: 1033–1036, 1962.
5. AGOSTONI, E., A. TAGLIETTI, AND I. SETNIKAR. Absorption force of the capillaries of the visceral pleura in determination of the intrapleural pressure. *Am. J. Physiol.* 191: 277–282, 1957.
6. ALBERT, R. K., S. LAKSHMINARAYAN, T. W. HUANG, AND J. BUTLER. Fluid leaks from extra-alveolar vessels in living dog lungs. *J. Appl. Physiol.: Respirat. Environ. Exercise Physiol.* 44: 759–762, 1978.
7. ANDERSON, R. R., R. L. HOLLIDAY, A. A. DRIEDGER, M. LEFCOE, B. REID, AND W. J. SIBBALD. Documentation of pulmonary capillary permeability in the adult respiratory distress syndrome accompanying human sepsis. *Am. Rev. Respir. Dis.* 119: 869–877, 1979.
8. ANDERSON, R. W., AND W. C. DEVRIES. Transvascular fluid and protein dynamics in the lung following hemorrhagic shock. *J. Surg. Res.* 20: 281–290, 1976.
9. ARFORS, K. E., G. RUTILI, AND E. SVENSJÖ. Microvascular transport of macromolecules in normal and inflammatory conditions. *Acta Physiol. Scand. Suppl.* 463: 93–103, 1979.
10. ASHBAUGH, D. C., AND T. UZAWA. Respiratory and hemodynamic changes after injection of free fatty acids. *J. Surg. Res.* 8: 417–423, 1968.
11. AUKLAND, K., AND G. NICOLAYSEN. Interstitial fluid volume: local regulatory mechanisms. *Physiol. Rev.* 61: 556–643, 1981.
12. BACHOFEN, H., P. GEHR, AND E. R. WEIBEL. Alterations of mechanical properties and morphology in excised rabbit lungs rinsed with a detergent. *J. Appl. Physiol.: Respirat. Environ. Exercise Physiol.* 47: 1002–1010, 1979.
13. BACHOFEN, M., H. BACHOFEN, AND E. R. WEIBEL. Lung edema in the adult respiratory distress syndrome. In: *Pulmonary Edema*, edited by A. P. Fishman and E. M. Renkin. Bethesda, MD: Am. Physiol. Soc., 1979, chapt. 18, p. 241–252.
14. BAILE, E. M., P. D. PARÉ, R. W. DAHLBY, AND J. C. HOGG. Regional distribution of extravascular water and hematocrit in the lung. *J. Appl. Physiol.: Respirat. Environ. Exercise Physiol.* 46: 937–942, 1979.
15. BARIE, P. S., F. L. MINNEAR, AND A. B. MALIK. Increased pulmonary vascular permeability after bone marrow injection in sheep. *Am. Rev. Respir. Dis.* 123: 648–653, 1981.
16. BARRIOS, R., S. INOUE, AND J. C. HOGG. Intercellular junctions in "shock lung." A freeze-fracture study. *Lab. Invest.* 36: 628–635, 1977.
17. BEAN, J. W., AND D. L. BECKMAN. Centrogenic pulmonary pathology in mechanical head injury. *J. Appl. Physiol.* 27: 807–812, 1969.
18. BEAN, J. W., D. ZEE, AND B. THOM. Pulmonary changes with convulsions induced by drugs and oxygen at high pressure. *J. Appl. Physiol.* 21: 865–872, 1966.
19. BENJAMIN, J. J., P. S. MURTAGH, D. F. PROCTOR, H. A. MENKES, AND S. PERMUTT. Pulmonary vascular interdependence in excised dog lobes. *J. Appl. Physiol.* 37: 887–894, 1974.
20. BENNETT, H. S., J. H. LUFT, AND J. C. HAMPTON. Morphological classifications of vertebrate blood capillaries. *Am. J. Physiol.* 196: 381–390, 1959.
21. BERGOFSKY, E. H., AND S. HOLTZMAN. A study of the mechanisms involved in the pulmonary arterial pressure response to hypoxia. *Circ. Res.* 20: 506–519, 1967.
22. BESSA, S. M., A. P. DALMASSO, AND R. L. GOODALE, JR. Studies on the mechanism of endotoxin-induced increase of alveolocapillary permeability. *Proc. Soc. Exp. Biol. Med.* 147: 701–705, 1974.
23. BEVAN, D. R. Colloid osmotic pressure. *Anaesthesia* 35: 263–270, 1980.
24. BHATTACHARYA, J., K. NAKAHARA, AND N. C. STAUB. Effect of edema on pulmonary blood flow in the isolated perfused dog lung lobe. *J. Appl. Physiol.: Respirat. Environ. Exercise Physiol.* 48: 444–449, 1980.
25. BHATTACHARYA, J., S. NANJO, AND N. C. STAUB. Effect of lung edema on vertical distribution of subpleural connective tissue fluid pressure in isolated perfused dog lung (Abstract). *Microvasc. Res.* 21: 236, 1981.
26. BHATTACHARYA, J., S. NANJO, AND N. C. STAUB. Micropuncture measurement of lung microvascular pressure during 5-HT infusion. *J. Appl. Physiol.: Respirat. Environ. Exercise Physiol.* 52: 634–637, 1982.
27. BHATTACHARYA, J., AND N. C. STAUB. Direct measurements of microvascular pressures in the isolated perfused dog lung. *Science* 210: 327–328, 1980.
28. BIDDLE, T. L., AND P. N. YU. Effect of furosemide on hemodynamics and lung water in acute pulmonary edema secondary to myocardial infarction. *Am. J. Cardiol.* 43: 86–90, 1979.
29. BILL, A. Plasma protein dynamics: albumin and IgG capillary permeability, extravascular movement and regional blood flow in unanesthetized rabbits. *Acta Physiol. Scand.* 101: 28–42, 1977.
30. BINDER, A. S., K. NAKAHARA, K. OHKUDA, W. KAGELER, AND N. C. STAUB. Effect of heparin or fibrinogen depletion on lung fluid balance in sheep after emboli. *J. Appl. Physiol.: Respirat. Environ. Exercise Physiol.* 47: 213–219, 1979.
31. BLAISDELL, F. W., AND R. M. SCHLOBOHM. The respiratory distress syndrome: a review. *Surgery* 74: 251–262, 1973.
32. BLAKE, L. H., AND N. C. STAUB. Pulmonary vascular transport in sheep. A mathematic model. *Microvasc. Res.* 12: 197–200, 1976.
33. BLAND, R. D., R. H. DEMLING, S. L. SELINGER, AND N. C. STAUB. Effects of alveolar hypoxia on lung fluid and protein transport in unanesthetized sheep. *Circ. Res.* 40: 269–274, 1977.
34. BØ, G., A. HAUGE, AND G. NICOLAYSEN. Alveolar pressure and lung volume as determinants of net transvascular fluid filtration. *J. Appl. Physiol.: Respirat. Environ. Exercise Physiol.* 42: 476–482, 1977.
35. BOLTON, C., AND E. H. STARLING. Note on the blood-pressure and lymph flow in the case of heart disease in the dog. *Heart* 1: 292–296, 1910.
36. BOONYAPRAKOB, U., P. M. TAYLOR, D. W. WATSON, V. WATERMAN, AND E. LOPATA. Hypoxia and protein clearance from the pulmonary vascular beds of adult dogs and pups. *Am. J. Physiol.* 216: 1013–1019, 1969.
37. BOWDEN, D. H., AND I. Y. R. ADAMSON. Endothelial regeneration as a marker of the differential vascular responses in oxygen-induced pulmonary edema. *Lab. Invest.* 30: 350–357, 1974.
38. BOWERS, R. E., K. L. BRIGHAM, AND P. J. OWEN. Salicylate pulmonary edema: the mechanism in sheep and review of the clinical literature. *Am. Rev. Respir. Dis.* 115: 261–268, 1977.

39. BOYD, R. D. H., J. R. HILL, P. W. HUMPHREYS, I. C. S. NORMAND, E. O. R. REYNOLDS, AND L. B. STRANG. Permeability of lung capillaries to macromolecules in fetal and newborn lambs and sheep. *J. Physiol. London* 201: 567-588, 1969.
40. BRACE, R. A. The chronically implanted capsule: interstitial fluid pressure and solute concentration measurements. In: *Tissue Fluid Pressure and Composition*, edited by A. R. Hargens. Baltimore, MD: Williams & Wilkins, 1981, chapt. 24, p. 233-246.
41. BRACE, R. A. Progress toward resolving the controversy of positive vs. negative interstitial fluid pressure. *Circ. Res.* 49: 281-297, 1981.
42. BRACE, R. A., D. N. GRANGER, AND A. E. TAYLOR. Analysis of lymphatic protein flux data. II. Effect of capillary heteroporosity on estimates of reflection coefficients and PS products. *Microvasc. Res.* 14: 215-226, 1977.
43. BRACE, R. A., D. N. GRANGER, AND A. E. TAYLOR. Analysis of lymphatic protein flux data. III. Use of the nonlinear flux equation to estimate σ and PS. *Microvasc. Res.* 16: 297-303, 1978.
44. BRACE, R. A., AND A. C. GUYTON. Interstitial pressure: capsule, free fluid, gel fluid, and gel absorption pressure in subcutaneous tissue. *Microvasc. Res.* 18: 217-228, 1979.
45. BRACE, R. A., A. C. GUYTON, AND A. E. TAYLOR. Reevaluation of the needle method for measuring interstitial fluid pressure. *Am. J. Physiol.* 229: 603-607, 1975.
46. BREDENBERG, C. E. The pulmonary response to hemorrhagic shock: differences between primate and dog. *Circ. Shock* 6: 165-171, 1979.
47. BREDENBERG, C. E., T. KAZUI, AND W. R. WEBB. Experimental pulmonary edema: the effect of positive end-expiratory pressure on lung water. *Ann. Thorac. Surg.* 26: 62-67, 1978.
48. BRENNAN, N. J., AND M. X. FITZGERALD. Anatomically localised re-expansion pulmonary oedema following pneumothorax drainage. Case report and literature review. *Respiration* 38: 233-237, 1979.
49. BRESLER, E. H., AND L. J. GROOME. On equations for combined convective and diffusive transport of neutral solute across porous membranes. *Am. J. Physiol.* 241 (*Renal Fluid Electrolyte Physiol.* 10): F469-F476, 1981.
50. BRESSACK, M. A., AND R. D. BLAND. Alveolar hypoxia increases lung fluid filtration in unanesthetized newborn lambs. *Circ. Res.* 45: 111-116, 1980.
51. BRESSACK, M. A., D. D. McMILLAN, AND R. D. BLAND. Pulmonary oxygen toxicity: increased microvascular permeability to protein in unanesthetized lambs. *Lymphology* 12: 133-139, 1979.
52. BRIGHAM, K. L. Pulmonary edema: cardiac and noncardiac. *Am. J. Surg.* 138: 361-367, 1979.
53. BRIGHAM, K. L., R. E. BOWERS, AND J. HAYNES. Increased sheep lung vascular permeability caused by *Escherichia coli* endotoxin. *Circ. Res.* 45: 292-297, 1979.
54. BRIGHAM, K. L., R. E. BOWERS, AND C. R. McKEEN. Methylprednisolone prevention of increased lung vascular permeability following endotoxemia in sheep. *J. Clin. Invest.* 67: 1103-1110, 1981.
55. BRIGHAM, K. L., R. E. BOWERS, AND P. J. OWEN. Effects of antihistamines on the lung vascular response to histamine in unanesthetized sheep. Diphenhydramine prevention of pulmonary edema and increased permeability. *J. Clin. Invest.* 58: 391-398, 1976.
56. BRIGHAM, K. L., T. R. HARRIS, AND P. J. OWEN. [^{14}C]urea and [^{14}C]sucrose as permeability indicators in histamine pulmonary edema. *J. Appl. Physiol.: Respirat. Environ. Exercise Physiol.* 43: 99-101, 1977.
57. BRIGHAM, K. L., AND P. J. OWEN. Mechanism of the serotonin effect on lung transvascular fluid and protein movement in awake sheep. *Circ. Res.* 36: 761-770, 1975.
58. BRIGHAM, K. L., W. C. WOOLVERTON, L. H. BLAKE, AND N. C. STAUB. Increased sheep lung vascular permeability caused by *Pseudomonas bacteremia*. *J. Clin. Invest.* 54: 792-804, 1974.
59. BRIGHAM, K. L., W. C. WOOLVERTON, AND N. C. STAUB. Effects of changing hemodynamics on the extra plasma space in the lungs of sheep. *Microvasc. Res.* 10: 352-359, 1975.
60. BRODERICK, T. W., R. T. REINKE, AND E. GOLDMAN. Salicylate-induced pulmonary edema. *Am. J. Roentgenol.* 127: 865-866, 1976.
61. BROE, P. J., T. J. K. TOUNG, S. MARGOLIS, S. PERMUTT, AND J. L. CAMERON. Pulmonary injury caused by free fatty acid: evaluation of steroid and albumin therapy. *Surgery* 89: 582-587, 1981.
62. BRUDERMAN, I., K. SOMERS, W. K. HAMILTON, W. H. TOOLEY, AND J. BUTLER. Effect of surface tension on circulation in the excised lungs of dogs. *J. Appl. Physiol.* 19: 707-712, 1964.
63. BRUNS, R. R., AND G. E. PALADE. Studies on blood capillaries. II. Transport of ferritin molecules across the wall of muscle capillaries. *J. Cell Biol.* 37: 277-299, 1968.
64. BURTON, A. C., AND D. J. PATEL. Effect on pulmonary vascular resistance of inflation of the rabbit lungs. *J. Appl. Physiol.* 12: 239-246, 1958.
65. BUTLER, J. Pulmonary edema. *Clin. Sci.* 60: 1-4, 1981.
66. CALDINI, P., J. D. LEITH, AND M. J. BRENNAN. Effect of continuous positive-pressure ventilation (CPPV) on edema formation in dog lung. *J. Appl. Physiol.* 39: 672-679, 1975.
67. CAMERON, J. L., P. CALDINI, J. K. TOUNG, AND G. D. ZUIDEMA. Aspiration pneumonia: physiologic data following experimental aspiration. *Surgery* 72: 238-245, 1972.
68. CAMPBELL, T., AND T. HEATH. Intrinsic contractility of lymphatics in sheep and in dogs. *Q. J. Exp. Physiol.* 58: 207-217, 1973.
69. CASABURI, R., K. WASSERMAN, AND R. M. EFFROS. Detection and measurement of pulmonary edema. In: *Lung Biology in Health and Disease. Lung Water and Solute Exchange*, edited by N. C. Staub. New York: Dekker, 1978, vol. 7, chapt. 11, p. 323-376.
70. CASLEY-SMITH, J. R. The fine structure of the tissues and tissue channels. In: *Tissue Fluid Pressure and Composition*, edited by A. R. Hargens. Baltimore, MD: Williams & Wilkins, 1981, chapt. 11, p. 99-112.
71. CASLEY-SMITH, J. R., P. J. O'DONOGHUE, AND K. W. J. CROCKER. The quantitative relationships between fenestrae in jejunal capillaries and connective tissue channels: proof of "tunnel capillaries." *Microvasc. Res.* 9: 78-100, 1975.
72. CHEN, H. I., AND C. Y. CHAI. Pulmonary edema and hemorrhage as a consequence of systemic vasoconstriction. *Am. J. Physiol.* 227: 144-151, 1974.
73. CHEN, H. I., H. J. GRANGER, AND A. E. TAYLOR. Lymph flow transients following elevation of venous pressure in the dog's hind paw. In: *Progress in Lymphology*, edited by R. C. Mayall and M. H. Witte. New York: Plenum, 1977, p. 19-26.
74. CHEN, H. I., J. D. LIN, AND J. F. LIAO. Participation of regional sympathetic outflows in the centrogenic pulmonary pathology. *Am. J. Physiol.* 240 (*Heart Circ. Physiol.* 9): H109-H115, 1981.
75. CHINARD, F. P. The alveolar-capillary barrier: some data and speculations. *Microvasc. Res.* 19: 1-17, 1980.
76. CHRISTY, J. H. Pathophysiology of gram-negative shock. *Am. Heart J.* 81: 694-701, 1971.
77. CINTORA, I., S. BESSA, R. L. GOODALE, G. W. MOTSAY, AND J. W. BORNER. Further studies of endotoxin and alveolocapillary permeability. *Ann. Surg.* 2: 372-375, 1974.
78. CLARK, J. M., AND C. J. LAMBERTSEN. Pulmonary oxygen toxicity: a review. *Pharmacol. Rev.* 23: 38-117, 1971.
79. CLEMENTI, F., AND G. PALADE. Intestinal capillaries. I. Permeability to peroxidase and ferritin. *J. Cell Biol.* 41: 33-58, 1969.
80. CLEMENTI, F., AND G. PALADE. Intestinal capillaries. II. Structural effects of EDTA and histamine. *J. Cell Biol.* 42: 706-714, 1969.
81. CLEMENTS, J. A. Pulmonary edema and permeability of alveolar membrane. *Arch. Environ. Health* 2: 280-283, 1961.
82. CLEMENTS, J. A., AND D. F. TIERNEY. Alveolar instability associated with altered surface tension. In: *Handbook of Phys-*

iology. Respiration, edited by W. O. Fenn and H. Rahn. Washington, DC: Am. Physiol. Soc., 1965, sect. 3, vol. 2, chapt. 69, p. 1565-1583.
83. COLLINS, J. C., T. R. HARRIS, C. R. MCKEEN, AND K. L. BRIGHAM. Increased lung lymph transport without heart failure after coronary ligation in sheep. *J. Appl. Physiol.: Respirat. Environ. Exercise Physiol.* 47: 792-797, 1979.
84. COMPER, W. D., AND T. C. LAURENT. Physiological function of connective tissue polysaccharides. *Physiol. Rev.* 58: 255-315, 1978.
85. COTTRELL, T. S., O. R. LEVINE, R. M. SENIOR, J. WIENER, D. SPIRO, AND A. P. FISHMAN. Electron microscopic alterations at the alveolar level in pulmonary edema. *Circ. Res.* 21: 783-797, 1967.
86. COURTICE, F., AND P. KORNER. Effect of anoxia on pulmonary oedema produced by massive intravenous infusions. *Aust. J. Exp. Biol. Med. Sci.* 30: 511-526, 1952.
87. COWAN, G. S. M., JR., N. C. STAUB, AND L. H. EDMUNDS, JR. Changes in the fluid compartments and dry weights of reimplanted dog lungs. *J. Appl. Physiol.* 40: 962-970, 1976.
88. CRADDOCK, P. R., J. FEHR, K. L. BRIGHAM, R. S. KRONENBERG, AND H. S. JACOB. Complement and leukocyte-mediated pulmonary dysfunction in hemodialysis. *N. Engl. J. Med.* 296: 769-774, 1977.
89. CRAPO, J. D., B. E. BARRY, H. A. FOSCUE, AND J. SHELBURNE. Structural and biochemical changes in rat lungs occurring during exposures to lethal and adaptive doses of oxygen. *Am. Rev. Respir. Dis.* 122: 123-143, 1980.
90. CRAPO, J. D., M. PETERS-GOLDEN, J. MARSH-SALIN, AND J. S. SHELBURNE. Pathologic changes in the lungs of oxygen-adapted rats: a morphometric analysis. *Lab. Invest.* 39: 640-653, 1978.
91. CRAPO, J. D., K. SJOSTROM, AND R. T. DREW. Tolerance and cross-tolerance using NO_2 and O_2. I. Toxicology and biochemistry. *J. Appl. Physiol.: Respirat. Environ. Exercise Physiol.* 44: 364-369, 1978.
92. CUNNINGHAM, A. L., AND J. V. HURLEY. Alpha-naphthylthiourea-induced pulmonary oedema in the rat: a topographical and electron-microscope study. *J. Pathol.* 106: 25-35, 1972.
93. CURRAN, P. F., AND J. R. MACINTOSH. A model system for biological water transport. *Nature London* 193: 347-348, 1962.
94. D'ANGELO, E., G. MISEROCCHI, S. MICHELINI, AND E. AGOSTONI. Local transpulmonary pressure after lobar occlusion. *Respir. Physiol.* 18: 328-337, 1973.
95. DAWSON, C. A., D. J. GRIMM, AND J. H. LINEHAN. Effects of lung inflation on longitudinal distribution of pulmonary vascular resistance. *J. Appl. Physiol.: Respirat. Environ. Exercise Physiol.* 43: 1089-1092, 1977.
96. DAWSON, C. A., D. J. GRIMM, AND J. H. LINEHAN. Influence of hypoxia on the longitudinal distribution of pulmonary vascular resistance. *J. Appl. Physiol.: Respirat. Environ. Exercise Physiol.* 44: 493-498, 1978.
97. DAWSON, C. A., R. L. JONES, AND L. H. HAMILTON. Hemodynamic responses of isolated cat lungs during forward and retrograde perfusion. *J. Appl. Physiol.* 35: 95-102, 1973.
98. DAWSON, C. A., J. H. LINEHAN, AND D. A. RICKABY. Pulmonary microcirculatory hemodynamics. *Ann. NY Acad. Sci.* 384: 90-106, 1982.
99. DEEN, W. M., AND B. SATVAT. Determinants of the glomerular filtration of proteins. *Am. J. Physiol.* 241 (*Renal Fluid Electrolyte Physiol.* 10): F162-F170, 1981.
100. DEFOUW, D. O. Morphologic study of the alveolar septa in normal and edematous isolated dog lungs fixed by vascular perfusion. *Lab. Invest.* 42: 413-419, 1980.
101. DEFOUW, D. O., AND P. D. BERENDSEN. Morphological changes in isolated perfused dog lungs after acute hydrostatic edema. *Circ. Res.* 43: 72-82, 1978.
102. DEL MAESTRO, R. F., H. H. THAW, J. BJORK, M. PLANKER, AND K. E. ARFORS. Free radicals as mediators of tissue injury. *Acta Physiol. Scand. Suppl.* 42: 43-58, 1980.
103. DEMLING, R. H., G. NIEHAUS, A. PEREA, AND J. A. WILL. Effect of burn-induced hypoproteinemia on pulmonary transvascular fluid filtration rate. *Surgery* 85: 339-343, 1979.
104. DEMLING, R. H., G. NIEHAUS, AND J. A. WILL. Pulmonary microvascular response to hemorrhagic shock, resuscitation, and recovery. *J. Appl. Physiol.: Respirat. Environ. Exercise Physiol.* 46: 498-503, 1979.
105. DEMLING, R. H., R. PROCTOR, N. DUY, AND J. R. STARLING. Lung lysosomal enzyme release during hemorrhagic shock and endotoxemia. *J. Surg. Res.* 28: 269-279, 1980.
106. DEMLING, R. H., S. L. SELINGER, R. D. BLAND, AND N. C. STAUB. Effect of acute hemorrhagic shock on pulmonary microvascular fluid filtration and protein permeability in sheep. *Surgery* 77: 512-519, 1975.
107. DEMLING, R. H., M. SMITH, R. GUNTHER, J. T. FLYNN, AND M. H. GEE. Pulmonary injury and prostaglandin production during endotoxemia in conscious sheep. *Am. J. Physiol.* 240 (*Heart Circ. Physiol.* 9): H348-H353, 1981.
108. DEMLING, R. H., N. C. STAUB, AND L. H. EDMUNDS, JR. Effect of end-expiratory airway pressure on accumulation of extravascular lung water. *J. Appl. Physiol.* 38: 907-912, 1975.
109. DERKS, C. M., AND D. JACOBVITZ-DERKS. Embolic pneumopathy induced by oleic acid: a systematic morphological study. *Am. J. Pathol.* 87: 143-158, 1977.
110. DIKSHIT, K., J. K. VYDEN, J. S. FORRESTER, K. CHATTERJEE, R. PRAKASH, AND H. J. C. SWAN. Renal and extrarenal hemodynamic effects of furosemide in congestive heart failure after acute myocardial infarction. *N. Engl. J. Med.* 288: 1087-1090, 1973.
111. DIKSHITH, T. S., K. K. DATTA, R. B. RAIZADA, AND H. S. KUSHWAH. Effects of paraquat dichloride in male rabbits. *Indian J. Exp. Biol.* 17: 926-928, 1979.
112. DRAKE, R. E. *Changes in Starling Forces During the Formation of Pulmonary Edema*. University: Univ. of Mississippi, 1975. Dissertation.
113. DRAKE, R., T. ADAIR, D. TRABER, AND J. GABEL. Contamination of caudal mediastinal node efferent lymph in sheep. *Am. J. Physiol.* 241 (*Heart Circ. Physiol.* 10): H354-H357, 1981.
114. DRAKE, R. E., AND E. DAVIS. A corrected equation for the calculation of reflection coefficients (Letter to the editor). *Microvasc. Res.* 15: 259, 1978.
115. DRAKE, R., K. A. GAAR, AND A. E. TAYLOR. Estimation of the filtration coefficient of pulmonary exchange vessels. *Am. J. Physiol.* 234 (*Heart Circ. Physiol.* 3): H266-H274, 1978.
116. DRAKE, R. E., AND J. C. GABEL. Effect of histamine and alloxan on canine pulmonary vascular permeability. *Am. J. Physiol.* 239 (*Heart Circ. Physiol.* 8): H96-H100, 1980.
117. DRAKE, R. E., J. H. SMITH, AND J. C. GABEL. Estimation of the filtration coefficient in intact dog lungs. *Am. J. Physiol.* 238 (*Heart Circ. Physiol.* 7): H430-H438, 1980.
118. DRAKE, R. E., AND A. E. TAYLOR. Tissue and capillary force changes during the formation of intra-alveolar edema. *Progress in Lymphology*, edited by R. C. Mayall and M. H. Witte. New York: Plenum, 1977, p. 13-17.
119. DRINKER, C. K. *Pulmonary Edema and Inflammation*. Cambridge, UK: Cambridge Univ. Press, 1945.
120. DRINKER, C. K., AND E. HARDENBERGH. Acute effects upon the lungs of dogs of large intravenous doses of alpha-naphthyl thiourea (ANTU). *Am. J. Physiol.* 156: 35-43, 1949.
121. DUMONT, A. E., R. H. CLAUSS, G. E. REED, AND D. A. TICE. Lymph drainage in patients with congestive heart failure: comparison with findings in hepatic cirrhosis. *N. Engl. J. Med.* 269: 949-952, 1963.
122. EGAN, E. A. Response of alveolar epithelial solute permeability to changes in lung inflation. *J. Appl. Physiol.: Respirat. Environ. Exercise Physiol.* 49: 1032-1036, 1980.
123. EGAN, E. A. Lung inflation, lung solute permeability, and alveolar edema. *J. Appl. Physiol.: Respirat. Environ. Exercise Physiol.* 53: 121-125, 1982.
124. EGAN, E. A., R. M. NELSON, AND I. H. GESSNER. Solute permeability of the alveolar epithelium in acute hemodynamic pulmonary edema in dogs. *Am. J. Physiol.* 233 (*Heart Circ. Physiol.* 2): H80-H86, 1977.

125. EHRHART, I. C., AND W. F. HOFMAN. Oleic acid dose-related edema in isolated canine lung perfused at constant pressure. *J. Appl. Physiol.: Respirat. Environ. Exercise Physiol.* 50: 1115–1120, 1981.
126. EHRLICH, K., P. SEETHANATHAN, AND P. TAYLOR. Isolation of proteoglycans from lung tissue (Abstract). *Federation Proc.* 38: 653, 1979.
127. ENJETI, S., P. B. TERRY, H. A. MENKES, AND R. J. TRAYSTMAN. Mechanical factors and the regulation of perfusion through atelectatic lung in pigs. *J. Appl. Physiol.: Respirat. Environ. Exercise Physiol.* 52: 647–654, 1982.
128. ERASLAN, S., M. D. TURNER, AND J. D. HARDY. Lymphatic regeneration following lung reimplantation in dogs. *Surgery* 56: 970–973, 1964.
129. ERDMANN, A. J., T. R. VAUGHAN, K. L. BRIGHAM, W. C. WOOLVERTON, AND N. C. STAUB. Effect of increased vascular pressure on lung fluid balance in unanesthetized sheep. *Circ. Res.* 37: 271–284, 1975.
130. EULER, U. S. VON, AND L. LILJESTRAND. Observations on the pulmonary arterial blood pressures in the cat. *Acta Physiol. Scand.* 12: 301–320, 1946.
131. EVEN, T., J. F. BOISVIEUX, AND A. LOCKHARD. Biophysical introduction to pulmonary edema. *Bull. Physiol-Pathol. Respir.* 7: 1019–1073, 1971.
132. FAIRMAN, R. P., F. L. GLAUSER, AND R. FALLS. Increases in lung lymph and albumin clearance with ethchlorvynol. *J. Appl. Physiol.: Respirat. Environ. Exercise Physiol.* 50: 1151–1155, 1981.
133. FEIN, A., R. F. GROSSMAN, J. G. JONES, E. OVERLAND, L. PITTS, J. F. MURRAY, AND N. C. STAUB. The value of edema fluid protein measurement in patients with pulmonary edema. *Am. J. Med.* 67: 32–38, 1979.
134. FISHMAN, A. P. Respiratory gases in the regulation of the pulmonary circulation. *Physiol. Rev.* 41: 214–280, 1961.
135. FISHMAN, A. P. Pulmonary edema. The water-exchanging function of the lung. *Circulation* 46: 390–408, 1972.
136. FISHMAN, A. P. Shock lung: a distinctive nonentity. *Circulation* 17: 921–923, 1973.
137. FISHMAN, A. P. Interstitial pulmonary edema. *Acta Cardiol.* 19: 177–180, 1974.
138. FISHMAN, A. P. (editor). *Pulmonary Diseases and Disorders.* New York: McGraw-Hill, 1980.
139. FISHMAN, A. P., AND G. G. PIETRA. Hemodynamic pulmonary edema. In: *Pulmonary Edema*, edited by A. P. Fishman and E. M. Renkin. Bethesda, MD: Am. Physiol. Soc., 1979, chapt. 6, p. 79–96.
140. FISHMAN, A. P., AND G. G. PIETRA. Stretched pores, blast injury and neurohemodynamic pulmonary edema. *Physiologist* 23: 53–56, 1980.
141. FLICK, M. R., J. M. HOEFFEL, AND N. C. STAUB. Superoxide dismutase with heparin prevents increased lung vascular permeability during air emboli in sheep. *J. Appl. Physiol.: Respirat. Environ. Exercise Physiol.* 55: 1284–1291, 1983.
142. FLICK, M. R., A. PEREL, W. KAGELER, AND N. C. STAUB. Regional extravascular lung water in normal sheep. *J. Appl. Physiol.: Respirat. Environ. Exercise Physiol.* 46: 932–936, 1979.
143. FLICK, M. R., A. PEREL, AND N. C. STAUB. Leukocytes are required for increased lung microvascular permeability after microembolization in sheep. *Circ. Res.* 48: 344–352, 1981.
144. FOLKOW, B., AND E. NEIL. *Circulation.* New York: Oxford Univ. Press, 1971, p. 399–416.
145. FOUNTAIN, S. W., B. A. MARTIN, C. E. MUSCLOW, AND J. C. COOPER. Pulmonary leukostasis and its relationship to pulmonary dysfunction in sheep and rabbits. *Circ. Res.* 46: 175–180, 1980.
146. FOX, R. B., J. R. HOIDAL, D. N. BROWN, AND J. E. REPINE. Pulmonary inflammation due to oxygen toxicity: involvement of chemotactic factors and polymorphonuclear leukocytes. *Am. Rev. Respir. Dis.* 123: 521–523, 1981.
147. FRANK, L., AND R. J. ROBERTS. Endotoxin protection against oxygen-induced acute and chronic lung injury. *J. Appl. Physiol.: Respirat. Environ. Exercise Physiol.* 47: 577–581, 1979.
148. FRANK, L., J. SUMMERVILLE, AND D. MASSARO. Protection from oxygen toxicity with endotoxin. Role of the endogenous antioxidant enzymes of the lung. *J. Clin. Invest.* 65: 1104–1110, 1980.
149. FRIEDERICI, H. H. R. Freeze-etch observations on interstitial connective tissue. *J. Ultrastruct. Res.* 24: 269–285, 1968.
150. FRØKJAER-JENSEN, J. Three-dimensional organization of plasmalemmal vesicles in endothelial cells. An analysis by serial sectioning of frog mesenteric capillaries. *J. Ultrastruct. Res.* 73: 9–20, 1980.
151. FULTON, R. L., AND C. E. JONES. The cause of post-traumatic pulmonary insufficiency in man. *Surg. Gynecol. Obstet.* 140: 176–186, 1975.
152. FUNG, Y. C., AND S. S. SOBIN. Theory of sheet flow in lung alveoli. *J. Appl. Physiol.* 26: 472–488, 1969.
153. GAAR, K. A., JR., A. E. TAYLOR, L. J. OWENS, AND A. C. GUYTON. Effect of capillary pressure and plasma protein on development of pulmonary edema. *Am. J. Physiol.* 213: 79–82, 1967.
154. GAAR, K. A., JR., A. E. TAYLOR, L. J. OWENS, AND A. C. GUYTON. Pulmonary capillary pressure and filtration coefficient in the isolated perfused lung. *Am. J. Physiol.* 213: 910–914, 1967.
155. GABEL, J. C., AND R. E. DRAKE. Pulmonary capillary pressure in intact dog lungs. *Am. J. Physiol.* 235 (*Heart Circ. Physiol.* 4): H569–H573, 1978.
156. GABEL, J. C., R. E. DRAKE, J. F. ARENS, AND A. E. TAYLOR. Unchanged pulmonary capillary filtration coefficients after *Escherichia coli* endotoxin infusion. *J. Surg. Res.* 25: 97–104, 1978.
157. GARDINER, T. H. Quantitative changes in permeability of rat lung epithelium in lung edema. *J. Appl. Physiol.: Respirat. Environ. Exercise Physiol.* 44: 576–580, 1978.
158. GEE, M. H., AND A. M. HAVILL. The relationship between pulmonary perivascular cuff fluid and lung lymph in dogs with edema. *Microvasc. Res.* 19: 209–216, 1980.
159. GEE, M. H., AND J. A. SPATH, JR. The dynamics of the lung fluid filtration systems in dogs with edema. *Circ. Res.* 46: 796–801, 1980.
160. GEE, M. H., AND N. C. STAUB. Role of bulk fluid flow in protein permeability of the dog lung alveolar membrane. *J. Appl. Physiol.: Respirat. Environ. Exercise Physiol.* 42: 144–149, 1977.
161. GEE, M. H., AND D. O. WILLIAMS. Effect of lung inflation on perivascular cuff fluid volume in isolated dog lung lobes. *Microvasc. Res.* 17: 192–201, 1979.
162. GEHR, P., AND E. R. WEIBEL. Morphometric estimation of regional differences in the dog lung. *J. Appl. Physiol.* 37: 648–653, 1974.
163. GIL, J. Improvements in demonstration of lining layer of lung alveoli by electron microscopy. *Respir. Physiol.* 8: 13–36, 1969.
164. GIL, J. Influence of surface forces on pulmonary circulation. In: *Pulmonary Edema*, edited by A. P. Fishman and E. M. Renkin. Bethesda, MD: Am. Physiol. Soc., 1979, chapt. 4, p. 53–64.
165. GIL, J., H. BACHOFEN, P. GEHR, AND E. R. WEIBEL. Alveolar volume-surface area relation in air- and saline-filled lungs fixed by vascular perfusion. *J. Appl. Physiol.: Respirat. Environ. Exercise Physiol.* 47: 990–1001, 1979.
166. GIL, J., AND E. R. WEIBEL. Morphologic study of pressure-volume hysteresis in rat lungs fixed by vascular perfusion. *Respir. Physiol.* 15: 190–213, 1972.
167. GILBERT, R. D., J. R. HESSLER, D. V. EITZMAN, AND S. CASSIN. Site of pulmonary vascular resistance in fetal goats. *J. Appl. Physiol.* 32: 47–53, 1972.
168. GLAUSER, F. L., W. R. SMITH, A. CALDWELL, M. HOSHIKO, G. S. DOLAN, H. BAER, AND N. OLSHER. Ethchlorvynol (Placidyl)-induced pulmonary edema. *Ann. Intern. Med.* 84: 46–48, 1976.

169. GLAZIER, J. B., J. M. B. HUGHES, J. E. MALONEY, AND J. B. WEST. Vertical gradient of alveolar size in lungs of dogs frozen intact. *J. Appl. Physiol.* 23: 694–705, 1967.
170. GLAZIER, J. B., J. M. B. HUGHES, J. E. MALONEY, AND J. B. WEST. Measurements of capillary dimensions and blood volume in rapidly frozen lungs. *J. Appl. Physiol.* 26: 65–76, 1969.
171. GOETZMAN, B. W., AND M. B. VISSCHER. The effects of alloxan and histamine on the permeability of the alveolar capillary barrier to albumin. *J. Physiol. London* 204: 51–61, 1969.
172. GOLDBERG, H. S. Effect of lung volume history on rate of edema formation in isolated canine lobe. *J. Appl. Physiol.: Respirat. Environ. Exercise Physiol.* 45: 880–884, 1978.
173. GOLDBERG, H. S. Pulmonary interstitial compliance and microvascular filtration coefficient. *Am. J. Physiol.* 239 (*Heart Circ. Physiol.* 8): H189–H198, 1980.
174. GOLDBERG, H. S., W. MITZNER, AND G. BATRA. Effect of transpulmonary and vascular pressures on rate of pulmonary edema formation. *J. Appl. Physiol.: Respirat. Environ. Exercise Physiol.* 43: 14–19, 1977.
175. GORIN, A. B., AND P. A. STEWART. Differential permeability of endothelial and epithelial barriers to albumin flux. *J. Appl. Physiol.: Respirat. Environ. Exercise Physiol.* 47: 1315–1324, 1979.
176. GORIN, A. B., W. J. WEIDNER, R. H. DEMLING, AND N. C. STAUB. Noninvasive measurement of pulmonary transvascular protein flux in sheep. *J. Appl. Physiol.: Respirat. Environ. Exercise Physiol.* 45: 225–233, 1978.
177. GOSHY, M., S. J. LAI-FOOK, AND R. E. HYATT. Perivascular pressure measurements by wick-catheter technique in isolated dog lobes. *J. Appl. Physiol.: Respirat. Environ. Exercise Physiol.* 46: 950–955, 1979.
178. GRANGER, D. N., R. E. PARKER, E. W. QUILLEN, R. A. BRACE, AND A. E. TAYLOR. Lymph flow transients. In: *Lymphology*, edited by P. Malek, V. Bartos, H. Weissleder, and M. H. Witte. Stuttgart: Thieme, 1979, p. 61–64.
179. GRANGER, D. N., G. RUTILI, AND J. M. MCCORD. Superoxide radicals in feline intestinal ischemia. *Gastroenterology* 81: 22–29, 1981.
180. GRANGER, D. N., AND A. E. TAYLOR. Permeability of intestinal capillaries to endogenous macromolecules. *Am. J. Physiol.* 238 (*Heart Circ. Physiol.* 7): H457–H464, 1980.
181. GRANGER, H. J. Role of the interstitial matrix and lymphatic pump in regulation of transcapillary fluid balance. *Microvasc. Res.* 18: 209–216, 1979.
182. GRANGER, H. J. Physicochemical properties of the extracellular matrix. In: *Tissue Fluid Pressure and Composition*, edited by A. Hargens. Baltimore, MD: Williams & Wilkins, 1981, chapt. 5, p. 43–62.
183. GRANGER, H. J., AND A. P. SHEPHERD. Dynamics and control of the microcirculation. *Adv. Biomed. Eng.* 7: 1–63, 1979.
184. GRANGER, H. J., AND A. E. TAYLOR. Permeability of connective tissue linings isolated from implanted capsules. *Circ. Res.* 36: 222–228, 1975.
185. GRAUER, S., B. T. PETERSON, M. KUENZIG, R. W. HYDE, AND S. I. SCHWARTZ. Effect of lung denervation on development of pulmonary edema. *Surgery* 89: 617–621, 1981.
186. GREENE, D. G. Pulmonary edema. In: *Handbook of Physiology. Respiration*, edited by W. O. Fenn and H. Rahn. Washington, DC: Am. Physiol. Soc., 1965, sect. 3, vol. II, chapt. 70, p. 1585–1600.
187. GREENFIELD, L. J., R. P. SINGLETON, D. R. MCCAFFREE, AND J. J. COALSON. Pulmonary effects of experimental graded aspiration of hydrochloric acid. *Ann. Surg.* 170: 74–86, 1969.
188. GREGA, G. J., R. M. DAUGHERTY, JR., J. B. SCOTT, D. P. RADAWSKI, AND F. J. HADDY. Effect of pressure, flow and vasoactive agents on vascular resistance and capillary filtration in canine fetal, newborn and adult lung. *Microvasc. Res.* 3: 297–307, 1971.
189. GRIFFITH, B. P., R. G. CARROLL, R. L. HARDESTY, R. L. PEEL, AND H. S. BOROVETZ. Selected lobar injury after infusion of oleic acid. *J. Appl. Physiol.: Respirat. Environ. Exercise Physiol.* 47: 706–711, 1979.
190. GRIMBERT, F. A., J. C. PARKER, AND A. E. TAYLOR. Increased pulmonary vascular permeability following acid aspiration. *J. Appl. Physiol.: Respirat. Environ. Exercise Physiol.* 51: 335–345, 1981.
191. GUMP, F. E. Lung fluid and solute compartments. In: *Lung Biology in Health and Disease. Lung Water and Solute Exchange*, edited by N. C. Staub. New York: Dekker, 1978, vol. 7, chapt. 4, p. 75–98.
192. GUYTON, A. C. A concept of negative interstitial pressure based on pressures in implanted perforated capsules. *Circ. Res.* 12: 399–414, 1963.
193. GUYTON, A. C. Interstitial fluid pressure. II. Pressure-volume curves of interstitial space. *Circ. Res.* 16: 452–460, 1965.
194. GUYTON, A. C., B. J. BARBER, AND D. S. MOFFATT. Theory of interstitial pressures. In: *Tissue Fluid Pressure and Composition*, edited by A. Hargens. Baltimore, MD: Williams & Wilkins, 1981, chapt. 2, p. 11–20.
195. GUYTON, A. C., H. J. GRANGER, AND A. E. TAYLOR. Interstitial fluid pressure. *Physiol. Rev.* 51: 527–563, 1971.
196. GUYTON, A. C., AND A. E. LINDSEY. Effect of elevated left atrial pressure and decreased plasma protein concentration on the development of pulmonary edema. *Circ. Res.* 7: 649–657, 1959.
197. GUYTON, A. C., K. SCHEEL, AND D. MURPHREE. Interstitial fluid pressure. III. Its effect on resistance to tissue fluid mobility. *Circ. Res.* 19: 412–419, 1966.
198. GUYTON, A. C., A. E. TAYLOR, AND R. A. BRACE. A synthesis of interstitial fluid regulation and lymph flow. *Federation Proc.* 35: 1881–1885, 1976.
199. GUYTON, A. C., A. E. TAYLOR, R. E. DRAKE, AND J. C. PARKER. Dynamics of subatmospheric pressure in the pulmonary interstitial fluid. In: *Lung Liquids*. Amsterdam: Excerpta Med., 1976, p. 77–100. (Ciba Found. Symp. 38.)
200. GUYTON, A. C., A. E. TAYLOR, AND H. J. GRANGER. Analysis of types of pressure in the pulmonary spaces: interstitial fluid pressure, solid tissue pressure, and total tissue pressure. In: *Central Hemodynamics and Gas Exchange*, edited by C. Guinini. Basel: Karger, 1971, p. 41–55.
201. GUYTON, A. C., A. E. TAYLOR, AND H. J. GRANGER. *Circulatory Physiology. Dynamics and Control of the Body Fluids*. Philadelphia, PA: Saunders, 1975, vol. II, p. 149–193.
202. HACKETT, P. H., C. E. CREAGH, R. F. GROVER, B. HONIGMAN, C. S. HOUSTON, J. T. REEVES, A. M. SOPHOCLES, AND M. VAN HARDENBROEK. High-altitude pulmonary edema in persons without the right pulmonary artery. *N. Engl. J. Med.* 302: 1070–1073, 1980.
203. HAKIM, T. S., C. A. DAWSON, AND J. H. LINEHAN. Hemodynamic responses of dog lung lobe to lobar venous occlusion. *J. Appl. Physiol.: Respirat. Environ. Exercise Physiol.* 47: 145–152, 1979.
204. HAKIM, T. S., R. P. MICHEL, AND H. K. CHANG. Partitioning of pulmonary vascular resistance in dogs by arterial and venous occlusion. *J. Appl. Physiol.: Respirat. Environ. Exercise Physiol.* 52: 710–715, 1982.
205. HAKIM, T. S., F. L. MINNEAR, H. VAN DER ZEE, P. S. BARIE, AND A. B. MALIK. Adrenoceptor control of lung fluid and protein exchange. *J. Appl. Physiol.: Respirat. Environ. Exercise Physiol.* 51: 68–72, 1981.
206. HAKIM, T. S., H. VAN DER ZEE, AND A. B. MALIK. Effects of sympathetic nerve stimulation on lung fluid and protein exchange. *J. Appl. Physiol.: Respirat. Environ. Exercise Physiol.* 47: 1025–1030, 1979.
207. HALES, C. A., D. J. KANAREK, B. AHLUWALIA, A. LATTY, J. ERDMANN, S. JAVAHERI, AND H. KAZEMI. Regional edema formation in isolated perfused dog lungs. *Circ. Res.* 48: 121–127, 1981.
208. HALES, C. A., L. SONNE, M. PETERSON, D. KONG, M. MILLER, AND W. D. WATKINS. Role of thromboxane and prostacyclin in pulmonary vasomotor changes after endotoxin in dogs. *J. Clin. Invest.* 68: 497–505, 1981.
209. HAMMEL, H. T., AND P. F. SCHOLANDER. *Osmosis and Tensile*

Solvent. New York: Springer-Verlag, 1976.
210. HAMMERSCHMIDT, D. E. Of lungs and leukocytes. *JAMA* 244: 2199-2200, 1980.
211. HANCE, A. I., AND R. G. CRYSTAL. The connective tissue of lung. *Am. Rev. Respir. Dis.* 112: 657-720, 1975.
212. HARGENS, A. R. Interstitial osmotic pressures associated with Donnan equilibria. In: *Tissue Fluid Pressure and Composition*, edited by A. R. Hargens. Baltimore, MD: Williams & Wilkins, 1981, chapt. 8, p. 77-86.
213. HARRIS, T. R., AND K. L. BRIGHAM. The exchange of small molecules as a measure of normal and abnormal lung microvascular function. *Ann. NY Acad. Sci.* 384: 417-434, 1982.
214. HARRIS, T. R., AND R. J. ROSELLI. A theoretical model of protein, fluid, and small molecule transport in the lung. *J. Appl. Physiol.: Respirat. Environ. Exercise Physiol.* 50: 1-14, 1981.
215. HARRISON, L. H., J. J. BELLER, L. B. HINSHAW, J. J. COALSON, AND L. J. GREENFIELD. Effects of endotoxin on pulmonary capillary permeability, ultrastructure and surfactant. *Surg. Gynecol. Obstet.* 129: 723-733, 1969.
216. HAUGE, A., P. K. M. LUNDE, AND B. A. WAALER. Bradykinin and pulmonary vascular permeability in isolated blood perfused rabbit lungs. In: *Hypotensive Peptides*, edited by E. G. Erdos, N. Bach, F. Sicuters, and A. F. Wilde. New York: Springer, 1966, p. 385-395.
217. HAUGE, A., AND G. NICOLAYSEN. Studies on transvascular fluid balance and capillary permeability in isolated lungs. *Bull. Physio-Pathol. Respir.* 7: 1197-1216, 1971.
218. HAYATDAVOUDI, G., J. J. O'NEIL, B. E. BARRY, B. A. FREEMAN, AND J. D. CRAPO. Pulmonary injury in rats following continuous exposure to 60% O_2 for 7 days. *J. Appl. Physiol.: Respirat. Environ. Exercise Physiol.* 51: 1220-1231, 1981.
219. HEFLIN, C., AND K. L. BRIGHAM. Prevention by granulocyte depletion of increased vascular permeability of sheep lung following endotoxemia. *J. Clin. Invest.* 68: 1253-1260, 1981.
220. HELLEMS, H. K., F. W. HAYNES, L. DEXTER, AND T. D. KINNEY. Pulmonary capillary pressure in animals estimated by venous and arterial catherization. *Am. J. Physiol.* 155: 98-105, 1948.
221. HENSON, P. M., K. MCCARTHY, G. L. LARSEN, R. O. WEBSTER, P. C. GICLAS, R. B. DREISIN, T. E. KING, AND J. O. SHAW. Complement fragments, alveolar macrophages, and alveolitis. *Am. J. Pathol.* 97: 93-110, 1979.
222. HIDA, W., H. INOUE, AND J. HILDEBRANDT. Lobe weight gain and vascular, alveolar, and peribronchial interstitial fluid pressures. *J. Appl. Physiol.: Respirat. Environ. Exercise Physiol.* 52: 173-183, 1982.
223. HILL, S. L., V. B. ELINGS, AND F. R. LEWIS. Changes in lung water and capillary permeability following sepsis and fluid overload. *J. Surg. Res.* 28: 140-150, 1980.
224. HOGG, J. C. Effect of pulmonary edema on distribution of blood flow in the lung. In: *Lung Biology in Health and Disease. Lung Water and Solute Exchange*, edited by N. C. Staub. New York: Dekker, 1978, vol. 7, chapt. 7, p. 167-182.
225. HOGG, J. C., AND S. NEPSZY. Regional lung volume and pleural pressure gradient estimated from lung density in dogs. *J. Appl. Physiol.* 27: 198-203, 1969.
226. HOLLOWAY, H., M. PERRY, J. DOWNEY, J. PARKER, AND A. TAYLOR. Estimation of effective pulmonary capillary pressure in intact lungs. *J. Appl. Physiol.: Respirat. Environ. Exercise Physiol.* 54: 846-851, 1983.
227. HOPEWELL, P. C., AND J. F. MURRAY. Effects of continuous positive-pressure ventilation in experimental pulmonary edema. *J. Appl. Physiol.: Respirat. Environ. Exercise Physiol.* 40: 568-574, 1976.
228. HOROVITZ, J. H., AND C. J. CARRICO. Lung colloid permeability in hemorrhagic shock. *Surg. Forum* 23: 6-8, 1972.
229. HORWITZ, A. L., AND R. G. CRYSTAL. Content and synthesis of glycosaminoglycans in the developing lung. *J. Clin. Invest.* 56: 1312-1318, 1975.
230. HOVIG, T., A. NICOLAYSEN, AND G. NICOLAYSEN. Ultrastructural studies of the alveolar-capillary barrier in isolated plasma-perfused rabbit lung. Effects of EDTA and increased pressure. *Acta Physiol. Scand.* 82: 417-432, 1971.
231. HOWELL, J. B. L., S. PERMUTT, D. F. PROCTOR, AND R. L. RILEY. Effect of inflation of the lung on different parts of pulmonary vascular bed. *J. Appl. Physiol.* 16: 71-76, 1961.
232. HUGHES, J. M. B. Pulmonary interstitial pressure. *Bull. Physio-Pathol. Respir.* 7: 1095-1123, 1971.
233. HUGHES, J. M. B. Pulmonary circulation and fluid balance. In: *Respiratory Physiology II*, edited by J. G. Widdicombe. Baltimore, MD: University Park, 1977, vol. 14, p. 135-184. (Int. Rev. Physiol. Ser.)
234. HUGHES, J. M. B., J. B. GLAZIER, J. E. MALONEY, AND J. B. WEST. Effect of extra-alveolar vessels on distribution of blood flow in the dog lung. *J. Appl. Physiol.* 25: 701-712, 1968.
235. HULTGREN, H. N. Furosemide for high altitude pulmonary edema. *JAMA* 234: 589-590, 1975.
236. HULTGREN, H. N., R. F. GROVER, AND L. H. HARTLEY. Abnormal circulatory responses to high altitude in subjects with a previous history of high-altitude pulmonary edema. *Circulation* 44: 759-770, 1971.
237. HULTGREN, H. N., AND E. A. MARTICORENA. High altitude pulmonary edema. Epidemiologic observations in Peru. *Chest* 74: 372-376, 1978.
238. HURLEY, J. V. Current views on the mechanisms of pulmonary oedema. *J. Pathol.* 125: 59-79, 1978.
239. HYMAN, A. L., AND P. J. KADOWITZ. Effects of alveolar and perfusion hypoxia and hypercapnia on pulmonary vascular resistance in the lamb. *Am. J. Physiol.* 228: 397-403, 1975.
240. ILIFF, L. D. Extra-alveolar vessels and edema development in excised dog lungs. *Circ. Res.* 28: 524-532, 1971.
241. ILIFF, L. D., R. E. GREENE, AND J. M. B. HUGHES. Effect of interstitial edema on distribution of ventilation and perfusion in isolated lung. *J. Appl. Physiol.* 33: 462-467, 1972.
242. INOUE, H., C. INOUE, AND J. HILDEBRANDT. Interstitial fluid pressure (Px(f)) gradients along bronchi in excised dog lobes (Abstract). *Federation Proc.* 38: 1265, 1979.
243. INOUE, H., C. INOUE, AND J. HILDEBRANDT. Vascular and airway pressures, and interstitial edema, affect peribronchial fluid pressure. *J. Appl. Physiol.: Respirat. Environ. Exercise Physiol.* 48: 177-185, 1980.
244. INOUE, S., R. P. MICHEL, AND J. C. HOGG. Zonulae occludentes in alveolar epithelium and capillary endothelium of dog lungs studied with the freeze-fracture technique. *J. Ultrastruct. Res.* 56: 215-225, 1976.
245. JOHNSON, A., AND A. B. MALIK. Effects of different-size microemboli on lung fluid and protein exchange. *J. Appl. Physiol.: Respirat. Environ. Exercise Physiol.* 51: 461-464, 1981.
246. JOHNSON, A., AND A. B. MALIK. Pulmonary edema after glass bead microembolization: protective effect of granulocytopenia. *J. Appl. Physiol.: Respirat. Environ. Exercise Physiol.* 52: 155-161, 1982.
247. JOHNSON, A., AND A. B. MALIK. Effect of defibrinogenation on lung fluid and protein exchange after glass bead embolization. *J. Appl. Physiol.: Respirat. Environ. Exercise Physiol.* 53: 895-900, 1982.
248. JOHNSON, A., M. V. TAHAMONT, J. E. KAPLAN, AND A. B. MALIK. Lung fluid balance after pulmonary embolization: effects of thrombin vs. fibrin aggregates. *J. Appl. Physiol.: Respirat. Environ. Exercise Physiol.* 52: 1565-1570, 1982.
249. JOHNSON, J. A. Capillary permeability, extracellular space estimation, and lymph flow. *Am. J. Physiol.* 211: 1261-1263, 1966.
250. JOHNSON, K. J., J. C. FANTONE III, J. KAPLAN, AND P. A. WARD. In vivo damage of rat lungs by oxygen metabolites. *J. Clin. Invest.* 67: 983-993, 1981.
251. JONES, J. G., M. BERRY, G. H. HULANDS, J. C. W. CRAWLEY. The time course and degree of change in alveolar capillary membrane permeability induced by aspiration of hydrochloric acid and hypotonic saline. *Am. Rev. Respir. Dis.* 118: 1007-

1013, 1978.
252. JONES, J. G., R. F. GROSSMAN, M. BERRY, G. SLAVIN, G. H. HULANDS, AND B. MINTY. Alveolar-capillary membrane permeability. *Am. Rev. Respir. Dis.* 120: 399–410, 1979.
253. JONES, J. G., P. LAWLER, J. C. W. LAWLER, B. D. MINTY, G. HULANDS, AND N. VEALL. Increased alveolar epithelial permeability in cigarette smokers. *Lancet* 1: 66–67, 1980.
254. JONES, T. A., M. I. TOWNSLEY, AND W. J. WEIDNER. Effects of intracranial and left atrial hypertension on lung fluid balance in sheep. *J. Appl. Physiol.: Respirat. Environ. Exercise Physiol.* 52: 1324–1329, 1982.
255. KADOWITZ, P. J., C. A. GRUETTER, E. W. SPANNHAKE, AND A. L. HYMAN. Pulmonary vascular responses to prostaglandins. *Federation Proc.* 40: 1991–1996, 1981.
256. KAPLAN, H. P., F. R. ROBINSON, Y. KAPANCI, AND E. R. WEIBEL. Pathogenesis and reversibility of the pulmonary lesions of oxygen toxicity in monkeys. *Lab. Invest.* 20: 44–100, 1969.
257. KARNOVSKY, M. J. The ultrastructural basis of transcapillary exchange. *J. Gen. Physiol.* 52: 641–696, 1968.
258. KATCHALSKY, A., AND P. F. CURRAN. *Nonequilibrium Thermodynamics in Biophysics.* Cambridge, MA: Harvard Univ. Press, 1965, chapt. 10, p. 113–132.
259. KATO, M., AND N. C. STAUB. Response of small pulmonary arteries to unilobar hypoxia and hypercapnia. *Circ. Res.* 19: 426–440, 1966.
260. KATZ, S., A. ABERMAN, U. FRAND, I. M. STEIN, AND M. FULOP. Heroin pulmonary edema. Evidence for increased pulmonary capillary permeability. *Am. Rev. Respir. Dis.* 106: 472–474, 1972.
261. KEDEM, O., AND A. KATCHALSKY. Thermodynamic analysis of the permeability of biological membranes to non-electrolytes. *Biochim. Biophys. Acta* 27: 229–246, 1958.
262. KERN, D. F. *Pulmonary Capillary Permeabilities and Reflection Coefficients.* Minneapolis: Univ. of Minnesota, 1981. Thesis.
263. KIM, K. J., A. M. CRITZ, AND E. E. CRANDALL. Transport of water and solutes across sheep visceral pleura. *Am. Rev. Respir. Dis.* 120: 883–892, 1979.
264. KIMURA, T., J. K. TOUNG, S. MARGOLIS, S. PERMUTT, AND J. L. CAMERON. Respiratory failure in acute pancreatitis: a possible role for triglycerides. *Ann. Surg.* 189: 509–514, 1979.
265. KINNEBREW, P. S., J. C. PARKER, H. J. FALGOUT, AND A. E. TAYLOR. Pulmonary microvascular permeability following *E. coli* endotoxin and hemorrhage. *J. Appl. Physiol.: Respirat. Environ. Exercise Physiol.* 52: 403–409, 1982.
266. KISTLER, G. S., P. R. B. CALDWELL, AND E. R. WEIBEL. Development of fine structural damage to alveolar and capillary lining cells in oxygen-poisoned rat lungs. *J. Cell Biol.* 32: 305–328, 1967.
267. KLEINER, J. P., AND W. P. NELSON. High altitude pulmonary edema—a rare disease? *JAMA* 234: 491–495, 1975.
268. KOHLER, J. P., C. L. RICE, G. S. MOSS, AND J. P. SZIDON. Alveolar pressure in fluid filled occluded lung segments (Abstract). *Federation Proc.* 40: 448, 1981.
269. KOPANIAK, M. M., A. C. ISSEKUTZ, AND H. Z. MOVAT. Kinetics of acute inflammation induced by *E. coli* in rabbits. *Am. J. Pathol.* 98: 485–498, 1980.
270. KRAHL, V. E. Anatomy of the mammalian lung. In: *Handbook of Physiology. Respiration,* edited by W. O. Fenn and H. Rahn. Washington, DC: Am. Physiol. Soc., 1964, sect. 3, vol. I, chapt. 6, p. 213–284.
271. KRAMER, G., B. A. HARMS, R. A. GUNTHER, E. M. RENKIN, AND R. H. DEMLING. The effects of hypoproteinemia on blood-to-lymph fluid transport in sheep lung. *Circ. Res.* 49: 1173–1180, 1981.
272. KRUS, S., B. MAMINSK, AND J. NIELUBOWICZ. Studies on acute lung lymphatic edema. *Pol. Med. Sci. Hist. Bull.* 18: 139–147, 1975.
273. KURAMOTO, K., AND S. RODBARD. Effects of blood flow and left atrial pressure on pulmonary venous resistance. *Circ. Res.* 11: 240–246, 1962.
274. KWATRA, S. K., AND R. VISWANATHAN. Effect of furosemide on altitude tolerance in experimental animals. *Respiration* 37: 109–113, 1979.
275. LAHNBORG, G., S. NYLEN, AND C. SYLVEN. Induced fat embolism in rabbits: effects of defibrinogenation and thrombocytopenia. *Eur. Surg. Res.* 8: 428–434, 1976.
276. LAI-FOOK, S. J. A continuum mechanics analysis of pulmonary vascular interdependence in isolated dog lobes. *J. Appl. Physiol.: Respirat. Environ. Exercise Physiol.* 46: 419–429, 1979.
277. LAI-FOOK, S. J. Interstitial pressure in the lung. In: *Tissue Fluid Pressure and Composition,* edited by A. R. Hargens. Baltimore, MD: Williams & Wilkins, 1981, chapt. 13, p. 125–134.
278. LAI-FOOK, S. J. Perivascular interstitial fluid pressure measured by micropipettes in isolated dog lung. *J. Appl. Physiol.: Respirat. Environ. Exercise Physiol.* 52: 9–15, 1982.
279. LAI-FOOK, S. J., AND K. C. BECK. Alveolar liquid pressure measured by micropipettes in isolated dog lung. *J. Appl. Physiol.: Respirat. Environ. Exercise Physiol.* 53: 737–743, 1982.
280. LAI-FOOK, S. J., AND R. E. HYATT. Effect of parenchyma and length changes on vessel pressure-diameter behavior in pig lungs. *J. Appl. Physiol.: Respirat. Environ. Exercise Physiol.* 47: 666–669, 1979.
281. LAI-FOOK, S. J., R. E. HYATT, AND J. R. RODARTE. Effect of parenchymal shear modulus and lung volume on bronchial pressure-diameter behavior. *J. Appl. Physiol.: Respirat. Environ. Exercise Physiol.* 44: 859–868, 1978.
282. LAI-FOOK, S. J., AND M. J. KALLOK. Bronchial-arterial interdependence in isolated dog lung. *J. Appl. Physiol.: Respirat. Environ. Exercise Physiol.* 52: 1000–1007, 1982.
283. LAI-FOOK, S. J., AND B. TOPOROFF. Pressure-volume behavior of perivascular interstitium measured in isolated dog lung. *J. Appl. Physiol.: Respirat. Environ. Exercise Physiol.* 48: 939–946, 1980.
284. LANDIS, E. M. Capillary pressure and capillary permeability. *Physiol. Rev.* 14: 404–481, 1934.
285. LANDIS, E. M., AND J. R. PAPPENHEIMER. Exchange of substances through the capillary walls. In: *Handbook of Physiology. Circulation,* edited by W. F. Hamilton. Washington, DC: Am. Physiol. Soc., 1963, sect. 2, vol. II, chapt. 29, p. 961–1034.
286. LATTA, H. Pulmonary edema and pleural effusion produced by acute α-naphthylthiourea poisoning in rats and dogs. *Bull. Johns Hopkins Hosp.* 80: 181–197, 1947.
287. LAURENT, T. C. The interaction between polysaccharides and other macromolecules. IX. The exclusion from hyaluronic acid gels and solutions. *Biochem. J.* 93: 106–112, 1964.
288. LAUWERYNS, J. M. The juxta-alveolar lymphatics in the human adult lung. *Am. Rev. Respir. Dis.* 102: 877–885, 1970.
289. LAUWERYNS, J. M., AND J. H. BAERT. Alveolar clearance and the role of the pulmonary lymphatics. *Am. Rev. Respir. Dis.* 115: 625–683, 1977.
290. LEE, B. C., A. B. MALIK, P. S. BARIE, AND F. L. MINNEAR. Affect of acute pancreatitis on pulmonary transvascular fluid and protein exchange. *Am. Rev. Respir. Dis.* 123: 618–621, 1981.
291. LEVINE, O. R., R. B. DELL, E. BONE, AND A. HYMAN. Pulmonary extravascular chloride space and albumin content in adult dogs and puppies. *Pediatr. Res.* 8: 270–274, 1974.
292. LEVINE, O. R., AND R. B. MELLINS. Effect of gravity on interstitial pressure of the lung in intact dogs. *J. Appl. Physiol.* 33: 357–361, 1972.
293. LEVINE, O. R., R. B. MELLINS, R. M. SENIOR, AND A. P. FISHMAN. The application of Starling's law of capillary exchange to the lungs. *J. Clin. Invest.* 46: 934–944, 1967.
294. LEVINE, O. R., F. RODRIGUEZ-MARTINEZ, AND R. B. MELLINS. Fluid filtration in the lung of the intact puppy. *J. Appl. Physiol.* 34: 683–686, 1973.
295. LINEHAN, J. H., C. A. DAWSON, AND D. A. RICKABY. Distribution of vascular resistance and compliance in a dog lung lobe. *J. Appl. Physiol.: Respirat. Environ. Exercise Physiol.* 53:

158–168, 1982.
296. LLOYD, T. C., JR. Effect of alveolar hypoxia on pulmonary vascular resistance. *J. Appl. Physiol.* 19: 1086–1094, 1964.
297. LOPEZ-MUNIZ, R., N. L. STEPHENS, B. BROMBERGER-BARNEA, S. PERMUTT, AND R. L. RILEY. Critical closure of pulmonary vessels analyzed in terms of Starling resistor model. *J. Appl. Physiol.* 24: 625–635, 1968.
298. LOW, F. N. Lung interstitium: development, morphology, fluid content. In: *Lung Biology in Health and Disease. Lung Water and Solute Exchange*, edited by N. C. Staub. New York: Dekker, 1978, vol. 7, chapt. 2, p. 17–48.
299. LUISADA, A. A. Mechanism of neurogenic pulmonary edema. *Am. J. Cardiol.* 20: 66–68, 1967.
300. LUNDE, P. K. M., AND B. A. WAALER. Transvascular fluid balance in the lung. *J. Physiol. London* 205: 1–18, 1969.
301. LUTERMAN, A., D. MANWARING, AND P. W. CURRERI. The role of fibrinogen degradation products in the pathogenesis of the respiratory distress syndrome. *Surgery* 82: 703–707, 1977.
302. MACHADO, D. C., G. M. BOHM, AND P. A. PADOVAN. Comparative study of the ultrastructural alterations in the pulmonary vessels of rats treated with alpha-naphthylthiourea (ANTU) and ammonium sulfate. *J. Pathol.* 121: 205–211, 1977.
303. MACHIEDO, G. W., C. S. BROWN, J. E. LAVIGNE, AND B. F. RUSH, JR. Beneficial effect of prostaglandin E$_1$ in experimental hemorrhagic shock. *Surg. Gynecol. Obstet.* 143: 433–436, 1976.
304. MAGNO, M., B. ATKINSON, A. KATZ, AND A. P. FISHMAN. Estimation of pulmonary interstitial fluid space compliance in isolated perfused rabbit lung. *J. Appl. Physiol.: Respirat. Environ. Exercise Physiol.* 48: 677–683, 1980.
305. MAGNO, M., AND J. P. SZIDON. Hemodynamic pulmonary edema in dogs with acute and chronic lymphatic ligation. *Am. J. Physiol.* 231: 1777–1782, 1976.
306. MAHAJAN, V. K., M. SIMON, AND G. L. HUBER. Re-expansion pulmonary edema. *Chest* 75: 192–194, 1979.
307. MAJNO, G., V. GILMORE, AND M. LEVENTHAL. On the mechanism of vascular leakage caused by histamine-type medications. *Circ. Res.* 21: 833–847, 1967.
308. MAJNO, G., S. M. SHEA, AND M. LEVENTHAL. Endothelial contraction induced by histamine-type mediators. An electron microscopy study. *J. Cell Biol.* 42: 647–672, 1969.
309. MALIK, A. B. Pulmonary vascular response to increase in intracranial pressure: role of sympathetic mechanisms. *J. Appl. Physiol.: Respirat. Environ. Exercise Physiol.* 42: 335–343, 1977.
310. MALIK, A. B., AND B. S. L. KIDD. Pulmonary arterial wedge and left atrial pressures and the site of hypoxic pulmonary vasoconstriction. *Respiration* 33: 123–132, 1976.
311. MALIK, A. B., B. C. LEE, H. VAN DER ZEE, AND A. JOHNSON. The role of fibrin in the genesis of pulmonary edema after embolization in dogs. *Circ. Res.* 45: 120–125, 1979.
312. MALIK, A. B., AND N. C. STAUB (editors). *Ann. NY Acad. Sci.* 384: 1–561, 1982.
313. MALIK, A. B., AND H. VAN DER ZEE. Mechanism of pulmonary edema induced by microembolization in dogs. *Circ. Res.* 42: 72–79, 1976.
314. MALIK, A. B., AND H. VAN DER ZEE. Time course of pulmonary vascular response to microembolization. *J. Appl. Physiol.: Respirat. Environ. Exercise Physiol.* 43: 51–58, 1977.
315. MALIK, A. B., AND H. VAN DER ZEE. Lung vascular permeability following progressive pulmonary embolization. *J. Appl. Physiol.: Respirat. Environ. Exercise Physiol.* 45: 590–597, 1978.
316. MALIK, A. B., H. VAN DER ZEE, AND B. C. LEE. Pulmonary transvascular fluid dynamics in sheep during hemorrhage. *Lymphology* 12: 149–157, 1979.
317. MANOHAR, M. What causes the microvascular permeability change in high altitude pulmonary edema? (Letter to the editor). *Circ. Res.* 44: 873–874, 1979.
318. MANWARING, D., D. THORNING, AND P. W. CURRERI. Mechanisms of acute pulmonary dysfunction induced by fibrinogen degradation product D. *Surgery* 84: 45–54, 1978.
319. MARON, M. B. Differential effects of histamine on protein permeability in dog lung and forelimb. *Am. J. Physiol.* 242 (*Heart Circ. Physiol.* 11): H565–H572, 1982.
320. MARON, M. B. Modification of lymph during passage through the lymph node: effect of histamine. *Am. J. Physiol.* 245 (*Heart Circ. Physiol.* 14): H553–H559, 1983.
321. MARTIN, B. A., R. DAHLBY, I. NICHOLLS, AND J. C. HOGG. Platelet sequestration in lung with hemorrhagic shock and reinfusion in dogs. *J. Appl. Physiol.: Respirat. Environ. Exercise Physiol.* 50: 1306–1312, 1981.
322. MARTIN, D. Mesure des variations de la filtration capillaire pulmonaire au cours de l'hypoxie par l'analyse de la lymphe intrathoracique. Grenoble, France: L'Univ. Scientifique et Medicale de Grenoble, 1981. Dissertation.
323. MARTIN, D. J., J. C. PARKER, AND A. E. TAYLOR. Simultaneous comparison of tracheobronchial and right duct lymph dynamics in dogs. *J. Appl. Physiol.: Respirat. Environ. Exercise Physiol.* 54: 199–207, 1983.
324. MATALON, S. V., AND O. D. WANGENSTEEN. Pulmonary capillary filtration and reflection coefficients in the newborn rabbit. *Microvasc. Res.* 14: 99–110, 1977.
325. MATTHAY, M. A., C. C. LANDOLT, AND N. C. STAUB. Differential liquid and protein clearance from the alveoli of anesthetized sheep. *J. Appl. Physiol.: Respirat. Environ. Exercise Physiol.* 53: 96–104, 1982.
326. MCCAFFREE, D. R., B. A. GRAY, B. E. PENNOCK, J. COALSON, C. BRIDGES, F. B. TAYLOR, AND R. M. ROGERS. Role of pulmonary edema in the acute pulmonary response to sepsis. *J. Appl. Physiol.: Respirat. Environ. Exercise Physiol.* 50: 1198–1205, 1981.
327. MCCORD, J. M. Free radicals and inflammation: protection of synovial fluid by superoxide dismutase. *Science* 185: 529, 1978.
328. MCCORD, J. M., AND I. FRIDOVICH. The biology and pathology of oxygen radicals. *Ann. Intern. Med.* 89: 122–127, 1978.
329. MCINTIRE, L. V., T. S. DEWITZ, AND P. R. MARTIN. Effect of antiplatelet drug dipyridamole (RAF) on leukocyte response to mechanical trauma. *Trans. Am. Soc. Artif. Intern. Organs* 24: 310–374, 1978.
330. MCINTOSH, M., AND A. SILBERGLEIT. Intravascular platelet neutrophil aggregation in staging of post-traumatic pulmonary insufficiency. *Surg. Forum* 27: 176–177, 1976.
331. MCKEEN, C. R., K. L. BRIGHAM, R. E. BOWERS, AND T. R. HARRIS. Pulmonary vascular effects of fat emulsion infusion in unanesthetized sheep. Prevention by indomethacin. *J. Clin. Invest.* 61: 1291–1297, 1978.
332. MCNAMEE, J. E. Restricted dextran transport in the sheep lung lymph preparation. *J. Appl. Physiol.: Respirat. Environ. Exercise Physiol.* 52: 585–590, 1982.
333. MCNAMEE, J. E., AND N. C. STAUB. Pore models of sheep lung microvascular barrier using new data on protein tracers. *Microvasc. Res.* 18: 229–244, 1979.
334. MEAD, J., T. TAKISHIMA, AND D. LEITH. Stress distribution in lungs: a model of pulmonary elasticity. *J. Appl. Physiol.* 28: 596–608, 1970.
335. MELLINS, R. B., O. R. LEVINE, R. SKALAK, AND A. P. FISHMAN. Interstitial pressure of the lung. *Circ. Res.* 24: 197–212, 1969.
336. MENKES, H., D. LINDSAY, L. WOOD, A. MUIR, AND P. T. MACKLEM. Interdependence of lung units in intact dog lungs. *J. Appl. Physiol.* 32: 681–686, 1972.
337. MENON, N. D. High altitude pulmonary edema: a clinical study. *J. Med.* 273: 66–73, 1965.
338. MEYER, B. J., A. MEYER, AND A. C. GUYTON. Interstitial fluid pressure. V. Negative pressure in the lung. *Circ. Res.* 22: 263–271, 1968.
339. MEYER, E. C., AND R. OTTAVIANO. Right duct distribution volume in dogs. Relationship to pulmonary interstitial volume. *Circ. Res.* 35: 197–203, 1974.
340. MEYER, E. C., AND R. OTTAVIANO. Fibrinogen clearance from pulmonary interstitium. *Lymphology* 12: 208–216, 1979.

341. MEYER, E. C., AND A. SILBERBERG. In vitro study of the influence of some factors important for any physicochemical characterization of connective tissue in the microcirculation. *Microvasc. Res.* 8: 263–273, 1974.
342. MEYRICK, B., J. MILLER, AND L. REID. Pulmonary oedema induced by ANTU, or by high or low oxygen concentration in rat—an electron microscopic study. *Br. J. Exp. Pathol.* 53: 347–358, 1972.
343. MICHEL, R. P., S. INOUE, AND J. C. HOGG. Pulmonary capillary permeability to HRP in dogs: a physiological and morphological study. *J. Appl. Physiol.: Respirat. Environ. Exercise Physiol.* 42: 13–21, 1977.
344. MICHEL, R. P., M. LAFORTE, AND J. C. HOGG. Physiology and morphology of pulmonary microvascular injury with shock and reinfusion. *J. Appl. Physiol.: Respirat. Environ. Exercise Physiol.* 50: 1227–1235, 1981.
345. MILLEN, J. E., F. L. GLAUSER, D. SMELTZER, P. EGAN, K. PROPST, P. FISCHER, L. DEARDEN, AND P. OTIS. The role of leukocytes in ethchlorvynol-induced pulmonary edema. *Chest* 73: 75–78, 1978.
346. MINNEAR, F. L., P. S. BARIE, AND A. B. MALIK. Effects of epinephrine and norepinephrine infusion on lung fluid balance in sheep. *J. Appl. Physiol.: Respirat. Environ. Exercise Physiol.* 50: 1353–1357, 1981.
347. MINNEAR, F. L., P. S. BARIE, AND A. B. MALIK. Lung fluid and protein exchange in the acute sheep preparation. *J. Appl. Physiol.: Respirat. Environ. Exercise Physiol.* 50: 1358–1361, 1981.
348. MITZNER, W., AND J. L. ROBOTHAM. Distribution of interstitial compliance and filtration coefficient in canine lung. *Lymphology* 12: 140–148, 1979.
349. MOLSTAD, L. S., AND A. E. TAYLOR. Effects of hydrostatic height on pulmonary lymph protein concentration (Abstract). *Microvasc. Res.* 11: 124, 1976.
350. MORRISS, A. W., R. E. DRAKE, AND J. C. GABEL. Comparison of microvascular filtration characteristics in isolated and intact lungs. *J. Appl. Physiol.: Respirat. Environ. Exercise Physiol.* 48: 438–443, 1980.
351. MUIR, A. L., D. L. HALL, P. DESPAS, AND J. C. HOGG. Distribution of blood flow in the lungs in acute pulmonary edema in dogs. *J. Appl. Physiol.* 33: 763–769, 1972.
352. NAIMARK, A., B. W. KIRK, AND W. CHERNECKI. Regional water volume, blood volume, and perfusion in the lung. In: *Central Hemodynamics and Gas Exchange*, edited by G. Giantini. Torino, Italy: Minerva Med., 1971, p. 144–160.
353. NAKAHARA, K., K. KIMURA, M. MAEDA, A. MASAOKA, AND H. MANABE. Quantitative assessment of pulmonary edema induced by ligation of lymphatics in dogs. *Med. J. Osaka Univ.* 23: 199–214, 1973.
354. NAVAR, P. D., AND L. G. NAVAR. Relationship between colloid osmotic pressure and plasma protein concentration in the dog. *Am. J. Physiol.* 233 (*Heart Circ. Physiol.* 2): H295–H298, 1977.
355. NEUFELD, G. R., J. J. WILLIAMS, D. J. GRAVES, L. R. SOMA, AND B. E. MARSHALL. Pulmonary capillary permeability in man and a canine model of chemical pulmonary edema. *Microvasc. Res.* 10: 192–207, 1975.
356. NICOLAYSEN, G. Intravascular concentrations of calcium and magnesium ions and edema formation in isolated lungs. *Acta Physiol. Scand.* 81: 325–339, 1971.
357. NICOLAYSEN, G. Increase in capillary filtration rate resulting from reduction in the intravascular calcium ion-concentration. *Acta Physiol. Scand.* 81: 517–527, 1971.
358. NICOLAYSEN, G., P. AARSETH, AND B. A. WAALER. Transvascular fluid filtration and intravascular volume in isolated perfused lungs (Abstract). *Acta Physiol. Scand.* 96: 25A–26A, 1976.
359. NICOLAYSEN, G., AND A. HAUGE. Fluid exchange in the isolated perfused lung. *Ann. NY Acad. Sci.* 384: 115–125, 1982.
360. NICOLAYSEN, G., A. NICOLAYSEN, AND N. STAUB. A quantitative radioautographic comparison of albumin concentration in different sized lymph vessels in normal mouse lungs. *Microvasc. Res.* 10: 138–152, 1975.
361. NICOLAYSEN, G., AND N. C. STAUB. Time course of albumin equilibration in interstitium and lymph of normal mouse lungs. *Microvasc. Res.* 9: 29–37, 1975.
362. NICOLAYSEN, G., B. A. WAALER, AND P. AARSETH. On the existence of stretchable pores in the exchange vessels of the isolated rabbit lung preparation. *Lymphology* 12: 201–207, 1979.
363. NICOLL, P. A., AND A. E. TAYLOR. Lymphatics and lymph flow. *Annu. Rev. Physiol.* 39: 73–95, 1977.
364. NITTA, S., AND N. C. STAUB. Lung fluids in acute ammonium chloride toxicity and edema in cats and guinea pigs. *Am. J. Physiol.* 224: 613–617, 1973.
365. NOBLE, W. H. Early changes in lung water after haemorrhagic shock in pigs and dogs. *Can. Anaesth. Soc. J.* 22: 39–49, 1975.
366. NOBLE, W. H. Pulmonary edema: a review. *Can. Anaesth. Soc. J.* 27: 286–302, 1980.
367. NORTHRUP, W. F., AND E. W. HUMPHREY. Albumin permeability in the pulmonary capillaries. *Surg. Forum* 28: 224–226, 1978.
368. NORTHRUP, W. F., AND E. W. HUMPHREY. Effect of hemorrhagic shock on pulmonary vascular permeability to plasma proteins. *Surgery* 83: 264–273, 1978.
369. OGLETREE, M. L. Pharmacology of prostaglandins in the pulmonary microcirculation. *Ann. NY Acad. Sci.* 384: 191–206, 1982.
370. OGLETREE, M. L., AND K. L. BRIGHAM. Arachidonate raises vascular resistance but not permeability in lungs of awake sheep. *J. Appl. Physiol.: Respirat. Environ. Exercise Physiol.* 48: 581–586, 1980.
371. OGSTON, A. G. The spaces in a uniform random suspension of fibers. *Trans. Faraday Soc.* 54: 1745–1757, 1958.
372. OGSTON, A. G., B. N. PRESTON, AND J. D. WELLS. On the transport of compact particles through solutions of chain-polymers. *Proc. R. Soc. London Ser. A* 333: 297–316, 1973.
373. OPPENHEIMER, L., H. W. UNRUH, C. SKOOG, AND H. S. GOLDBERG. Transvascular fluid flux measured from intravascular water concentration changes. *J. Appl. Physiol.: Respirat. Environ. Exercise Physiol.* 54: 64–72, 1983.
374. PAIN, M. C. F., AND J. B. WEST. Effect of the volume history of the isolated lung on distribution of blood flow. *J. Appl. Physiol.* 21: 1545–1550, 1966.
375. PALADE, G. E., AND R. R. BRUNS. Structural modulations of plasmalemmal vesicles. *J. Cell Biol.* 37: 633–649, 1968.
376. PALADE, G. E., M. SIMIONESCU, AND N. SIMIONESCU. Structural aspects of the permeability of the microvascular endothelium. *Acta Physiol. Scand.* 463: 11–32, 1979.
377. PANG, L. M., R. B. MELLINS, AND F. RODRIQUEZ-MARTINEZ. Effect of acute lymphatic obstruction on fluid accumulation in the chest in dogs. *J. Appl. Physiol.* 39: 985–989, 1975.
378. PAPPENHEIMER, J. R., E. M. RENKIN, AND L. M. BORRERO. Filtration, diffusion and molecular sieving through peripheral capillary membranes. A contribution to the pore theory of capillary permeability. *Am. J. Physiol.* 167: 13–46, 1951.
379. PAPPENHEIMER, J. R., AND A. SOTO-RIVERA. Effective osmotic pressure of the plasma proteins and other quantities associated with the capillary circulation in the hindlimbs of cats and dogs. *Am. J. Physiol.* 152: 471–491, 1948.
380. PARKER, J. C., R. C. ALLISON, AND A. E. TAYLOR. Edema affects intra-alveolar fluid pressures and interdependence in dog lungs. *J. Appl. Physiol.: Respirat. Environ. Exercise Physiol.* 51: 911–921, 1981.
381. PARKER, J. C., M. CRAIN, F. GRIMBERT, G. RUTILI, AND A. E. TAYLOR. Total lung lymph flow and fluid compartmentation in edematous dog lungs. *J. Appl. Physiol.: Respirat. Environ. Exercise Physiol.* 51: 1268–1277, 1981.
382. PARKER, J. C., H. J. FALGOUT, F. A. GRIMBERT, AND A. E. TAYLOR. The effect of increased vascular pressure on albumin excluded volume and lymph flow in the dog lung. *Circ. Res.* 47: 866–875, 1980.
383. PARKER, J. C., H. J. FALGOUT, R. E. PARKER, D. N. GRANGER,

AND A. E. TAYLOR. The effect of fluid volume loading on exclusion of interstitial albumin and lymph flow in the dog lung. *Circ. Res.* 45: 440–450, 1979.

384. PARKER, J. C., A. C. GUYTON, AND A. E. TAYLOR. Pulmonary interstitial and capillary pressures estimated from intra-alveolar fluid pressures. *J. Appl. Physiol.: Respirat. Environ. Exercise Physiol.* 44: 267–276, 1978.

385. PARKER, J. C., A. C. GUYTON, AND A. E. TAYLOR. Pulmonary transcapillary exchange and pulmonary edema. In: *Cardiovascular Physiology III*, edited by A. C. Guyton and D. B. Young. Baltimore, MD: University Park, 1979, vol. 18, chapt. 7, p. 261–316. (Int. Rev. Physiol. Ser.)

385a. PARKER, J. C., P. R. KVIETYS, K. P. RYAN, AND A. E. TAYLOR. Comparison of isogravimetric and venous occlusion capillary pressures in isolated dog lungs. *J. Appl. Physiol.: Respirat. Environ. Exercise Physiol.* 55: 964–968, 1983.

386. PARKER, J. C., D. J. MARTIN, G. RUTILI, J. MCCORD, AND A. E. TAYLOR. Prevention of free radical mediated vascular permeability increases in lung using superoxide dismutase. *Chest Suppl.* 83: 52S–53S, 1983.

387. PARKER, J. C., R. E. PARKER, D. N. GRANGER, AND A. E. TAYLOR. Vertical gradient in regional vascular resistance and pre- to postcapillary resistance ratios in the dog lung. *Lymphology* 12: 191–200, 1979.

388. PARKER, J. C., R. E. PARKER, D. N. GRANGER, AND A. E. TAYLOR. Vascular permeability and transvascular fluid and protein transport in the dog lung. *Circ. Res.* 48: 549–561, 1981.

389. PARKER, J. C., AND A. E. TAYLOR. Comparison of capsular and intra-alveolar fluid pressures in the lung. *J. Appl. Physiol.: Respirat. Environ. Exercise Physiol.* 52: 1444–1452, 1982.

390. PARKER, R. E., D. N. GRANGER, AND A. E. TAYLOR. Estimates of isogravimetric capillary pressures during alveolar hypoxia. *Am. J. Physiol.* 241 (*Heart Circ. Physiol.* 10): H732–H739, 1981.

391. PARKER, R. E., R. J. ROSSELI, T. R. HARRIS, AND K. L. BRIGHAM. Effect of graded increases in pulmonary vascular pressures on lung fluid balance in unanesthetized sheep. *Circ. Res.* 49: 1164–1172, 1981.

392. PATLAK, C. S., D. A. GOLDSTEIN, AND J. F. HOFFMAN. The flow of solute and solvents across a two-membrane system. *J. Theor. Biol.* 5: 426–442, 1963.

393. PATTLE, R. E. Surface lining of lung alveoli. *Physiol. Rev.* 45: 48–79, 1965.

394. PATTLE, R. E. The relation between surface tension and area in the alveolar lining film. *J. Physiol. London* 269: 591–604, 1977.

395. PERL, W., P. CHOWDHURY, AND F. P. CHINARD. Reflection coefficients of dog lung endothelium to small hydrophilic solutes. *Am. J. Physiol.* 228: 797–809, 1975.

396. PERMUTT, S. Effect of interstitial pressure in the lung on pulmonary circulation. *Med. Thorac.* 22: 118–131, 1965.

397. PERMUTT, S. Mechanical influences on water accumulation in the lungs. In: *Pulmonary Edema*, edited by A. P. Fishman and E. M. Renkin. Bethesda, MD: Am. Physiol. Soc., 1979, chapt. 13, p. 175–193.

398. PERMUTT, S., AND P. CALDINI. Tissue pressures and fluid dynamics of the lung. *Federation Proc.* 35: 1876–1880, 1976.

399. PERMUTT, S., P. CALDINI, H. N. BANE, P. HOWARD, AND R. L. RILEY. Liquid pressure versus surface pressure of the esophagus. *J. Appl. Physiol.* 23: 927–933, 1967.

400. PERMUTT, S., J. B. L. HOWELL, D. F. PROCTER, AND R. L. RILEY. Effect of lung inflation on static pressure-volume characteristics of pulmonary vessels. *J. Appl. Physiol.* 16: 64–70, 1961.

401. PERMUTT, S., AND R. L. RILEY. Hemodynamics of collapsible vessels with tone: the vascular waterfall. *J. Appl. Physiol.* 18: 924–932, 1963.

402. PERRY, M. A. Capillary filtration and permeability coefficients calculated from measurements of interendothelial cell junctions in rabbit lung and skeletal muscle. *Microvasc. Res.* 19: 142–157, 1980.

403. PERRY, M. A., AND D. G. GARLICK. Permeability and pore radii of pulmonary capillaries in rabbits of different ages. *Clin. Exp. Pharmacol. Physiol.* 5: 361–377, 1978.

404. PIETRA, G. G., M. MAGNO, AND L. JOHNS. Morphological and physiological study of the effect of histamine on the isolated perfused rabbit lung. *Lymphology* 12: 165–176, 1979.

405. PIETRA, G. G., M. MAGNO, L. JOHNS, AND A. P. FISHMAN. Bronchial veins and pulmonary edema. In: *Pulmonary Edema*, edited by A. P. Fishman and E. M. Renkin. Bethesda, MD: Am. Physiol. Soc., 1979, chapt. 14, p. 195–206.

406. PIETRA, G. G., J. P. SZIDON, H. A. CARPENTER, AND A. P. FISHMAN. Bronchial venular leakage during endotoxin shock. *Am. J. Pathol.* 77: 387–406, 1974.

407. PIETRA, G. G., J. P. SZIDON, M. M. LEVENTHAL, AND A. P. FISHMAN. Hemoglobin as a tracer in hemodynamic pulmonary edema. *Science* 166: 1643–1646, 1969.

408. PIETRA, G. G., J. P. SZIDON, M. M. LEVENTHAL, AND A. P. FISHMAN. Histamine and interstitial pulmonary edema in the dog. *Circ. Res.* 29: 323–337, 1971.

409. PINE, M. B., P. M. BEACH, T. S. COTTRELL, M. SCOLA, AND G. M. TURINO. The relationship between right duct lymph flow and extravascular lung water in dogs given α-naphthylthiourea. *J. Clin. Invest.* 58: 482–492, 1976.

410. PINGLETON, W. W., J. J. COALSON, AND C. A. GUENTER. Significance of leukocytes in endotoxic shock. *Exp. Mol. Pathol.* 22: 183–194, 1975.

411. POWNER, D., J. V. SNYDER, AND A. GRENVIK. Altered pulmonary capillary permeability complicating recovery from diabetic ketoacidosis. *Chest* 68: 253–255, 1975.

412. PRATHER, J. W., D. N. BOWES, D. A. WARRELL, AND B. W. ZWEIFACH. Comparison of capsule and wick techniques for measurement of interstitial fluid pressure. *J. Appl. Physiol.* 31: 942–945, 1971.

413. PRATHER, J. W., K. A. GAAR, JR., AND A. C. GUYTON. Direct continuous recording of plasma colloid osmotic pressure of whole blood. *J. Appl. Physiol.* 24: 602–605, 1968.

414. PRICHARD, J. S., AND G. DE J. LEE. Measurement of water distribution and transcapillary solute flux in dog lung by external radioactivity counting. *Clin. Sci.* 57: 145–154, 1979.

415. PRICHARD, J. S., B. RAJAGOPALAN, AND G. DE J. LEE. Transvascular albumin flux and the interstitial water volume in experimental pulmonary oedema in dogs. *Clin. Sci.* 59: 105–113, 1980.

416. PROCKOP, D. J. Collagen, elastin, and proteoglycans: matrix for fluid accumulation in the lung. In: *Pulmonary Edema*, edited by A. P. Fishman and E. M. Renkin. Bethesda, MD: Am. Physiol. Soc., 1979, chapt. 9, p. 125–135.

417. PROPST, K., J. E. MILLEN, AND F. L. GLAUSER. The effects of endogenous and exogenous histamine on pulmonary alveolar membrane permeability. *Am. Rev. Respir. Dis.* 117: 1063–1068, 1978.

418. RABIN, E. R., AND E. C. MEYER. Cardiopulmonary effects of pulmonary venous hypertension with special reference to pulmonary lymphatic flow. *Circ. Res.* 8: 324–335, 1960.

419. RAFFIN, T. A., AND E. D. ROBIN. Paraquat ingestion and pulmonary injury. *West. J. Med.* 128: 26–34, 1978.

420. REESE, T. S., AND M. J. KARNOVSKY. Fine structural localization of a blood-brain barrier to exogenous peroxidase. *J. Cell Biol.* 34: 207–217, 1969.

421. REIFENRATH, R. The significance of alveolar geometry and surface tension in the respiratory mechanics of the lung. *Respir. Physiol.* 24: 115–137, 1975.

422. RENKIN, E. M. Lymph as a measure of the composition of interstitial fluid. In: *Pulmonary Edema*, edited by A. P. Fishman and E. M. Renkin. Bethesda, MD: Am. Physiol. Soc., 1979, chapt. 11, p. 145–159.

423. RENKIN, E. M., P. D. WATSON, C. H. SLOOP, W. M. JOYNER, AND F. E. CURRY. Transport pathways for fluid and large molecules in microvascular endothelium of the dog's paw. *Microvasc. Res.* 14: 205–214, 1977.

424. RENNARD, S. I., V. J. FERRANS, K. H. BRADLEY, AND R. G.

CRYSTAL. Lung connective tissue. In: *Mechanisms in Pulmonary Toxicology*, edited by H. Witschi. Cleveland, OH: CRC, 1981.
425. REPINE, J. E., J. W. EATON, M. W. ANDERS, J. R. HOIDAL, AND R. B. FOX. Generation of hydroxyl radical by enzymes, chemicals, and human phagocytes in vitro. Detection with the anti-inflammatory agent, dimethyl sulfoxide. *J. Clin. Invest.* 64: 1642–1651, 1979.
426. REPINE, J. E., J. G. WHITE, C. C. CLAWSON, AND B. M. HOLMES. Effects of phorbol myristate acetate on the metabolism and ultrastructure of neutrophils in chronic granulomatous disease. *J. Clin. Invest.* 54: 83–90, 1974.
427. RHODES, M. L., D. C. ZAVALA, AND D. BROWN. Hypoxic protection in paraquat poisoning. *Lab. Invest.* 35: 496–500, 1976.
428. RICE, C. L., C. F. HOBELMAN, D. A. JOHN, D. E. SMITH, J. D. MALLEY, B. F. CAMMACK, D. R. JAMES, R. M. PETERS, AND R. W. VIRGILIO. Central venous pressure or pulmonary capillary wedge pressure as the determinant of fluid replacement in aortic surgery. *Surgery* 84: 437–440, 1978.
429. RICHTER, C. P. The physiology and cytology of pulmonary edema and pleural effusion produced in rats by ANTU. *J. Thorac. Cardiovasc. Surg.* 23: 66–91, 1952.
429a.RIPPE, B., R. C. ALLISON, J. C. PARKER, AND A. E. TAYLOR. Effects of histamine, serotonin, and norepinephrine on circulation of dog lungs. *J. Appl. Physiol.: Respirat. Environ. Exercise Physiol.* 57: 223–232, 1984.
430. RIPPE, B., A. KAMIYA, AND B. FOLKOW. Transcapillary passage of albumin, effects of tissue cooling, and of increases in filtration and plasma colloid osmotic pressure. *Acta Physiol. Scand.* 105: 171–187, 1979.
431. ROBIN, E., L. CAREY, A. GRENVICK, F. GLAUSER, AND K. GAUDIO. Capillary leak syndrome with pulmonary edema. *Arch. Intern. Med.* 130: 66–71, 1972.
432. ROBIN, E., C. CROSS, AND R. ZELIS. Pulmonary edema. *N. Engl. J. Med.* 288: 239–304, 1973.
433. ROOS, A., L. J. THOMAS, JR., E. L. NAGEL, AND D. C. PROMMAS. Pulmonary vascular resistance as determined by lung inflation and vascular pressures. *J. Appl. Physiol.* 16: 77–84, 1961.
434. ROSENZWEIG, D. Y., J. M. B. HUGHES, AND J. B. GLAZIER. Effects of transpulmonary and vascular pressures on pulmonary blood volume in isolated lung. *J. Appl. Physiol.* 28: 553–560, 1970.
435. RUSSELL, J. A., J. HOEFFEL, AND J. F. MURRAY. Effect of different levels of positive end-expiratory pressure on lung water content. *J. Appl. Physiol.: Respirat. Environ. Exercise Physiol.* 53: 9–15, 1982.
436. RUTILI, G. Transport of Macromolecules in Subcutaneous Tissue Studied by FITC-Dextrans. Uppsala, Sweden: Univ. of Uppsala, 1978. Dissertation.
437. RUTILI, G., P. KVIETYS, D. MARTIN, J. C. PARKER, AND A. E. TAYLOR. Increased pulmonary microvascular permeability induced by α-naphthylthiourea. *J. Appl. Physiol.: Respirat. Environ. Exercise Physiol.* 52: 1316–1323, 1982.
438. SACKS, T., C. F. MOLDOW, P. R. CRADDOCK, T. K. BOWERS, AND H. S. JACOB. Oxygen radicals mediate endothelial cell damage by complement-stimulated granulocytes. *J. Clin. Invest.* 62: 1161–1167, 1978.
439. SALDEEN, T. Trends in microvascular research. The microembolism syndrome. *Microvasc. Res.* 11: 227–259, 1976.
440. SARNOFF, S. J., AND L. C. SARNOFF. Neurohemodynamics of pulmonary edema. *Circulation* 6: 51–62, 1952.
441. SCHERZER, H., AND P. A. WARD. Lung injury produced by immune complexes of varying composition. *J. Immunol.* 121: 947–952, 1978.
442. SCHNEEBERGER, E. E. Ultrastructural basis for alveolar-capillary permeability to protein. In: *Lung Liquids*. Amsterdam: Excerpta Med., 1976, p. 3–21. (Ciba Found. Symp. 38.)
443. SCHNEEBERGER, E. E. Segmental differentiation of endothelial intercellular junctions in intra-acinar arteries and veins of the rat lung. *Circ. Res.* 49: 1102–1111, 1981.
444. SCHNEEBERGER, E. E., AND M. J. KARNOVSKY. The influence of intravascular fluid volume on the permeability of newborn and adult mouse lungs to ultrastructural protein tracers. *J. Cell Biol.* 49: 319–334, 1971.
445. SCHNEEBERGER, E. E., AND M. J. KARNOVSKY. Substructure of intracellular junctions in freeze-fractured alveolar-capillary membranes of mouse lung. *Circ. Res.* 38: 404–411, 1976.
446. SCHOLANDER, P. F., A. R. HARGENS, AND S. L. MILLER. Negative pressure in the interstitial fluid of animals. *Science* 161: 321–328, 1968.
447. SCHÜRCH, S., J. GOERKE, AND J. A. CLEMENTS. Direct determination of surface tension in the lung. *Proc. Natl. Acad. Sci. USA* 73: 4698–4702, 1976.
448. SCOGGIN, C. H., T. M. HYERS, J. T. REEVES, AND R. F. GROVER. High altitude pulmonary edema in children and young adults of Leadville, Colorado. *N. Engl. J. Med.* 297: 1269–1272, 1977.
449. SELINGER, S. L., R. D. BLAND, R. H. DEMLING, AND N. C. STAUB. Distribution volumes of [^{131}I]albumin, [^{14}C]sucrose, and ^{36}Cl in sheep lung. *J. Appl. Physiol.* 39: 773–779, 1975.
450. SEWELL, R. W., J. G. FEWEL, F. L. GROVER, AND K. V. AROM. Experimental evaluation of re-expansion pulmonary edema. *Ann. Thorac. Surg.* 26: 126–132, 1978.
451. SHASBY, D. M., R. B. FOX, R. N. HARADA, AND J. E. REPINE. Reduction of the edema of acute hyperoxic lung injury by granulocyte depletion. *J. Appl. Physiol.: Respirat. Environ. Exercise Physiol.* 52: 1237–1244, 1982.
452. SHIRLEY, H. H., JR., C. G. WOLFRAM, K. WASSERMAN, AND H. S. MAYERSON. Capillary permeability to macromolecules: stretched pore phenomenon. *Am. J. Physiol.* 190: 189–193, 1957.
453. SHU, H., R. E. TALCOTT, S. A. RICE, AND E. T. WEI. Lipid peroxidation and paraquat toxicity. *Biochem. Pharmacol.* 28: 327–331, 1979.
454. SIBBALD, W. J., A. A. DRIEDGER, J. D. MOFFAT, M. L. MYERS, B. A. REID, AND R. L. HOLLIDAY. Pulmonary microvascular clearance of radiotracers in human cardiac and noncardiac pulmonary edema. *J. Appl. Physiol.: Respirat. Environ. Exercise Physiol.* 50: 1337–1347, 1981.
455. SIDEL, V. W., AND A. K. SOLOMON. Entrance of water into human red cells under an osmotic gradient. *J. Gen. Physiol.* 41: 243–257, 1957.
456. SILBERBERG, A. The significance of hydrostatic pressure in the fluid phase of a structural tissue. In: *Tissue Fluid Pressure and Composition*, edited by A. R. Hargens. Baltimore, MD: Williams & Wilkins, 1981, chapt. 7, p. 71–76.
457. SIMIONESCU, M., N. SIMIONESCU, AND G. E. PALADE. Morphometric data on the endothelium of blood capillaries. *J. Cell Biol.* 60: 128–137, 1974.
458. SIMIONESCU, N., M. SIMIONESCU, AND G. E. PALADE. Permeability of intestinal capillaries. Pathway followed by dextrans and glycogens. *J. Cell Biol.* 53: 365–392, 1972.
459. SIMIONESCU, N., M. SIMIONESCU, AND G. E. PALADE. Structural-functional correlates in the transendothelial exchange of water soluble macromolecules. *Thromb. Res.* 8: 257–269, 1976.
460. SIMIONESCU, N., M. SIMIONESCU, AND G. E. PALADE. Structural basis of permeability in sequential segments of the microvasculature. II. Pathways followed by microperoxidase across the endothelium. *Microvasc. Res.* 15: 17–36, 1978.
461. SIMMONS, R. L., A. M. MARTIN, JR., C. A. HEISTERKAMP, AND T. B. DUCKER. Respiratory insufficiency in combat casualties. II. Pulmonary edema following head injury. *Ann. Surg.* 170: 39–44, 1969.
462. SIMON, R. P., L. L. BAYNE, R. F. TRANBAUGH, AND F. R. LEWIS. Elevated pulmonary lymph flow and protein content during status epilepticus in sheep. *J. Appl. Physiol.: Respirat. Environ. Exercise Physiol.* 52: 91–95, 1982.
463. SINGH, I., C. C. KAPILA, P. K. KHANNA, R. B. NANDA, AND B. D. P. RAO. High altitude pulmonary edema. *Lancet* 1: 229–234, 1965.

464. SMITH, H. C., V. F. GOULD, F. W. CHENEY, AND J. BUTLER. Pathogenesis of hemodynamic pulmonary edema in excised dog lungs. *J. Appl. Physiol.* 37: 904–911, 1974.
465. SMITH, J. C., AND W. MITZNER. Analysis of pulmonary vascular interdependence in excised dog lobes. *J. Appl. Physiol.: Respirat. Environ. Exercise Physiol.* 48: 450–467, 1980.
466. SMITH, L. L., AND M. S. ROSE. A comparison of the effects of paraquat and diquat on the water content of rat lung and the incorporation of thymidine into lung DNA. *Toxicology* 8: 223–230, 1977.
467. SMITH-ERICHSEN, N., AND G. BØ. Airway closure and fluid filtration in the lung. *Br. J. Anaesth.* 51: 475–479, 1979.
468. SNASHALL, P. D. Mucopolysaccharide osmotic pressure in the measurement of interstitial pressure. *Am. J. Physiol.* 232 (*Heart Circ. Physiol.* 1): H608–H616, 1977.
469. SNASHALL, P. D. Pulmonary edema. *Br. J. Dis. Chest* 74: 2–22, 1980.
470. SNASHALL, P. D. Mucopolysaccharide osmotic pressure in the measurement of interstitial pressure. In: *Tissue Fluid Pressure and Composition*, edited by A. R. Hargens. Baltimore, MD: Williams & Wilkins, 1981, chapt. 6, p. 63–70.
471. SNASHALL, P. D., AND J. M. B. HUGHES. Lung water balance. *Rev. Physiol. Biochem. Pharmacol.* 89: 5–62, 1981.
472. SNASHALL, P. D., S. J. KEYES, B. MORGAN, B. JONES, AND K. MURPHY. Regional extravascular and interstitial lung water in normal dogs. *J. Appl. Physiol.: Respirat. Environ. Exercise Physiol.* 49: 547–551, 1980.
473. SNASHALL, P. D., K. NAKAHARA, AND N. C. STAUB. Estimation of perimicrovascular fluid pressure in isolated perfused dog lung lobes. *J. Appl. Physiol.: Respirat. Environ. Exercise Physiol.* 46: 1003–1010, 1979.
474. SNASHALL, P. D., W. J. WEIDNER, AND N. C. STAUB. Extravascular lung water after extracellular fluid volume expansion in dogs. *J. Appl. Physiol.: Respirat. Environ. Exercise Physiol.* 42: 624–629, 1977.
475. STARLING, E. H. The influence of mechanical factors on lymph production. *J. Physiol. London* 10: 14–155, 1894.
476. STARLING, E. H. On the absorption of fluid from the connective tissue spaces. *J. Physiol. London* 19: 312–326, 1896.
477. STAUB, N. C. Pulmonary edema. *Physiol. Rev.* 54: 678–811, 1974.
478. STAUB, N. C. The forces regulating fluid filtration in the lungs. *Microvasc. Res.* 14: 45–55, 1978.
479. STAUB, N. C. Pathways for fluid and solute fluxes in pulmonary edema. In: *Pulmonary Edema*, edited by A. P. Fishman and E. M. Renkin. Bethesda, MD: Am. Physiol. Soc., 1979, chapt. 8, p. 113–124.
480. STAUB, N. C. Pulmonary edema—hypoxia and overperfusion. *N. Engl. J. Med.* 201: 1085–1087, 1980.
481. STAUB, N. C. Pulmonary edema due to increased microvascular permeability. *Annu. Rev. Med.* 32: 291–312, 1981.
482. STAUB, N. C., R. D. BLAND, K. L. BRIGHAM, R. ERDMANN III, AND W. C. WOLVERTON. Preparation of chronic lung lymph fistulas in sheep. *J. Surg. Res.* 19: 315–320, 1975.
483. STAUB, N. C., M. FLICK, A. PEREL, C. LANDOLT, AND T. R. VAUGHAN, JR. Lung lymph as a reflection of interstitial fluid. In: *Tissue Fluid Pressure and Composition*, edited by A. R. Hargens. Baltimore, MD: Williams & Wilkins, 1981, chapt. 12, p. 113–123.
484. STAUB, N. C., H. NAGANO, AND M. L. PEARCE. Pulmonary edema in dogs, especially the sequence of fluid accumulation in lungs. *J. Appl. Physiol.* 22: 227–240, 1967.
485. STOTHERT, J. C., J. WEAVER, AND C. J. CARRICO. Lung albumin content after acid aspiration pulmonary injury. *J. Surg. Res.* 30: 256–261, 1981.
486. SUTTON, J. R., AND N. LASSEN. Pathophysiology of acute mountain sickness and high altitude pulmonary edema: an hypothesis. *Bull. Eur. Physiolpathol. Respir.* 15: 1042–1052, 1979.
487. SZABÓ, G., AND Z. MAGYAR. Effect of increased systemic venous pressure on lymph pressure and flow. *Am. J. Physiol.* 212: 1469–1474, 1967.
488. SZIDON, J. P., G. G. PIETRA, AND A. P. FISHMAN. The alveolar-capillary membrane and pulmonary edema. *N. Engl. J. Med.* 286: 1200–1208, 1972.
489. TAYLOR, A. E. Capillary fluid filtration. Starling forces and lymph flow. *Circ. Res.* 49: 557–575, 1981.
490. TAYLOR, A. E., V. S. BISHOP, AND A. C. GUYTON. Permeability of the alveolar membrane to solutes. *Circ. Res.* 16: 353–362, 1965.
491. TAYLOR, A. E., AND R. E. DRAKE. Fluid and protein exchange. In: *Lung Biology in Health and Disease. Lung Water and Solute Exchange*, edited by N. C. Staub. New York: Dekker, 1978, vol. 7, chapt. 6, p. 129–166.
492. TAYLOR, A. E., AND K. A. GAAR. Calculation of equivalent pore radii of pulmonary capillary and alveolar membranes. *Rev. Argent. Angiol.* 111: 25–40, 1969.
493. TAYLOR, A. E., AND K. A. GAAR, JR. Estimation of equivalent pore radii of pulmonary capillary and alveolar membranes. *Am. J. Physiol.* 218: 1133–1140, 1970.
494. TAYLOR, A. E., AND H. GIBSON. Concentrating ability of lymphatic vessels. *Lymphology* 8: 43–49, 1975.
495. TAYLOR, A. E., H. GIBSON, H. J. GRANGER, AND A. C. GUYTON. The interaction between intracapillary and tissue forces in the overall regulation of interstitial fluid volume. *Lymphology* 6: 192–208, 1973.
496. TAYLOR, A. E., AND D. N. GRANGER. Equivalent pore modelling: vesicles, channels, and charge. *Federation Proc.* 42: 2440–2445, 1983.
497. TAYLOR, A. E., AND D. N. GRANGER. Exchange of macromolecules across the microcirculation. In: *Handbook of Physiology. The Cardiovascular System. Microcirculation*, edited by E. M. Renkin and C. C. Michel. Bethesda, MD: Am. Physiol. Soc., 1984, sect. 2, vol. IV, pt. 1, chapt. 11, p. 467–520.
498. TAYLOR, A. E., D. N. GRANGER, AND R. A. BRACE. Analysis of lymphatic protein flux data. I. Estimation of the reflection coefficient and permeability surface area product for total protein. *Microvasc. Res.* 13: 297–313, 1977.
499. TAYLOR, A. E., D. N. GRANGER, AND R. A. BRACE. Estimation of the reflection coefficient and permeability surface area product using lymphatic protein flux data: problems created by axial pressure gradients (Abstract). *Microvasc. Res.* 15: 33, 1978.
500. TAYLOR, A. E., F. GRIMBERT, G. RUTILI, P. R. KVIETYS, AND J. C. PARKER. Pulmonary edema. In: *Tissue Fluid Pressure and Composition*, edited by A. R. Hargens. Baltimore, MD: Williams & Wilkins, 1981, chapt. 14, p. 135–143.
500a. TAYLOR, A. E., AND D. MARTIN. Oxygen radicals and the microcirculation. *Physiologist* 26: 152–155, 1983.
501. TAYLOR, A. E., J. C. PARKER, D. N. GRANGER, N. A. MORTILLARO, AND G. RUTILI. Assessment of capillary permeability using lymphatic protein flux: estimation of the osmotic reflection coefficient. In: *The Microcirculation*, edited by R. Effros, H. Schmid-Shonbein, and J. Ditzel. New York: Academic, 1981, p. 19–32.
502. TAYLOR, A. E., J. C. PARKER, P. R. KVIETYS, AND M. PERRY. Pulmonary interstitium in capillary exchange. *Ann. NY Acad. Sci.* 384: 148–168, 1982.
503. TAYLOR, P. M., U. BOONYAPRAKOB, V. WATERMAN, D. WATSON, AND E. LOPATA. Clearances of plasma proteins from pulmonary vascular beds of adult dogs and pups. *Am. J. Physiol.* 213: 441–449, 1967.
504. TAYLOR, P. M., U. BOONYAPRAKOB, D. W. WATSON, AND P. FIREMAN. Relative efflux of native proteins from the canine pulmonary vascular bed. *Am. J. Physiol.* 214: 1310–1314, 1968.
505. THEODORE, J., AND E. D. ROBIN. Speculations on neurogenic pulmonary edema. *Am. Rev. Respir. Dis.* 113: 405–411, 1976.
506. TIERNEY, D. F., L. AYERS, AND R. S. KASUYAMA. Altered sensitivity to oxygen toxicity. *Am. Rev. Respir. Dis.* 115: 59–66, 1977.
507. TODD, T. R. J., E. BAILE, AND J. C. HOGG. Pulmonary capillary permeability during hemorrhagic shock. *J. Appl.*

Physiol.: Respirat. Environ. Exercise Physiol. 45: 298–306, 1978.
508. TOUNG, T. J. K., D. BORDOS, D. W. BENSON, D. CARTER, G. D. ZUIDEMA, S. PERMUTT, AND J. L. CAMERON. Aspiration pneumonia: experimental evaluation of albumin and steroid therapy. *Ann. Surg.* 183: 179–184, 1976.
509. TOUNG, T. J., J. L. CAMERON, T. KIMURA, AND S. PERMUTT. Aspiration pneumonia: treatment with osmotically active agents. *Surgery* 89: 588–593, 1981.
510. TOUNG, T., P. SAHARIA, S. PERMUTT, G. D. ZUIDEMA, AND J. L. CAMERON. Aspiration pneumonia: beneficial and harmful effects of positive end-expiratory pressure. *Surgery* 82: 279–283, 1979.
511. UHLEY, H. N., S. E. LEEDS, J. J. SAMPSON, AND M. FRIEDMAN. Role of pulmonary lymphatics in chronic pulmonary edema. *Circ. Res.* 11: 966–970, 1962.
512. VAAGE, J., G. NICOLAYSEN, AND B. A. WAALER. Aggregation of blood platelets and increased hydraulic conductivity of pulmonary exchange vessels. *Acta Physiol. Scand.* 98: 175–184, 1976.
513. VAN DER ZEE, H., A. B. MALIK, B. C. LEE, AND T. S. HAKIM. Lung fluid and protein exchange during intracranial hypertension and role of sympathetic mechanisms. *J. Appl. Physiol.: Respirat. Environ. Exercise Physiol.* 48: 273–280, 1980.
514. VAUGHAN, T. R., A. J. ERDMANN, K. L. BRIGHAM, W. C. WOOLVERTON, W. J. WEIDNER, AND N. C. STAUB. Equilibration of intravascular albumin with lung lymph in unanesthetized sheep. *Lymphology* 12: 217–223, 1979.
515. VIJEYARATHNAM, G. S., AND B. CORRIN. Fine structural alterations in the lungs of iprindole-treated rats. *J. Pathol.* 114: 233–239, 1974.
516. VISSCHER, M. D., F. J. HADDY, AND G. STEPHENS. The physiology and pharmacology of lung edema. *Pharmacol. Rev.* 8: 389–394, 1956.
517. VISWANATHAN, R., S. K. JAIN, AND S. SUBRAMANIAN. Pulmonary edema of high altitude. *Am. Rev. Respir. Dis.* 100: 342–349, 1969.
518. VISWANATHAN, R., S. K. JAIN, S. SUBRAMANIAN, T. A. V. SUBRAMANIAN, G. L. DUA, AND J. GIRI. Pulmonary edema of high altitude. II. Clinical, aerohemodynamic and biochemical studies in a group with history of pulmonary edema at high altitude. *Am. Rev. Respir. Dis.* 100: 327–341, 1969.
519. VOELKEL, N. F., S. WORTHEN, J. T. REEVES, P. M. HENSON, AND R. C. MURPHY. Nonimmunological production of leukotrienes induced by platelet-activating factor. *Science* 218: 286–288, 1982.
520. VOSS, T. How to get your "juice" flowing. In: *Prevention* 33: 57–62, 1981.
521. VREIM, C. E., K. OHKUDA, AND N. C. STAUB. Proportions of dog lung lymph in the thoracic and right lymph ducts. *J. Appl. Physiol.: Respirat. Environ. Exercise Physiol.* 43: 894–898, 1977.
522. VREIM, C. E., P. D. SNASHALL, R. H. DEMLING, AND N. C. STAUB. Lung lymph and free interstitial fluid protein composition in sheep with edema. *Am. J. Physiol.* 230: 1650–1653, 1976.
523. VREIM, C. E., P. D. SNASHALL, AND N. C. STAUB. Protein composition of lung fluids in anesthetized dogs with acute cardiogenic edema. *Am. J. Physiol.* 231: 1466–1469, 1976.
524. VREIM, C. E., AND N. C. STAUB. Protein composition of lung fluids in acute alloxan edema in dogs. *Am. J. Physiol.* 230: 376–379, 1976.
525. WAGNER, E., P. A. RIEBENS, K. KATSUKARA, AND P. SALISBURY. Influence of airway pressures on edema in the isolated dog's lung. *Circ. Res.* 9: 382–386, 1961.
526. WAGNER, W. W., JR., L. P. LATHAM, AND R. L. CAPEN. Capillary recruitment during airway hypoxia: role of pulmonary artery pressure. *J. Appl. Physiol.: Respirat. Environ. Exercise Physiol.* 47: 383–387, 1979.
527. WANGENSTEEN, O. D., E. LYSAKER, AND P. SAVARYN. Pulmonary capillary filtration and reflection coefficients in the adult rabbit. *Microvasc. Res.* 14: 81–97, 1977.
528. WARREN, M. F., AND C. K. DRINKER. The flow of lymph from the lungs of the dog. *Am. J. Physiol.* 136: 207–221, 1942.
529. WARREN, M. F., D. K. PETERSON, AND C. K. DRINKER. The effects of heightened negative pressure in the chest, together with further experiments upon anoxia in increasing the flow of lung lymph. *Am. J. Physiol.* 137: 641–648, 1942.
530. WASIUTYNSKI, A., J. KACKI, AND W. OLSZEWSKI. Studies on acute lung lymphatic edema. *Pol. Med. Sci. Hist. Bull.* 18: 139–147, 1975.
531. WEBB, W. R., S. D. WAX, K. KUSAJIMA, AND T. M. KAMIYAMA. Microscopic studies of the pulmonary circulation in situ. *Surg. Clin. North Am.* 54: 1067–1076, 1974.
532. WÉGRIA, R., H. ZEKERT, K. E. WALTER, R. W. ENTRUP, C. DE SCHRYVER, W. KENNEDY, AND D. PAIEWONSKY. Effect of systemic venous pressure on drainage of lymph from thoracic duct. *Am. J. Physiol.* 204: 284–288, 1963.
533. WEIBEL, E. R., AND H. BACHOFEN. Structural design of the alveolar septum and fluid exchange. In: *Pulmonary Edema*, edited by A. P. Fishman and E. M. Renkin. Bethesda, MD: Am. Physiol. Soc., 1979, chapt. 1, p. 1–20.
534. WEIL, M. H., R. J. HENNING, M. MORRISSETTE, AND S. MICHAELS. Relationship between colloid osmotic pressure and pulmonary artery wedge pressure in patients with acute cardiorespiratory failure. *Am. J. Med.* 64: 643–650, 1978.
535. WEISER, P. C., AND F. GRANDE. Estimation of fluid shifts and protein permeability during pulmonary edemagenesis. *Am. J. Physiol.* 227: 1028–1034, 1974.
536. WENDT, R. P., E. KLEIN, E. H. BRESLER, F. F. HOLLAND, R. M. SERINO, AND H. VILLA. Sieving properties of hemodialysis membranes. *J. Membr. Sci.* 5: 23–49, 1979.
537. WEST, J. B., AND C. T. DOLLERY. Distribution of blood flow and ventilation-perfusion ratio in the lung, measured with radioactive CO_2. *J. Appl. Physiol.* 15: 405–410, 1960.
538. WEST, J. B., C. T. DOLLERY, AND B. E. HEARD. Increased pulmonary vascular resistance in the dependent zone of isolated dog lung caused by perivascular edema. *Circ. Res.* 17: 191–206, 1965.
539. WHAYNE, T. F., JR., AND J. W. SEVERINGHAUS. Experimental hypoxic pulmonary edema in the rat. *J. Appl. Physiol.* 25: 729–732, 1968.
540. WIEDERHIELM, C. A. The interstitial space. In: *Biomechanics: Its Foundations and Objectives*, edited by Y. C. Fung, N. Perrone, and M. Anliker. Englewood Cliffs, NJ: Prentice-Hall, 1972, p. 273–286.
541. WIEDERHIELM, C. A. The tissue pressure controversy, a semantic dilemma. In: *Tissue Fluid Pressure and Composition*, edited by A. R. Hargens. Baltimore, MD: Williams & Wilkins, 1981, chapt. 3, p. 21–34.
542. WIEDERHIELM, C. A., J. R. FOX, AND D. R. LEE. Ground substance mucopolysaccharides and plasma proteins: their role in capillary water balance. *Am. J. Physiol.* 230: 1121–1125, 1976.
543. WILLIAMS, M. C., AND S. L. WISSIG. The permeability of muscle capillaries to horseradish peroxidase. *J. Cell Biol.* 66: 531–555, 1975.
544. WILSON, T. A. Parenchymal mechanics at the alveolar level. *Federation Proc.* 38: 7–10, 1979.
545. WILSON, T. A. Effect of alveolar wall shape on alveolar water stability (Letter to the editor). *J. Appl. Physiol.: Respirat. Environ. Exercise Physiol.* 50: 222–224, 1981.
546. WILSON, T. A. Relations among recoil pressure, surface area, and surface tension in the lung. *J. Appl. Physiol.: Respirat. Environ. Exercise Physiol.* 50: 921–926, 1981.
547. WINN, R., B. NADIR, J. GLEISNER, AND J. HILDEBRANDT. Chronic lung lymph fistula in the goat. *J. Appl. Physiol.: Respirat. Environ. Exercise Physiol.* 48: 399–402, 1980.
548. WITTMERS, L. E. Permeability Characteristics of the Blood-Gas Barrier. Duluth: Univ. of Minnesota, 1974, p. 164–165. Dissertation.
549. WOLFE, W. G., AND W. C. DEVRIES. Oxygen toxicity. *Annu.*

Rev. Med. 26: 203–217, 1975.
550. WOOLVERTON, W. C., K. L. BRIGHAM, AND N. C. STAUB. Effect of positive pressure breathing on lung lymph flow and water content in sheep. Circ. Res. 42: 550–557, 1978.
551. YOFFEY, J. M., AND F. C. COURTICE. Lymphatics, Lymph and the Lymphomyeloid Complex. London: Academic, 1970.
552. YONEDA, K. Anatomic pathway of fluid leakage in fluid-overload pulmonary edema in mice. Am. J. Pathol. 101: 7–16, 1980.
553. ZARINS, C. K., C. L. RICE, R. M. PETERS, AND R. W. VIRGILIO. Lymph and pulmonary response to isobaric reduction in plasma oncotic pressure in baboons. Circ. Res. 43: 925–930, 1978.
554. ZIDULKA, A., M. DEMEDTS, S. NADLER, AND N. R. ANTHONISEN. Pleural pressure with lobar obstruction in dogs. Respir. Physiol. 26: 239–248, 1976.
555. ZWEIFACH, V. W., AND A. SILBERBERG. The interstitial-lymphatic flow system. In: Cardiovascular Physiology III, edited by A. C. Guyton and D. B. Young. Baltimore, MD: University Park, 1979, vol. 18, chapt. 6, p. 215–260. (Int. Rev. Physiol. Ser.)

CHAPTER 5

Oxygen utilization and toxicity in the lungs

ARON B. FISHER
HENRY J. FORMAN

Department of Physiology, University of Pennsylvania School of Medicine, Philadelphia, Pennsylvania

CHAPTER CONTENTS

Bioenergetics
  General concepts
    Energy conservation
    Generation of reduced pyridine and flavin nucleotides
    Substrate-level phosphorylation
    Electron-transport chain
    Oxidative phosphorylation
    Inhibitors and uncouplers of mitochondrial bioenergetics
    Control of ATP synthesis
  Lung bioenergetics
    Oxygen uptake
    Energy state and ATP generation
    Lung mitochondria
Oxygen-Dependent Metabolic Reactions
  Pathways of O_2 utilization
  Pulmonary O_2-dependent metabolic reactions
    Cytochrome P-450–linked monooxygenase
    Inactivation of vasoactive amines
    Synthesis of connective tissue components
    Synthesis of eicosanoids
    Bactericidal activity
Oxygen Toxicity
  Pathological effects of O_2
    General aspects of toxicity
    Pulmonary O_2 toxicity
  Mechanisms of O_2 toxicity
    Free-radical production
    Oxidation of tissue components
    Alterations of metabolic function
  Antioxidant defenses
    Enzymatic defenses
    Nonenzymatic defenses
    Protection against pulmonary O_2 toxicity
Conclusion

GAS EXCHANGE IN THE LUNG is the O_2 source for reactions throughout the body that use O_2 for metabolism. The pulmonary gas-exchange process will be covered in detail in another volume in this *Handbook* section on the respiratory system. Our discussion focuses on O_2 utilization at the cellular level, with emphasis on ATP generation, nonmitochondrial pathways for O_2 utilization, and the toxic effects of O_2-reduction products. Many O_2-consuming reactions were considered in detail in the chapter by Jöbsis (104) in the 1964 edition and in the chapter by Davies and Davies (41) in the 1965 edition of the *Handbook* section on respiration. This chapter supplements these earlier discussions by reviewing recent developments and emphasizing lung metabolism.

BIOENERGETICS

General Concepts

ENERGY CONSERVATION. Energy generation is the consequence of catabolism of nutrients that supply the reducing power required for generation of ATP in mitochondria through oxidative phosphorylation. The oxidation of glucose and other carbon substrates produces CO_2 and H_2O and releases energy in an overall reaction analogous to combustion. Unlike combustion the indirect stepwise process of biological oxidation allows available energy from these reactions to be conserved through production of relatively stable high-energy compounds. The term *high energy* refers to the presence of chemical bonds, e.g., acyl phosphate bonds in ATP, that on hydrolysis yield relatively large quantities of free energy, which may then be used in productive work. Through this mechanism the cell can effectively regulate production and utilization of energy derived from oxidation, whereas the energy generated during combustion would be immediately lost as heat. The catabolic reactions that provide substrates for energy generation are covered elsewhere [(104); see the chapter by Tierney and Young in this *Handbook*]. This section concentrates on the connection between the reactions of intermediary metabolism and O_2-dependent reactions in mitochondria.

GENERATION OF REDUCED PYRIDINE AND FLAVIN NUCLEOTIDES. A major step in the conservation of energy released from biological oxidations is the chemical reduction of nucleotide cofactors: NAD to NADH and FAD to $FADH_2$. The reductive power of these nucleotides can drive ATP generation in mitochondria. These nucleotides may be reduced through the catabolic reactions of intermediary metabolism occurring in both cytoplasmic and mitochondrial compartments of the cell. Much of the NADH derived from catabolism is generated in the mitochondrial matrix, where it can be directly oxidized by mitochondrial enzymes. Because mitochondrial membrane is not permeable to these compounds, NADH produced in the cytosol cannot be directly oxidized. However, "shuttle" mechanisms are present to transfer reducing equivalents through the inner mitochondrial membrane to the mitochondrial matrix. The carrier in these shuttles is a metabolite that can be reduced in the cytoplasm and dehydrogenated in the mitochondrion to generate NADH or $FADH_2$ plus the original metabolite. To function as a carrier, both the reduced and oxidized forms of the metabolite must be able to cross the mitochondrial membranes. The best-characterized hydrogen shuttle mechanisms are the redox pairs, aspartate and malate and glycerol 3-phosphate and dihydroxyacetone phosphate.

In contrast to NADH, NADPH is not used directly by the electron-transport chain. The major physiological role of NADPH is to provide reducing potential for biosynthetic reactions rather than to generate ATP. Although the standard redox midpoint potentials for $NADP^+/NADPH$ and $NAD^+/NADH$ are identical, the redox pairs do not equilibrate because reducing equivalents are not transferred directly between them. In most cells the $NADP^+/NADPH$ is balanced toward the reduced form, whereas the $NAD^+/NADH$ is usually poised toward the oxidized state. However, a transhydrogenase is present in mitochondria that catalyzes the essentially irreversible energy-dependent reduction of $NADP^+$ by NADH

$$NADH + NADP^+ + ATP \quad\quad\quad (1)$$
$$\rightarrow ADP + P_i + NAD^+ + NADPH$$

Presumably Reaction 1 maintains an intramitochondrial pool of NADPH when ATP requirements are satisfied.

Both FAD and FMN are cofactors of several dehydrogenases and are generally bound to enzymes. For example, FAD is physically bound to fatty acyl coenzyme A (acyl-CoA) dehydrogenase, whereas FAD of succinate dehydrogenase is actually covalently bound to the protein (183). This is significant because the same molecule of FAD is involved in repetitive redox cycles of the enzyme. Flavin-containing proteins function in electron transfer from dehydrogenases to the respiratory chain and also in many oxygenase reactions.

SUBSTRATE-LEVEL PHOSPHORYLATION. Although oxidative phosphorylation in mitochondria is the major source of ATP in most mammalian cells, the stoichiometric production of ATP by two of the enzyme-catalyzed reactions in glycolysis (phosphoglycerate kinase and pyruvate kinase) contributes to the total energy pool of the cell and provides most of the energy in red blood cells and some skeletal muscle cells. These reactions involve the transfer of phosphate from an acyl phosphate compound to a high-energy enzyme-phosphate intermediate. The high-energy bond is then transferred to ADP, the acceptor molecule, to form ATP

$$Enz\text{-}O\text{-}P_i + ADP \rightarrow Enz\text{-}OH + ATP \quad (2)$$

Substrate-level phosphorylation does not consume NADH or $FADH_2$ or require O_2. An additional substrate-level phosphorylation (with GDP as an acceptor to produce GTP) occurs in the mitochondria in the succinyl-CoA synthetase reaction of the tricarboxylic acid cycle.

Adenylate kinase (Reaction 3) and creatine kinase (Reaction 4) can also generate ATP in the cytosol of some cells

$$2ADP \rightarrow ATP + AMP \quad\quad (3)$$
$$phosphocreatine + ADP \rightarrow creatine + ATP \quad (4)$$

Reactions 3 and 4 do not increase the number of high-energy bonds in the cell but rather convert them into a more usable form.

ELECTRON-TRANSPORT CHAIN. The electron-transport chain is a group of carriers located in the mitochondrial inner membrane (Fig. 1). A series of redox reactions are linked to allow the flow of electrons from NADH to O_2. The net reaction is

$$NADH + \tfrac{1}{2}O_2 + H^+ \rightarrow NAD^+ + H_2O \quad (5)$$

Electrons enter the chain through oxidation of NADH by a dehydrogenase or beyond the NADH step through FAD-bound dehydrogenases. Both FMN- and FAD-containing flavoproteins transfer electrons to the ubiquinone–cytochrome b–cytochrome c_1 complex through intermediary iron-sulfur centers (3, 152). The ubiquinone–cytochrome b–cytochrome c_1 complex is composed of ubiquinone, two type b cytochromes ($b_T[566]$ and $b_K[561]$), and cytochrome c_1 (51). Electrons are transferred from this complex to cytochrome c, then to cytochrome c oxidase (i.e., cytochrome a–cytochrome a_3 complex), and finally to O_2 (Fig. 1).

Electron transport in the respiratory chain involves transferring two electrons from substrates to carriers. Some can only accept one electron. Flavin and ubiquinone can undergo both one- and two-electron transfer and either could be the point at which the change from two-electron to one-electron transfer occurs in the chain. Four electrons accumulate in the terminal oxidase and are transferred nearly simultaneously to O_2, forming two H_2O molecules. Reduction of O_2 by cytochrome c oxidase probably involves the formation of an O_2 bridge between cytochrome a_3 and one of the Cu atoms, with rapid transfer of electrons from cytochrome a and the other Cu atom to the bound O_2. Thus there is no release of intermediates in the reduction of O_2 to H_2O by cytochrome c oxidase (29).

Since publication of the earlier edition of the *Handbook* on respiration, the role of ubiquinone reduction in electron transport has been clarified. Ubiquinone

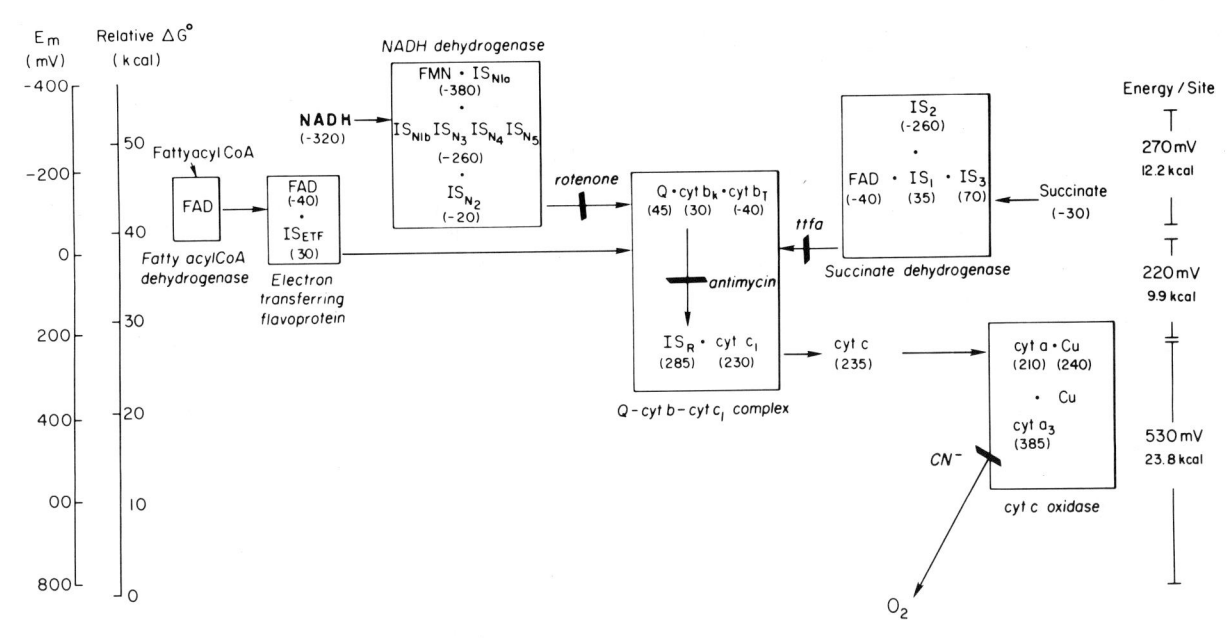

FIG. 1. Scheme for mitochondrial electron-transport chain showing pathway for electrons from substrate (NADH, fatty acyl-CoA, or succinate) to O_2. Components are shown with their midpoint redox potentials in parentheses. Components of complexes are grouped together. *Arrows*, direction of electron flow between complexes. *Left*, scales for redox potential (Em) and relative standard free-energy changes (ΔG^0). *Right*, summation of energy (ΔG^0) available per phosphorylation site. Energy available at each site exceeds the ΔG^0 required for ATP synthesis (7 kcal/mol); ΔG^0 required for ATP synthesis under physiological conditions exceeds the ΔG^0 by ~50%. *Heavy bars*, sites of inhibition by electron-transport inhibitors. IS, iron-sulfur center; ttfa, thenoyltrifluoroacetone.

reduction was thought to be on a bypass or "blind alley" of the respiratory chain rather than an obligatory component (104). However, it was shown that the kinetics of the redox reactions of ubiquinone are consistent with direct participation in the chain between the dehydrogenases and cytochrome b (122). Ubiquinone can be reduced in two steps to form the ubisemiquinone free radical (QH·) after addition of the first electron and reduced ubiquinone (QH_2) after addition of the second. Mitchell (143) suggested that the involvement of ubiquinone in the electron-transport chain is a cyclic reaction with cytochromes b_T and b_K and a nonheme-iron center (Fig. 2, ubiquinone cycle). In this scheme the quinone must be physically separated into two pools, and the two redox potentials (Q → QH· and QH· → QH_2) must be different in one pool and similar in the other. This concept is supported by measurements with electron paramagnetic resonance that indicated the presence of QH· in two different environments and suggested that QH· is more stable (i.e., less likely to dismute to Q + QH_2) in one site than in the other (147, 153). Kinetic studies also support two sites of ubiquinone reduction and indicate that QH· is produced in at least one (69). Measurement of the two midpoint potentials for ubiquinone in its interactions with dehydrogenase and cytochrome b_K suggest that they are very close and can satisfy the requirements for half of the cycle (51).

The separation of the two midpoint potentials involved with the other half of the cycle (i.e., nonheme iron and cytochrome b_T) could occur if ubiquinone binds to protein during electron transfers (144, 147). However, definitive confirmation that this cycle is operative is still lacking.

OXIDATIVE PHOSPHORYLATION. The stepwise process of electron transport permits efficient coupling between the exergonic transfer of electrons from NADH (or $FADH_2$) to O_2 and the production of ATP. Three of the reactions in the respiratory chain generate sufficient energy to allow phosphorylation of ADP [change in free energy under physiological conditions (ΔG) ~ 11 kcal/mol]: *1)* NADH → Q, *2)* cytochrome b → cytochrome c_1, and *3)* cytochrome c → O_2 (Fig. 1). When electrons enter the chain through succinate dehydrogenase or the $FADH_2$ reactions, only the latter two sites of ADP phosphorylation are available for ATP synthesis.

The identification of the precise redox reactions within each site that are coupled to ATP production is complicated by insufficient understanding of the mechanism of oxidative phosphorylation. One approach to solving this problem has been to assume that shifts in phosphate potential (see CONTROL OF ATP SYNTHESIS, p. 235) alter the midpoint potentials of the components of the respiratory chain associated

FIG. 2. Postulated scheme for ubiquinone (Q) cycle, indicating movements of electrons and protons across mitochondrial inner membrane in cyclic reduction and oxidation of ubiquinone. Associated components of electron-transport chain are shown with midpoint potentials (in mV) in parentheses. Scheme provides both a mechanism for involvement of ubiquinone in electron-transport chain and movement of protons from mitochondrial matrix through inner membrane into intermembrane space.

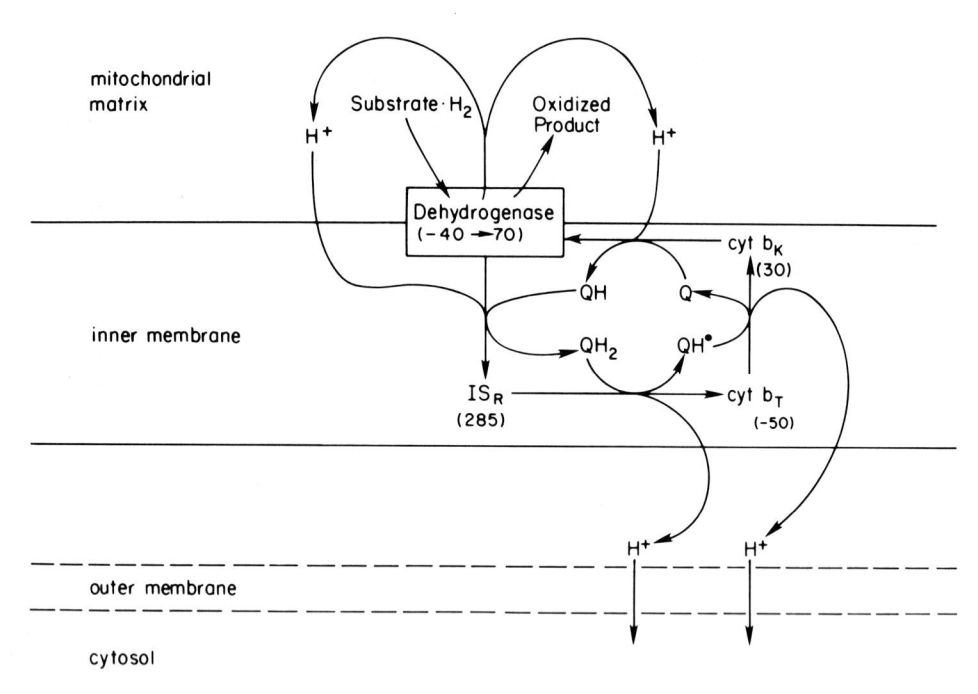

with ATP production. This analysis suggested that the probable steps that supply energy for ATP production are electron transfers between nonheme-iron centers in NADH oxidase (site 1) and oxidation of cytochrome b_T by cytochrome c_1 (site 2) (29). The reaction for energy transduction at site 3 is between cytochromes a and a_3, but the precise step remains unidentified.

Several hypotheses have been advanced for the actual mechanism of oxidative phosphorylation, although none has been proven. One hypothesis applied the concept of substrate-level phosphorylation to the three sites of phosphorylation in the electron-transport chain. However, the search for the required high-energy intermediates between the electron-transport chain and ATP has been unsuccessful. A second hypothesis is conformation coupling (24), in which redox energy produces a conformational change in an ATP synthetase, which then catalyzes phosphorylation through release of energy in returning to its original state. This hypothesis does not explain how the energy available from the electron-transport chain is coupled to changes in conformation of the ATP synthetase. A third hypothesis, which has been formalized in the chemiosmotic hypothesis of Mitchell (142), attributes oxidative phosphorylation to generation of localized proton gradients. This theory proposes that the energy of electron transport drives protons out of the mitochondrion, thereby establishing a transmembrane electrochemical potential (negative inside). Reverse flow of protons through the ATP synthetase (i.e., down the electrochemical gradient) drives the phosphorylation of ADP. This hypothesis requires a mechanism for coupling the transfer of H^+ out of the mitochondrion and the establishment of a transmembrane potential across a membrane essentially impermeable to H^+. Possibly the ubiquinone cycle (see ELECTRON-TRANSPORT CHAIN, p. 232) may simultaneously transport protons across the mitochondrial membrane (143). Although this could provide the proton gradient for oxidative phosphorylation at site 2, the possible reactions associated with proton movements at sites 1 and 3 are unknown. Furthermore the stoichiometric relationship between the proton motive force (transmembrane pH gradient plus membrane potential) and ATP synthesis varies with metabolic conditions (202, 209), suggesting that this mechanism for oxidative phosphorylation requires additional coupling factors.

INHIBITORS AND UNCOUPLERS OF MITOCHONDRIAL BIOENERGETICS. Several inhibitors of mitochondrial ATP synthesis are useful for studying mitochondrial bioenergetics. These compounds fall into three major groups: 1) inhibitors of the redox steps of electron transport, 2) inhibitors of electron transport when coupled to phosphorylation, and 3) uncoupling agents. The first group blocks specific sites along the chain (Fig. 1); for example, cyanide blocks the terminal oxidase (site 3), antimycin A blocks oxidation of cytochrome b by cytochrome c_1 (site 2), thenoyltrifluoroacetone blocks oxidation of succinate (195), and rotenone blocks NADH dehydrogenase (site 1). The second group blocks the transfer of energy between oxidation and phosphorylation, although the energy from electron transport may still be used for other mitochondrial processes, such as uptake of cations into the mitochondrial matrix. This group includes oligomycin, which interferes with energy transduction to ADP, and atractylate, which blocks the transfer of

ADP into the mitochondrion by the adenylate translocase (see next section). The third group (e.g., dinitrophenol), called uncouplers of oxidative phosphorylation, release the energy of oxidation in ways that allow neither phosphorylation nor energy-dependent ion uptake by mitochondria. Uncoupling agents produce large increases in O_2 consumption without a corresponding increase in ATP synthesis, contrary to the normal situation, in which phosphorylation and oxidation are coordinated so that inhibition or acceleration of one has a parallel effect on the other.

CONTROL OF ATP SYNTHESIS. In the steady state of cellular metabolism, the ATP synthesis rate is coupled to ATP utilization. Presumably the coupling between utilization and synthesis depends ultimately on the energy state of the cell. Two formulations for expressing the energy state are the equations for the adenylate energy charge (9)

$$\text{energy charge} = \frac{[\text{ATP}] + 0.5[\text{ADP}]}{[\text{ATP}] + [\text{ADP}] + [\text{AMP}]} \quad (6)$$

and the phosphate potential

$$\Gamma = \frac{[\text{ATP}]}{[\text{ADP}][\text{P}_i]} \quad (7)$$

Equation 6 essentially considers the number of high-energy bonds in the adenylate compounds as a fraction of the total possible number. Equation 7 is based on the mass-action formulation for ATP synthesis. The phosphate-potential formulation may more sensitively describe changes in the energy state because the energy-charge formulation is always dominated by the ATP concentration and consequently shows little numerical variation with altered metabolic conditions.

The mechanism for coupling the energy state of the cell to the regulation of ATP generation is unclear. With isolated mitochondria the ATP synthesis rate has been shown to vary with availability of substrate (i.e., reducing equivalents), ADP, P_i, O_2, and coupling between the respiratory chain and ADP phosphorylation. Each of these factors can be rate limiting under appropriate conditions, and their limitations have been described as mitochondrial states [(32); see also the discussion in the chapter by Jöbsis (104) in the 1964 edition of the *Handbook* section on respiration]. Under normal resting conditions in the cell the major regulator of mitochondrial respiratory activity is probably ADP generated from ATP hydrolysis.

In the intact cell, ATP synthesis is coordinated between mitochondrial and cytosolic compartments through allosteric regulation of the activity of some enzymes in the glycolytic pathway by concentrations of the adenine nucleotides (see the chapter by Tierney and Young in this *Handbook*). Regulation of glycolysis affects not only substrate-level phosphorylation but also substrate availability for mitochondrial oxidation.

In most cells, ATP synthesis occurs predominantly in the mitochondrion, whereas most ATP utilization occurs outside the mitochondrion. Because the inner mitochondrial membrane is not permeable to adenine nucleotides, they must be transferred from the mitochondrial to the cytosolic space. This is accomplished by exchange of mitochondrial ATP for cytosolic ADP by a protein translocation (118)

$$[\text{ATP}]_{\text{in}} + [\text{ADP}]_{\text{out}} \rightarrow [\text{ATP}]_{\text{out}} + [\text{ADP}]_{\text{in}} \quad (8)$$

It has been proposed that ATP synthesis might be regulated in cells by the rate of ADP translocation into the mitochondrion (31, 42, 123). Oxidative phosphorylation can be regulated by this mechanism in isolated mitochondria when the concentration of ADP is below the Michaelis constant (K_m) for the translocase, but it is likely that this condition occurs physiologically only under extreme conditions (42).

The availability of O_2 is not a major factor in the regulation of mitochondrial ATP synthesis when the intracellular partial pressure of O_2 (P_{O_2}) is above a critical value. However, O_2 concentration becomes increasingly important in regulation as O_2 availability is decreased below the value required to saturate cytochrome c oxidase. This critical P_{O_2} is not precisely known, although experiments with isolated mitochondria suggest it is <0.5 mmHg (31, 193). However, studies with some isolated cell preparations have indicated a critical P_{O_2} ~1 order of magnitude greater (50, 107, 208, 210). One possible explanation for this discrepancy is the existence of a diffusion gradient for O_2 within the cell. Recent studies of *Amoeba proteus* with quenching of pyrene fluorescence as an O_2 indicator suggested the presence of intracellular O_2 gradients (160). Furthermore studies with two endogenous indicators with differing O_2 affinity in perfused liver during hypoxia are compatible with intracellular P_{O_2} gradients (181). This gradient presumably is generated through mitochondrial O_2 consumption. Jones and Kennedy (106) suggested that in the isolated hepatocyte the P_{O_2} gradient actually occurs between the endoplasmic reticulum and mitochondrion. However, this concept of intracellular O_2 gradients requires further evaluation before the mechanism for the apparent difference in O_2 affinity for cytochrome c oxidase in vivo versus in vitro is clarified.

Forman and Wilson (78) and Erecińska et al. (50) recently suggested that a progressive decrease in cellular P_{O_2} may result in alterations of the mitochondrial redox state that precede a measurable decrease in O_2 utilization. They showed that the first two sites of oxidative phosphorylation are in near equilibrium, as defined by the relationship

$$K_{eq} = \frac{[\text{NAD}^+][\text{Cyt } c^{2+}]^2[\text{ATP}]^2}{[\text{NADH}][\text{Cyt } c^{3+}]^2[\text{ADP}]^2[\text{P}_i]^2} \quad (9)$$

They also showed that net oxidative phosphorylation depends on the irreversible O_2-dependent reaction catalyzed by cytochrome c oxidase (50)

$$4\text{Cyt } c^{2+} + O_2 + 4H^+ + 2ADP + 2P_i \quad (10)$$
$$\rightarrow 4\text{Cyt } c^{3+} + 2H_2O + 2ADP$$

Consequently a decrease in O_2 concentration can result in alteration of cytochrome c^{2+}/cytochrome c^{3+}, NAD^+/NADH, and $ATP/ADP \cdot P_i$. These redox changes result in an increased flux through the respiratory chain that essentially restores O_2 utilization and ATP synthesis to nearly normal levels. However, the new set point for the cell energy level (defined by the phosphate potential) will be somewhat lower. This slight change in the cellular energy state might stimulate glycolysis, contributing to overall cellular ATP production. Consequently changes in the redox state, energy state, and glycolytic activity might occur despite essentially normal O_2 consumption and cellular ATP turnover. This mechanism does not define the range of P_{O_2} at which O_2 availability becomes limiting for saturation of cytochrome c oxidase, but this might occur at 1–2 orders of magnitude above the generally accepted critical P_{O_2}. These redox changes may explain the apparent stimulation of glycolysis prior to the change in the ATP content of the isolated perfused lung as alveolar P_{O_2} is decreased toward the critical value (61, 168).

Lung Bioenergetics

The lung is unique among mammalian organs in situ because O_2 is added to the arterial blood during its passage through the capillaries. The amount of O_2 added under steady-state conditions equals the rest of the body's O_2 consumption. However, it is now appreciated that the constituent cells of the lung have metabolic requirements that must be satisfied to maintain structural integrity of this organ. Therefore these metabolic requirements, although small in quantity, in a sense determine the metabolic fate of the entire organism. This section examines the bioenergetics of the lung tissue.

Although techniques developed for metabolic studies of other organs are suitable for study of the lung, their applicability is frequently limited, largely because of the peculiar structure-function relationships of the organ. First, despite its relatively large volume the tissue mass of the lung is only ~0.5% of body wt. Second, a sizable percentage (~33%) of lung weight is due to its blood content. The problems that small size and large vascularity introduce for studying lung metabolism are compounded because the lung is cellularly heterogeneous and no single cell type normally constitutes >40% of the total cell population. Third, the lung tissue is perfused by two very different vascular supplies: bronchial and pulmonary circulations. Finally, the normally huge perfusion (100% of cardiac output) in relation to tissue mass means that differences in metabolite concentration across the organ are difficult to measure. Despite these difficulties, considerable information has recently become available on lung metabolism. Moreover the lung presents a unique opportunity to evaluate oxidative metabolism in an intact organ in which diffusion limitation of O_2 availability is not a factor.

OXYGEN UPTAKE. The lung slice preparation has provided most of the information on tissue O_2 consumption because of the difficulties in accurately making this measurement in the intact lung. The O_2 uptake by lungs is ~1% of the total O_2 uptake (54). Because lung weight is ~0.5% of body wt, the O_2 uptake by the lungs is about twice the average O_2 consumption by body tissues. For example, O_2 consumption by the intact rat is ~60 $\mu l \cdot min^{-1} \cdot g^{-1}$ dry wt (214), whereas O_2 consumption by rat lung slices is 109 $\mu l \cdot min^{-1} \cdot g^{-1}$ dry wt [mean value of eight published reports (12, 27, 48, 49, 121, 128, 182, 185); range of mean values 48–148 $\mu l \cdot min^{-1} \cdot g^{-1}$ dry wt]. The large variations in the results are largely unexplained, although O'Neil et al. (154) described sources of variability and indicated conditions for obtaining maximal rates of O_2 uptake. Comparison of O_2 uptake by various rat organs per unit weight indicates that the lung is less active metabolically than the brain, kidney, liver, or heart but as active as the spleen, diaphragm, intestine, and pancreas (Table 1).

It has been observed that O_2 uptake by lung slices (and slices from other organs) of various mammalian species decreases in an approximately semilogarithmic relationship as a function of body weight (Fig. 3). Thus O_2 uptake by mouse lung slice is approximately twice as great per unit weight as O_2 uptake by horse or cow lung slice. This species effect for lung slices has been attributed partly to a higher proportion of slowly metabolizing connective tissue in lungs of larger animals, although differences in intrinsic metabolic rates may also be a factor. Evidence supporting the latter mechanism indicates that the volume density of mitochondria in granular pneumocytes from various species is directly proportional to O_2 consump-

TABLE 1. *Oxygen Consumption of Tissue Slices From Various Rat Organs*

	O_2 Uptake, $\mu l \cdot min^{-1} \cdot g^{-1}$ dry wt*					
	Ref. 48	Ref. 185†	Ref. 121	Ref. 27	Ref. 49	Mean
Kidney cortex	289		623	387	321	405
Brain cortex		310	429	243		327
Heart muscle				279	130	204
Liver		119	280	248	127	193
Spleen			207		124	166
Diaphragm	90	120		148		119
Intestine	116					116
Lung	129	107	140	45	96	103
Pancreas	60					60

Mean values are for selected reports including measurements with lung slices. * 1 $\mu l \cdot min^{-1} \cdot g^{-1}$ dry wt $\cong$ 0.045 $\mu mol \cdot min^{-1} \cdot g^{-1}$ dry wt $\cong$ 2.7 $\mu mol \cdot h^{-1} \cdot g^{-1}$ dry wt. † Assuming that dry/wet = 0.22.

tion by lung tissue (134). Furthermore intraspecies variation of lung metabolism may also reflect intrinsic tissue differences, as suggested by the higher O_2 consumption by lungs from waltzing as compared with normal mice (85).

The physiological factors regulating O_2 consumption by lung tissue have not been defined well. Clearly the lung has no major energy-consuming functions compared with the heart or other very metabolically active tissues. Because energy demands for lung inflation are supplied by respiratory muscles, lung ventilation per se should not increase O_2 utilization of lung tissue. Because the lung is cellularly diverse its O_2 uptake represents the aggregate contributions of the heterogeneous lung cell population. Therefore O_2 requirements for the lung are related to general cell maintenance and energy requirements for specialized functions of individual cell types. These specialized functions include tracheobronchial clearance, regulation of the distribution of air flow and blood flow, surfactant turnover, and regulation of vasoactive amine concentration in arterial blood (Table 2). Some of these energy-dependent processes may be indirectly stimulated by lung inflation, with resultant increased O_2 uptake (53).

Examination of lung ultrastructure reveals considerable disparity in the mitochondrial volume density among cell types, supporting the suggestion that O_2 uptake of different cell types varies considerably. A morphometric analysis of rat lung indicates that the fraction of cell volume accounted for by mitochondria is ~3 times greater for the granular pneumocyte compared with the combined value for endothelial cells and membranous pneumocytes (134). This observation is compatible with the presumed energy-requiring functions of the granular pneumocyte in surfactant metabolism. It seems likely that O_2 utilization by the granular pneumocytes contributes a disproportionately large share to the total O_2 uptake by the lung. Based on their functions and morphological characteristics, bronchial Clara and ciliated cells and alveolar macrophages also appear metabolically more active than the average lung cell.

ENERGY STATE AND ATP GENERATION. Coupling between O_2 consumption and energy-dependent functions is provided by lung energy stores that can be estimated from measurement of tissue adenine nucleotide content. Like other organs, adenine nucleotides in the lung are present mainly as ATP [Table 3; (13, 14, 16, 55, 61); see also Table 10 in the chapter by Tierney and Young in this *Handbook*]. The ATP content of the lung is less than that of the heart but similar to many other actively metabolizing tissues. The mean intracellular ATP concentration for rat lung is ~5 mM, assuming that intracellular H_2O is ~50% of lung wet wt. Lung tissue shows a high ATP/ADP ratio and a high energy charge, indicating that

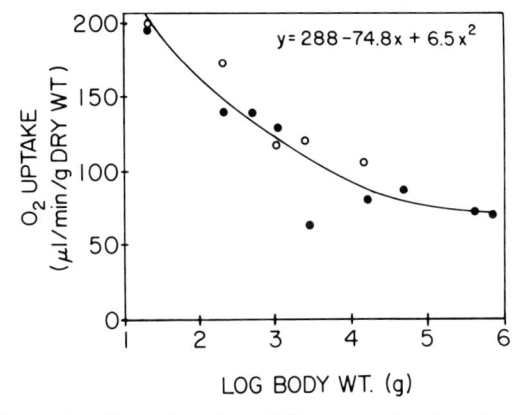

FIG. 3. O_2 uptake of lung slices from different species plotted as a function of body weight. *Closed circles*, results for mouse, rat, guinea pig, rabbit, cat, dog, sheep, cow, and horse. *Open circles*, results for mouse, rat, cat, rabbit, and dog. *Line*, least mean square regression for a second-degree polynomial ($r = 0.936$). [*Closed circles*, data from Krebs (121). *Open circles*, data from Massaro et al. (134).]

TABLE 2. *Proposed Specialized Energy-Dependent Functions of Lung Cells*

Function	Cell	Reaction	Ref.*
Secretion			
Mucus	Bronchial gland epithelium	Cytoskeletal elements	
Chloride	Tracheobronchial epithelium	Linked to Na^+-K^+-ATPase	206
Surfactant	Granular pneumocyte	Cytoskeletal elements	132
O_2^-· release	Alveolar macrophage	Activation of NADPH oxidase	35
Synthesis			
Surfactant	Granular pneumocyte	Generation of fatty acyl-CoA and CDP choline	16
Collagen	Fibroblast	Activation of amino acyl-tRNA	5
Transport			
Amine uptake	Capillary endothelium	Linked to Na^+-K^+-ATPase	108, 187
Sodium absorption	Alveolar epithelium	Linked to Na^+-K^+-ATPase	90, 133
Motility			
Phagocytosis	Alveolar macrophages	Cytoskeletal elements	155
Ciliary clearance	Ciliated bronchial cell	Actin-tubulin interaction	40
Bronchoconstriction	Bronchial smooth muscle	Actin-myosin cross-bridge cycling	188
Vasoconstriction	Vascular smooth muscle	Actin-myosin cross-bridge cycling	130

* Studies in which a presumed energy-dependent reaction has been demonstrated for the lung.

TABLE 3. *Typical Values for Adenine Nucleotide Content of Rat Organs*

	ATP	ADP	AMP	ATP/ADP	Energy Charge
	μmol/g dry wt				
Heart*	21.7	2.5	0.35	8.7	0.94
Brain	13.3	1.5	0.23	8.9	0.94
Liver	10.5	2.5	0.40	4.2	0.88
Kidney	9.7	1.7	0.35	5.7	0.90
Lung*	11.0	1.3	0.39	8.5	0.92

* Perfused organ. Other values from organs in vivo. [Lung values from Bassett and Fisher (13); other values from Williamson and Corkey (207).]

the normal balance between energy utilization and generation maintains the tissue in a highly energized state. Because the phosphate concentration in lung cells is not known, phosphate potential cannot be calculated. The concentration of phosphocreatine in the lung is 2.2 μmol per g dry wt or 20% of the ATP content (25). It is possible that the bulk of the phosphocreatine in the lung is contained in smooth muscle.

The relationship between O_2 uptake by lung tissue and mitochondrial oxidative phosphorylation and ATP synthesis has been demonstrated by measuring the metabolic response of the lung to the addition of inhibitors of mitochondrial respiration (62). In the presence of CO, cyanide, or amytal, lung content of the reduced component for several NADH-dependent reactions was increased, resulting in increased ratios of lactate/pyruvate, glycerol 3-phosphate/dihydroxyacetone phosphate, and glutamate/α-ketoglutarate. The increased ratios are compatible with the increased cellular content of reduced pyridine nucleotides due to the inhibition of their oxidation by the mitochondrial respiratory chain. Increased lung tissue NADH (measured from surface fluorescence) provided further evidence for the metabolic effect of mitochondrial inhibitors (62). Furthermore ventilation of isolated lung with CO led to a marked decrease in glucose oxidation and tissue content of ATP and ATP/ADP, whereas perfusion with an uncoupler of oxidative phosphorylation (dinitrophenol) resulted in a large increase of glucose oxidation but decreased cellular ATP and ATP/ADP (13, 14).

Alveolar hypoxia also results in a shift of the lung's pyridine nucleotide redox state toward reduction and decreased tissue ATP content. However, these effects are more difficult to demonstrate than the effects with mitochondrial inhibitors because of the difficulties in producing sufficiently low alveolar P_{O_2} for inhibition of the respiratory chain. Because of the high affinity of cytochrome c oxidase for O_2, severe alveolar hypoxia is required to inhibit oxidative phosphorylation (61). For the isolated lung the alveolar P_{O_2} required to produce 50% of the maximal increase in glycolysis (defined by the response to CO) is ~0.055 mmHg P_{O_2}, and no major change in metabolic parameters is seen until the alveolar P_{O_2} approaches 1 mmHg (Fig. 4).

Lung ATP content (Fig. 5) and ATP/ADP are also unaffected until P_{O_2} is reduced to these low values (61). These extremely low values for P_{O_2} cannot occur in the normal lung because severe systemic hypoxemia would preclude survival of the organism. Thus lung cells, by virtue of the short diffusion distances in the lung and the large reservoir of O_2 at relatively constant P_{O_2} in the alveolar space, can maintain normal metabolic function even in the presence of marked alveolar hypoxia. The critical P_{O_2} for the intact perfused lung is intermediate between values obtained with isolated mitochondria and isolated cells from various sources.

Relative contributions of cytoplasmic and mitochondrial pathways to overall ATP production by the lung have been estimated by tracing the metabolism of radiolabeled glucose. Mitochondrial pathways [pyruvate dehydrogenase (cytochrome) and tricarboxylic cycle] accounted for 86% of total ATP produced from glucose by normal isolated perfused rat lung (Table 4). With inhibition of the mitochondrial respiratory chain by CO, cytoplasmic ATP production increased threefold, but cellular ATP concentration was not maintained at normal levels (13). Thus substrate-level phosphorylation in the cytoplasm can compensate only partly for inhibition of lung mitochondrial function.

Shuttle mechanisms used by the lung for transport of reducing equivalents between cytoplasmic and mitochondrial spaces have not been well characterized, although it is likely that both the glycerol 3-phosphate–dihydroxyacetone phosphate and the aspartate-malate shuttles are operative. Evidence for this comes from several sources. Isolated rat lungs perfused with a transaminase inhibitor (aminooxyacetic acid) show

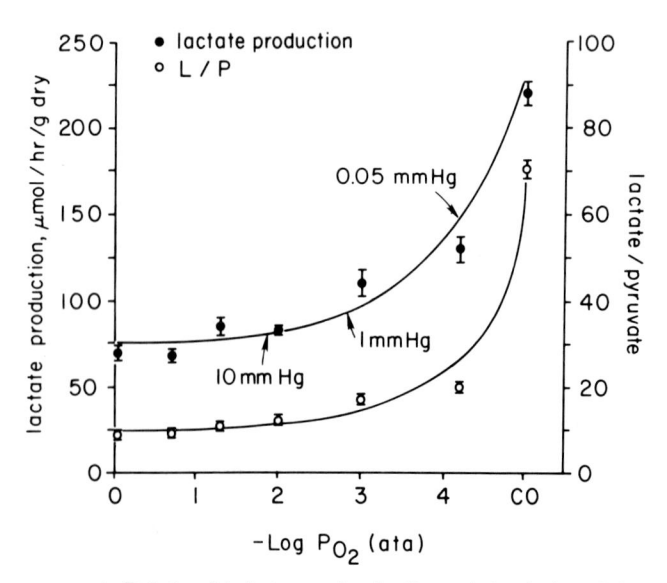

FIG. 4. Relationship between alveolar P_{O_2} and glycolytic activity of the isolated perfused rat lung. Lactate (L) production and lactate to pyruvate (P) ratios are plotted as a function of log P_{O_2}. Arrows, approximate values for alveolar P_{O_2} of 10 mmHg, 1 mmHg, and 0.05 mmHg. [Data from Fisher and Dodia (61).]

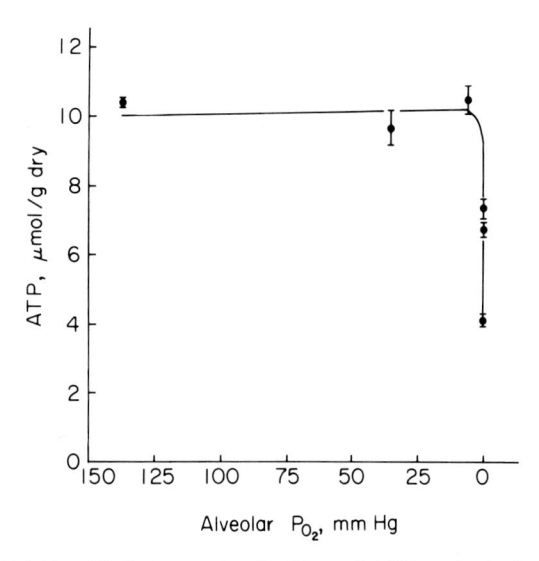

FIG. 5. Relationship between alveolar P_{O_2} and ATP content of isolated perfused rat lung. Effect of hypoxia on lung ATP content occurs well below the physiological range of alveolar P_{O_2}. [Data from Fisher and Dodia (61).]

TABLE 4. *Effect of Mitochondrial Inhibition on ATP Content and Generation of ATP in Cytoplasmic and Mitochondrial Compartments by Perfused Rat Lung*

	ATP Content, μmol/g dry wt	ATP Synthesis,* μmol·h^{-1}·g^{-1} dry wt		
		Cyto	Mito	Total
Control	10.4	45	267	312
CO†	4.9	135	49	184

* Estimated from production rates for lactate, pyruvate, and CO_2 from glucose. Cyto, substrate-level phosphorylation in cytoplasm; mito, pyruvate dehydrogenase and tricarboxylic acid cycle reactions; total = cyto + mito.   † Lungs were ventilated with 95% CO-5% CO_2. [Data calculated from Bassett and Fisher (13).]

increased lactate-to-pyruvate production ratios, suggesting interference with the malate-aspartate shuttle, which depends on transamination (62). The presence of both mitochondrial and cytoplasmic glycerol 3-phosphate dehydrogenases in lung cells provides enzyme systems required for the glycerol 3-phosphate shuttle (60, 63, 67, 145). The K_m for glycerol 3-phosphate oxidation by lung mitochondria is ~0.6 mM (63), whereas the intracellular concentration of the substrate in normal isolated rat lungs is ~0.5 mM (62). Therefore this pathway should be operative. Activity of mitochondrial glycerol 3-phosphate dehydrogenase is modulated by external calcium ion concentration over a range (~10^{-7}–10^{-9} M) that may approximate physiological values for intracellular concentration of this ion [Fig. 6; (67)]. Consequently Ca^{2+} may regulate activity of the glycerol 3-phosphate–dihydroxyacetone phosphate shuttle for the intramitochondrial transfer of reducing equivalents and thereby help coordinate cytoplasmic and mitochondrial ATP synthesis.

LUNG MITOCHONDRIA. Preparations of intact respiring mitochondria from the lung have been used to evaluate substrate utilization and metabolic requirements of these organelles (63, 67, 124, 145, 167, 177, 184). Characteristics of lung mitochondrial preparations are qualitatively comparable with those from other tissues. Furthermore lung mitochondria from a variety of mammalian species indicate generally similar properties (63): lung mitochondria generate ATP, show O_2 consumption linked to oxidative phosphorylation, and demonstrate energy-dependent accumulation of divalent cations (67). Oxygen concentration does not become rate limiting for O_2 uptake until medium concentration is in the range of 1 μM, indicating high affinity of the mitochondrial cytochrome c oxidase for O_2 (67). Lung mitochondria have the enzymes that are required to oxidize a wide variety of substrates, including pyruvate, fatty acids, tricarboxylic acid cycle intermediates (e.g., succinate, malate, isocitrate, and α-ketoglutarate), glutamate (indicating the presence of transamination pathways), and glycerol 3-phosphate. Ketone bodies (acetoacetate, β-hydroxybutyrate) are relatively poor substrates, at least for rat lung mitochondria (67, 145), but may be oxidized more readily by mitochondria from lungs of other species (63). Although rates of substrate oxidation, degree of coupling between oxidation and phosphorylation, and content of cytochromes with mitochondrial preparations from the lung have been somewhat less than those observed with preparations from the liver, the difference may be related primarily to the greater contamination of lung preparations with nonmitochondrial protein and the greater difficulty in homogenizing the lung. Recently methods were described to obtain lung mitochondria with a relatively

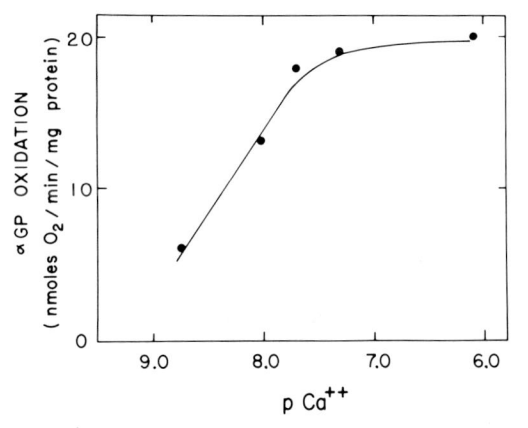

FIG. 6. Relationship between concentration of free Ca^{2+} in incubation medium and rate of glycerol 3-phosphate oxidation by isolated rat lung mitochondria. Glycerol 3-phosphate concentration was 3 mM. Free Ca^{2+} is plotted as minus log free Ca^{2+} (p Ca^{++}). [From Fisher et al. (67). Copyright 1973 American Chemical Society.]

high degree of coupling between oxidation and phosphorylation (184). Preparations and properties of lung mitochondria are discussed in greater detail in the chapter by Tierney and Young in this *Handbook*.

OXYGEN-DEPENDENT METABOLIC REACTIONS

Pathways of O_2 Utilization

Although the cytochrome c oxidase reaction of the mitochondria accounts for the greatest fraction of O_2 utilization in most cells, a wide variety of other metabolic reactions utilize O_2 as a reactant. Mason classified over 200 oxidases into three general groups of reactions, as reviewed in the chapter by Jöbsis (104) in the 1964 edition of the *Handbook* section on respiration and more recently by Keevil and Mason (112). These general groups are O_2 transferases (dioxygenases), in which the O_2 molecule is incorporated into the substrate; electron-transfer oxidases, in which the O_2 is reduced to superoxide anion ($O_2^-\cdot$), hydrogen peroxide (H_2O_2), or H_2O; and the mixed-function oxidases, which share the properties of the other two groups (one atom of the O_2 molecule is incorporated into the substrate while the other atom is reduced). Examples of these reactions are illustrated in Table 5.

In most cells the electron-transfer reactions quantitatively account for the bulk of O_2 consumption because this category includes reduction of O_2 to H_2O by mitochondrial cytochrome c oxidase. Other electron-transfer enzymes include urate oxidase, which generates H_2O_2, and plasma membrane NADPH oxidase of phagocytic cells, which generates $O_2^-\cdot$. A special class in this category is illustrated by amine oxidase (flavin-containing), which results in transfer of electrons to a nucleotide acceptor and incorporation of O_2 derived from H_2O into the substrate.

Mixed-function oxidase reactions require one or more cosubstrates in addition to O_2 and the organic substrate. The reactions catalyzed by these enzymes result in the incorporation of O_2 into the organic product with concomitant production of H_2O and oxidation of the cosubstrate (most commonly NADPH). Examples are cytochrome P-450–dependent steroid (or drug) hydroxylases and demethylases (88) and phenylalanine 4-monooxygenase, which generates tyrosine. Another group of mixed-function oxidases uses ascorbate instead of NADPH as cosubstrate. An example is dopamine β-monooxygenase, which converts dopamine to norepinephrine (110). The mixed-function prolyl and lysyl hydroxylases that generate peptide-bound hydroxyproline and hydroxylysine use α-ketoglutarate plus CoA as cosubstrates (163).

Dioxygenases incorporate O_2 into an organic product without production of additional reduced O_2 products. For example, tryptophan 2,3-dioxygenase oxidizes tryptophan to formylkynurenine (O_2 is incorporated into both aldehyde and keto groups in the product), and cyclooxygenase oxidizes arachidonic acid to an unstable cyclic O_2 adduct in the first oxidative step in the production of prostaglandins.

The prosthetic cofactors that participate in oxygenase reactions by binding O_2 and serving to transfer electrons have been classified into four groups: copper-containing sites, iron-porphyrin sites, nonheme-iron sites, and flavin sites, including the similar tetrahydrobiopterin, a pteridine derivative (112). Nonheme iron can serve as a prosthetic group through iron bound directly to protein amino acid moieties or in an iron-sulfur center in which iron is bound to inorganic sulfur. The cofactors that participate in the mitochondrial electron-transport chain have been described in Figure 1. The cytochrome P-450–containing mixed-function oxidases actually are composed of a small version of an electron-transport chain (Fig. 7). The enzymes xanthine oxidase (dehydrogenase) and aldehyde oxidase are flavoproteins that also require molybdenum and an iron-sulfur center for their catalytic function (164, 165). Dopamine β-monooxygenase and prolyl hydroxylase contain, respectively, copper and nonheme iron as the prosthetic group (110, 117). Phenylalanine hydroxylase requires participation of

TABLE 5. *Classification and Examples of O_2-Dependent Oxidoreductase Reactions*

Type	Example	Reaction
Oxidase (electron-transfer oxidase)	Cytochrome c oxidase	$2Fe^{2+}Cyt\ ox + \frac{1}{2}O_2 + 2H^+ \rightarrow 2Fe^{3+}Cyt\ ox + H_2O$
	Urate oxidase	Urate + H_2O + O_2 $\rightarrow$ allantoin + CO_2 + H_2O_2
	NADPH oxidase*	NADPH + $2O_2$ $\rightarrow$ NADP$^+$ + H$^+$ + $2O_2^-\cdot$
	Amine oxidase, flavin-containing	5-Hydroxytryptamine + FAD + H_2O $\rightarrow$ 5-hydroxyindoleacetaldehyde + FADH$_2$ + NH$_3$
Hydroxylase (mixed-function oxidase)	Phenylalanine 4-monooxygenase	L-Phenylalanine + O_2 + NADPH + H$^+$ $\rightarrow$ L-tyrosine + NADP$^+$ + H_2O
	Cytochrome P-450–linked demethylase	p-Nitroanisole + O_2 + NADPH + H$^+$ $\rightarrow$ p-nitrophenol + NADP$^+$ + HCHO + H_2O
	Prolyl hydroxylase	Peptide-proline + O_2 + α-ketoglutarate + CoA $\rightarrow$ peptide-4-OHproline + succinyl-CoA + CO_2 + H_2O
	Dopamine β-hydroxylase	Dopamine + 2 ascorbate + O_2 $\rightarrow$ norepinephrine + 2 semidehydroascorbate + H_2O
Dioxygenase (O_2 transferase)	Tryptophan 2,3-dioxygenase	L-Tryptophan + O_2 $\rightarrow$ N-formyl-L-kynurenine
	Cyclooxygenase	Arachidonic acid + O_2 $\rightarrow$ arachidonate endoperoxide

Cyt ox, cytochrome oxidase.   * Plasma membrane enzyme of phagocytic cells.

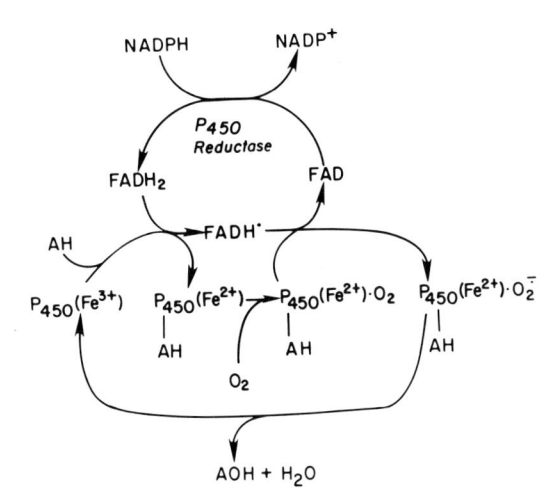

FIG. 7. Scheme for mixed-function oxidation by cytochrome P-450 system. Flow of electrons from NADPH to O_2 and an organic substrate (AH_2) through the NADPH–cytochrome P-450 reductase–cytochrome P-450 complex.

biopterin (110). The common role for these cofactors is their ability to undergo cyclic oxidation and reduction.

Like most enzymes, oxygenases can be competitively inhibited by analogues of their organic substrates or noncompetitively inhibited by substances that bind in positions other than the active site. Oxygenases are unique because they may be strongly inhibited by small molecules or ions such as CO, cyanide, or sulfite, depending on the relative affinities of the cofactor in the enzyme for O_2 versus these inhibitors. This property of the oxygenases results from their necessary interaction with O_2, which requires either a transition metal or a highly efficient electron-transferring cofactor like flavin. Because of the large variation in the reactions catalyzed by oxygenases with the same or similar cofactors, these inhibitors exhibit essentially no specificity despite their considerable potency.

Non-ATP-generating oxidases and oxygenases catalyze important cellular functions, although their overall contribution to O_2 uptake is relatively small. Their quantitative contribution has been estimated by measuring O_2 uptake in the presence of an inhibitor of cytochrome c oxidase–dependent O_2 uptake (e.g., cyanide). Although cyanide-insensitive respiration approximates O_2 utilization by non–cytochrome c oxidase pathways, quantitation is imprecise: 1) cyanide may inhibit other oxygenases, and 2) the altered energy state and inhibition of cytochrome c oxidase may modify other pathways. For example, the rate of ubiquinone reduction and autoxidation may be accelerated (with an increased rate of $O_2^-\cdot$ generation) when cytochrome c oxidase is inhibited (69). Cyanide-insensitive respiration has been estimated at 14% of total O_2 utilization in lung homogenates, similar to values obtained with liver homogenates (172).

Pulmonary O_2-Dependent Metabolic Reactions

Some physiologically important oxygenases in the lung include cytochrome P-450–linked monooxygenases, which are important for metabolism of steroids and drug detoxification; amine oxidase (flavin-containing), important for metabolism of vasoactive amines (see the chapter by Junod in this *Handbook*); prolyl and lysyl hydroxylases, for synthesis of connective tissue components (see the chapter by Massaro in this *Handbook*); cyclo- and lipoxygenases, for synthesis of eicosanoids (see the chapter by Bakhle and Ferreira in this *Handbook*); and NADPH oxidase, for bactericidal activity (see the chapter by Brain in this *Handbook*).

CYTOCHROME P-450–LINKED MONOOXYGENASE. Cytochrome P-450 refers to a group of enzymes that use NADPH as a cofactor while O_2 is both incorporated into substrate and reduced to H_2O (i.e., mixed-function oxidation). This enzyme system shows activity toward a wide variety of organic substrates, and common reactions include hydroxylation, *N*-oxidation, sulfoxidation, and dealkylation (of both *O*- and *N*-alkyl groups) (88). The *N*-oxidation (e.g., oxidation of tertiary amines to *N*-oxides) may also occur in lungs (and other tissues) by non–cytochrome P-450 pathways (45, 131). The dealkylation reactions result in generation of an aldehyde product from the alkyl side chain, as illustrated by *p*-nitroanisole demethylase (Table 5). Common substrates for these reactions include aryl hydrocarbons [aryl hydrocarbon hydroxylase (88)], steroids [steroid hydroxylase (178)], and possibly unsaturated fatty acids (28). Physiologically this system is of major importance in adrenal glands (178), where it functions in steroid biosynthesis, and in the liver, where hydroxylation of hydrocarbons results in increased H_2O solubility, facilitating their excretion (88). The enzymes for this system are generally located in the endoplasmic reticulum.

The binding of O_2 to the heme of cytochrome P-450 is affected by both the oxidation and spin state of the heme iron (205). Oxygen will not bind to oxidized cytochrome P-450 (Fe^{3+}) whether substrate is present or not. In the reduced state, substrates alter the spin state, which markedly enhances the affinity for O_2. The amount of this enhancement and consequently the affinity for O_2 should depend on the substrate. This can explain the observation that the K_m for O_2 for the enzyme from *Pseudomonas putida* or mammalian liver varies severalfold with different substrates (18, 107).

The lung is one of the major extrahepatic sites of cytochrome P-450 activity (54, 158). However, activity in the lung is only 5%–10% per unit weight of the corresponding value for liver and compared with the liver shows relatively limited inducibility during pretreatment of the animal with most drug substrates (17, 158). [An exception is aryl hydrocarbon hydroxylase activity, which may be induced up to 15-fold in rat lung microsomes by pretreatment with 3-methylcholanthrene (135).] Because normal liver weight is about three times lung weight, the contribution of the lungs to total body cytochrome P-450 activity is negligible. Nevertheless the role of the lung in metabolism may be selectively important for those agents that reach the lung directly from the airways by inhalation or through the pulmonary circulation after injection or absorption through the skin. Furthermore for some chemicals (e.g., benzphetamine, benzene, and p-xylene) the specific oxidase activity of lung cytochrome P-450 (per unit microsomal protein) exceeds that of the liver enzyme (158).

The general characteristics of lung and liver enzyme systems are similar regarding cosubstrate (NADPH) and flavin (NADPH–cytochrome c reductase) requirements, localization to the endoplasmic reticulum, and inhibition by CO and metyrapone (17, 99, 158, 159, 212). At least two isoenzymes of the cytochrome P-450 class are identified in the lung. One appears similar to phenobarbital-inducible cytochrome P-450 of the liver (179, 212, 213). Specific drugs metabolized by the intact lung include methadone, pentobarbital, lidocaine, carbaryl, and several steroids (e.g., testosterone, cortisone) (20, 96, 127, 148, 156, 162). Oxidation of a broad range of other chemicals has also been demonstrated with the intact lung or lung microsomal preparations (158).

Metabolic characteristics of the P-450–linked mixed-function oxidation reaction in the intact system have been studied with isolated perfused rabbit or rat lung (101). Maximal activity of the enzyme requires glucose, presumably to provide NADPH through reactions of the pentose shunt pathway (66). Mitochondrial substrates can substitute for glucose, suggesting a role for the intramitochondrial energy-linked transhydrogenation reaction in the generation of cytoplasmic reducing equivalents (66). The lung enzyme with p-nitroanisole as a model substrate has a high affinity for O_2, and the reaction rate is decreased by 50% only when the alveolar P_{O_2} is reduced to ~0.3 mmHg (65). The enzyme is inhibited by CO (competitively with O_2), and the reaction rate is decreased by 50% when the ratio of CO to O_2 is 0.5 (65). This contrasts with the mitochondrial respiratory chain, where 50% inhibition of respiration requires a CO-to-O_2 ratio of ~15 (61).

The principal sites of cytochrome P-450 activity have been identified in rabbit lung as the nonciliated, bronchiolar, epithelial cell (Clara cell) and the cuboidal, alveolar, epithelial cell (granular pneumocyte or type II cell) (46, 180). Although the Clara cell has higher specific activity, the type II cell may contribute more to the overall lung activity because of its greater cell number. There is little activity in alveolar macrophages (64, 98).

The precise role for the cytochrome P-450 system in the lung has not been defined. The most likely physiological role is a metabolic one, perhaps related to metabolism of steroids and/or unsaturated fatty acids or detoxification of inhaled agents. The suggestion that cytochrome P-450 facilitates transport of O_2 through lung cells (92) is unconvincing because of the high affinity of the cytochrome P-450–substrate complex for O_2, and the dissociation of molecular O_2 from the cytochrome P-450–substrate complex would be negligible because of the rapid incorporation of O_2 into the product (205). Furthermore oxidized cytochrome P-450 (Fe^{3+}) does not bind O_2, and the enzyme reduced in the absence of substrate does not reversibly release molecular O_2 but rather decomposes slowly to the Fe^{3+} form with the release of $O_2^-\cdot$ (178). Involvement of cytochrome P-450 in hypoxic pulmonary vasoconstriction has also been proposed based on inhibition of vasoconstriction in the presence of inhibitors of cytochrome P-450 activity (139, 194). It seems likely that the high affinity of cytochrome P-450 for O_2 precludes a function as an O_2 sensor for this system but does not rule out the possibility that the true sensor or transducer of the hypoxic effect is activated through metabolism by the cytochrome P-450 system.

From a toxicological standpoint the cytochrome P-450 system may be important in the lung, because it can generate carcinogenic or toxic agents from less reactive compounds (23, 44, 166, 203). Thus pulmonary toxicity of some organic compounds may be directly related to their metabolic activation.

INACTIVATION OF VASOACTIVE AMINES. Pulmonary endothelium can accumulate both 5-hydroxytryptamine (5-HT) and norepinephrine by an active transport process that may serve to regulate arterial concentration of these amines (100, 108, 187). Intracellularly the amines are metabolized through a series of reactions catalyzed by oxidases to produce biologically inactive products. The 5-HT is converted by amine oxidase (flavin-containing) to 5-hydroxyindoleacetaldehyde and then by aldehyde oxidase to 5-hydroxyindoleacetic acid (5-HIAA). These enzymes, which are located in the outer membranes of mitochondria, transfer electrons to FAD. The O_2 that is incorporated into products is derived from H_2O. Molecular O_2 is used in these overall reactions to reoxidize the flavin cofactor with production of H_2O_2. The net reaction is O_2-dependent oxidation of 5-HT to 5-HIAA plus NH_3. This enzyme system oxidizes norepinephrine to vanillylmandelic acid. Lungs also contain the isoenzyme of amine oxidase (flavin-containing type B) that shows specificity for phenylethylamine (11, 173).

SYNTHESIS OF CONNECTIVE TISSUE COMPONENTS. Lung fibroblasts or fibroblast-like cells synthesize and secrete the interstitial tissue components (principally collagen and elastin) that account largely for the lung's elastic properties (95). Furthermore lung epithelial and probably endothelial cells synthesize type IV collagen as a component of their basement membranes (175). A requisite step in biosynthesis of collagen is the hydroxylation of prolyl and lysyl residues in the collagen fragments (163). These reactions are catalyzed by three mixed-function oxidases that utilize α-ketoglutarate plus CoA as a source of reducing potential (see *Pathways of O_2 Utilization*, p. 240). Ascorbate is also necessary for these reactions to maintain the prosthetic Fe^{2+} in the reduced state. The enzymes involved are prolyl-4-hydroxylase, prolyl-3-hydroxylase, and lysyl hydroxylase; these enzymes generate peptide-bound 4-hydroxyproline, 3-hydroxyproline, and hydroxylysine, respectively. If activity of these enzymes is inhibited (e.g., by lack of O_2 as substrate), the collagen molecules generated do not form a stable triple helix and remain in a gelatinlike state (163). The alveolar P_{O_2} at which proline hydroxylation in the lung is decreased by 50% has been estimated at 5 mmHg (5).

The extracellular processing of collagen (and elastin) fibrils to form the mature protein requires activity of lysyl oxidase, a copper-containing enzyme of the oxidase (flavin-containing) class (163). This deaminating enzyme generates in some lysine and hydroxylysine residues an aldehyde group that is required for the cross-linking reaction.

SYNTHESIS OF EICOSANOIDS. Lung tissue synthesizes prostaglandins, thromboxanes, and leukotrienes, and they appear in the lung effluent (see the chapter by Bakhle and Ferreira in this *Handbook*). The precise physiological roles for pumonary synthesis are still under investigation, but it may be involved in regulation of bronchomotor and vasomotor tone as well as hemofluidity (e.g., platelet adhesion). The synthesis of prostaglandins and thromboxanes requires formation of an endoperoxide peroxide free-radical intermediate from arachidonic acid through two sequential dioxygenase reactions catalyzed by a cyclooxygenase (prostaglandin synthase). This intermediate is reduced (possibly with glutathione and glutathione peroxidase) to produce endoperoxide and peroxide derivatives, including prostaglandins H_2, E_2, and $F_{2\alpha}$. Lipoxygenase (another dioxygenase) generates 12-L-hydroperoxy-5, 8,10,14-eicosatetraenoic acid (12-HPETE) or the 5-hydroperoxides, which then give rise to leukotrienes.

BACTERICIDAL ACTIVITY. The plasma membranes of phagocytes, including alveolar macrophages, contain a flavoprotein NADPH oxidase that catalyzes the oxidation of NADPH with reduction of O_2 to $O_2^-\cdot$ (74, 84). Activity of this enzyme can be readily demonstrated after stimulation of the plasma membrane with various agents. This phenomenon is termed *respiratory burst* because it is manifested by increased O_2 uptake. Activation of the oxidase requires receptor binding and is energy dependent (35). The mechanism that mediates the respiratory burst may involve membrane depolarization, Ca^{2+} mobilization, and calmodulin binding (129, 138). Physiologically this process is associated with recognition of a target agent. The superoxide produced during phagocytosis may mediate microbicidal activity (105).

OXYGEN TOXICITY

Pathological Effects of O_2

GENERAL ASPECTS OF TOXICITY. The metabolism of O_2 for generation of ATP and oxidation of cellular components is necessary for mammalian life. This dependence on O_2 is not without risk because O_2 is a toxin that can cause pulmonary damage and death at concentrations not even 1 order of magnitude higher than normal. The manifestations of O_2 toxicity have been presented in detail in the chapter by Davies and Davies (41) and the chapter by Lambertsen (125) in the 1965 edition of this *Handbook* section on respiration and several recent reviews (33, 56, 97, 126, 137, 146, 211). This chapter presents recent developments related to pathophysiology, emphasizing proposed mechanisms for O_2 toxicity and the mechanisms used by cells to cope with this hazard. The focus is on the lung, although other organs are susceptible to O_2 poisoning and at O_2 pressures >2.5 ATA, central nervous system (CNS) manifestations predominate.

PULMONARY O_2 TOXICITY. The lungs are the major site of damage during breathing of O_2 at normobaric pressures. This likely reflects the direct exposure of lung cells to relatively high alveolar P_{O_2} (in contrast to most systemic organs, where mean P_{O_2} is considerably lower) rather than an intrinsic sensitivity of these cells to O_2. Overt pulmonary damage occurs at ~0.6 ATA O_2, although individual susceptibility may vary greatly and more subtle pulmonary changes may occur at lower P_{O_2}. If sensitivity to O_2 damage is expressed as time to death during exposure to a fixed concentration of O_2, species susceptibility shows wide variation. For example, the time to death for 50% of normal adult animals exposed to 1 ATA O_2 is ~72 h for most laboratory species, whereas primates may survive for up to 7 days (33). However, the mean lethal concentration of O_2 for all species probably lies between 0.8 and 1.2 ATA O_2, suggesting that differences in species susceptibility to O_2 are relatively trivial.

Apparently the earliest manifestation of pulmonary toxicity during O_2 exposure is tracheobronchitis related to the interactions of O_2 with the tracheobronchial mucosa. The associated physiological alterations are decreased tracheobronchial clearance and (in studies with humans) chest pain, cough, and decreased vital capacity (33, 174). These changes occur within the initial 24 h of breathing 1 ATA O_2.

In the approximate period between 24 and 48 h of exposure to 100% O_2, functional and morphological changes occur in cells of the alveolar septum. Alveolar macrophages show decreased capacity to develop a respiratory burst and impairment of chemotaxis and phagocytosis (76, 169, 170). Pulmonary endothelium shows decreased capacity to remove amines from perfusate (21, 47, 59) and swelling and blebbing of endothelial cell membranes (36, 116). Membranous (type I) epithelium develops ultrastructural alterations that generally follow and are less prominent than endothelial changes but may be more extensive, depending on species and exposure conditions (109). However, granular pneumocytes (type II epithelium) are relatively resistant to the toxic effects of O_2. Ultrastructural changes that have been described for type II cell mitochondria and lamellar bodies generally appear relatively late (2) or may be adaptive rather than toxic (171).

Between 48 and 72 h of O_2 exposure, cellular changes progress and areas of capillary endothelium and alveolar epithelium may be denuded (36, 109, 116). Apparently cell division at this state is inhibited (52). These cellular changes are accompanied by fluid accumulation in the interstitium, physiological alterations in lung compliance and gas transfer, and infiltration of polymorphonuclear leukocytes and macrophages. Death at ~72 h is generally ascribed to pulmonary edema and respiratory failure.

With exposure to sublethal concentrations of O_2, repair processes and chronic pulmonary changes are superimposed on the changes of acute injury. In addition to cellular toxicity and subacute lung edema, this stage is characterized by cellular proliferation (22, 94). Proliferation of interstitial fibroblasts and increased collagen formation are prominent (36, 201). Proliferation of granular pneumocytes occurs to restore the epithelial surface (1, 2, 52). Endothelial regeneration may also occur (22). These repair processes are presumably similar to those that occur after other acute injuries to the alveolar septum.

Mechanisms of O_2 Toxicity

FREE-RADICAL PRODUCTION. Evidence has now accumulated to implicate by-products of O_2 metabolism rather than the O_2 molecule as the toxic agent. The nature of these products was initially obscure because studies on O_2 metabolism were focused on its complete reduction to H_2O. Subsequently the two-electron reduction product, H_2O_2, was shown to be the primary product of some cellular reactions and was proposed as the major mediator of O_2-induced tissue damage (30). Recently attention has been directed toward the cellular production of $O_2^-\cdot$, the one-electron reduction product of O_2. (Actually O_2 reacts more readily through one-electron or free-radical processes than through direct two-electron transfer reactions because of the relatively long duration in the high-energy transition state required to invert the spin of one electron.) Protonation of $O_2^-\cdot$ generates the hydroperoxy radical ($HO_2\cdot$). Furthermore secondary reactions involving these primary products may generate hydroxyl radical ($HO\cdot$) or singlet O_2 (O_2^*). The $O_2^-\cdot$, $HO_2\cdot$, and $HO\cdot$ are free radicals (i.e., their outer orbital has an unpaired electron). The O_2^* is a higher-energy form of molecular O_2 resulting from spin inversion of one electron in the outer orbital. The relationship of these species is shown in Figure 8. The O_2^*, $HO_2\cdot$, and $HO\cdot$ are extremely potent electrophiles that through interaction with tissue components can result in chain free-radical reactions and subsequent tissue damage. These concepts form the basis for the free-radical theory of O_2 toxicity first proposed by Gerschman (87), who noted the similarity of tissue effects from X irradiation and elevated P_{O_2}.

Earlier in this chapter (see *Pathways of O_2 Utilization*, p. 240) some of the enzymatic reactions that produce $O_2^-\cdot$ and H_2O_2 through direct one- and two-electron reduction were presented. The $O_2^-\cdot$ is also produced through autoxidation of cellular components such as epinephrine (141), sulfhydryl compounds (140), and ubisemiquinone (69)

$$UQ^-\cdot + O_2 \rightarrow UQ + O_2^-\cdot \qquad (11)$$

The $O_2^-\cdot$ has a pK of 4.8 so that the steady-state concentration of the protonated relative to the nonprotonated form is <1% at physiological pH. Dismutation of superoxide generates H_2O_2

$$2O_2^-\cdot + 2H^+ \rightarrow H_2O_2 + O_2 \qquad (12)$$

This is a spontaneous reaction that can be greatly accelerated by superoxide dismutases (see ENZYMATIC DEFENSES, p. 246). The reactions that may generate $HO\cdot$ in the cell have not been well defined. Those that have been proposed are part of the Haber-Weiss (93) cycle

$$O_2^-\cdot + Fe^{3+}X \rightarrow O_2 + Fe^{2+}X \qquad (13)$$
$$Fe^{2+}X + H_2O_2 + H^+ \rightarrow Fe^{3+}X + H_2O + HO\cdot \qquad (14)$$

where X is a chelator of iron. There is debate about the requirement of $O_2^-\cdot$ for generation of $HO\cdot$, as other reductants can reduce iron. Possible mechanisms for producing O_2^* are even less certain, but $O_2^-\cdot$ participation as an intermediate has been proposed (114).

Potential subcellular sites for production of O_2-reduction products include cytoplasm and several organelles. Potential sources in the cytoplasmic compartment include soluble oxidases, such as xanthine oxidase and autoxidizable catechols. In the endoplasmic reticulum, $O_2^-\cdot$ production may result largely from leakage of electrons from the enzyme-substrate complex of cytochrome P-450 [see Fig. 3; (192)]. Apparently mitochondrial $O_2^-\cdot$ production is primarily due to autoxidation of ubisemiquinone (69). Peroxisomes generate H_2O_2 primarily by the urate oxidase reaction. The $HO\cdot$ is presumably generated where the concentrations of $O_2^-\cdot$ and H_2O_2 are greatest, near their production sites. Recently research on pulmonary O_2 toxicity has focused on the extracellular generation of $O_2^-\cdot$ by phagocytes (polymorphonuclear leukocytes and pulmonary macrophages) as a manifestation of the respiratory burst (79). Although this mechanism would increase the total oxidant load in the lung, this is apparently not as important as intracellular reactions (89).

The free-radical theory of O_2 toxicity predicts that $O_2^-\cdot$ production is increased with elevated P_{O_2}. Although many oxygenases are saturated by O_2 in normoxia, some have affinities for O_2 in the range where elevated P_{O_2} would increase the rate of O_2 reaction (83). Perhaps more significant is that autoxidation rates yielding $O_2^-\cdot$ increase proportionately with P_{O_2}. For example, the rate of mitochondrial production of $O_2^-\cdot$ is proportional to P_{O_2} (69). In recent studies with isolated organelles from lung, cyanide-insensitive respiration is used as an index of potential $O_2^-\cdot$ production and indicated that increased $O_2^-\cdot$ generation as a function of P_{O_2} is primarily mitochondrial in origin (199, 200).

OXIDATION OF TISSUE COMPONENTS. Presumably the mechanisms of tissue damage in O_2 toxicity involve interaction of O_2-reduction products with tissue components. Lipids and proteins may be the primary targets, but oxidation of nucleic acid bases and carbohydrates may also occur. Oxygen (i.e., ground state or triplet O_2) is relatively unreactive, as indicated by the large positive free-energy change for reduction. However, both $O_2^-\cdot$ and H_2O_2 may be involved in the oxidation of cellular constituents and the generation of more potent oxidizing agents. Because $O_2^-\cdot$ is a negatively charged electrophile, its reactivity is limited by electrostatic repulsion. However, electrically neutral $HO_2\cdot$ is more reactive, so that essentially all oxidation by $O_2^-\cdot$ may be through its protonated form (86). Although intracellular concentration of $HO\cdot$ and O_2^* is extremely low, their great reactivity as electrophiles ensures almost complete efficiency in their oxidation reactions.

$$O_2 + e^- \longrightarrow O_2^-$$

$$O_2^- + e^- + 2H^+ \longrightarrow H_2O_2$$

$$H_2O_2 + e^- + H^+ \longrightarrow HO\cdot + H_2O$$

$$HO\cdot + e^- + H^+ \longrightarrow H_2O$$

$$O_2 + 22\text{ kcal} \longrightarrow O_2^*$$

FIG. 8. Relationships of active O_2 species formed from reduction of molecular O_2. Electrons, if added one at a time, result in sequential formation of superoxide ($O_2^-\cdot$), hydrogen peroxide (H_2O_2), hydroxyl radical ($HO\cdot$), and finally H_2O. Addition of 22 kcal of energy to O_2 (e.g., through photoactivation with methylene blue) can form metastable singlet oxygen (O_2^*). Not shown are protonation of $O_2^-\cdot$ to form hydroperoxy radical ($HO_2\cdot$) or addition of 37 kcal to O_2 to form a higher but very labile O_2^* state.

Lipid peroxidation. The combination of $O_2^-\cdot$ and H_2O_2 has been shown in model systems to peroxidize lipids, but details of the process remain controversial (113, 157). Initiation of lipid peroxidation requires iron (157) and may involve formation of $HO\cdot$

$$RH + HO\cdot \xrightarrow{Fe^{2+}} R\cdot + H_2O \qquad (15)$$

In some lipid peroxidation systems there is no evidence of $HO\cdot$ involvement (10), but ferryl-iron complexes have been proposed as the initiator. Singlet O_2 can also initiate lipid peroxidation in model systems, although its physiological role is controversial. Recent studies suggest that $HO_2\cdot$ reacts specifically with polyunsaturated fatty acids (PUFA) (required structure: —CH=CH—CH=CH—), whereas $O_2^-\cdot$ is unreactive (19). The second-order rate constant for the reaction of $HO_2\cdot$ with the methylene group is $\sim 10^3 \cdot M^{-1}\cdot s^{-1}$ for each reactive site. For comparison, rate constants for reactions with unsaturated lipids are $\sim 10^9 \cdot M^{-1}\cdot s^{-1}$ for $HO\cdot$ and $\sim 10^6 \cdot M^{-1}\cdot s^{-1}$ for O_2^* (111).

Propagation of lipid peroxidation may involve a cyclic process in which RH (a lipid) and O_2 yield ROOH (a lipid peroxide), but $ROO\cdot$ is regenerated in each cycle

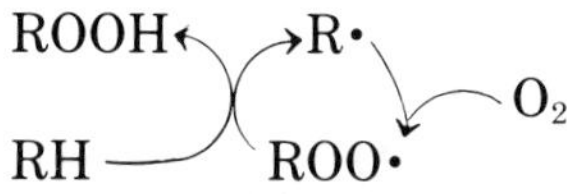

$$\begin{array}{c} ROOH \leftarrow \quad \rightarrow R\cdot \\ \qquad \qquad \qquad \qquad \searrow O_2 \\ RH \longrightarrow ROO\cdot \end{array} \qquad (16)$$

Consequently, once initiated by activated O_2 species, a chain reaction in the presence of molecular O_2 results in progressive lipid peroxidation. Furthermore the lipid peroxides react like H_2O_2 and may give rise to toxic radicals such as $RO\cdot$ and $HO\cdot$. Although lipid peroxidation has been proposed as an important manifestation of O_2 toxicity, actual proof with intact systems has remained elusive.

Protein oxidation. Several side-chain moieties of proteins are susceptible to oxidation by reduced O_2 products, and inactivation of key enzymes in the cell has long been regarded as one of the possible major effects of exposure to hyperoxia (97). The primary interaction of O_2 radicals with proteins may be with the sulfhydryl portion of cysteine.

$$HO_2\cdot + RSH \rightarrow RS\cdot + H_2O_2 \qquad (17)$$

$$2RS\cdot \rightarrow RSSR \qquad (18)$$

The formation of the protein disulfide is reversible. However, reactions with $HO\cdot$ or O_2^* may disrupt peptide bonds and irreversibly oxidize amino acids such as histidine, tryptophan, tyrosine, methionine, and cysteine, resulting in irreversible protein inactivation (161).

Oxidation of other components. Probably most free radicals produced from O_2 react with low-molecular-weight metabolites and cofactors in the cell, such as glutathione, ascorbic acid, and vitamin E. Reduced pyridine nucleotides are oxidized during the enzymatic reduction of oxidized products. Oxidation of these low-molecular-weight cellular components can be reflected in a shift of the cellular redox state (15). Because these cofactors can be rereduced or rapidly replaced through diet or synthesis, their oxidation in hyperoxia may be more of a defense than a loss to the cell.

ALTERATIONS OF METABOLIC FUNCTION. The biochemical alterations resulting from hyperoxic exposure are likely to be multiple and diffuse because of the broad spectrum of possible reactions between tissue components and O_2-reduction products. Thus late manifestations of O_2 poisoning probably include widespread alterations in cell protein, nucleic acid, and lipid components, with disruptions of cellular membranes and organelles and inhibition of diverse metabolic pathways. There has been some interest in defining the earliest metabolic alterations during O_2 exposure because these reactions could serve as an index of poisoning or indicate directions for altering O_2 tolerance. The metabolic pathways in lung cells that are most sensitive to alteration as a result of interactions with O_2-reduction products have not been adequately defined and may vary with the cell type under consideration. One generalized metabolic effect of hyperoxia that has been proposed is inhibition of cellular respiration, possibly due to inactivation of key dehydrogenases of the tricarboxylic acid cycle and electron-transport pathway (97, 103, 176). However, there is little evidence that significant depression of mitochondrial ATP generation occurs early in the course of O_2 poisoning (15, 55, 57). It is more likely that the earliest toxic effect of O_2 is interference with membrane transport phenomena, possibly due to inactivation of Na^+-K^+-ATPase, inactivation of membrane transport proteins, peroxidation of lipids comprising the membrane matrix, or oxidation of the carbohydrate moiety of cell surface receptors (4, 119). In addition the altered redox state may disrupt cellular processes linked to redox potentials, e.g., the intracellular Ca^{2+} distribution (particularly between cytosol and mitochondria) may be related to cellular NADPH/NADP (69).

Antioxidant Defenses

Antioxidant defenses of the cell can be categorized into three general schemes (see ref. 70 for review): *1*) limit production or accelerate removal of toxic free radicals, *2*) quench the accelerative (chain) reactions of lipid peroxidation, and *3*) rereduce or replace compounds that have been subjected to oxidative attack. Antioxidant defenses of the organ include mechanisms to replace damaged cells or other components.

A number of enzymes and low-molecular-weight compounds may contribute to these cellular mechanisms of antioxidant defense. First the proposed biochemical defenses are described and then some of the supporting evidence regarding the lung is presented. Figure 9 summarizes the interaction between free-radical generation and antioxidant defense.

ENZYMATIC DEFENSES. Removal of $O_2^-\cdot$, principally by dismutation, represents the first line of defense against free-radical toxicity (83)

$$2O_2^-\cdot + 2H^+ \rightarrow H_2O_2 + O_2 \quad (19)$$

The noncatalyzed (spontaneous) reaction probably requires the protonation of one of the $O_2^-\cdot$ molecules. The reaction can be catalyzed by either of two superoxide dismutase enzymes (mitochondrial and cytosolic) that at physiological pH increase the noncatalyzed rate by ~7 orders of magnitude to ~$2 \times 10^9 \cdot M^{-1} \cdot s^{-1}$ (73). One enzyme contains manganese as its cofactor and is found primarily in the mitochondrial matrix (204). The second enzyme is cytosolic and contains both copper, which functions in catalysis, and zinc, which maintains structural stability (72, 136). In removing $O_2^-\cdot$, H_2O_2 is generated. However, H_2O_2 is less reactive than $O_2^-\cdot$ and cells contain several enzymes for H_2O_2 removal.

Catalase and peroxidase remove H_2O_2. Catalase, a heme protein located in peroxisomes, catalyzes the dismutation of H_2O_2 by $>10^8$-fold (30)

$$2H_2O_2 \rightarrow 2H_2O + O_2 \quad (20)$$

Peroxidase (and catalase in its peroxidatic function) removes H_2O_2 at the expense of organic molecules such as aliphatic alcohols (189)

$$H_2O_2 + RCH_2OH \rightarrow 2H_2O + RCHO \quad (21)$$

or formic acid

$$H_2O_2 + HCOOH \rightarrow 2H_2O + CO_2 \quad (22)$$

Glutathione peroxidase is a particular peroxidase that removes H_2O_2 specifically with GSH (34)

$$H_2O_2 + 2GSH \rightarrow 2H_2O + GSSG \quad (23)$$

Glutathione peroxidase also catalyzes removal of ROOH, which the lipid alcohol rather than H_2O is formed

$$ROOH + 2GSH \rightarrow ROH + H_2O + GSSG \quad (24)$$

Two forms of glutathione peroxidase are found in mammalian cells (26). One is a selenium-containing enzyme found in both the cytosol and mitochondrial matrix. Because of its distribution throughout the cell and apparent greater affinity for H_2O_2, it has been proposed that this enzyme may be actually more important than catalase for H_2O_2 removal (34). The second form of glutathione peroxidase is a group of non-selenium-containing proteins that has lower affinity for H_2O_2 than ROOH and functions primarily as thioltransferase rather than peroxidase (102). Enzymes of this latter group are able to reduce disulfide bonds in proteins

$$RSSR + 2GSH \rightarrow 2RSH + GSSG \quad (25)$$

and can replace the oxidized sulfur of cysteic acid

$$RSO_3 + GSH \rightarrow RSH + GSSO_3 \quad (26)$$

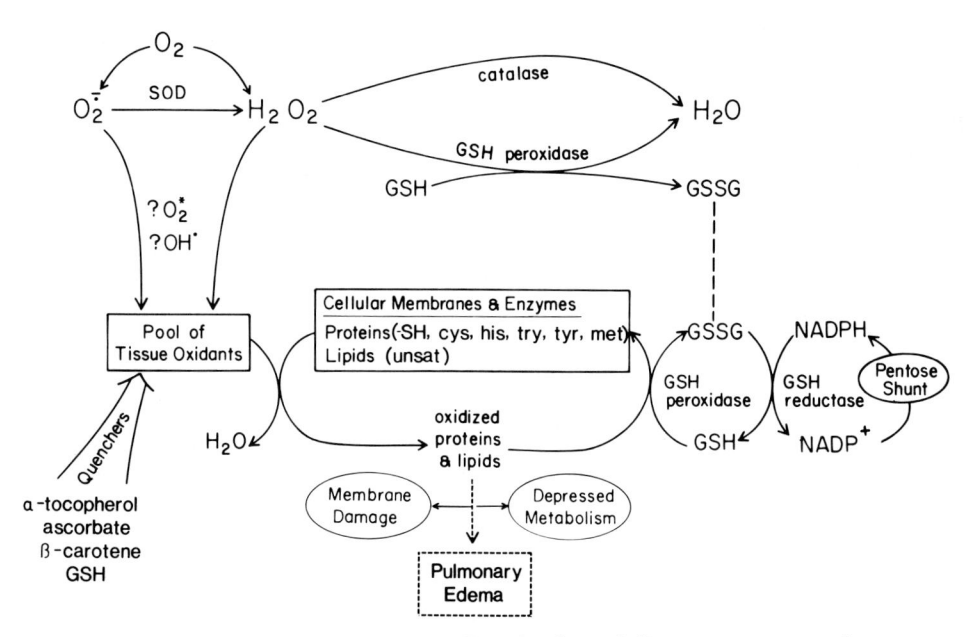

FIG. 9. Postulated metabolic events accompanying exposure to elevated partial pressures of O_2. Primary event is an increased rate of generation of superoxide anion, H_2O_2, and possibly O_2^* and $HO\cdot$. These and perhaps other agents form tissue pool of oxidants. Interaction of these oxidants with tissue components may oxidize tissue proteins and lipids, resulting in damage to cell membranes and intracellular enzymes. Interaction of quenchers with oxidizing agents and with tissue-oxidized components decreases size of tissue oxidant pool and terminates free-radical chain reactions. Oxidized tissue components (including H_2O_2 and oxidized quenchers) can be reduced through action of glutathione system, which in turn is in equilibrium with cytoplasmic $NADP^+/NADPH$. In the lung, NADPH is generated primarily through activity of pentose shunt pathway of glucose metabolism. Degree of lung damage during O_2 exposure may depend on outcome of interaction between radical-generating and radical-quenching pathways and tissue-damaging and tissue-repairing processes. Increased oxidation of tissue components may become manifest by damage to tissue membranes and depression of tissue metabolism due to inactivation of enzymes. This process may eventuate in pulmonary edema, but the precise mechanisms remain to be defined. GSH, reduced glutathione; GSSG, oxidized glutathione; SOD, superoxide dismutase. [From Fisher, Bassett, and Forman (58).]

Thus this latter enzyme may function in the restoration of oxidized sulfhydryls.

The GSH required as substrate for glutathione peroxidase can be regenerated enzymatically by the action of glutathione reductase

$$GSSG + NADPH + H^+ \rightarrow 2GSH + NADPH^+ \quad (27)$$

The NADPH required as a cofactor in this reaction can be regenerated primarily through the action of the enzymes of the pentose phosphate shunt (glucose-6-phosphate dehydrogenase and phosphogluconate dehydrogenase) but also by cytoplasmic isocitrate dehydrogenase, malic enzyme, and the mitochondrial transhydrogenase (described in GENERATION OF REDUCED PYRIDINE AND FLAVIN NUCLEOTIDES, p. 231; see also the chapter by Tierney and Young in this *Handbook*). Consequently the reactions of intermediary metabolism are ultimately involved in generation of reducing potential for enzymatic removal of O_2-reduction products. Thus the removal of $O_2^-\cdot$, $HO_2^-\cdot$, and H_2O_2 and the reduction of lipid peroxides and sulfhydryls can be accomplished by enzymatic processes at little expense to the cell. However, note that there are no enzymatic defenses against either O_2^* or $HO\cdot$.

NONENZYMATIC DEFENSES. Several low-molecular-weight compounds function specifically in antioxidant defense. These are referred to in Figure 9 as free-radical quenchers. Agents that received special attention include glutathione, α-tocopherol (the most active form of vitamin E), ascorbic acid (vitamin C), and β-carotene (vitamin A). In addition PUFA, through its oxidation, can function as a trap for $HO\cdot$ and O_2^*. These factors can be replaced from the diet or synthesized from dietary amino acids.

Glutathione can react with $O_2^-\cdot$, $HO_2^\cdot$, H_2O_2, $HO\cdot$, and O_2^* without catalysis by enzymes. For example

$$GSH + O_2^-\cdot + H^+ \rightarrow GS\cdot + H_2O_2 \quad (28)$$

In tissues glutathione acts as a major source of reducing power because it is present in relatively high intracellular concentration (~0.1–5 mM) and is maintained in its reduced form by an enzyme-catalyzed reaction (see Reaction 27 and ref. 7).

α-Tocopherol is a potent scavenger of O_2^*. Vitamin E also reacts with $HO_2^{\bullet}$ ~100 times faster than the reaction between $HO_2^{\bullet}$ and polyunsaturated lipids. Consequently vitamin E, even at relatively low concentrations, can protect lipids against peroxidation by $HO_2^{\bullet}$ (8). Furthermore its solubility in lipid permits it to act effectively in competing with lipids for oxidation by lipid (R·) and lipid oxide (RO·) free radicals

$$\text{vitamin E} + RO\cdot \rightarrow \text{vitamin E}\cdot + ROH \quad (29)$$

Thus vitamin E can function to terminate lipid peroxidation chain reactions (196).

Vitamin C, although an essential nutrient for humans and guinea pigs, is synthesized by most plants and animals. It may scavenge $O_2^-\cdot$ in vitro to produce semidehydroascorbate· (dehydroascorbate radical) (150)

$$O_2^-\cdot + H^+ + \text{ascorbate} \quad (30)$$
$$\rightarrow \text{semidehydroascorbate}\cdot + H_2O_2$$

Interactions of these quenching molecules with $O_2^-\cdot$ or other free radicals generates a free-radical product, i.e., GS·, vitamin E·, or semidehydroascorbate·. These radicals may act as pro-oxidants. However, it is likely that they are less destructive than the O_2-derived radicals because they are either less reactive or there are specific mechanisms for their removal. These radicals can spontaneously dismute

$$2 \text{ semidehydroascorbate}\cdot \quad (31)$$
$$\rightarrow \text{ascorbate} + \text{dehydroascorbate}$$

or associate

$$2GS\cdot \rightarrow GSSG \quad (32)$$

or react with other radical scavengers

$$\text{vitamin E}\cdot + \text{ascorbate} \quad (33)$$
$$\rightarrow \text{vitamin E} + \text{semidehydroascorbate}\cdot$$

Some mammalian cells can reduce oxidized ascorbate enzymatically by a semidehydroascorbate reductase (186)

$$2 \text{ semidehydroascorbate}\cdot + H^+ + NADH \quad (34)$$
$$\rightarrow 2 \text{ ascorbate} + NAD^+$$

or by dehydroascorbate reductase (91)

$$\text{dehydroascorbate} + 2GSH \quad (35)$$
$$\rightarrow GSSG + \text{ascorbate}$$

The β-carotene is an effective scavenger for O_2^* through a reaction in which it absorbs energy and/or undergoes a conformational change but is not oxidized

$$O_2^* + \beta\text{-carotene} \rightarrow O_2 + \beta\text{-carotene}^* \quad (36)$$

$$\beta\text{-carotene}^* \rightarrow \beta\text{-carotene} + \text{energy (heat)} \quad (37)$$

$$\beta\text{-carotene}^* \rightarrow \text{all-}trans\text{-}\beta\text{-carotene} \quad (38)$$

One mole of β-carotene can quench 1,000 mol of O_2^* with a rate constant of 3×10^{10} $M^{-1} \cdot s^{-1}$, ~4 orders of magnitude greater than the reaction rate of unsaturated lipids with O_2^* (68).

PROTECTION AGAINST PULMONARY O_2 TOXICITY. The role of antioxidant defenses has been elucidated through studies with diverse tissues and model systems. Evidence for the role of these pathways in lung defense has been obtained by analysis of the effects of O_2 on metabolic flux, of the nutritional factors in pulmonary O_2 toxicity, and by the study of mechanisms of O_2 adaptation and tolerance.

Metabolic flux. Oxidant stress has been observed to produce alterations in metabolic flux that could be predicted from models of antioxidant defense outlined in *Antioxidant Defenses*, p. 246. Perfused rat lungs released increased amounts of GSSG into the perfusate in hyperbaric O_2, presumably because the GSH oxidation rate exceeded the ability of glutathione reductase to convert the somewhat permeable GSSG to impermeable GSH (149). Exposure of guinea pigs to 1 ATA O_2 caused a marked decrease in both lung and plasma ascorbate contents, presumably reflecting increased oxidation of this compound (6). Perfused rat lungs showed an 81% increase in glucose utilization through the pentose shunt when the ventilating gas was changed from 0.2 to 5 ATA O_2 (15). These reports suggest increased oxidation of GSH, ascorbate, and NADPH during O_2 exposure. Thus studies of metabolic flux in lungs during O_2 exposure support the importance of the proposed antioxidant pathways.

Nutritional factors. The adverse effects of vitamin E deficiency in hyperoxic exposure have been well documented. Vitamin E deficiency increased the effect of hyperbaric O_2 on release of GSSG from lungs (149), accelerated the loss due to O_2 exposure of the ability of lungs to clear 5-HT (21), and decreased the survival time of rats in O_2 (198). Lungs from vitamin E–deficient rats show increased glucose-6-phosphate dehydrogenase and glutathione peroxidase activities compared with controls (149), possibly to compensate for loss of antioxidant capacity.

A selenium-deficient diet leads to decreased glutathione peroxidase activity in the tissue and decreased survival of rats in O_2 (39, 75). Catalase activity may increase in the lungs of selenium-deficient rats, perhaps as a partial compensation for the loss of H_2O_2-removing capacity (26), although this was not confirmed in a subsequent study (75). Dietary deficiency of sulfur-containing amino acids (methionine, cystine) also decreases survival time in O_2, which correlates with lung tissue GSH content (43, 75).

Adaptation and tolerance to O_2. Exposure to 1 ATA O_2 is lethal in 66–80 h for adult rats (and most mammals). Adult rats preexposed to 0.8–0.85 ATA O_2 for 5 to 7 days sustain lung damage (36) but usually survive subsequent exposure to 1 ATA O_2 (171) and have increased tolerance to hyperbaric O_2 (120). Tierney et al. (197) showed that the lungs of these adapted rats had twice the glucose-6-phosphate dehydrogenase activity as control animals, suggesting increased cellular demand for NADPH. Subsequent studies have indicated increased superoxide dismutases, glutathione peroxidase, glutathione reductase, and catalase in lungs of O_2-adapted rats (37, 38, 115). Furthermore lungs from species that do not develop tolerance to O_2 do not show increases in these enzymes with exposure to 0.85 ATA O_2 (38). Neonatal rats, mice, and rabbits inherently tolerant to O_2 show increases in lung antioxidant enzyme contents after 1 day in O_2 at 1 ATA, whereas neonatal hamsters and guinea pigs not tolerant to O_2 fail to increase lung enzyme content under similar exposure conditions (80). Thus an increase in the antioxidant enzyme content of the lung on exposure to O_2 correlates with tolerance and adaptation to hyperoxia.

Further evidence that lung antioxidant enzyme levels are correlated with tolerance to O_2 is provided by studies with agents that induce or block these enzymes. Administration of lipopolysaccharide from *Salmonella typhimurium* (endotoxin) to rats results in increased lung superoxide dismutase and increased O_2 tolerance (81). However, injection of diethyldithiocarbamate or its oxidized form disulfiram leads to inhibition of cytosolic superoxide dismutase in the lung and greatly decreases time to mortality in O_2 (77, 82).

The increases in lung enzyme activities of O_2-adapted and O_2-tolerant animals apparently reflect changes in the antioxidant capacity of individual cells but may also reflect partly a shift in composition of lungs toward cells (36), such as granular pneumocytes and alveolar macrophages, that have constitutively high activities of antioxidant enzymes (71). The effect of hyperoxia on the enzyme content of lung cell types has been investigated in alveolar macrophages, granular pneumocytes, and endothelial cells isolated from animals exposed to hyperoxia or incubated in vitro under a hyperoxic atmosphere. Increases due to O_2 exposure have been observed for superoxide dismutase in alveolar macrophages from neonatal (but not adult) rats exposed either to O_2 in vivo or in vitro (190), in the granular pneumocyte (type II epithelial cell) from rats exposed in vivo (71), and in cultured pig pulmonary arterial (and aortic) endothelial cells exposed in vitro (151). High constitutive activities of antioxidant enzymes in lung cells or induction with hyperoxia may correlate with intrinsic cellular tolerance to O_2 toxicity. Investigation of methods to increase tolerance to O_2 represents the forefront of research in O_2 toxicity and may lead to significant improvement in the ability to administer O_2 therapeutically.

CONCLUSION

This article reviewed the pathways of O_2 utilization for energy generation and incorporation of molecular O_2 into substrates. As an unavoidable consequence some of these reactions may generate toxic intermediates that under usual metabolic conditions may be partly responsible for the aging process, and during breathing of elevated O_2 concentrations may result in damage to vital organs. Despite these difficulties life with O_2 is better than life without it.

We thank B. Storey, A. Kleinzeller, D. Massaro, and N. G. Forman for critical review of the manuscript.

REFERENCES

1. ADAMSON, I. Y. R., AND D. H. BOWDEN. The type II cells as progenitor of alveolar epithelial regeneration. *Lab. Invest.* 30: 35–42, 1974.
2. ADAMSON, I. Y. R., D. H. BOWDEN, AND J. P. WYATT. Oxygen poisoning in mice, ultrastructural and surfactant studies during exposure and recovery. *Arch. Pathol.* 90: 463–472, 1970.
3. ALBRACHT, S. P. J., H. VAN HEERIKHUIZEN, AND E. C. SLATER. Iron-sulfur proteins in the succinate oxidase system. *Biochim. Biophys. Acta* 256: 1–13, 1972.
4. ALLEN, J. E., D. B. GOODMAN, A. BESARAB, AND H. RASMUSSEN. Studies on the biochemical basis of oxygen toxicity. *Biochim. Biophys. Acta* 320: 708–728, 1973.
5. ALPER, R., J. S. KERR, N. A. KEFALIDES, AND A. B. FISHER. Relation between alveolar P_{O_2} and collagen biosynthesis in the perfused rat lung. *J. Lab. Clin. Med.* 99: 442–450, 1982.
6. ARAD, I. D., H. J. FORMAN, AND A. B. FISHER. Ascorbate efflux from guinea pig and rat lungs. Effect of starvation and O_2 exposure. *J. Lab. Clin. Med.* 96: 673–681, 1980.
7. ARIAS, I. M., AND W. B. JAKOBY (editors). *Glutathione: Metabolism and Function.* New York: Raven, 1976.
8. ARUDI, R. L., M. W. SUTHERLAND, AND B. H. J. BIELSKI. Reaction of $HO_2^{\cdot}/O_2^{-\cdot}$ with α-tocopherol in ethanolic solutions. In: *Oxy Radicals and Their Scavenger Systems,* edited by G. Cohen and R. Greenwald. Amsterdam: Elsevier, 1983, p. 26–31.
9. ATKINSON, D. E. Adenine nucleotides as universal stoichiometric metabolic coupling agents. *Adv. Enzyme Regul.* 9: 207–219, 1971.
10. AUST, S. D., AND B. A. SVINGEN. The role of iron in enzymatic lipid peroxidation: In: *Free Radicals in Biology,* edited by W. A. Pyror. New York: Academic, vol. 5, 1982, p. 1–28.
11. BAKHLE, Y. S., AND M. B. H. YOUDIM. Metabolism of phenylethylamine in rat isolated perfused lung: evidence for monoamine oxidase 'type B' in lung. *Br. J. Pharmacol.* 56: 125–127, 1976.
12. BARRON, E. S. G., Z. B. MILLER, AND G. R. BARTLETT. Studies of biological oxidations. XXI. The metabolism of lung as determined by study of slices and ground tissue. *J. Biol. Chem.* 171: 791–800, 1947.
13. BASSETT, D. J. P., AND A. B. FISHER. Metabolic response to carbon monoxide by isolated rat lungs. *Am J. Physiol.* 230: 658–663, 1976.
14. BASSETT, D. J. P., AND A. B. FISHER. Stimulation of rat lung metabolism with 2,4-dinitrophenol and phenazine methosulfate. *Am. J. Physiol.* 231: 898–902, 1976.
15. BASSETT, D. J. P., AND A. B. FISHER. Glucose metabolism in rat lung during exposure to hyperbaric O_2. *J. Appl. Physiol.: Respirat. Environ. Exercise Physiol.* 46: 943–949, 1979.
16. BASSETT, D. J. P., A. B. FISHER, AND J. L. RABINOWITZ. Effect of hypoxia on incorporation of glucose carbons into lipids by isolated rat lung. *Am. J. Physiol.* 227: 1103–1108, 1974.

17. Bend, J. R., G. E. R. Hook, R. E. Easterling, T. E. Gram, and J. R. Fouts. A comparative study of the hepatic and pulmonary microsomal mixed-function oxidase systems in the rabbit. *J. Pharmacol. Exp. Ther.* 183: 206–217, 1972.
18. Bernhardt, F. H., N. Erdin, H. Staudinger, and V. Ullrich. Interactions of substrates with purified 4-methyl-benzoate monooxygenase system (o-demethylating) from *Pseudomonas putida*. *Eur. J. Biochem.* 35: 126–134, 1973.
19. Bielski, B. H. J., R. L. Arudi, and M. W. Sutherland. A study of the reactivity of $HO_2^{\bullet}/O_2^{-\bullet}$ with unsaturated fatty acids. *J. Biol. Chem.* 258: 4759–4761, 1983.
20. Blase, B. W., and T. A. Loomis. The uptake and metabolism of carbaryl by isolated perfused rabbit lung. *Toxicol. Appl. Pharmacol.* 37: 481–490, 1976.
21. Block, E. R., and A. B. Fisher. Depression of serotonin clearance by rat lungs during oxygen exposure. *J. Appl. Physiol.: Respirat. Environ. Exercise Physiol.* 42: 33–38, 1977.
22. Bowden, D. H., and I. Y. R. Adamson. Endothelial regeneration as a marker of the differential vascular responses in oxygen-induced pulmonary edema. *Lab. Invest.* 30: 350–357, 1974.
23. Boyd, M. R., C. N. Statham, and N. S. Longo. The pulmonary Clara cell as a target for toxic chemicals requiring metabolic activation: studies with carbon tetrachloride. *J. Pharmacol. Exp. Ther.* 212: 109–114, 1980.
24. Boyer, P. D. Conformational coupling in oxidative phosphorylation and photophosphorylation. *Trend Biochem. Sci.* 2: 35–41, 1977.
25. Buechler, K. F., and R. A. Rhoades. Fatty acid synthesis in the perfused rat lung. *Biochim. Biophys. Acta* 619: 186–195, 1980.
26. Burk, R. F., K. Nishiki, R. A. Lawrence, and B. Chance. Peroxide removal by selenium-dependent and selenium-independent glutathione peroxidases in hemoglobin-free perfused rat liver. *J. Biol. Chem.* 253: 43–46, 1978.
27. Caldwell, P. R. B., and B. A. Wittenberg. The oxygen dependency of mammalian tissue. *Am. J. Med.* 57: 447–452, 1974.
28. Capdevila, J., N. Chacos, J. Werringloer, R. A. Prough, and R. Estabrook. Liver microsomal cytochrome P-450 and the oxidative metabolism of arachidonic acid. *Proc. Natl. Acad. Sci. USA* 78: 5362–5366, 1981.
29. Chance, B. The nature of electron transfer and energy coupling reactions. *FEBS Lett.* 23: 3–20, 1972.
30. Chance, B., H. Sies, and A. Boveris. Hydroperoxide metabolism in mammalian organs. *Physiol. Rev.* 59: 527–605, 1979.
31. Chance, B., and G. R. Williams. Respiratory enzymes of oxidative phosphorylation. I. Kinetics of O_2 utilization. *J. Biol. Chem.* 217: 385–393, 1955.
32. Chance, B., and G. R. Williams. Respiratory enzymes in oxidative phosphorylation. III. The steady state. *J. Biol. Chem.* 217: 409–427, 1955.
33. Clark, J. M., and C. J. Lambertsen. Pulmonary oxygen toxicity: a review. *Pharmacol. Rev.* 23: 37–133, 1971.
34. Cohen, G., and P. Hochstein. Glutathione peroxidase: the primary agent for the elimination of hydrogen peroxide in erythrocytes. *Biochemistry* 2: 1420–1428, 1963.
35. Cohen, H. J., and M. E. Chovaniec. Superoxide production by digitonin-stimulated guinea pig granulocytes. The effects of N-ethyl maleimide, divalent cations, and glycolytic and mitochondrial inhibitors on the activation of the superoxide generating system. *J. Clin. Invest.* 61: 1088–1096, 1978.
36. Crapo, J. D., B. E. Barry, H. A. Foscue, and J. Shelburne. Structural and biochemical changes in rat lungs occurring during exposures to lethal and adaptive doses of oxygen. *Am. Rev. Respir. Dis.* 112: 123–143, 1980.
37. Crapo, J. D., K. Sjostrom, and R. T. Drew. Tolerance and cross-tolerance using NO_2 and O_2. I. Toxicology and biochemistry. *J. Appl. Physiol.: Respirat. Environ. Exercise Physiol.* 44: 364–369, 1978.
38. Crapo, J. D., and D. F. Tierney. Superoxide dismutase and pulmonary oxygen toxicity. *Am. J. Physiol.* 226: 1401–1407, 1974.
39. Cross, C. E., G. Hasegawa, K. A. Reddy, and S. T. Omaye. Enhanced lung toxicity of O_2 in selenium-deficient rats. *Res. Commun. Chem. Pathol. Pharmacol.* 16: 695–706, 1977.
40. Dalhamn, T., and A. Rosengren. The effect of oxygen lack on the tracheal ciliary activity. *Arch. Environ. Health* 16: 371–373, 1968.
41. Davies, H. C., and R. E. Davies. Biochemical aspects of oxygen poisoning. In: *Handbook of Physiology. Respiration*, edited by W. O. Fenn and H. Rahn. Washington, DC: Am. Physiol. Soc., 1965, sect. 3, vol. II, chapt. 40, p. 1047–1058.
42. Davis, E. J., and L. Lumeng. Relationship between the phosphorylation potentials generated by liver mitochondria and respiratory state under conditions of adenosine diphosphate control. *J. Biol. Chem.* 250: 2275–2282, 1975.
43. Deneke, S. M., S. N. Gershoff, and B. L. Fanburg. Potentiation of oxygen toxicity in rats by dietary protein or amino acid deficiency. *J. Appl. Physiol.: Respirat. Environ. Exercise Physiol.* 54: 147–151, 1983.
44. Den Engelse, L., M. Gebbink, and P. Emmelot. Studies on lung tumours. III. Oxidative metabolism of dimethylnitrosamine by rodent and human lung tissue. *Chem. Biol. Interact.* 11: 535–544, 1975.
45. Devereux, T. R., and J. R. Fouts. N-oxidation and demethylation of N,N-dimethylaniline by rabbit liver and lung microsomes. Effects of age and metals. *Chem. Biol. Interact.* 8: 91–105, 1974.
46. Devereux, T. R., C. J. Serabjit-Singh, S. R. Slaughter, C. R. Wolf, R. M. Philpot, and J. R. Fouts. Identification of P-450 isozymes in non-ciliated bronchiolar epithelial (Clara) and alveolar type II cells isolated from rabbit lung. *Exp. Lung Res.* 2: 221–230, 1981.
47. Dobuler, K. J., J. D. Catravas, and C. N. Gillis. Early detection of oxygen-induced lung injury in conscious rabbits. *Am. Rev. Respir. Dis.* 126: 534–539, 1982.
48. Edson, N. L., and L. F. Leloir. Ketogenesis-antiketogenesis. V. Metabolism of ketone bodies. *Biochem. J.* 30: 2319–2332, 1936.
49. Engelbrecht, F. M., and G. Maritz. Influence of substrate composition on in vitro oxygen consumption of lung slices. *S. Afr. Med. J.* 48: 1882–1884, 1974.
50. Erecińska, M., R. L. Veech, and D. F. Wilson. Thermodynamic relationships between the oxidation-reduction reactions and the ATP synthesis in suspensions of isolated pigeon heart mitochondria. *Arch. Biochem. Biophys.* 160: 412–421, 1974.
51. Erecińska, M., and D. F. Wilson. The effect of antimycin A on cytochromes b_{561}, b_{566}, and their relationship to ubiquinone and the iron-sulfur centers S-1 (+N-2) and S-3. *Arch. Biochem. Biophys.* 174: 143–157, 1976.
52. Evans, M. J., J. D. Hackney, and R. F. Bills. Effects of a high concentration of oxygen on cell renewal in the pulmonary alveoli. *Aerosp. Med.* 40: 1365–1368, 1969.
53. Faridy, E. E., and A. Naimark. Effect of distension on metabolism of excised dog lung. *J. Appl. Physiol.* 31: 31–37, 1971.
54. Fisher, A. B. Oxygen utilization and energy production. In: *Lung Biology in Health and Disease. The Biochemical Basis of Pulmonary Function*, edited by R. Crystal. New York: Dekker, 1976, vol. 2, chapt. 3, p. 75–104.
55. Fisher, A. B. Energy status of the rat lung after exposure to elevated P_{O_2}. *J. Appl. Physiol.: Respirat. Environ. Exercise Physiol.* 45: 56–59, 1978.
56. Fisher, A. B. Oxygen therapy. Side effects and toxicity. *Am. Rev. Respir. Dis.* 122: 61–69, 1980.
57. Fisher, A. B., and D. J. P. Bassett. Lung ATP turnover during oxidant stress. In: *Underwater Physiology VII*, edited by A. J. Bachrach and M. M. Matzen. Bethesda, MD: Undersea Med. Soc., 1981, p. 55–63. (Proc. 7th Symp. Underwater Physiol.)

58. FISHER, A. B., D. J. P. BASSETT, AND H. J. FORMAN. Oxygen toxicity of the lung: biochemical aspects. In: *Pulmonary Edema*, edited by A. P. Fishman and E. M. Renkin. Bethesda, MD: Am. Physiol. Soc., 1979, chapt. 15, p. 207–216.
59. FISHER, A. B., E. R. BLOCK, AND G. G. PIETRA. Environmental influences on uptake of serotonin and other amines. *Environ. Health Perspect.* 35: 191–198, 1980.
60. FISHER, A. B., AND A. CHANDER. Glycerol kinase activity and glycerol metabolism of rat granular pneumocytes in primary culture. *Biochim. Biophys. Acta* 711: 128–133, 1982.
61. FISHER, A. B., AND C. DODIA. Lung as a model for evaluation of critical intracellular P_{O_2} and P_{CO}. *Am. J. Physiol.* 241 (*Endocrinol. Metab.* 4): E47–E50, 1981.
62. FISHER, A. B., L. FURIA, AND B. CHANCE. Evaluation of redox state of isolated perfused rat lung. *Am. J. Physiol.* 230: 1198–1204, 1976.
63. FISHER, A. B., G. A. HUBER, AND D. J. P. BASSETT. Oxidation of alpha-glycerophosphate by mitochondria from lungs of rabbits, sheep, and pigeons. *Comp. Biochem. Physiol.* 50B: 5–8, 1975.
64. FISHER, A. B., G. A. HUBER, AND L. FURIA. Cytochrome P-450 content and mixed function oxidation by microsomes from rabbit alveolar macrophages. *J. Lab. Clin. Med.* 90: 101–108, 1977.
65. FISHER, A. B., N. ITAKURA, C. DODIA, AND R. G. THURMAN. Relationship between alveolar P_{O_2} and the rate of *p*-nitroanisole O-demethylation by the cytochrome P-450 pathway in isolated rabbit lungs. *J. Clin. Invest.* 64: 770–774, 1979.
66. FISHER, A. B., N. ITAKURA, C. DODIA, AND R. G. THURMAN. Pulmonary mixed-function oxidation: stimulation by glucose and the effects of metabolic inhibitors. *Biochem. Pharmacol.* 30: 379–383, 1981.
67. FISHER, A. B., A. SCARPA, K. F. LANOUE, D. J. P. BASSETT, AND J. R. WILLIAMSON. Respiration of rat lung mitochondria and the influence of Ca^{2+} on substrate utilization. *Biochemistry* 12: 1438–1445, 1973.
68. FOOTE, C. S., R. W. DENNY, L. WEAVER, Y. CHONG, AND J. PETERS. Quenching of singlet oxygen. *Ann. NY Acad. Sci.* 171: 139–148, 1970.
69. FORMAN, H. J., AND A. BOVERIS. Superoxide radical and hydrogen peroxide in mitochondria. In: *Free Radicals in Biology*, edited by W. A. Pryor. New York: Academic, 1982, vol. 5, p. 65–90.
70. FORMAN, H. J., AND A. B. FISHER. Antioxidant defenses. In: *Oxygen and Living Processes*, edited by D. L. Gilbert. New York: Springer-Verlag, 1981, p. 235–249.
71. FORMAN, H. J., AND A. B. FISHER. Antioxidant enzymes of rat granular pneumocytes: constitutive levels and effect of hyperoxia. *Lab. Invest.* 45: 1–6, 1981.
72. FORMAN, H. J., AND I. FRIDOVICH. On the stability of bovine superoxide dismutase: the effects of metals. *J. Biol. Chem.* 248: 2645–2649, 1973.
73. FORMAN, H. J., AND I. FRIDOVICH. Superoxide dismutase: a comparison of rate constants. *Arch. Biochem. Biophys.* 158: 396–400, 1973.
74. FORMAN, H. J., J. NELSON, AND A. B. FISHER. Rat alveolar macrophages require NADPH for superoxide production in the respiratory burst. Effect of NADPH depletion by paraquat. *J. Biol. Chem.* 255: 9879–9883, 1980.
75. FORMAN, H. J., E. I. ROTMAN, AND A. B. FISHER. The roles of selenium and sulfur-containing amino acids in protection against oxygen toxicity. *Lab. Invest.* 49: 148–153, 1983.
76. FORMAN, H. J., J. J. WILLIAMS, J. NELSON, R. P. DANIELE, AND A. B. FISHER. Hyperoxia inhibits stimulated superoxide release by rat alveolar macrophages. *J. Appl. Physiol.: Respirat. Environ. Exercise Physiol.* 53: 685–689, 1982.
77. FORMAN, H. J., J. L. YORK, AND A. B. FISHER. Mechanism for the potentiation of oxygen toxicity by disulfiram. *J. Pharmacol. Exp. Ther.* 212: 452–455, 1980.
78. FORMAN, N. G., AND D. F. WILSON. Energetics and stoichiometry of oxidative phosphorylation from NADH to cytochrome *c* in isolated rat liver mitochondria. *J. Biol. Chem.* 257: 12908–12915, 1982.
79. FOX, R. B., J. R. HOIDAL, D. M. BROWN, AND J. E. REPINE. Pulmonary inflammation due to oxygen toxicity: involvement of chemotactic factors and polymorphonuclear leukocytes. *Am. Rev. Respir. Dis.* 123: 521–523, 1981.
80. FRANK, L., J. R. BUCHER, AND R. J. ROBERTS. Oxygen toxicity in neonatal and adult animals of various species. *J. Appl. Physiol.: Respirat. Environ. Exercise Physiol.* 45: 699–704, 1978.
81. FRANK, L., J. SUMMERVILLE, AND D. MASSARO. Protection from oxygen toxicity with endotoxin: the role of the endogenous antioxidant enzymes of the lung. *J. Clin. Invest.* 65: 1104–1110, 1980.
82. FRANK, L., D. L. WOOD, AND R. J. ROBERTS. Effect of diethyldithiocarbamate on oxygen toxicity and lung enzyme activity in immature and adult rats. *Biochem. Pharmacol.* 27: 251–254, 1978.
83. FRIDOVICH, I. Superoxide radical and superoxide dismutases. In: *Oxygen and Living Processes*, edited by D. L. Gilbert. New York: Springer-Verlag, 1981, p. 250–272.
84. GABIG, T. G., R. S. KIPNES, AND B. M. BABIOR. Solubilization of the O_2^--forming activity responsible for the respiratory burst in human neutrophils. *J. Biol. Chem.* 253: 6663–6665, 1978.
85. GAIL, D. B., G. D. MASSARO, AND D. MASSARO. Intraspecies differences in lung metabolism and granular pneumocyte mitochondria. *Respir. Physiol.* 23: 175–180, 1975.
86. GEBICKI, J. M., AND B. H. J. BIELSKI. Comparison of the capacities of the perhydroxyl and the superoxide radicals to initiate chain oxidation of linoleic acid. *J. Am. Chem. Soc.* 103: 7020–7022, 1981.
87. GERSCHMAN, R. Biological effects of oxygen. In: *Oxygen in the Animal Organism*, edited by F. Dickens and E. Neil. New York: Macmillan, 1964, p. 475–494.
88. GILLETTE, J. R., D. C. DAVIS, AND H. A. SASAME. Cytochrome P-450 and its role in drug metabolism. *Annu. Rev. Pharmacol.* 12: 57–84, 1972.
89. GLASS, M., H. J. FORMAN, E. I. ROTMAN, J. M. CLARK, G. G. PIETRA, AND A. B. FISHER. Cellular composition of lung lavage in oxygen toxicity (Abstract). *Federation Proc.* In press.
90. GOODMAN, B. E., AND E. D. CRANDALL. Dome formation in primary cultured monolayers of alveolar epithelial cells. *Am. J. Physiol.* 243 (*Cell Physiol.* 12): C96–C100, 1982.
91. GRIMBLE, R. F., AND R. E. HUGHES. A 'dehydroascorbic acid reductase' factor in guinea pig tissues. *Experientia* 23: 362, 1967.
92. GURTNER, G. H., H. PEARY, W. SUMMER, AND B. BURNS. Physiological evidence for carrier mediated O_2 and CO_2 transport in lung and placenta. *Prog. Respir. Res.* 8: 166–176, 1975.
93. HABER, F., AND J. WEISS. The catalytic decomposition of hydrogen peroxide by iron salts. *Proc. R. Soc. London Ser. A* 147: 332–349, 1934.
94. HACKNEY, J. D., M. J. EVANS, AND B. R. CHRISTIE. Effects of 60 and 80% oxygen on cell division in lung alveoli of squirrel monkeys. *Aviat. Space Environ. Med.* 46: 791–794, 1975.
95. HANCE, A. J., K. BRADLEY, AND R. G. CRYSTAL. Lung collagen heterogeneity. II. Synthesis of type I and type II collagen by rabbit and human lung cells in culture. *J. Clin. Invest.* 57: 102–111, 1976.
96. HARTIALA, J. Steroid metabolism in adult lung. *Agents Actions* 6: 522–526, 1976.
97. HAUGAARD, N. Cellular mechanisms of oxygen toxicity. *Physiol. Rev.* 48: 311–373, 1968.
98. HOOK, G. E. R., J. R. BEND, AND J. R. FOUTS. Mixed-function oxidases and the alveolar macrophage. *Biochem. Pharmacol.* 21: 3267–3277, 1972.
99. HOOK, G. E. R., J. R. BEND, D. HOEL, J. R. FOUTS, AND T. E. GRAM. Preparation of lung microsomes and a comparison of the distribution of enzymes between subcellular fractions of rabbit lung and liver. *J. Pharmacol. Exp. Ther.* 182: 474–490, 1972.

100. HUGHES, J., C. N. GILLIS, AND F. E. BLOOM. Uptake and disposition of norepinephrine in perfused rat lung. *J. Pharmacol. Exp. Ther.* 169: 237–248, 1969.
101. ITAKURA, N., A. B. FISHER, AND R. G. THURMAN. Cytochrome P450-linked *p*-nitroanisole *O*-demethylation in the perfused lung. *J. Appl. Physiol.: Respirat. Environ. Exercise Physiol.* 43: 238–245, 1977.
102. JAKOBY, W. B., AND J. H. KEEN. A triple treat in detoxification: the glutathionine-*S*-transferases. *Trends Biochem. Sci.* 2: 229, 1977.
103. JAMIESON, D., K. LADNER, AND H. A. S. VAN DEN BRENK. Pulmonary damage due to high pressure oxygen breathing in rats. IV. Quantitative analysis of sulfhydryl and disulphide groups in rat lungs. *Aust. J. Exp. Biol. Med. Sci.* 41: 491–497, 1963.
104. JÖBSIS, F. F. Basic processes in cellular respiration. In: *Handbook of Physiology. Respiration*, edited by W. O. Fenn and H. Rahn. Washington, DC: Am. Physiol. Soc., 1964, sect. 3, vol. I, chapt. 2, p. 63–124.
105. JOHNSTON, R. B., JR. Oxygen metabolism and the microbicidal action of macrophages. *Federation Proc.* 37: 2759–2764, 1978.
106. JONES, D. P., AND F. G. KENNEDY. Intracellular oxygen supply during hypoxia. *Am. J. Physiol.* 243 (*Cell Physiol.* 12): C247–C253, 1982.
107. JONES, D. P., AND H. S. MASON. Gradients of O_2 concentration in hepatocytes. *J. Biol. Chem.* 253: 4874–4880, 1978.
108. JUNOD, A. F. Uptake, metabolism, and efflux of ^{14}C-5-hydroxytryptamine in isolated perfused rat lungs. *J. Pharmacol. Exp. Ther.* 183: 341–355, 1973.
109. KAPANCI, Y., E. R. WEIBEL, H. P. KAPLAN, AND F. R. ROBINSON. Pathogenesis and reversibility of the pulmonary lesions of oxygen toxicity in monkeys. II. Ultrastructural and morphometric studies. *Lab. Invest.* 20: 101–118, 1969.
110. KAUFMAN, S. D. Coenzymes and hydroxylases: ascorbate and dopamine beta-hydroxylase; tetrahydropteridines and phenylalanine and tyrosine hydroxylases. *Pharmacol. Rev.* 18: 61–69, 1966.
111. KEARNS, D. R. Physical and chemical properties of singlet oxygen. *Chem. Rev.* 71: 395–427, 1971.
112. KEEVIL, T., AND H. S. MASON. Molecular oxygen in biological oxidations—an overview. *Methods Enzymol.* 52: 3–40, 1978.
113. KELLOGG, E. W., III, AND I. FRIDOVICH. Superoxide, hydrogen peroxide and singlet oxygen in lipid peroxidation by a xanthine oxidase system. *J. Biol. Chem.* 250: 8812–8817, 1975.
114. KHAN, A. U. Singlet molecular oxygen from superoxide anion and sensitized fluorescence of organic molecules. *Science* 168: 474–477, 1970.
115. KIMBALL, R. E., K. REDDY, T. H. PEIRCE, L. W. SCHWARTZ, M. G. MUSTAFA, AND C. E. CROSS. Oxygen toxicity: augmentation of antioxidant defense mechanisms in rat lung. *Am. J. Physiol.* 230: 1425–1431, 1976.
116. KISTLER, G. S., P. R. B. CALDWELL, AND E. R. WEIBEL. Development of fine structural damage to alveolar and capillary lining cells in oxygen-poisoned rat lungs. *J. Cell Biol.* 32: 605–628, 1967.
117. KIVIRIKKO, K. I., AND D. J. PROKOP. Hydroxylation of proline in synthetic polypeptides with purified protocollagen hydroxylase. *J. Biol. Chem.* 242: 4007–4012, 1967.
118. KLINGENBERG, M. The ADP-ATP translocation in mitochondria, a membrane potential controlled transport. *J. Membr. Biol.* 56: 97–105, 1980.
119. KOVACHICH, G. B., AND N. HAUGAARD. Biochemical aspects of oxygen toxicity in the metazoa. In: *Oxygen and Living Processes*, edited by D. L. Gilbert. New York: Springer-Verlag, 1981, p. 210–234.
120. KRAVETZ, G., A. B. FISHER, AND H. J. FORMAN. The oxygen adapted rat model: tolerance to oxygen at 1.5 and 2 ATA. *Aviat. Space Environ. Med.* 51: 775–777, 1980.
121. KREBS, H. A. Body size and tissue respiration. *Biochim. Biophys. Acta* 4: 249–269, 1950.
122. KROGER, A., AND M. KLINGENBERG. The kinetics of the redox reactions of ubiquinone related to the electron-transport activity in the respiratory chain. *Eur. J. Biochem.* 34: 358–368, 1973.
123. KUNZ, W., R. BOHNENSACK, G. BOHME, U. KUNSTER, G. LETKO, AND P. SCHONFELD. Relations between extramitochondrial and intramitochondrial adenine nucleotide systems. *Arch. Biochem. Biophys.* 209: 219–229, 1981.
124. KYLE, J. L., AND W. H. REISSEN. Stress and cigarette smoke effects on lung mitochondrial phosphorylation. *Arch. Environ. Health* 21: 492–497, 1970.
125. LAMBERTSEN, C. J. Effects of oxygen at high partial pressure. In: *Handbook of Physiology. Respiration*, edited by W. O. Fenn and H. Rahn. Washington, DC: Am. Physiol. Soc., 1965, sect. 3, vol. II, chapt. 39, p. 1027–1046.
126. LAMBERTSEN, C. J. Effects of hyperoxia on organs and their tissues. In: *Lung Biology in Health and Disease. Extrapulmonary Manifestations of Respiratory Disease*, edited by E. D. Robin. New York: Dekker, 1978, vol. 8, chapt. 8, p. 239–303.
127. LAW, F. C. P., T. E. ELING, J. R. BEND, AND J. R. FOUTS. Metabolism of xenobiotics by the isolated perfused lung. *Drug Metab. Dispos.* 2: 433–442, 1974.
128. LEVY, S. E., AND E. HARVEY. Effect of tissue slicing on rat lung metabolism. *J. Appl. Physiol.* 37: 239–240, 1974.
129. LEW, P. D., AND T. P. STOSSEL. Effect of calcium on superoxide production by phagocytic vesicles from rabbit alveolar macrophages. *J. Clin. Invest.* 67: 1–9, 1981.
130. LLOYD, T. C., JR. Effect of alveolar hypoxia on pulmonary vascular resistance. *J. Appl. Physiol.* 19: 1086–1094, 1964.
131. MACHINIST, J. M., E. W. DEHNER, AND D. M. ZIEGLER. Microsomal oxidases. III. Comparison of species and organ distribution of dialkylarylamine *N*-oxide dealkylase and dialkylarylamine *N*-oxidase. *Arch. Biochem. Biophys.* 125: 858–864, 1968.
132. MARINO, P. A., AND S. A. ROONEY. Surfactant secretion in a newborn rabbit lung slice model. *Biochim. Biophys. Acta* 620: 509–519, 1980.
133. MASON, R. J., M. C. WILLIAMS, J. H. WIDDICOMBE, M. J. SANDERS, D. S. MISFELDT, AND L. C. BERRY, JR. Transepithelial transport by pulmonary alveolar type II cells in primary culture. *Proc. Natl. Acad. Sci. USA* 79: 6033–6037, 1982.
134. MASSARO, G. D., D. B. GAIL, AND D. MASSARO. Lung oxygen consumption and mitochondria of alveolar epithelial and endothelial cells. *J. Appl. Physiol.* 38: 588–592, 1975.
135. MATSUBARA, T., R. A. PROUGH, M. D. BURKE, AND R. W. ESTABROOK. The preparation of microsomal fractions of rodent respiratory tract and their characterization. *Cancer Res.* 34: 2196–2203, 1974.
136. McCORD, J. M., AND I. FRIDOVICH. Superoxide dismutase. An enzymic function for erythrocuprein (hemocuprein). *J. Biol. Chem.* 244: 6049–6055, 1969.
137. MENZEL, D. B. Toxicity of ozone, oxygen, and radiation. *Annu. Rev. Pharmacol.* 10: 379–394, 1970.
138. MILES, P. R., L. BOWMAN, AND V. CASTRANOVA. Transmembrane potential changes during phagocytosis in rat alveolar macrophages. *J. Cell. Physiol.* 106: 109–117, 1981.
139. MILLER, M. A., AND C. A. HALES. Role of cytochrome P-450 in alveolar hypoxic vasoconstriction in dogs. *J. Clin. Invest.* 64: 666–673, 1979.
140. MISRA, H. P. Generation of superoxide free radical during the autoxidation of thiols. *J. Biol. Chem.* 249: 2151–2155, 1974.
141. MISRA, H. P., AND I. FRIDOVICH. The role of superoxide anion in the autoxidation of epinephrine and a simple assay for superoxide dismutase. *J. Biol. Chem.* 247: 3170–3175, 1972.
142. MITCHELL, P. Chemiosmotic coupling in oxidative and photosynthetic phosphorylation. *Biol. Rev. Cambridge Philos. Soc.* 41: 445–502, 1966.
143. MITCHELL, P. Protonmotive redox mechanism of the cytochrome *b-c*₁ complex in the respiratory chain: protonmotive ubiquinone cycle. *FEBS Lett.* 56: 1–6, 1975.
144. MITCHELL, P. Possible molecular mechanisms of the proton-

motive function of cytochrome systems. *J. Theor. Biol.* 62: 327-367, 1976.
145. MUSTAFA, M. G., AND C. E. CROSS. Lung cell mitochondria: rapid oxidation of glycerol-1-phosphate but slow oxidation of 3-hydroxybutyrate. *Am. Rev. Respir. Dis.* 109: 301-303, 1974.
146. MUSTAFA, M. G., AND D. F. TIERNEY. Biochemical and metabolic changes in the lung with oxygen, ozone, and nitrogen dioxide toxicity. *Am. Rev. Respir. Dis.* 118: 1061-1090, 1978.
147. NAGAOKA, S., L. YU, AND T. E. KING. Characterization of ubisemiquinone radical in the cytochrome b-c_1 segment of the mitochondrial respiratory chain. *Arch. Biochem. Biophys.* 208: 334-343, 1981.
148. NICHOLAS, T. E., AND P. A. KIM. The metabolism of ^{3}H-cortisol by the isolated perfused rat and guinea pig lungs. *Steroids* 25: 387-402, 1975.
149. NISHIKI, K., D. JAMIESON, N. OSHINO, AND B. CHANCE. Oxygen toxicity in the perfused rat liver and lung under hyperbaric conditions. *Biochem. J.* 160: 343-355, 1976.
150. NISHIKIMI, M. Oxidation of ascorbic acid with superoxide ion generated by the xanthine-oxidase system. *Biochem. Biophys. Res. Commun.* 63: 463-468, 1975.
151. ODY, C., Y. BACH-DIETERLE, I. WAND, AND A. F. JUNOD. The effect of hyperoxia on superoxide dismutase content of pig pulmonary artery and aortic endothelial cells in culture. *Exp. Lung Res.* 1: 271-279, 1980.
152. OHNISHI, T. Mitochondrial iron-sulfur flavodehydrogenases. In: *Membrane Proteins in Energy Transduction*, edited by R. A. Capaldi. New York: Dekker, 1979, p. 1-87.
153. OHNISHI, T., AND B. L. TRUMPOWER. Differential effects of antimycin on ubisemiquinone bound in different environments in isolated succinate·cytochrome c reductase complex. *J. Biol. Chem.* 255: 3278-3284, 1980.
154. O'NEIL, J. J., R. L. SANFORD, S. WASSERMAN, AND D. F. TIERNEY. Metabolism in rat lung tissue slices: technical factors. *J. Appl. Physiol.: Respirat. Environ. Exercise Physiol.* 43: 902-906, 1977.
155. OREN, R., A. E. FARNHAM, K. SAITO, E. MILOFSKY, AND M. L. KARNOVSKY. Metabolic patterns in three types of phagocytizing cells. *J. Cell Biol.* 17: 487-501, 1963.
156. ORTON, T. C., M. W. ANDERSON, R. D. PICKETT, T. E. ELING, AND J. R. FOUTS. Xenobiotic accumulation and metabolism by isolated perfused rabbit lungs. *J. Pharmacol. Exp. Ther.* 186: 482-497, 1973.
157. PEDERSEN, T. C., AND S. D. AUST. The role of superoxide and singlet oxygen in lipid peroxidation promoted by xanthine oxidase. *Biochem. Biophys. Res. Commun.* 82: 1071-1078, 1973.
158. PHILPOT, R. M., M. W. ANDERSON, AND T. E. ELING. Uptake, accumulation and metabolism of chemicals by the lung. In: *Lung Biology in Health and Disease. Metabolic Functions of the Lung*, edited by Y. S. Bakhle and J. R. Vane. New York: Dekker, 1977, vol. 4, chapt. 5, p. 123-171.
159. PHILPOT, R. M., E. ARINIC, AND J. R. FOUTS. Reconstitution of the rabbit pulmonary microsomal mixed-function oxidase system from solubilized components. *Drug Metab. Dispos.* 3: 118-126, 1975.
160. PODGORSKI, G. T., I. S. LONGMUIR, J. A. KNOPP, AND D. M. BENSON. Use of encapsulated fluorescent probe to measure intracellular Po_2. *J. Cell. Physiol.* 107: 329-333, 1981.
161. POLITZER, I. R., G. W. GRIFFIN, AND J. L. LASETER. Singlet oxygen and biological systems. *Chem. Biol. Interact.* 3: 73-93, 1971.
162. POST, C., R. G. G. ANDERSSON, A. RYRFELDT, AND E. NILSSON. Transport and binding of lidocaine by lung slices and perfused lung of rats. *Acta Pharmacol. Toxicol.* 43: 156-163, 1978.
163. PROKOP, D. J., K. I. KIVIRIKKO, L. TUDERMAN, AND N. A. GUZMAN. The biosynthesis of collagen and its disorders. *N. Engl. J. Med.* 301: 13-23, 1979.
164. RAJAGOPALAN, K. V., I. FRIDOVICH, AND P. HANDLER. Hepatic aldehyde oxidase. *J. Biol. Chem.* 237: 922-928, 1962.
165. RAJAGOPALAN, K. V., AND P. HANDLER. Purification and properties of chicken liver xanthine dehydrogenase. *J. Biol. Chem.* 242: 4097-4107, 1967.
166. REID, W. D., K. F. ILETT, J. M. GLICK, AND G. KRISHNA. Metabolism and binding of aromatic hydrocarbons in the lung. *Am. Rev. Respir. Dis.* 107: 539-551, 1973.
167. REISS, O. K. Studies in lung metabolism. I. Isolation and properties of subcellular fractions from rabbit lung. *J. Cell Biol.* 30: 45-58, 1966.
168. RHOADES, R. A., M. E. SHAW, AND M. L. ESKEW. Influence of altered O_2 tension on substrate metabolism in perfused rat lung. *Am. J. Physiol.* 229: 1476-1479, 1975.
169. RISTER, M. Effects of hyperoxia on phagocytosis. *Blut* 45: 157-166, 1982.
170. RISTER, M., AND R. L. BAEHNER. Effect of hyperoxia on superoxide anion and hydrogen peroxide production of polymorphonuclear leukocytes and alveolar macrophages. *Br. J. Haematol.* 36: 241-248, 1977.
171. ROSENBAUM, R. M., M. WITTNER, AND M. LENGER. Mitochondrial and other ultrastructural changes in great alveolar cells of oxygen-adapted and poisoned rats. *Lab. Invest.* 20: 516-528, 1969.
172. ROSSOUW, D. J., AND F. M. ENGELBRECHT. The effect of paraquat on the respiration of lung cell fractions. *S. Afr. Med. J.* 54: 1101-1104, 1978.
173. ROTH, J. A., AND C. N. GILLIS. Multiple forms of amine oxidases in perfused rabbit lung. *J. Pharmacol. Exp. Ther.* 194: 537-544, 1975.
174. SACKNER, M. A., J. LANDA, J. HIRSCH, AND A. ZAPATA. Pulmonary effects of oxygen breathing. A 6-hour study in normal men. *Ann. Intern. Med.* 82: 40-43, 1975.
175. SAGE, H., F. M. FARIN, G. E. STRIKER, AND A. B. FISHER. Granular pneumocytes in primary culture secrete several major components of the extracellular matrix. *Biochemistry* 22: 2148-2155, 1983.
176. SANDERS, A. P., AND W. D. CURRIE. Pulmonary O_2 toxicity: energy metabolism and data analysis. *Proc. Soc. Exp. Biol. Med.* 164: 82-88, 1980.
177. SAYEED, M. M., AND A. E. BAUE. Mitochondrial metabolism of succinate, β-hydroxybutyrate, and α-ketoglutarate in hemorrhagic shock. *Am. J. Physiol.* 220: 1275-1281, 1971.
178. SCHLEYER, H., D. Y. COOPER, AND O. ROSENTHAL. Cytochrome P-450 from the adrenal cortex: studies of its chemical and physical properties. In: *Oxidases and Related Redox Systems*, edited by T. E. King, H. S. Mason, and M. Morrison. Baltimore, MD: University Park, 1973, vol. 2, p. 469-491.
179. SERABJIT-SINGH, C. J., C. R. WOLF, AND R. M. PHILPOT. The rabbit pulmonary monooxygenase system. Immunological and biochemical characterization of enzyme components. *J. Biol. Chem.* 254: 9902-9907, 1979.
180. SERABJIT-SINGH, C. J., C. R. WOLF, R. M. PHILPOT, AND C. G. PLOPPER. Cytochrome P-450: localization in rabbit lung. *Science* 207: 1469-1470, 1980.
181. SIES, H. Oxygen gradients during hypoxic steady states in liver. Urate oxidase and cytochrome oxidase as intracellular O_2 indicators. *Hoppe-Seyler's Z. Physiol. Chem.* 358: 1021-1032, 1977.
182. SIMON, F. P., A. M. POTTS, AND R. W. GERRARD. Metabolism of isolated lung tissue: normal and in phosgene poisoning. *J. Biol. Chem.* 167: 303-311, 1947.
183. SINGER, T. P., E. B. KEARNEY, AND W. C. KENNEY. Succinate dehydrogenase. *Adv. Enzymol.* 37: 189-272, 1973.
184. SPEAR, R. K., AND L. LUMENG. A method for isolating lung mitochondria from rabbits, rats, and mice with improved respiratory characteristics. *Anal. Biochem.* 90: 211-219, 1978.
185. STADIE, W. C., B. C. RIGGS, AND N. HAUGAARD. Oxygen poisoning. IV. The effects of high oxygen pressures upon the metabolism of liver, kidney, lung, and muscle tissue. *J. Biol. Chem.* 160: 209-216, 1945.
186. STAUDINGER, H., K. KRISCH, AND S. LEONHAUSER. Role of ascorbic acid in microsomal electron transport and the possible relationship to hydroxylation reactions. *Ann. NY Acad. Sci.*

92: 195–207, 1961.
187. STEINBERG, H., D. J. P. BASSETT, AND A. B. FISHER. Depression of pulmonary 5-hydroxytryptamine uptake by metabolic inhibitors. *Am. J. Physiol.* 228: 1298–1303, 1975.
188. STEPHENS, N. L., J. L. MEYERS, AND R. M. CHERNIACK. Oxygen, carbon dioxide, H$^+$ ion, and bronchial length-tension relationships. *J. Appl. Physiol.* 25: 376–383, 1968.
189. STERN, K. G. On the mechanisms of enzyme action: a study of the decomposition of monoethyl hydrogen peroxide by catalase and of an intermediate enzyme substrate compound. *J. Biol. Chem.* 114: 473–494, 1936.
190. STEVENS, J. B., AND A. P. AUTOR. Oxygen-induced synthesis of superoxide dismutase and catalase in pulmonary macrophages of neonatal rats. *Lab. Invest.* 37: 470–478, 1977.
191. STOSSEL, T. P. The mechanism of phagocytosis. *J. Reticuloendothel. Soc.* 19: 237–245, 1976.
192. STROBEL, H. W., AND M. J. COON. Effect of superoxide generation and dismutation on hydroxylation reactions catalyzed by liver microsomal cytochrome P-450. *J. Biol. Chem.* 246: 7826–7829, 1971.
193. SUGANO, T., N. OSHINO, AND B. CHANCE. Mitochondrial function under hypoxic conditions. The steady states of cytochrome c reduction and energy metabolism. *Biochim. Biophys. Acta* 347: 340–358, 1974.
194. SYLVESTER, J. T., AND C. MCGOWAN. The effects of agents that bind to cytochrome P-450 on hypoxic pulmonary vasoconstriction. *Circ. Res.* 43: 429–437, 1978.
195. TAPPEL, A. Inhibition of electron transport by antimycin A. Alkyl hydroxyl napthoquinone and metal coordination compounds. *Biochem. Pharmacol.* 3: 289–296, 1960.
196. TAPPEL, A. L. Vitamin E as the biological lipid antioxidant. *Vitam. Horm. NY* 20: 493–510, 1969.
197. TIERNEY, D., L. AYERS, S. HERZOG, AND J. YANG. Pentose pathway and production of reduced nicotinamide adenine dinucleotide phosphate. A mechanism that may protect lungs from oxidants. *Am. Rev. Respir. Dis.* 108: 1348–1351, 1973.
198. TIERNEY, D. F., L. AYERS, AND R. S. KASUYAMA. Altered sensitivity to oxygen toxicity. *Am. Rev. Respir. Dis.* 115: 59–65, 1977.
199. TURRENS, J. F., B. A. FREEMAN, AND J. D. CRAPO. Hyperoxia increases H$_2$O$_2$ release by lung mitochondria and microsomes. *Arch. Biochem. Biophys.* 217: 411–421, 1982.
200. TURRENS, J. F., B. A. FREEMAN, J. G. LEVITT, AND J. D. CRAPO. The effect of hyperoxia on superoxide production by lung submitochondrial particles. *Arch. Biochem. Biophys.* 217: 401–410, 1982.
201. VALIMAKI, M., K. JUVA, J. RANTANEN, T. EKFORS, AND J. NIINIKOSKI. Collagen metabolism in rat lungs during chronic intermittent exposure to oxygen. *Aviat. Space Environ. Med.* 46: 684–690, 1975.
202. VILLALOBO, A., AND A. L. LEHNINGER. The proton stoichiometry of electron transport in Ehrlich ascites tumor mitochondria. *J. Biol. Chem.* 254: 4352–4358, 1979.
203. WARREN, D. L., D. L. BROWN, JR., AND A. R. BUCKPITT. Evidence for cytochrome P-450 mediation in the bronchiolar damage by naphthalene. *Chem. Biol. Interact.* 40: 287–303, 1982.
204. WEISINGER, R. A., AND I. FRIDOVICH. Superoxide dismutase: organelle specificity. *J. Biol. Chem.* 248: 3582–3592, 1973.
205. WHITE, R. E., AND M. J. COON. Oxygen activation by cytochrome P-450. *Annu. Rev. Biochem.* 49: 315–356, 1980.
206. WIDDICOMBE, J. H., AND M. J. WELSH. Anion selectivity of the chloride-transport process in dog tracheal epithelium. *Am. J. Physiol.* 239 (*Cell Physiol.* 8): C112–C117, 1980.
207. WILLIAMSON, J. R., AND B. E. CORKEY. Assays of intermediates of the citric acid cycle and related compounds by fluorometric enzyme methods. *Methods Enzymol.* 13: 434–513, 1969.
208. WILSON, D. F., M. ERENCINSKA, C. DROWN, AND I. A. SILVER. The oxygen dependence of cellular energy metabolism. *Arch. Biochem. Biophys.* 195: 485–493, 1979.
209. WILSON, D. F., AND N. G. FORMAN. Mitochondrial transmembrane pH and electrical gradients: evaluation of their energy relationships with respiratory rate and adenosine 5′-triphosphate synthesis. *Biochemistry* 21: 1438–1444, 1982.
210. WILSON, D. F., M. STUBBS, N. OSHINO, AND M. ERECINSKA. Thermodynamic relationships between the mitochondrial oxidation-reduction reactions and cellular ATP levels in ascites tumor cells and perfused rat liver. *Biochemistry* 13: 5303–5311, 1974.
211. WINTER, P. M., AND G. SMITH. The toxicity of oxygen. *Anesthesiology* 37: 210–241, 1972.
212. WOLF, C. R., S. R. SLAUGHTER, J. P. MARCINISZYN, AND R. M. PHILPOT. Purification and structural comparison of pulmonary and hepatic cytochrome P-450 from rabbits. *Biochim. Biophys. Acta* 624: 409–419, 1980.
213. WOLF, C. R., B. R. SMITH, L. M. BALL, C. SERABJIT-SINGH, J. R. BEND, AND R. M. PHILPOT. The rabbit pulmonary monooxygenase system. Catalytic differences between two purified forms of cytochrome P-450 in the metabolism of benzo(a)pyrene. *J. Biol. Chem.* 254: 3658–3663, 1979.
214. WOSTMANN, B. S., E. BRUCKNER-KARDOSS, AND P. L. KNIGHT, JR. Cecal enlargement, cardiac output, and O$_2$ consumption in germfree rats. *Proc. Soc. Exp. Biol. Med.* 128: 137–141, 1968.

CHAPTER 6

Glucose and intermediary metabolism of the lungs

DONALD F. TIERNEY | Department of Medicine, University of California, Los Angeles, California

STEPHEN L. YOUNG | Department of Medicine, Duke University, Durham, North Carolina

CHAPTER CONTENTS

Major Pathways of Glucose Metabolism
   Glycolysis
   Cellular respiration
Physiological Significance of Lung Carbohydrate Metabolism
Methods of Study of Lung Carbohydrate Metabolism
   Isotopic tracer techniques
   Compartmentation
   Isolated lung mitochondria
Glucose Transport by Lung Tissue
Glucose Consumption by Lung Tissue
Glycogenesis and Gluconeogenesis
Regulation of Pulmonary Carbohydrate Metabolism
   Hypoxia
   Nutrition
   Insulin and diabetes
Major Products of Lung Glucose Metabolism
   Lactate
   Lactate production in vivo
   Lactate metabolism by perfused lung
   Generation of reducing equivalents
   Pentose phosphate pathway
Lung Energy Production
   Substrates
   Oxygen as substrate
   Nucleotide pools
Pathophysiology and Toxicology
   Oxidants and carbohydrate metabolism
   Glucose consumption during pulmonary edema

IF INTERMEDIARY METABOLISM is defined as the sum of all enzymatic reactions and if carbohydrate metabolism is broadly interpreted to include all possible pathways for any of the carbohydrate atoms, this topic has almost no limits. By necessity we have focused on selected aspects of intermediary metabolism that depend on carbohydrates and aspects of energy metabolism most relevant to the lung. We have also concentrated on lung parenchyma and left the discussion of metabolism in airways to other chapters.

This first brief section provides some background for those readers unfamiliar with the fundamental information necessary to make the rest of the chapter easier to follow.

MAJOR PATHWAYS OF GLUCOSE METABOLISM

Glycolysis

Glucose is the major carbohydrate available to the lung. We discuss the distribution of its carbon atoms and also of its hydrogen atoms into reducing equivalents in the form of NADH or NADPH. We also consider some related aspects of ATP production. Generally pulmonary metabolism is assumed to follow major pathways described for other tissues, and many of these pathways have been studied in the lung. One such pathway is glycolysis, the anaerobic degradation of glucose to lactate with the production of ATP. The ATP content in part controls glycolysis; when ATP consumption exceeds production, the lower ATP content accelerates glycolysis and produces more ATP. For instance, transient demands for ATP production (e.g., during muscle contraction) can be met by glycolysis. Mitochondria produce most of the ATP, and when their production falls (e.g., during anoxia) glycolysis may increase and partially compensate by producing more ATP. Some cells (e.g., erythrocytes) use glycolysis as a major source of ATP even under normal resting conditions, and they release lactate, the final product, into their environment.

Because glycolysis to pyruvate consumes NAD^+ and the process cannot continue without it, the cell must have mechanisms to replenish NAD^+ from NADH. The most direct means is to convert the pyruvate to lactate with the concomitant conversion of NADH back to NAD^+. Under anaerobic conditions when mitochondria cannot contribute to NAD^+ regeneration, glycolysis would eventually be limited by depleting NAD^+ if lactate were not produced (Fig. 1). Other mechanisms for converting cytosolic NADH back to NAD^+ are also discussed.

There is remarkable coordination of the glycolytic enzymes, and glycolysis is controlled primarily at the phosphofructokinase reaction (Fig. 2). However, in some circumstances hexokinase or pyruvate kinase are also sites of control. Such allosteric enzymes can

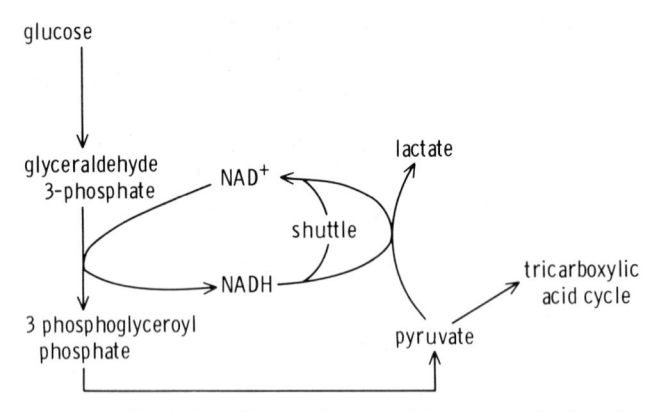

FIG. 1. NAD⁺, NADH, glycolysis, and lactate production. In cytoplasm, glycolysis converts NAD⁺ to NADH. Reconversion uses either a shuttle mechanism through mitochondria or lactate production.

be inhibited by the products of their own reactions and thus prevent an accumulation of these products (11). Characteristics of these enzymes differ from organ to organ, but if lung phosphofructokinases are similar to those in other organs (60), they can be inhibited by several products of glycolysis and by products of related pathways, including high concentrations of ATP. Conversely this enzyme generally is activated by AMP and ADP, which usually accumulate when ATP is consumed. Consequently it permits greater glycolysis and ATP production when ATP content falls and removes its inhibition and when ATP is consumed and releases AMP and ADP. Hexokinase from most tissues is inhibited by its own product, glucose 6-phosphate, which otherwise would accumulate if phosphofructokinase slowed glycolysis. Furthermore the product from phosphofructokinase, fructose 1,6-diphosphate, activates pyruvate kinase and thus prevents its own accumulation. Continued metabolism of pyruvate in mitochondria can produce citrate and other products that inhibit pyruvate kinase and phosphofructokinase and thus can stop excessive flow of pyruvate from glycolysis into systems such as the tricarboxylic acid (TCA) cycle. These interrelationships illustrate the coordination of this multienzyme system. Generation of ATP by glycolysis in the cytosol and by oxidative phosphorylation in the mitochondria is highly coordinated and regulated. Only glycolysis can generate ATP under anaerobic conditions, but it generates only 2 ATP molecules from a molecule of glucose, whereas complete aerobic oxidation of glucose generates 36 ATP molecules. Therefore during anoxia 18 times as much glycolysis would be required to produce the same quantity of ATP from glucose. To the extent that mitochondria receive carbon products from fatty acid or amino acid catabolism, glycolysis would need to increase even more than 18-fold to produce sufficient ATP for the cell during anoxia. Glucose entry into the cells generally cannot increase to this extent, and therefore few tissues or cells can generate sufficient ATP by anaerobic glycolysis alone.

One can therefore predict that in an aerobic environment most cells would consume less glucose and produce less lactate than when they have no oxidative phosphorylation. Pasteur first observed that the products of glycolysis accumulated faster in an anaerobic environment, and the Pasteur effect refers to the inhibition of glucose consumption and lactate production when O_2 is consumed (62, 130). Many investigators have demonstrated that the lung does have a Pasteur effect (5, 9, 68, 87, 97, 118, 125).

Hydrogen from glucose and its intermediates is transferred to NAD⁺ and NADP⁺ to form NADH and NADPH, which then retain the potential of transferring hydrogen in reduction reactions. The NADH is produced by glycolysis, and it may be converted back to NAD⁺ when pyruvate is converted to lactate or when its hydrogen is transferred into mitochondria and participates in oxidative phosphorylation. A tissue as highly perfused as the lung could release lactate into the circulation to provide a mechanism to convert NADH back to NAD⁺ without local accumulation of

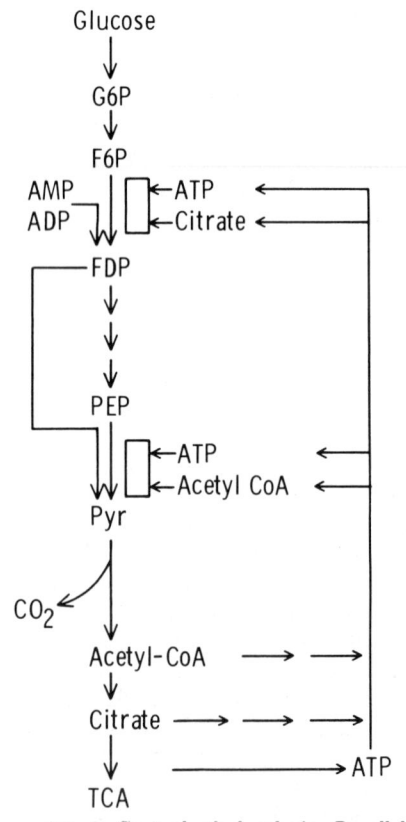

FIG. 2. Control of glycolysis. *Parallel arrows*, reaction rate is promoted; *rectangles*, reaction rate is slowed. G6P, glucose 6-phosphate; F6P, fructose 6-phosphate; FDP, fructose 1,6-diphosphate; PEP, phosphoenolpyruvate; Pyr, pyruvate; TCA, tricarboxylic acid cycle. Plentiful supply of ATP slows glycolysis at 2 steps indicated, whereas accumulation of ADP and AMP when ATP is consumed accelerates glycolysis; net result is a system highly responsive to changes of ATP concentration in cytoplasm.

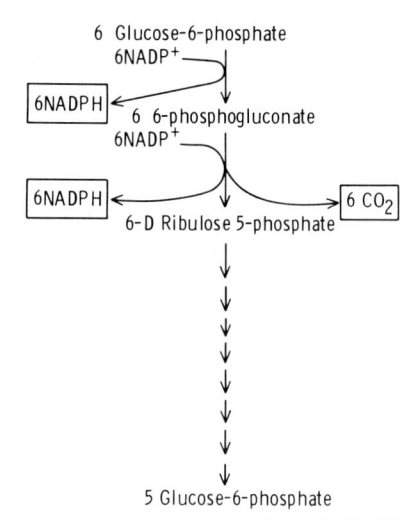

FIG. 3. Pentose phosphate cycle. This cycle contributes NADPH to cytoplasm at steps indicated with production of a pentose (D-ribulose 5-phosphate); 6 molecules of the pentose can then reappear as 5 molecules of a hexose or in pools of various carbohydrates. In this cycle the 1st carbon atom is released as CO_2; therefore [1-^{14}C]glucose loses its ^{14}C and does not pass it to other carbohydrates as it progresses through the cycle. All other labeled carbon atoms in glucose reenter carbohydrate pool, however. D-Ribulose 5-phosphate may be utilized for nucleotide synthesis, but cycle activity is generally controlled by NADPH requirements.

lactate; the lactate could then be consumed by other organs. The pentose phosphate cycle in the cytosol generates NADPH (Fig. 3), which can participate in many reactions, including some relating to toxins and oxidants in the lung (54, 75).

Cellular Respiration

A detailed review of cellular energetics has been presented by Lehninger (64). Although a complete restatement of this field is beyond the scope of this chapter, some general comments on lung bioenergetics are appropriate.

Energy from glycolysis and oxidative processes can be conserved in the phosphate bonds of adenine nucleotides for use elsewhere. The intermediate value for the standard free energy of the phosphate bond, −7.3 kcal/mol, permits the conservation of energy released by exergonic (energy-producing) chemical reactions but can still provide the necessary chemical motive force for endergonic (energy-consuming) reactions. Two moles of ATP (net) are released for each mole of glucose degraded to lactate. Some carbons from glucose are then oxidized to CO_2, whereas others are transferred, two carbon units at a time, to mitochondria. These acetyl units are fully oxidized in mitochondria to CO_2; when coupled with efficient electron transfer to molecular O_2, 36 mol of ATP are generated for each mole of glucose oxidized. Each of the major substrates (carbohydrates, lipids, and amino acids) can serve as fuels for lung mitochondrial respiration. Mitochondria from lungs are difficult to isolate, and

differences were initially reported when they were compared with those from other tissues (39, 80, 92, 93). Lung mitochondria appear to behave qualitatively much like those from other tissues.

Ultrastructural studies of the lung have repeatedly emphasized its great cellular heterogeneity (109), and it is apparent that lung cells as different as the huge but flat alveolar type I epithelium and the cuboidal alveolar type II epithelium contain mitochondria that are dramatically different in size and shape as well as in number per unit volume of cell cytoplasm (73, 74). Now that some cell types can be isolated from the lung, it may be possible to detect quantitative differences between different cell types, but currently we can only describe lung mitochondria as they are isolated from the many cell types of lung tissue.

PHYSIOLOGICAL SIGNIFICANCE OF LUNG CARBOHYDRATE METABOLISM

Carbohydrate intermediary metabolism is the linchpin for much of cellular metabolism, including those aspects discussed in the chapter by Fisher and Forman in this *Handbook*. Carbohydrates are indispensable for energy metabolism, and they provide reducing equivalents for biosynthesis of proteins and lipids and carbon atoms for lipid synthesis. Despite its central role, few physiological events in the lung have been directly attributed to carbohydrate metabolism. This contrasts with the great physiological significance of lipid metabolism in the pulmonary surfactant or of protein metabolism in the synthesis of collagen or elastin. However, abnormal conditions related to carbohydrate metabolism probably exist but are undetected because their manifestations are not specific. Many abnormalities of the lung have the same or similar clinical presentations. Except for infections and neoplasms, lung abnormalities manifest themselves in a limited number of syndromes and generally are grouped as obstructive airway disease, emphysema, interstitial lung disease, or acute alveolar injury. Any abnormalities of carbohydrate intermediary metabolism in the lung would probably present as one of these conditions, and a few cases due to abnormal carbohydrate metabolism would be unrecognized as different from those attributed to other etiologies. For instance, if glucose-6-phosphate dehydrogenase activity were abnormal in some lungs, as it is in some erythrocytes that lyse during oxidative stresses, acute oxidative stresses could result in diffuse alveolar damage. However, with chronic or repeated stresses, emphysema might result if glucose-6-phosphate dehydrogenase could not maintain sufficient reducing equivalents to protect proteases and other molecules. Thus alveolar damage could result acutely or chronically if glucose-6-phosphate dehydrogenase were unable to provide sufficient NADPH for mechanisms that protect the lung from oxidants (see PATHOPHYSIOLOGY

AND TOXICOLOGY, p. 270). Until enzyme activities of human lung tissue are studied, uncommon enzyme defects limited to the lung probably will not be detected. It is likely that abnormalities of carbohydrate metabolism do occur in some lungs simply because most other organs have been found to have such abnormalities when these enzymes were evaluated in uncommon diseases.

METHODS OF STUDY OF LUNG CARBOHYDRATE METABOLISM

Because freshly removed lung tissue is required for study of carbohydrate metabolism, most of our information derives from animals and little is known about carbohydrate metabolism in human lungs. Except for gluconeogenesis, however, the pathways for carbohydrate metabolism are remarkably similar in different organs and species. Clearly the extrapolation of animal data to humans must be done with caution, but at least there are some good clues and a fair probability that most of these pathways are similar in both.

Isotopic Tracer Techniques

Net production or consumption of carbohydrates and their metabolites can be obtained relatively simply by determining their quantities in a closed system before and after the metabolic process. Most methods used to measure glucose consumption by lung tissue depend on depletion of glucose from a closed system, such as a flask containing tissue slices (4, 67, 83, 85). However, the utilization of glucose atoms must be determined by tracer methods. Tracers have been used for many years to determine pathways of carbohydrate metabolism, but only recently has enough information been amassed to use them for quantitative estimates of metabolism (53). Not all reports separate these two uses of tracers, and some confuse changes of tracers in a metabolite with net changes of quantities of that metabolite. For instance, after [^{14}C]lactate is added to tissue in a flask, it may be metabolized to $^{14}CO_2$ and other products, and the ^{14}C in lactate decreases even if lactate accumulates through glycolysis. On the other hand, entry of a tracer into a metabolic pool such as glycogen does not necessarily indicate a net synthesis of that pool from the original tracer because an exchange of the labeled atoms for the unlabeled atoms during metabolic reactions may have occurred. To measure the total flux of lactate or other metabolites with labeled carbon, all carbon atoms entering and leaving the lactate pool must be accounted for. The complexity extends well beyond that of knowing the sources of carbon atoms from the classic pathways, because frequently molecular fragments, such as acetyl coenzyme A (acetyl-CoA), from one pathway undergo exchange with other pathways without contributing a net increase of carbon atoms. Therefore it does not necessarily follow, as some investigators have assumed, that lung tissue prefers lactate over glucose even if more $^{14}CO_2$ is derived from lactate than from labeled glucose under comparable conditions (98). Steady-state conditions with equilibration of ^{14}C in all the carbon pools where it might exchange may not occur during the incubation, and the specific activity of carbon in a pool may be changing for several hours. When comparing glucose and lactate utilization one must consider that ^{14}C from glucose will be diluted by carbon pools preceding lactate in glycolysis. Gluconeogenesis and glycogenesis cannot be determined quantitatively simply by the entry of a tracer from ^{14}C-labeled precursor into glucose and glycogen. One must consider exchange of ^{14}C-labeled molecules and isotope dilution by the TCA cycle; for instance, ^{14}C from an intermediate in the TCA cycle may appear in glucose simply by carbon exchange but no net synthesis of glucose may have occurred. [For a thorough discussion see the symposium on tracer methodology to measure glycogenesis and gluconeogenesis (91).]

Compartmentation

The metabolism of a whole organ is of course the sum of the metabolism of different cell types with different metabolic activities. In the lung the alveolar epithelium consists of two cell types that may have markedly different metabolism. The structure of type II alveolar cells suggests that they are very active metabolically, and it is known that they are oriented toward synthesis of pulmonary surfactant. These cells would be expected to have a very active pentose phosphate cycle to contribute NADPH for reductive biosynthesis of the surfactant and for reducing oxidants. In contrast, type I alveolar cells have few structural characteristics of metabolically active cells, and it is assumed they would have a less active pentose phosphate cycle that would be oriented to reduce oxidants but presumably not to synthesize the surfactant. Such compartmentation can lead to discrepant results when different methods are used to evaluate metabolism. For instance, if the activity of the pentose phosphate cycle is estimated by detecting radioactivity from glucose that appears in fatty acids presumably synthesized largely in type II cells, the results are different from those obtained by methods that use lactate or other products (5, 7, 9) and do not focus on the role of the pentose phosphate cycle in fatty acid synthesis. An excellent example of compartmentation that can be detected morphologically is the distribution of glycogen in some but not all cells of the fetal lung. Therefore fetal lung cells that contain glycogen may use it as a source of glucose 6-phosphate, whereas other cells utilize glucose from the medium. Tracers from this glucose could be diluted in the cells containing glycogen, and the tracer would underestimate the total glucose 6-phosphate metabolism. It may be very difficult to compare glucose metabolism in fetal lungs if some cells channeling it into the pentose phosphate cycle use glycogen during one stage of development and exogenous glucose during another. We do not know whether [^{14}C]glucose in a medium would have equal access to intermediary pools in all cells or be displaced by glucose 6-phosphate from glycogen in some cells. For instance, $^{14}CO_2$ production from [1-^{14}C]glucose and [6-^{14}C]glucose has been used to estimate the activity of the pentose phosphate cycle in the fetal lung. Although this approach is appropriate with adult lungs, which contain almost no glycogen, it may be impossible to interpret the differences of $^{14}CO_2$ production from [1-^{14}C]glucose and [6-^{14}C]-glucose if glucose 6-phosphate from glycolysis is preferentially channeled by glycogen-containing cells into one pathway.

Compartmentation exists within as well as among cells. For instance, the NAD^+/NADH ratio may not be the same in mitochondria and in the cytoplasm, although there are mechanisms that promote an equilibrium of these redox couples in these two compartments (127). Furthermore compounds may bind to proteins; NAD^+ and NADH as coenzymes bind to these enzymes, and to the extent they are not readily exchangeable they are compartmented. In lung cells the most commonly mentioned candidate for a discrepancy between cytoplasm and mitochondrial compartments is the type I alveolar cell, which has a very extensive cytoplasm distributed over a huge surface area and presumably considerable distances between mitochondria (73, 126). If diffusion distances to mitochondria in such a cell are sufficiently great, the redox couples might be significantly different at sites close to the mitochondria than at sites great distances from the mitochondria. Furthermore lactate produced at considerable distances from the mitochondria might diffuse into the blood before its metabolic counterpart from glycolysis (NADH) could diffuse to the mitochondria.

An apparent solution to the problems presented by compartmentation between different cell types would be to isolate these specific cell types and then study them. However, such isolated cells may not retain the same characteristics they had in situ because the process of isolation requires rather extensive digestion of the tissue and other procedures that might change them. Furthermore there is increasing evidence that adjacent cells influence each other, and it may be impossible to reproduce a comparable environment with isolated cells. Currently the glucose metabolism of isolated type II cells has been reported by excellent investigators to differ by a factor of 10 or more (36, 71); this unresolved disparity may be a result of these problems and illustrates that results cannot be extrapolated from isolated cells directly to the intact organ until more is known about the condition of these isolated cells.

One of the least discussed but important methodological problems relates to the expression of lung metabolism to its mass. Does it matter if glucose consumption is expressed per gram of wet lung, per gram of dry lung, per milligram of DNA, per milligram of protein, or per whole lung? Comparisons between laboratories may be impossible if one report is expressed per gram wet weight but the other is per milligram of protein. For instance, the wet weight might double if pulmonary edema occurs, and the protein content in the lung may increase significantly with vascular congestion and edema because of the protein in blood. However, the metabolism of lung cells may not change under these circumstances even though the metabolism expressed per gram wet weight or per milligram of protein may drop by half. Because DNA relates only to cells in the lung it may be the best measurement to use, but there are major discrepancies among laboratories in the reported DNA content of normal lungs. Also inflammation might recruit leukocytes into the lung and moderately increase the DNA content. It may be best to compare several of these values, because each indicates a somewhat different characteristic of lung mass. Even the same expression of lung mass may vary with the details of the methods used; the dry weight of a lung tissue slice may be 30% less if determined after incubation in a medium instead of before (85).

Isolated Lung Mitochondria

Methods that are adequate to isolate mitochondria for other tissues may not be adequate for the lung, which has structural differences from other organs, including air spaces, a huge vascular bed, and many attenuated cells. Isolation of intact mitochondria from the lung first received detailed attention in 1966 when Reiss (92, 93) identified several unique characteristics that have troubled investigators ever since. The lung is so fibrous that methods commonly used to disrupt cells of other tissues required modification or the lung mitochondria were obtained in unacceptably low yields with poor coupling between substrate utilization and ADP phosphorylation. Reiss improved the yield and respiration characteristics of lung mitochondria by milling the Potter-Elvehjem Teflon pestle to a clearance of 0.4 mm and by employing low-speed prolonged homogenization, a method subsequently adopted by some investigators. Reiss recognized that some lipids of lung tissue, presumably the pulmonary surfactant, sedimented with mitochondria and activated mitochondrial ATPase with resulting poor coupling between substrate oxidation and ADP phosphorylation. He also recognized that the addition of a divalent cation chelator was necessary to achieve maximal rates of lung mitochondrial respiration; Ca^{2+} is reported to decrease respiration of lung mitochondrial preparations (39), and Mg^{2+} may have similar effects (10, 18). The problem of ATPase activation by divalent cations in lung mitochondria has not yet been solved. Tables 1 and 2 abstract the most detailed

TABLE 1. *Techniques for Preparation of Lung Mitochondria*

Animal	Homogenization	Homogenization Medium	Isolation	Ref.
Rabbit, both sexes, 1.6–2.8 kg	Potter-Elvehjem, 0.4-mm clearance, 150 rpm × 2 min, then increase to 250 rpm × 2 min	0.25 M sucrose, 10 mM Tris-HCl, 1 mM EDTA, pH 7.2–7.4	500 g × 10 min, decant; 1,600 g × 5 min, decant; 12,500 g × 10 min, wash mitochondria × 2, repellet at 25,000 g × 10 min	93
Rat, male, 180–220 g	Polytron 10 s, Potter-Elvehjem 0.16-mm clearance, 2 passes	0.225 M mannitol, 75 mM sucrose, 2 mM EDTA, 5 mM MOPS, 1%–2% fatty acid–free BSA, pH 7.3	13,000 g × 10 min, wash pellet × 2 in homogenate without MOPS or BSA	39
Rat, male, 300–400 g	Potter-Elvehjem, 0.4-mm clearance, homogenize with standard pestle	0.25 M sucrose, 10 mM Tris-HCl, 1 mM dithiothreitol, 1 mM EDTA, pH 7.4	600 g × 15 min × 2, 12,000 g × 20 min, wash mitochondria × 1	30
Rabbit, male, 1.4–1.8 kg Rat male, 180–220 g Mouse, male, 20–30 g	Potter-Elvehjem unmilled 2 strokes at 1,000 rpm	0.25 M sucrose, 2 mM EDTA, 5 mM Tris-HCl, 0.5% fatty acid–free BSA, pH 7.4	2,000 g × 5 min, 17,800 g × 5 min, wash mitochondria × 3	110

BSA, bovine serum albumin; EDTA, ethylenediaminetetraacetic acid; MOPS, morpholinopropanesulfonic acid; Tris-HCl, Tris-(hydroxymethyl)aminomethane HCl.

TABLE 2. *Respiration by Isolated Lung Mitochondria*

Incubation Conditions, State 3	FAD-Linked Succinate Oxidation State 3, nmol $O_2 \cdot mg^{-1}$ protein $\cdot min^{-1}$	RCR	Substrate	NAD-Linked Substrate Oxidation State 3, nmol $O_2 \cdot mg^{-1}$ protein $\cdot min^{-1}$	RCR	Ref.
34°C, Warburg apparatus. 100–150 mM KCl, 12.5 mM KH$_2$PO$_4$, 5 mM MgCl$_2$, 10 mM Tris-HCl, 10 mM NaF, 0.84 μM cytochrome c, 0.9 mM ATP, hexokinase, D-glucose, pH 7.4	67	1.2				93
28°C, Clark electrode. 145 mM KCl, 5 mM KH$_2$PO$_4$, 20 mM Tris-HCl, 0.2–0.4 mM ADP, pH 7.2	53	2.1	Pyruvate Isocitrate Glutamate Malate β-Hydroxybutyrate	40 38 25 20 7	2.9 2.5 3.0 1.8 1.4	39
30°C, Clark electrode. 125 mM KCl, 4 mM KH$_2$PO$_4$, 30 mM Tris-HCl, 2 mM MgCl$_2$, 12.5 mM KHCO$_3$, 2 mM EDTA, 0.3 mM ADP, pH 7.4	69	2.9	Isocitrate Malate	42 35	4.2 2.9	30
30°C, Clark electrode. 105 mM KCl, 2 mM KH$_2$PO$_4$, 30 mM Tris-HCl, 0.1 mM EDTA, 0.5% BSA, 0.3 mM ADP, pH 7.2	176	5.6	Glutamate Malate Glutamate + malate	146 70 208	9.8 3.8 6.2	110

State 3 mitochondrial respiration, O_2 utilization by mitochondria in the presence of substrate and ADP. State 4 mitochondrial respiration, O_2 utilization by mitochondria in the presence of substrate but without ADP. RCR, respiratory control ratio (state 3/state 4 respiration).

recent reports of methods to isolate lung mitochondria. None has entirely overcome the difficulties, and these results are presented for initial comparison only. The choice of experimental animal has an effect because of the known relationship between mitochondrial respiration and body size (63), but major differences have not been reported between mice and rabbits (110) and other small animals (38). To avoid possible depressant effects of anesthetics that have high initial lung concentrations after either parenteral administration or inhalation, animals have been killed by cervical dislocation (31, 32) or decapitation (39). Perfusion of the lungs in situ removes most erythrocytes that cosediment with mitochondria (31). Electron micrographs of lung mitochondrial fractions commonly show swelling of the cristae and contamination with membranous and lamellar material, some of which is probably surfactant. Repeated washing and recentrifugation on sucrose density gradients (92, 93) can improve purity but substantially decrease yield with no demonstrable improvement in respiratory control ratio. Mitochondrial yields for the methods listed in Table 1 are in the range of 1–4 mg mitochondrial protein per gram of lung with 25%–30% of the initial tissue succinate oxidase activity.

Isolated lung mitochondria can oxidize succinate through FAD-linked dehydrogenase with ADP/O ratios (ratio of moles of added ADP to extra O_2 consumed) close to the predicted value of 2.0, but the respiratory control ratios (ratio of O_2 consumption with added ADP to O_2 consumption without added ADP) are generally lower than those reported for liver and heart mitochondria (Table 2). Lung mitochondria can oxidize NAD-linked substrates with ADP/O ratios between 2 and 3, but again with relatively poor respiratory control ratios. The substantially improved respiratory control ratios reported by Spear and Lumeng (110) are in contrast to those of most other workers and must be confirmed, but their results indicate that lung mitochondria may be as tightly coupled as mitochondria from other tissues.

All these workers have evaluated their isolated mitochondria (18, 29) by testing their lack of increased oxidation to exogenous NADH and by showing higher ADP/O ratios with NAD-linked substrates compared with succinate. All the preparations demonstrate Mg^{2+}-dependent ATPase activity, although Spear and Lumeng suggest that this activity is present in the contaminating microsomes and does not represent damaged mitochondria. Turrens et al. (122) found that addition of Mg^{2+} increased the respiratory control ratio of porcine lung mitochondria, and they added 3 mM $MgCl_2$ for maximal respiratory control. This effect is likely due to a greater effect of Mg^{2+} on state 4 respiration than on state 3 respiration.

GLUCOSE TRANSPORT BY LUNG TISSUE

Perhaps because early reports indicated no direct effect of insulin on lung tissue in vitro, glucose transport into lung cells was not systematically determined until experimental diabetes was found to affect glucose metabolism of the lung (77, 78) and the structure of type II cells (88) and Clara cells (89). Subsequently several groups of investigators have reported that lung tissue has both active transport and facilitated diffusion of glucose with transport systems that are stereospecific for D-glucose (46, 87). These different transport mechanisms may be in different cell types, but some cells, including alveolar macrophages, have membranes with geographically separate transport sites (121) that may permit several mechanisms of glucose transport in the same cell. Facilitated diffusion of glucose can accelerate glucose transport into a cell, leading to equilibration of glucose across cell membranes. However, by this mechanism alone glucose concentration within the cell cannot exceed that outside the cell. Active transport of glucose with higher concentrations inside the cell, i.e., transfer against a chemical gradient, occurs in some epithelial tissues (e.g., kidney and intestine) and requires metabolic energy. Kerr et al. (59) reported that one glucose analogue, methyl-α-D-[U-^{14}C]glucopyranoside, can accumulate to a higher concentration in the isolated perfused lung than in extracellular areas, thus indicating active transport. However, other glucose analogues are apparently transported by facilitated diffusion or by other means. The authors suggest, by analogy with other tissues, that active transport may be limited to the epithelial cells of the lung. Another glucose analogue, 2-deoxy-D-glucose (DG), is taken up by lung tissue and phosphorylated but is not metabolized beyond that step (16). Fricke and Longmore (46) reported that the apparent kinetic constants for DG uptake by isolated perfused lungs from control, insulin-treated, and diabetic rats were Michaelis constant (K_m) values of 1.55, 2.87, and 3.57 mM and maximal velocity (V_{max}) values of 0.94, 2.02, and 0.53 μmol·g^{-1} dry wt·min^{-1}, respectively. The marked effect of insulin and diabetes on glucose transport into the lung had not been fully appreciated before such studies.

During hypoxia, when glycolysis increases, glucose transport into lung tissue has been reported to only double (34, 68, 97), and it may be a limiting factor in glucose consumption. Pérez-Díaz et al. (87) noted that isolated lung cells have glycolytic enzymes with much greater capacities for glucose utilization than are used to metabolize glucose from extracellular sources. However, when fructose is also in the medium these cells have greater maximum lactate production. Because fructose and glucose are transported into the cell by different systems, these results suggest that glycolytic control mechanisms below fructose, but including phosphofructokinase and pyruvate kinase, do not limit glucose consumption because they accommodate more flux to lactate when fructose is transported into the cells (87). Glucose transport into cells has been studied more extensively in some other tissues and can be classified as described by Elbrink and Bihler (27). Erythrocytes, the lens of the eye, and probably other tissues with relatively fixed glucose requirements only utilize facilitated diffusion and are insensitive to factors such as insulin that regulate glucose transport. Tissues containing substantial quantities of free glucose within the cell, including liver and erythrocytes, do not have glucose utilization limited by its penetration into the cell. Elbrink and Bihler (27) concluded that cells that use insulin and other factors to regulate glucose metabolism contain very low concentrations of glucose, have variable rates of glucose metabolism, usually respond to insulin, contain energy reserves in the form of glycogen and triglycerides, and have a capacity for both aerobic and anaerobic metabolism. At least some lung cells have characteristics suggesting that they fit these criteria and are responsive to insulin, as judged by studies with isolated cells as well as the whole lung (46, 49, 77, 82, 87, 88, 103, 108, 113).

GLUCOSE CONSUMPTION BY LUNG TISSUE

Glucose serves as a precursor for glycogen, lactate, nucleic acids, lipids, and proteins, as a source of reducing equivalents (NADH, NADPH), and as a source of energy under anaerobic or aerobic conditions. After entering a cell, glucose is rapidly phosphorylated to glucose 6-phosphate, which subsequently can follow several pathways of intermediary metabolism. In gluconeogenic tissues such as the liver and perhaps the fetal lung, glucose 6-phosphate can be hydrolyzed to glucose or converted to yield glycogen. In glycolytic tissues such as the adult lung, however, it either enters the Embden-Meyerhof pathway of glycolysis or is oxidized to phosphogluconate and ribulose 5-phosphate by the pentose cycle. The quantity of glucose consumed by lung tissue depends on nutrition, species, concentrations of many intermediates (including glucose), the presence of hormones, and technical factors. In addition comparisons between laboratories may be difficult because different units have been used to express lung mass: per gram wet weight, dry weight, and whole lung, milligram of protein, or milligram of DNA. To make comparisons for this chapter, we converted results expressed per gram wet weight to per gram dry weight by assuming a ratio of dry weight to wet weight of 0.20 and a DNA content of 6.2 mg/g wet wt (83, 120).

Methodological differences between laboratories can lead to significantly different results. Rat lungs sliced 1.0 mm thick consume less glucose but more O_2 than slices only 0.3 mm thick (67, 83). This difference may be related to greater cellular injury when the lung is sliced at short intervals and less O_2 consumption and consequently greater glycolysis when the cells are disrupted by the blade. However, 1.0-mm lung slices consume slightly more glucose (75 $\mu mol \cdot g^{-1}$ dry wt·h^{-1}; Table 3) than do isolated perfused lungs (55 $\mu mol \cdot g^{-1}$ dry wt·h^{-1}; Table 4) (84). These results were obtained by direct measurement of glucose concentrations before and after incubation. In contrast, Bassett and Fisher (5, 7) used [^{3}H]glucose and then determined the tritium-containing metabolic products, including ^3H_2O. After initial experiments in which Bassett and Fisher (5) measured tritium in all the products, they subsequently determined only the tritiated H_2O and applied a correction factor for the fraction of tritium that would be in other products. The results from this laboratory are generally lower than those from other laboratories and range between 30 and 49 $\mu mol \cdot g^{-1}$ dry wt·h^{-1} (5, 7). Other differences in method that may be related to the differences in glucose consumption noted in Tables 3 and 4 include fatty acid and amino acid concentrations, the presence of insulin, and the nutritional state of the animal. Clearly, however, no single value of glucose consumption would apply to all lungs.

Change of glucose consumption with hypoxia can be determined better with the isolated perfused lung than with any other preparation because the O_2 supply is most similar to lungs in vivo. The remarkable access of lung cells to O_2 from gas-filled alveoli and from the pulmonary vascular bed provides diffusion distances as short as 2–3 μm for much of the lung, although a small proportion of the isolated perfused lung may have greater diffusion distances. Tissue slices incubated in a medium lack both gas-filled air spaces and perfusion of the vascular bed, and the greater diffusion distances for O_2 may make the interior of some slices hypoxic, with consequent greater glycolysis and lactate production. In contrast to the high partial pressure of O_2 (P_{O_2}) required to avoid increased glycolysis with tissue slices, the isolated perfused lung has only slight increases of glycolysis and lactate production when it is ventilated with 5% O_2 instead of 95% O_2 (84). Bassett and Fisher (5) reported that it may be difficult to rid the isolated perfused lung of sufficient O_2 to obtain maximal anaerobic metabolism as reflected by glucose consumption and lactate production. They found that ventilation with 95% CO-5% CO_2 to prevent oxidative metabolism increased lactate production three- to fourfold, yet glucose consumption increased only 50% with hypoxia (95% N_2-5% CO_2). The lung thus has a significant Pasteur effect, and glucose transport into some lung cells is regulated. The critical P_{O_2} for oxidative metabolism of the lung is very low (34, 37) and is close to the critical P_{O_2} reported for isolated mitochondria (17).

Isolated lung cells, prepared with trypsin to release them from the tissue but not to separate them into specific cell types, have been reported to consume glucose at a rate of 212 nmol·h^{-1}·(10^6 cells)$^{-1}$ (2, 87),

TABLE 3. *Glucose Consumption by Slices of Rat Lungs*

Glucose Consumption, $\mu mol \cdot g^{-1}$ dry wt·h^{-1}	Ref.
75	131
70*	84
85†	124

Slices 1 mm thick, glucose concentration 4–6 mM, $P_{O_2} > 100$ Torr. *Calculated from assumption that wet wt/dry wt ratio = 5.0. †Slices 0.1 mm thick.

TABLE 4. *Glucose Consumption by Isolated Perfused Rat Lungs*

Glucose Consumption, $\mu mol \cdot g^{-1}$ dry wt·h^{-1}	Ref.
55, 78*†	84, 120
30, 37, 44‡	5, 6, 8
132	94
57§	111
54†§	125

Initial glucose concentration 4–6 mM, $P_{O_2} > 100$ Torr. *Calculated from assumption that wet wt/dry wt ratio = 5.0; 0.7 mM palmitate added to medium. †Amino acids in medium. ‡Insulin added to medium. §Perfused in situ.

TABLE 5. *Glucose Consumption and Lactate Production by Isolated Rat Lung Cells*

Cell Type	Glucose Consumption	Lactate Production	Ref.
	$nmol \cdot h^{-1} \cdot (10^6\ cells)^{-1}$		
Type II	104*	58	36
Type II	10†	0.5	72
Alveolar macrophages	127†	10.3	72
Mixed cells	212		3
Mixed cells	19*	9.5	2
Mixed cells	220*	2.7	87
Cloned type II	‡	1,000	107

*Glucose concentration 5 mM, $P_{O_2} >$ 100 Torr. †Glucose concentration 2.7 mM, $P_{O_2} >$ 100 Torr. ‡Glucose concentration 10 mM, $P_{O_2} >$ 100 Torr.

which is very high compared with results obtained with isolated type II cells (Table 5). Type II cells appear to be very active metabolically, but Mason et al. (71) and Fisher et al. (36) reported lower and discrepant values of glucose consumption by this cell type. Mason et al. found glucose consumption of only 10 $nmol \cdot h^{-1} \cdot (10^6\ cells)^{-1}$, whereas Fisher et al. found 104 $nmol \cdot h^{-1} \cdot (10^6\ cells)^{-1}$. Although many assumptions are required, these values may be compared with the glucose consumption of the whole lung by use of the number of type II cells in rat lungs estimated by morphometry (20). Assuming 125×10^6 type II cells for a 1.4-g rat lung (20) and the estimate of glucose consumption by the cells of Fisher et al., ~50 $\mu mol \cdot g^{-1}$ dry wt $\cdot h^{-1}$ would be consumed by these cells, which would nearly equal the glucose consumption of the whole lung. The value of Mason et al. would lead to an estimated 5 $\mu mol \cdot g^{-1}$ dry wt $\cdot h^{-1}$. These calculations illustrate that data from isolated cells may not reflect values of these cell types in vivo, and extrapolation from isolated cells to the whole lung cannot yet be done for quantitative results.

GLYCOGENESIS AND GLUCONEOGENESIS

Glycogenesis barely occurs in the adult lung, if it occurs at all. Glycogen is an important metabolite for the fetal lung, however, and changes in glycogen content parallel lung maturation. Between days 17 and 20 of rat gestation, glycogen content (expressed per milligram of DNA) doubles and equals 2%–3% of the lung weight (69, 70). By the end of gestation (day 22) the glycogen content decreases to about one-third of the peak value, and 1 day after birth the glycogen content drops to one-eighth of the peak value. Glycogen synthase activity peaks at about day 21 of gestation and then falls rapidly.

Quantitative determination of glycogen synthesis by isotopic studies is very complex (91), but ^{14}C from glucose has been reported to appear in the small quantity of glycogen in the adult rat lung. Although it amounts to <1% of all ^{14}C taken up from glucose (131), these results suggest that glycogen in the adult lung may be metabolically active.

Glycogen metabolism requires separate pathways for synthesis and degradation and involves only five or six enzymes other than those used for glucose metabolism. [Details of glycogen metabolism as determined with other tissues are given by Huijing (52) and Lehninger (65).]

REGULATION OF PULMONARY CARBOHYDRATE METABOLISM

Hypoxia

Although Pasteur observed that hypoxia increased carbohydrate metabolism in some systems, the isolated lung requires such severe hypoxia before lung carbohydrate metabolism changes significantly that other tissues or the entire organism would die if such hypoxia existed thoughout the lung in vivo. Although tissue slices cannot be used to approximate the effects of hypoxia on lung tissue in vivo, they can be used to demonstrate a Pasteur effect. These results and those with isolated lungs indicate that lung tissue produces lactate even when the P_{O_2} is high (Table 6) and has a definite Pasteur effect and produces more lactate when the tissue P_{O_2} is low. Overwhelming evidence indicates that lung tissue can vary the quantity of lactate produced two- to fourfold, depending on the cellular P_{O_2}. Fisher and Dodia (34) found that isolated and perfused rat lungs did not have maximum lactate production with 95% N_2-5% CO_2; only when they were ventilated with CO to compete with O_2 and eliminate oxidative metabolism by the mitochondria did lactate production reach a peak. These investigators reported that lactate production increased by 23% when the lung was ventilated with 5% O_2, by 60% with 0.1% O_2, by 100% with 0.006% O_2, but by 200% with 95% CO-5% CO_2 (34). The glucose consumption increased by 55% with hypoxia and by 153% with 95% CO-5% CO_2 (9). Others have reported similar percentage increases (125).

Agents that uncouple oxidative phosphorylation,

TABLE 6. *Lactate Production by Isolated Perfused Rat Lungs*

Lactate Production, $\mu mol \cdot g^{-1}$ dry wt $\cdot h^{-1}$	Ref.
64*	84
33–46	5, 9, 34, 40, 58
54	68
52–121†	97, 98
57–137	111, 112
22	23

Initial glucose concentration 4–6 mM, $P_{O_2} >$ 100 Torr. *Calculated from assumption that wet wt/dry wt ratio = 5.0. Palmitate and amino acids added to medium; lactate <1.0 mM. †Methodological correction in later study led to lower values.

such as dinitrophenol, also increase lactate production, presumably by removing the inhibitory effects of ATP and ADP on glycolysis. Bassett and Fisher (6) found that 0.8 mM dinitrophenol increased glucose consumption by 60% and lactate production by 70%. This is considerably less than results with CO and CO_2 ventilation but nearly as much as with N_2 and CO_2 ventilation. J. Turner and D. F. Tierney (unpublished observations) used 0.6 mM dinitrophenol and O_2 toxicity to determine whether the maximal O_2 consumption, expressed per milligram of DNA, was a sensitive index of lung injury during O_2 toxicity. Tissue slices of unexposed rat lungs increased O_2 consumption by 70% with dinitrophenol. However, after 24 and 48 h of exposure to 1.0 atm O_2, O_2 consumption was 20% less than the unexposed control and was increased by dinitrophenol only 40%–50%. Furthermore, by 48 h, glucose consumption doubled and lactate production tripled, indicating greater glucose entry into lung cells and greater glycolysis. After 96 h of exposure, O_2 consumption per milligram of DNA had increased by 35% without added dinitrophenol and by only 32% more when dinitrophenol was added. However, by this time the glucose consumption had increased fourfold and lactate production fivefold. These results indicate that the lung can increase O_2 consumption by 70% immediately and can markedly increase glucose consumption and lactate production after several days of lung injury and repair.

Hypoxia produces acute and chronic increases of glycolysis by increasing activity of existing enzymes or by increasing enzyme content. Acute hypoxia must rely on rapidly acting control mechanisms, such as the allosteric controls manifested in the Pasteur effect and increased glucose transport into the cell. However, other enzymatic changes appear responsible for the chronic effects of hypoxia. To determine enzyme content and not just activity, Hance et al. (50) used monoclonal antibodies with cloned lung cells and fibroblasts before and after 96 h of hypoxia. Based on their observation that the content of pyruvate kinase increases with hypoxia, these investigators proposed that the availability of O_2 modulates the content of key glycolytic enzymes that in turn regulate the generation of ATP through glycolysis. This observation may also explain some of the enzymatic differences found between cells in the lung exposed to a high P_{O_2} and similar cells in other organs exposed to lower P_{O_2}. For instance, macrophages obtained by lung lavage have different activities of glycolytic enzymes than those obtained from peritoneal washings. However, alveolar macrophages exposed to hypoxia for several days develop increased pyruvate kinase (15) and phosphofructokinase activities (106) that resemble the enzyme patterns of peritoneal macrophages. Thus there can be very rapid changes in flux through glycolysis due to allosteric effects that increase the activity of existing enzymes, and there can be slower changes of glycolysis related to enzyme content with chronic hypoxia.

Nutrition

Fasting for 48–72 h has been reported to increase lactate production by the lung by 40% (96), to have no effect (94), or to decrease production by ~25% (24). Some of the apparent change with fasting may be due to a loss of lung weight; this is one circumstance where it may matter whether the metabolism is expressed per wet weight, dry weight, milligram of DNA, or whole lung. The wet lung weight and protein content are 10% less in rats fasted 3 days than in fed controls (113), whereas the DNA content changes relatively little during fasting (86, 95). Therefore the O_2 consumption would appear to increase when expressed per wet or dry weight even if there had been no change when expressed per milligram of DNA or whole lung. A 3-day fast of pregnant rats near term produced fetuses with decreased body weight (30%), lung weight (30%), and lung glycogen but not decreased DNA (96). Therefore the glycogen content of the lung would be considered decreased if expressed per milligram of DNA but not if expressed per gram of lung.

Insulin and Diabetes

Insulin added directly to lung slices has little or no effect on carbohydrate metabolism. Such observations led early investigators to assume that the lung did not respond to insulin, but subsequently several differences of carbohydrate metabolism in lungs of diabetic animals were noted. Morishige et al. (77) injected streptozocin into adult rats. Coincident with other changes of diabetes, the lung had a decreased ability to oxidize glucose; this effect was reversed by insulin injections. Although tissue slices from lungs of both diabetic and normal rats had Michaelis-Menten saturation kinetics with glucose concentrations between 0 and 22 mM, the lungs of diabetic animals had a decreased capacity to oxidize glucose and a 50% increased production of lactate. The balance between glucose oxidation to CO_2 or to lactate production shifted toward lactate production in lungs from diabetic rats. Furthermore the V_{max} of glucose oxidation by lung slices from normal rats was 436 ± 35 nmol but only 300 ± 26 nmol by lung slices from diabetic rats.

Morishige and colleagues (76, 77) confirmed earlier reports that insulin had no significant effect on glucose metabolism when added directly to slices of normal lungs and observed it had no significant effect even when added to slices from diabetic rats. This apparent resistance to insulin in vitro is unlikely to be the result of destruction by the insulin-degrading activity reported for lung subcellular fractions because very high concentrations of insulin can be measured in the medium and because there are detectable effects of insulin on leucine uptake by lung slices from diabetic rats (76). The lung has high-affinity receptor sites specific for insulin (77), and it has been proposed that these may be on the type II alveolar cells and Clara cells because these cells develop structural changes with diabetes (88, 89). However, the lung reportedly has relatively few insulin receptors (12).

In contrast to the lack of response to insulin when added directly to lung slices, there is a marked effect when insulin is injected intravenously into diabetic rats; glucose oxidation and lactate production of lung slices revert to normal within minutes after the injection (46, 78). Moxley and Longmore (78) found that within 15–30 min after injecting insulin into diabetic rats the incorporation of [U-^{14}C]glucose into phosphatidylcholine and phosphatidylglycerol doubled. This central role of carbohydrate intermediary metabolism and insulin is supported by the observations that acetyl-CoA carboxylase and fatty acid synthetase activities were reduced in lung homogenates from diabetic rats. Furthermore the clinical observation that fetuses of diabetic mothers are at increased risk for respiratory distress may be related to disturbed surfactant metabolism associated with altered carbohydrate metabolism. Such fetuses respond to the high maternal glucose with hyperinsulinism, and Neufeld et al. (82) found that insulin added to lung slices of fetal rabbits caused less [^{14}C]glucose to be incorporated into phosphatidylcholine. Although conclusions regarding the total synthesis of phosphatidylcholine based on such isotopic incorporation data are tentative at best, this report is one of the few to indicate a direct effect of insulin on lung tissue slices and may reflect differences between fetal and mature lungs.

Cortisol has marked effects on the surfactant metabolism of fetal lung cells, and insulin can antagonize some of these effects. In addition to its role in carbohydrate metabolism, insulin is a growth promoter, and its reported capacity to block phosphatidylcholine synthesis by fetal lung cells may be distinct from its role in carbohydrate metabolism. Nevertheless insulin concentration in vivo is largely regulated through carbohydrate metabolism, which may therefore influence tissue growth indirectly. These studies promote speculation that hyperinsulinism in the fetus may affect lung development and contribute to the respiratory distress syndrome seen in some infants of diabetic mothers.

MAJOR PRODUCTS OF LUNG GLUCOSE METABOLISM

Yeager and Massaro (132) were the first to report products of [^{14}C]glucose metabolism as shown in Table 7. We emphasize one of the most puzzling aspects of

TABLE 7. *Major Products of Lung [^{14}C]Glucose Metabolism*

Glycogen	Lactate	CO$_2$	Lipid	Amino Acid	Protein	Ref.
	30	19	4.4		1.4	132
1	40	23	5	9	2	66

Values are percent of ^{14}C taken up by tissue that was accounted for by ^{14}C in each pool.

glucose metabolism in the lung: the unusually large percentage converted to lactate.

Lactate

Lungs contain large quantities of lactate dehydrogenase, which catalyzes the reaction

$$\text{pyruvate} + \text{NADH} \rightleftharpoons \text{lactate} + \text{NAD}^+$$

This reaction is thought to be close to an equilibrium in cells containing high activities of lactate deydrogenase, and generally the lactate concentration is 5–10 times the pyruvate concentration; this lactate/pyruvate ratio has been used to estimate the corresponding NAD$^+$/NADH ratio. During glycolysis, NAD$^+$ is converted to NADH; because NAD$^+$ is essential for glycolysis to continue, NADH must be reconverted to NAD$^+$. Generally other mechanisms can be used to convert NADH back to NAD$^+$, and lactate does not accumulate. An alternative possibility that may utilize lactate production but avoid its accumulation in tissues as greatly perfused as the lung is that lactate rapidly diffuses across the short distance to the blood and is metabolized elsewhere. When the lung is normally perfused, NADH may be converted back to NAD$^+$ by the production of lactate, which immediately leaves the lung. Because lung glucose metabolism represents ~1% of glucose utilization by the total body, the lung's production of lactate would not represent a major fraction of the body's lactate metabolism.

Most physiologists associate lactate production with anaerobiosis, probably because they are familiar with the Pasteur effect. However, many cells produce lactate even in aerobic environments, and their lactate production may be linked to ATP and NADP metabolism. When pyruvate is fully oxidized instead of converted to lactate, 18 times as much ATP becomes available as would have been produced from glycolysis only. Because the lung has such a high P$_{O_2}$ available from the air spaces and from its great blood supply, one might expect it to oxidize pyruvate rather than produce lactate. With few exceptions, however, reports indicate that the lung can oxidize pyruvate yet produce lactate (98, 99, 114, 124, 125, 129).

Lactate dehydrogenase is essential if lactate is to be further metabolized. Of the many isomeric forms of lactate dehydrogenase, the H and M types dominate (25, 65). The H type is inhibited by high concentrations of pyruvate, an effect that should lead to increasingly higher concentrations of pyruvate as it accumulates and by mass-action effects should force the pyruvate toward the citric acid cycle and increase its aerobic metabolism. Oxidation to CO_2 and H_2O also inhibit it. This H type is generally present in tissues where aerobic metabolism predominates, as in heart muscle. The M type generally is present in tissues with a low P_{O_2} or with sudden demands for energy, such as skeletal muscle, where sudden contraction may require more ATP than its mitochondria can produce quickly but glycolysis would be a ready source of ATP. Although the lung is highly aerobic and would be expected to have the H type by analogy with the distribution of H-type lactate dehydrogenase in other tissues, it also contains M-type lactate dehydrogenase (19). The presence of the M type may explain the rapid production of lactate even if pyruvate accumulates and inhibits the H type. Whether these two types coexist in the same cells of the lung is not yet known.

About half of the glucose consumed by the lung is released as lactate under most in vitro conditions. However, it is much more difficult to estimate lactate production of the lung in vivo; it can be determined for most organs by the Fick principle, which requires a measurable difference in lactate concentration in the arterial and venous blood. Compared with other organs, the lung's small mass and huge blood flow dilute this concentration difference and generally make such measurements impossible; the calculated concentration gradients are so small that sampling and analytical errors can easily exceed the true differences (115).

The initial findings of high lactate production by lung tissue in vitro were often assumed to be misleading or the result of anaerobic conditions. The results were eventually accepted, however, and a spate of questions regarding the significance and mechanisms of lactate production resulted. Does lactate production affect the pH of lung tissue and partially mediate the hypoxic vasomotor response that occurs with hypoxia? When the lung is poorly perfused will enough lactate accumulate to injure the tissue by acidosis? During diabetic ketoacidosis can lactate from the lung be utilized by other tissues in lieu of glucose? Do some lung cells have a relative deficiency of mitochondria that might limit their capacity to oxidize pyruvate? Do lung cells have different controls of phosphofructokinase and other key enzymes of glycolysis? Are the shuttle mechanisms to exchange reducing equivalents for NADH in the cytoplasm to the mitochondria relatively inactive? Many of these questions have been partly answered, but none has been conclusively decided.

To understand the possible mechanisms for lung lactate production, comparisons have been attempted with other lactate-producing tissues. Erythrocytes release lactate into the blood because they require glycolysis for energy, but without mitochondria they cannot metabolize pyruvate to CO_2 and H_2O. Erythrocytes therefore depend on glycolysis for ATP production, but NADH does not accumulate because it is converted back to NAD^+ as pyruvate is converted to lactate, which is then released into the blood and metabolized elsewhere. Some lung cells may have a relatively great diffusion distance to mitochondria (126) and produce lactate, as does the erythrocyte. Type I alveolar epithelial cells are the most likely candidates for this effect; although the volume density of mitochondria is not particularly low in these cells (73), they are so flat and have such thin cytoplasm that intramitochondrial distances in some parts of the cell may be relatively great. Skeletal muscle also produces lactate but requires bursts of energy when it contracts, and glycolysis can be an excellent source of ATP in response to such sudden, intermittent energy demands. It seems unlikely that two different systems adjacent to each other could be regulated by ATP content; however, glycolysis might contribute ATP and lactate in those portions of the cytoplasm far from mitochondria, whereas near mitochondria the ATP supply may be sufficient to limit glycolysis.

Lactate accumulates in malignant cells partly because they lack alternative means to convert NADH back to NAD^+ without conversion of pyruvate to lactate. These alterations involve NAD^+ and NADH, which normally do not enter mitochondrial membranes because there are shuttle mechanisms that transport reducing equivalents into the mitochondrial membranes and in effect convert cytoplasmic NADH to NAD^+. For instance, the glycerol phosphate shuttle in many cells can transfer reducing equivalents from NADH to the mitochondria and release NAD^+ (see *Generation of Reducing Equivalents*, p. 267). However, the lung contains the enzymes necessary for this shuttle mechanism, although some malignant cells do not.

Significant lactate accumulation from pathways other than glycolysis appears unlikely. Lactate can be produced from amino acids such as alanine, but this source appears relatively inactive in the lung (98). Rat lungs perfused with a solution containing 5 mM alanine released relatively little lactate, and presumably alanine aminotransferase activity was low (22, 111). Furthermore Longmore and Mourning (68) found using tracers that nearly 100% of lactate formed by the lung was derived from glucose under aerobic conditions and that alternative pathways must therefore contribute very little.

Lactate Production In Vivo

Generally the great blood flow through the lungs so greatly dilutes the lactate released that differences of lactate concentration in arterial and venous blood cannot be determined accurately; therefore the Fick principle cannot be used to determine lactate production in most mammals. However, the Weddell seal decreases its pulmonary blood flow to about one-sixth of its resting value when it dives (51, 79), and the arteriovenous concentration differences would increase sixfold if lactate release remained the same under these circumstances. One might question whether the entire lung is perfused when the blood flow decreases so dramatically and whether lactate accumulates in nonperfused lung tissue instead of being released. Hochachka et al. (51) reported that the lung of a diving Weddell seal has a net consumption of lactate, unlike the results from in vitro studies of lungs from other species. Prior to diving the arteriovenous difference for lactate was +0.090 ± 0.159 μmol/ml, indicating a slight net lactate release from the lung, although the arteriovenous differences were not statistically significant. During the simulated dive the average arteriovenous differences for lactate fell to −0.1630 ± 0.1756 μmol, indicating net lactate consumption ($P < 0.02$). The authors note that the arteriovenous gradients across the lung are the mirror image of those across the brain: during a dive the lungs utilize lactate that may have been formed by the brain. This is an interesting teleological explanation, because the lung stores most of the body's O_2 supply and may have a very high P_{O_2} during a dive, whereas other tissues have a low P_{O_2}. Conceivably this high P_{O_2} permits aerobiosis in the lung, which may utilize the products of anaerobiosis (lactate) from other organs. Other in vivo studies of lactate release or consumption have reported conflicting results (99).

Lactate Metabolism by Perfused Lung

Lactate production by the isolated perfused lung varies with factors such as the concentration of glucose, lactate, and other substrates in the media; the P_{O_2}; the presence of lung injury, such as O_2 toxicity; the presence of lung edema; and methodological problems, including bacterial growth in the perfusate (Table 8). With an initial glucose concentration of 4–6 mM and an O_2 tension that is high but not toxic, lactate production has been reported to be as low as 30 (5) and as high as 137 $\mu mol \cdot h^{-1} \cdot g^{-1}$ dry wt (94). Most reported values are between 33 and 64 $\mu mol \cdot h^{-1} \cdot g^{-1}$ dry wt (84, 98, 125). The explanation for the wide range is not apparent, but at least one laboratory subsequently reported that technical differences were responsible for some of their high values (98). With rare exceptions the isolated perfused lungs produce more lactate than they consume even with high lactate concentrations that might suppress lactate production in some tissue. Apparently nearly all lactate is derived from glucose (68, 133); although Kerr et al. (58) estimated that only 46% was from glucose, they may not have permitted radioactivity in the various pools to reach an equilibrium. Insulin had little or no effect on lactate production at a glucose concentration of 5.6 mM or higher, but insulin reportedly increased the lactate released by nearly 50% with 1.5 mM glucose (58).

TABLE 8. *Lactate Production by Isolated Perfused Rat Lungs*

Lactate Production, $\mu mol \cdot g^{-1}$ dry wt $\cdot h^{-1}$	Glucose, mM	Lactate, mM	Palmitate, mM	Ref.
52	5.6	0	0*	
53	5.6	0.2	0*	
52	5.6	0.5	0*	68
54	5.6	1.0	0*	
14.5	0	0.5	0*	
19	0	0†	0*	
41	1.5	0†	0*	58
50	5.6	0†	0*	
67	10	0†	0*	
68	2	0†	0.7	
86	6	0†	0.7	
132	18	0†	0.7	105
99	6	0†	0.2	
86	6	0†	0.7	
91	6	0†	1.8	

$P_{O_2} > 100$ Torr. *Palmitate was not added to medium but may have been present with albumin and other compounds. †Lactate was not added to medium initially.

Hypoxia must be severe to increase lung lactate production, but lungs ventilated with N_2 and CO_2 and perfused with 5.6 mM glucose doubled their lactate production from 52.3 $\mu mol \cdot h^{-1} \cdot g^{-1}$ dry wt and decreased the fraction of lactate derived from [U-^{14}C]-glucose from nearly 100% to ~57% (68). Kerr et al. (58) found a comparable increase in net lactate production when the lung was ventilated with CO and perfused with 5.6 mM glucose but found a slight increase in lactate derived from [U-^{14}C]glucose (from 46% when ventilated with a high P_{O_2} to 61% when ventilated with CO). These somewhat conflicting reports indicate that most (but perhaps not all) lactate is derived from glucose and that under conditions of stress (such as hypoxia) other sources of lactate may increase. Although the isolated perfused lung oxidizes lactate readily, it also releases lactate into the medium under nearly all conditions when glucose is present, and the net balance is lactate release.

Generation of Reducing Equivalents

Pyridine nucleotides (NAD^+ and $NADP^+$) serve as coenzymes by transferring reducing equivalents. Many dehydrogenases, including lactate dehydrogenase and glucose-6-phosphate dehydrogenase, selectivity bind either NAD^+ or $NADP^+$ but not both. Although these two couples (NAD^+-NADH and $NADP^+$-NADPH) have the same standard oxidation-reduction potential and are similar in many ways, the specificity of the enzymes for one couple but not the other indicates their different roles in oxidation-reduction reactions. In this section we focus on the oxidized form of NAD^+-NADH and the reduced form of $NADP^+$-NADPH. We emphasize NAD^+ because it is essential for glycolysis; if the resulting NADH were not rapidly converted back to NAD$^+$, glycolysis would slow and be limited by the availability of NAD$^+$. However, NADPH in the lung cytosol has a variety of roles, ranging from lipid synthesis to protection from inhaled oxidants.

Because these pyridine nucleotides play such a vital role in oxidation-reduction reactions, the ratios of the oxidized form to the reduced form have been used to approximate the redox state of the cell. At least three approaches have been used to estimate these ratios: *1*) direct measurement with rapidly frozen tissue, *2*) indirect estimates by fluorescence and absorbance of the whole organ with wavelengths considered to be specific for these pyridine nucleotides, and *3*) indirect estimates by determining the concentration of other related reactants, such as lactate and pyruvate, in a tissue and then calculating the ratio of oxidized to reduced pyridine nucleotides by the mass law.

Pyridine nucleotide contents have been determined directly from isolated perfused lungs (37). The NAD$^+$ content was 1,771 ± 263 nmol/g dry wt, but the NADH content was only 18.2 ± 3.5 nmol/g dry wt; the resulting NAD$^+$/NADH ratio was 97. In contrast the NADP$^+$ content of lungs was only 35 ± 9 nmol/g dry wt with an NAD$^+$/NADH ratio <2. Other studies report higher values for the rat lung, with NADP$^+$/NADPH ratios as high as 5 (119, 128). Therefore the lung has a much greater proportion of the NAD$^+$/NADH couple in the oxidized form, and the redox state is not the same for both couples.

Pyridine nucleotide ratios of the isolated perfused lung have also been determined with fluorescence from the lung's surface used to detect changes in the reduced pyridine nucleotides (37). This method indicates the direction of changes of these redox states but is not quantitative. Such studies have led to an appreciation that if the enzymes are compartmentalized then the loosely bound coenzyme may also be compartmentalized. During the catalytic reaction the coenzymes are bound, but they may rapidly dissociate afterward and release the pyridine nucleotide as a dissociable carrier of electrons (64). Bucher et al. (14) estimated that under specific conditions only 1% of cytosolic NADH in the isolated perfused rat liver may be in the free form and the rest may be bound to enzymes or other proteins.

The third method to estimate redox potential of NAD$^+$/NADH uses ratios of substrates such as lactate and pyruvate that are involved in reactions with NAD$^+$ and NADH, for example

$$AH_2 + NAD^+ \rightleftharpoons B + NADH + H_2^+$$

The ratio of NAD$^+$ to NADH can be calculated if one knows the ratio of B to A and the equilibrium constant. The calculation assumes that an equilibrium exists, that the intracellular pH is known (thus selecting the correct rate constant is possible), and that compartmentation within the cell and between different cells is not significant. Clearly these are major

TABLE 9. *Redox Couples Measured in Isolated Perfused Rat Lungs*

	Lactate/Pyruvate	Glycerol 3-P/Dihydroxyacetone-P	Glutamate/α-Ketoglutarate
Control	14	3.0	36
95% N$_2$-5% CO$_2$	32	7.2	69
95% CO-5% CO$_2$	82	12.9	73

Data from Fisher et al. (37).

assumptions, and significant compartmentation probably occurs in the lung with its variety of cell types. Nevertheless this approach has frequently been used to indicate the direction of changes and the general state of the tissue under different conditions. For instance, Table 9 shows the changes in redox couples that occur in isolated perfused rat lungs under different conditions. If severe enough, hypoxia should lead to accumulation of the reduced forms, but even at a P$_{O_2}$ of only 1-2 Torr the ratio is only twice the control value. When CO is used to inhibit oxidative metabolism the ratio increases nearly sixfold. The metabolism of the ventilated lung changes relatively little with severe hypoxia, and there is severe hypoxia in vivo except in unusual situations when the lung tissue is neither ventilated nor perfused.

The NADH conserves reducing equivalents released in the cytosol and eventually passes electrons into the mitochondrial electron-transport chains where ATP can be generated. However, the mitochondrial membrane in most tissue is impermeable to NADH, and the hydrogen therefore must be transferred to other molecules without significant energy loss before it enters mitochondria. Lung tissue can use several shuttle mechanisms to transfer electrons derived from NADH into the mitochondria. The glycerol phosphate shuttle is relatively simple, requiring only two enzymes. In the cytosol, glycerol-3-phosphate dehydrogenase converts NADH and dihydroxyacetone phosphate to NAD$^+$ and glycerol phosphate. Glycerol phosphate, containing the reducing equivalent, can then pass through the outer membrane of the mitochondria and release the reducing equivalent as it is converted back to dihydroxyacetone phosphate, which can then return to the cytosol and complete the shuttle. The mitochondrial glycerol-3-phosphate dehydrogenase is not limited to NAD$^+$ as a coenzyme but is a flavin-containing dehydrogenase; both enzymes must be present for this shuttle to function.

Lungs of rats, rabbits, sheep, and pigeons contain relatively high activity of flavin-linked glycerol-3-phosphate dehydrogenase (38, 39, 80). Therefore the potential for this shuttle mechanism exists in lungs, but it may not be distributed to all lung cells. In most tissues glycerol-3-phosphate dehydrogenase activity can be increased severalfold by producing a hyperthyroid state with thyroid hormones (63a). Hyperthyroidism might alter lung metabolism and its lactate production, but such studies have not yet been reported.

Another more complicated shuttle uses malate and aspartate and requires malate dehydrogenase in the cytosol and mitochondria as well as aspartate aminotransferase. Aminooxyacetic acid inhibits aspartate transaminase; when it is infused into isolated perfused rat lungs, the lactate/pyruvate ratio increases two- to threefold, which is evidence that this shuttle can also operate in the lung (37).

Although shuttle mechanisms exist in the lung tissue, they may not be capable of converting all NADH back to NAD^+. The great production of lactate by lung tissue and the evidence that the major source is from pyruvate indicate that not all NADH produced in the cytosol has ready access to a shuttle mechanism, perhaps because of compartmentation.

Pentose Phosphate Pathway

Some of the many roles of NADPH may be particularly important in the lung. During biosynthesis NADPH transfers chemical energy yielded by catabolism to energy-requiring reactions. Synthesis of pulmonary surfactant, for example, probably requires such transfer of energy through NADPH. In addition NADPH protects the cell from many oxidative reactions, and its participation in processes that alter drugs and other compounds is discussed in *Oxidants and Carbohydrate Metabolism*, p. 270. In some tissues cytosolic NADPH can be generated from succinate and malate. However, the low activity of the required enzyme in lung tissue indicates that this is a minor source of NADPH in the lung.

Although the pentose phosphate cycle (Fig. 3) generates precursors for the pentoses of nucleotides and nucleic acids, its major physiological function is to generate NADPH; the pentose phosphates are mostly reconverted to fructose 6-phosphate, which readily cycles back to glucose 6-phosphate. This source of NADPH is important, and Katz and his colleagues (55–57) have published a series of papers that refine their original analyses of methods to determine its activity. In a single passage of the initial glucose molecule through the pentose phosphate cycle, only the first carbon is removed and oxidized to CO_2. Thus, if the first carbon of glucose is labeled with ^{14}C, it may yield $^{14}CO_2$ either by passage through the pentose cycle or by entry into the Embden-Meyerhof pathway and subsequent oxidation in the TCA cycle. If the sixth carbon of glucose is labeled with ^{14}C, it can produce $^{14}CO_2$ only from the TCA cycle as long as rearrangement of glucose carbons does not occur. Consequently the activity of the pentose cycle is frequently estimated by noting the difference between $^{14}CO_2$ produced by glucose labeled in the first carbon compared with $^{14}CO_2$ produced by glucose labeled in the sixth carbon. That difference in $^{14}CO_2$ production from the two carbons indicates the difference between the $^{14}CO_2$ produced from the pentose cycle plus the TCA cycle (1st carbon) versus the TCA cycle only (6th carbon).

At least two other methods have been used to estimate pentose phosphate cycle activity; if the tissue has the same cell type, all methods should give the same result. However, in tissues with diverse cell types such as the lung, different methods may yield discrepant values if the glucose is utilized differently in the various cell types. Bassett and Fisher (7) found higher estimates for pentose phosphate cycle activity in isolated perfused rat lungs when they determined ^{14}C in the fatty acids instead of in $^{14}CO_2$. Although most estimates of the pentose phosphate cycle activity in lung tissue have used $^{14}CO_2$ yields, the results of Bassett and Fisher (7) suggest that cells in the lung that synthesize fatty acids have a very active pentose phosphate cycle, whereas other cells in the lung do not. The best candidates for such fatty acid synthesis are the type II cells. The $^{14}CO_2$ yields reflect the pentose phosphate cycle for the entire lung, whereas the fatty acid values indicate pentose phosphate cycle activity for the type II cells and other cells involved in fatty acid synthesis.

Estimated pentose phosphate cycle activity derived from $^{14}CO_2$ yields is ~5%–10% of all glucose utilized. Before comparing this percentage with other tissues, however, one should consider that the total glucose consumption for the lung is relatively high because ~50% of all glucose consumed is converted to lactate and is not immediately oxidized to $^{14}CO_2$. Therefore the pentose phosphate cycle activity in the lung is ~10%–20% of all glucose utilized for purposes other than lactate production.

The activity of the pentose cycle and presumably the production of NADPH in the cytosol can vary considerably, depending on the presence or absence of conditions such as O_2 toxicity and the consumption of reducing equivalents by drugs and other toxic agents such as paraquat. These topics are discussed in PATHOPHYSIOLOGY AND TOXICOLOGY, p. 270.

LUNG ENERGY PRODUCTION

Adenine nucleotides (ATP, ADP, and AMP) and guanosine nucleotides (GTP, GDP, and GMP) store chemical energy and control the rates of many cellular reactions. The cyclic nucleotides (3′,5′-cAMP and 3′,5′-cGMP) regulate a variety of cellular functions in other tissues and presumably have similar roles in lung cells. The lung content of cyclic nucleotides increases when drugs such as dibutryl cGMP or isoproterenol are added or if the lung is maximally inflated (61). Once again the heterogeneity of lung cells limits the interpretation of quantitative changes in whole lung tissue, and isolated cells and cell cultures have not yet provided reliable data. Unless the information from isolated cells is consistent with the information obtained from the whole lung, the interpretations are not reliable; currently nearly all the available information is from studies of whole lungs. We discuss only those aspects of lung energy metabolism relating to its parenchyma.

Substrates

Although glycolysis yields some ATP directly and the lung produces large quantities of lactate, most of the ATP derived from glucose when O_2 is available depends on oxidative phosphorylation in mitochondria. Fisher et al. (40) have estimated mitochondrial ATP generation by CO_2 production plus NADH shuttle mechanisms in the lung to be ~ 360 $\mu mol \cdot h^{-1} \cdot g^{-1}$ dry wt in the cytosol. The consequences of complete inhibition of oxidative metabolism with anoxia plus CO ventilation (5) were to double cytosolic ATP production by glycolysis (from 60 $\mu mol \cdot h^{-1} \cdot g^{-1}$ dry wt to 120 $\mu mol \cdot h^{-1} \cdot g^{-1}$ dry wt), whereas total ATP production was reduced (from 430 $\mu mol \cdot h^{-1} \cdot g^{-1}$ dry wt to 170 $\mu mol \cdot h^{-1} \cdot g^{-1}$ dry wt). As do other tissues, the lung depends on aerobic metabolism for optimal rates of ATP production, although under anaerobic conditions glycolysis can provide $\sim 25\%$ of the required ATP. Under anaerobic conditions ATP levels fall because the increased ATP production from glycolysis cannot compensate for the loss of mitochondrial ATP production.

Other substrates utilized by lung mitochondria include fatty acids, glycerol, citrate, and amino acids, but their quantitative importance is less well known and their omission does not appear to result in the same serious consequences as does the lack of glucose (35), at least in studies of short duration.

Oxygen as Substrate

The P_{O_2} needed to maintain cytochrome aa_3 in an oxidized state is extremely low in isolated mitochondria (17). The very thin alveolar septa with short diffusion paths suggests that the minimal alveolar P_{O_2} necessary for oxidative metabolism is a close estimate of the corresponding lung parenchymal P_{O_2}. Fisher and Dodia (34) found little change in lung ATP pools or reduction of mitochondrial cytochromes until the alveolar P_{O_2} fell below 0.4 Torr in the isolated perfused rat lung. Full reduction of the cytochromes requires the addition of CO in sufficiently high concentrations to effectively compete for cytochrome aa_3-binding sites. Their report utilizes the physiology of the lung to support the concept that mitochondria normally exist in a highly oxidized state (17), a concept based primarily on in vitro studies.

Nucleotide Pools

Representative values for rat tissue high-energy phosphate pools calculated by using the most complete reports are given in Table 10. Absolute values typically vary among laboratories measuring these highly labile compounds. The reported values for lung ATP have been increasing over the past decade, presumably as techniques of freezing and analyzing nucleotides have improved. The lung contains substantial amounts of adenine nucleotides even after isolation and perfusion for 60 min. Furthermore these are in a high-energy state as expressed by ATP/ADP ratios or by the value $E = (ATP + \frac{1}{2}ADP)/(ATP + ADP + AMP)$. The importance of these two calculated values in the metabolic regulation of enzymes is discussed by Atkinson (1). Phosphocreatine content of lung tissue appears to be very small compared with that in heart muscle but is higher than in liver, where it was not detectable (90). Together these high-energy phosphate pools would be able to provide the calculated ATP requirements of the lung for only a few minutes if ATP production were drastically reduced.

TABLE 10. *Lung High-Energy Phosphate Pools*

Preparation*	ATP	ADP	AMP	Total†	ATP/ADP	E‡	Ref.
	\multicolumn{4}{c}{$\mu mol/g$ wet wt§}			
Rabbit lung							
Fresh, unfrozen	1.5	0.44	0.15	2.1	3.5	0.83	123
Rat lung							
IPL, 95% O_2	1.7	0.24	0.07	2.0	7.3	0.92	9
Fresh, frozen	2.9	0.37	0.48	3.7	8.5	0.82	101
IPL, 95% O_2	2.2	0.26	0.08	2.5	8.6	0.92	5
IPL, 95% CO	1.0	0.37	0.16	1.5	2.7	0.75	5
Fresh, frozen	4.0	0.56	0.23	4.8	7.1	0.89	90
IPL, 95% O_2	3.8	0.56	0.17	4.5	6.6	0.90	90

* Fresh, taken directly from anesthetized animal. Frozen, freeze clamped between blocks of precooled metal. IPL, isolated perfused lung after 60 min of perfusion. †ATP + ADP + AMP. ‡E = (ATP + ½ADP)/(ATP + ADP + AMP). §Calculated from original reports with 6.2 mg DNA/g wet wt or dry wt/wet wt ratio of 0.2.

PATHOPHYSIOLOGY AND TOXICOLOGY

The pathophysiology of intermediary glucose metabolism in the lung parenchyma may include many conditions not yet known, including abnormal metabolism in some humans. The areas currently studied most intensively concern metabolic mechanisms of protection from toxic substances (generally oxidants) or energy-dependent fluid transport across epithelium. Fluid transport across the conducting airways is an important clinical topic (discussed in the chapter by Nadel, Widdicombe, and Peatfield in this *Handbook*). However, we discuss the relationship of glucose metabolism to pulmonary edema and of energy-related fluid transport across alveolar epithelial cells to pulmonary edema.

Oxidants and Carbohydrate Metabolism

Many inhaled substances, including oxidants, react in the lung with reducing equivalents generated from glucose such as glutathione; when the product is less toxic than the inhaled substance, the reaction can be considered a protective mechanism. For example, glutathione peroxidase reduces peroxides to less toxic compounds, and this enzymatic system may be considered a protective mechanism. In other cases, however, the product may have even greater toxicity (44). Some toxic substances are endogenously produced; Freeman and Crapo (45) demonstrated increased free-radical formation from oxidative metabolism when the lung tissue was exposed to elevated P_{O_2}. Metabolic mechanisms that protect against such free radicals include superoxide dismutase (21), which is not related to carbohydrate intermediary metabolism, and glutathione peroxidase, which utilizes NADPH and depends on the pentose phosphate cycle for regeneration. Figure 3 illustrates this dependency on the pentose phosphate cycle. In effect the reducing equivalents generated by the pentose phosphate cycle are passed to NADPH and then to glutathione, which can react with many oxidants, including peroxides. The same mechanisms utilizing reduced glutathione are responsible for protecting sulfhydryl groups in a wide variety of proteins and enzymes.

An interesting and important phenomenon that may be related to increased activities of such protective reactions in some species has been called tolerance or adaptation. This condition develops hours to days after an initial lung injury from a variety of agents. For example, rats exposed to toxic but not lethal P_{O_2} for several days can then survive exposures to P_{O_2} that would otherwise be lethal (20, 21, 81). The activities of several enzyme systems, including superoxide dismutase and those of the pentose phosphate cycle and glutathione metabolism, increase as the lungs become relatively resistant or tolerant to the toxic agent. Under such conditions the activity of pentose phosphate cycle enzymes (glucose-6-phosphate dehydrogenase and 6-phosphogluconate dehydrogenase) nearly doubles (116, 117), and presumably the pentose phosphate cycle thereby is capable of providing more reducing equivalents as NADPH. This phenomenon may be a nonspecific reaction to injury, because it also occurs with ozone and NO_2 exposure and with injections of α-naphthylthiourea (117). Although the acute effects of a toxin or O_2 are decreased, there is evidence that chronic injury and lung destruction occurs; these lungs are not completely tolerant (117). The increased activity of enzymes in the pentose phosphate cycle may reflect increased use of NADPH for tissue repair or for the glutathione system. A report (28) that indicates that the increased activity of enzymes in the pentose phosphate cycle depends on the activity of glutathione peroxidase suggests that this response is related to glutathione metabolism and not to tissue repair. It is perhaps not surprising that pentose phosphate cycle activity could be affected by concentrations of its products, and there is evidence that oxidized glutathione or NADPH can activate and NADPH can acutely suppress the enzymes of the pentose phosphate cycle (26).

Cellular NADPH also participates in many other reactions with compounds (54) that can damage membranes and may be mutagens. In many reactions the reducing equivalents are transferred from NADPH to glutathione, which can react with O_2, for instance, and lead to a chain reaction that could injure membranes (44). In addition NADPH may react as a cofactor with NADPH–cytochrome c reductase to reduce substances that subsequently can activate O_2 by electron transfer and eventually generate superoxide anion radicals (75). Drugs and toxins that may react in this fashion include alloxan (54), which is a diabetogenic drug that can also injure the lung and produce pulmonary edema; anticancer drugs such as adriamycin (54); and possibly the herbicide paraquat (128), which is highly toxic to the lung. Paraquat stimulates the pentose phosphate cycle activity of lung slices (42) or isolated perfused rat lungs (8), presumably because NADPH is being rapidly oxidized to $NADP^+$. In lungs of rats given paraquat, NADPH and $NADP^+$ decreased 20%–25% and the $NADP^+$/NADPH ratio decreased 45%, suggesting that these pyridine nucleotides play a major role in paraquat toxicity (128). Paraquat toxicity has been studied extensively because it appears to be a good model of oxidant lung injury and accidental ingestion has led to severe and often fatal lung injury. Furthermore lung injury frequently requires that patients receive O_2 therapy, but the combined toxic effects of paraquat and 100% O_2 are lethal to rats 1–2 days before the lethal effect of either agent alone (43). Such studies have led to the conclusion that even ambient air may have a P_{O_2} high enough to contribute to paraquat toxicity. High P_{O_2} levels (1.0 and 5.0 atm) also increase the pentose phosphate cycle activity of rat lungs (33), and a common mechanism for toxicity of O_2 and paraquat may exist.

It is not clear whether the increased activity of the pentose phosphate pathway when paraquat is present with lung tissue reflects a protective mechanism or an unimportant side reaction. Consumption of NADPH may not be important in protecting against toxicity. For instance, other compounds, including diquat (128), alter the lung NADPH and $NADP^+$ content and ratio but do not injure the lung to the same extent as does paraquat. Furthermore paraquat accelerates the decline of O_2 consumption by lung slices to the same extent whether or not glucose is present to provide NADPH (117).

Glucose Consumption During Pulmonary Edema

Pulmonary edema is associated with marked changes in glucose consumption and lactate production (133). Edema produced by elevated left atrial pressures in the isolated perfused rat lung doubles glucose consumption and lactate production. Similar changes occur when tissue slices are prepared from lungs made edematous in vivo (120, 133), and under these conditions the $^{14}CO_2$ production from [^{14}C]-glucose is not different from that of control lungs.

These changes are not due solely to fluid in the air spaces because glucose consumption and lactate production increase only 15%–20% when fluid is injected into the airways and air spaces of the isolated perfused rat lung (120). Additional studies by Postlethwait and Young (90) demonstrated decreased ATP concentrations in edematous lungs, a condition that should increase glycolysis. Furthermore dinitrophenol decreases ATP content in isolated perfused rat lungs and produces pulmonary edema (6). These studies suggest a relationship between glucose utilization and pulmonary edema that may depend on decreased ATP content in the lung tissue.

Recently a possible explanation for the association of pulmonary edema, ATP content, and glycolysis became apparent from studies of lung cell cultures. As with other epithelial cells, alveolar type II cells in cultures form small fluid-filled domes that appear to be produced by active transport of fluid across these cells (72) and require ATP. Dome formation is suppressed by dinitrophenol (48, 72), an effect consistent with the concept that relatively normal concentrations of ATP are required to maintain active transport of fluid. If these cells function similarly in vivo, pulmonary edema may be avoided by active transport of fluid from the air space into the interstitium and may be related to ATP content and requirements. If ATP content decreases, glycolysis would be expected to increase.

Many conditions with increased glucose consumption and lactate production may result from a common mechanism associated with coincident pulmonary edema. For instance, increased glucose consumption occurring with O_2 toxicity (33) or distensions of isolated lung (120) may be related to the pulmonary edema that occurs in these conditions.

There are other reports that glucose metabolism may be related to pulmonary edema. Edema develops in isolated perfused lungs if no glucose is added to the perfusion medium (35) or if iodoacetate is used to block glucose utilization (47). In addition to the energy-dependent reabsorption of fluid by alveolar type II epithelial cells, at least two other (perhaps overlapping) mechanisms are possible. The permeability of membranes between the capillary and alveolar space may depend on energy and intermediary metabolism. Altered alveolocapillary permeability has been reported as a consequence of hemorrhagic shock, endotoxin, histamine, and drugs such as heroin (13, 100–102). Some of these agents can interfere with mitochondrial oxidative phosphorylation and suggest a common link between energy metabolism and alveolocapillary permeability. The close cell-to-cell contacts of endothelial cells that may regulate permeability may in turn depend on microfilaments. Shasby and co-workers (104) have recently suggested such a relationship in a cultured cell model of endothelial permeability.

REFERENCES

1. ATKINSON, D. E. The energy charge of the adenylate pool as a regulatory parameter. Interaction with feedback modifiers. *Biochemistry* 7: 4030–4034, 1968.
2. AYUSO, M. S., A. B. FISHER, R. PARILLA, AND J. R. WILLIAMSON. Glucose metabolism by isolated rat lung cells. *Am. J. Physiol.* 225: 1153–1160, 1973.
3. AYUSO-PARRILLA, M. S., J. PÉREZ-DÍAZ, AND R. PARRILLA. Glucose inhibition of oxygen utilization by isolated rat lung cells. *Biochimie* 60: 823–862, 1978.
4. BARRON, E. S. G., Z. B. MILLER, AND G. R. BARTLETT. Studies in biological oxidations. XXI. The metabolism of lung as determined by a study of slices and ground tissue. *J. Biol. Chem.* 171: 791–800, 1947.
5. BASSETT, D. J. P., AND A. B. FISHER. Metabolic response to carbon monoxide by isolated rat lungs. *Am. J. Physiol.* 230: 658–663, 1976.
6. BASSETT, D. J. P., AND A. B. FISHER. Stimulation of rat lung metabolism with 2,4-dinitrophenol and phenazine methosulfate. *Am. J. Physiol.* 231: 898–902, 1976.
7. BASSETT, D. J. P., AND A. B. FISHER. Pentose cycle activity of the isolated perfused rat lung. *Am. J. Physiol.* 231: 1527–1532, 1976.
8. BASSETT, D. J. P., AND A. B. FISHER. Alterations of glucose metabolism during perfusion of rat lung with paraquat. *Am. J. Physiol.* 234 (*Endocrinol. Metab. Gastrointest. Physiol.* 3): E653–E659, 1978.
9. BASSETT, D. J. P., A. B. FISHER, AND J. L. RABINOWITZ. Effect of hypoxia on incorporation of glucose carbons into lipids by isolated rat lung. *Am. J. Physiol.* 227: 1103–1108, 1974.
10. BLAIR, P. V. Induction of mitochondrial contraction and concomitant inhibition of succinate oxidation by magnesium ions. *Arch. Biochem. Biophys.* 181: 550–568, 1977.
11. BLOXHAM, D. P. Metabolic flux through phosphofructokinase and fructose 1,6-diphosphatase. *Int. J. Biochem.* 5: 429–434, 1974.
12. BONNEVIE-NIELSEN, V., AND E. F. GEPPERT. Presence of surface receptors for insulin and absence of glucagon receptors on rat alveolar type II cells (Abstract). *Am. Rev. Respir. Dis.* 125, Suppl.: 229, 1982.
13. BRIGHAM, K. L., AND P. J. OWEN. Increased sheep lung vascular permeability caused by histamine. *Circ. Res.* 37: 647–657, 1975.
14. BUCHER, T., B. BRAUSER, A. CONZE, F. KLEIN, O. LANGGUTH, AND H. SIES. State of oxidation-reduction and state of binding in the cytosolic NADH-system as disclosed by equilibration with extracellular lactate/pyruvate in hemoglobin-free perfused rat liver. *Eur. J. Biochem.* 27: 301–317, 1972.
15. BUTTERICK, C. J., D. A. WILLIAMS, L. A. BOXER, R. A. JERSILD, JR., N. MANTICH, C. HIGGINS, AND R. L. BAEHNER. Changes in energy metabolism, structure and function in alveolar macrophages under anaerobic conditions. *Br. J. Haematol.* 48: 523–532, 1981.
16. CHAISSON, C. F., AND D. MASSARO. 2-Deoxy-D-glucose uptake by lung slices from fed and fasted rats. *J. Appl. Physiol.: Respirat. Environ. Exercise Physiol.* 44: 380–383, 1978.
17. CHANCE, B., AND J. R. WILLIAMS. The respiratory chain and oxidative phosphorylation. *Adv. Enzymol. Relat. Subj. Biochem.* 17: 65–134, 1956.
18. CHAO, D. L. S., AND E. J. DAVIS. Studies on the role of Mg^{2+} and the Mg^{2+}-stimulated adenosine triphosphatase in oxidative phosphorylation. *Biochemistry* 11: 1943–1952, 1972.
19. CHVAPIL, M. Lactate dehydrogenase isoenzyme pattern and total LDH activity in the lung and liver of rats chronically exposed to low and high oxygen concentrations. *Life Sci.* 17: 761–766, 1975.

20. CRAPO, J. D., M. PETERS-GOLDEN, J. MARSH-SALIN, AND J. S. SHELBURNE. Pathologic changes in lungs of oxygen adapted rats: a morphometric analysis. *Lab. Invest.* 39: 640–653, 1978.
21. CRAPO, J. D., AND D. F. TIERNEY. Superoxide dismutase and pulmonary oxygen toxicity. *Am. J. Physiol.* 226: 1401–1407, 1974.
22. DATTA, H., AND K. G. G. M. ALBERTI. Substrate utilization by the isolated perfused rat lung. *Biochem. Soc. Trans.* 5: 1312–1316, 1977.
23. DATTA, H., AND K. G. G. M. ALBERTI. Substrate utilization by the isolated perfused rat lung. *Biochem. Soc. Trans.* 7: 1026–1028, 1979.
24. DATTA, H., W. A. STUBBS, AND K. G. G. M. ALBERTI. Substrate utilization by the lung. In: *Metabolic Activities of the Lung*, edited by R. Porter and J. Whelan. Amsterdam: Excerpta Med., 1980, p. 85–104. (Ciba Found. Symp. 78.)
25. DAWSON, D. D., T. L. GOODFRIEND, AND N. O. KAPLAN. Lactic dehydrogenases: function of the two types. *Science* 143: 929–933, 1964.
26. EGGLESTON, L. V., AND H. A. KREBS. Regulation of the pentose phosphate cycle. *Biochem. J.* 138: 425–435, 1974.
27. ELBRINK, J., AND I. BIHLER. Membrane transport: its relation to cellular metabolic rates. *Science* 188: 1177–1184, 1975.
28. ELSAYED, N., A. HACKER, M. MUSTAFA, K. KUEHN, AND G. SCHRAUZER. Effects of decreased glutathione peroxidase activity on the pentose phosphate cycle in mouse lung. *Biochem. Biophys. Res. Commun.* 104: 564–569, 1982.
29. ESTABROOK, R. W. Mitochondrial respiratory control and the polarographic measurement of ADP:O ratios. *Methods Enzymol.* 10: 41–47, 1967.
30. EVANS, R. M., AND R. W. SCHOLZ. Phosphopyruvate carboxylase of rat lung. *Biochim. Biophys. Acta* 321: 671–680, 1973.
31. EVANS, R. M., AND R. W. SCHOLZ. Citrate formation by rat lung mitochondrial preparations. *Biochim. Biophys. Acta* 381: 278–291, 1975.
32. EVANS, R. M., AND R. W. SCHOLZ. Pulmonary fatty acid synthesis. I. Mitochondrial acetyl transfer by rat lung in vitro. *Am. J. Physiol.* 232 (*Endocrinol. Metab. Gastrointest. Physiol.* 1): E358–E363, 1977.
33. FISHER, A. B. Energy status of the rat lung after exposure to elevated P_{O_2}. *J. Appl. Physiol.: Respirat. Environ. Exercise Physiol.* 45: 56–59, 1978.
34. FISHER, A. B., AND C. DODIA. Lung as a model for evaluation of critical intracellular P_{O_2} and P_{CO}. *Am. J. Physiol.* 241 (*Endocrinol. Metab.* 4): E47–E50, 1981.
35. FISHER, A. B., C. DODIA, AND J. LINASK. Perfusate composition and edema formation in isolated rat lungs. *Exp. Lung Res.* 1: 13–21, 1980.
36. FISHER, A. B., L. FURIA, AND H. BERMAN. Metabolism of rat granular pneumocytes isolated in primary culture. *J. Appl. Physiol.: Respirat. Environ. Exercise Physiol.* 49: 743–750, 1980.
37. FISHER, A. B., L. FURIA, AND B. CHANCE. Evaluation of redox state of isolated perfused rat lung. *Am. J. Physiol.* 230: 1198–1204, 1976.
38. FISHER, A. B., G. A. HUBER, AND D. J. P. BASSETT. Oxidation of α-glycophosphate by mitochondria from lungs of rabbits, sheep and pigeons. *Comp. Biochem. Physiol.* 50: 5–8, 1975.
39. FISHER, A. B., A. SCARPA, K. F. LANOUE, D. BASSETT, AND J. R. WILLIAMSON. Respiration of rat lung mitochondria and the influence of Ca^{2+} on substrate utilization. *Biochemistry* 12: 1438–1445, 1973.
40. FISHER, A. B., H. STEINBERG, AND D. BASSETT. Energy utilization by the lung. *Am. J. Med.* 57: 437–446, 1974.
41. FISHER, A. B., H. STEINBERG, AND C. DODIA. Reversal of 2-deoxyglucose inhibition of serotonin uptake in isolated guinea pig lung. *J. Appl. Physiol.: Respirat. Environ. Exercise Physiol.* 46: 447–450, 1979.
42. FISHER, H. K., J. A. CLEMENTS, D. F. TIERNEY, AND R. R. WRIGHT. Pulmonary effects of paraquat in the first day after injection. *Am. J. Physiol.* 228: 1217–1223, 1975.
43. FISHER, H. K., J. A. CLEMENTS, AND R. R. WRIGHT. Enhancement of oxygen toxicity by the herbicide paraquat. *Am. Rev. Respir. Dis.* 107: 246–252, 1973.
44. FLOHE, L. Glutathione peroxidase brought into focus. In: *Free Radicals in Biology*, edited by W. A. Pryor. New York: Academic, 1982, vol. 5, p. 223–254.
45. FREEMAN, B. A., AND J. D. CRAPO. Hyperoxia increases oxygen radical production in rat lungs and lung mitochondria. *J. Biol. Chem.* 256: 10986–10992, 1981.
46. FRICKE, R. F., AND W. J. LONGMORE. Effects of insulin and diabetes on 2-deoxy-D-glucose uptake by the isolated perfused rat lung. *J. Biol. Chem.* 254: 5092–5098, 1979.
47. GOODALE, R. L., B. GOETZMAN, AND M. B. VISSCHER. Hypoxia and iodoacetic acid and alveolocapillary barrier permeability to albumin. *Am. J. Physiol.* 219: 1226–1230, 1970.
48. GOODMAN, B. E., AND E. D. CRANDALL. Dome formation in primary cultured monolayers of alveolar epithelial cells. *Am. J. Physiol.* 243 (*Cell Physiol.* 12): C96–C100, 1982.
49. GREGORIO, C. A., AND D. MASSARO. Influence of insulin on amino acid uptake by lung slices. *J. Appl. Physiol.: Respirat. Environ. Exercise Physiol.* 42: 216–220, 1977.
50. HANCE, A. J., E. D. ROBIN, L. M. SIMON, S. ALEXANDER, L. A. HERZENBERG, AND J. THEODORE. Regulation of glycolytic enzyme activity during chronic hypoxia by changes in rate-limiting enzyme content. *J. Clin. Invest.* 66: 1258–1264, 1980.
51. HOCHACHKA, P. W., G. C. LIGGINS, J. QVIST, R. SCHNEIDER, M. Y. SNIDER, T. R. WONDERS, AND W. M. ZAPOL. Pulmonary metabolism during diving: conditioning blood for the brain. *Science* 198: 831–834, 1977.
52. HUIJING, F. Glycogen metabolism and glycogen-storage diseases. *Physiol. Rev.* 55: 609–658, 1975.
53. KAMEN, M. D. *Isotopic Tracers in Biology: An Introduction to Tracer Methodology* (3rd ed.), edited by L. F. Fieser and M. Fieser. New York: Academic, 1957.
54. KAPPUS, H., AND H. SIES. Toxic drug effects associated with oxygen metabolism: redox cycling and lipid peroxidation. *Experientia* 37: 1233–1358, 1981.
55. KATZ, J. Use of isotopes for the study of glucose metabolism in vivo. In: *Techniques in the Life Sciences. Techniques in Metabolic Research*, edited by H. L. Kornberg, J. C. Metcalf, D. H. Northcote, C. I. Pogson, and K. F. Tipton. Amsterdam: Elsevier/North-Holland, 1979, vol. B207, p. 1–22.
56. KATZ, J., AND N. GRUNNET. Estimation of metabolic pathways in steady state in vitro. Rates of tricarboxylic and pentose cycles. In: *Techniques in the Life Sciences. Techniques in Metabolic Research*, edited by H. L. Kornberg, J. C. Metcalf, D. H. Northcote, C. I. Pogson, and K. F. Tipton. Amsterdam: Elsevier/North-Holland, 1979, vol. B208, p. 1–18.
57. KATZ, J., AND R. ROGNSTAD. Futile cycles in the metabolism of glucose. *Curr. Top. Cell. Regul.* 10: 237–289, 1976.
58. KERR, J. S., N. J. BAKER, D. J. P. BASSETT, AND A. B. FISHER. Effect of perfusate glucose concentration on rat lung glycolysis. *Am. J. Physiol.* 236 (*Endocrinol. Metab. Gastrointest. Physiol.* 5): E229–E233, 1979.
59. KERR, J. S., A. B. FISHER, AND A. KLEINZELLER. Transport of glucose analogues in rat lung. *Am. J. Physiol.* 241 (*Endocrinol. Metab.* 4): E191–E195, 1981.
60. KIRBY, W., AND C. B. TAYLOR. Multiple forms of phosphofructokinase in rat tissue. *Int. J. Biochem.* 5: 89–93, 1974.
61. KLASS, D. J. Dibutyryl cyclic GMP and hyperventilation promote rat lung phospholipid release. *J. Appl. Physiol.: Respirat. Environ. Exercise Physiol.* 47: 285–289, 1979.
62. KOOBS, D. H. Phosphate mediation of the Crabtree and Pasteur effects. *Science* 178: 127–133, 1972.
63. KREBS, H. A. Body size and tissue respiration. *Biochim. Biophys. Acta* 4: 249–269, 1950.
63a. LEE, Y. P., AND H. A. LARDY. Influence of thyroid hormones on L-α-glycerophosphate dehydrogenases and other dehydrogenases in various organs of the rat. *J. Biol. Chem.* 240: 1427–1436, 1965.
64. LEHNINGER, A. L. *Bioenergetics* (2nd ed.). Menlo Park, CA: Benjamin, 1972.
65. LEHNINGER, A. L. *Biochemistry* (2nd ed.). New York: Worth, 1975.

66. LEVY, S. E. The role of glucose in lung metabolism (Abstract). *Clin. Res.* 19: 145, 1971.
67. LEVY, S. E., AND E. HARVEY. Effect of tissue slicing on rat lung metabolism. *J. Appl. Physiol.* 37: 239–240, 1974.
68. LONGMORE, W. J., AND J. T. MOURNING. Lactate production in isolated perfused rat lung. *Am. J. Physiol.* 231: 351–354, 1976.
69. MANISCALCO, W. M., C. M. WILSON, AND I. GROSS. Influence of aminophylline and cyclic AMP of glycogen metabolism in fetal rat lung in organ culture. *Pediatr. Res.* 13: 1319–1322, 1979.
70. MANISCALCO, W. M., C. M. WILSON, I. GROSS, L. GOBRAN, S. A. ROONEY, AND J. B. WARSHAW. Development of glycogen and phospholipid metabolism in fetal and newborn rat lung. *Biochim. Biophys. Acta* 530: 333–346, 1978.
71. MASON, R. J., M. C. WILLIAMS, R. D. GREENLEAF, AND J. A. CLEMENTS. Isolation and properties of type II alveolar cells from rat lung. *Am. Rev. Respir. Dis.* 115: 1015–1026, 1977.
72. MASON, R. J., M. C. WILLIAMS, J. H. WIDDICOMBE, M. J. SANDERS, D. S. MISFELDT, AND L. C. BERRY, JR. Transepithelial transport by pulmonary alveolar type II cells in primary culture. *Proc. Natl. Acad. Sci. USA* 79: 6033–6037, 1982.
73. MASSARO, G. D., D. B. GAIL, AND D. MASSARO. Lung oxygen consumption and mitochondria of alveolar epithelial and endothelial cells. *J. Appl. Physiol.* 38: 588–592, 1975.
74. MASSARO, G. D., AND D. MASSARO. Mitochondria of the pulmonary granular pneumocyte in different species. *Am. Rev. Respir. Dis.* 115: 359–361, 1977.
75. MISRA, H. P., AND L. D. GORSKY. Paraquat and NADPH-dependent lipid peroxidation in lung microsomes. *J. Biol. Chem.* 256: 9994–9998, 1981.
76. MORISHIGE, W. K. Endocrine influences on aspects of lung biochemistry. In: *Metabolic Activities of the Lung*, edited by R. Porter and J. Whelan. Amsterdam: Excerpta Med., 1980, p. 239–250. (Ciba Found. Symp. 78.)
77. MORISHIGE, W. K., C. A. UETAKE, F. C. GREENWOOD, AND J. AKAKA. Pulmonary insulin responsivity: in vivo effects of insulin on the diabetic rat lung and specific insulin binding to lung receptors in normal rats. *Endocrinology* 100: 1710–1722, 1977.
78. MOXLEY, M. A., AND W. J. LONGMORE. Effect of experimental diabetes and insulin on lipid metabolism in the isolated perfused rat lung. *Biochim. Biophys. Acta* 488: 218–224, 1977.
79. MURPHY, B., W. M. ZAPOL, AND P. W. HOCHACHKA. Metabolic activities of heart, lung, and brain during diving and recovery in the Weddell seal. *J. Appl. Physiol.: Respirat. Environ. Exercise Physiol.* 48: 596–605, 1980.
80. MUSTAFA, M. G., AND C. E. CROSS. Lung cell mitochondria: rapid oxidation of glycerol-1-phosphate but slow oxidation of 3-hydroxybutyrate. *Am. Rev. Respir. Dis.* 109: 301–303, 1974.
81. MUSTAFA, M. G., AND D. F. TIERNEY. Biochemical and metabolic changes in the lung with oxygen, ozone and nitrogen dioxide toxicity. *Am. Rev. Respir. Dis.* 118: 1061–1090, 1978.
82. NEUFELD, N. D., A. SEVANIAN, C. T. BARRETT, AND S. A. KAPLAN. Inhibition of surfactant production by insulin in fetal rabbit lung slices. *Pediatr. Res.* 13: 752–754, 1979.
83. O'NEIL, J. J., R. L. SANFORD, S. WASSERMAN, AND D. F. TIERNEY. Metabolism in rat lung tissue slices: technical factors. *J. Appl. Physiol.: Respirat. Environ. Exercise Physiol.* 43: 902–906, 1977.
84. O'NEIL, J. J., AND D. F. TIERNEY. Rat lung metabolism: glucose utilization by isolated perfused lungs and tissue slices. *Am. J. Physiol.* 226: 867–873, 1974.
85. O'NEIL, J. J., AND S. L. YOUNG. Tissue slices in the study of lung metabolism. In: *Lung Development: Biological and Clinical Perspectives*, edited by P. M. Farrell. New York: Academic, 1982, p. 87–99.
86. PATHAK, R. M., A. MAHMOOD, AND D. SUBRAHMAYAM. The effect of undernutrition on lipid metabolism in lung: in vivo incorporation of labeled glucose into lipids. *Biochem. Med.* 24: 268–273, 1980.
87. PÉREZ-DÍAZ, J., A. MARTÍN-REQUERO, M. S. AYUSO-PARRILLA, AND R. PARRILLA. Metabolic features of isolated rat lung cells. I. Factors controlling glucose utilization. *Am. J. Physiol.* 232 (*Endocrinol. Metab. Gastrointest. Physiol.* 1): E394–E400, 1977.
88. PLOPPER, C. G., AND W. K. MORISHIGE. Alterations in granular (type II) pneumocyte ultrastructure by streptozotocin-induced diabetes in the rat. *Lab. Invest.* 38: 143–184, 1978.
89. PLOPPER, C. G., AND W. K. MORISHIGE. Alterations in the ultrastructure of nonciliated bronchiolar epithelial (Clara) cells by streptozotocin-induced diabetes in rats. *Am. Rev. Respir. Dis.* 120: 1137–1143, 1979.
90. POSTLETHWAIT, E. M., AND S. L. YOUNG. Alteration of rat lung adenine nucleotide content after pulmonary edema. *Lung* 158: 157–164, 1980.
91. RADZIUK, J. Developments in the tracer measurement of gluconeogenesis and glycogenesis in vivo: an overview. *Federation Proc.* 41: 88–90, 1982.
92. REISS, O. K. Properties of mitochondrial preparations from rabbit lung. *Med. Thorac.* 22: 100–103, 1965.
93. REISS, O. K. Studies of lung metabolism. I. Isolation and properties of subcellular fractions from rabbit lung. *J. Cell Biol.* 30: 45–57, 1966.
94. RHOADES, R. A. Net uptake of glucose, glycerol, and fatty acids by the isolated perfused rat lung. *Am. J. Physiol.* 226: 144–149, 1974.
95. RHOADES, R. A. Influence of starvation on the lung: effect on glucose and palmitate utilization. *J. Appl. Physiol.* 38: 513–516, 1975.
96. RHOADES, R. A., AND D. A. RYDER. Fetal lung metabolism response to maternal fasting. *Biochim. Biophys. Acta* 663: 621–629, 1981.
97. RHOADES, R. A., M. E. SHAW, AND M. L. ESKEW. Influence of altered O_2 tension on substrate metabolism in perfused rat lung. *Am. J. Physiol.* 229: 1476–1479, 1975.
98. RHOADES, R. A., M. E. SHAW, M. L. ESKEW, AND S. WALI. Lactate metabolism in perfused rat lung. *Am. J. Physiol.* 235 (*Endocrinol. Metab. Gastrointest. Physiol.* 4): E619–E623, 1978.
99. ROCHESTER, D. F., W. A. WICHERN, JR., H. W. FRITTS, JR., P. R. B. CALDWELL, M. L. LEWIS, C. GUINTINI, AND J. W. GARFIELD. Arteriovenous differences of lactate and pyruvate across healthy and diseased human lung. *Am. Rev. Respir. Dis.* 107: 442–448, 1973.
100. SAYEED, M. M., AND A. E. BAUE. Mitochondrial metabolism of succinate, β-hydroxybutyrate, and α-ketogluturate in hemorrhagic shock. *Am. J. Physiol.* 220: 1275–1281, 1971.
101. SAYEED, M. M., I. H. CHAUDRY, AND A. E. BAUE. Na^+-K^+ transport and adenosine nucleotides in the lung in hemorrhagic shock. *Surgery* 77: 395–402, 1975.
102. SAYEED, M. M., R. M. SENIOR, I. H. CHAUDRY, AND A. E. BAUE. Characteristics of sodium and potassium transport in the lung. *Am. J. Physiol.* 229: 1073–1079, 1975.
103. SCHUYLER, M. R., D. E. NIEWOEHNER, S. R. INKLEY, AND R. KOHN. Abnormal lung elasticity in juvenile diabetes mellitus. *Am. Rev. Respir. Dis.* 113: 37–41, 1976.
104. SHASBY, D. M., S. S. SHASBY, J. M. SULLIVAN, AND M. J. PEACH. Role of endothelial cell cytoskeleton in control of endothelial permeability. *Circ. Res.* 51: 657–661, 1982.
105. SHAW, M. E., AND R. A. RHOADES. Substrate metabolism in the perfused lung: response to changes in circulating glucose and palmitate levels. *Lipids* 12: 930–935, 1977.
106. SIMON, L. M., E. D. ROBIN, J. R. PHILLIPS, J. ACEVEDO, S. G. AXLINE, AND J. THEODORE. Enzymatic bases for bioenergetic differences of alveolar versus peritoneal macrophages and enzyme regulation by molecular O_2. *J. Clin. Invest.* 59: 443–448, 1977.
107. SIMON, L. M., E. D. ROBIN, T. RAFFIN, J. THEODORE, AND W. H. J. DOUGLAS. Bioenergetic pattern of isolated type II pneumocytes in air and during hypoxia. *J. Clin. Invest.* 61: 1232–1239, 1978.

108. SMITH, B. T., C. J. GIROUD, M. ROBERT, AND M. E. AVERY. Insulin antagonism of cortisol action on lecithin synthesis by cultured fetal lung cells. *J. Pediatr.* 87: 953–955, 1975.
109. SOROKIN, S. P. Cells of the lung. In: *Morphology of Experimental Respiratory Carcinogenesis*, edited by P. Nettesheim, M. G. Hanna, Jr., and J. W. Deatherage, Jr. Oak Ridge, TN: USAEC, Div. Tech. Info., 1970, p. 3–41.
110. SPEAR, R. K., AND L. LUMENG. A method for isolating lung mitochondria from rabbits, rats and mice with improved respiratory characteristics. *Anal. Biochem.* 90: 211–219, 1978.
111. STUBBS, W. A., D. M. KELLY, F. J. WALTERS, AND K. G. M. M. ALBERTI. The metabolic characteristics of the ventilated and non-ventilated perfused rat lung. *Biochem. Soc. Trans.* 5: 1312–1314, 1977.
112. STUBBS, W. A., I. MORGAN, B. LLOYD, AND K. G. M. M. ALBERTI. The effect of insulin on lung metabolism in the rat. *Clin. Endocrinol.* 7: 181–184, 1977.
113. THET, L. A., M. D. DELANEY, C. A. GREGORIO, AND D. MASSARO. Protein metabolism by rat lung: influence of fasting, glucose, and insulin. *J. Appl. Physiol.: Respirat. Environ. Exercise Physiol.* 43: 463–467, 1977.
114. TIERNEY, D. F. Lactate metabolism in rat lung tissue. *Arch. Intern. Med.* 127: 858–860, 1971.
115. TIERNEY, D. F. Intermediary metabolism of the lung. *Federation Proc.* 33: 2232–2237, 1974.
116. TIERNEY, D. F., L. AYERS, S. HERZOG, AND J. YANG. Pentose pathway and production of reduced nicotinamide adenine dinucleotide phosphate. *Am. Rev. Respir. Dis.* 108: 1348–1351, 1973.
117. TIERNEY, D. F., L. AYERS, AND R. S. KASUYAMA. Altered sensitivity to oxygen toxicity. *Am. Rev. Respir. Dis.* 115: 59–65, 1977.
118. TIERNEY, D. F., AND S. E. LEVY. Glucose metabolism. In: *Lung Biology in Health and Disease. The Biochemical Basis of Pulmonary Function*, edited by R. G. Crystal. New York: Dekker, 1976, vol. 2, chapt. 4, p. 105–126.
119. TIERNEY, D. F., J. YANG, AND L. AYERS. Enzymatic activity in rat lungs: some changes with exposure to 1 ATM oxygen. *Chest* 67, Suppl.: 40–42, 1975.
120. TIERNEY, D. F., S. L. YOUNG, J. J. O'NEIL, AND M. ABE. Isolated perfused lung-substrate utilization. *Federation Proc.* 36: 161–165, 1977.
121. TSAN, M. F. Effect of phagocytosis by human polymorphonuclear leukocytes and rabbit alveolar macrophages on 2-deoxyglucose transport. *J. Cell. Physiol.* 99: 23–30, 1979.
122. TURRENS, J., B. A. FREEMAN, AND J. D. CRAPO. Hyperoxia increases H_2O_2 release by lung mitochondria and microsomes. *Arch. Biochem. Biophys.* 217: 411–421, 1982.
123. VON WICHERT, P. Studies on the metabolism of ischemic rabbit lungs. Conclusions for lung transplantation. *J. Thorac. Cardiovasc. Surg.* 63: 284–291, 1972.
124. WALLACE, H. W., T. P. STEIN, AND E. M. LIQUORI. Lactate and lung metabolism. *J. Thorac. Cardiovasc. Surg.* 68: 810–814, 1974.
125. WATKINS, C. A., AND D. E. RANNELS. In situ perfusion of rat lungs: stability and effects of oxygen tension. *J. Appl. Physiol.: Respirat. Environ. Exercise Physiol.* 47: 325–329, 1979.
126. WEIBEL, E. R. Morphological basis of alveolar-capillary gas exchange. *Physiol. Rev.* 53: 419–495, 1973.
127. WILLIAMSON, D. H., P. LUND, AND H. A. KREBS. The redox state of free nicotinamide-adenine dinucleotide in the cytoplasm and mitochondria of rat liver. *Biochem. J.* 103: 514–527, 1967.
128. WITSCHI, H., S. KACEW, K. I. HIRAI, AND M. G. CÔTÉ. In vitro oxidation of reduced nicotinamide-adenine dinucleotide phosphate by paraquat and diquat in rat lung. *Chem. Biol. Interact.* 19: 143–160, 1977.
129. WOLFE, R. R., P. W. HOCKACHKA, R. L. TRELSTAD, AND J. F. BURKE. Lactate oxidation in perfused rat lung. *Am. J. Physiol.* 236 (*Endocrinol. Metab. Gastrointest. Physiol.* 5): E276–E282, 1979.
130. WU, R., AND E. RACKER. IV. Pasteur effect and Crabtree effect in ascites tumor cells. Regulatory mechanisms in carbohydrate metabolism. *J. Biol. Chem.* 234: 1036–1041, 1959.
131. YEAGER, H., JR., AND P. S. HICKS. Glucose metabolism in lung slices of late fetal, newborn, and adult rats. *Proc. Soc. Exp. Biol. Med.* 141: 1–3, 1972.
132. YEAGER, H., JR., AND D. MASSARO. Glucose metabolism and glycoprotein synthesis by lung slices. *J. Appl. Physiol.* 32: 477–482, 1972.
133. YOUNG, S. L., J. J. O'NEIL, R. S. KASUYAMA, AND D. F. TIERNEY. Glucose utilization by edematous rat lungs. *Lung* 157: 165–177, 1980.

CHAPTER 7

Protein turnover in the lungs

DONALD MASSARO | *Veterans Administration and Pulmonary Division, University of Miami School of Medicine, Miami, Florida*

CHAPTER CONTENTS

Protein Turnover in Nonpulmonary Tissues and Cells
Physiological Importance of Protein Turnover
Methods of Studying Protein Turnover in the Lung
Precursor Pools
Effect of Proteolysis on Extracellular Specific Radioactivity
Amino Acid Compartmentation in Perfused Lung
Protein Turnover Rates
Regulation of General Protein Turnover
　Diet
　Hormones
Degradation of General Lung Proteins
Regulation of Protein Degradation
　Exogenous amino acids
　Hypoxia
　Interaction between exogenous amino acids and hypoxia
　Potential physiological importance of interaction between amino acids and hypoxia
　Glucose and insulin
Connective Tissue Proteins of the Lung
　Collagen
　　Composition and synthesis of lung collagen
　　Changes in collagen content of the lung
　Elastin
　　Elastin content of the lung
　　Elastin turnover
Pulmonary Fibrosis
Proteases and Protease Inhibitors
Hyperoxia and Protein Synthesis
Protein Turnover in Pulmonary Macrophages
　Choice of precursor amino acid
　Precursor pools
　Protein degradation
　Phagocytosis and protein turnover
　Substrates and protein turnover
　Other factors affecting protein turnover in pulmonary macrophages

BORSOOK AND KEIGHLEY (16) in 1935 proposed the important concept that proteins in mammalian tissues are continually synthesized and degraded. When isotopes became available, this concept was supported by experiments showing that isotopic compounds were incorporated into and released from proteins in a wide variety of tissues [Schoenheimer's "dynamic state of body constituents" (247)]. The term *protein turnover* is now generally used to identify the combined phenomena of protein synthesis and degradation. Where possible in this chapter, I identify the synthetic and degradative processes separately and discuss the rate of synthesis or degradation. Several extensive, useful, and excellent reviews of these topics have recently been published (90–92, 241–244, 251, 273, 287), but these reviews contain virtually no information about protein turnover in the lung or in cells of the lung.

The study of protein turnover can be approached from different points of interest. To examine the molecular and subcellular mechanisms and processes of protein synthesis and degradation, investigators usually seek the most appropriate experimental model rather than confining their efforts to a particular organ or cell system. Because of its small size and cellular heterogeneity, the lung is not likely to be useful for experiments designed to shed new light on molecular or subcellular mechanisms of protein turnover.

Protein turnover can be studied to understand how specific cells or organs become specialized and contain different kinds of proteins (242). For example, Figure 1 shows the time course of changes in certain lung proteins and in lung structure in the neonatal rat. It seems reasonable to suppose that some of the biochemical changes are due to the extensive shift in cell population during the time of the study (27a). However, alterations in cell population are not a likely explanation for the different time course of the activity of angiotensin-converting enzyme and carbonic anhydrase (carbonate dehydratase) because these enzymes seem to be localized to the same cell—the pulmonary capillary endothelial cell (167).

Protein turnover can be studied in a particular organism, cell, tissue, or organ to gain insight into mechanisms by which these systems respond to environmental changes encountered under normal conditions, during periods of stress, or in disease. These studies provide information on the kinds of responses cells can make to various perturbations and characterize the manner in which particular systems "solve" the problem of survival and maintenance of function in the face of various conditions.

Most research on protein turnover has dealt with cellular proteins (90, 92). There is less information available on the turnover of extracellular proteins under normal conditions (288). Furthermore there is

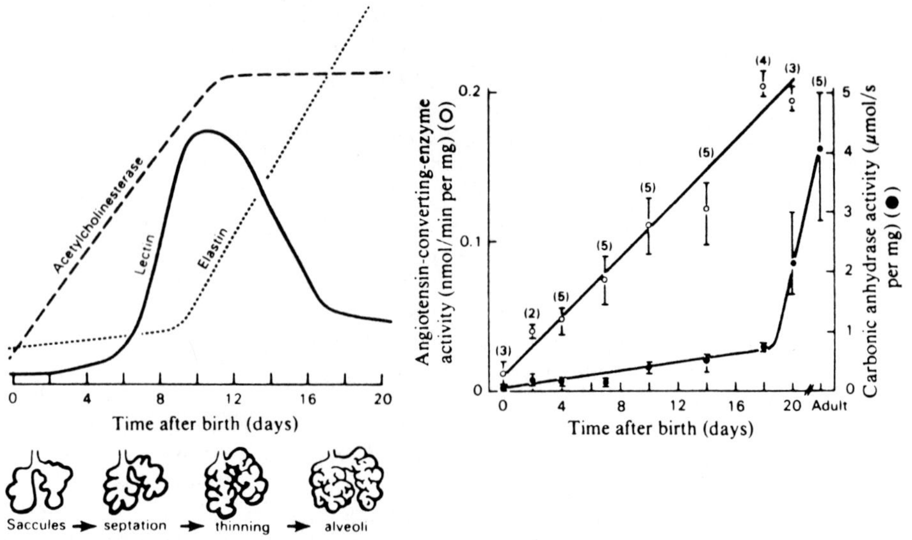

FIG. 1. Correlation of enzymes, lectin, and elastin with postnatal anatomical development of rat lung. *Left*: acetylcholinesterase, lectin, and elastin. *Right*: angiotensin-converting enzyme and carbonic anhydrase activity. [From Powell and Whitney (220).]

relatively little specific information on the mechanisms by which extracellular proteins such as collagen and elastin are protected from proteolytic attack in particular tissues under normal conditions or in disease. This topic is particularly interesting to respiratory physiologists and physicians because elastin and collagen are important to normal lung function (136, 141, 266, 276) and because evidence suggests that excessive proteolysis of extracellular elastin plays a major role in the development of emphysema (150). This chapter deals with aspects of protein turnover in the lung, particularly the contribution that protein synthesis and protein degradation make in maintaining the lung as an efficient organ for gas exchange. To provide background and perspective, I will begin with salient features of protein turnover learned from work on nonpulmonary tissues and systems.

PROTEIN TURNOVER IN NONPULMONARY TISSUES AND CELLS

After the groundbreaking efforts of Schoenheimer (247), studies on general tissue proteins (189, 197), specific proteins (23, 24, 64, 77, 164, 178) [including the same enzymes in different tissues (77)], and proteins of various subcellular organelles or subcellular sites (6, 89, 277) showed that protein turnover may be rapid and extensive and that rates of protein turnover vary widely (244). The studies also showed that protein turnover may be modulated by nutrition (170, 176, 189, 240), hormones (8, 52, 66, 79, 93, 135, 142, 192, 230, 264, 301), age (18, 19, 184, 254), substrates (50, 54, 160, 194, 222, 300), development (7, 112, 208, 249, 297), genetic factors (86, 224, 304), energy depletion and metabolite accumulation (35, 45), antigenic stimuli (187), and physical activity (193). Protein turnover may be altered by complementary changes in the rate of synthesis and degradation (301) or by a change in only the rate of synthesis or of degradation (176). In some cases the tissue level of a given enzyme may be altered by changes in the rates of both synthesis and degradation under certain circumstances and by changes in either its rate of synthesis or degradation under other conditions (89).

The importance of protein synthesis to an organism has long been appreciated, and protein synthesis is well recognized as a highly regulated process. However, interest in the degradative aspect of protein turnover lagged until the past decade, although studies 20–30 years ago indicated that proteolysis requires energy and hence is not likely to be simply an accompaniment of cell death (12, 26, 35, 148, 218, 257, 269). Since then, studies of many different tissues and systems have shown that protein degradation is mainly a highly regulated intracellular event and that there is a wide variation in the degradation rate of proteins (90, 92, 218, 242, 244, 288).

The enzyme proteins that regulate the flux of substrates through metabolic pathways seem to degrade the fastest (90). Large (51a), negatively charged (51b), or abnormal proteins, which occur in genetic defects (86, 224, 304) or when amino acid analogues have been incorporated into proteins (22, 254), are degraded faster than other proteins. Proteins most sensitive to proteases in vitro tend to be more rapidly degraded in vivo than proteins less sensitive to in vitro proteolysis (15a, 89a, 245). Protein degradation is also influenced by the subunit composition and by the protein's isoelectric point (51b) and seems to require ongoing protein synthesis (56, 298a, 298b).

PHYSIOLOGICAL IMPORTANCE OF PROTEIN TURNOVER

Some aspects of the physiological importance of protein degradation are obvious or inferred, e.g., its contribution to the level of proteins within the cell. In addition, Schimke (241) pointed out that the faster an enzyme or a protein is degraded the faster its concentration in cells can change. Goldberg and Dice (90) have amplified this concept by pointing out that in rat liver where half-lives for ~40 enzymes have been measured, the 12 enzymes with the shortest half-lives catalyze either the first or the rate-limiting step in metabolic pathways. Because changes in the concentration of key regulatory enzymes can be expected to alter flux through the metabolic pathway in which the enzyme participates, the ability to rapidly change the level of regulatory enzymes must offer the organism survival advantages.

This advantage to the lung and hence to the organism of rapid changes in enzyme levels may be illustrated by the response of the lung to a hyperoxic environment. A substantial amount of evidence supports the idea that the damaging effects of hyperoxia are due to highly reactive metabolites of O_2. These free radicals are products of normal cellular oxidation-reduction processes, but under hyperoxic conditions their production markedly increases (75, 76, 190). Cells have various antioxidant enzymes that defend the tissue by converting free radicals to less toxic forms (74, 75). Neonates of the rat, mouse, and rabbit are extremely tolerant to hyperoxia, but the adults succumb within days after being placed in >95% O_2 (69). The specific activity of antioxidant enzymes is not higher in the lungs of newborn than adult animals when they breathe air (69, 302). However, the newborn is able to rapidly increase the activity of antioxidant enzyme in its lung when exposed to hyperoxia; the untreated adult does not increase these enzymes (69). If the increase in activity of superoxide dismutase (SOD) is pharmacologically blocked, newborn rats succumb to hyperoxia, as do adult rats (72). Administering small doses of endotoxin can make adult rats tolerant to hyperoxia (70–73). Endotoxin does not increase the antioxidant content in lungs of rats breathing room air, but its administration to rats exposed to >95% O_2 results in an absolute increase in the amount of SOD as measured by immunoprecipitation (108). The endotoxin-treated adult rats show virtually 100% survival in >95% O_2 with almost no lung damage but behave as untreated rats if the rise in SOD is blocked by pharmacological means (72). Thus the survival of newborn and adult rats to a major change in environment clearly depends on the organism's ability to mount a rapid increase in the lung's antioxidant enzymes before fatal alveolar flooding occurs. With an atmosphere increasingly altered by industrialization and with forays into unknown atmospheres, the protective aspects of adaptive changes in lung protein turnover may assume great importance to the survival of air-breathing organisms.

The lung may face special problems in maintaining cellular homeostasis. Unlike other organs, it receives substrates and O_2 by different routes, i.e., perfusion and ventilation, respectively, thereby increasing the possibilities for local perturbations in the environment of lung cells. Changes in ventilation and perfusion and imbalances between these processes occur under normal conditions and are accentuated in disease. Because O_2 tension, H^+, lactate, and other substrates and components of the blood (e.g., hormones) have profound effects on protein metabolism in other tissues, local changes in the concentration of these moieties (consequent to changes in ventilation or perfusion) clearly require or lead to shifts in the lung's metabolism to maintain cellular integrity and thus allow the lung to function efficiently in gas exchange. Changes in cellular metabolism undoubtedly require changes in protein turnover.

Protein degradation per se may be important to the lung for the removal of abnormal, potentially harmful proteins that might arise from errors in gene expression or by denaturation or chemical modification brought about by inhaled toxins or even chemotherapeutic agents. As in other tissues, protein degradation in the lung may effectively remove or lower the content of unneeded proteins. In addition the degradation of unneeded proteins could provide amino acids for the synthesis of different newly needed proteins.

METHODS OF STUDYING PROTEIN TURNOVER IN THE LUNG

The half-lives of most proteins are too long to permit their net accumulation to be determined under most in vitro conditions. Furthermore the use of the net accumulation of protein to study protein turnover does not allow differentiation between contributions from protein synthesis and protein degradation to the accumulation of proteins or to changes in the rate of protein accumulation. These constraints and the commercial availability of pure amino acids of high specific radioactivity and of sensitive detectors of radioactivity resulted in the widespread use of isotopic amino acids to study protein turnover. The methods involved in the use of isotopes to measure protein turnover, including their advantages and disadvantages, have recently been reviewed in depth (90, 241, 244, 306). This chapter discusses the results of methods used to study protein turnover in the lung and its cells.

Several requirements should be met when choosing an isotopic amino acid to use in the study of protein turnover. Chemical purity is important. The presence of other amino acids or of compounds that can be metabolized to other amino acids can mislead. In this situation the accumulation of radioactivity in protein would reflect the incorporation of two or more amino acids. If the specific radioactivity of these contaminating amino acids in the pool of amino acids serving as the immediate precursors for protein synthesis (see next section) is high, their contribution to the radioactivity accumulated in protein could be great and hence the error or artifact large. Furthermore amino acids used to study rates of protein turnover should not be metabolized to any great degree by the cell or tissue under study, except in pathways of protein synthesis or degradation. Failure to meet this condition leads to the accumulation of radioactivity in protein, which represents the incorporation of more than one amino acid and the same potential artifact as could occur if the original amino acid was of low chemical purity.

The specific radioactivity of an amino acid used to study rates of protein metabolism should be high enough that its presence in proteins or in other moieties can be easily detected with an available means of measuring radioactivity. In addition the amino acid chosen should have a concentration that can be measured with reasonable ease and sufficient sensitivity. This is especially true in experiments where the specific radioactivity of tRNA-bound amino acids is being measured in a small number of cells. The amino acid should rapidly reach the cellular site of tRNA charging and should maintain a stable intracellular concentration.

Phenylalanine has thus far met these criteria in rat lung and rabbit pulmonary macrophages. Initially phenylalanine was chosen to study protein turnover in the lung because it is an essential amino acid in rats (11, 233) and rabbits (65) and because phenylalanine hydroxylase (phenylalanine 4-monooxygenase) is absent in the lungs of these species (275, 279). Its essentiality indicates that it will not be synthesized by the lung or other organs, and hence potential changes in de novo synthesis are excluded as a cause of variation in the intracellular concentration of this amino acid. The failure to detect phenylalanine hydroxylase activity in the lung suggests that phenylalanine is not metabolized to other amino acids and hence that its metabolism would mainly reflect processes of protein turnover. Recent studies show that phenylalanine is not metabolized to CO_2 by rat lung slices (270), isolated perfused rat lung (289), or rabbit pulmonary macrophages (105, 299). In these systems virtually no phenylalanine is converted to other metabolites, as indicated by the observation that >95% of the acid-soluble radioactivity in lung tissue or in pulmonary macrophages and of radioactivity released by hydrolysis of lung proteins coelutes with known phenylalanine when these materials are subjected to ion-exchange chromatography (33, 272, 289, 299). This amino acid is also useful when prolonged exposure to radioactive label is required, as shown by experiments where [^{14}C]phenylalanine was administered to intact rats and the lungs excised 5 h later; >90% of the acid-soluble and the acid-insoluble radioactivity in the lung coeluted from ion-exchange resins with known phenylalanine (33).

Studies with lung slices (272), in situ ventilated perfused rat lung (289), and pulmonary macrophages (62, 106) show that phenylalanine rapidly enters lung cells. In the in vitro perfused rat lung, phenylalanine equilibration between perfusate and tissue is a first-order process with a half time of 81 s (289). The tissue concentration of phenylalanine is stable for at least 3 h (272), and phenylalanine is rapidly incorporated into protein in both lung slices (272) and the perfused lung (289); in both systems its incorporation into protein remains linear with time for at least 3 h. Where it has been directly examined, i.e., in attached pulmonary macrophages, there is rapid charging of tRNA by phenylalanine (62), although controversy exists about the extent of charging from the extracellular pool of phenylalanine compared with phenylalanine derived from protein degradation (see next section). Experiments show the absence of a lag, at early time points, in incorporating phenylalanine into protein (289). This indirect evidence indicates that the pool of phenylalanine, which provides precursors for charging tRNA, rapidly reaches a steady-state specific radioactivity in the lung.

Phenylalanine can be measured by a variety of means, including ion-exchange chromatography (69, 191, 272), fluorometry (5), isotope dilution (236), and thin-layer chromatography of the dansyl derivative of phenylalanine (2). The latter method has been successfully used to measure picomole amounts of phenylalanine in small numbers of lung cells (2, 62).

PRECURSOR POOLS

Using isotopic amino acids to measure rates of protein synthesis implies that cells do not discriminate between radioactive and nonradioactive amino acids. With this assumption, the rate at which labeled amino acids are incorporated into protein depends not only on the actual rate of protein synthesis but also on the relative proportion of radioactive and nonradioactive amino acids present at the sites of tRNA charging. Thus the rate at which radioactive amino acids are incorporated into proteins is not necessarily a true reflection of the absolute rate of protein synthesis. To be sure if a particular perturbation or experimental condition has or has not altered protein synthesis, the absolute rate of protein synthesis must be measured. The use of isotopic amino acids for this purpose requires knowledge of the specific radioactivity of the tRNA-bound amino acids. If this information is not available or if it cannot be safely inferred, changes in the rate of protein synthesis cannot be distinguished from alterations in the rate of isotope incorporation into protein that reflect only changes in the relative proportion of isotopic and nonisotopic amino acids.

Cellular amino acids are supplied in vivo by constituents of the blood (55) and in vitro by the perfusate or medium. However, it is now recognized that a substantial percentage of the intracellular pool of free amino acids is derived from the intracellular degradation of proteins (3, 115, 144, 197). During most experiments involving isotope incorporation into protein, these degraded proteins are predominantly nonradioactive, because the life of the cell before the experiment is usually long compared with the period of exposure to the isotope. The pool of isotopic amino acids is therefore diluted by nonradioactive amino acids derived from protein degradation. Because many factors influence rates of proteolysis, the contribution from this source may vary widely and in some instances unpredictably from system to system (90, 92).

The problem of the specific radioactivity of the precursor pool could be dealt with easily if intracellular amino acids were the sole precursors used for protein synthesis and if intracellular amino acids existed as a single, rapidly and well-mixed pool. However, heterogeneity of intracellular pools of amino acids for protein synthesis exists in many tissues (1, 3, 34, 105, 111, 115, 127, 144, 147, 165, 185, 226, 229, 231, 246, 283, 287). The nature of the precursor pool of amino acids used for protein synthesis in the lung had been neglected until the systematic study by Watkins and Rannels (289) in the rat lung perfused in situ. They increased the concentration of perfusate phenylalanine 50-fold at constant specific radioactivity and found a 4-fold increase in the rate of incorporation of [^{14}C]phenylalanine into lung protein (Fig. 2A). The concentration of perfusate phenylalanine used does not seem to alter the rate of protein synthesis per se because the rate at which a different amino

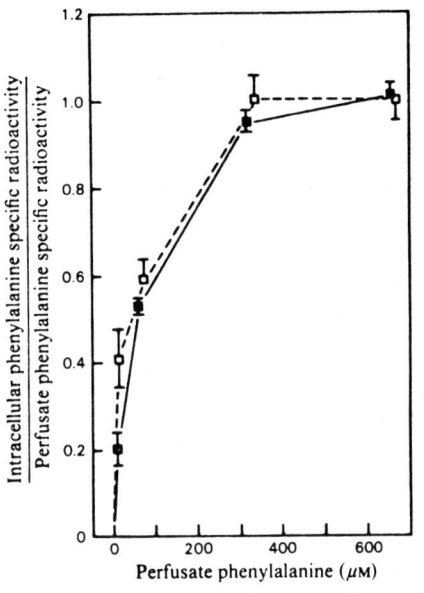

FIG. 3. Effect of perfusate phenylalanine concentration on specific radioactivity of intracellular phenylalanine in perfused lungs. Rat lungs were perfused in situ for 60 (■) or 180 (□) min. Data were plotted with perfusate phenylalanine concentration measured at end of perfusion period. [From Watkins and Rannels (289).]

acid, [^{14}C]histidine, is incorporated into protein is the same at low and high concentrations of phenylalanine (Fig. 2B). The changes in the incorporation of [^{14}C]-phenylalanine into protein as the concentration of perfusate phenylalanine is varied probably do not represent differences in the rate of protein synthesis; instead they seem to result from the effect the concentration of medium phenylalanine has on the specific radioactivity of phenylalanine in the pools supplying precursor amino acids for protein synthesis.

The mechanism for this effect can be gleaned from experiments in which intracellular concentration of phenylalanine was measured as the concentration of perfusate phenylalanine was increased (289). These experiments revealed a linear relationship between the intracellular and extracellular (perfusate) concentration of phenylalanine. Furthermore extrapolation of this relationship to an extracellular phenylalanine concentration of zero indicates that the intracellular concentration of phenylalanine would be 31 μM if no phenylalanine were present in the perfusate. Note that 31 μM represents ~50% of the intracellular concentration of phenylalanine in the lung when the perfusate concentration of phenylalanine is 69 μM (concentration of phenylalanine in normal rat plasma). Increasing the concentration of phenylalanine in the perfusate expands the total intracellular pool so that it becomes many times bigger than the pool derived from proteolysis. This expansion would markedly diminish the influence that amino acids from proteolysis have on the specific radioactivity of the total intracellular pool of phenylalanine.

Figure 3 shows that at a low concentration of per-

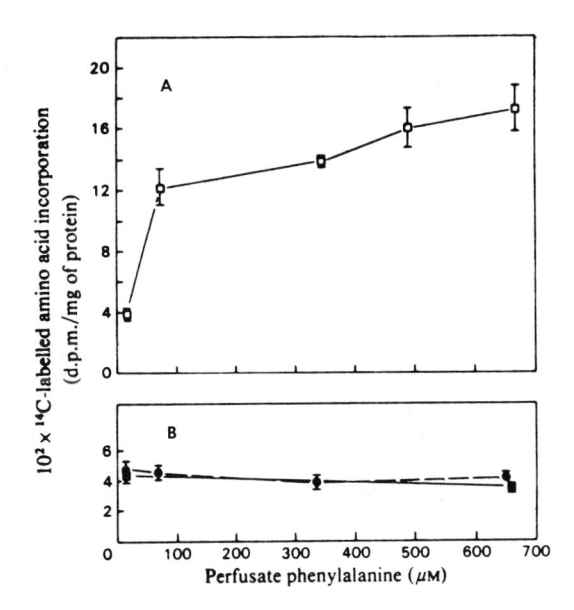

FIG. 2. Effect of perfusate phenylalanine concentration on incorporation of radioactive amino acids into protein by rat lung perfused in situ. Perfusate contained 10–690 μM phenylalanine and either (A) [^{14}C]phenylalanine (specific radioactivity 320 dpm/nmol; perfusions of 180 min) or (B) [^{14}C]histidine (specific radioactivity 850 dpm/nmol; perfusions of 60 min). ●, Perfusate equilibrated with O$_2$:CO$_2$ (19:1). ■, □, Perfusate equilibrated with O$_2$:N$_2$:CO$_2$ (4:15:1). [From Watkins and Rannels (289).]

fusate phenylalanine the specific radioactivity of intracellular phenylalanine is only ~20%–60% of that in the perfusate. This ratio reaches unity at higher concentrations of medium phenylalanine. The differences at low concentrations of extracellular phenylalanine indicate that at those concentrations the apparent rate of protein synthesis depends on which value is used in calculating the rate of protein synthesis. Figure 4 illustrates this. At low concentrations of perfusate phenylalanine, the apparent rates of protein synthesis are much higher when the specific radioactivity of intracellular phenylalanine is used to calculate the rate of protein synthesis than when the specific radioactivity of extracellular phenylalanine is used for calculation. These differences are absent when there is a high concentration of perfusate phenylalanine, i.e., levels at which the specific radioactivity of intracellular and extracellular phenylalanine is equal. These experiments indicate that neither the extracellular nor the intracellular pool serves as the sole source of amino acids for protein synthesis, an observation similar to that made in other tissues (3, 115, 144, 231).

For all practical purposes, amino acids bound to tRNA serve as the most immediate precursors for peptide-bond formation. Note that the rates of protein synthesis determined with the specific radioactivity of tRNA-bound phenylalanine is the same at very low and very high concentrations of perfusate phenylalanine (Fig. 4). This observation and finding that high levels of perfusate phenylalanine do not impair the incorporation of [^{14}C]histidine into protein [Fig. 2B; (70)] support the conclusion that high concentrations of a single amino acid do not in themselves alter the rate of protein synthesis. The information in Figures 3 and 4 indicates that when the concentration of perfusate phenylalanine is high enough that intracellular and extracellular specific radioactivity are equal, the latter, more easily obtainable value may be used to determine absolute rates of protein synthesis. However, in some tissues (231, 246), including lung fibroblasts (111) and possibly pulmonary macrophages (1, 106), the specific radioactivity of tRNA-bound amino acids may differ from that of the same amino acids in the intracellular or extracellular pool even when the ratio of the latter two specific radioactivities is unity. These relationships must be established in the system being studied and under the conditions of the experiment.

EFFECT OF PROTEOLYSIS ON EXTRACELLULAR SPECIFIC RADIOACTIVITY

Protein degradation can significantly influence the specific radioactivity of extracellular and intracellular amino acids. The amount of phenylalanine in sliced lung tissue remains constant over at least 3 h, whereas phenylalanine in the surrounding medium increases linearly (Fig. 5). Because phenylalanine is an essential amino acid in rats, it is not synthesized by the lung. The phenylalanine that accumulates in the medium in the face of a constant tissue concentration of phenylalanine must be derived from protein degradation. Because most amino acids derived from proteolysis during short-term studies are nonradioactive, their release into the medium should decrease the specific radioactivity of the extracellular amino acids, especially if the medium concentration of the exogenous amino acid is low. Figure 6 plots data from studies of perfused rat lungs by Watkins and Rannels (289). There is a progressive fall with time of the specific radioactivity of phenylalanine in the perfusate at low but not at high concentrations of medium

FIG. 4. Effect of perfusate phenylalanine concentration on estimates of protein synthesis. Rat lungs were perfused in situ for 60 min with [^{14}C]phenylalanine. Rates of protein synthesis were calculated with specific radioactivity of intracellular or extracellular perfusate phenylalanine or of tRNA-bound phenylalanine at the end of perfusion period. [Data from Watkins and Rannels (289).]

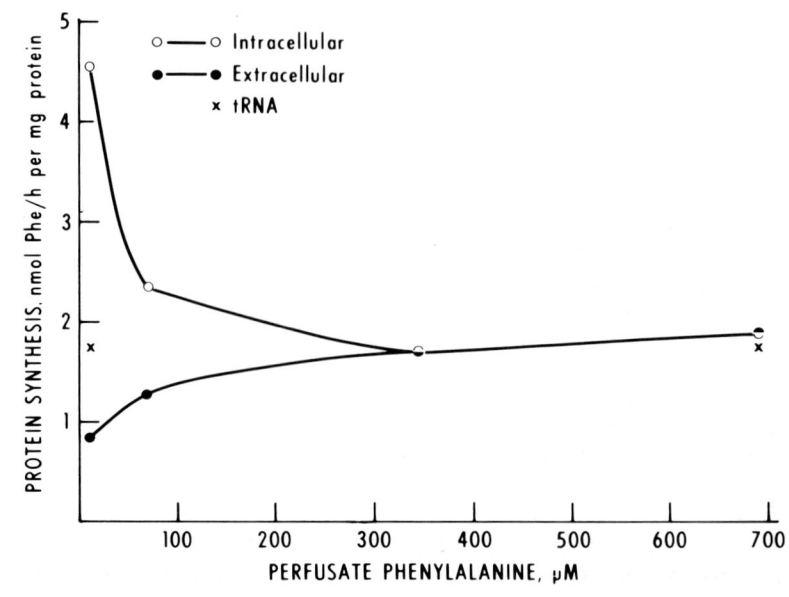

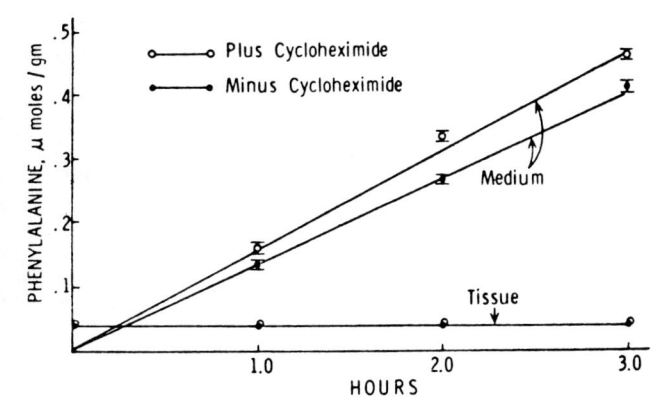

FIG. 5. Time course of intracellular and medium concentration of phenylalanine. In each experiment lung slices were incubated with or without enough cycloheximide to inhibit protein synthesis by >90%. [From Thet et al. (272).]

phenylalanine. The effect of proteolysis on the specific radioactivity of extracellular phenylalanine affects the apparent rate of protein synthesis if the rate is calculated by use of the specific radioactivity of extracellular phenylalanine.

AMINO ACID COMPARTMENTATION IN PERFUSED LUNG

Observations on protein metabolism in the lung suggest the model shown in Figure 7 for amino acid compartmentation in the lung. This is the most rudimentary scheme consistent with available information about the lung. The pool from proteolysis is considered to comprise amino acids derived from protein degradation that have not yet mixed with the main pool of intracellular amino acids. This pool could be made of intralysosomal amino acids and possibly of amino acids just released from proteins by intracytoplasmic proteolysis; in fact there may be multiple pools. In any case most of the cell proteins have long turnover times compared with the duration of most in vitro experiments of protein turnover. This pool, derived mainly from endogenous proteolysis, will contain mostly nonradioactive amino acids; hence the specific radioactivity of the amino acids in this compartment will be low. Measurements of the specific radioactivity of the total intracellular pool of a particular free amino acid include amino acids derived from proteolysis. Thus the specific radioactivity used in calculating rates of protein synthesis is influenced by both intracellular and extracellular pools. At low concentrations of extracellular phenylalanine the specific radioactivity of the entire pool of free intracellular phenylalanine is lower than that of the pool of amino acids serving as the immediate precursors for protein synthesis. This results in overestimation of the rate of protein synthesis (Fig. 4, curve formed by the open circles). At low concentrations of medium phenylala-

nine, especially over short times, the specific radioactivity of extracellular phenylalanine is high compared with that of the most immediate precursors to peptide-bond formation, and hence the rate of protein synthesis is underestimated (see Fig. 4, curve formed by closed circles). As the extracellular concentration of phenylalanine increases, the total intracellular pool enlarges, thereby diminishing the effect of phenylalanine of low specific radioactivity derived from protein degradation. Expanding the pools leads to equal specific radioactivity of intracellular and extracellular phenylalanine and hence equal rates of protein synthesis calculated from these two parameters. As shown in Figure 4, when this equality is achieved in the in

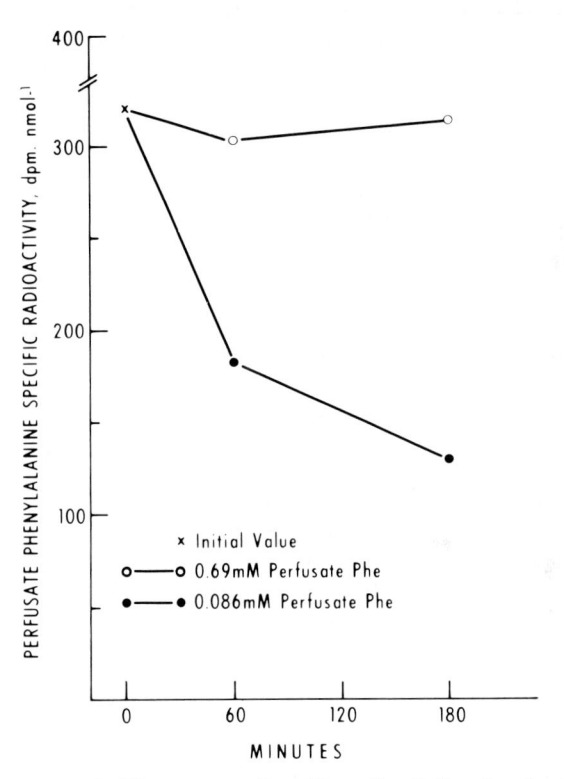

FIG. 6. Time course of specific radioactivity of perfusate phenylalanine. Rat lungs were perfused in situ with either 0.086 or 0.69 mM perfusate phenylalanine. [Data from Watkins and Rannels (289).]

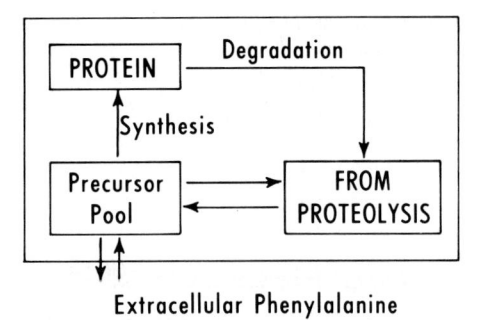

FIG. 7. Scheme for compartmentation of extracellular phenylalanine in lung tissue.

situ perfused lung, the rates of protein synthesis calculated from the specific radioactivity of intracellular or extracellular phenylalanine are equal to the rates calculated from the specific radioactivity of tRNA-bound phenylalanine. The rates calculated with the latter parameter are independent of the extracellular concentration of phenylalanine.

PROTEIN TURNOVER RATES

For many years the lung has been viewed as metabolically inert compared with other tissues. However, studies on the turnover of lung proteins and on many other areas of lung metabolism show that the lung is metabolically very active. For example, when pellets of radioactive tyrosine were implanted in unanesthetized mice to maintain the specific radioactivity of free tyrosine fairly constant, protein turnover in the lung was among the fastest of the organs studied (154). Garlick et al. (87) used a similar method, the continuous intravenous infusion of [^{14}C]tyrosine into unanesthetized pigs, and measured the fractional rate of protein synthesis and the RNA concentration of different tissues. This showed that the fractional rate of protein synthesis in pig lung is among the most rapid in the organs studied (Table 1); the proportion of the lung protein that is renewed each day corresponds to a half-life for lung proteins of ~3 days.

Munro (199) proposed that the capacity of a tissue for protein synthesis is related to its RNA concentration. This was confirmed by Garlick et al. (87), who found good correlation between tissue RNA concentration and its fractional rate of protein synthesis (Fig. 8); the lung's position falls on a straight line that can be drawn through these points. When the rate of

TABLE 1. *Fractional Rates of Protein Synthesis in Pig and Rat Tissues*

	Fractional Rate of Synthesis, %/day	
	Pig	Rat
Viscera		
Liver	23.2 ± 8.3	67.5
Kidney cortex	24.5 ± 5.7	
Kidney medulla	15.6 ± 3.7	47.9
Lung	18.3 ± 5.2	
Spleen	30.6 ± 3.1	
Brain		
Cerebellum	8.8 ± 1.2	
Cerebrum	8.3 ± 0.9	17.0
Pons	6.6 ± 1.4	
Muscle		
Leg	4.8 ± 1.6	13.0
Abdomen	3.7 ± 0.8	
Diaphragm	4.1 ± 0.6	
Heart, right	6.7 ± 1.4	
Heart, left	6.9 ± 1.4	17.2

Values are means ± SD of 6 pigs weighing 60–90 kg. Fractional rate of protein synthesis was calculated from specific radioactivity of free and protein-bound tyrosine in each tissue after [U-^{14}C]-tyrosine infusion lasting 6 h. [From Garlick et al. (87).]

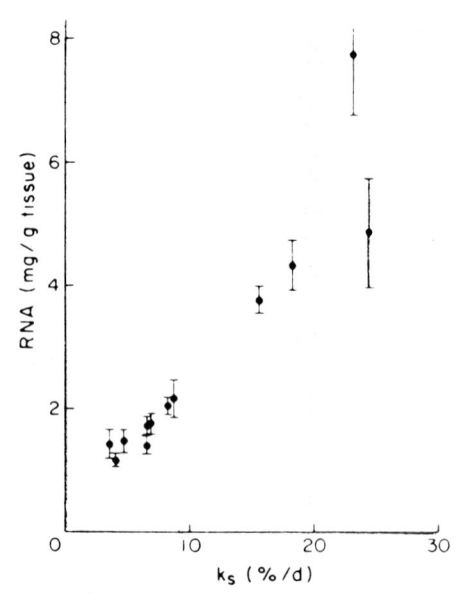

FIG. 8. RNA concentration of pig tissues plotted against fractional rate of protein synthesis (k_s) of these tissues. Pig lung is 4th value from right. d, Day. [From Garlick et al. (87).]

TABLE 2. *Protein Synthesis and Degradation*

	Phenylalanine, nmol·h^{-1}·mg^{-1} protein	
	Incorporated	Released
Rat lung, slices	2.1 (179a)	1.5 (270)
Rat lung, in situ, perfused	1.8 (287)	1.7 (287)
Rat heart, perfused	0.9 (193)	1.3 (193)
Rat skeletal muscle, perfused	0.3 (163)	0.8 (87)
Pig lung, in vivo	2.4 (87)	

References in parentheses.

phenylalanine incorporated by the lung is calculated per milligram of RNA, the rate in pig lung (65 nmol/h) (87) is virtually identical to the rate for the rat lung perfused in situ (69 nmol/h) (289). Apparently the efficiency of protein synthesis is equal in the lungs of the two species.

The in vivo studies showing that protein turnover in the lung is as rapid as it is in other tissues are supported by in vitro experiments (Table 2). This table demonstrates that under conditions where the specific radioactivity of extracellular phenylalanine is likely to equal that of tRNA-bound phenylalanine, the rate of protein synthesis in lung slices is about the same as in the perfused lung. In the latter preparation the specific radioactivity of tRNA-bound phenylalanine was measured. These rates of protein synthesis are higher than those observed in the perfused heart (193) and perfused skeletal muscle of the rat (164). In these organs the rates of protein synthesis were also measured at concentrations (0.4 mM) of perfusate phenylalanine where the intracellular or extracellular phenylalanine specific radioactivity equals that of tRNA-bound phenylalanine (164, 185). The rate of protein breakdown observed in lung slices is remarkably similar to the rate found in the in situ perfused lung (Table 2). Note that rat lung slices and in situ perfused lung are not in a catabolic state, as are perfused heart and skeletal muscle (Table 2).

It is unclear to what extent the rates of protein turnover measured in the in vitro rat lung systems approximate in vivo protein turnover in rat lung. For example, the protein content of the left lung of rats with an initial body weight of ~230 g is 34.6 mg; rats of equal initial body weight weigh ~250 g 3 days later, and the protein content of the left lung of these rats is ~41 mg (272). The protein concentration in these lungs is ~90 mg/g of lung, similar to the 118 mg/g of lung reported by others (222). Thus the protein concentration increased ~14 mg/g of wet lung over 3 days. Lung protein contains 308 nmol of phenylalanine per milligram of protein (221). With this figure for the phenylalanine content of lung protein and the rates of protein synthesis and degradation reported for in situ perfused rat lung (289), a net gain is calculated over 3 days of ~9 mg of protein per gram of wet lung. The discrepancy is not large between the measured increase (14 mg) and the calculated increase of protein (9 mg) when all the variables are considered, especially the different sizes of the rats used in the studies. This gives some confidence that the turnover rates measured in vitro are reasonable approximations of those occurring in vivo.

REGULATION OF GENERAL PROTEIN TURNOVER

Diet

The effect of food intake on protein turnover has been studied extensively in a wide variety of tissues (see ref. 288 for review) except the lung. The observation that complete food deprivation increases both the retractive forces of the lung and the minimal surface tension of lung extracts stimulated interest in the effect of nutrition on protein metabolism in the lung (63). The connection between these observations and lung proteins is the presence of apoproteins in lung surfactant (146). Additional potential relations between food intake and protein metabolism may be physiologically and clinically important. These include the observations that food deprivation diminishes the amount of dipalmitoyl phosphatidylcholine in lung tissue and lavage returns (85) and diminishes the enzyme activity required for the synthesis of phospholipid components of pulmonary surfactant (97); partial food restriction leads to an increase in alveolar surface forces and a loss of tissue elastic recoil (237). Diminished food intake has also been reported to increase the extent of enzyme-induced emphysema in rats (236) and to decrease lysyl oxidase activity of rat lungs (171).

Three days of total fasting decreases the rate at which protein accumulates in the lung from ~4 mg/day to ~1.5 mg/day (272). This degree of food deprivation decreases the RNA content of the lung by ~20% (80), indicating that a decreased capacity for protein synthesis probably contributes to the change in protein metabolism. Early studies showed that the incorporation of radioactive leucine into lung proteins was substantially diminished after 48 h of food deprivation (80). Because tracer amounts of labeled leucine were used in this study and the specific radioactivity of tRNA-bound leucine was not measured, the results reflect only apparent rates of protein synthesis. In view of the tracer levels of $[^{14}C]$leucine used, the rate of isotope incorporation into protein could be substantially altered by starvation-induced changes in the proteolysis rate, which was shown to occur by subsequent studies (272). However, despite these provisos the lower RNA content of the lungs from starved rats indicates that these lungs did indeed have a diminished capacity for protein synthesis (80).

Rannels et al. (223) resolved the issue of the effect of starvation on protein synthesis in the lung. They fasted rats for 3 days and measured protein synthesis in the in situ perfused rat lung with 0.69 mM radioactive phenylalanine in the perfusate. At this concentration of phenylalanine (10 times the normal rat plasma level) the specific radioactivity of intracellular and perfusate phenylalanine are equal, and in this system both are equal to the specific radioactivity of tRNA-bound phenylalanine (289). They found that the rate of protein synthesis diminished ~22% in starved rats, similar to the 20% decrease reported by Thet et al. (272) in the apparent rate of protein synthesis.

The decreased rate of protein synthesis in lungs of starved rats occurs without a change in the profile that lung ribosomes develop when centrifuged in a sucrose gradient (223). This finding, together with the reduced amount of RNA in the lungs of starved rats, and the observation that protein synthesis per milligram of RNA is the same in lungs from fed rats as in fasted rats (223) indicate that the capacity but not the efficiency of protein synthesis is decreased by food deprivation.

The effect of tryptophan on protein synthesis in lungs of starved animals is unresolved. Tryptophan was studied because fasting decreases the amount of polyribosomes and increases the amount of lighter RNA aggregates in rat and mouse liver. The administration of a complete mixture of amino acids or of tryptophan alone rapidly reverses the ribosomal pattern to that in fed animals (67, 256). Presumably these changes result in a decreased then increased rate of protein synthesis (see ref. 286 for a discussion of the problem of interpreting the effect of fasting in protein synthesis in the liver). Administering tryptophan intraperitoneally to fasting rabbits 45 min before they are killed results in a return to control values in the rate of incorporation of $[^{14}C]$leucine into protein by lung slices (80). Note that these studies also used only trace amounts of leucine, and hence the specific radioactivity of the precursor pool may have been substantially diluted by nonradioactive amino acids from accelerated protein degradation. Rannels et al. (223) carefully attempted to reproduce the conditions of tryptophan dose in fasted rats and were not able to confirm the effect found in rabbits (i.e., the administration of tryptophan did not increase the rate of lung protein synthesis in fasted rats). The data are internally consistent (i.e., fasting did not shift the pattern of lung ribosomes to lighter aggregates, and tryptophan did not increase the rate of protein synthesis). It is possible that the discrepancy is due to different species, but it is more likely that the earlier report (80) was flawed because of undetected changes in precursor specific radioactivity.

Hormones

It is now clear that the lung contains receptors for many powerful hormones and that those hormones influence important processes in the lung. Insulin increases the uptake of amino acids by lung slices (96). Diabetes may predispose to a loss of elastic recoil of human lungs (248), but this has not been confirmed (102).

Untreated diabetic rats do not increase their body weight normally and in fact seem to lose weight. The lungs of diabetic rats grow less rapidly and have less protein than those of normal rats (223). These findings are similar to the effects of food deprivation on the lung (272). However, unlike fasted rats the RNA content of the lungs of diabetic rats and nondiabetic rats is the same. Furthermore, lungs from diabetic rats synthesize protein at the same rate as normal rats (223). Insulin does not increase protein synthesis when added to lung slices from nondiabetic rats (272). The equal rates of protein synthesis suggest that the smaller amount of protein in lungs of diabetic rats must be due to increased proteolysis rates. The observation that insulin diminishes the proteolysis rate in lung slices supports this (272).

DEGRADATION OF GENERAL LUNG PROTEINS

Studies of protein turnover in the lung reviewed so far have focused on understanding protein synthesis. The importance of protein degradation to the level of tissue and cellular proteins, the possibility that protein degradation may be a means of removing abnormal potentially damaging proteins from cells, and the almost total lack of information on the regulation of the degradation of lung proteins led to a series of studies designed to examine protein degradation by the lung. The isolated perfused and ventilated rat lung has been used extensively for these studies, and the accumulation of a labeled amino acid in the perfusate has served as an index of the rate of protein degradation (31–33).

Phenylalanine, because of its essentiality for rats and its virtual lack of metabolism by the lung except in the pathways of protein turnover, was chosen as an amino acid that might be useful for the study of protein degradation in the isolated perfused rat lung. It proved to be a good choice. Radioactive phenylalanine can be injected into the intact rat at least 5 h before excising the lung. Despite this long exposure to all cells of the body, ~92% of the radioactivity released by acid hydrolysis of lung proteins labeled during 5 h is phenylalanine, as determined by ion-exchange chromatography, and >95% of the acid-soluble radioactivity appearing in the medium that is used to perfuse the lung elutes with the phenylalanine peak from an ion-exchange resin (33). Similarly >90% of the radioactivity added to the perfusate is recovered in the combined acid-soluble and acid-insoluble fractions after 60 min of perfusing and ventilating the isolated lung (Table 3). Furthermore the phenylalanine space, the intracellular concentration of phenylalanine, and the ratio of intracellular to extracellular radioactivity remain constant between at least min 15 and 90 of perfusion (33, 234).

When radioactive amino acids are used in the measurement of protein degradation, it is important to consider the reutilization for protein synthesis of amino acids released by proteolysis. This problem may be overcome by the addition of high concentrations of the nonradioactive form of the amino acid to the perfusate or medium after proteins are labeled with the isotopic amino acid. This is effective in the isolated perfused lung, where the presence of 10 mM nonradioactive phenylalanine in the medium results in the incorporation into proteins of only 0.02%–0.03% of [^{14}C]phenylalanine present in the perfusate; this represents only ~0.03% of the isotope usually present in protein at the beginning of perfusion (33). The high concentration (10 mM) of phenylalanine does not per se alter the proteolysis rate, as shown in studies in which lung proteins are labeled with [^{14}C]leucine. In these experiments the proteolysis rate is 13.4%/h without and 14.0%/h with 10 mM L-phenylalanine in the perfusate.

When the lung is preexposed to [^{14}C]phenylalanine for 10 min or 5 h and then excised, ventilated, and

TABLE 3. *Recovery of Radioactivity*

Fraction	Radioactivity Recovered, %	
	Experiment 1	Experiment 2
Trichloroacetic acid soluble		
Lung	2.1	2.5
Perfusate	67.6	71.9
Trichloroacetic acid insoluble		
Lung	21.2	17.3
Perfusate	1.4	1.04
Total	92.3	92.74

Lungs were perfused for 60 min with L-[U-^{14}C]phenylalanine. [From Chiang, Whitney, and Massaro (33).]

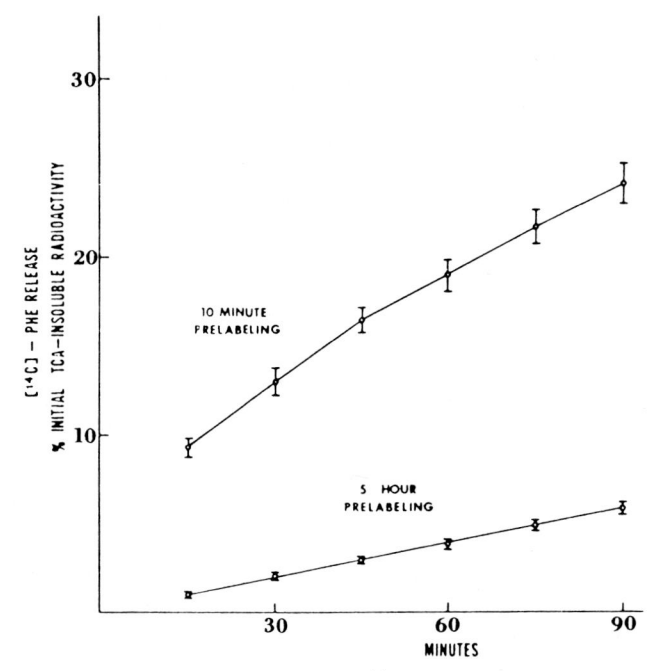

FIG. 9. Time course of release of [^{14}C]phenylalanine into perfusate by isolated perfused rat lung. Amounts of released label are expressed as percent of initial acid-insoluble radioactivity. [From Chiang et al. (33).]

perfused for 90 min, measurable amounts of free [^{14}C]phenylalanine appear in the perfusate (33). The amount of acid-soluble [^{14}C]phenylalanine accumulating in the perfusate represents a 240% increase in total free [^{14}C]phenylalanine between 15 and 90 min. During this time the absolute amount of acid-soluble phenylalanine in the tissue does not change (Table 3). Hence the appearance of [^{14}C]phenylalanine in the perfusate cannot be due to a simple shift of free [^{14}C]phenylalanine from lung tissue pools to the perfusion medium. Furthermore, because the intracellular concentration of phenylalanine remains unchanged and the phenylalanine is not synthesized or metabolized by the lung (except in the pathways of protein turnover), the [^{14}C]phenylalanine accumulating in the perfusate can only be derived from protein degradation. The time course of release of [^{14}C]phenylalanine expressed as a percent of the initial acid-insoluble radioactivity is shown in Figure 9. The proteolysis rate represents the difference in the percent of the radioactivity released between two time points and is expressed as percent released per hour. The proteolysis rate between 15 and 45 min and between 45 and 90 min for the proteins labeled for 10 min is ~16% and 11%/h. The rate for the proteins labeled for 5 h is only 3%/h. Proteins labeled during 10 min probably represent only a small fraction of lung proteins (49), and hence the high degradation rates for this group of proteins probably has little influence on the overall rate of protein degradation in the lung.

REGULATION OF PROTEIN DEGRADATION

Exogenous Amino Acids

In the isolated ventilated perfused rat lung the degradation rate of proteins labeled during 10 min is not altered during min 15–45 of perfusion by the absence of exogenous amino acids, but in their absence the proteolysis rate is diminished ~30% during min 45–90 of perfusion [Table 4; (32)]. This decreased proteolysis rate is reversed by adding sufficient exogenous amino acids to the perfusate after 45 min to achieve amino acid concentrations present in normal rat plasma. These effects of exogenous amino acids apparently are not due to changes in the ATP content of the lung, the intracellular concentration of phenylalanine, or the ratio of intracellular to extracellular phenylalanine (32). By contrast the degradation rate of proteins labeled for 5 h is not altered by the absence of exogenous amino acids (32).

The effects of exogenous amino acids indicate that, as with other systems (219, 285), the degradation of proteins that turn over slowly and proteins that turn over rapidly is independently regulated in the lung. However, the lung responds differently than other organs to exogenous amino acids. Thus in most other systems exogenous amino acids affect the degradation of proteins that turn over slowly (4, 79, 121, 300) and, when studied, have had little or no effect on the degradation of proteins that turn over rapidly (219, 285). By contrast the presence or absence of exogenous amino acids alters the degradation of proteins that turn over rapidly but not that of proteins that turn over slowly in the lung (32). The lung also differs in that the absence of exogenous amino acids produces a decrease in the proteolysis rate, whereas in other tissues the absence of exogenous amino acids leads to an increase in proteolysis. In this respect the lung behaves like hepatoma cells (56). However, a strict

TABLE 4. *Effects of Exogenous Amino Acids on Protein Degradation*

Condition	Proteolysis Rate, %/h	
	15–45 min*	45–90 min*
Labeled 10 min		
Control	14.3 ± 0.6 (32)	9.9 ± 0.7 (28)
Minus amino acids	13.1 ± 0.9 (17)	6.9 ± 0.5† (9)
Minus-plus amino acids		10.5 ± 0.9‡ (8)
Labeled 5 h		
Control	4.1 ± 0.5 (6)	3.5 ± 0.4 (6)
Minus amino acids	4.0 ± 0.4 (8)	3.3 ± 0.2 (8)

Values are means ± SE; number of experiments in parentheses. Lungs were perfused for 90 min. Minus-plus amino acids indicate that, after perfusing for 45 min without exogenous amino acids except for 10 mM L-phenylalanine, amino acids were added to perfusate to achieve levels of normal rat plasma. * Perfusion time. † $P < 0.025$ compared with control at 45–90 min. ‡ $P < 0.025$ compared with minus amino acids at 45–90 min, not significant compared with control at 45–90 min. [From Chiang and Massaro (32).]

comparison with proteins that turn over rapidly in other tissues may not be appropriate because the labeling period in the lung (10 min) is shorter than usually used in other systems (60 min) and hence might have resulted in the labeling of a group of proteins with different regulatory characteristics from those labeled in 60 min.

Most studies of the effect of amino acids on proteolysis have used levels of exogenous amino acids far different from those existing in plasma (32, 79, 219, 285). Although there is little reason to doubt the reported effects of amino acids on proteolysis rates, the physiological significance of the findings has not been established. However, it is possible that the lung may be exposed to more extreme variations in substrate deprivation than organs that receive both substrates and O_2 from the circulation, because lung oxygenation can continue when a diminution of blood flow limits delivery of substrates. Continued oxygenation may maintain relatively high levels of metabolism, which by fostering the uptake of materials from the interstitium might rapidly deplete substrates, thereby mimicking conditions in the lung perfused without exogenous amino acids. Under those conditions protein metabolism may mainly be influenced by cellular stores of substrates. If so amino acids may play a physiological role in the regulation of proteolysis in the lung, as Chiang et al. suggested (31, 32, 33a).

It is not known if the absence of exogenous amino acids or their replacement in the perfusate after 45 min results in changes in the intracellular concentration of amino acids. A lack of change in the intracellular concentration of amino acids in response to these maneuvers would suggest that changes in the transmembrane flux of amino acids serve as a signal to alter protein metabolism. The rates of amino acid flux might be especially sensitive to rates of blood flow and the concentration of amino acids in the blood.

Hypoxia

The differences between the isolated perfused rat lung and other tissues, with respect to the effect of exogenous amino acids on the proteolysis rate, led to studies designed to test the influence of hypoxia on protein degradation in the perfused lung. Hypoxia was chosen for study because it uniformly depresses proteolysis in other tissues, although the mechanism by which it acts is unclear (26, 35, 257, 269). Hypoxia also decreases the rate of protein degradation in the lung (Fig. 10). Only severe hypoxia (0% O_2) alters the proteolysis rate for proteins labeled for 10 min during min 15–45 of perfusion, but there is a concentration-related decrease in the proteolysis rate during min 45–90 of perfusion as the O_2 concentration is lowered. The onset of the hypoxia-associated decrease in the proteolysis rate is more rapid for proteins labeled during 5 h than for proteins with shorter half-lives;

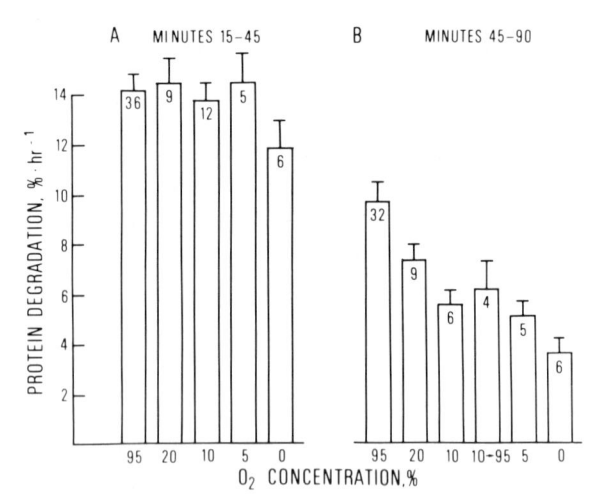

FIG. 10. Protein degradation at different O_2 concentrations. Lungs of rats were exposed in vivo during room air breathing to [^{14}C]phenylalanine for 10 min and then perfused and ventilated for 90 min with concentrations of O_2 indicated and in presence of rat plasma concentrations of amino acids plus 10 mM nonradioactive phenylalanine and 5.5 mM glucose. In A, bars represent rates of protein degradation during min 15–45. In B, bars represent rates of protein degradation during min 45–90. 10 → 95, Lungs were ventilated with 10% O_2 during 0–45 min and 95% O_2 during 45–90 min. [From Chiang et al. (31).]

the proteolysis rate is diminished within min 15–45 in the presence of 10% O_2 (Fig. 11). These findings indicate that with respect to hypoxia, protein degradation in the lung is diminished as in other tissues.

The diminished proteolysis rate found under hypoxic conditions has been generally attributed to the energy-poor state of the hypoxic tissues. However, unlike protein synthesis (where energy deficiency results in an immediate fall in the synthesis rate) there may be a lag between the onset of a low-energy state and a fall in the proteolysis rate (31). The lag between the onset of hypoxia and the beginning of a decrease in the proteolysis rate has led to the suggestion that metabolite accumulation alone, or with the low-energy state, is responsible for the diminished proteolysis rate that occurs during hypoxia. Metabolite accumulation was suspected as a cause for the decreased proteolysis rate by the isolated perfused lung for three reasons: *1*) the onset of changes in the proteolysis rate occurs well after the ATP content of the lung has fallen, *2*) the institution of ventilation with >95% O_2 after 45 min of ventilation with 10% O_2 does not increase the proteolysis rate (Fig. 10), and *3*) lactate and hydrogen ions decrease the rate of protein degradation in the heart (35).

These considerations led to a series of experiments that tested the effect on proteolysis of medium that had previously been used to perfuse nonradioactive lungs ventilated for 90 min with 95% O_2 or 0% O_2 (31). Figure 12 shows that the proteolysis rate in fresh lung perfused with medium previously used to perfuse nonhypoxic lungs is decreased ~20% during min 45–90 compared with control lungs. In contrast the proteolysis rate is decreased ~60% during min 45–90 in lungs perfused with medium previously used to perfuse lungs ventilated with 0% O_2. The magnitude of this decrease in the proteolysis rate (60%) is identical to the extent to which 0% O_2 diminishes the proteolysis rate, but the former occurs under nonhypoxic conditions and in lungs in which the ATP content is not diminished (31).

The depressant effect of used perfusate from hypoxic lungs on proteolysis cannot be accounted for by the accumulation of lactate or hydrogen ions. Thus 50 mM exogenous lactate depresses the proteolysis rate of nonhypoxic lungs only ~20% (Fig. 12); this concentration of lactate is higher than the concentration reached in the perfusate of hypoxic (0% O_2) isolated ventilated perfused rat lung (165). In addition dialysis of used medium or adjustment of its pH to the pH of fresh perfusate does not alter the diminished proteolysis rate produced by used medium from hypoxic lungs (Fig. 12). The possibility that small inhibitor molecules are retained in the dialysis bag because they become bound to albumin seems to be excluded by experiments in which hypoxic lungs were perfused with medium that did not contain exogenous albumin; this medium also lowers the proteolysis rate when it is then used to perfuse fresh nonhypoxic lungs [Fig. 12; (31)]. Boiling the used medium does not diminish its ability to lower the proteolysis rate (31).

Studies with a cell-free system with either radioactive lung proteins or radioactive hemoglobin as a substrate show that used perfusate contains a heat-stable inhibitor of cathepsin D (31). The nature of this is not yet known in detail, but its activity in cell-free homogenates shows that its interaction with plasma membranes is not required for its inhibition of proteolysis (31). Boiled extracts from nonhypoxic lungs inhibit the proteolysis rate of lung proteins by cathepsin D (31), indicating that the inhibitor may be present in lungs with normal proteolysis rates. If the inhibitor is normally present, it apparently undergoes translocation under hypoxic conditions from its usual site to a site where it may more effectively inhibit proteolysis. Alternatively the inhibitory action of the boiled lung extract on the proteolysis rate may reflect the action of a protease inhibitor that is normally bound to a heat-labile protease; boiling, thus destroying the protease, may allow the inhibitor to express itself.

Interaction Between Exogenous Amino Acids and Hypoxia

By virtue of matched or unmatched changes in ventilation and perfusion, the concentration of O_2, substrates, and products of cell metabolism may be maintained at optimal or suboptimal levels in the lung. This led to studies examining the interaction between exogenous amino acids and hypoxia on the proteolysis

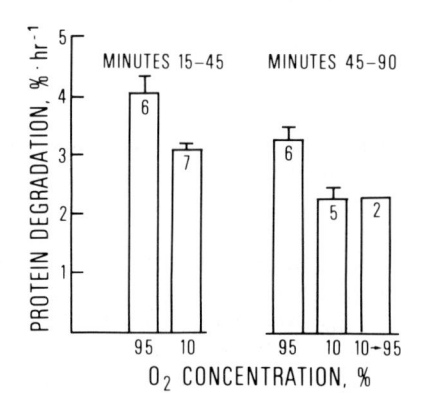

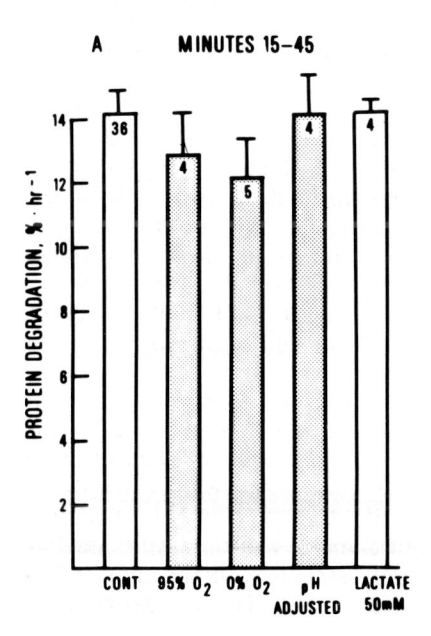

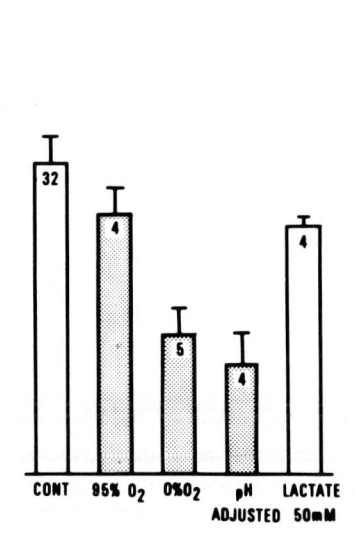

FIG. 11. Degradation in vitro at different O_2 concentrations of proteins labeled in vivo during 5 h. [From Chiang et al. (31).]

FIG. 12. Effect of used perfusate and lactate on protein degradation. Rat lungs were labeled with [^{14}C]phenylalanine as described in legend of Fig. 10. Cont., control; lungs perfused with fresh medium and ventilated with 95% O_2. *Shaded bars*, values from lungs perfused with used medium, i.e., medium initially used to perfuse unlabeled lungs for 90 min that were ventilated with 0% O_2 or 95% O_2. In some experiments the pH of used medium from hypoxic lungs was adjusted to 7.4 before it was used to study proteolysis (designated *pH adjusted*). Lactate, fresh medium identical to control medium but with exogenous (50 mM) lactate. In all experiments, regardless of medium used, lungs were ventilated with 95% O_2. [From Chiang et al. (31).]

rate in the isolated perfused rat lung. In the absence of exogenous amino acids the proteolysis rate was found to be less sensitive to the depressing effect of hypoxia than it is to the presence of exogenous amino acids (33a). In addition, during moderate hypoxia, amino acid deprivation does not impair proteolysis beyond the impairment caused by hypoxia alone (33a). Thus these regulators of proteolysis in the isolated perfused lung seem to buffer the effect of each other.

Potential Physiological Importance of Interaction Between Amino Acids and Hypoxia

If hypoxia causes a decreased rate of lung protein degradation in vivo and if in vivo hypoxia results in the accumulation within the lung of an inhibitor of proteolysis, what is the physiological relevance of these effects? Consider the current paradigm regarding the result of protease-antiprotease imbalance in the lung for the production of emphysema (130, 134, 150). It suggests that conditions favoring proteolysis (increased numbers of protease-releasing cells in the lung, genetic deficiency of protease inhibitors, or oxidant inactivation of protease inhibitors) lead to destruction of lung tissue. However, pneumococcal pneumonia is a common disorder that fills the affected area of the lung with large numbers of protease-releasing cells, yet tissue destruction in this and many other forms of pneumonia is uncommon. Is it possible that because of local hypoxia in fluid-filled alveoli an inhibitor of proteolysis accumulates and helps protect the lung from the extracellular proteases that must be present?

I also wonder if the inhibitor of proteolysis, which accumulates in the medium perfusing the hypoxic lung, may play a role in the alveolar proliferation and in the increased size of alveolar type I, type II, and capillary endothelial cells that occur when animals are maintained in an hypoxic environment (210). Is the increase in lung protein, which must accompany cellular hyperplasia and hypertrophy, mediated partly or mainly by a decreased rate of proteolysis rather than an increased rate of protein synthesis?

These are obviously speculations. Furthermore the accumulation of inhibitors of proteolysis in the medium perfusing hypoxic lungs may be an artifact of the recirculating system used in those studies. If protease inhibitors were released into the pulmonary circulation in vivo, they would pass through other organs before returning to the lung and might be destroyed or inactivated and hence not affect the degradation of lung proteins.

Hypoxia and the absence of exogenous amino acids buffer each other's depression of the proteolysis rate, within the constraints imposed on the physiological relevance by the use of unphysiological concentrations of amino acids in the perfusate (33a). If this also occurs under less extreme conditions, the avoidance of severe depression of proteolysis would provide more intracellular amino acids from degraded proteins than would be provided if proteolysis were more severely decreased. The increased availability of intracellular amino acids resulting from greater rates of proteolysis should allow lung cells to maintain higher rates of protein synthesis. Higher rates of protein synthesis would allow the cells to adapt to the new metabolic demands imposed when both ventilation (hypoxia) and perfusion (substrate deprivation) are impaired. This might help explain the excellent preservation of function in lungs collapsed for long periods (139, 291).

Glucose and Insulin

The effect of glucose on protein degradation in the lung has been studied in two systems and by two methods. In lung slices, protein degradation was studied by measuring the accumulation of nonradioactive phenylalanine in the medium in the absence and the presence of cycloheximide at a concentration that blocked protein synthesis by >90%, thereby virtually eliminating the reincorporation into protein of phenylalanine derived from proteolysis (272). The rate of protein degradation was also studied in the isolated perfused lung by measuring the accumulation of radioactive phenylalanine in the presence of sufficient nonradioactive phenylalanine to almost completely prevent the reincorporation of [^{14}C]phenylalanine into protein (32). These methods allow the study of different classes of proteins. The release of nonradioactive phenylalanine into the medium reflects mainly the degradation of proteins with slow rates of degradation; [^{14}C]phenylalanine released into the perfusate from proteins labeled during 5 h mainly reflects the degradation of proteins with intermediate rates of turnover; radioactive phenylalanine released into the medium from proteins labeled during a 10-min exposure to [^{14}C]phenylalanine mainly reflects the very rapid degradation of proteins. The absence of glucose and insulin accelerates the degradation rate of proteins with slow rates of degradation (32), and in this regard the lung behaves like most tissues (90). The absence of glucose also accelerates the proteolysis rate of proteins that undergo very rapid breakdown, but the absence of glucose decreases the proteolysis rate of proteins with intermediate rates of degradation. Thus glucose has different effects on the degradation of different classes of proteins in the lung (32, 272).

CONNECTIVE TISSUE PROTEINS OF THE LUNG

Collagen

Collagen is a protein composed of three polypeptide subunits called α-chains. These subunits wind together as a right-handed helix to form the collagen molecule, which is rod shaped, ~300 nm long and 1.4 nm wide, and consists of slightly more than 1,000 amino acid residues. A nomenclature has evolved based on the subunit composition of the collagen molecules. The subunit composition for the three most common collagens follows: type I, $[\alpha 1(I)_2]\alpha 2$; type II, $[\alpha 1(II)]_3$; and type III, $[\alpha 1(III)]_3$. The five chains have different amino acid sequences and are therefore products of different structural genes; type I collagen with two different α-chains is the product of two structural genes (for an excellent review of the molecular diversity of collagen see ref. 59). Every third residue of each α-chain within the triple helix is a glycine residue. The terminal sequences—termed *telopeptides*—at each end do not form a triple helix; they lack glycine at every third residue and are the primary sites of cross-linking. Proline and hydroxyproline account for 25% of the total amino acids in collagen, and the ring structures of these two amino acids place restrictions on chain formation, thereby strengthening the triple helix and stiffening the molecule (221).

Collagen comprises ~10%–15% of the dry weight of the adult lung (17, 47, 117, 138, 217). In the conducting zone of the lung, collagen is found in cartilage, the connective tissue surrounding airways and blood vessels, and the media and adventitia of pulmonary arteries and veins (120). In the gas-exchange region of the lung, collagen is present in the interstitium, the basal laminae, and the whorls around the mouths of alveoli (216).

COMPOSITION AND SYNTHESIS OF LUNG COLLAGEN. A problem facing investigators examining the composition and synthesis of collagen is its insolubility. This is especially true in the adult lung where only ~1%–2% of the collagen present can be extracted with solvents that remove considerably more collagen in other tissues (20). Covalent cross-linking of tropocollagen molecules is a major cause of this insolubility. However, the development of cross-links during the synthesis of collagen can be blocked by feeding rats agents such as α-aminoproprionitrile. This results in a substantial increase of soluble collagen in tissues in which collagen turnover is fairly rapid. These agents do not work as well in adult lungs because collagen turnover is slow; most lung collagen is synthesized in early life (19). Crystal and associates (19) nevertheless used lathrogens in a series of studies that have considerably expanded our knowledge of collagen in the lung. They approached the problem of insolubility two ways: *1*) they used α-aminoproprionitrile to double the amount of collagen extracted by neutral salt solutions or by acetic acid (20–22), and *2*) they studied the incorporation of radioactive amino acids into collagen by lung slices; isotopic labeling permitted the identification of small amounts of α-chains by cochromatography of the radiolabeled collagen with known carrier collagen α-chains from rabbit skin. This approach also made it possible to use relatively small amounts of tissue, thereby permitting studies of the synthesis and composition of collagen to be performed on tissue obtained by biopsy of human lungs. These techniques and more direct biochemical analysis with large amounts of lung tissue have provided an important beginning to the understanding of the synthesis and composition of lung collagen.

Peripheral lung tissue, free of large conducting airways and blood vessels, synthesizes type I collagen, as evidenced by the incorporation of radioactive proline into collagenase-sensitive material that coelutes with carrier $\alpha 1$ and $\alpha 2$ collagen chains (18–20). Type I collagen has been chemically identified by CNBr digestion of peripheral human lung tissue and isolation of CNBr peptides of $[\alpha 1(I)_2]\alpha 2$ collagen (57, 253). Seyer et al. (253) found that type I collagen makes up about two-thirds of the collagen present in the periphery of normal human lung and type III collagen comprises most of the remaining collagen. Type I collagen seems to be the collagen molecule present at sites where great tensile strength is needed and hence may be mainly responsible for collagen's contribution to the lung's tensile strength.

Type II collagen is present in most mammalian hyaline cartilages (188). Apparently this is true for cartilage of the conducting airways, as evidenced by studies on proline incorporation into collagen by minced tracheal tissue and tissue from large bronchi. These tissues incorporate radioactive proline into collagenase-sensitive material that elutes with carrier $\alpha 1(II)$ chains from carboxymethyl cellulose columns and has the same electrophoretic mobility as $\alpha 1(II)$ chains isolated from rabbit sternal cartilage (21).

Fibroblasts from lungs of newborn rabbits and human fetal lung (WI-38 fibroblasts) incorporate radioactive proline into type III collagen (107). This suggests that the lung synthesizes and hence contains type III collagen. This interpretation must be drawn with some caution because cells isolated in culture may synthesize different types of collagen than they do when they are part of whole organs (159, 198). However, confirmation that the biosynthetic studies reflect the presence of type III collagen in the lung was obtained when type III collagen was isolated from human lungs (57). These investigators isolated and identified CNBr peptides of collagen and confirmed their chromatographic identification by amino acid analysis. They demonstrated that the hydroxylysine content of hydroxylysine $\alpha 1(III)$ is higher than that of $\alpha 1(III)$ isolated from the skin (186). The high content of hydroxylysine could reflect a greater proportion of hydroxylysine-derived cross-links, and this might in part contribute to the great insolubility of lung collagen (186).

Type IV collagen, which is found in basement membranes, is probably present in the lung because the lungs contain considerable amounts of basement membrane. In addition electron-microscope studies have shown that the basement membrane lamina of the lung is removed by collagenase (296). With the use of so-called affinity-purified type-specific collagen antibodies, the presence of immunofluorescence has been observed in lungs reacted with type IV collagen antibody (171, 172).

A recent report indicates that two newly discovered collagen chains (αA and αB) are present in the lung (36). Because of the reported widespread nature of this form of collagen (frequently termed *AB collagen type V*) (59) it is likely that it is present in the lung. However, more rigorous evidence is required to establish this with certainty.

CHANGES IN COLLAGEN CONTENT OF THE LUNG. Changes in the collagen content of the lung during normal development have been extensively studied in rabbits. Figure 13 shows the alterations in body and lung weight and in lung collagen content that take place as rabbits mature. The ratio of total protein to dry lung mass remains constant as lung mass increases some 100-fold (20). By contrast the quantity of collagen per milligram of dry lung increases markedly in late gestation. In the early postnatal period it contin-

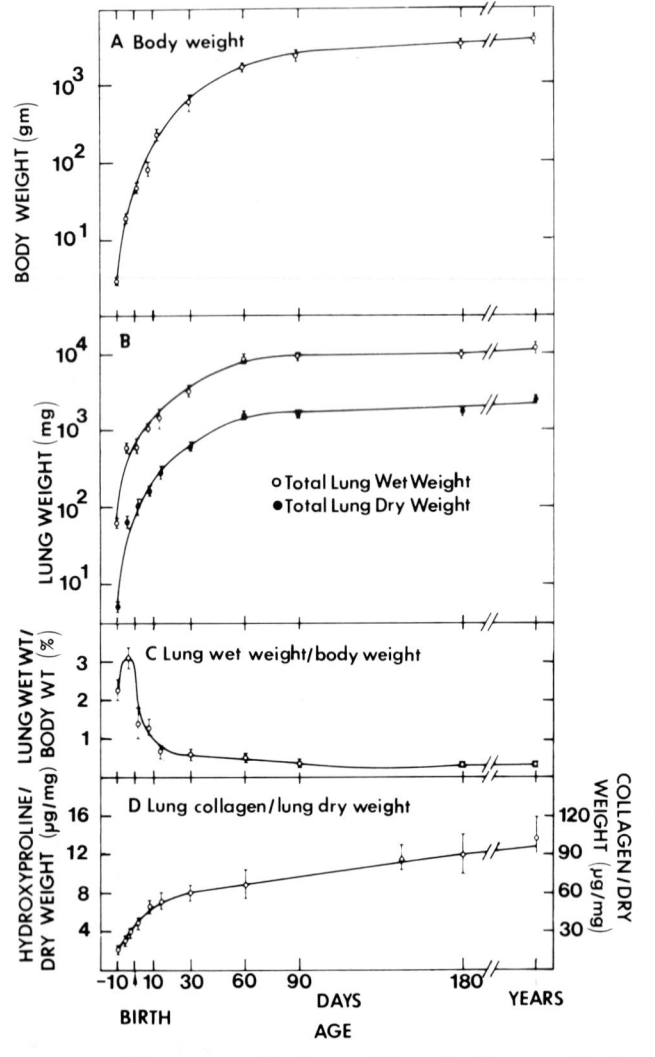

FIG. 13. Changes in rabbit lung weight and collagen and body weight with age. [From Crystal (46).]

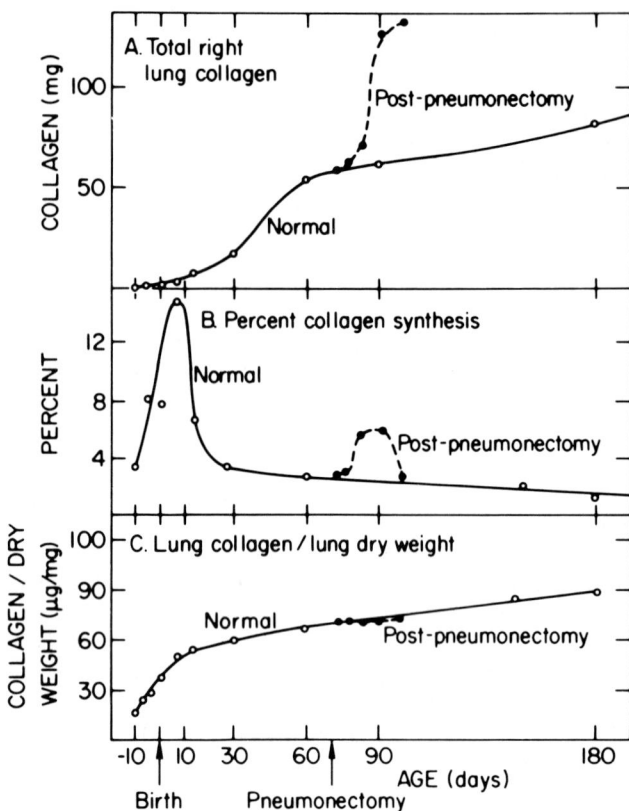

FIG. 14. Effect of right pneumonectomy in rabbits on collagen in remaining left lung. [From Cowan and Crystal (44).]

ues to increase but at a slower rate until around day 180 and then remains stable (Fig. 13). Thus the late prenatal and early postnatal periods are characterized by an increase in the concentration of collagen and the total amount of collagen in the lung.

These changes during normal lung development may be compared with those occurring in the lung remaining after pneumonectomy. Total lung protein increases ~1.7 times, and the collagen content doubles in the right lung of rabbits by ~28 days after removal of the left lung (Fig. 14). Thus during normal development and after pneumonectomy, total proteins and collagen increase. However, the concentration of collagen increases only during normal development and not as part of the growth of the remaining lung after pneumonectomy (20, 44); the protein concentration of the lung does not increase in either situation. In both circumstances (normal development and postpneumonectomy) there is an increased rate of incorporation of radioactive proline into total protein and into collagen. The increase in collagen synthesis is much greater than the increase of total protein synthesis and precedes it by 1–2 wk (Fig. 15). In both conditions the percent of total protein synthesis that is due to collagen synthesis is increased (20, 44).

These reports of the incorporation of amino acids into collagen and into total protein are useful but must

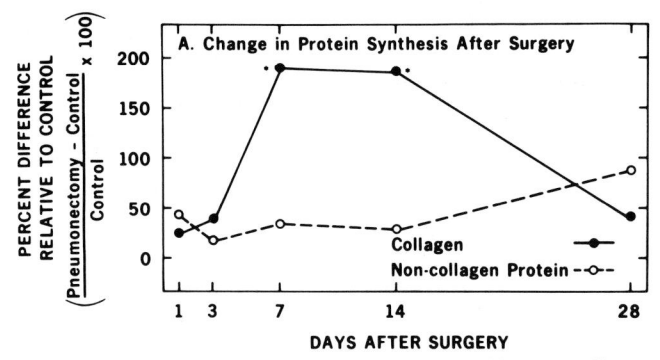

FIG. 15. Effect of right pneumonectomy in rabbits on collagen and protein synthesis in remaining left lung. [From Cowan and Crystal (44).]

not be overinterpreted. Caution is required because the specific radioactivity of tRNA-bound precursor amino acids was not measured, and therefore only apparent rates of synthesis were determined. The use of only trace amounts of precursor amino acids (usually proline) in the studies mentioned means that relatively small changes in proteolysis rates can alter the rate of incorporation of isotope into protein by changing the specific radioactivity of the precursor amino acids. Thus changes in the rate of isotope incorporation into protein can occur that do not reflect changes in the absolute rate of protein synthesis. The effect of proteolysis on the specific radioactivity of the amino acids serving as precursors for protein synthesis may be especially pronounced in studies of collagen synthesis because ~30% of collagen newly synthesized in vitro is reported to be degraded intracellularly in ~8 min (13). Because this process also occurs in vivo it is ongoing at the start of in vitro studies and should result in considerable dilution of the precursor pool by nonradioactive amino acids derived from the breakdown of collagen. This is particularly true for proline, the most common precursor used in studies of collagen synthesis, because the number of proline molecules per 1,000 total residues in collagen is large (20).

Nevertheless there are reasons to believe that the increased rate of incorporation of radioactive amino acids into collagen and into total lung proteins during periods of lung growth do reflect increased synthesis rates of these macromolecules. The reasons include the observations that 1) in otherwise identical cell-free systems the synthesis of collagen and of total lung protein directed by polyribosomes from fetal lung is twice as rapid as synthesis directed by polyribosomes isolated from adult lung (42), 2) the developmental and postpneumonectomy changes in the incorporation of amino acids into collagen are associated with concordant changes in the activity of enzymes involved in collagen synthesis (25, 307), and 3) the increased rate of incorporation of isotopic amino acids measured in vitro occurs at a time when the similar lungs are accumulating increased amounts of total protein and

collagen in vivo. However, the relative contribution of changes in rates of synthesis and degradation to the accumulation of collagen cannot be ascertained from these studies.

Elastin

Elastin contains ~800 amino acid residues of which the nonpolar amino acids (glycine, proline, alanine, valine, phenylalanine, isoleucine, and leucine) make up >85%. Extracellular elastin exists as two major forms: mature elastin and its precursor tropoelastin. Their amino acid compositions are very similar except for the amount of lysine present. Tropoelastin has much more lysine than mature elastin; this probably reflects the use of lysine to form the cross-linking amino acids desmosine and isodesmosine that are present in elastin. Desmosine and isodesmosine have not been found in any proteins other than elastin. The sequence of amino acids in elastin has two unusual features: *1*) lysine residues always occur in pairs in the tropoelastin chain, and *2*) alanine molecules are concentrated near the lysine pairs. As a consequence of this sequence and as lysine molecules become involved in cross-linking, alanine is concentrated near the cross-links in mature elastin.

Foster et al. (68) have recently reported that mRNA isolated from chick embryonic lung or aortic tissue and translated in an mRNA-dependent reticulocyte lysate directs the synthesis of two elastin proteins. The 70,000-dalton protein (tropoelastin b) and the 73,000-dalton protein (tropoelastin a) are precipitated by antibody directed against chick aortic tropoelastin. The 70,000-dalton protein has been isolated from lathyritic chick lungs and is probably identical to conventional tropoelastin, as indicated by amino acid analysis, electrophoretic mobility, and amino acid sequence. Furthermore embryonic chick lung in organ culture incorporates [^{3}H]valine into two immunoreactive elastins similar to those synthesized by the cell-free system. This observation indicated that the translation of the lung mRNA in the reticulocyte system faithfully reflects elastin synthesis in the intact lung. The proportion of tropoelastin b to tropoelastin a differs significantly between lung and aortic tissues during chick embryonic development. This has led Foster et al. (68) to speculate that the ratio of tropoelastin b to tropoelastin a may differ between tissues in a manner that reflects or contributes to the different molecular organization of elastic fibers seen in various tissues. The different molecular organization may of course be the basis for the elastic characteristics of the tissues.

The problems of isolating elastin from tissues are even more severe than those encountered with collagen. The painstaking studies of Paz et al. (209) are therefore particularly useful. They compared methods to isolate elastin from pleural-free lung parenchyma, large conducting airways and vessels, and visceral pleura and aorta. For lung parenchyma they compared the following methods of extraction: procedure B—hot alkali extraction; procedure A_2—hot alkali extraction plus pyridine and $CaCl_2$ to remove cell membranes and other tissue components and treatment with hot trichloracetic acid to remove some collagen and to denature the remaining collagen, thereby making subsequent digestions with collagenase more efficient; procedure A_1—similar to A_2 but omitting the use of pyridine and $CaCl_2$; a method similar to procedure A_2 but without the extraction with pyridine; and procedure A_2 without the step using $CaCl_2$. Procedure A_2 gave the lowest yield of elastin, but the extracted elastin, when compared with elastin isolated by procedure B from ligamentum nuchae, was most pure as determined by amino acid analysis. Procedure A_2 also seems to best conserve elastin cross-links as indicated by the desmosine and isodesmosine content of the purified elastin. Procedure A_1 resulted in the most pure elastin isolated from pleura. Procedure B, extraction with hot alkali (207), resulted in a loss of some cross-links in elastin from both lung parenchyma and pleura compared with elastin extracted by method A_1. Analysis of the cross-linking profiles of elastins isolated from calf pleura, calf ligamentum nuchae, dog aorta, and calf parenchyma revealed differences in the type, distribution, and quality of the cross-links (209). However, these results should be viewed with some caution because only about half of the lysine residues could be accounted for as lysine and lysine-derived cross-links and intermediates.

ELASTIN CONTENT OF THE LUNG. The reported content of elastin varies widely and undoubtedly reflects differences in the assay procedures used, whether or not visceral pleura was included when lung parenchyma was extracted, and probably varies with the extent to which large conducting vessels were removed prior to assay. Nevertheless certain things seem reasonably clear. First, the concentration of elastin in the visceral pleura is as high as or in most reports higher than it is in pleura-free lung parenchyma or in bronchioles (137, 215, 250); this is true in several species. Second, the amount of elastin in the pleura increases with age during adult life, whereas its concentration in the parenchyma remains unchanged (137). The elastin content of conducting airways and vessels has not been measured in animals of widely different ages.

The time course of changes in the postnatal concentration of elastin in the lung (assayed as desmosine + isodesmosine per gram of wet lung) differs from that of collagen. Collagen increases parabolically from birth, its concentration increasing ~4-fold in the first 3 wk after birth (220). By contrast the elastin concentration in the lung increases <2-fold during the first postpartum week, but then the concentration increases ~10-fold, reaching its adult levels over the next 2 wk (220). The rapid postnatal increase in elastin concentration in the lung seems to have as its major anatomical correlate the thinning of the alveolar septa and the transformation of the alveolar vessels from a double- to a single-capillary network. However, the meaning of this relationship, if any, is not clear.

ELASTIN TURNOVER. Despite the many studies on the elastin content of the lung very few have examined elastin turnover (53, 109, 151, 215, 305). Pierce et al. (215) administered radioactive proline to suckling rats from about the 10th to the 31st postpartum day. This period encompasses the time of rapid increase in lung elastin concentration (220). They found that the specific radioactivity of lung elastin decreases by about one-third during the 13 mo between the 122nd and 510th postpartum day. Although these experiments did not account for the reincorporation of radioactive amino acids into protein, they do indicate that elastin turns over very slowly in rats of the age studied; recent work has confirmed these findings (151, 305). Furthermore Dubick et al. (53) showed that the specific radioactivity of desmosine in elastin remains constant for ~25 wk, whereas the specific radioactivity of total lung proteins falls ~10-fold over 5 wk. Because radioactive amino acids available for reutilization in the synthesis of proteins should be equally available for the synthesis of elastin and other proteins, the virtually constant specific radioactivity of desmosine must indicate an almost complete lack of synthesis of elastin in the relatively mature normal lung.

Compared with elastin synthesis in the normal lung, evidence shows that elastin synthesis in the damaged adult lung is markedly increased. There is a marked fall in the elastin content of hamster lung within 24 h of the intratracheal administration of elastase (151, 305). The evidence for the increased rate of de novo elastin synthesis in damaged lungs includes a return to control amounts of elastin per lung by 60 days after the damage in the absence of a change in the elastin content of undamaged lungs. Additionally Kuhn and Senior (150) labeled lung elastin by injecting [^{14}C]-proline before administering elastase. During the 118 days after the administration of elastase, the specific radioactivity of elastin from undamaged lungs fell little, if at all; the specific radioactivity of elastin isolated from damaged lungs fell ~50% during this time. The fall in specific radioactivity reflects the incorporation of unlabeled proline into elastin, thereby signifying increased rates of elastin synthesis. In addition the rate of incorporation of radioactive proline into elastin increased in elastase-treated hamsters compared with control animals. This probably reflects an increased rate of elastin synthesis because the total amount of elastin was increasing when the isotope studies were performed. It is possible that the accelerated breakdown of tissue proteins by elastase resulted in an increased intracellular pool of nonradioactive amino acids, thereby diluting the intracellular radioactive proline and leading to an underestimation of the rate of protein synthesis. A factor that is difficult to evaluate is the effect of lung damage on the delivery and distribution of radioactive proline in the lung and hence on its availability for protein synthesis. Nevertheless the results of the experiments of Kuhn and Senior (150) taken together clearly indicate that the rates of elastin synthesis are increased in the damaged lung. It is unclear if the rate of elastin degradation was altered after the initial effect of elastase was completed.

PULMONARY FIBROSIS

Diffuse pulmonary fibrosis can develop spontaneously in otherwise healthy individuals, can occur in association with systemic and hereditable diseases, can develop during granulomatous diseases involving the lung, and can be caused by various therapeutic agents or by several atmospheric and environmental constituents or pollutants (41, 152, 238). These forms of abnormality were discovered by a histological examination of the lungs. Recently further insight into the pathogenesis of these disorders has been sought with chemical means to quantitate and identify the types of fibrous tissue that appear by histological examination to be present in increased amounts. These studies have shown that, where tested, all forms of histologically documented experimental pulmonary fibrosis have an increased amount of collagen per lung, and in several forms the concentration of collagen is also increased (38, 143, 267, 273). The concentration of collagen in the human lung with diffuse interstitial pulmonary fibrosis and in baboons with bleomycin-induced fibrosis (43) was not increased in one study in which tissue was obtained by lung biopsy (79a). In a separate human study the concentration of collagen increased (172). There seems to be rather good evidence that the ratio of type I to type III collagen is increased above normal in human lungs with diffuse interstitial fibrosis (253), but the significance of this is not clear. There have been fewer studies of the elastin content of the lung in experimental fibrosis. However, experimental forms of pulmonary fibrosis result in an increased content of elastin and increased apparent rates of elastin synthesis (43, 267).

The documented increase in lung collagen in experimental animals has led to attempts to measure its synthesis rate mainly by use of the incorporation of radioactive proline into collagen. Although these studies suffer from certain defects, particularly the failure to measure the specific radioactivity of the appropriate precursor pool of amino acids, taken with the increase of total collagen, they provide useful information. Some have measured fractional incorporation of the isotopic amino acid (compared with total proteins) into collagen or into the different collagen types. The results and interpretations of these comparisons are less dependent on the measurement of precursor specific radioactivity. The virtually universal finding has been an increased rate of radioactive proline incorporation into collagen in experimental conditions that result in the accumulation of increased amounts of collagen in the lung (37–39, 43, 88, 95, 104, 110, 125, 145, 155). These increased rates usually precede the detection by chemical means of increased amounts of collagen. During the development of pulmonary fibrosis the fractional incorporation of isotope into collagen assumes a substantially greater percentage of the isotope incorporated into total protein. However, it is not known if this indicates a greater capacity for collagen synthesis (i.e., a greater proportion of the protein synthetic apparatus being devoted to collagen synthesis) or if the synthesis of collagen relative to total lung protein is more efficient.

What is particularly interesting about the above normal increase in the ratio of type I to type III collagen found in fibrotic human lungs is that in two instances tested (ozone- and paraquat-induced lung fibrosis) the relative incorporation of proline into type I collagen compared with type III collagen is increased above that of control lungs (110, 228). The evidence shows that in the experimental models the rate of collagen degradation is increased. This is consistent with the recent discovery of increased collagenase activity in lavage returns from humans with pulmonary fibrosis (83a). However, because the total amount of collagen is increased in experimentally produced lung fibrosis the rate of collagen synthesis must exceed the degradation rate, at least during the time collagen is accumulating in the lungs. Now that the experimental models that produce pulmonary fibrosis are well established it may be very informative to study absolute rates of collagen synthesis (and to study degradation in ways that minimize isotope reutilization) over a prolonged portion of the course of pulmonary fibrosis.

PROTEASES AND PROTEASE INHIBITORS

Proteases, protease inhibitors, and the interaction between them are obviously important to protein turnover as it occurs under normal and abnormal conditions. The demonstration by Gross et al. (98, 99) that the inhalation of a proteolytic enzyme causes emphysema in animals, when most other attempted methods failed, and the observation of the high prevalence of emphysema in individuals deficient in α_1-antitrypsin (58, 157) led to a recrudescence of interest in the interaction of proteases and protease inhibitors in the development of diseases of the lung, and to a search for the cellular sources of these enzymes as well as for clues regarding the stimulus for cells with large amounts of proteases to enter the lung.

These studies began early in the history of lung research. Nye (201) in 1922 cited several articles published between 1877 and 1901 in which it was observed that sputum from cases of lung gangrene [Nye (201, ref. 1)], bronchitis, pneumonia, and phthisis [Nye

(201, refs. 2 and 3)] dissolved coagulated egg white; leukocytes were considered to be the source of these proteolytic enzymes [Nye (201, ref. 4)]. Nye performed experiments in which he concluded that proteases present in the lung were mainly in free cells as opposed to the "true lung substance" and that this proteolytic activity was increased in lungs from a patient with lobar pneumonia caused by type I pneumococcus (201). Other experimental work indicates that the liquefaction of tubercles in the lung is associated with increased proteolytic activity in the tissue and that "the rate of proteinase action is proportional to the intensity of cellular infiltration"—again relating the protease activity to inflammatory cells (201). A role for protease inhibitors in protecting the lung was suggested many years ago: "decreases in proteinase activity may be due... to the presence of inhibitors which inactivate or denature these enzymes" (290). Work in Dannenberg's laboratory (261) showed that cathepsin D from lung and pulmonary macrophages can produce C5a from C5; the C5a fragment was very chemotactic for polymorphonuclear leukocytes and pulmonary macrophages (255, 286). More recent work has indicated that elastin breakdown products are chemotactic for monocytes (122). Thus degradative products of proteases may attract more cells rich in proteases into an area of ongoing damage.

Fruton (78) reported the presence of proteolytic activity in extracts of normal lungs and, like earlier workers, attributed this activity to leukocytes or lymphocytes rather than to cells specific to the lung, because similar proteolytic activity was present in a wide variety of tissues. Dannenberg and Smith (48, 49), attempting to understand the liquefaction process of tuberculosis, studied protease activity in the lung and identified two proteases: one with optimal activity at pH 4 and one with optimal activity at pH 8.4. They were probably describing the activity of lysosomal proteases and cytoplasmic proteases, respectively (40). Recently it has been shown that nonspecific proteolytic activity present over a pH range of 3–10 exists in lung homogenates. Blood components can inhibit this proteolytic activity by ~60%–80% throughout the pH range tested, 2.2–9.9 (126). Unfortunately dose-response studies to determine if all the proteolytic activity could be inhibited by serum were not reported. More recent work has concentrated on the isolation and purification of specific proteases from the lung, in particular, lysosomal proteases such as cathepsins (195, 258, 259, 262, 263). These lysosomal proteases are undoubtedly associated with the regulation of normal intracellular proteolysis as evidenced by studies showing that the lysosomotropic agent NH_4Cl (33a) and pepstatin (206) inhibit proteolysis by lung cells.

There is now substantial evidence that elastase delivered by aerosol to animal lung can produce emphysema (14, 129, 133, 140, 177, 179, 227, 252, 260) and a loss of elastic recoil as in human emphysema (115a). Other purified enzymes (e.g., trypsin and collagenase) do not produce emphysema (136, 141, 150). These observations have led to attempts to identify cells that might serve as sources of elastase in the lung. Current evidence indicates that polymorphonuclear leukocytes and pulmonary macrophages are the major sources of elastase present in the lung (133, 162, 177, 179, 227, 232). Leukocyte elastase is inhibited by α_1-antitrypsin (9, 128, 202, 203, 271, 278), and in nonsmokers without a genetic deficiency of the protease inhibitor, lung damage due to this enzyme should be minimal. However, oxidizing agents, including those in cigarette smoke (268, 274), inactivate this protease inhibitor (10, 28, 29, 41, 51), probably resulting in a functional though not quantitative deficiency of α_1-antitrypsin in the lungs of smokers (82, 131). This finding provides an important link between the relationship of smoking and emphysema in individuals without a genetic defiency of circulating protease inhibitors.

Pulmonary macrophages produce elastase but in smaller amounts than leukocytes (132, 163, 232). However, pulmonary macrophages from human smokers release elastase at a more rapid rate than macrophages from nonsmokers (232). Furthermore elastase from mouse pulmonary macrophages is only partially inhibited by α_1-proteinase inhibitor (295). This suggests that intrapulmonary inhibitors may be responsible for inhibiting pulmonary macrophage elastase. Evidence indicating the presence of such an inhibitor was presented by Weinbaum et al. (292), who identified a heat-labile, high-molecular-weight substance in lung lavage returns that inhibits pancreatic elastase; when mixed with pancreatic elastase before the elastase is administered intratracheally, it prevents the development of emphysema. In addition pulmonary macrophages release an inhibitor of elastase (15) like the hypoxic perfused rat lung (M.-J. Chiang, P. Whitney, and D. Massaro, unpublished observations). Thus evidence suggests that inhibitors of elastase may arise from cells in the lung. The possibility that lung cells produce inhibitors of elastase and that these inhibitors play a role in preventing emphysema has not been explored significantly.

Although elastase (but not collagenase) can produce experimental pulmonary emphysema, it is not known if this is true for human emphysema. Considering this and the protein turnover of connective tissue two recent observations seem important: 1) purified leukocyte elastase can degrade human type III collagen (83, 175) and type IV collagen, which is present in basement membranes (174); and 2) treatment of rabbit synovial fibroblasts with a variety of proteolytic enzymes induces the secretion of collagenase by the fibroblasts (294). This secretion, once begun, is maintained in the absence of the protease. Thus it is possible that proteases secreted by macrophages or leukocytes could induce the prolonged secretion of a collagenase by fibroblasts in the lung, with resultant damage.

In the early 1970s Hochstrasser and co-workers identified an acid-stable protease inhibitor in normal nasal (113) and bronchial secretions (114). This inhibitor has a molecular weight of ~10,000 and inhibits leukocyte elastase and cathepsin G; it does not inhibit human granulocyte collagenase (204, 205). Within the tracheobronchial tree it has been localized in serous cells of bronchial glands (149). The inhibitor is not in the serum. It is inactivated by cigarette smoke and phagocyte-derived oxidants (30). These findings have naturally led to the suggestion that the inhibitor protects conducting airways against leukocyte proteases; its inactivation by cigarette smoke suggests smoke may exert its harmful effect on the airway by this mechanism. Apparently this protease inhibitor is not unique to the lung; it is also found in uterine cervical mucus (284) and seminal plasma (239). It is not known if this protease inhibitor plays a role in intracellular proteolysis.

HYPEROXIA AND PROTEIN SYNTHESIS

Studies of the effect of hyperoxia on protein synthesis by the lung have been undertaken for two major reasons: *1*) earlier studies tried to assess the damaging effects of hyperoxia on an important biosynthetic process and to correlate changes in biosynthesis with the ultrastructure of alveolar type 2 cells and with the lung's mechanical properties, and *2*) more recent studies were undertaken to examine mechanisms by which the lung adapts to hyperoxia. Most of the studies of protein synthesis used only trace amounts of radiolabeled amino acids and did not measure the specific radioactivity of the precursor tRNA-bound acid. Therefore the results provide only apparent rates of protein synthesis. They must also be interpreted recognizing that differences in the proteolysis rate could have resulted in serious discrepancies between the true and the apparent rate of protein synthesis.

The rate of incorporation of [^{14}C]leucine into protein by lung slices is diminished by ~25% after exposing adult rats to >95% O_2 for 24 h (182). This effect is not due to a diminution in the uptake of [^{14}C]leucine by lung cells because it also occurs in a cell-free system (D. Massaro, unpublished observations). The decreased incorporation of [^{14}C]leucine into protein takes place without a change in the total RNA content of the lung (84); it is associated with a diminution in the amount of polyribosomal RNA, indicating that after 24-48 h of hyperoxia the lungs from nontolerant rats have a diminished capacity for protein synthesis (60). Hyperoxia lowers the amount of polyribosomal RNA, which provides some reassurance that the decreased apparent rate of protein synthesis does in fact reflect an actual decrease in the rate of protein synthesis.

Hyperoxia does not equally decrease the rate of incorporation of [^{14}C]leucine into all proteins. The incorporation of [^{14}C]leucine into protein in a surface-active lung fraction is inhibited to a greater extent than the incorporation of ^{14}C[leucine] into general lung proteins (84). These differences could reflect changes in the rate at which proteins in these fractions are degraded. They could also represent a different susceptibility of the protein-synthesizing structures of the cell (i.e., the rough endoplasmic reticulum vs. the free polyribosomes) to the toxic effects of hyperoxia. The latter concept is supported by studies suggesting that hyperoxia decreases the synthesis by lymph nodes of secretory proteins more than the synthesis of nonsecretory proteins (101). Because surfactant proteins are made for secretion, this effect may also be occurring in the lung.

The decreased incorporation of [^{14}C]leucine into proteins of the surface-active lung fraction is associated with compatible changes in the lamellar bodies (surfactant storage granules) of alveolar type 2 cells. After 48 h of hyperoxia the lamellar bodies are smaller and occupy a smaller fraction of the cytoplasm of type 2 cells than in air-breathing rats (182). The changes in fractional volume could reflect greater rates of secretion in the O_2-exposed rats unrelated to protein synthesis rates. However, because exocytosis seems to be an all-or-nothing phenomenon it is more likely that the lower fractional volume and the smaller size of the storage granules reflect decreased synthesis rather than increased secretion of the secretory product.

After 48 h of >95% O_2 followed by 4 h of room air breathing, the apparent rate of protein synthesis by rat lung slices is still diminished by ~30%-40% (180). When 24 h of breathing room air follows 48 h of breathing >95% O_2, the apparent rate of protein synthesis by rat lung slices is about twice as fast as in lungs from rats not exposed to hyperoxia. The results for proteins in a surface-active fraction compared with total lung proteins are the reverse of the effects noted after 48 h of continuous hyperoxia. During recovery the apparent rate of synthesis of total lung proteins is augmented ~2.2-fold compared with a 1.6-fold augmentation of [^{14}C]leucine incorporation into protein of a surface-active lung fraction. The difference between the apparent rates of synthesis of structural and secretory proteins during recovery is similar to the reparative response to injury found in other tissues (27).

Adult rats tolerate hyperoxia poorly. More than 70%-80% die within 72 h of the onset of continuous exposure to >95% O_2 (69-71, 73). Young adult rats sustain lung damage during exposure to >95% O_2, but most live for extended periods; this permits studies on the effect of more prolonged hyperoxia on protein synthesis (183). In young rats there is an initial fall in the incorporation of [^{14}C]leucine into protein followed by a return to the rate of incorporation present in air-breathing rats; after 96 h of exposure there is a marked increase in the incorporation of [^{14}C]leucine into protein above that seen in air-breathing rats [Fig. 16; (183)]. The difference in the incorporation of [^{14}C]-leucine into protein after 96 h, between air- and O_2-breathing rats, is greatest for total lung protein and least for protein in a surface-active lung fraction (183). In these studies (183) trace amounts of [^{14}C]leucine were used, and the specific activity of tRNA-bound leucine was not measured. Therefore undetected differences in the size of the precursor pool of leucine, perhaps due to differences in proteolysis rates, render it impossible to make claims about the effect of hypoxia on absolute rates of protein synthesis. However, two ancillary findings support an interpretation that the differences in the rate of [^{14}C]leucine incorporation into protein do indeed reflect differences in the rate of protein synthesis. The concentration of RNA (RNA/DNA) in the lung is 25%–30% higher in the lungs of rats exposed to >95% O_2 for 96 h than in air-breathing rats (84). In addition (and consistent with the increased incorporation of [^{14}C]leucine in protein of a surface-active lung fraction after 96 h of hyperoxia) there is the 37% greater surface density of the rough endoplasmic reticulum of type 2 alveolar cells of the O_2-exposed rats compared with air-breathing rats (183).

There is now substantial evidence that O_2 toxicity is mediated by the accelerated generation of O_2 free radicals, and antioxidant enzymes (e.g., SOD, catalase, and glutathione reductase) scavenge these free radicals and convert them to a less harmful or nonharmful form (76). Frank et al. (69–73) have shown that the administration of small amounts of endotoxin from gram-negative bacteria confers marked protection to adult rats against the lethality and lung-damaging effects of >95% O_2. Apparently this tolerance is due to an early increase in the activity of antioxidant enzymes in the lungs of O_2-exposed, endotoxin-treated adult rats (71).

Studies of lung protein metabolism in endotoxin-treated rats exposed to hyperoxia indicate that the increased activity of SOD is associated with an absolute increase in SOD as measured by immunoprecipitation (108). This increased concentration of SOD is at least partly due to an absolute increase in the rate of protein synthesis (108). Furthermore the increased synthesis rate of SOD in endotoxin-treated rats exposed to >95% O_2 is at least partly due to an increased capacity for protein synthesis. This is evidenced by an increased amount of polyribosomal RNA in these rats compared with rats breathing >95% O_2 but not given endotoxin or compared with rats breathing room air (D. Fan, L. Frank, and D. Massaro, unpublished observations).

Neonatal rats exhibit endogenous tolerance to hyperoxia (302). As in endotoxin-treated adult rats this tolerance seems to be mediated by a rapid rise in the activity of antioxidant enzymes, but the enzyme increase in neonatal rats does not require endotoxin. Elevations of antioxidant enzyme activity in neonatal lungs can be produced by in vitro exposure to hyperoxia. Because this increased enzyme activity requires protein synthesis it probably represents at least partly an increased rate of de novo synthesis of antioxidant enzymes (270).

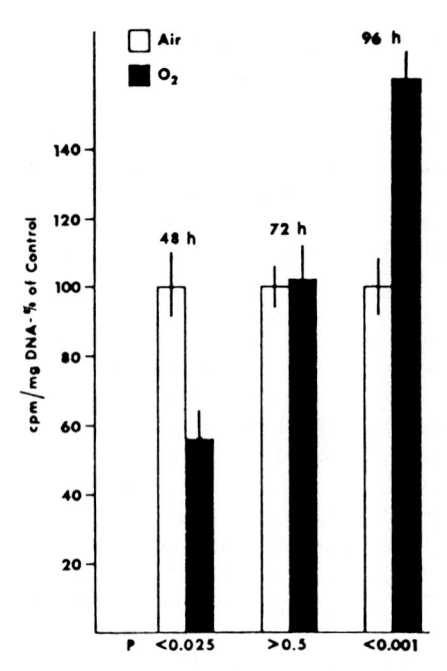

FIG. 16. Time course of effect of in vivo hyperoxia on L-[U-^{14}C]leucine incorporation into protein by rat lung slices. [From Massaro and Massaro (183).]

PROTEIN TURNOVER IN PULMONARY MACROPHAGES

Pulmonary macrophages obtained by lung lavage are the only cells of the several varieties of lung cells in which protein metabolism has been seriously studied. These studies, as with the whole lung, have mainly involved the use of isotopic precursors to study synthesis and degradation rates generally, rather than specifically.

Choice of Precursor Amino Acid

Phenylalanine is the amino acid most extensively evaluated for its suitability in the study of protein turnover in pulmonary macrophages. Phenylalanine is essential for rabbits (65); their lungs do not have detectable phenylalanine hydroxylase activity (275, 279). However, because macrophages constitute a relatively small percentage of lung cells (103) it is possible that phenylalanine hydroxylase in these cells could go undetected when measured in whole lung homogenates. This is unlikely because recent work indicates that phenylalanine is used by rabbit pulmonary macrophages almost exclusively in pathways of protein metabolism. This evidence includes the following: 1) when rabbit pulmonary macrophages are incubated with [^{14}C]phenylalanine, virtually all the intracellular and extracellular acid-soluble radioactivity is in free phenylalanine (299); 2) similarly all the acid-insoluble radioactivity of pulmonary macrophages is phenylalanine (299); 3) no radioactivity is detected in the supernatant fraction when macrophage acid-insoluble radioactivity is exposed to lipid solvents (299); and 4) virtually no radioactivity appears as ^{14}CO$_2$ when [^{14}C]phenylalanine is incubated with pulmonary macrophages for 2 h (105, 299). The evidence that pulmonary macrophages do not metabolize phenylalanine to other substrates to any significant degree was extended by Hammer and Rannels (105). Other investigators observed that phenylalanine is metabolized in perfused heart by a mitochondrial aminotransferase as indicated by the production of ^{3}H$_2$O from phenyl-[2,3-^{3}H]alanine (298); if this pathway were present in pulmonary macrophages it could lead to a significant underestimation of the proteolysis rate as measured by the release of phenylalanine into the medium. When tested it was found that pulmonary macrophages did not generate significant amounts of ^{3}H$_2$O from phenylalanine (105). As final evidence of its suitability for the study of protein turnover the phenylalanine space in pulmonary macrophages attains, within 60 s, a level that is maintained for at least 2 h (105).

Precursor Pools

Regarding protein metabolism it seems clear that the intracellular amino acid pools in pulmonary macrophages are compartmented. Thus the apparent rate of protein synthesis at low extracellular concentrations of phenylalanine (i.e., 0.01–0.02 mM) is widely different when the synthesis rates calculated with the specific radioactivity of extracellular phenylalanine are compared with the rates of synthesis calculated with the specific radioactivity of intracellular phenylalanine. The former rates are lower, suggesting that nonradioactive phenylalanine derived from endogenous proteolysis is added to the intracellular pool of amino acids (62). When the concentration of extracellular phenylalanine is raised from low to high levels, the rate of incorporation of phenylalanine into protein increases until an extracellular concentration of phenylalanine of 345 μM is reached. There is no further increase in the rate of incorporation when the extracellular concentration of phenylalanine is raised from 345 μM to 5 mM (105). Such a response has usually signified for the amino acid under study the achievement of equal specific radioactivity of the extracellular, intracellular, and tRNA-bound amino acid. This equality has permitted the use of the more easily determined specific radioactivity of the extracellular amino acid as a basis for calculating the absolute rate of protein synthesis (105). This is the case for phenylalanine in the in situ perfused rat lung (289). Similar observations have been made in perfused liver (144), heart (184), HeLa cells (265), and cultured hepatocytes (265). The attainment of equal specific radioactivity between the three pools of phenylalanine or other amino acid has been taken as an indication that virtually no amino acid derived from protein degradation is being reutilized for protein synthesis at the high extracellular concentrations of the amino acid under study.

There is disagreement about the effect an increased concentration of extracellular amino acids has on intracellular amino acid pools in pulmonary macrophages. Two reports indicate that even at high concentrations of medium amino acids substantial differences exist between the specific radioactivity of a particular amino acid in the medium and the specific radioactivity of the same species of amino acid bound to tRNA (1, 105). Thus Hammer and Rannels (105) found that at an extracellular phenylalanine concentration of 345 μM (the concentration beyond which the apparent rate of protein synthesis is unchanged as the concentration of phenylalanine is increased) the rate of protein synthesis calculated with the specific radioactivity of extracellular phenylalanine is >40% below that calculated with the specific radioactivity of phenylalanyl-tRNA. Airhart et al. (1) have made a similar observation. They found that at an extracellular leucine concentration of 5 mM the specific radioactivity of intracellular and extracellular leucine is the same, but the specific radioactivity of tRNA-bound leucine is only ~50% that of the extracellular value. These findings are consistent with the concept that a substantial portion of amino acids used to charge tRNA are derived from the breakdown of protein and that they charge tRNA before they equilibrate with the rest of the cellular pool of amino acids. These studies differ from another report in which it was found that even at the concentration of phenylalanine found in plasma (~65 μM) the rates of protein synthesis calculated on the basis of the specific radioactivity of intracellular and extracellular phenylalanine and/or phenylalanine released from tRNA are equal (62). The reason for these differences is not clear. However, reports by Hammer and Rannels (105) and Airhart et al. (1) make it clear that raising the extracellular concentrations so that the intracellular and extracellular specific radioactivities of an amino acid are equal cannot be used as an approach to simplify determinations of the absolute rate of protein synthesis. That is, when the ratio of intra- to extracellular phenylalanine specific radioactivity is one it cannot be assumed that the specific radioactivity of tRNA-bound amino acid is identical to that of the extracellular or intracellular specific radioactivity. This assumption must be verified in each system.

Protein Degradation

The degradation of endogenous proteins by pulmonary macrophages has been studied by isotopic and nonisotopic methods. The use of isotopes allows one to measure the degradation of two general classes of proteins—those with rapid and those with slow degradation rates. For example, one can allow pulmonary macrophages to incorporate [^{14}C]phenylalanine into protein for 1 or 20 h, wash the cells to remove all extracellular radioactivity, and then measure the appearance of [^{14}C]phenylalanine in the medium in the presence of sufficient nonradioactive phenylalanine to almost completely prevent reincorporation of [^{14}C]-phenylalanine into protein. When this is done proteins labeled during 1 or 20 h are degraded 8%/h and 3%/h, respectively (299); Hammer and Rannels (105) reported a similar proteolysis rate (2.2%/h) for proteins labeled during 18 h. Decreases in cell viability slow the proteolysis rate, indicating that proteolysis is not a reflection of cell disintegration or death (296).

Phagocytosis and Protein Turnover

Studies on protein turnover during phagocytosis have been undertaken because many of the metabolic and morphological events associated with the phagocytic process seem to require changes in protein metabolism. Early reports indicated that phagocytosis by pulmonary macrophages in suspension is associated with a decreased rate of incorporation of [^{14}C]leucine into protein (181). However, studies in attached pulmonary macrophages found an increased incorporation of radioactive leucine into protein (169). Both studies used only trace amounts of precursor amino acids in the medium, and neither assessed the specific radioactivity of the tRNA-bound precursor amino acid (169, 181). Recently, specific radioactivity of phenylalanine released from tRNA was measured in attached pulmonary macrophages during phagocytosis of latex beads; phagocytosis results in an absolute increase in the rate of protein synthesis (62). In phagocytizing macrophages, the rate of protein synthesis increases per microgram of polyribosomal RNA, indicating that phagocytosis increases the efficiency of protein synthesis. Because the amount of polyribosomal RNA is the same in both groups of cells, phagocytosis does not increase the capacity for protein synthesis during the 1-h incubation (62).

The greater efficiency of protein synthesis during phagocytosis seems to be due to the faster rate of polypeptide chain elongation and/or termination. This conclusion is based on the observations that the increased rate of protein synthesis during phagocytosis (1.4-fold) is almost identical to the increased rate of polypeptide chain elongation and/or termination (1.3-fold) and that the decreased ribosome transit time during phagocytosis occurs without a fall in the average molecular weight of macrophage proteins (62). In fact during phagocytosis pulmonary macrophages synthesize more large proteins than when they are not involved in phagocytosis (62).

After it was found that phagocytosis by attached macrophages results in an increase in the absolute rate of protein synthesis, the effect of phagocytosis by pulmonary macrophages in suspension was tested. The rate of protein synthesis in pulmonary macrophages in suspension is decreased during phagocytosis (D. Fan and D. Massaro, unpublished observations). The reason for the different effect of phagocytosis on protein synthesis between suspended and attached pulmonary macrophages is unclear. However, it seems to be related to the state of the cell (suspended or attached) at the time protein synthesis is measured rather than the state of the cell during the process of bead uptake. Thus experiments were performed in which pulmonary macrophages were allowed to ingest beads while other macrophages were similarly incubated but without beads; the beads were removed and both groups of macrophages were allowed to attach to plastic. The rate of protein synthesis is more rapid in attached macrophages preloaded with beads while in suspension than in macrophages not preloaded with beads (62). Finally, the rate of protein synthesis is greater in attached macrophages than in suspended macrophages, even in the absence of beads (62). The reasons for the differences are unclear. Macrophages in suspension tend to clump together despite rather vigorous agitation of the incubation reactions. It is possible that clumping impairs dilution by the suspending medium of potentially harmful metabolites, resulting in a less than optimal microenvironment immediately around the suspended cells. This may be especially true during phagocytosis if toxic free radicals are released (119).

Apparently there are no reports on the effect of phagocytosis on protein degradation in attached pulmonary macrophages. The degradation rate of endogenous proteins in suspended pulmonary macrophages is diminished during phagocytosis of latex beads (299). It is possible that clumping of suspended macrophages leads to an adverse local microenvironment about the cell and that the decrease in the proteolysis rate is a reflection of this event. The fact that the fall in the proteolysis rate is greatest late rather than early in the phagocytic process (299) is consistent with the progressive development of a poor local environment in suspended cells, although there are certainly other explanations for this time course of changes in proteolysis rate. The observation that the degradation rate of proteins that turn over rapidly is diminished about two-thirds, whereas the degradation rate of proteins that turn over slowly is diminished by only one-third argues against the concept that an adverse microenvironment is responsible for the diminished proteolysis rate during phagocytosis.

Hammer and Rannels (105) studied protein degradation by suspended pulmonary macrophages in the presence and absence of bovine serum albumin. The presence of albumin in the medium markedly increases the flux of phenylalanine out of the cells. This increased flux represents phenylalanine produced by the degradation of albumin, because the release of [^{14}C]phenylalanine from macrophage proteins prelabeled during 3 or 18 h was not altered by the subsequent presence of albumin in the medium (105). Thus pinocytosis, unlike phagocytosis (62), does not alter the degradation rate of endogenous proteins by suspended pulmonary macrophages.

Substrates and Protein Turnover

The absence of exogenous glucose does not diminish the rate of protein synthesis in attached pulmonary macrophages during a 3-h incubation (D. Fan and D. Massaro, unpublished observations); its absence does diminish the degradation rate of proteins that turn over rapidly (20% decrease) but not of proteins that turn over slowly (296). Insulin does not alter the degradation rate of proteins that turn over rapidly or slowly (299).

The absence of exogenous amino acids decreases the rate of protein synthesis in suspended (105) and attached pulmonary macrophages (62). Interestingly amino acids supplied by the degradation of albumin taken up by pulmonary macrophages prevent the fall in protein synthesis that occurs in the absence of exogenous free amino acids (105). The decreased rate of protein synthesis that occurs in the absence of exogenous amino acids during short times (3 h) is mainly due to a decreased rate of polypeptide chain elongation and/or termination rather than a diminished capacity for protein synthesis (62).

Other Factors Affecting Protein Turnover in Pulmonary Macrophages

The synthesis of macrophage proteins as evidenced by decreased rates of incorporation of radioactive amino acids into general cell proteins is decreased by cigarette smoke extracts (168, 303), trypsin treatment (280), and washing by centrifugation (281). However, these studies used trace amounts of isotopic precursor and did not assess the specific radioactivity of tRNA-bound amino acids or of potential changes in the proteolysis rate during the study. Changes in the proteolysis rate could significantly alter the specific radioactivity of the precursor amino acids and hence lead to erroneous conclusions.

In contrast to these reports, Hammer and Rannels (106) studied the effect of the volatile anesthetic halothane on protein turnover in suspended pulmonary macrophages. They found that in vitro preexposure of macrophages to halothane causes a reversible decrease in the incorporation of [^{14}C]phenylalanine into protein but does not alter the rate at which macrophages degrade endogenous or exogenous proteins. In this study the medium concentration of phenylalanine was 690 μM; the specific radioactivity of tRNA-bound phenylalanine was not reported, and on the basis of a separate report by these authors (105) it is not certain if the specific radioactivity of tRNA-bound phenylalanine equals that of medium phenylalanine when the concentration of the latter is 690 μM. Thus the rates of protein synthesis must be considered apparent rather than absolute. However, because halothane did not alter the proteolysis rate it is likely, if the cellular uptake of phenylalanine by halothane-treated cells is equal to that of unexposed cells, that the specific radioactivity of tRNA-bound phenylalanine is the same in both groups and that the results represent a valid comparison of apparent rates of protein synthesis between halothane-exposed and halothane-unexposed cells.

Research from the author's laboratory was supported by the Veterans Administration, the National Heart, Lung, and Blood Institute (Grants HL-20366, HL-22333, and HL-07283), and the Parker B. Francis Foundation.

REFERENCES

1. AIRHART, J., J. A. ARNOLD, C. A. BULMAN, AND R. B. LOW. Protein synthesis in pulmonary macrophages. Source of amino acids for leucyl-tRNA. *Biochim. Biophys. Acta* 653: 108–117, 1981.
2. AIRHART, J., J. KELLEY, J. E. BRAYDEN, R. B. LOW, AND W. S. STIREWALT. An ultramicromethod of amino acid analysis: application to studies of protein metabolism in cultured cells. *Anal. Biochem.* 96: 45–55, 1979.
3. AIRHART, J., A. VIDRICH, AND E. A. KHAIRALLAH. Compartmentation of free amino acids for protein synthesis in rat liver. *Biochem. J.* 140: 539–548, 1974.
4. AMENTA, J. S., F. M. BACCINO, AND M. J. SARGUS. Cell protein degradation in cultured rat embryo fibroblasts. Suppression by vinblastine of the enhanced proteolysis by serum-deficient media. *Biochim. Biophys. Acta* 451: 511–516, 1976.
4a. AMENTA, J. S., M. J. SARGUS, AND S. C. BROCHER. Protein synthesis and degradation in growth regulation in rat embryo fibroblasts: role of fast-turnover and slow-turnover protein. *J. Cell. Physiol.* 105: 51–61, 1980.
5. ANDREWS, T. M., R. GOLDTHORP, AND R. W. E. WATTS. Fluorometric measurement of the phenylalanine content of human granulocytes. *Clin. Chim. Acta* 43: 379–387, 1973.
6. ARIAS, I. M., D. DOYLE, AND R. T. SCHIMKE. Studies on the synthesis and degradation of proteins of the endoplasmic reticulum of rat liver. *J. Biol. Chem.* 244: 3303–3315, 1969.
7. AUGUSTINE, S. L., AND R. W. SWICK. Turnover of total proteins and ornithine aminotransferase during liver regeneration in rats. *Am. J. Physiol.* 238 (*Endocrinol. Metab.* 1): E46–E52, 1980.
8. AYUSO-PARRILLA, M. S., A. MARTÍN-REGUERO, J. PÉREZ-DÍAZ, AND R. PARRILLA. Role of glucagon on the control of hepatic protein synthesis and degradation in the rat in vivo. *J. Biol. Chem.* 251: 7785–7790, 1976.
9. BAUGH, R. J., AND J. TRAVIS. Human leukocyte granule elastase: rapid isolation and characterization. *Biochemistry* 15: 836–841, 1976.
10. BEATTY, K., J. DIETH, AND J. TRAVIS. Kinetics of association of serine proteinases with native and oxidized α-1-proteinase inhibitor and α-1-antichymotrypsin. *J. Biol. Chem.* 255: 3931–3934, 1980.

11. BENDITT, E. P., W. S. BURROUGHS, C. H. STEFFEE, AND L. E. FRAZIER. Studies in amino acid utilization. IV. The minimum requirements of the indispensable amino acids for maintenance of the adult well nourished male albino rat. *J. Nutr.* 40: 335–350, 1950.
12. BERNHEIM, F., AND M. L. C. BERNHEIM. The nitrogen metabolism of rat tissue slices under various conditions. *J. Biol. Chem.* 163: 203–209, 1946.
13. BIENKOWSKI, R. S., M. J. COWAN, J. A. MCDONALD, AND R. G. CRYSTAL. Degradation of newly synthesized collagen. *J. Biol. Chem.* 253: 4356–4363, 1978.
14. BLACKWOOD, C. E., Y. HOSANNAH, E. PERMAN, S. KELLER, AND I. MANDL. Experimental emphysema in rats: elastolytic titer of inducing enzyme as determinant of the response. *Proc. Soc. Exp. Biol. Med.* 114: 450–454, 1973.
15. BLONDIN, J., R. ROSENBERG, AND A. JANOFF. An inhibitor in human lung macrophages active against human neutrophil elastase. *Am. Rev. Respir. Dis.* 106: 477–479, 1972.
15a. BOND, J. S. Relationship between inactivation of an enzyme by acid or lysosomal extracts and its in vivo degradation rate (Abstract). *Federation Proc.* 34: 651, 1975.
16. BORSOOK, H., AND G. L. KEIGHLEY. The "continuing" metabolism of nitrogen in animals. *Proc. R. Soc. London Ser. B* 118: 488–521, 1935.
17. BOUCEK, R. J., N. L. NOBLE, AND A. MARKS. Age and the fibrous proteins of the human lung. *Gerontologia* 5: 150–157, 1961.
18. BRADLEY, K., S. MCCONNELL-BREUL, AND R. G. CRYSTAL. Lung collagen heterogeneity. *Proc. Natl. Acad. Sci. USA* 71: 2828–2832, 1974.
19. BRADLEY, K., S. MCCONNELL-BREUL, AND R. G. CRYSTAL. Collagen in the human lung. Quantitation of rates of synthesis and partial characterization of composition. *J. Clin. Invest.* 55: 543–550, 1975.
20. BRADLEY, K. H., S. D. MCCONNELL, AND R. G. CRYSTAL. Lung collagen composition and synthesis. Characterization and changes with age. *J. Biol. Chem.* 249: 2674–2683, 1974.
21. BRADLEY, M. O., J. F. DICE, L. HAYFLICK, AND R. T. SCHIMKE. Protein alterations in aging WI-38 cells as determined by proteolytic susceptibility. *Exp. Cell Res.* 96: 103–112, 1975.
22. BRADLEY, M. O., L. HAYFLICK, AND R. T. SCHIMKE. Protein degradation in human fibroblasts (WI-38). Effects of aging, viral transformation, and amino acid analogs. *J. Biol. Chem.* 251: 3521–3529, 1976.
23. BRESNICK, E., E. D. MAYFIELD, AND H. MOSSÉ. Increased activity of enzymes for de novo pyrimidine biosynthesis after orotic acid administration. *Mol. Pharmacol.* 4: 173–180, 1968.
24. BRESNICK, E., S. S. WILLIAMS, AND H. MOSSÉ. Rates of turnover of deoxythymidine kinase and of its template RNA in regenerating and control liver. *Cancer Res.* 27: 469–475, 1967.
25. BRODY, J. S., H. KAGAN, AND A. MANALO. Lung lysyl oxidase activity: relation to lung growth. *Am. Rev. Respir. Dis.* 120: 1289–1295, 1979.
26. BROSTROM, C. O., AND H. JEFFAY. Protein catabolism in rat liver homogenates. A re-evaluation of the energy requirement for protein catabolism. *J. Biol. Chem.* 245: 4001–4008, 1970.
27. BUCKER, N. L. R. Regeneration of mammalian liver. *Int. Rev. Cytol.* 15: 245–300, 1963.
27a. BURRI, P. H., AND E. R. WEIBEL. Ultrastructure and morphometry of the developing lung. In: *Lung Biology in Health and Disease. Development of the Lung*, edited by W. A. Hodson. New York: Dekker, 1977, vol. 6, p. 215–268.
28. CARP, H., AND A. JANOFF. Possible mechanisms of emphysema in smokers. In vitro suppression of serum elastase-inhibitory capacity by fresh cigarette smoke and its prevention by antioxidants. *Am. Rev. Respir. Dis.* 118: 617–621, 1978.
29. CARP, H., AND A. JANOFF. In vitro suppression of serum elastase-inhibitory capacity by phagocytosing polymorphonuclear leukocytes. *J. Clin. Invest.* 63: 793–797, 1979.
30. CARP, H., AND A. JANOFF. Inactivation of bronchial mucous proteinase inhibitor by cigarette smoke and phagocyte-derived oxidants. *Exp. Lung Res.* 1: 225–237, 1980.
31. CHIANG, M.-J., F. KISHI, P. WHITNEY, AND D. MASSARO. Proteolysis in the rat lung: hypoxia and evidence for an inhibitor of proteolysis. *Am. J. Physiol.* 241 (*Endocrinol. Metab.* 4): E101–E107, 1981.
32. CHIANG, M.-J., AND D. MASSARO. Protein metabolism in lung. II. Influence of amino acids and glucose on protein degradation. *J. Appl. Physiol.: Respirat. Environ. Exercise Physiol.* 47: 1058–1061, 1979.
33. CHIANG, M.-J., P. WHITNEY, JR., AND D. MASSARO. Protein metabolism in lung: use of isolated perfused lung to study protein degradation. *J. Appl. Physiol.: Respirat. Environ. Exercise Physiol.* 47: 72–78, 1979.
33a. CHIANG, M.-J., P. WHITNEY, JR., AND D. MASSARO. Proteolysis in the lung: modulation by amino acids and hypoxia (Abstract). *Am. Rev. Respir. Dis.* 123: 216A, 1981.
34. CHRISTENSEN, H. N., AND A. M. CULLER. Effects of nonmetabolizable analogs on the distribution of amino acids in the rat. *Biochim. Biophys. Acta* 150: 237–252, 1968.
35. CHUA, B., R. L. KAO, D. E. RANNELS, AND H. E. MORGAN. Inhibition of protein degradation by anoxia and ischemia in perfused rat hearts. *J. Biol. Chem.* 254: 6617–6623, 1979.
36. CHUNG, E., E. M. KEELE, AND E. J. MILLER. Isolation and characterization of the cyanogen bromide peptides from $\alpha 1$ (III) chain of human collagen. *Biochemistry* 13: 3459–3464, 1974.
37. CHVAPIL, M., C. D. ESKELSON, V. STIFFEL, AND J. A. OWEN. Early changes in the chemical composition of the rat lung after silica administration. *Arch. Environ. Health* 34: 402–406, 1979.
38. CLARK, J. G., J. E. OVERTON, B. A. MARINO, J. UITTO, AND B. C. STARCHER. Collagen biosynthesis in bleomycin-induced pulmonary fibrosis in hamsters. *J. Lab. Clin. Med.* 96: 943–953, 1980.
39. CLARK, J. G., B. C. STARCHER, AND J. UITTO. Bleomycin-induced synthesis of type I procollagen by human lung and skin fibroblasts. *Biochim. Biophys. Acta* 631: 359–370, 1980.
40. CLARK, M. G., C. J. BEINLICH, E. E. MCKEE, J. A. LINS, AND H. E. MORGAN. Relationship between alkaline proteolytic activity and protein degradation in rat heart. *Federation Proc.* 39: 26–30, 1980.
41. COHEN, A. B. The effects of in vivo and in vitro oxidative damage to purified alpha$_1$-antitrypsin and to the enzyme-inhibiting activity of plasma. *Am. Rev. Respir. Dis.* 119: 953–960, 1979.
42. COLLINS, J. F., AND R. G. CRYSTAL. Characterization of cell-free synthesis of collagen by lung polysomes in a heterologous system. *J. Biol. Chem.* 250: 7332–7342, 1975.
43. COLLINS, J. F., B. MCCULLOUGH, J. J. COALSON, AND W. G. JOHANSON, JR. Bleomycin-induced diffuse interstitial pulmonary fibrosis in baboons. II. Further studies on connective tissue changes. *Am. Rev. Respir. Dis.* 123: 305–312, 1981.
44. COWAN, M. J., AND R. G. CRYSTAL. Lung growth after unilateral pneumonectomy: quantitation of collagen synthesis and content. *Am. Rev. Respir. Dis.* 111: 267–277, 1975.
45. CRIE, J. S., AND K. WILDENTHAL. Influence of acidosis and lactate on protein degradation in adult and fetal hearts. *J. Mol. Cell. Cardiol.* 12: 1065–1074, 1980.
46. CRYSTAL, R. G. Lung collagen: definition, diversity, and development. *Federation Proc.* 33: 2248–2255, 1974.
47. CRYSTAL, R. G., J. E. GADEK, V. J. FERRNAS, J. D. FULMER, B. R. LINE, AND G. W. HUNNINGHAKE. Interstitial lung disease: current concepts of pathogenesis, staging and therapy. *Am. J. Med.* 70: 542–568, 1981.
48. DANNENBERG, A. M., JR., AND E. L. SMITH. Proteolytic enzymes of lung. *J. Biol. Chem.* 215: 45–54, 1955.
49. DANNENBERG, A. M., JR., AND E. L. SMITH. Action of proteinase I of bovine lung. Hydrolysis of the oxidized β chain of insulin; polymer formation from amino acid esters. *J. Biol.*

Chem. 215: 55–66, 1955.
50. DAVID, M., AND Y. AVI-DOR. Stimulation of protein synthesis in cultured heart muscle cells by glucose. *Biochem. J.* 150: 405–411, 1975.
51. DEL MAR, E. G., J. W. BRODICK, M. C. GEOKAS, AND C. LARGMAN. Effect of oxidation of methionine in a peptide substrate for human elastase. A model for inactivation of α_1-protease inhibitor. *Biochem. Biophys. Res. Commun.* 88: 346–350, 1979.
51a. DICE, J. F., P. J. DEHLINGER, AND R. T. SCHIMKE. Studies on the correlation between size and relative degradation rate of soluble proteins. *J. Biol. Chem.* 248: 4220–4228, 1973.
51b. DICE, J. F., AND A. L. GOLDBERG. Degradative rates of proteins are related to their isoelectric points (Abstract). *Federation Proc.* 34: 651, 1975.
51c. DICE, J. F., AND A. L. GOLDBERG. Relationship between in vivo degradative rates and isoelectric points of proteins. *Proc. Natl. Acad. Sci. USA* 72: 3893–3897, 1975.
52. DICE, J. F., C. D. WALKER, B. BYRNE, AND A. CARDIEL. General characteristics of protein degradation in diabetes and starvation. *Proc. Natl. Acad. Sci. USA* 75: 2093–2097, 1979.
53. DUBICK, M. A., R. B. RUCKER, J. A. LAST, L. O. LOLLINI, AND C. E. CROSS. Elastin turnover in murine lung after repeated ozone exposure. *Toxicol. Appl. Pharmacol.* 58: 203–210, 1981.
54. EAGLE, H., K. A. PIEZ, AND M. LEVY. The intracellular amino acid concentrations required for protein synthesis in cultured human cells. *J. Biol. Chem.* 236: 2039–2042, 1961.
55. ELWYN, D. H., W. J. LAUNDER, H. C. PARIKH, AND E. M. WISE, JR. Roles of plasma and erythrocytes in interorgan transport of amino acids in dogs. *Am. J. Physiol.* 222: 1333–1342, 1972.
56. EPSTEIN, D., S. ELIAS-BISHKO, AND A. HERSHKO. Requirement for protein synthesis in the regulation of protein breakdown in cultured hepatoma cells. *Biochemistry* 14: 5199–5204, 1975.
57. EPSTEIN, E. H., JR., AND N. H. MUNDERLOH. Isolation and characterization of CNBr peptides of human $\alpha 1(III)_3$ collagen and tissue distribution of $\alpha 1(I)_2 \alpha 2$ and $\alpha 1(III)_3$ collagens. *J. Biol. Chem.* 250: 9304–9312, 1975.
58. ERIKSSON, S. Studies in alpha-1-antitrypsin deficiency. *Acta Med. Scand. Suppl.* 432: 1–85, 1965.
59. EYRE, D. R. Collagen: molecular diversity in the body's protein scaffold. *Science* 207: 1315–1322, 1980.
62. FAN, D., P. PARKER, AND D. MASSARO. Protein synthesis by attached pulmonary macrophages. Effect of phagocytosis. *Biochim. Biophys. Acta* 699: 98–109, 1982.
63. FARIDY, E. E. Effect of food and water deprivation on surface activity of lungs of rats. *J. Appl. Physiol.* 29: 493–498, 1970.
64. FEIGELSON, P., T. DASHMAN, AND F. MARGOLIS. The half-lifetime of induced tryptophan peroxidase in vivo. *Arch. Biochem. Biophys.* 85: 478–482, 1959.
65. FISHER, H. Protein and amino acid requirements of the laboratory rabbit. *Lab. Anim. Sci.* 26: 659–663, 1976.
66. FLAIM, K. E., J. B. LI, AND L. S. JEFFERSON. Protein turnover in rat skeletal muscle: effects of hypophysectomy and growth hormone. *Am. J. Physiol.* 234 (*Endocrinol. Metab. Gastrointest. Physiol.* 3): E38–E43, 1978.
67. FLECK, A., J. SHEPHERD, AND H. N. MUNRO. Protein synthesis in rat liver: influence of amino acids in diet on microsomes and polysomes. *Science* 150: 628–629, 1965.
68. FOSTER, J. A., C. B. RICH, S. FLETCHER, S. R. KARR, M. D. DESA, T. OLIVER, AND A. PRZYBYLA. Elastin biosynthesis in chick embryonic lung tissue. Comparison to chick aortic elastin. *Biochemistry* 20: 3528–3535, 1981.
69. FRANK, L., J. R. BUCHER, AND R. J. ROBERTS. Oxygen toxicity in neonatal and adult animals of various species. *J. Appl. Physiol.: Respirat. Environ. Exercise Physiol.* 45: 699–704, 1978.
70. FRANK, L., AND R. J. ROBERTS. Endotoxin protection against oxygen-induced acute and chronic lung injury. *J. Appl. Physiol.: Respirat. Environ. Exercise Physiol.* 47: 577–581, 1979.
71. FRANK, L., J. SUMMERVILLE, AND D. MASSARO. Protection from oxygen toxicity with endotoxin. *J. Clin. Invest.* 65: 1104–1110, 1980.
72. FRANK, L., D. WOOD, AND R. J. ROBERTS. Effect of diethyldithiocarbamate on oxygen toxicity and lung enzyme activity in immature and adult rats. *Biochem. Pharmacol.* 27: 251–254, 1978.
73. FRANK, L., J. YAM, AND R. J. ROBERTS. The role of endotoxin in protection of adult rats from oxygen-induced lung toxicity. *J. Clin. Invest.* 61: 269–275, 1978.
74. FRIDOVICH, I. Superoxide dismutases. *Adv. Enzymol.* 41: 35–97, 1974.
75. FRIDOVICH, I. Oxygen radicals, hydrogen peroxide and oxygen toxicity. In: *Free Radicals in Biology*, edited by W. A. Pryor. New York: Academic, 1976, vol. I, p. 239–277.
76. FRIDOVICH, I. The biology of oxygen radicals. *Science* 201: 875–880, 1978.
77. FRITZ, P. J., E. S. VESELL, E. L. WHITE, AND K. M. PRUITT. The role of synthesis and degradation in determining tissue concentrations of lactase dehydrogenase-5. *Proc. Natl. Acad. Sci. USA* 62: 558–565, 1969.
78. FRUTON, J. S. On the proteolytic enzymes of animal tissues. V. Peptidases of skin, lung and serum. *J. Biol. Chem.* 166: 721–738, 1946.
79. FULKS, R. M., J. B. LI, AND A. L. GOLDBERG. Effects of insulin, glucose, and amino acids on protein turnover in rat diaphragm. *J. Biol. Chem.* 250: 290–298, 1975.
79a. FULMER, J. D., R. S. BIENKOWSKI, M. J. COWAN, S. D. BREUL, K. M. BRADLEY, V. J. FERRANS, W. C. ROBERTS, AND R. G. CRYSTAL. Collagen concentration and rates of synthesis in idiopathic pulmonary fibrosis. *Am. Rev. Respir. Dis.* 122: 289–301, 1980.
80. GACAD, G., K. DICKIE, AND D. MASSARO. Protein synthesis in lung: influence of starvation on amino acid incorporation into protein. *J. Appl. Physiol.* 33: 381–384, 1972.
81. GACAD, G., AND D. MASSARO. Hyperoxia: influence on lung mechanics and protein synthesis. *J. Clin. Invest.* 52: 559–565, 1973.
82. GADEK, J. E., G. A. FELLS, AND R. G. CRYSTAL. Cigarette smoking induces functional antiprotease deficiency in the lower respiratory tract of humans. *Science* 206: 1315–1316, 1979.
83. GADEK, J. E., G. A. FELLS, D. G. WRIGHT, AND R. G. CRYSTAL. Human neutrophil elastase functions as a type III collagen "collagenase." *Biochem. Biophys. Res. Commun.* 95: 1815–1822, 1980.
83a. GADEK, J. E., J. A. KELMAN, G. A. FELLS, S. E. WEINBERGER, A. L. HORWITZ, H. Y. REYNOLDS, J. D. FULMER, AND R. G. CRYSTAL. Collagenase in the lower respiratory tract of patients with idiopathic pulmonary fibrosis. *N. Engl. J. Med.* 301: 737–742, 1979.
84. GAIL, D. B., AND D. MASSARO. Oxygen consumption by rat lung after in vivo hyperoxia. *Am. Rev. Respir. Dis.* 113: 889–892, 1976.
85. GAIL, D. B., G. D. MASSARO, AND D. MASSARO. Influence of fasting on the lung. *J. Appl. Physiol.: Respirat. Environ. Exercise Physiol.* 42: 88–92, 1977.
86. GANSCHOW, R., AND R. T. SCHIMKE. Independent genetic control of the catalytic activity and the rate of degradation of catalase in mice. *J. Biol. Chem.* 244: 4649–4658, 1969.
87. GARLICK, P. J., T. L. BURK, AND R. W. SWICK. Protein synthesis and RNA in tissues of the pig. *Am. J. Physiol.* 230: 1108–1112, 1976.
88. GIRI, S. N., L. W. SCHWARTZ, M. A. HOLLINGER, M. E. FREYWALD, M. J. SCHIEDT, AND J. E. ZUCKERMAN. Biochemical and structural alterations of hamster lungs in response to intratracheal administration of bleomycin. *Exp. Mol. Pathol.* 33: 1–14, 1980.
89. GLASS, R. D., AND D. DOYLE. On the measurement of protein turnover in animal cells. *J. Biol. Chem.* 247: 5234–5242, 1972.

89a. GOLDBERG, A. L. Correlation between rates of degradation of bacterial proteins in vivo and their sensitivity to proteases. *Proc. Natl. Acad. Sci. USA* 69: 2640–2644, 1972.
90. GOLDBERG, A. L., AND J. F. DICE. Intracellular protein degradation in mammalian and bacterial cells. *Annu. Rev. Biochem.* 43: 835–869, 1974.
91. GOLDBERG, A. L., E. M. HOWELL, J. B. LI, S. B. MARTEL, AND W. F. PROUTY. Physiological significance of protein degradation in animal and bacterial cells. *Federation Proc.* 33: 1112–1120, 1974.
92. GOLDBERG, A. L., AND A. C. ST. JOHN. Intracellular protein degradation in mammalian and bacterial cells. Pt. 2. *Annu. Rev. Biochem.* 45: 747–803, 1976.
93. GOODRIDGE, A. G., AND T. G. ADELMAN. Regulation of malic enzyme synthesis by insulin, triiodothyronine and glucagon in liver cells in culture. *J. Biol. Chem.* 251: 3027–3032, 1976.
94. GRAND, R. J., AND P. R. GROSS. Independent stimulation of secretion and protein synthesis in rat parotid glands. *J. Biol. Chem.* 244: 5608–5615, 1969.
95. GREENBERG, D., S. A. LYONS, AND J. LAST. Paraquat-induced changes in the rate of collagen biosynthesis by rat lung explants. *J. Lab. Clin. Med.* 92: 1033–1042, 1978.
96. GREGORIO, C. A., AND D. MASSARO. Influence of insulin on amino acid uptake by lung slices. *J. Appl. Physiol.: Respirat. Environ. Exercise Physiol.* 42: 216–220, 1977.
97. GROSS, I., S. A. ROONEY, AND J. B. WARSHAR. The inhibition of enzymes related to pulmonary fatty acid and phospholipid synthesis by dietary deprivation in the rat. *Biochem. Biophys. Res. Commun.* 64: 59–63, 1975.
98. GROSS, P., M. A. BABYAK, E. TOLKER, AND M. KASCHAK. Enzymatically produced pulmonary emphysema. A preliminary report. *J. Occup. Med.* 6: 481–484, 1964.
99. GROSS, P., E. A. PFITZER, E. TOLKER, M. A. BABYAK, AND M. KASCHAK. Experimental emphysema. Its production with papain in normal and silicotic rats. *Arch. Environ. Health* 11: 50–58, 1965.
100. GUNN, J. M., F. J. BALLARD, AND R. W. HANSON. Influence of hormones and medium composition on the degradation of phosphoenolpyruvate carboxykinase (GTP) and total protein in Reuber H35 cells. *J. Biol. Chem.* 251: 3586–3593, 1976.
101. GUTTMAN, H. N. Oxygen inhibition of antibody synthesis (Abstract). *J. Cell Biol.* 55: 100a, 1972.
102. HABER, P., F. KUMMER, AND H. LUDWIG. Lung elasticity in juvenile-onset diabetes mellitus. *Am. Rev. Respir. Dis.* 116: 544–546, 1977.
103. HAIES, D. M., J. GIL, AND E. R. WEIBEL. Morphometric study of rat lung cells. I. Numerical and dimensional characteristics of parenchymal cell population. *Am. Rev. Respir. Dis.* 123: 533–541, 1981.
104. HALME, J., J. UITTO, K. KAHANPÄÄ, P. KARHUNEN, AND S. LINDY. Protocollagen proline hydroxylase activity in experimental pulmonary fibrosis of rats. *J. Lab. Clin. Med.* 75: 535–541, 1970.
105. HAMMER, J. A., III, AND D. E. RANNELS. Effects of halothane on protein synthesis and degradation in rabbit pulmonary macrophages. *Am. Rev. Respir. Dis.* 124: 50–55, 1981.
106. HAMMER, J. A., III, AND D. E. RANNELS. Protein turnover in pulmonary macrophages. *Biochem. J.* 198: 53–65, 1981.
107. HANCE, A. J., K. BRADLEY, AND R. G. CRYSTAL. Lung collagen heterogeneity. Synthesis of type I and type III collagen by rabbit and human lung cells in culture. *J. Clin. Invest.* 57: 102–111, 1976.
108. HASS, M. A., L. FRANK, AND D. MASSARO. The effect of bacterial endotoxin on synthesis of (Cu,Zn) superoxide dismutase in lungs of oxygen-exposed rats. *J. Biol. Chem.* 257: 9379–9383, 1982.
109. HAUSCHKA, P. V., AND P. M. GALLOP. Elastin biosynthesis in mouse lung (Abstract). *Federation Proc.* 33: 1536, 1974.
110. HESTERBERG, T. W., AND J. A. LAST. Ozone-induced acute pulmonary fibrosis in rats. Prevention of increased rates of collagen synthesis by methylprednisolone. *Am. Rev. Respir. Dis.* 123: 47–54, 1981.
111. HILDEBRAN, J., J. AIRHART, W. S. STIREWALT, AND R. B. LOW. Absolute rates of protein and collagen synthesis in cultured human lung fibroblasts (Abstract). *Am. Rev. Respir. Dis.* 121, Suppl.: 353A, 1980.
112. HILL, J. M., AND D. MALAMUD. Decreased protein catabolism during stimulated growth. *FEBS Lett.* 46: 308–311, 1974.
113. HOCHSTRASSER, K., H. HAENDLE, R. REICHERT, E. WERLE, AND S. SCHWARZ. Über Vorkommen und Eigenschaften eines Proteaseninhibitors in menschlichen Nasensekret. *Hoppe-Seyler's Z. Physiol. Chem.* 352: 954–958, 1971.
114. HOCHSTRASSER, K., R. REICHERT, S. SCHWARZ, AND E. WERLE. Isolierung und Charakterisierung eines Proteaseninhibitors aus menschlichen Bronchialsekret. *Hoppe-Seyler's Z. Physiol. Chem.* 353: 221–226, 1972.
115. HOD, Y., AND A. HERSHKO. Relationship of the pool of intracellular valine to protein synthesis and degradation in cultured cells. *J. Biol. Chem.* 251: 4458–4467, 1976.
116. HOFFMAN, L., O. O. BLUMENFELD, R. B. MONDSHINE, AND S. S. PARK. Effect of DL-penicillamine on fibrous proteins of rat lung. *J. Appl. Physiol.* 33: 42–46, 1972.
117. HOFFMAN, L., R. B. MONDSHINE, AND S. S. PARK. Effect of DL-penicillamine on elastic properties of rat lung. *J. Appl. Physiol.* 30: 508–511, 1971.
118. HOGG, J. C., S. J. NEPAZY, P. T. MACKLEM, AND W. M. THURLBECK. Elastic properties of the centrilobular emphysematous space. *N. Engl. J. Med.* 48: 1306–1312, 1969.
119. HOLIAN, A., AND R. P. DANIELE. Release of oxygen products from lung macrophages by N-formyl peptides. *J. Appl. Physiol.: Respirat. Environ. Exercise Physiol.* 50: 736–740, 1981.
120. HOLZER, H., AND P. C. HEINRICH. Control of proteolysis. *Annu. Rev. Biochem.* 49: 63–92, 1980.
121. HOPGOOD, M. F., M. C. CLARK, AND F. J. BALLARD. Inhibition of protein degradation in isolated hepatocytes. *Biochem. J.* 164: 399–407, 1977.
122. HUNNINGHAKE, G. W., J. M. DAVIDSON, S. RENNARD, S. SZAPIEL, J. E. GADEK, AND R. G. CRYSTAL. Elastin fragments attract macrophage precursors to diseased site in pulmonary emphysema. *Science* 212: 925–927, 1981.
123. HUSSAIN, M. Z., J. C. BELTON, AND R. S. BHATNAGAR. Macromolecular synthesis in organ cultures of neonatal rat lung. *In Vitro* 14: 740–745, 1978.
124. HUSSAIN, M. Z., AND R. S. BHATNAGAR. Involvement of superoxide in the paraquat-induced enhancement of lung collagen synthesis in organ culture. *Biochem. Biophys. Res. Commun.* 89: 71–76, 1979.
125. HUSSAIN, M. Z., C. E. CROSS, M. G. MUSTAFA, AND R. S. BHATNAGAR. Hydroxyproline contents and prolyl hydroxylase activities in lungs of rats exposed to low levels of ozone. *Life Sci.* 18: 897–904, 1976.
126. IHNEN, J., AND G. KALNITSKY. Lung proteases and protease inhibitors. In: *Intracellular Protein Catabolism*, edited by V. Turk and N. Marks. New York: Plenum, 1977, vol. II, p. 259–269.
127. ILAN, J., AND M. SINGER. Sampling of the leucine pool from the growing peptide chain: difference in leucine specific activity of peptidyl-transfer RNA from free and membrane-bound polysomes. *J. Mol. Biol.* 91: 39–51, 1975.
128. JANOFF, A. Anatomic emphysema produced in mice by lysosome-containing fractions from human alveolar macrophages (Abstract). *Federation Proc.* 31: 254, 1972.
129. JANOFF, A. Inhibition of human granulocyte elastase by serum α_1-antitrypsin. *Am. Rev. Respir. Dis.* 105: 121–122, 1972.
130. JANOFF, A. Granulocyte elastase: role in arthritis and in pulmonary emphysema. In: *Neutral Proteases of Human Polymorphonuclear Leukocytes. Biochemistry, Physiology, and Clinical Significance*, edited by K. Havemann and A. Janoff. Baltimore, MD: Urban & Schwarzenberg, 1978, p. 390–418.
131. JANOFF, A., H. CARP, D. K. LEE, AND R. T. DREW. Cigarette smoke inhalation decreased α_1-antitrypsin activity in rat lung. *Science* 206: 1313–1314, 1979.
132. JANOFF, A., R. ROSENBERG, AND M. GALDSTON. Elastase-like esteroprotease activity in human and rabbit alveolar macro-

phage granules. *Proc. Soc. Exp. Biol. Med.* 136: 1054–1058, 1971.

133. JANOFF, A., B. SLOAN, G. WEINBAUM, B. DAMIANO, R. A. SANDHAUS, J. ELIAS, AND P. KIMBEL. Experimental emphysema induced by human neutrophil elastase. *Am. Rev. Respir. Dis.* 115: 461–478, 1977.

134. JANOFF, A., R. WHITE, H. CARP, S. HAREL, R. DEARING, AND D. LEE. Lung injury induced by leukocytic proteases. *Am. J. Pathol.* 97: 111–136, 1979.

135. JEFFERSON, L. S., D. E. RANNELS, B. L. MUNGER, AND H. E. MORGAN. Insulin in the regulation of protein turnover in heart and skeletal muscle. *Federation Proc.* 33: 1098–1104, 1974.

136. JOHANSON, W., JR., AND A. K. PIERCE. Effects of elastase, collagenase, and papain on structure and function of rat lungs in vitro. *J. Clin. Invest.* 51: 288–293, 1972.

137. JOHN, R., AND J. THOMAS. Chemical compositions of elastins isolated from aortas and pulmonary tissues of humans of different ages. *Biochem. J.* 127: 261–269, 1972.

138. JOHNSON, A., AND F. A. ANDREWS. Lung scleroproteins in age and emphysema. *Chest* 57: 239–244, 1970.

139. JOYNER, L. R., AND D. MASSARO. The oxygen consumption of rabbit lung slices after pneumothorax. *Am. Rev. Respir. Dis.* 116: 537–540, 1977.

140. KAPLAN, P. D., C. KUHN, AND J. A. PIERCE. The induction of emphysema with elastase. I. The evolution of the lesion and influence of serum. *J. Lab. Clin. Med.* 82: 349–356, 1973.

141. KARLINSKY, J. B., G. L. SNIDER, C. FRANZBLAU, P. J. STONE, AND F. G. HOPPIN, JR. In vitro effects of elastase and collagenase on mechanical properties of hamster lungs. *Am. Rev. Respir. Dis.* 113: 769–777, 1976.

142. KELLER, G. H., AND J. M. TAYLOR. Effect of hypophysectomy on the synthesis of rat liver albumin. *J. Biol. Chem.* 251: 3768–3773, 1976.

143. KELLEY, J., R. A. NEWMAN, AND J. N. EVANS. Bleomycin-induced pulmonary fibrosis in the rat. *J. Lab. Clin. Med.* 96: 954–964, 1980.

144. KHAIRALLAH, E. A., AND G. E. MORTIMORE. Assessment of protein turnover in perfused rat liver. *J. Biol. Chem.* 251: 1375–1384, 1976.

145. KHURANA, M., AND A. H. NIDEN. Experimental model to study the development of pulmonary fibrosis (Abstract). *Am. Rev. Respir. Dis.* 113: 245A, 1976.

146. KING, R. J., AND J. A. CLEMENTS. Surface active materials from dog lung. II. Composition and physiological correlations. *Am. J. Physiol.* 223: 715–726, 1972.

147. KIPNIS, D. M., E. REISS, AND E. HELMREICH. Functional heterogeneity of the intracellular amino acid pool in mammalian cells. *Biochim. Biophys. Acta* 51: 519–524, 1961.

148. KLINE, D. L. A procedure for the study of factors which affect the nitrogen metabolism of isolated tissues: hormonal influences. *Endocrinology* 45: 596–604, 1949.

149. KRAMPS, J. A., C. FRANKEN, C. J. L. M. MEIJER, AND J. H. DIJKMAN. Localization of low molecular weight protease inhibitor in serous secretory cells of the respiratory tract. *J. Histochem. Cytochem.* 29: 712–719, 1981.

150. KUHN, C., III, AND R. M. SENIOR. The role of elastases in the development of emphysema. *Lung* 155: 185–197, 1978.

151. KUHN, C., III, Y. SHIU-YEH, M. CHRAPLYVY, H. E. LINDER, AND R. M. SENIOR. The induction of emphysema with elastase. II. Changes in connective tissue. *Lab. Invest.* 34: 372–380, 1976.

152. KUNSTLING, T. R., R. A. GOODWIN, JR., AND R. M. DES PREZ. Diffuse interstitial pulmonary fibrosis (cryptogenic fibrosing alveolitis). *South. Med. J.* 69: 479–487, 1976.

153. KUTTAN, R., M. LAFRANCONI, I. G. SIPES, E. MEEZAN, AND K. BRENDEL. Effect of paraquat treatment on prolyl hydroxylase activity and collagen synthesis of rat lung and kidney. *Res. Commun. Chem. Pathol. Pharmacol.* 25: 257–268, 1979.

154. LAJTHA, A., J. TOTH, K. FUMIMOTO, AND H. C. AGRAWAL. Turnover of myelin proteins in mouse brain in vivo. *Biochem. J.* 164: 323–329, 1977.

155. LAST, J. A., AND D. B. GREENBERG. Ozone-induced alterations in collagen metabolism of rat lungs. II. Long-term exposures. *Toxicol. Appl. Pharmacol.* 55: 108–114, 1980.

156. LAST, J. A., D. B. GREENBERG, AND W. L. CASTLEMAN. Ozone-induced alterations in collagen metabolism of rat lungs. *Toxicol. Appl. Pharmacol.* 51: 247–258, 1979.

157. LAURELL, C. B., AND S. ERIKSSON. The electrophoretical α_1-globulin pattern of serum in alpha$_1$ antitrypsin deficiency. *Scand. J. Clin. Lab. Invest.* 15: 132–140, 1963.

158. LAW, M. P., S. HORNSEY, AND S. B. FIELD. Collagen content of lungs of mice after x-ray irradiation. *Radiat. Res.* 65: 60–70, 1976.

159. LAYMAN, D. L., L. SOKOLOFF, AND E. J. MILLER. Collagen synthesis by articular chondrocytes in monolayer culture. *Exp. Cell Res.* 73: 107–112, 1972.

160. LEDFORD, B. E., R. W. WARNER, AND R. A. COCHRAN. Albumin synthesis in cultured hepatoma cells. Regulation by essential amino acids. *Biochim. Biophys. Acta* 475: 90–95, 1977.

161. LEFFINGWELL, C. M., AND R. B. LOW. Protein biosynthesis by the pulmonary alveolar macrophage. *Am. Rev. Respir. Dis.* 112: 349–359, 1975.

162. LEVINE, E. A., R. M. SENIOR, AND J. V. BUTLER. The elastase activity of alveolar macrophages: measurements using synthesis substrates and elastin. *Am. Rev. Respir. Dis.* 112: 349–359, 1975.

163. LI, J. B., J. E. HIGGINS, AND L. S. JEFFERSON. Changes in protein turnover in skeletal muscle in response to fasting. *Am. J. Physiol.* 236 (*Endocrinol. Metab. Gastrointest. Physiol.* 5): E222–E228, 1979.

164. LIN, E. C. C., AND W. E. KNOX. Adaption of the rat liver tyrosine-α-ketoglutarate transaminase. *Biochim. Biophys. Acta* 26: 85–88, 1957.

165. LOFTFIELD, R. B., AND A. HARRIS. Participation of free amino acids in protein synthesis. *J. Biol. Chem.* 219: 151–159, 1956.

166. LONGMORE, W. J., AND J. T. MOURNING. Lactate production in isolated perfused rat lung. *Am. J. Physiol.* 231: 351–354, 1976.

167. LÖNNERHOLM, G. Carbonic anhydrase in the lung. *Acta Physiol. Scand.* 108: 197–199, 1980.

168. LOW, R. B. Protein biosynthesis by the pulmonary alveolar macrophage: conditions of assay and the effects of cigarette smoke extracts. *Am. Rev. Respir. Dis.* 110: 466–477, 1974.

169. LOW, R. B. Macromolecule synthesis by alveolar macrophages: response to a phagocytic load. *J. Reticuloendothel. Soc.* 22: 99–109, 1977.

170. MACDONALD, M. L., AND R. W. SWOCK. The effect of protein depletion and repletion in muscle-protein turnover in the chick. *Biochem. J.* 194: 811–819, 1981.

171. MADIA, A. M., S. J. ROZOVSKI, AND H. M. KAGAN. Changes in lung lysyl oxidase activity in streptozotocin-diabetes and in starvation. *Biochim. Biophys. Acta* 585: 481–487, 1979.

172. MADRI, J. A., AND H. FURTHMAYR. Isolation and tissue location of type AB collagen from normal lung parenchyma. *Am. J. Pathol.* 94: 323–331, 1979.

173. MADRI, J. A., AND H. FURTHMAYR. Collagen polymorphism in the lung. *Human Pathol.* 11: 353–366, 1980.

174. MAINARDI, C. L., S. N. DIXIT, AND A. H. KANG. Degradation of type IV (basement membrane) collagen by a proteinase isolated from human polymorphonuclear leukocyte granules. *J. Biol. Chem.* 255: 5435–5441, 1980.

175. MAINARDI, C. L., D. L. HASTY, J. M. SEYER, AND A. H. KANG. Specific cleavage of human type III collagen by human polymorphonuclear leukocyte elastase. *J. Biol. Chem.* 255: 12006–12010, 1980.

176. MAJERUS, P. W., AND R. KOLBURN. Acetyl coenzyme A carboxylase. The roles of synthesis and degradation in regulation of enzyme levels in rat liver. *J. Biol. Chem.* 244: 6254–6262, 1969.

177. MARCO, V., B. MASS, D. R. MERANZE, G. WEINBAUM, AND P. KIMBEL. Induction of experimental emphysema in dogs using leukocyte homogenates. *Am. Rev. Respir. Dis.* 104: 595–598, 1971.

178. MARVER, H. S., A. COLLINS, D. P. TSCHUDY, AND M. RE-

CHEIGL, JR. δ-Aminolaevulinic acid synthetase. II. Induction in rat liver. *J. Biol. Chem.* 241: 4323–4329, 1966.
179. MASS, B., T. IKEDA, D. R. MERANZE, G. WEINBAUM, AND P. KIMBEL. Deduction of experimental emphysema cellular and species specificity. *Am. Rev. Respir. Dis.* 106: 308–391, 1972.
180. MASSARO, D. Protein synthesis in lung: recovery from exposure to hyperoxia. *J. Appl. Physiol.* 35: 32–34, 1973.
181. MASSARO, D., K. KELLEHER, G. MASSARO, AND H. YEAGER, JR. Alveolar macrophages: depression of protein synthesis during phagocytosis. *Am. J. Physiol.* 218: 1533–1539, 1970.
182. MASSARO, G. D., AND D. MASSARO. Hyperoxia: a stereological ultrastructural examination of its influence on cytoplasmic components of the pulmonary granular pneumocyte. *J. Clin. Invest.* 52: 566–570, 1973.
183. MASSARO, G. D., AND D. MASSARO. Adaption to hyperoxia. Influence on protein synthesis by lung and on granular pneumocyte ultrastructure. *J. Clin. Invest.* 53: 705–709, 1974.
184. MATIORRI, D., AND R. RUSCITTO. Age-related changes of accuracy and efficiency of protein synthesis machinery in rat. *Biochim. Biophys. Acta* 475: 96–102, 1977.
185. MCKEE, E. E., J. V. CHEUNG, D. E. RANNELS, AND H. E. MORGAN. Measurement of the rate of protein synthesis and compartmentation of heart phenylalanine. *J. Biol. Chem.* 253: 1030–1040, 1978.
186. MCLEES, B. D., G. SCHLEITER, AND S. R. PINNEL. Isolation of type III collagen from human adult parenchymal lung tissue. *Biochemistry* 16: 185–190, 1977.
187. MERLIE, J. P., S. HEINEMANN, B. EINARSON, AND J. M. LINDSTROM. Degradation of acetylcholine receptor in diaphragms of rats with experimental autoimmune myasthenia gravis. *J. Biol. Chem.* 254: 6328–6332, 1979.
188. MILLER, E. J. Biochemical characteristics and biological significance of the genetically-distinct collagens. *Mol. Cell. Biochem.* 13: 165–192, 1976.
189. MILLWARD, D. J., AND P. J. GARLICK. The pattern of protein turnover in the whole animal and the effect of dietary variations. *Proc. Nutr. Soc.* 31: 257–263, 1972.
190. MISRA, H. P., AND I. FRIDOVICH. The generation of superoxide radical during the autoxidation of ferredoxins. *J. Biol. Chem.* 246: 6886–6890, 1971.
191. MOORE, S., AND W. H. STEIN. Procedures for the chromatographic determination of amino acids on four per cent cross-linked sulfonated polystyrene resins. *J. Biol. Chem.* 211: 893–906, 1954.
192. MORGAN, H. E. Effects of hypophysectomy, growth hormone and thyroid on protein turnover in heart. *J. Biol. Chem.* 250: 4556–4561, 1975.
193. MORGAN, H. E., B. H. L. CHUA, E. O. FULLER, AND D. SIEHL. Regulation of protein synthesis and degradation during in vitro cardiac work. *Am. J. Physiol.* 238 (*Endocrinol. Metab.* 1): E431–E442, 1980.
194. MORGAN, H. E., D. C. N. EARL, A. BROADUS, E. B. WOLPERT, K. E. GIGER, AND L. S. JEFFERSON. Regulation of protein synthesis in heart muscle. I. Effect of amino acid levels on protein synthesis. *J. Biol. Chem.* 246: 2152–2162, 1971.
195. MORIYAMA, A., AND T. TAKAHASHI. Studies on the distribution of acid proteases in primate lungs and other tissues by diethylaminoethyl-cellulose chromatography. *J. Biochem. Tokyo* 87: 737–743, 1980.
196. MORTIMORE, G. E., AND C. E. MONDON. Inhibition by insulin of valine turnover in liver. Evidence for a general control of proteolysis. *J. Biol. Chem.* 245: 2375–2383, 1970.
197. MORTIMORE, G. E., K. H. WOODSIDE, AND J. E. HENRY. Compartmentation of free valine and its relation to protein turnover in perfused rat liver. *J. Biol. Chem.* 247: 2776–2784, 1972.
198. MUELLER, P., C. LEMMEN, S. GAY, K. VON DER MARK, AND K. KUHN. Biosynthesis of collagen by chondrocytes in vitro. In: *Extracellular Matrix Influences on Gene Expression*, edited by H. C. Slavkin and R. C. Gruelich. New York: Academic, 1975, p. 293–302.
199. MUNRO, H. N. Evolution of protein metabolism in mammals. In: *Mammalian Protein Metabolism*, edited by H. N. Munro. New York: Academic, 1969, vol. III, chapt. 25, p. 133–182.
200. NAGAISHI, C. *Functional Anatomy and Histology of the Lung.* Baltimore, MD: University Park, 1972.
201. NYE, R. N. Studies on the pneumonic exudate. V. The relation of pneumonic lung protease activity to hydrogen ion concentration, and a consideration of the origin of the enzyme. *J. Exp. Med.* 35: 153–160, 1922.
202. OHLSSON, K. Neutral leukocyte proteases and elastase inhibited by plasma alpha-1-antitrypsin. *Scand. J. Lab. Clin. Med.* 28: 251–253, 1971.
203. OHLSSON, K., AND I. OLSSON. The neutral proteases of human granulocytes. Isolation and partial characterization of granulocyte elastases. *Eur. J. Biochem.* 42: 519–527, 1974.
204. OHLSSON, K., AND H. TEGNER. Inhibition of elastase from granulocytes by the low molecular weight bronchial protease inhibitor. *Scand. J. Clin. Lab. Invest.* 36: 437–445, 1976.
205. OHLSSON, K., H. TEGNER, AND U. AKESSON. Isolation and partial characterization of a low molecular weight acid-stable protease inhibitor from human bronchial secretion. *Hoppe-Seyler's Z. Physiol. Chem.* 358: 583–589, 1977.
206. OWENS, R. A., L. WU-SCHYONG, G. I. GLOVER, AND J. M. GUNN. Inhibition of protein turnover in human lung cells by pepstatin and tripeptide analogs of pepstatin. *Biochem. Pharmacol.* 28: 1263–1266, 1979.
207. PARTRIDGE, S. M., H. F. DAVIS, AND G. S. ADAIR. The chemistry of connective tissues. 3. Composition of the soluble proteins derived from elastin. *Biochem. J.* 61: 21–30, 1955.
208. PASKIN, N., AND R. J. MAYER. The role of enzyme degradation in enzyme turnover during tissue differentiation. *Biochim. Biophys. Acta* 47: 1–10, 1977.
209. PAZ, M. A., D. A. KEITH, H. P. TRAVERSO, AND P. M. GALLOP. Isolation, purification, and cross-linking profiles of elastin from lung and aorta. *Biochemistry* 15: 4912–4918, 1976.
210. PEARSON, O. P., AND A. K. PEARSON. A stereological analysis of the ultrastructure of the lungs of wild mice living at low and high altitude. *J. Morphol.* 150: 359–368, 1976.
211. PHAN, S. M., R. S. THRALL, AND P. WARD. Bleomycin-induced pulmonary fibrosis in rats: biochemical demonstration of increased rate of collagen synthesis. *Am. Rev. Respir. Dis.* 121: 501–506, 1980.
212. PICKRELL, J. A., D. V. HARRIS, S. A. BENJAMIN, R. C. CUDDIHY, R. C. PFLEGER, AND J. L. MAUDERLY. Pulmonary collagen metabolism after lung injury from inhaled 90y in fused clay particles. *Exp. Mol. Pathol.* 25: 70–81, 1976.
213. PICKRELL, J. A., D. V. HARRIS, F. F. HAHN, J. J. BELASICH, AND R. J. JONES. Biological alterations resulting from chronic lung irradiation. III. Effect of partial [30]CO thoracic irradiation upon pulmonary collagen metabolism and fractionation in Syrian hamsters. *Radiat. Res.* 62: 133–144, 1975.
214. PICKRELL, J. A., D. V. HARRIS, R. C. PFLEGER, S. A. BENJAMIN, J. J. BELASICH, R. K. JONES, AND R. D. MCCLELLAN. Biological alterations resulting from chronic lung irradiation. II. Connective tissue alterations following inhalation of [144]Ce fused clay aerosol in beagle dogs. *Radiat. Res.* 63: 299–309, 1975.
215. PIERCE, J. A., H. BESNICK, AND P. H. HENRY. Collagen and elastin metabolism in the lungs, skin, and bones of adult rats. *J. Lab. Clin. Med.* 69: 485–493, 1967.
216. PIERCE, J. A., AND R. V. EBERT. Fibrous network of the lung and its change with age. *Thorax* 20: 469–475, 1965.
217. PIERCE, J. A., AND J. B. HOCOTT. Studies on the collagen and elastin content of the human lung. *J. Clin. Invest.* 39: 8–14, 1960.
218. PINE, M. J. Turnover intracellular proteins. *Annu. Rev. Microbiol.* 26: 103–126, 1972.
219. POOLE, D. B., AND M. WIBO. Protein degradation in culture cells. *J. Biol. Chem.* 248: 6221–6226, 1973.
220. POWELL, J. T., AND P. L. WHITNEY. Postnatal development of rat lung. Changes in lung lectin, elastin, acetylcholinesterase and other enzymes. *Biochem. J.* 188: 1–8, 1980.
221. RAMACHANDRAN, G. N., AND C. RAMAKRISHNAN. Molecular

structure. In: *Biochemistry of Collagen*, edited by G. N. Ramachandran and C. Ramakrishnan. New York: Plenum, 1976, p. 45-84.
222. RANNELS, D. E., A. C. HJALMARSON, AND H. E. MORGAN. Effects of noncarbohydrate substrates on protein synthesis in muscle. *Am. J. Physiol.* 226: 528-539, 1974.
223. RANNELS, D. E., R. H. SAHMS, AND C. A. WATKINS. Effects of starvation and diabetes on protein synthesis in lung. *Am. J. Physiol.:* 236 (*Endocrinol. Metab. Gastrointest. Physiol.* 5): E421-E428, 1979.
224. RECHCIGL, M., JR., AND W. E. HESTON. Genetic regulation of enzyme activity in mammalian system by the alteration of the rates of enzyme degradation. *Biochem. Biophys. Res. Commun.* 27: 119-124, 1967.
225. REGIER, J. C., AND F. C. KAFATOS. Microtechnique for determining the specific activity of radioactive intracellular leucine and applications to in vivo studies of protein synthesis. *J. Biol. Chem.* 246: 6480-6488, 1971.
226. REGIER, J. C., AND F. C. KAFATOS. Absolute rates of protein synthesis in sea urchins with specific activity measurements of radioactive leucine and leucyl-tRNA. *Dev. Biol.* 57: 270-283, 1977.
227. REILLY, C. F., AND J. TRAVIS. The degradation of human lung elastin by neutrophil proteinases. *Biochim. Biophys. Acta* 621: 147-157, 1980.
228. REISER, K. M., AND J. A. LAST. Pulmonary fibrosis in experimental acute respiratory disease. *Am. Rev. Respir. Dis.* 123: 58-63, 1981.
229. RIGHETTI, P., E. P. LITTLE, AND G. WOLF. Reutilization of amino acids in protein synthesis by HeLa cells. *J. Biol. Chem.* 246: 5724-5732, 1971.
230. RILLEMA, J. A., AND B. E. LINEBAUGH. Characteristics of the insulin stimulation of DNA, RNA, and protein metabolism in cultured human mammary carcinoma cells. *Biochim. Biophys. Acta* 475: 74-89, 1977.
231. ROBINSON, J. G. The nature of the amino acid pool used for protein synthesis in cultured, androgen-responsive tumor cells. *Exp. Cell Res.* 106: 239-246, 1977.
232. RODRIGUEZ, R. J., R. R. WHITE, R. M. SENIOR, AND E. A. LEVINE. Elastase release from human alveolar macrophages. Comparison between smokers and nonsmokers. *Science* 198: 313-314, 1977.
233. ROSE, W. C., M. J. OESTERLING, AND M. WOMACK. Comparative growth on diets containing ten and nineteen amino acids, with further observations upon the role of glutamic and aspartic acids. *J. Biol. Chem.* 176: 753-762, 1948.
234. ROSENBERG, L. E., S. J. DOWNING, AND S. SEGAL. Extracellular space estimation in rat kidney slices using C^{14} saccharides and phlorizin. *Am. J. Physiol.* 202: 800-804, 1962.
235. RUBIN, I. B., AND G. GOLDSTEIN. An ultrasensitive isotope dilution method for the determination of L-amino acids. *Anal. Biochem.* 33: 244-254, 1970.
236. SAHEBJAMI, H., AND C. L. VASSALLO. Influence of starvation on enzyme-induced emphysema. *J. Appl. Physiol.: Respirat. Environ. Exercise Physiol.* 48: 284-288, 1980.
237. SAHEBJAMI, H., C. L. VASSALLO, AND J. A. WIRMAN. Lung mechanics and ultrastructure in prolonged starvation. *Am. Rev. Respir. Dis.* 117: 77-83, 1978.
238. SCADDING, J. G. Diffuse pulmonary alveolar fibrosis. *Thorax* 29: 271-281, 1974.
239. SCHIESSLER, H., E. FINK, AND H. FRITZ. Acid-stable proteinase inhibitors from human seminal plasma. *Methods Enzymol.* 45: 847-859, 1976.
240. SCHIMKE, R. T. The importance of both synthesis and degradation in the control of arginase levels in rat liver. *J. Biol. Chem.* 239: 3808-3817, 1964.
241. SCHIMKE, R. T. Regulation of protein degradation in mammalian tissues. In: *Mammalian Protein Metabolism*, edited by H. N. Munro and J. B. Allison. New York: Academic, 1970, vol. 4, p. 177-228.
242. SCHIMKE, R. T. Control of enzyme levels in animal tissues. *Adv. Enzymol.* 37: 135-187, 1973.
243. SCHIMKE, R. T. The synthesis and degradation of membrane proteins. In: *Advances in Cytopharmacology*, edited by B. Ceccarelli, F. Clements, and J. Meldolesi. New York: Raven, 1974, vol. 2, p. 63-69.
244. SCHIMKE, R. T., AND D. DOYLE. Control of enzyme levels in animal tissues. *Annu. Rev. Biochem.* 39: 929-976, 1970.
245. SCHIMKE, R. T., E. W. SWEENEY, AND C. M. BERLIN. Studies on the stability in vivo and in vitro of rat liver tryptophan pyrrolase. *J. Biol. Chem.* 240: 4609-4620, 1965.
246. SCHNEIBLE, P. A., J. AIRHART, AND R. B. LOW. Differential compartmentation of leucine for oxidation and for protein synthesis in cultured skeletal muscle. *J. Biol. Chem.* 256: 4888-4894, 1981.
247. SCHOENHEIMER, R. *The Dynamic State of Body Constituents*. Cambridge, MA: Harvard Univ. Press, 1949.
248. SCHUYLER, M. R., D. E. NIEWOEHNER, S. R. INKLEY, AND R. KOHN. Abnormal lung elasticity in juvenile diabetes mellitus. *Am. Rev. Respir. Dis.* 113: 37-41, 1976.
249. SCORNIK, O. A., AND V. BOTBOL. Role of changes in protein degradation in the growth of regenerating livers. *J. Biol. Chem.* 251: 2891-2897, 1976.
250. SEETHANATHAN, P., B. RADHARKRISHNAMURTHY, E. R. DALFERES, JR., AND G. S. BERENSON. The composition of connective tissue macromolecules from bovine respiratory system. *Respir. Physiol.* 24: 347-354, 1975.
251. SEGAL, H. L. Mechanism and regulation of protein turnover in animal cells. *Curr. Top. Cell. Regul.* 11: 183-210, 1976.
252. SENIOR, R. M., P. D. KAPLAN, C. KUHN, AND H. E. LINDER. Enzyme-induced emphysema. In: *Fundamental Problems of Cystic Fibrosis and Related Diseases*, edited by J. A. Mangos and R. C. Talamo. New York: Stratton, 1973, p. 183-194.
253. SEYER, J. M., E. T. HUTCHESON, AND A. H. KANG. Collagen polymorphism in idiopathic chronic pulmonary fibrosis. *J. Clin. Invest.* 57: 1498-1507, 1976.
254. SHAKESPEARE, V., AND J. H. BUCHANAN. Increased degradation rates of protein in aging human fibroblasts and in cells treated with an amino acid analog. *Exp. Cell Res.* 100: 1-8, 1976.
255. SHIN, H. S., R. SNYDERMAN, E. FRIEDMAN, A. MELLORS, AND M. M. MAYER. Chemotactic and anaphylatoxic fragment cleaved from the fifth component of guinea pig complement. *Science* 162: 361-363, 1968.
256. SIDRANSKY, H., D. S. SARMA, M. BONGIONO, AND E. VERNEY. Effect of dietary tryptophan on hepatic polysomes and protein synthesis in fasted mice. *J. Biol. Chem.* 243: 1123-1132, 1968.
257. SIMPSON, M. V. The release of labeled amino acids from the proteins of rat liver slices. *J. Biol. Chem.* 201: 143-154, 1953.
258. SINGH, H., AND G. KALNITSKY. Separation of a new α-N-benzoylarginine-β-naphthylamide hydrolase from cathepsin B_1. *J. Biol. Chem.* 253: 4319-4326, 1978.
259. SINGH, H., AND G. KALNITSKY. α-N-benzoylarginine-β-naphthylamide hydrolase, an aminoendopeptidase from rabbit lung. *J. Biol. Chem.* 255: 369-374, 1980.
260. SNIDER, G. L., J. A. HAYES, C. FRANZBLAU, H. M. KAGAVY, P. S. STONE, AND A. L. KORTHY. Relationship between elastolytic activity and experimental emphysema-inducing properties of papain preparations. *Am. Rev. Respir. Dis.* 110: 254-262, 1974.
261. SNYDERMAN, R., H. S. SHIN, AND A. M. DANNENBERG, JR. Macrophage proteinase and inflammation: the production of chemotactic activity from the fifth component of complement by macrophage proteinase. *J. Immunol.* 109: 896-898, 1972.
262. SOGAWA, K., AND K. TAKAHASHI. The structure and function of acid protease. VII. Distribution and some properties of acid protease in monkey tissues. *J. Biochem.* 81: 423-429, 1977.
263. SOGAWA, K., AND K. TAKAHASHI. Cathepsins D from rhesus monkey lung: purification and characterization. *J. Biochem.* 88: 619-633, 1980.
264. SPEAKE, B. K., R. DILS, AND R. J. MAYER. Regulation of enzyme turnover during tissue differentiation. Studies on the effects of hormones on the turnover of fatty acid synthetase in rabbit mammary gland in organ culture. *Biochem. J.* 148: 309-320, 1975.

265. STACHFIELD, J. E., AND J. D. YAGER. Insulin effects on protein synthesis and secretion in primary cultures of amphibian hepatocytes. *J. Cell. Physiol.* 100: 279-290, 1979.
266. STANLEY, N. N., R. ALPER, E. L. CUNNINGHAM, N. S. CHERNIAK, AND N. A. KEFALIDES. Effects of a molecular change in collagen on lung structure and mechanical function. *J. Clin. Invest.* 55: 1195-1201, 1975.
267. STARCHER, B. C., C. KUHN, AND J. E. OVERTON. Increased elastin and collagen content in the lungs of hamsters receiving an intratracheal injection of bleomycin. *Am. Rev. Respir. Dis.* 117: 299-305, 1978.
268. STEDMAN, R. L. The chemical composition of tobacco and tobacco smoke. *Chem. Rev.* 68: 153-207, 1968.
269. STEINBERG, D., AND M. VAUGHAN. Intracellular protein degradation in vitro. *Biochim. Biophys. Acta* 19: 584-585, 1956.
270. STEVENS, J. B., AND A. P. AUTOR. Induction of superoxide dismutase by oxygen in neonatal rat lung. *J. Biol. Chem.* 252: 3509-3514, 1974.
271. TAYLOR, J. C., AND J. P. CRAWFORD. Purification and preliminary characterization of human leukocyte elastase. *Arch. Biochem. Biophys.* 169: 91-101, 1975.
272. THET, L. A., M. D. DELANEY, C. A. GREGORIO, AND D. MASSARO. Protein metabolism by rat lung: influence of fasting, glucose, and insulin. *J. Appl. Physiol.: Respirat. Environ. Exercise Physiol.* 43: 463-467, 1977.
273. THRALL, R. S., J. R. MCCORMICK, R. M. JACK, R. A. MCREYNOLDS, AND P. A. WARD. Bleomycin-induced pulmonary fibrosis in the rat. Inhibition by indomethacin. *Am. J. Pathol.* 95: 117-127, 1979.
274. TONGE, B. L. Effect of tobacco smoke condensate on the aerial oxidation of cysteine. *Nature London* 194: 284-285, 1962.
275. TOURIAN, A., J. GODDARD, AND T. T. PUCK. Phenylalanine hydroxylase activity in mammalian cells. *J. Cell. Physiol.* 73: 159-170, 1969.
276. TURINO, G. M., R. V. LOURENÇO, AND G. H. MCCRACKEN. Role of connective tissues in large pulmonary airways. *J. Appl. Physiol.* 25: 645-653, 1968.
277. TWETO, J., AND D. DOYLE. Turnover of iodinated plasma membrane proteins of hepatoma tissue cultured cells. In: *Intracellular Protein Turnover*, edited by R. T. Schimke and N. Katunuma. New York: Academic, 1975, p. 295-308.
278. TWUMASI, D. Y., AND I. E. LIENER. Proteases from purulent sputum. Purification and properties of the elastase and chymotrypsin-like enzymes. *J. Biol. Chem.* 252: 1917-1926, 1977.
279. UDENFRIEND, S., AND J. R. COOPER. The enzymatic conversion of phenylalanine to tyrosine. *J. Biol. Chem.* 194: 503-511, 1952.
280. ULRICH, F. Effects of trypsin on protein synthesis in macrophages. *Exp. Cell Res.* 101: 267-277, 1976.
281. ULRICH, F. Washing macrophage suspensions inhibits protein synthesis. *Proc. Soc. Exp. Biol. Med.* 155: 13-18, 1977.
282. VAN VENROOIJ, W. J., H. MOONEN, AND L. VAN LOONKLAASEN. Source of amino acids used for protein synthesis in HeLa cells. *Eur. J. Biochem.* 50: 297-304, 1974.
283. VIDRICH, A., J. AIRHART, M. K. BRUNO, AND E. A. KHAIRALLAH. Compartmentation of free amino acids for protein biosynthesis. Influence of diurnal changes in hepatic amino acid concentrations on the composition of the precursor pool charging aminoacyltransfer ribonucleic acid. *Biochem. J.* 162: 257-266, 1977.
284. WALLNER, O., AND H. FRITZ. Characterization of an acid-stable proteinase inhibitor in human cervical mucus. *Hoppe-Seyler's Z. Physiol. Chem.* 355: 709-715, 1974.
285. WARBURTON, M. J., AND B. POOLE. Effect of medium composition on protein degradation and DNA synthesis in rat embryo fibroblasts. *Proc. Natl. Acad. Sci. USA* 74: 2427-2431, 1977.
286. WARD, P. A., AND L. J. NEWMAN. A neutrophil chemotactic factor from human C_5. *J. Immunol.* 102: 93-99, 1969.
287. WARD, W. F., AND G. E. MORTIMORE. Compartmentation of intracellular amino acids in rat liver. *J. Biol. Chem.* 253: 3581-3587, 1978.
288. WATERLOW, J. C., P. J. GARLICK, AND D. J. MILLWARD. *Protein Turnover in Mammalian Tissues and in the Whole Body.* Amsterdam: North-Holland, 1978.
289. WATKINS, C. A., AND D. E. RANNELS. Measurement of protein synthesis in rat lungs perfused in situ. *Biochem. J.* 188: 269-278, 1980.
290. WATKINS, S., M. G. CLARK, A. W. ROGERS, M. F. HOPGOOD, AND F. J. BALLARD. Degradation of extracellular protein by the isolated perfused rat liver. A biochemical and autoradiographic study. *Exp. Cell Res.* 119: 111-117, 1979.
291. WEBB, W. R., AND T. H. BURFORD. Studies on the reexpanded lung after prolonged atelectasis. *Arch. Surg. Chicago* 66: 801-809, 1953.
292. WEINBAUM, G., M. TAKAMOTO, B. SLOAN, AND P. KIMBEL. Lung antiproteinase: a potential defense against emphysema development. *Am. Rev. Respir. Dis.* 113: 245-248, 1976.
293. WEISS, C., AND M. L. BOYAR-MANSTEIN. On the mechanism of liquefaction of tubercles. I. The behavior of endocellular proteinases in tubercles developing in the lungs of rabbits. *Am. Rev. Tuberc.* 63: 694-705, 1961.
294. WERB, A., AND J. AGGELER. Proteases induce secretion of collagenase and plasminogen activator by fibroblasts. *Proc. Natl. Acad. Sci. USA* 75: 1839-1843, 1978.
295. WERB, Z., AND S. GORDAN. Elastase secretion by stimulated macrophages. Characterization and regulation. *J. Exp. Med.* 142: 361-377, 1975.
296. WESSELS, N. K., AND J. H. COHEN. Effects of collagenase on developing epithelia in vitro: lung, ureteric bud, and pancreas. *Dev. Biol.* 18: 294-309, 1968.
297. WILDE, C. J., N. PASKIN, J. SAXTON, AND R. J. MAYER. Protein degradation during terminal cytodifferentiation. *Biochem. J.* 192: 311-320, 1980.
298. WILLIAMS, I. H., P. H. SUGDEN, AND H. E. MORGAN. Use of aromatic amino acids as monitors of protein turnover. *Am. J. Physiol.* 240 (*Endocrinol. Metab.* 3): E677-E681, 1981.
298a. WOODSIDE, K. H. Inhibition of liver protein degradation by cycloheximide (Abstract). *Federation Proc.* 34: 651, 1975.
298b. WOODSIDE, K. H. Inhibition of hepatic protein degradation by inhibitors of macromolecular assembly (Abstract). *Federation Proc.* 35: 283, 1976.
299. WOODSIDE, K. H., AND D. MASSARO. Degradation of endogenous protein by rabbit pulmonary macrophages. *J. Appl. Physiol.: Respirat. Environ. Exercise Physiol.* 47: 79-86, 1979.
300. WOODSIDE, K. H., AND G. E. MORTIMORE. Suppression of protein turnover by amino acids in the perfused rat liver. *J. Biol. Chem.* 247: 6474-6481, 1972.
301. WOODSIDE, K. H., W. F. WARD, AND G. E. MORTIMORE. Effects of glucagon on general protein degradation and synthesis in perfused rat liver. *J. Biol. Chem.* 249: 5458-5463, 1974.
302. YAM, J., L. FRANK, AND R. J. ROBERTS. Oxygen toxicity: comparison of lung biochemical responses in neonatal and adult rats. *Pediatr. Res.* 12: 115-119, 1978.
303. YEAGER, H., JR. Alveolar cells: depressant effect of cigarette smoke on protein synthesis. *Proc. Soc. Exp. Biol. Med.* 131: 247-250, 1969.
304. YOSHIDA, A., G. STAMATOYANNOPOULOS, AND A. G. MOTULSKY. Negro variant of glucose-6-phosphate dehydrogenase deficiency (A-) in man. *Science* 155: 97-99, 1967.
305. YU, S. Y., N. R. KELLER, AND A. YOXHIDA. Biosynthesis of insoluble elastin in hamster lungs during elastase-emphysema. *Proc. Soc. Exp. Biol. Med.* 157: 369-373, 1978.
306. ZAK, R., A. F. MARTIN, AND R. BLOUGH. Assessment of protein turnover by use of radioisotopic tracers. *Physiol. Rev.* 59: 407-447, 1979.
307. ZIMMERBERG, J., O. GREENGARD, AND W. E. KNOX. Peptidyl proline hydroxylase in adult, developing, and neoplastic rat tissues. *Cancer Res.* 35: 1009-1014, 1975.
308. ZUCKERMAN, J. E., M. A. HOLLINGER, AND S. N. GIRI. Evaluation of antifibrotic drugs in bleomycin-induced pulmonary fibrosis in hamsters. *J. Pharmacol. Exp. Ther.* 213: 425-431, 1980.

CHAPTER 8

Lipid synthesis and surfactant turnover in the lungs

RICHARD J. KING | *Department of Physiology, University of Texas Health Science Center, San Antonio, Texas*

JOHN A. CLEMENTS | *Cardiovascular Research Institute, University of California, San Francisco, California*

CHAPTER CONTENTS

Lipid Composition of Lung Tissue
  Parenchyma
  Alveolar type II cells
  Pulmonary surfactant
    Extracellular surfactant lipids
    Lamellar bodies
    Apolipoproteins of surfactant
Metabolic Pathways of Lipids in Lung Tissue
  Phosphatidylcholine
  Phosphatidylglycerol
  Other lipids in surfactant
  Enzymes of lipid synthesis
    Choline kinase
    Cholinephosphate cytidylyltransferase
    Phosphatidic acid phosphohydrolase
    Cholinephosphotransferase
    Phosphatidylcholine remodeling enzymes
Regulation of Surfactant Metabolism
  Regulation of synthesis and storage of surfactant components
  Regulation of secretion of surfactant components
  Regulation of clearance of surfactant components
  Relationship between protein and lipid metabolism
Compartmental Analysis in Studies of Surfactant Turnover

LIKE OTHER ORGANS, the lungs must perform a variety of functions to maintain their own architecture and serve the organism as a whole. This chapter is concerned with lung functions associated with cellular lipids and secreted lipoprotein, especially pulmonary surface-active material. Lipids account for 10%–20% of the dry weight of lung tissue, and their metabolic turnover is brisk (see REGULATION OF SURFACTANT METABOLISM, p. 322). Thus the synthetic reactions required to offset lipid catabolism place a significant energy demand on lung cells and must be appropriately controlled. Maintenance of proper stoichiometric relationships among the lipid classes in cellular and subcellular membranes and within the secretory products also implies efficient coregulation of anabolic and degradative reactions. In the normal lung such regulation must operate effectively despite major changes in substrate availability, blood flow, ventilatory state of the lung, cell turnover, environmental influences, growth, age, and performance of other organ systems. Virtually nothing is now known about how such controls operate at the molecular level in lung cells. Consequently this chapter provides only a descriptive treatment of this subject.

The marked cellular heterogeneity of lung tissue introduces a further set of complications. Just as lipid composition varies substantially from tissue to tissue, important differences must also be expected among the lipids of the various pulmonary cells. Little information about such differences is currently available to guide our thinking, except by analogy with other cell systems. Conclusions based on studies of lipids in intact lung tissue must remain correspondingly ambiguous until methods are available that can determine the components of the various cells.

Despite these difficulties pulmonary lipids, lipoproteins, and their derivatives exhibit many interesting characteristics. This chapter emphasizes information on the role of lipids in maintaining lung architecture. Other important topics, e.g., transmethylation of phospholipids and phospholipase activation in stimulus-response coupling, prostaglandin and leukotriene metabolism, phospholipid turnover connected with transmembrane transport, and contributions of lipids to energy metabolism, are not discussed. Even so the material that should be covered is extensive and has occupied hundreds of investigators in recent decades; we can only consider illustrative results, however, and have selected material mainly pertaining to the surfactant system.

LIPID COMPOSITION OF LUNG TISSUE

Parenchyma

Several studies have analyzed the composition of the lung tissue lipids of several species (1, 3, 13, 37, 133, 151, 207). The primary emphasis of most of this work has been on the phospholipids, because they

TABLE 1. *Phospholipid Composition of Lung Tissue of Various Species*

	Percent of Total Phosphorus Recovered								
	Rat[a]	Rat[b]	Human[b]	Mouse[b]	Dog[c]	Rabbit[d]	Bovine[a]	Frog[a]	Turtle[e]
Phosphatidylcholine	54.3	44.9	47.5	43.7	48	54.1	39.5	42.6	55.5
Phosphatidylethanolamine	20.2	22.2	17.5	20.1	24	17.8	21.2	21.2	25.9
Phosphatidylserine	5.5	9.0	7.0	8.1	8	4.6	9.4	7.8	
Phosphatidylinositol		3.9	3.2	4.1	4	4.4	3.3	3.4	
Phosphatidylglycerol	3.9	2.2	2.5	2.4	3	3.2	2.0	1.8	
Lyso-bis-phosphatidic acid		0.3	1.5	0.3			0.5	0.3	
Diphosphatidylglycerol	3.9	1.1	1.0	1.1			1.0	0.9	
Phosphatidic acid		0.3	0.5	0.4			1.4	0.3	
Lysophosphatidylcholine		1.3	2.0	1.1			0.3	0.7	1.6
Lysophosphatidylethanolamine		0.5	0.6				0.2	0.2	
Sphingomyelin	12.6	10.0	11.1	9.3	7	13.7	16.1	10.8	17.0

[a] Data from Godinez et al. (70). [b] Data from Baxter et al. (13). [c] Data from Pfleger and Thomas (163). [d] Data from Rooney et al. (170). [e] Data from Clements et al. (37).

comprise 70%–80% of the total lipid pool. The results of this work are summarized in Table 1. Phosphatidylcholine is the predominant lipid, comprising ~50% of the phospholipids. Phosphatidylethanolamine makes up ~20% of the lipids, and three acidic phospholipids (phosphatidylserine, phosphatidylinositol, and phosphatidylglycerol) constitute 12%–15% of the total. The differences in composition of these classes of phospholipids among vertebrate species are relatively minor, even when the analyses are extended to the lungs of some amphibians (13, 37). This is not true, however, when examining the distribution of phosphatidylcholines between fully saturated and unsaturated molecules (Tables 2 and 3). The lungs of turtles and frogs contain less fully saturated phosphatidylcholine than do mammalian lungs (37), marking a breaking point in the phylogenetic trend. Saturated phosphatidylcholines occur in relatively high concentrations in mammalian lung tissue and in even greater amounts in purified surfactant. Saturated and monoenoic phosphatidylcholines comprise ~32% and ~27% of the phosphatidylcholines of rat lung, respectively, or ~60% of the total phosphatidylcholine pool. The remaining 40% are species with fatty acids of greater unsaturation. Surfactant phosphatidylcholine consists almost entirely of saturated and monoenoic phosphatidylcholines (47, 111). Not all of the saturated phosphatidylcholine found in lung tissue is associated with surfactant, however; recent studies indicate that multiple metabolic pools of dipalmitoyl phosphatidylcholine exist in mammalian lung, not all of which are secreted to the alveolar surface as part of the surfactant complex. Best estimates (26, 218) suggest that only 30%–40% of the saturated phosphatidylcholine pool in mammalian lung tissue is associated with intracellular or extracellular stores of surfactant.

The molecular species of the phosphatidylethanolamines and the diacylglycerols are shown in Table 4. The phosphatidylethanolamines are highly unsaturated, and >63% contain six double bonds each. No appreciable amounts of saturated phosphatidylethanolamines are found in lung tissue. These compositional data suggest that the phosphatidylcholines and phosphatidylethanolamines do not derive from a common diglyceride pool through their reaction with either cytidine 5′-diphosphocholine (CDPcholine) or CDPethanolamine, respectively (103). Likewise, according to these data it is unlikely that the stepwise methylation of phosphatidylethanolamine (23) forms appreciable amounts of phosphatidylcholine, unless the resulting phosphatidylcholine undergoes extensive fatty acid remodeling by acyltransferase reactions (207).

TABLE 2. *Percent Distribution of Saturated and Unsaturated Phosphatidylcholines in Lung Tissue of Various Species*

	Percent of Total Phosphatidylcholines	
	Saturated	Unsaturated
Rat*	32	68
Rat†	33.5	66.5
Rat	32.6	67.4
Mouse	38.4	61.6
Guinea pig	41.5	58.5
Rabbit	35.1	64.9
Sea lion	57.5	42.5
Chicken	41.8	58.2
Dog	34.4	65.6
Human	54.9	45.1
Bovine	19.8	80.2
Turtle	6.3	93.7
Frog	6.6	93.4

All data from Clements et al. (37) unless other refs. noted.
* Data from Van Golde (207).   † Data from Akino and Abe (3).

Alveolar Type II Cells

Convincing evidence now exists that the synthesis of lipids of pulmonary surfactant (and probably other components as well) occurs in the alveolar epithelial type II cell (122). The details of the subcellular organization associated with this activity are only presently being clarified, but it seems reasonably certain that the lamellar inclusion body, an intracellular organelle of the type II cell (Fig. 1), contains the pulmonary surfactant lipids arranged in densely packed lamellar leaflets. Investigators have therefore predicted that the composition of lipids in type II cells should more closely approximate that of surfactant than would the composition of whole lung. This appears to be the case. Type II cells are now routinely recovered in purities of 80%–90% with yields adequate for compositional studies (106, 136). The results of studies on rat cells (73) and rabbit cells (190) are given in Table 5. Compared with whole lung tissue, type II cells are richer in phosphatidylcholine and phosphatidylglycerol and poorer in phosphatidylethanolamine. Over 40% of the total phosphatidylcholine in rat type II cells is saturated, a distribution containing more of this lipid than that of the phosphatidylcholines of whole lung tissue. Rabbit cells have a lower saturated phosphatidylcholine content, reflecting either a genuine species difference or heterogeneity of the respective cellular preparation. The relatively high concentrations of both saturated phosphatidylcholine and saturated phosphatidylglycerol in rat type II cells are consistent with the cell's purported function as the metabolic source of pulmonary surfactant. A significant proportion of the total saturated phosphatidylcholine in whole lung is contained in other lung cells, however, because the amount of saturated phosphatidylcholine in type II cells represents only 30% of the total in lung tissue (26). The identification of these other cells with significant amounts of saturated phosphatidylcholine, and how they use it, is generally unknown. Alveolar macrophages contain saturated phosphatidylcholines and even synthesize small amounts of them (135), but other intracellular sources probably also exist.

TABLE 3. *Percent Distribution of Molecular Species of Phosphatidylcholines in Rat Lung Tissue*

	Van Golde (207)	Akino and Abe (3)
Saturated		
16:0/14:0*		6.7
16:0/16:0	28	25.1
16:0/18:0 and 18:0/16:0	4	1.7
Monoenoic		
14:0/16:1		0.5
16:0/16:1	7	11.7
16:0/18:1 and 18:1/16:0	19	9.5
18:0/18:1	1	1.4
Dienoic		
16:0/18:2 and 18:2/16:0	17	10.4
18:0/18:2	3	2.4
16:1/16:1		1.0
18:1/18:1		1.9
Trienoic	4	
16:1/18:2		0.9
18:1/18:2		2.0
18:0/20:3		1.3
Tetraenoic		
16:0/20:4	6	6.9
18:0/20:4	3	4.3
Polyenoic	4	
16:0/20:5		2.2
16:0/22:6		4.7
18:0/22:6		1.3

* Chain length and number of ethylenic bonds.

TABLE 4. *Percent Distribution of Molecular Species of Phospholipids in Rat Lung Tissue*

	Phosphatidylcholine,* %	Diacylglycerol,* %	Phosphatidylglycerol,* %	Phosphatidylethanolamine,† %
Saturated				
16:0/14:0	6.7	5.1	3.0	
16:0/16:0	25.1	17.3	18.5	
16:0/18:0	1.7	1.8	0.7	
Total	33.5	24.2	22.2	0
Monoenoic				
14:0/16:1	0.5	0.5	0.2	
16:0/16:1	11.7	6.7	9.6	
16:0/18:1	9.5	11.0	17.6	
18:0/18:1	1.4	1.1	1.1	
Total	23.1	19.3	28.5	9
Dienoic				
16:1/16:1	1.0	0.7	0.7	
16:0/18:2	10.4	11.5	17.5	
18:1/18:1	1.9	1.5	1.6	
18:0/18:2	2.4	2.2	1.4	
Total	15.7	15.9	21.2	13
Trienoic				
16:1/18:2	0.9	1.6	2.7	
18:1/18:2	2.0	6.3	4.8	
18:0/20:3	1.3	0.9		
Total	4.2	8.8	7.5	0
Tetraenoic				
16:0/20:4	6.9	5.5	8.0	
18:0/20:4	4.3	15.8	3.1	
Total	11.2	21.3	11.1	15
Polyenoic				
16:0/20:5	2.2	1.0	2.5	
16:0/22:6	4.7	6.1	6.5	
18:0/22:6	1.3	0.4	0.2	
Total	8.2	7.5	9.2	63

* Data from Akino and Abe (3). † Data from Abe and Akino (1).

Pulmonary Surfactant

Two major pools of pulmonary surfactant exist: *1)* an extracellular pool associated with the material adsorbed at the alveolar air-liquid interface or in the alveolar subphase fluid, and *2)* an intracellular pool in type II cells, concentrated in lamellar inclusion bodies. Most studies have used extracellular surfactant, because it is easier to isolate and identify than the intracellular surfactant. Several reports on purifying the lamellar bodies have appeared recently, and a description of their chemical and physical properties is being developed.

EXTRACELLULAR SURFACTANT LIPIDS. Several methods have been developed to isolate surfactant from the alveolar lumen, thereby increasing this procedure's

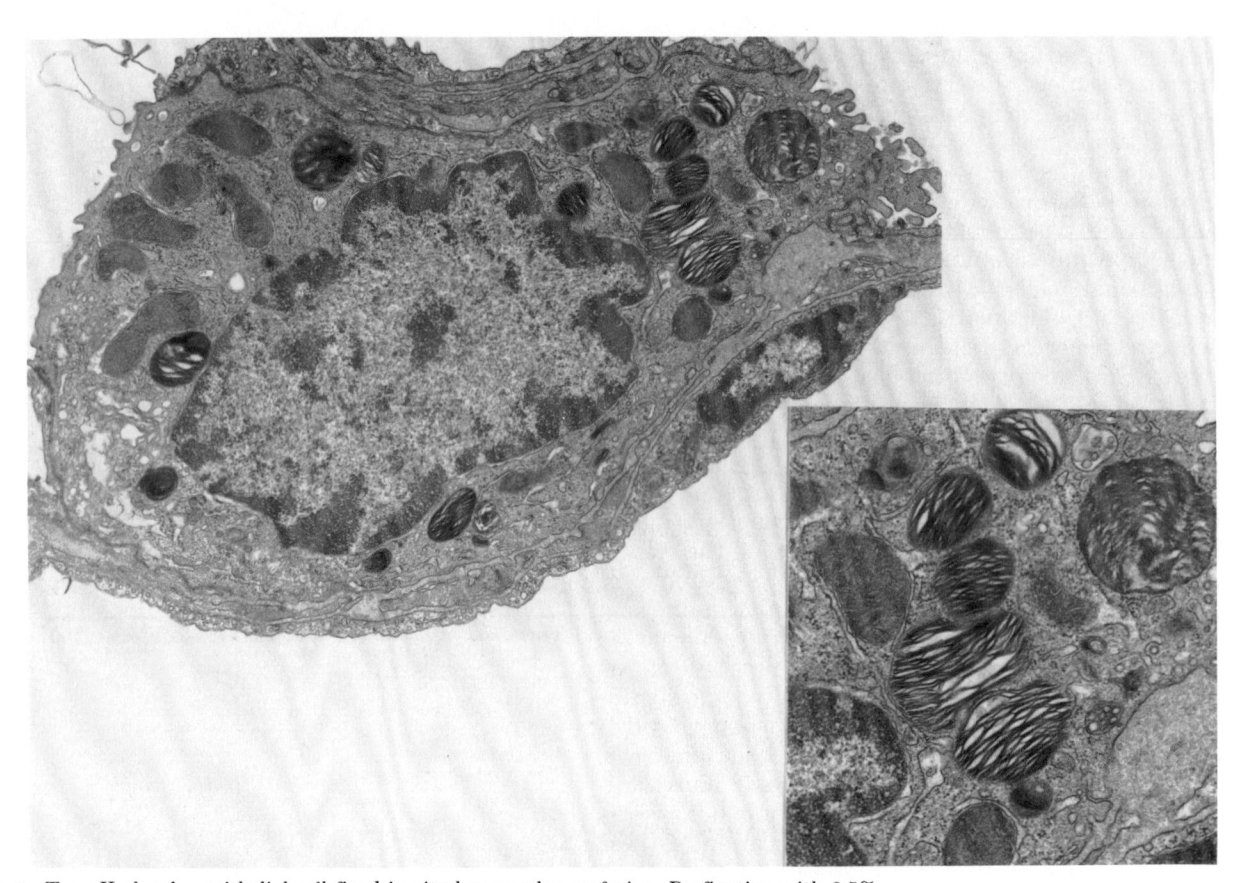

FIG. 1. Type II alveolar epithelial cell fixed in situ by vascular perfusion. Prefixation with 2.5% glutaraldehyde in 0.2 M sodium cacadylate, pH 7.4, followed by postfixation with 1% osmium tetroxide. × 14,250. *Inset*: cytoplasmic region containing several lamellar bodies. × 26,400.

TABLE 5. *Phospholipid Composition of Alveolar Epithelial Type II Cells*

	Phosphorus, %	
	Rat[a,b]	Rabbit[c]
Phosphatidylcholine	71.8	63.3
Saturated	39.6[d]	16.1[e]
Unsaturated	32.2[d]	47.2[e]
Phosphatidylethanolamine	12.6	16.9
Phosphatidylserine	0.3	
Phosphatidylinositol	0.5	
Phosphatidylglycerol	10.3	4.2
Saturated	4.4[d]	0.9[e]
Unsaturated	5.9[d]	3.3[e]

[a] Data from Greenleaf et al. (73). [b] Data from Mason and Dobbs (134). [c] Data from Smith and Kikkawa (190). [d] Values estimated from distribution of radioactive glycerol. [e] Values estimated from fatty acid composition (minimum amount of saturated species possible).

reliability since it was first attempted 18 years ago (2). Pulmonary surfactant is a complex material composed of lipids, proteins, and carbohydrates that forms lamellar bilayers in an aqueous environment. The physical and chemical properties of the complex may be affected by the solvents used to disperse the material, and its size distribution is markedly heterogeneous. These properties severely limit the techniques that may be applied to isolate this substance. Consequently electrophoresis and gel filtration are not useful preparative procedures. Density-gradient centrifugation is a satisfactory method used extensively to segregate this material from other constituents in lung lavage fluid. Figure 2 outlines a procedure resulting in a product with reproducible composition that does not change after further centrifugation (110). Other procedures, some of which require less time, have also been reported (39, 56, 60, 64, 69, 120, 163, 178, 186).

The lipid composition of pulmonary surfactants isolated from dog, rat, and rabbit lavage fluids is shown in Table 6. Dipalmitoyl phosphatidylcholine is the predominant lipid, constituting ~50% (all percents by weight) of the total lipid content in rat and dog surfactants. Unsaturated phosphatidylcholines, most of which are of the *cis*-monoenoic type, comprise 10%–56% of the lipid content, depending on species. Thus 70%–80% of the material is made up of phosphatidylcholines. The next most abundant phospholipid is phosphatidylglycerol, comprising 3%–11% of the lipid content. Cholesterol is found in 2%–10% (69, 111), with the larger amount occurring in canine surfactant (not shown in Table 6). Because of cholesterol's lower molecular weight it constitutes nearly 20 mol % of this surfactant.

Numerous physiological and physicochemical stud-

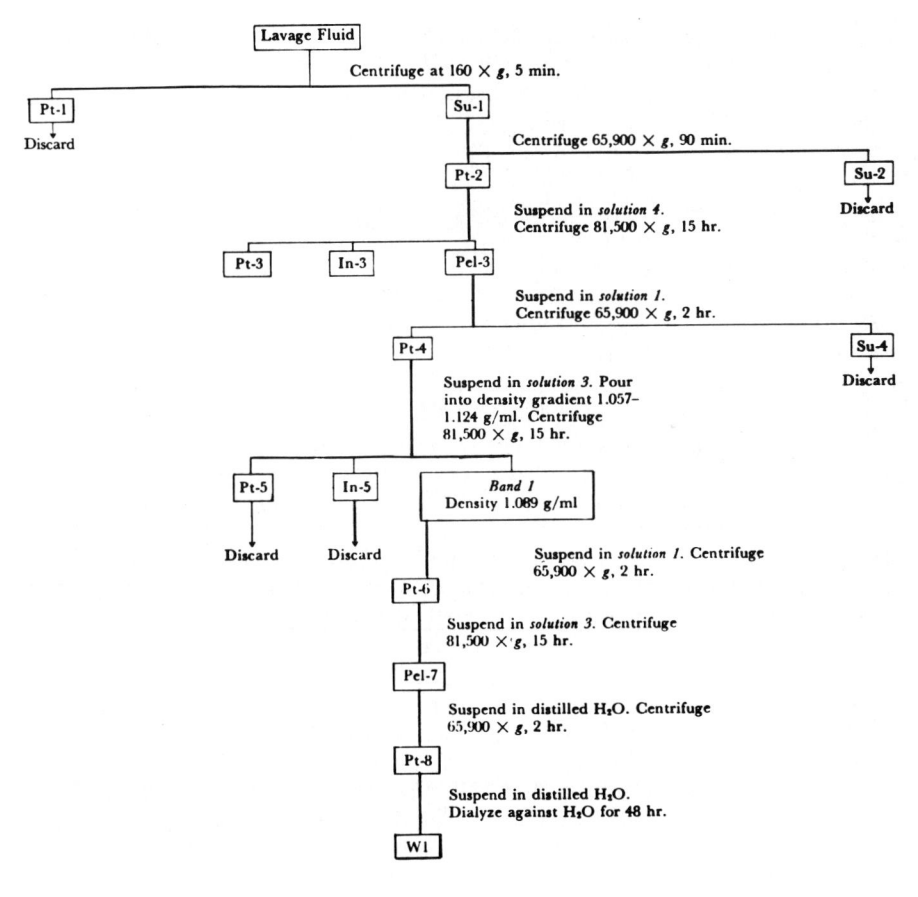

FIG. 2. Schema for isolation of pulmonary surfactant from alveolar lavage fluid. Extracellular fluid is recovered from lung by gently instilling 0.1 M NaCl containing 3 mM Ca^{2+} and Mg^{2+} buffered to pH 7.4 into tracheobronchial tree. [From King and Clements (110).]

TABLE 6. *Phospholipid Composition in Pulmonary Surfactants Purified From Lavage Fluids of Various Species*

	Rat[a]	Rat[b]	Dog[c]	Dog[d]	Rabbit[e]
Phosphatidylcholine	68.8	75.5	74	87	86.2
Saturated	59.0[f]		33[f]	55	30.2[f]
Unsaturated	9.8[f]		41[f]	32	56.0[f]
Phosphatidylserine	6.1	1.9	2	1	3.4
Phosphatidylinositol		3.0	3		
Phosphatidylglycerol	6.7	11.0	10	3	6.2
Saturated	6.1[f]		4.4[f]		0[f]
Unsaturated	0.6[f]		5.6[f]		6.2[f]
Phosphatidylethanolamine	9.8	4.6	4	6	3.0
Sphingomyelin	5.0	1.5	5	2	1.7
Lysophosphatidylcholine		0.2		1	
Phosphatidic acid		0.5			
Diphosphatidylglycerol		0.1			
Other	3.6	1.7	1.3		1.2

[a] Data from Engle et al. (47). [b] Data from Hallman and Gluck (78). [c] Data from Pfleger and Thomas (163). [d] Data from King et al. (113). [e] Data from Rooney et al. (173). [f] Values estimated from fatty acid composition (minimum amount of saturated species possible).

ies have indicated that alveolar surfactant is required to maintain alveolar stability and to prevent atelectasis [see the chapter by Goerke and Clements (70a) in the volume on the mechanics of breathing in this *Handbook* section on the respiratory system]. Both experimental and theoretical considerations have shown that pulmonary surfactant must be able to lower alveolar surface tension to <10 dyn/cm (35). Dipalmitoyl phosphatidylcholine has the physicochemical properties needed to do this (24). Pulmonary surfactant, however, must do more. It must also rapidly lower surface tension to <10 dyn/cm, adsorbing from the alveolar subphase fluid into the alveolar interface, spreading in the interface as a monomolecular lipid film, and then forming a transiently stable interfacial film. At low surface tensions it has a low surface compressibility (35, 111), which is defined as the rate of change of the logarithm of surface area with respect to surface tension (43). A film with low surface compressibility demonstrates a large change in surface tension with small changes in molecular surface area. Structure-function studies (33, 35, 86, 111) show that the mixture of lipids and proteins in surfactant, rather than any single component, provides these properties. Dipalmitoyl phosphatidylcholine lowers surface tension to <10 dyn/cm, provides film stability, and has a very low film compressibility. The unsaturated phosphatidylcholines, and perhaps the proteins (114, 115), provide appropriate physicochemical properties for rapid adsorption and spreading. Phosphatidylglycerol's function is uncertain, but lipid-protein recombination experiments suggest it may be required to facilitate maximal interaction between the lipid and protein (115). The stoichiometry of the lipid components may change as the material enters the alveolar interface and undergoes several respiratory cycles. Unsaturated lipids, present in relatively high concentrations in surfactant as it adsorbs to the surface, are apparently "squeezed" from the surface during breathing, leaving a surface film enriched in dipalmitoyl phosphatidylcholine (86). This interfacial film is considerably more stable than that obtained by the complete mixture of lipids found in surfactant and has a tendency to collapse that is similar to that of the alveoli, as determined from pressure-volume experiments (33). For more information on these processes see the chapter by Goerke and Clements (70a) in the volume on the mechanics of breathing in this *Handbook* section on the respiratory system.

LAMELLAR BODIES. Lamellar bodies have been purified from a homogenate of lung tissue in continuous or discontinuous density gradients (46, 69, 82, 91, 160). Lamellar bodies from rat lung had an isopycnic density of ~1.06 g/ml and were isolated in sucrose gradients containing 0.45 M and 0.58 M sucrose (82). The osmotic effects of these concentrations of sucrose apparently did not have a detrimental effect on the membrane integrity of the lamellar bodies, because electron microscopy indicated well-preserved organelle structure. The homogenization of the tissue, however, may be a critical step. Lung tissue is difficult to disrupt because it contains a large amount of connective tissue, and vigorous homogenization may greatly damage the limiting membranes of the lamellar bodies.

The morphology of lamellar bodies, shown in Figure 1, has been described extensively elsewhere (189, 197, 211, 212). Lamellar bodies are spherical subcellular organelles about the size of a mitochondrion and bound by a trilaminar limiting membrane of the usual thickness. The body is densely packed with a lamellar material that has a repeat distance of ~60–80 Å and that apparently contains phospholipid bilayers of surfactant. In some sections a "core" can be observed; in other sections this core may contain a small number of vesicles ~0.1 μm in diameter. Freeze-fracture experiments differ on whether the lamellar membranes are particulate (189) or smooth (211), indicating the presence or absence, respectively, of protein embedded in the bilayers. During secretion the limiting membrane of the lamellar body and the outer membrane of the type II cell fuse and a lamellar material extrudes into the alveolar space. The lamellae interact in this process of exocytosis, forming an unusual material with long-range order (Fig. 3). This material is called tubular myelin and is found only in alveoli. Freeze-fracture electron microscopy shows that the lamellar bilayers of tubular myelin are particulate (189, 211), suggesting that protein is integrated within the bilayers. Tubular myelin contains an apolipoprotein of surfactant that is probably specific for this substance (212). Because of technical problems, it has not been determined whether this protein is also present in lamellar bodies (212). This protein is found in type II cells and alveolar macrophages, however, and only in the subcellular sites associated with protein synthesis in the type II cells. Thus the question of where the protein and lipid components of surfactant are integrated remains unanswered.

The composition of lipids isolated from the lamellar bodies closely resembles that of extracellular surfactant purified from alveolar material, supporting the concept that these bodies transport surfactant from intracellular depots to the alveolar lumen. Representative results are presented in Table 7. Lamellar body lipid is rich in phosphatidylcholine and contains a substantial amount of phosphatidylglycerol. The fatty acid distribution of phosphatidylcholines in the lamellar bodies and alveolar surfactant is very similar, and most investigations indicate that the phosphatidylcholine in both depots is composed of >50% fully saturated species. There is less uniformity in the results reported for phosphatidylglycerol. Engle et al. (47) reported that the phosphatidylglycerol fraction in lamellar bodies had a higher percentage of esterified stearic acid than did that in alveolar lavage fluid, but both were highly enriched in fully saturated constituents. Hallman and Gluck (78) found that only ~60% of the fatty acid residues in the phosphatidylglycerol fraction were saturated. Rooney et al. (170, 173) showed that the phosphatidylglycerols in both lamellar bodies and lavage fluid principally contained unsaturated components. Esterified palmitic acid made up 7% and 27% of the fatty acid composition of lamellar body and lavage phosphatidylglycerol, respectively. These results may partially reflect species differences, as Engle et al. (47) and Hallman and Gluck (78) analyzed lamellar bodies isolated from rat lung, whereas Rooney et al. (173) used rabbit lung, and phosphatidylglycerol content varies widely among species. It is present in lung tissue derived from bullfrog (79), rat (78, 79, 134, 170, 173), adult rabbit (170, 173), newborn rabbit 1 h after parturition (79), adult monkey (170), adult human (170), seal (78), and healthy newborn human (79). It is absent in surfactant

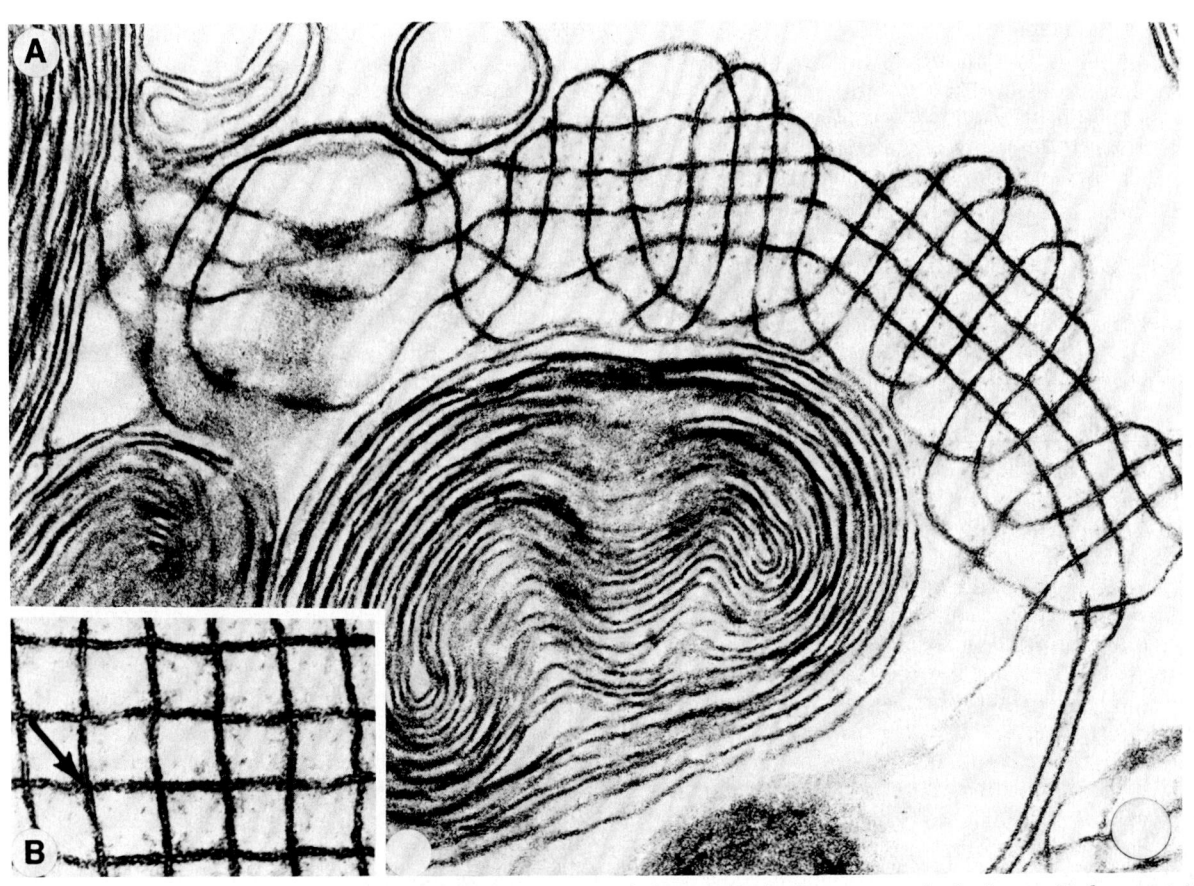

FIG. 3. *A*: formation of tubular myelin lattice structure in fetal rats, 21 days gestational age. Particles are seen on membrane layers extending into regular lattice. × 81,000. *B*: small particles (*arrow*) present within many corners of lattice; however, structures connecting them to membranes are not resolved. × 138,000. [From Williams (210).]

TABLE 7. *Phospholipid Composition of Lamellar Bodies*

	Rat*	Rat†	Rabbit‡
Phosphatidylcholine	75.0	77.0	73.0
Saturated§	65.8		25.3
Unsaturated§	9.2		47.7
Phosphatidylserine }	2.9	1.2	7.7
Phosphatidylinositol }		3.2	
Phosphatidylglycerol	11.7	11.2	8.1
Saturated§	10.1	2.1	0.0
Unsaturated§	1.6	9.1	8.1
Phosphatidylethanolamine	6.1	4.2	6.8
Sphingomyelin	0.7	0.7	
Diphosphatidylglycerol			0.3
Phosphatidic acid			0.3
Lysophosphatidylcholine			0.4
Other	3.5	1.5	4.5

* Data from Engle et al. (47). † Data from Hallman and Gluck (78). ‡ Data from Rooney et al. (173). § Values estimated from fatty acid composition (minimum amount of saturated species possible).

from chicken (79), newborn human with respiratory distress (79), or fetal rabbit 30 days of gestational age (79). Thus it is reasonable to think that its fatty acid composition among different species may also vary.

The different results of Engle et al. (47) and Hallman and Gluck (78), however, probably represent experimental variation, as both used rats in their studies. These researchers (47, 78, 170, 173) reported <10% mitochondrial contamination of their preparations, as judged by enzyme markers, the only means available to judge purity. We expect the fatty acid composition of the phospholipids in lamellar bodies and alveolar surfactant to be very similar, and all reports support this expectation. More work needs to be done before definitive conclusions can be made on the content and composition of the phosphatidylglycerol in lamellar bodies, however.

The physiological role of surfactant phosphatidylglycerol is still hypothetical. The species and/or experimental variations observed in content and composition (if that is what actually is being observed) suggest its role may be secondary to the function of other constituents of surfactant or that other components may substitute for it in the expression of surface activity.

APOLIPOPROTEINS OF SURFACTANT. *Composition.* Pulmonary surfactant contains 8%–10% protein

(110). Researchers disagree on the composition and importance of the protein content and are concerned that it may actually be an artifact of preparation (36, 107). The method used to isolate a surfactant fraction can alter its protein composition. Rigorous methods involving multiple centrifugations of surfactant can isolate a surface-active fraction whose protein composition is relatively simple (107). Such procedures may conceivably also be capable of dissociating lipid and protein complexes, resulting in the loss of some of the constituents present in the original material. Less rigorous methods may be able to separate a surface-active fraction but be unable to segregate serum and other proteins that interact nonspecifically with surfactant lipids, particularly when some pathological process leads to a transudation of intravascular and interstitial fluids into the alveolar spaces. The fundamental problem is that surfactant can be recognized only by its physicochemical properties. These are, for the most part, determined by the constituent lipids. Many investigators must therefore accept the proteins tagging along with the lipids of a surfactant fraction that has the appropriate physicochemical properties and then attempt to describe their composition, metabolism, and physical properties. They might then use these results to predict whether the proteins are specific to surfactant or whether they are contaminants from other sources. This indirect approach is time consuming, and progress has been slow compared with that of workers investigating the lipid moiety.

The protein composition of the "most purified" (i.e., containing fewest proteins) preparations of dog lung pulmonary surfactant consisted of three major proteins ($M_r \sim 70,000$, $\sim 35,000$, and $\sim 10,000$) that migrated in polyacrylamide gel electrophoresis under reducing conditions. Immunological methods showed that the 70,000-M_r band was partly albumin. Similarly sensitive methods showed that the other two proteins were not found in serum. Therefore most of the work focused on these peptides.

The lower-molecular-weight peptide was isolated from surfactant by precipitation from alcohol solutions and was purified by gel filtration chromatography (113). This protein had a high percentage of hydrophobic amino acid residues and only dissolved in aqueous solutions containing detergent. The low-molecular-weight protein migrated in electrophoresis as a low-molecular-weight peptide and generally appeared in this system as one band. However, the resolution in polyacrylamide gel electrophoresis is not good for small proteins, and it may be heterogeneous, composed of several small ($M_r < 10,000$) peptides. The 35,000-M_r protein was less hydrophobic (198), dissolved in buffers as an isotropic solution (114), and represented the principal nonserum antigen in surfactant purified by extensive centrifugation (107). The 10,000-M_r protein cross-reacted weakly with the 35,000-M_r protein in immunoprecipitation tests when it was reacted against antiserum to whole surfactant (107). Thus the two proteins might possibly share antigenic determinants. In recent publications we named the larger protein apolipoprotein A and the smaller, apolipoprotein B (names we retain in this review). This terminology is new, however, and may not be unique. Other investigators, possibly studying these same proteins, use other terms.

Because apolipoprotein A is a principal nonserum antigen in pulmonary surfactant, major emphasis has been given to its study. Information has been compiled on its specificity to surfactant (36), its presence in different species (107), its interaction with lipids (114), and its metabolic turnover (116, 118). Sueishi and Benson (198) purified this protein to near homogeneity and described some of its chemical properties. In addition, King (107), Gikas et al. (68), and Sueishi and Benson (198) have developed quantitative immunoassays to help identify it.

The results of all studies on apolipoprotein A indicate that it is uniquely associated with pulmonary surfactant (36). Apolipoprotein A was found with surfactant lipids even after repeated attempts at purification with methods designed to remove soluble protein. It was not found in serum or in membrane preparations of lung parenchyma or trachea. It could not come from contaminating bacteria because it was found in surfactant from nonbreathing fetuses delivered by cesarean section. It was concentrated by >50-fold in purified surfactant compared with its content in whole lung tissue. It was found in human (119) and ovine (68) tracheal and amniotic fluids at times in their gestational development when surfactant lipids are synthesized and secreted, and it was precociously stimulated in fetal development by synthetic corticosteroids. It is probably also present in the lamellar bodies (R. J. King and H. Martin, unpublished observations). Immunohistochemistry (212) and quantitative immunoassay (108) localized it in two cell types within the lung (alveolar epithelial type II cell and alveolar macrophage), in extracellular sites bordering the airway, and in the alveolar subphase fluid. Within type II cells the antigen was found in the subcellular organelles associated with synthetic activities; in alveolar macrophages it was found in the secondary lysosomes (212). Recent work showed that apolipoprotein A was secreted into the alveoli of both rats and dogs with nearly the same time course as that found for the major lipids of surfactant (112, 116). It readily interacted with the lipids of surfactant and altered their physicochemical properties (114). Thus this protein is found at the right times and in the right places to be a component with a central role in surfactant function. Unfortunately it is this last crucial aspect of the evidence for specificity that is still uncertain. The physiological function and importance of apolipoprotein A remains open to speculation.

Proteins with molecular weights similar to that of apolipoprotein A from canine surfactant have now been observed in surfactants isolated from rat (108, 198), sheep (68, 112), human (102, 119) and monkey (102). In addition, immunological cross-reaction has been observed between some of these species in double-diffusion precipitation reactions (107). Thus apolipoprotein A may be widely distributed among surfactants of differing species, reinforcing other circumstantial evidence suggesting specificity. Presumably a specific protein would have a unique physiological function. Considering the physiological functions attributed to other apolipoproteins we would predict that surfactant apolipoprotein might be involved in either the enzymatic regulation of some biological activity (the organization of the lipid moiety and modulation of the physicochemical properties of the complex) or the control of the turnover of the protein-lipid complex. Nothing points to this protein having any enzymatic properties, but no wide-ranging survey has been reported. We know something of the effects of apolipoprotein A on the physicochemical properties of the lipid complex and on its metabolism compared with that of surfactant lipids.

Bhattacharyya, Lynn, and co-workers (17–19, 131) published extensively on certain proteins that they found in type II cells and the alveolar lavage fluid. They called the principal protein ($M_r \sim 250,000$) alveolyn (131). A high concentration of this protein was found in the lavage returns from patients with alveolar proteinosis (17). Antiserum against this protein cross-reacted with smaller peptides with molecular weights of 80,000, 62,000, and 36,000 (18, 19). These proteins were found in the lamellar bodies of two different species (18, 19) and in extracellular surfactant (18). Other proteins with molecular weights of 130,000, 80,000, and 26,000 were also found in the lavage fluid from normal humans and animals, but only in small quantities. In contrast, a high concentration of the 80,000-M_r protein was found in the soluble fraction of lavage fluid from patients with alveolar proteinosis (17). The authors suggest that all of these proteins were fragments of the parent 250,000-M_r protein with the smaller peptides caused by protease(s) in the lamellar bodies and alveolar fluid (131). Their function, however, is not known. The 36,000-M_r protein bound phosphatidylcholine, but the 62,000-M_r protein did not (131). Although they were found in cells and subcellular compartments associated with pulmonary surfactant, the authors did not suggest any association between these proteins and surfactant. The intriguing and still unexplained observations of Lynn and colleagues (131) provide an additional impetus to uncover this protein's physiological function. Its unusual amino acid composition, containing collagenlike sequences (Gly-Pro-OHPro) with high concentrations of hydrophobic amino acids could suggest a special function.

Lipid-protein interactions. Apolipoprotein A has been copurified with its lipids under relatively rigorous centrifugation and is probably found exclusively with surfactant (111). Consistency dictates then that this protein should have unique qualities allowing it to interact with surfactant lipids. To date our own results suggest this is true. We examined the ability of apolipoprotein A to interact with multilamellar, highly aggregated dispersions of pure dipalmitoyl phosphatidylcholine at room temperature (114) and with vesicles prepared from mixtures of lipids approximating the lipid composition of those found in natural surfactant (115). We found that apolipoprotein A interacted with the lipids of surfactant at both 25°C and 37°C. Contrary to the behavior of most other proteins, apolipoprotein A could bind lamellar phospholipids that were in a gel-crystalline array, i.e., lipids in which the movement of the fatty acyl moiety was considerably restricted. Thus apolipoprotein A bound pure dipalmitoyl phosphatidylcholine at both 25°C (114) and 37°C (115); both temperatures were below the phase transition temperature of the phospholipid (30). However, maximum lipid binding did not occur unless both phosphatidylglycerol and Ca^{2+} were present (115). Monoenoic phosphatidylcholine, mixed with the saturated phosphatidylcholine and phosphatidylglycerol at 20 mol %, induced domains in the lipid bilayer with a more liquid character than that of pure saturated phospholipids. Lipids containing monoenoic phosphatidylcholine interacted with apolipoprotein A, but the amount of bound lipid per mole of protein was less than that achieved with gel-crystalline lipids (115). Pure dioleoyl (18:1) phosphatidylcholine was not bound by apolipoprotein at 37°C (unpublished observations). These results may reflect the physicochemical demands placed on a protein interacting with the special lipids of surfactant. The physiological function of surfactant requires that its composition include a large amount of dipalmitoyl phosphatidylcholine, a gel-crystalline lipid at physiological temperature. Most other biological materials are composed of lipids rich in unsaturated phospholipid and are liquid-crystalline at physiological temperatures. These systems require a fluid physical state for optimal function. Thus this apolipoprotein's unusual binding properties may reflect its association with a substance having an uncommon complement of lipids highly enriched in fully saturated phosphatidylcholines. None of the molecular details of this lipid-protein interaction are known, however.

Do the physical properties of the lipid complex change after its interaction with apolipoprotein A? Early experiments with purified surfactant (111) suggested that they might. Adsorption experiments showed that surfactant (containing protein) in dilute suspension in an aqueous subphase reached the interface, spread there, and lowered the interfacial tension at rates compatible with those required to support lung ventilation. The lipids of this same material (extracted with chloroform-methanol) were dried, then resuspended in the aqueous subphase at the same concentration, and had a delay of 3–5 min in their adsorption to the interface. The adsorption of pure dipalmitoyl phosphatidylcholine was extremely slow. Thus both the protein and unsaturated lipids in surfactant appeared to have a demonstrable effect on the ability of the saturated components to reach the interface. These results should be interpreted cautiously though. Surfactant concentrations in the alveolar subphase must be much greater than the experimental level. In addition the form and physical properties of the lipid suspension depend on the dispersal technique used and sometimes on their concentration. The recent results of Metcalfe et al. (142) show no differences in the surface properties of protein-containing and protein-free surfactants evaluated by an oscillating bubble technique.

Recent in vitro studies (114) showed that the physical properties of a lipid complex could be modified after interaction with apolipoprotein A. Pure dipalmitoyl phosphatidylcholine at 25°C adsorbed to an air-liquid interface very slowly. After its interaction with apolipoprotein A, however, its rate of adsorption was markedly increased. Dipalmitoyl phosphatidylcholine has a change in properties at 41°C–42°C associated with its transition from gel to liquid state. When apolipoprotein and this lipid interacted at a lipid-to-protein molar ratio of <1,000:1, this abrupt transition disappeared. Thus the apolipoprotein may be a perturbant to the lipid's lamellar structure, producing altered domains around the disturbing sites and thereby accelerating the adsorption rate.

METABOLIC PATHWAYS OF LIPIDS IN LUNG TISSUE

Phosphatidylcholine

Phosphatidylcholine is ubiquitous in tissues and is the principal lipid of most membranes and circulating lipoproteins. The compound is amphipathic, consisting of a charged and highly polar backbone of glycerol phosphorylcholine, and a much less polar portion composed of long-chain acyl groups 12–24 carbons long. The charged polar portion is neutral at physiological pH, with equal numbers of positive and negative charges provided by the strongly ionized choline and phosphate groups. Because the compound is amphipathic it can lower surface tension when it orients itself at an air-liquid interface with its polar backbone immersed in the aqueous subphase and its hydrocarbon chains extended toward the air. As monomers in aqueous solutions these compounds are virtually insoluble and form highly aggregated units (micelles) when the monomeric concentration exceeds $\sim 10^{-10}$ M (192). The usual micellar form assumed by aggregated phosphatidylcholines is that of an extended planar bilayer, but these bilayers often interact to form very large multilamellar structures. Both the kinetics of the movement of such units to an interface and their subsequent spreading depend on their size and physical properties. The latter are governed, in large part, by the chain lengths, degree of unsaturation, and the homogeneity of the fatty acid composition. Saturated phosphatidylcholines, e.g., dipalmitoyl phosphatidylcholine, adsorb to an air-liquid interface rather slowly below their endothermal phase-transition temperatures (107). Egg phosphatidylcholine, which has a large monoenoic species content, adsorbs more rapidly than saturated phosphatidylcholine, but not as fast as phosphatidylcholine (saturated or monoenoic) containing a small amount of a perturbing impurity, such as phosphatidylglycerol or certain (but not all) proteins (114, 115). The physical properties conveyed by these relatively small amounts of lipids and proteins are described in EXTRACELLULAR SURFACTANT LIPIDS, p. 311, and their importance to the physiological functions of surfactant are treated in the chapter by Goerke and Clements (70a) in the volume on the mechanics of breathing in this *Handbook* section on the respiratory system.

Figure 4 shows the major pathways of phosphatidylcholine synthesis. Glycolysis generates glycerol 3-phosphate by reducing dihydroxyacetone phosphate. The observation of a direct phosphorylation of small amounts of exogenous glycerol indicates that lung tissue contains a glycerol kinase. Apparently this is not the major pathway, however (183). Glycerol 3-phosphate is acylated at the 1 and 2 positions with the coenzyme A (CoA) derivative of long-chain fatty acids to form phosphatidic acid, which is subsequently hydrolyzed to yield 1,2-diacylglycerol. The CDPcholine, formed from choline phosphate and cytidine 5′-triphosphate (CTP), combines with 1,2-diacylglycerol to form phosphatidylcholine. These reactions, which form most of the lung's newly synthesized phosphatidylcholine (207), are found in many mammalian tissues. In normal lung tissue of either the adult or fetus the methylation of phosphatidylethanolamine (23) generates little phosphatidylcholine (207). The enzymes of this pathway are present in lung tissue (144), however, and the pathway might be quantitatively important under pathological conditions (e.g., severe dietary choline deficiency) (101). The small amount of phosphatidylcholines normally formed in lung tissue by methylation may, of course, have significant physiological functions of their own (90).

Both pulmonary surfactant and lung tissue contain a high percentage of saturated phosphatidylcholine (whereas most other tissues do not). The pathways regulating this unusual phosphatidylcholine composition have generated much interest. Two alternatives have been explored: *1)* the saturated species are synthesized de novo by the CDPcholine pathway and are regulated by the specificities of the acyl-CoA transferases, adding saturated fatty acids directly to glycerol 3-phosphate; and *2)* both saturated and unsaturated phosphatidylcholines are formed de novo without

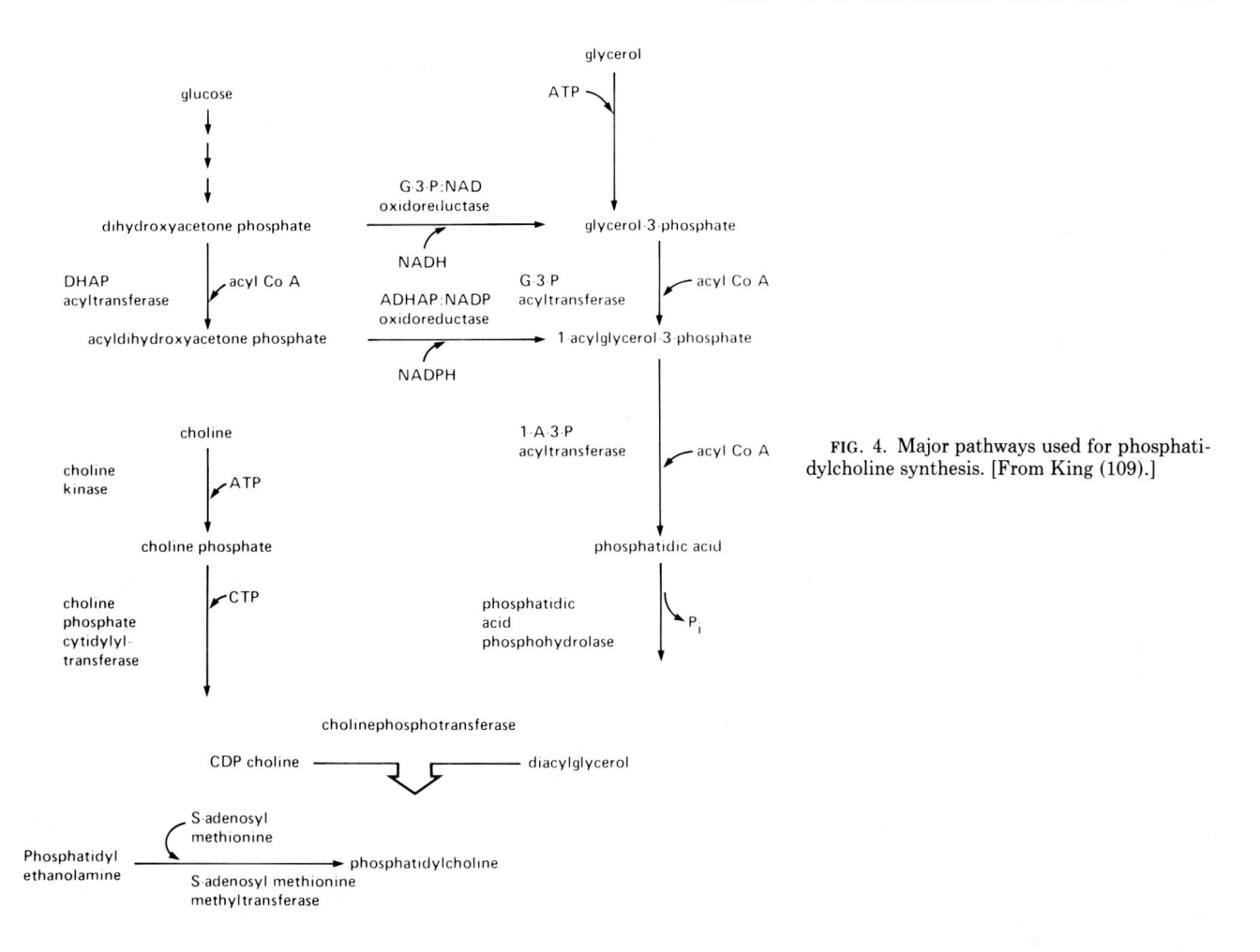

FIG. 4. Major pathways used for phosphatidylcholine synthesis. [From King (109).]

specificity and are subsequently remodeled by acyltransferase reactions. In this manner, a phospholipase A₂ hydrolyzes the phosphatidylcholines (Fig. 5) to 1-acyl, 2-lysophosphatidylcholine. The saturated phosphatidylcholine re-forms from the lyso derivative either by a lysophosphatidylcholine:acyl-CoA acyltransferase transferring the appropriate fatty acid directly to the lyso receptor (125) or by the condensation of two saturated lysophosphatidylcholines to form saturated phosphatidylcholine and glycerol 3-phosphate (48). Several studies clearly show that acyl rearrangement reactions proceed actively in lung tissue (2) and in type II cells (12, 134). Much of the saturated phosphatidylcholine found in surfactant is probably first synthesized de novo as an unsaturated species and is then remodeled to the saturated compound. Apparently the direct acylation of lysophosphatidylcholine is the preferred pathway in type II cells (12, 134).

Phosphatidylglycerol

Interest in pulmonary phosphatidylglycerol stems from its relatively high concentration in the surfactant. Low concentrations of phosphatidylglycerol are found in most mammalian tissues (13), but it comprises as much as 10% of purified pulmonary surfactant (133). Figure 6 shows the pathways leading to the synthesis of this phospholipid in other tissues. There is no evidence that other pathways exist in lung tissue. The CDPdiacylglycerol reacts with glycerol 3-phosphate to form phosphatidylglycerol 3-phosphate, which is then cleaved by a phosphatase to form phosphatidylglycerol. These reactions proceed actively in perfused lung (70) and isolated alveolar type II cells (134, 191). Radioactive palmitate is incorporated evenly into the 1 and 2 fatty acid positions in the saturated phosphatidylglycerols in type II cells (134), suggesting that remodeling reactions are not needed to obtain this species. The composition of the phosphatidylglycerols in alveolar surfactant and the relative percentage of saturated forms it contains are still in doubt (see *Pulmonary Surfactant*, p. 311). In type II cells radioactive glycerol is distributed among the phosphatidylglycerols as follows: 42% saturated, 39% monoenoic, 7% dienoic, and 12% polyenoic (134). If the near-equilibrium distribution of this label reflects the pool sizes of these phosphatidylglycerols, and if much of this phosphatidylglycerol is destined for ex-

FIG. 5. Proposed lung cell pathways for restructuring unsaturated phosphatidylcholines to dipalmitoyl phosphatidylcholine. [From King (109).]

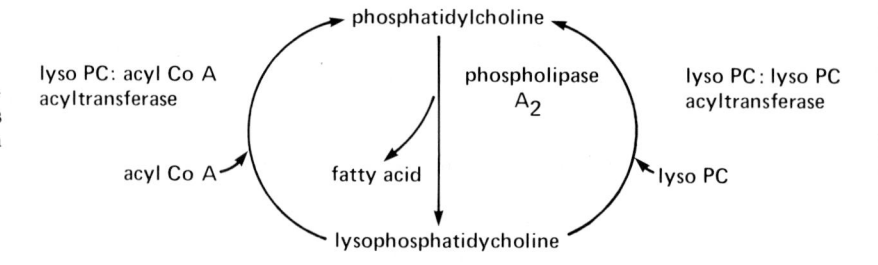

port as pulmonary surfactant, then these results suggest that there should be more saturated acyl groups in these surfactant phosphatidylglycerols than Hallman and Gluck (78) and Rooney et al. (173) have reported. These findings are more consistent with those of Engle et al. (47).

Other Lipids in Surfactant

Over 85% of the pulmonary surfactant lipids contain phosphorus (107), and practically all studies on surfactant metabolism have concentrated on them. Cholesterol is the major neutral (nonphosphorous) lipid in surfactant, comprising ~10% of the total material (by weight) in canine surfactant; information on its metabolism is limited, however. Apparently most of the cholesterol found in surfactant derives from circulating lipoproteins (81), and endogenous synthesis from acetate accounts for only ~1% in the isolated perfused lung of the fed rat.

At least three major pools of pulmonary surfactant are found in the lungs: *1*) an intracellular locus of synthesis, probably exclusively associated with type II epithelial cells; *2*) the extracellular surfactant within the alveolar region; and *3*) a poorly defined pool associated with surfactant in various states of clearance from the alveolar lumen. Estimates of the intracellular surfactant pool's composition have been made with the composition of either purified populations of type II cells (see Table 5) or isolated lamellar bodies (see Table 7). The data obtained to date are less reproducible than one might like, probably because the techniques required to isolate pure type II cells or well-preserved lamellar bodies are still formidable. The compositions of lamellar body lipids and alveolar surfactant are similar, and this is consistent with the probability that this is the intracellular precursor pool to the secreted material. There is probably little metabolic activity carried out within the lamellar bodies, because they contain few of the key enzymes for lipid synthesis (7); this opinion is still controversial, however (194). The compositions of the other intracellular pools are unknown, and it is not understood how the cell regulates the defined stoichiometry of the surfactant lipids.

The alveolar pool has been the most extensively studied, and its composition was described previously (see EXTRACELLULAR SURFACTANT LIPIDS, p. 311).

Even this pool may not be homogeneous, however. Surfactant probably exists in more than one form in the alveolar space, and it may have an enriched dipalmitoyl phosphatidylcholine content after its adsorption to the alveolar surface (86).

Extracellular surfactant must be removed at a rate comparable to its intracellular synthesis and secretion to maintain a steady state between the intracellular and extracellular pools. Both dipalmitoyl phosphatidylcholine (118, 133) and apolipoprotein A (108, 212) are found in alveolar macrophages, principally in secondary lysosomes (212), and the macrophages likely ingest some surfactant and participate in its clearance. Other clearance pathways have been discussed (58, 67), but their importance to the metabolism of surfactant is unclear. Only small amounts of surfactant are removed up the airways by mucociliary action (58). Surfactant lipid may be reabsorbed into the circulation, presumably through lymphatic drainage, as radioactive derivatives of [^{14}C]dipalmitoyl phosphatidylcholine aerosolized into the lung are found in blood, urine, and lung tissue (67). The [^{14}C]dipalmitoyl phosphatidylcholine deposited in liposomes in the lungs of adult rabbits disappears from the alveoli quickly (7%–14%/h), as measured by lavaging the lungs at intervals, but leaves the lungs slowly (2%–3%/h)(158).

Formidable problems face the investigator studying the metabolism of the lipids in pulmonary surfactant. The lung contains many different cell types and many of them, if not all, contain lipids common to those found in surfactant. Intracellular pools of surfactant

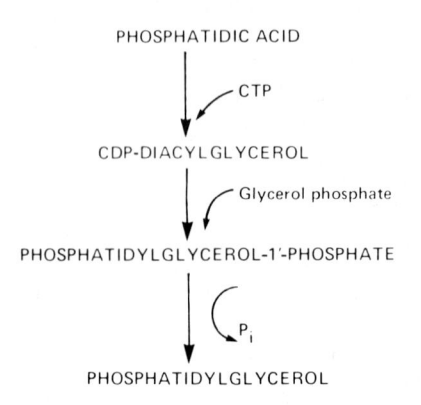

FIG. 6. Proposed metabolic pathway used by type II cells to synthesize phosphatidylglycerol in pulmonary surfactant.

lipids, even in type II cells, may be distributed among several subcellular sites, and we might expect a temporal difference in both isotopic uptake and precursor incorporation as the lipid moves from the cytosol to membrane-associated sites of the endoplasmic reticulum, Golgi apparatus, and lamellar bodies. Extracellular surfactant may be heterogeneous, as the processes of adsorption to the interface, spreading, film compression, and clearance could result in multiple pools of surfactant with differing compositions. Finally the pathways for the clearance and catabolism of surfactant may involve several different types of cells in the lungs, and the labeled components may be recycled, thereby confusing the interpretation of experiments. Using purified preparations of lung cells overcomes some of these problems and has led to some interesting results (109). In some cases, however, the advantages of purified cell types are negated by the damage caused by the dissociation and purification procedures. Thus finding the answers to difficult questions on metabolic pathways and their control will require studies conducted under both in vitro and in vivo conditions.

Enzymes of Lipid Synthesis

Four enzymes have received primary emphasis as potential regulators of the rate of de novo synthesis and composition of the phosphatidylcholine of lung surfactant: *1)* choline kinase (EC 2.7.1.32), ATP + choline → ADP + O-phosphocholine; *2)* cholinephosphate cytidylyltransferase (EC 2.7.7.15), CTP + choline phosphate → pyrophosphate + CDPcholine; *3)* phosphatidate phosphatase (EC 3.1.3.4), L-α-phosphatidate + H$_2$O → L-1,2-diglyceride + orthophosphate; and *4)* cholinephosphotransferase (EC 2.7.8.2), CDPcholine + 1,2-diacylglycerol → CMP + phosphatidylcholine.

The first two enzymes are involved in the synthesis of a "high energy" form of choline, and the last two prepare suitable intermediates for the terminal reactions. These reactions therefore represent the first and last steps in the overall pathway and would seem logical control points in its regulation. It is difficult to design experiments that directly measure the rate-limiting steps in a complicated synthetic pathway, but some results exist for tissues other than lung (206). Conclusions concerning regulation in lung tissue have come from indirect experiments. Thus it is known that several hormones stimulate the synthesis of lung phosphatidylcholine. Simultaneously measuring the changes in enzymatic activities provides circumstantial evidence for their involvement in controlling this pathway. Another approach has been to follow the gestational development of key enzymes in an attempt to correlate the appearance of an enzymatic activity with the known ontogeny of the surfactant system. The results of these studies have not always agreed and the assignment of rate-limiting step(s) in the phosphatidylcholine pathway is still in question.

CHOLINE KINASE. Choline kinase does not change significantly in the last 4 days of gestation in fetal mouse (153) or rabbit lung (174), suggesting that it does not control the rate of phosphatidylcholine synthesis in the developing lung of these species. Farrell and his colleagues (53), however, showed that this activity reaches a sharp maximum 3 days before term in rat lung. The enzyme in fetal rabbit lungs is not stimulated by glucocorticoids (171), although these hormones precociously increase the saturated phosphatidylcholine content (121). These results do not strongly indicate that choline kinase assumes a primary role in the regulation of phosphatidylcholine synthesis in fetal lung tissue. Similar conclusions were drawn from results in HeLa cells (206), protozoa (28), and rat liver (182).

CHOLINEPHOSPHATE CYTIDYLYLTRANSFERASE. This enzyme, which catalyzes the formation of CDPcholine, has been shown to be regulatory and rate limiting in HeLa cells (206). It is found in both soluble and membrane-bound fractions and is activated by diacylglycerol and certain acidic phospholipids (205). Vance and Choy (205) suggest that its regulatory role extends to phosphatidylcholine synthesis in tissues other than HeLa cells.

Cytidylyltransferase has been found both in rat microsomes and the soluble portions of adult rat lung tissue, but its distribution apparently varies with fetal age, parturition, and species. Thus it has been reported to be predominantly in the supernatant fractions of fetal rat lung (196) but was associated with both soluble and membrane fractions in the fetal mouse lung (153). During gestation its activity increased from 4 to 2 days before term in rat (52) and mouse lung (153), with peak activity 1 day before parturition. The activity in fetal rabbit lung at 25 days of gestation was modestly stimulated by glucocorticoid (171); it was unaffected in mouse lung, however (153).

Feldman et al. (54) reported some interesting physical properties of cytidylyltransferase in the lungs of near-term fetal rats and studied the relationship of its physical state to the modulation of its activity by phosphatidylglycerol and other acidic phospholipids. The enzyme was found in fetal lung in an inactive form ($M_r \sim 190,000$). During fetal maturation these inactive enzyme units aggregated, perhaps into an enzyme-membrane unit, and unsaturated phosphatidylglycerol increased this association. Increased enzymatic activity occurs during these changes in physical state. The authors suggested that the increase in lung phosphatidylglycerol in late gestation may partly be associated with the regulation of this enzymatic activity. If confirmed these findings offer support for speculation on the physiological role of phosphatidylglycerol in lung surfactant.

The diverse findings on the gestational development of this enzyme and its reaction to glucocorticoids complicate evaluations of its regulatory role in the synthesis of phosphatidylcholine in fetal lung tissue. We would not expect that the regulation of fetal phosphatidylcholine synthesis is controlled differently in species as phylogenetically similar as the mouse, rat, and rabbit. This argument, however, probably has only limited validity. Moreover, most studies measured the synthesis of the total phosphatidylcholine pool in lung tissue; therefore changes specifically associated with the synthesis of saturated phosphatidylcholine destined for export in the surfactant may be masked by changes in the synthesis of the other phosphatidylcholines. The search for more definitive results requires the use of fetal type II cells and improvements in the methods involved make such studies more feasible.

PHOSPHATIDIC ACID PHOSPHOHYDROLASE. This enzyme has probably received more attention than any enzyme in the de novo pathway in the lung. Jimenez and Johnston (97), Benson (15), and their co-workers found it in the amniotic fluid at times when they expected that the fetal lung produced surfactant. Brehier et al. (22) showed that synthetic glucocorticoid activity nearly doubles in fetal rabbits 22–26 days of gestation. Possmayer et al. (165), however, reported lesser effects. This enzyme was found in the microsomal and supernatant fractions of lung homogenate (29) and in the surfactant lipids obtained from alveolar fluid (15). Spitzer and Johnston (194) consider this enzyme to be an integral part of the lamellar body, whereas others definitively attribute its activity in the lamellar body fraction to microsomal contamination (7). This enzyme hydrolyzes phosphatidylglycerol phosphate to phosphatidylglycerol (15, 194), and it has been postulated that its physiological activity may be associated with its synthesis. Direct evidence for a regulatory role in either pathway has not been presented.

CHOLINEPHOSPHOTRANSFERASE. According to most studies, cholinephosphotransferase is neither regulatory nor rate limiting. This enzyme reached maximal activity 2 days before term in fetal rat (53) and mouse lung (152) but not in rabbit lung (174). Glucocorticoids did not stimulate its activity (165, 171).

PHOSPHATIDYLCHOLINE REMODELING ENZYMES. These enzymes may be of great importance in determining the surface activity of lung surfactant. Van Golde (207) has summarized evidence suggesting that a large proportion of the phosphatidylcholine synthesized de novo through the CDPcholine pathway is unsaturated. This indicates that the large proportion of saturated phosphatidylcholine found in lung tissue (and pulmonary surfactant) must use auxiliary enzymatic pathways to produce this type of phosphatidylcholine. Two pathways have been described: *1*) lysolecithin acyltransferase (EC 2.3.1.23), acyl-CoA + 1-acylglycero-3-phosphocholine → CoA + 1,2-diacyl-glycero-3-phosphocholine; and *2*) lysophosphatidylcholine: lysophosphatidylcholine acyltransferase, lysophosphatidylcholine + lysophosphatidylcholine → phosphatidylcholine + glycerophosphocholine.

Hydrolysis of the unsaturated phosphatidylcholine at the *sn*-2 position initiates the remodeling pathways, producing 1-saturated acyl, 2-lyso-*sn*-glycerophosphocholine. Phospholipase A_2 (EC 3.1.1.4) catalyzes this reaction and is found in lung tissue (83, 130). Both remodeling enzymes are active in whole-lung tissue, but only the lyso:acyl-CoA transferase has been demonstrated in isolated type II cells (12). Moreover this enzyme showed some specificity for saturated acyl groups (12).

There is still controversy over whether or not remodeling enzymes exist in the lamellar bodies. Some investigators reported finding a phospholipase A_2 (83) in lamellar bodies and suggested that the final site of synthesis of the saturated phosphatidylcholine lies within this organelle. Others, however, attributed this enzyme's activity in the lamellar body preparation to contamination from other cellular organelles (130). Neither a lysolecithin acyltransferase nor a lysolecithin:lysolecithin acyltransferase (7) were found in lamellar bodies. Engle et al. (47) suggested that a direct acyl exchange between palmitoyl CoA and unsaturated phosphatidylcholine could occur in lamellar bodies without intermediate deacylation by a phospholipase A_2 and the reacylation by specific acyltransferase enzymes. This interesting speculation, however, has not been confirmed.

REGULATION OF SURFACTANT METABOLISM

In the first two sections of this chapter (see *Parenchyma*, p. 309, and *Alveolar Type II Cells*, p. 310) the composition and metabolic pathways of the prominent lipids and proteins in lung surfactant were discussed, and it was evident that in the surfactant system, synthetic reactions have been studied more intensely than catabolic reactions. This is also true for the physiological regulation of these reactions. Factors affecting the synthetic and secretory processes are better known than those regulating the clearing and degradative reactions. In both cases they are poorly understood at the molecular level, and the information summarized here is largely phenomenological.

Regulation of Synthesis and Storage of Surfactant Components

Biosynthesis of the glycerolipids that constitute the main mass of lung surfactant requires metabolic energy and precursors (e.g., fatty acids, glycerol, phosphate, and the bases choline, glycerol, ethanolamine, inositol, serine, etc.). Normally the ratio of blood flow to lung mass is so large that substrate availability is not limiting. Several workers (49, 169) have studied the restriction of substrates that may occur during starvation. Although pressure-volume measurements indicated a small degree of instability (49, 169) and a lavage assay of alveolar saturated phosphatidylcholine (63) showed a substantial decrease (40%) in rats starved for 2–3 days, the labeling half-life of whole-lung phosphatidylcholines did not change measurably in similarly treated animals (66). Essential fatty acid deficiency in weanling rats (27, 124) resulted in decreased saturated phosphatidylcholine and decreased surface activity in lung lavage fluid. This was due possibly to a release of inhibition of fatty acid Δ9 desaturase activity, caused by a deficiency of unsaturated fatty acids (5).

Several workers (57, 185, 188) have used unilateral pulmonary artery occlusion in dogs to test the dependence of alveolar stability on blood flow. Almost immediately after occlusion (within 2 min), compliance in the occluded lung fell while ventilatory resistance rose. Because adding 5% CO_2 to the gas inspired by the occluded lung prevented these effects, it was felt that altering the alveolar surface tension did not explain them (185). With chronic occlusion, however, the occluded lung extract showed a minimal surface tension increase over that of the perfused lung as early as 2 h after occlusion; this difference persisted until collateral circulation developed in the occluded lung (57). The mechanism causing this change was not demonstrated. In more recent experiments (188) electron-microscopic examination performed 2, 4, and 8 h after occlusion showed a marked depletion of lamellar bodies from type II epithelial cells. In lungs in which blood flow was restored for 6 h after a period of occlusion, many small (new?) lamellar bodies were seen. Adding 5% CO_2 to the inspired gas prevented these changes. The authors concluded that lamellar bodies are dynamic organelles, capable of rapid responses to changes in alveolar capillary blood flow. Recent experiments in rabbits (8) demonstrated a temporary (1–2 h) rise in alveolar saturated phosphatidylcholine, determined by lung lavage, after occlusion of one pulmonary artery. After 7 h the saturated phosphatidylcholine level in the occluded lung decreased below that in the unoccluded lung, suggesting that a burst of secretion was followed by the depletion of intracellular stores. This interpretation is consistent with the loss of lamellar bodies observed in dogs by electron microscopy 2–8 h postocclusion (188). In experiments in which pulmonary capillary blood flow was decreased in steps down to very low levels (147, 148), the uptake and incorporation of [^{14}C]palmitate into phospholipids was hardly affected, whereas glucose uptake significantly diminished. It was concluded that even when blood flow limitation is extreme, the effects are more likely related to limited availability of glucose rather than free fatty acids (148).

Excessive substrate supply may also alter lung lipid metabolism. Baritussio et al. (9, 10), stimulated by reports of decreased partial pressure of arterial O_2, decreased pulmonary diffusing capacity, and abnormal ventilation/blood flow distribution in hyperlipemic patients (9, 10), induced hyperlipemia in rats through diets rich in glycerol, triglycerides, or cholesterol. The total amount of alveolar phospholipid estimated by lung lavage was not significantly changed in the hyperlipemic animals, but there was a 50% increase in phosphatidylglycerol and a 50% decrease in phosphatidylethanolamine compared with control values. Neutral lipid composition was not reported. The lungs expanded maximally at lower pressures and retained more air at a transpulmonary pressure of 5 cmH$_2$O. Because the pressure-volume characteristics with saline filling were not altered, the authors concluded that hyperlipemia can significantly change the surface properties of the alveoli, probably through changes in phospholipid composition. Changes in turnover rates of surfactant components, however, were not specifically implicated.

Administering large amounts of myoinositol to adult rabbits caused a marked decrease in phosphatidylglycerol and an increase in phosphatidylinositol in lung surfactant (obtained by lavage) (76). The compositions of other surfactant and tissue phospholipids were little affected.

Extreme changes in caloric intake or precursor levels in these experiments were used to perturb surfactant composition. There is little reason to believe that commonly occurring fluctuations in diet or blood levels of precursors affect surfactant composition significantly.

Changes of environmental temperature can cause changes in tissue lipid composition in poikilotherms. The lipids of lung surfactant (obtained by lavage) from map turtles acclimated to 5°C, 14°C, 22°C, and 32°C changed in a way that tended to maintain the fluidity of the complex constant at different temperatures (126). Compared with 5°C values, at 32°C the amount of lipid increased 74%, the proportion of phosphatidylcholine increased 9.8%, and the fraction of saturated fatty acids in the lipids increased 13%. Comparable adjustments in the lung surfactant of homeotherms are not likely, because of the relatively narrow variance of their body temperatures. Nonetheless it seems likely that the synthetic system that generates surfactant components possesses feedback characteristics that maintain the proper fluidity of the product despite changes in diet, substrate availability, level of lung activity, and environmental conditions.

Increased ventilation of isolated perfused lungs elevated the incorporation of radioactive palmitate into tissue phospholipids linearly with ventilatory frequency (65). The fraction of this increase caused by surfactant synthesis was not determined. The lungs, however, are active in prostaglandin metabolism, and some workers report that hyperventilation increased prostaglandin release from guinea pig (16) and dog

(179) lungs. Because aspirin inhibited this effect, it was concluded that distension of the lung stimulated prostaglandin synthesis. Mechanical distortion of mouse BALB/3T3 cells in culture also stimulates the formation of both prostaglandin E_2 and $F_{2\alpha}$, and indomethacin apparently blocks this response (93). Evidence has been presented that prostaglandins E_2 and $F_{2\alpha}$ stimulate biosynthesis of phosphatidylcholine in cell line A549 (38), cells derived from human lung carcinoma that have some characteristics of type II alveolar cells. It seems likely therefore that ventilation of the lungs stimulates increased surfactant component synthesis in type II cells. The secretion rate also increases, as is discussed in the next section. Prostaglandins might possibly be mediators of the response to ventilation.

Factors other than substrate availability, lung activity, and environmental conditions affect the synthesis and storage of surfactant components. Certain hormones, especially glucocorticoids, have profound effects on the fetal lung, e.g., alveolarization, induction of enzyme activities, decrease in glycogen content, type II cell differentiation with lamellar body formation, and enhanced synthesis and secretion of surfactant components (22, 52, 53, 121, 128, 129, 153, 164, 165, 171). On the other hand, insulin appears to inhibit maturation. Organ-cultured fetal rat lung showed increased glycogen content and both fewer and earlier forms of lamellar bodies when insulin was added to the medium (74).

High doses of 17β-estradiol increased the incorporation of choline into phosphatidylcholine by 150% (compared with controls) in rabbit lung slices prepared from treated fetuses (104). Similar results were obtained with fetal rat lung in organ culture. These results indicated that estrogen could act directly on the lung to enhance the formation of phospholipids (75).

On the other hand, androgens apparently slow fetal pulmonary maturation, and this may account for the higher incidence of respiratory distress syndrome in male infants (203). When the phosphatidylcholine-to-sphingomyelin ratio in lung lavage fluid was used as a measure of surfactant production, female rabbit fetuses were more mature than males in the transitional period from 26 to 28 days of gestation (149). In recent experiments, administering testosterone to rabbit fetuses from day 12 to day 26 of gestation eliminated the difference by lowering female maturation to male levels (150).

Several investigators (6, 80, 172) have considered the role of other hormones (e.g., prolactin, growth hormone, thyroid hormones) in regulating the synthesis of surfactant components. Further studies are needed to fully elucidate the role of these and other hormones in both fetal and adult lungs.

Several kinds of drugs have been shown to influence the surfactant system by stimulating or inhibiting secretion. Such responses imply concurrent effects on synthesis, but these have usually not been independently demonstrated. For this reason drug effects are discussed in the next section.

How the individual processes involved in the synthesis, translocation through the cell, packaging, storage (in lamellar bodies), and exocytosis of surfactant components are regulated is not known. Presumably, as in other secretory cells, many organelles of type II cells are involved. The Chediak-Higashi syndrome demonstrates that the components of the system do not always function optimally. This syndrome is an autosomal recessive genetic disease occurring in humans, mice, mink, cattle, and other species of mammals. It is characterized by large inclusion bodies in several cell types. The lamellar bodies of type II cells are immense in this syndrome (32, 193), but abnormalities of pulmonary function have not been documented. The amount of surfactant found in lung tissue was threefold greater than that of the controls. The increased fusion of organelles containing hydrolytic enzymes is apparently the common denominator in the affected cells. After cholinergic stimulation and the discharge of granules, the newly formed organelles were of normal size but were subsequently enlarged. The molecular defect(s) responsible for this have not been described.

Regulation of Secretion of Surfactant Components

Translocating surface-active material from its storage sites in type II cells to the alveolar lumina is a vital process that must be regulated and attuned to the requirements of the lungs in varying states of physiological activity. Lung ventilation is the most obvious variable that might influence the secretion, and several investigations of its influence have been conducted (50, 51, 59, 87, 139, 156, 157, 213).

These studies indicate that lung distension increases the alveolar pool of surfactant components (usually estimated by lavage) but that continued hyperventilation lowers lung compliance, perhaps by surfactant inactivation (213). Because chronic hyperventilation can cause pulmonary edema (208), we are not sure to what extent these results were influenced by this. On the other hand, shallow breathing also diminished lung compliance (140, 199) and increased the fraction of saturated phosphatidylcholine yielded as sediment by low-speed centrifugation from lavage fluid, without changing the total amount of saturated phosphatidylcholine recovered. Both effects were reversed by a single maximal inflation (199). In one study of the effects of increased ventilation (156), special attention was paid to the prevention of pulmonary edema and the increase in surfactant obtained by lavage (alveolar pool) was confirmed. In addition it was demonstrated that the alveolar pool of surfactant rose for 2 h and then fell after 4 h of increased ventilation. This data did not directly distinguish between a decrease in surfactant due to a gradual increase in the removal rate, the exhaustion of surfactant secretion, or both. Extrapolation of the raw rates of change of alveolar pool size toward zero time suggested that the initial (unsustained) secretory response may have been as high as 80%–100% of the alveolar pool size per hour. Without more direct information, however, the true explanation for these rather dramatic changes remains uncertain. Experiments with exogenous radioactive saturated phosphatidylcholine (158) showed its increased clearance from the alveoli with increased ventilation. Whether the same effect occurs in endogenous saturated phosphatidylcholine in lung surfactant is unproved. If it does, then the initial secretion rates provoked by increased ventilation may be even higher than the crude estimates suggest and intracellular surfactant-pool depletion may be anticipated, unless surfactant synthesis was comparably accelerated.

The possible mechanisms of such responses have received some attention. Cholinergic mediation was first investigated because of the well-known atelectasis after vagotomy in rats or guinea pigs (20, 71, 202). Loss of surface activity in lung extracts and depletion of lamellar bodies in alveolar type II cells have been shown (20, 202). Injecting pilocarpine appeared to cause the release of surfactant components (72, 137, 145, 154), and these effects were blocked by atropine, suggesting a cholinergic mediation of secretion. Atropine also blocked the rise in alveolar surfactant components accompanying increased ventilation (156). Later work (42) showed that propranolol and phenoxybenzamine could also block the effect of pilocarpine on the pressure-volume characteristics of fetal rabbit lungs. Isolated rat type II cells secreted saturated phosphatidylcholine in response to several secretogogues but not to carbamylcholine, methacholine, or pilocarpine (45). In another study (25) isolated type II cells secreted 340% more saturated phosphatidylcholine in response to isoproterenol (1 μM) and the cAMP level increased 4.9-fold. Acetylcholine (100 μM) increased cellular cGMP levels 8.7-fold but caused only a 46% increase in saturated phosphatidylcholine secretion. Atropine blocked the nucleotide response but not the secretory effect. Because of these findings, it appears that the rise in alveolar pool size caused by administering either pilocarpine or acetylcholine (156) may be indirect, possibly via the adrenal medulla. Atropine's effectiveness in blocking the response to increased ventilation in vivo (156) and to lung distension in vitro (87) suggests that cholinergic mechanism(s) may play a significant role in these responses in intact animals.

Several investigators (14, 42, 45, 127, 154, 157, 214, 215) have examined the adrenergic mediation of surfactant control with mainly concordant results: β-adrenergic stimulation increased both lung compliance and the size of the alveolar surfactant pool and released saturated phosphatidylcholine from isolated type II cells, whereas β-blockers inhibited these effects; α-adrenergic stimulation either decreased or had no measurable effect on compliance, and α-blockers prevented this change when it was expected. The increase in alveolar pool size due to increased ventilation was stopped by β-blockers but not by α-blockers (157). Thus the weight of current evidence supports the existence of a prominent, direct β-adrenergic pathway that stimulates surfactant secretion from type II cells and a less effective, probably indirect, cholinergic pathway. The role of α-adrenergic mediation remains uncertain.

As mentioned above, the evidence indicates that lung ventilation enhances prostaglandin formation (16, 179). Therefore the possible involvement of prostaglandins in the ventilatory control of surfactant secretion was examined (157). It was found that both prostaglandin synthetase inhibitors indomethacin and meclofenamate blocked the increase in alveolar surfactant expected with increased ventilation but did not decrease the pool size with normal ventilation. When we tried to stimulate a rise in the alveolar pool size by intravenously infusing prostaglandin E_1, E_2, or $F_{2\alpha}$ in normally breathing animals, the changes were not statistically significant. On the average, however, the pool size was lower with prostaglandin E_2 and higher with $F_{2\alpha}$ than in the control animals. These differences agree with the effects of these agents on adrenergic responses in some other systems (84). The small responses we observed may reflect the presence of the highly active prostaglandin-metabolizing system of pulmonary capillary endothelial cells (55, 176). Despite these problems of interpretation, the evidence implicates prostaglandins in the effect of ventilation on the size of the alveolar surfactant pool.

Evidence for the participation of neural reflexes in modulating surfactant secretion is more tenuous, however. The lungs contain autonomic nerve fibers, and electron-microscopic evidence indicates that nerve endings reach into alveolar membranes (94, 143). The fibers are probably efferents, but these images do not permit a more definite identification of them. Occasionally one is seen near a type II cell. Stimulation of the distal end of the cut left cervical vagus nerve in rabbits for 1 h at a frequency and intensity sufficient to lower the heart rate by 25% was associated with a 31% average increase in the alveolar surfactant pool (156). No attempt was made to block the response with atropine, indomethacin, or adrenergic blockers, so the effect cannot be ascribed to a direct, cholinergic mechanism. These results nonetheless suggest that a signal operating via efferent fibers in the vagus nerves could play a modest role in surfactant control, possibly through catecholamine release from the adrenal medulla.

We discussed earlier (see *Regulation of Synthesis and Storage of Surfactant Components*, p. 322) the effects unilateral pulmonary artery occlusion has on the surfactant system, i.e., a decrease in lamellar bodies in type II cells and a transient rise in alveolar saturated phosphatidylcholine (8, 187). These effects and the rise in specific activity of alveolar phospholipid after occlusion (180) indicate at least a temporary increase in surfactant secretion. The fact that maintaining normal CO_2 tension in the alveoli of the occluded lung prevents these acute effects of occlusion suggests that CO_2 and pH levels in and around the type II cells are important determinants of secretion. Whether small changes in CO_2 and pH levels might significantly modulate secretion, however, cannot be deduced.

One of the most dramatic physiological changes in surfactant secretion occurs during fetal development. Fluid produced continually by the lung can be collected from the fetus in utero via an indwelling tracheal catheter and the concentration of surfactant assayed (141). Multiplying the volume rate of fluid efflux by concentration and then dividing by the fetal weight gives a normalized surfactant production rate ($\mu g \cdot h^{-1} \cdot kg^{-1}$). Over the interval from 125 to 147 days of gestation, surfactant output increased ~20-fold (Fig. 7). If proportional reabsorption of surfactant components also occurred in the alveoli, the actual increase in secretion would be larger than Figure 7 indicates. Apparently the system is capable of even greater output rates, however. Infusing epinephrine into the fetal lamb reduced the flow of tracheal fluid by 50%–60% during a period of 6–12 h. Despite this the efflux of surfactant increased over the basal rates ~3-fold at 129 days of gestation and ~10-fold at 142 days of gestation (127). The highest rate exceeded steady-state rates calculated from tracer studies in normal adult animals (217). The experiments did not show how long such high efflux rates could be sustained. Obviously, however, the surfactant flux can be adjusted over an enormous range.

Regulation of Clearance of Surfactant Components

In the normal steady state the rate of alveolar surfactant removal must equal its secretion rate. Several clearance pathways have been suggested: ingestion by macrophages, propulsion up airways, enzymatic degradation at the surface of the alveolar epithelium, absorption into alveolar epithelial cells, and uptake into interstitial spaces and lymphatics (34, 100, 148, 181). After intravenous injection of [^{14}C]palmitate, the saturated phosphatidylcholine of alveolar macrophages showed a specific activity–time curve almost identical to, but slightly lagging behind, the curve for free saturated phosphatidylcholine in the lavage fluid (148). Provided that palmitate did not reach the macrophages directly, this result would be compatible with the role these cells play in surfactant clearance, as would the observation (with electron microscopy) that they contain occasional lamellar body contents and myelinic inclusions (166). How quantitatively significant this role is in normal animals cannot be deduced from this report. Other inves-

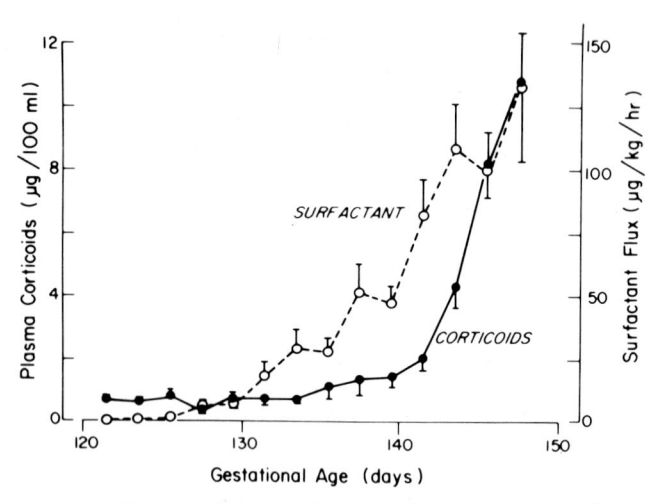

FIG. 7. Tracheal flux of surfactant and plasma corticoid levels in fetal lambs as functions of gestational age. [From Mescher et al. (141).]

tigators (11, 58, 156, 157) suggest that a very small fraction of the phospholipids secreted by type II cells is either cleared by the macrophages in the first pass or moves up the airways. If extensive reabsorption and recycling of these materials between the alveolar epithelium and lumen occurs (67, 77, 158), the amount cleared by macrophages might still account for an important fraction of the actual throughput of surfactant components. In experiments carried out with fetal lambs (181), a mixture of [^{14}C]phosphatidylcholines bound to albumin was introduced via the trachea into the lung fluid and the loss of label from the fluid determined for a period of 90 min. Loss was extremely rapid, with a half-life between 15 and 60 min, but simultaneously administered radioiodinated albumin was almost completely retained in the lung fluid. The authors concluded that the epithelial surface membranes of the lung were the primary barrier to absorption. They suggested that enzymatic hydrolysis occurred at the plasma membranes with the split products rapidly absorbed into circulating blood and the label principally contained in free fatty acids. Geiger et al. (67) gave 2-[9,10-^{3}H]palmitoyl-saturated phosphatidylcholine to young rats by aerosol inhalation. The animals were anesthetized, tracheotomized, and allowed to breathe the aerosol for 3 min. Clearance of label was followed by autoradiography on frozen sections and biochemical analysis. The authors concluded that the label remained in saturated phosphatidylcholine in the lung, that the saturated phosphatidylcholine was taken up very rapidly (within 4 min) by type I and type II alveolar epithelial cells, that type II cells stored saturated phosphatidylcholine for several hours but type I cells released label quickly into the circulating blood, and that a significant number of alveolar macrophages were labeled after 2 h (in a ratio of ~1 macrophage to 4 type I and type II cells). The half-life of the saturated phosphatidylcholine was estimated to be ~1 h in the alveolar lumina and ~3 h in the lung tissue, and it was felt that little saturated phosphatidylcholine was cleared via the airways.

Anesthetized rabbits were used to examine the clearance of radioactive L-dipalmitoyl phosphatidylcholine delivered to the alveoli by catheter as 40–60 nm unilamellar liposomes in half-strength Ringer's solution (158). The solution was rapidly absorbed from the alveoli and apparently caused little disturbance, as measured by respiratory and circulatory criteria, electron microscopy, alveolar-to-arterial O_2 gradient, and protein, cells, and lactate dehydrogenase content in sequential samples of lavage fluid. The liposomes remained in the alveolar lumina much longer and were cleared at a rate of ~7%/h in normally breathing animals. Doubling ventilation raised the clearance rate to ~14%/h. Label was lost from the lung as a whole at a rate of ~3.5%/h. Negligible amounts of label appeared in the trachea even after 7 h. When D-[^{3}H]dipalmitoyl phosphatidylcholine was also incorporated in the liposomes, the D-isomer label was cleared from the lumina at the same rate as the L-isomer label. With 20% phosphatidylglycerol added to the liposomes, clearance rates of tracers of both isomers were ~14%/h in normally breathing animals. Because phospholipases in lung homogenate hydrolyzed the L- but not the D-dipalmitoyl phosphatidylcholine in these liposomes (as might be expected from the stereospecificity of phospholipase A from porcine pancreas) (21) and because D- and L-dipalmitoyl phosphatidylcholine were cleared at the same rate, the clearance of the dipalmitoyl phosphatidylcholine liposomes from alveolar lumina did not seem to be mediated by an enzymatic process. Interestingly clearance times for the dipalmitoyl phosphatidylcholine liposomes administered in these experiments were much longer than those previously measured with exogenous phosphatidylcholines but agreed more closely with estimates based on endogenously labeled dipalmitoyl phosphatidylcholine. Our observations (lack of stereospecificity, acceleration of clearance by ventilation and by addition of phosphatidylglycerol to liposomes) suggest that a physical rather than chemical process(es) limits the clearance of dipalmitoyl phosphatidylcholine liposomes from the alveoli in these circumstances. Phagocytosis by alveolar macrophages, endocytosis by epithelial cells (44), the penetration of liposomes between epithelial cells, and the fusion of liposomes with the plasma membranes (159, 161) of surface cells are all apparently compatible with these results. Methods with resolution at the subcellular level are needed, however, to sort out these possibilities.

In recent experiments radioactively labeled surfactant phospholipids from one set of rabbits were deposited in the alveoli of other (unlabeled) rabbits and the clearance rate was measured (77). The labeled components (phosphatidylcholine, saturated phosphatidylcholine, phosphatidylglycerol, phosphatidylinositol) were largely cleared from the alveolar lumina in 1–2 h. Interestingly the labels quickly appeared in lamellar bodies prepared by subcellular fractionation (see ref. 67). The time courses of both labeling and control experiments indicate that simple contamination could not explain the appearance of label in the lamellar bodies. The fraction of alveolar label incorporated into lamellar bodies cannot be calculated precisely from these data.

Infusing the very potent stable cyclic endoperoxide analogue U 46619 into adult rabbits for only 15 min caused a precipitous 37% fall in the alveolar phospholipid pool (157). Pulmonary hypertension, occasional hemorrhage, and a doubling of total protein in the lavage fluid complicated but could not directly explain this result. The possibility that cyclic endoperoxides may significantly influence surfactant clearance or reabsorption must be considered.

Several papers (85, 123, 175) imply that interference with alveolar clearance may lead to serious consequences. Although the initial description of alveolar proteinosis (175) called attention to the enormous accumulation of lipid in the lung and presented microscopic evidence of cholesterol deposits (in addition to protein), 8 years passed before a study was performed that suggested any impairment of alveolar clearance. Kuhn et al. (123) suggested that alveolar proteinosis was a disease of defective clearance rather than surfactant oversecretion; they based their suggestion on histochemical findings, ultrastructural observations, and surface tension measurements indicating that extracts of affected tissue inhibited the surface activity of normal extracts.

Further studies with biochemical and tracer techniques (167) indicated that no enhancement of pulmonary lipid synthesis occurred in the biopsy tissue from the cases studied, whereas there was impaired removal or degradation of alveolar phospholipid as sampled by lavage. The authors theorized that alveolar proteinosis resulted from prolonged retention of the metabolic products and by-products of the alveolar lining. Phospholipids (especially saturated phosphatidylcholine) and cholesterol were found by direct analysis of lavage returns in amounts far greater than were found in control subjects, and radioactive palmitate incorporated into phospholipids persisted for several weeks rather than just a few days. A definite etiology for the suspected defect in clearance was not demonstrated, however. Similar studies with more extensive subfractionation of lipids (177) again showed the preponderance of phosphatidylcholine in lavage fluid but called attention to the presence of other phospholipids and of glycolipids in small amounts. Two glycoproteins similar to those found in the lamellar bodies were also present (162). We have found (unpublished observations) very large quantities of immunoreactive surfactant apoprotein in lavage returns from a patient with alveolar proteinosis. Though not definitive, these results are also consistent with the theorized impaired clearance in this syndrome.

When specific pathogen-free rats were made to inhale quartz dust for 8 wk, they developed lesions that resembled alveolar proteinosis rather than fibrosis (85). Neutral and polar lipid levels increased, and enormous amounts of saturated phosphatidylcholine and cholesterol accumulated in the lungs. Type II alveolar cells exhibited hyperplasia, but it was unclear whether oversecretion rather than impaired removal of surfactant components was responsible for this lipid accumulation. The possible roles played by alveolar macrophages in this unexpected response to quartz dust are also unknown, but whether the dust causes fibrosis or lipid deposition may be partly related to whether or not it activates phospholipolysis in the macrophages (146), causing the formation of large amounts of lysophospholipids.

The relationship of cholesterol and phospholipid metabolism in surfactant has been studied in isolated perfused rat lungs (81). Virtually all surfactant cholesterol apparently came from exogenous cholesterol supplied in serum lipoproteins, with only 1% arising by de novo synthesis from acetate. These results suggested that most or all of the cholesterol in alveolar surfactant was derived from lamellar bodies. The tracer studies indicated that the metabolism of lamellar body and alveolar surfactant cholesterol parallels that of phosphatidylcholine.

Administering AY 9944, which decreases tissue cholesterol and increases its precursor 7-dehydrocholesterol, resulted in increased levels of saturated phosphatidylcholine and sphingomyelin in the lung (88), with at least part of the increase probably due to intra-alveolar accumulation (105). Interestingly another inhibitor of cholesterol synthesis, triparanol, which causes a reduction of the tissue cholesterol level and the accumulation of a different cholesterol precursor (desmosterol), did not cause phospholipid accumulation in the lung (89). Neither of these studies completely characterized the sterol intermediates, however. Sterols, such as cholesterol and lanosterol (which is a precursor of both 7-dehydrocholesterol and desmosterol), differ considerably in their ability to interact with phosphatidylcholines, apparently largely because of the presence or absence of the 14α-methyl group (216). Cholesterol binds very firmly and is capable of strongly modifying physical properties, permeability, enzymatic reaction rates, and fusibility in natural and artificial membranes (96, 155, 159, 161, 216). Obviously then, alterations in sterol metabolism in the lung might affect synthesis, secretion, and surface activity, as well as the clearance of surfactant components, in many different ways and possibly to a functionally significant extent. Alternatively the effects on lung phospholipids seen with AY 9944 and triparanol might be secondary to other actions of the drugs and might therefore be unrelated to sterol metabolism. Nevertheless these results and cholesterol's abundance in surfactant purified from normal lungs (~15 mol %) suggest that sterols may have a significant influence on the turnover of surfactant components.

So far we have shed little light on clearance regulation. The possibility that most surfactant components (or at least lipid components) are reabsorbed into type II cells and then recycled implies that the rates of material exchange between epithelial cells and alveolar lumina may greatly exceed the net alveolar throughput. Before attempting to define the control of both the quality and quantity of intra-alveolar surfactant, future experiments must separate recycling from the true clearance processes.

Relationship Between Protein and Lipid Metabolism

The lung actively synthesizes proteins (41), some of which are released into the alveolar lumen (138). Radioautographic studies (31) show that radioactive leucine is incorporated into subcellular organelles, including lamellar bodies, and the time course of the appearance of this radioactivity suggests a transfer of components (presumably protein) from the rough endoplasmic reticulum to the multivesicular bodies and then to the lamellar bodies. This morphological evidence, together with that derived from metabolic (116, 118) and immunological studies (212), suggests that the intracellular metabolism of surfactant may involve the elaboration of specific proteins.

The time course of synthesis and secretion of apolipoproteins A and B has been compared with that of dipalmitoyl phosphatidylcholine in newborn dogs (118) and adult rats (116) to ascertain whether surfactant is assembled intracellularly as a lipoprotein package and then secreted into the extracellular space. The results suggested that it is. Both apolipoprotein A and the saturated phosphatidylcholine in type II cells were maximally labeled within 1 h after intravenous injection of isotopic precursors (Fig. 8). Both components showed decreased labeling throughout 9 h with similar kinetics. The labeling of the apolipoprotein increased from 9 to 21 h, possibly because of intracellular and/or vascular compartment recycling of the labeled proteins, and this caused ambiguity in quantitative estimates of turnover rates. Thus the calculation of metabolic half-life with the slope of the labeling curve likely overestimates it, because the catabolism and relabeling of the immediate precursor pool is not considered.

Figure 9 illustrates the labeling of these components in alveolar surfactant. The data shown were obtained from experiments on adult rats (116), but the general pattern and conclusions were reinforced with results from newborn dogs (118). Detectable activities of both apolipoprotein A and dipalmitoyl phosphatidylcholine were found in surfactant obtained by lung lavage within 1 h after injection, and both specific activities

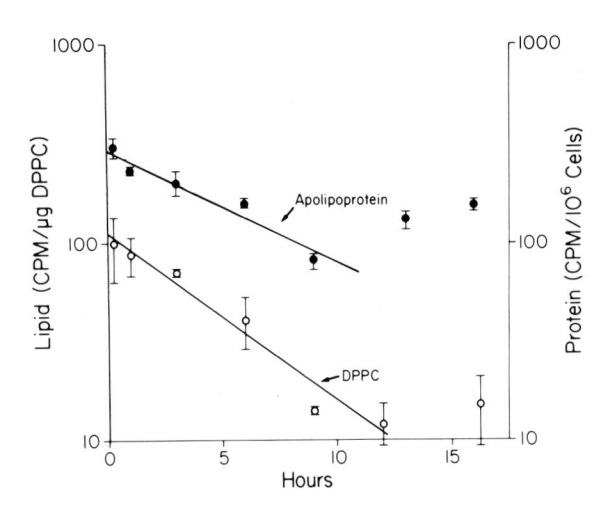

FIG. 8. Specific activities of dipalmitoyl phosphatidylcholine (○) and apolipoprotein A (●) in alveolar epithelial type II cells from rat lung. [From King and Martin (116).]

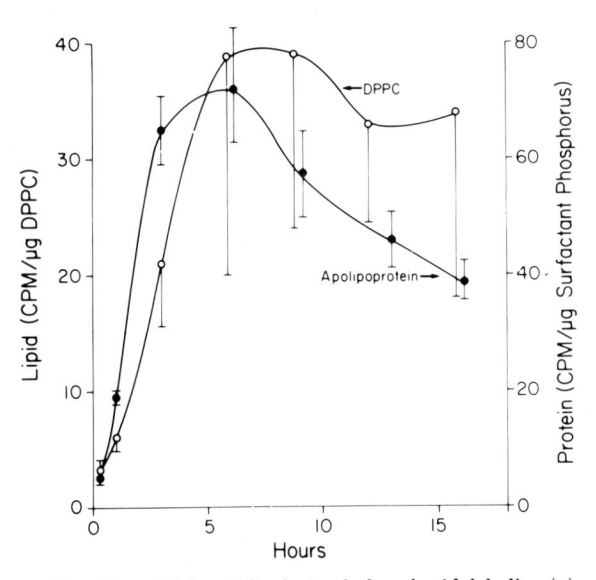

FIG. 9. Specific activities of dipalmitoyl phosphatidylcholine (○) and apolipoprotein A (●) in surfactant purified from alveolar lavage fluid. [From King and Martin (116).]

rate chemical components of surfactant. The variation in these data was great, however, and there were no statistically significant differences between the rates of clearance of the protein and lipid. The routes of clearance of surfactant from the alveolar lumen are poorly understood, with little more than speculation available concerning the details. Alveolar macrophages take up both components (108, 118, 212), but other pathways for clearance may also exist (67, 77).

The relationship of apolipoprotein B to apolipoprotein A is still in doubt. Both proteins react with antiserum against purified surfactant, but the reaction of apolipoprotein B is always weaker than that of apolipoprotein A. The two proteins form an immunological precipitation pattern of partial identity that suggests a sharing of antigenic determinants. The results of metabolic experiments, however, present complexities that make discerning the exact relationship between the two apolipoproteins difficult; hypotheses in that regard have not been rigorously verified (116). The labeling of apolipoprotein A in lavage fluid is always greater than apolipoprotein B early in the experiment and always lesser at later times (Fig. 10). This behavior is consistent with a precursor-product relationship (219), but these data do not fit all criteria for this model (219). Thus the curves do not cross at exactly the peak activity of apolipoprotein B, nor do the kinetics of decay fit a more sophisticated analysis (168) of a simple first- or higher-order relationship between the precursor and the product. Several explanations of these results exist, and they were

increased with similar kinetics. Maximum labeling of both components occurred ~6 h postinjection, reinforcing the information obtained from experiments on intracellular metabolism, which indicated that both components are secreted at similar rates. The kinetics of the catabolism of saturated phosphatidylcholine and apolipoprotein A may be different, however. The amount of labeled apolipoprotein A decreased to ~75% of maximum after 9 h, whereas the amount of saturated phosphatidylcholine was practically unchanged. By 16 h postinjection the specific activity of apolipoprotein A was ~50% of maximum and was still 85% for saturated phosphatidylcholine. Thus there may be alternative pathways for the catabolism of the sepa-

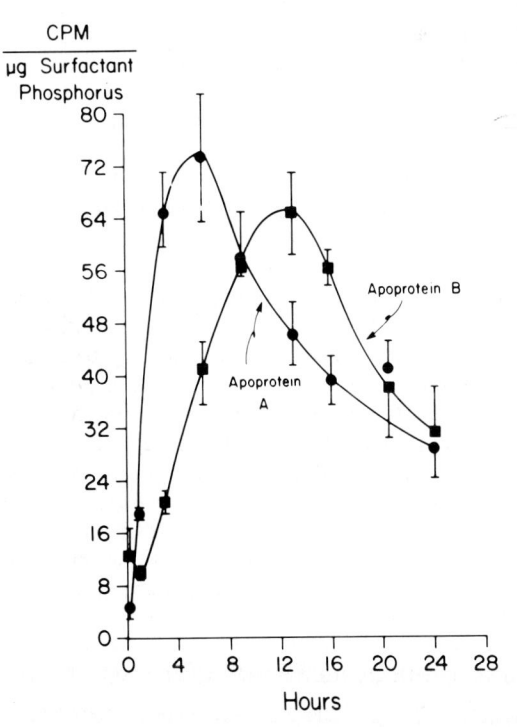

FIG. 10. Labeling of 2 principal proteins in alveolar lavage fluid of rat pulmonary surfactant by radioactive leucine. [From King and Martin (116).]

discussed in detail previously (116). It does appear probable, however, that apolipoprotein B is not metabolized by type II cells in the same manner as other lipid and protein components of surfactant, if indeed it is synthesized by these cells at all (116). It does not appear therefore as an identifiable part of the lipoprotein unit that is secreted into the alveolar subphase. These data do not exclude the possibility that it may be generated within the alveolar lumen from apolipoprotein A.

The results of recent studies (117) indicate that the secretion of lamellar body material did not require the ongoing synthesis of new cellular protein. Near-complete inhibition of cellular protein did not affect either the synthesis or the secretion of surfactant lipid by type II cells in primary culture over an 8-h period. Apparently the content of enzymes required for the synthesis of the lipid components of surfactant was relatively stable over this period, and continual enzyme synthesis was not required. Collet and Chevalier (40) observed some morphological changes in the lamellar bodies in animals given puromycin. Lamellar bodies were smaller and multivesicular bodies were virtually absent. Gail et al. (62) were unable to find functional changes in the pressure-volume characteristics of the lungs of animals 6 h after intraperitoneal injection of cycloheximide; likewise, Holden et al. (92) could not demonstrate any physiological effects 24 h after injecting puromycin. The intracellular residence of lamellar bodies may, however, be longer than 6 h. Extended inhibition of protein synthesis is likely to result in perturbations of synthesis and secretion, even though short-term inhibition can be tolerated. Naturally these effects may reflect nonspecific cell injury, rather than specialized processes associated with the interaction of surfactant lipids and proteins.

COMPARTMENTAL ANALYSIS IN STUDIES OF SURFACTANT TURNOVER

Investigations of the metabolic turnover of surfactant components often require the use of radioactive tracers. The usual protocol used in these studies (184, 188) calls for intravenous injection of a precursor that is then incorporated into one or more surfactant components. Animals are killed at various times after injection, the intracellular and extracellular surfactant components are isolated, and the concentration of isotope in each component (specific activity) measured. The wave of tracer moving through the pools of surfactant is visualized by plotting the specific activities against time. Mathematical analysis of the data allows testing of the precursor-product relationships and the estimation of turnover times.

Many studies of the metabolism of saturated phosphatidylcholine and other surfactant components have used these methods mentioned above (4, 61, 65, 98, 148, 195, 200, 201, 204, 218). Though they vary in details, these investigations conveyed a uniform message: that turnover of surfactant components is rapid, with rates of 10–15 h commonly estimated. One of these studies (218) pointed out the important fact that although saturated phosphatidylcholine is the principal component of lung surfactant, only ~50% of the saturated phosphatidylcholine in lung tissue is apparently associated with surfactant. The interpretation of specific activity–time curves for saturated phosphatidylcholine in lung tissue is therefore correspondingly complex.

As mentioned earlier (see *Relationship Between Protein and Lipid Metabolism*, p. 328) the turnover of two surfactant apoproteins in young dogs was compared with that of saturated phosphatidylcholine in surfactant obtained by lung lavage (118). This study indicated that the 35,000-M_r apoprotein may be the precursor of the 10,000-M_r apoprotein and suggested that the latter, rather hydrophobic protein might be cleared in a complex with surfactant phospholipid, as its half-life rather closely matched that of saturated phosphatidylcholine. Again the turnover time for saturated phosphatidylcholine in alveolar surfactant in dogs was estimated to be ~15 h.

Jobe et al. (99) analyzed specific activity–time curves for phospholipids other than saturated phosphatidylcholine in subcellular fractions and lavage fluid surfactant from rabbit lungs. Half-life values, calculated on the assumption of a pulse-labeled, single-compartment alveolar surfactant pool, were rather long for phosphatidylethanolamine, phosphatidylserine, and phosphatidylinositol, but phosphatidylglycerol and phosphatidylcholine species had shorter half-lives that agreed with the values found by other authors (148, 201) for saturated phosphatidylcholine. Jobe (98) and Young et al. (217) used specific activity–time graphs to determine the half-life of alveolar phospholipids, but they pointed out that alveolar phosphatidylcholines are not pulse labeled and that therefore their calculated half-life values would be too large. This also applies to previous studies of this kind.

To avoid this problem, the specific activity of the precursors to alveolar phospholipids must be accounted for. We modified the method used by Zilversmit et al. (219) for this analysis (11, 132) and applied it to specific activity–time data for lamellar body and alveolar phospholipids. We conclude from this analysis, as did Jacobs et al. (95), that the turnover times of alveolar phospholipids in rabbit lungs are much shorter than previously estimated, ranging from 2 to 7 h. The graphic analysis used in this work makes deviations from simple precursor-product relationships very obvious, and such deviations appear in the plots for lamellar body–alveolar components (11). The most probable explanation for such deviations is that surfactant compartments are stratified, rather than well mixed by diffusion, and consist of various forms of surfactant evolving continuously in a metabolic sequence. For example, lamellar bodies, once started, appear to grow by the accretion of lamellae; in addition alveolar surfactant is observed as tubular myelin, surface film, and vesicular structures under electron microscopy. Separating these forms might facilitate finding the direct precursor-product relationships among them, defining the turnover times of the individual forms, and determining the effects of changes in physiological state on the sizes and compositions of the various forms. Such information would greatly improve our understanding of both the nature and control of surfactant functions. Experiments designed to provide this information must take into account the possibility of extensive recycling of surfactant components, recycling that could make firmly establishing the precursor-product relationships among surfactant forms very difficult. One principal problem would be explaining how type II cells, which occupy only ~3% of the alveolar surface area (209), manage to reabsorb most of the secreted surfactant lipids.

We thank Barbara Ehrlich, Maureen Gallant, and Margaret Moran for their help in preparing this manuscript.

This work was supported in part by grants from the Public Health Service (HL-24075, HL-16725, and HL-19676). John A. Clements is a Career Investigator with the American Heart Association.

REFERENCES

1. ABE, M., AND T. AKINO. Comparison of metabolic heterogeneity of glycerolipids in rat lung and liver. *Tohoku J. Exp. Med.* 106: 343–355, 1972.
2. ABRAMS, M. E. Isolation and quantitative estimation of pulmonary surface-active lipoprotein. *J. Appl. Physiol.* 21: 718–720, 1966.
3. AKINO, T., AND M. ABE. Recent advances on the phospholipid metabolism of the lung: biosynthetic pathways of dipalmitoyl lecithin. A review. *J. Jpn. Med. Soc. Biol. Interface* 8: 2–18, 1977.
4. BALINT, J. A., D. A. BEELER, E. C. KYRIAKIDES, AND D. H. TREBLE. Studies on the biosynthesis of pulmonary surfactant lecithin. *Chest* 67, Suppl. 2: 21S–22S, 1975.
5. BALINT, J. A., E. C. KYRIAKIDES, AND D. A. BEELER. Fatty acid desaturation in lung: inhibition by unsaturated fatty acids. *J. Lipid Res.* 21: 868–873, 1980.
6. BALLARD, P. L., B. J. BENSON, A. BREHIER, J. P. CARTER, B. M. KRIZ, AND E. C. JORGENSEN. Transplacental stimulation of lung development in the fetal rabbit by 3,5-dimethyl-3′-isopropyl-L-thyronine. *J. Clin. Invest.* 65: 1407–1417, 1980.
7. BARANSKA, J., AND L. M. G. VAN GOLDE. Role of lamellar bodies in the biosynthesis of phosphatidylcholine in mouse lung. *Biochim. Biophys. Acta* 488: 285–293, 1977.
8. BARITUSSIO, A., AND J. A. CLEMENTS. Acute effects of pulmonary artery occlusion on the pool of alveolar surfactant. *Respir. Physiol.* 45: 323–331, 1981.
9. BARITUSSIO, A., G. ENZI, D. DE BIASI, M. SCHIAVON, L. ALLEGRA, AND E. M. INELMEN. The elastic properties of the lung in hyperlipidemias. In: *Diabetes, Obesity and Hyperlipidemias*, edited by G. Crepaldi, P. J. Lefebvre, and K. L. M. M. Alberti. London: Academic, 1978, p. 325–329.
10. BARITUSSIO, A., G. ENZI, E. M. INELMAN, M. SCHIAVON, F. DE BIASI, L. ALLEGRA, F. URSINI, AND G. BALDO. Altered surfactant synthesis and function in rats with diet-induced hyperlipidemia. *Metabolism* 29: 503–510, 1980.
11. BARITUSSIO, A. G., M. W. MAGOON, J. GOERKE, AND J. A. CLEMENTS. Precursor-product relationship between rabbit type II cell lamellar bodies and alveolar surface-active material. Surfactant turnover time. *Biochim. Biophys. Acta* 666: 382–393, 1981.
12. BATENBURG, J. J., W. J. LONGMORE, AND L. M. G. VAN GOLDE. The synthesis of phosphatidylcholine by adult rat lung alveolar type II epithelial cells in primary culture. *Biochim. Biophys. Acta* 529: 160–170, 1978.
13. BAXTER, C. F., G. ROUSER, AND G. SIMON. Variations among vertebrates of lung phospholipid class composition. *Lipids* 4: 243–244, 1968.
14. BECKMAN, D. L., AND K. F. MASON. Sympathetic influence on the dynamic lung compliance. *Life Sci.* 12: 43–48, 1973.
15. BENSON, B. J. Properties of an acid phosphatase in pulmonary surfactant. *Proc. Natl. Acad. Sci. USA* 77: 808–811, 1980.
16. BERRY, E. M., J. R. EDMUNDS, AND J. H. WYLLIE. Release of prostaglandin E$_2$ and unidentified factors from ventilated lungs. *Br. J. Surg.* 58: 189–192, 1971.
17. BHATTACHARYYA, S. N., AND W. S. LYNN. Structural characterization of a glycoprotein isolated from alveoli of patients with alveolar proteinosis. *J. Biol. Chem.* 254: 5191–5198, 1979.
18. BHATTACHARYYA, S. N., M. A. PASSERO, R. P. DiAUGUSTINE, AND W. S. LYNN. Isolation and characterization of two hydroxyproline-containing glycoproteins from normal animal lung lavage and lamellar bodies. *J. Clin. Invest.* 55: 914–920, 1975.
19. BHATTACHARYYA, S. N., M. C. ROSE, M. G. LYNN, C. MACLEOD, M. ALBERTS, AND W. S. LYNN. Isolation and characterization of a unique glycoprotein from lavage of chicken lungs and lamellar organelles. *Am. Rev. Respir. Dis.* 114: 843–850, 1976.
20. BOLANDE, R. P., AND M. H. KLAUS. The morphologic demonstration of an alveolar lining layer and its relationship to pulmonary surfactant. *Am. J. Pathol.* 45: 449–463, 1964.
21. BONSEN, P. P. M., G. H. DE HAAS, W. A. PIETERSON, AND L. L. M. VAN DEENEN. Studies on phospholipase A and its zymogen from porcine pancreas. IV. The influence of chemical modification of the lecithin structure on substrate properties. *Biochim. Biophys. Acta* 270: 364–382, 1972.
22. BREHIER, A., B. J. BENSON, M. C. WILLIAMS, R. J. MASON, AND P. L. BALLARD. Corticosteroid induction of phosphatidic acid phosphatase in fetal rabbit lung. *Biochem. Biophys. Res. Commun.* 77: 883–890, 1977.
23. BREMER, J., AND D. M. GREENBERG. Methyl transferring enzyme system of microsomes in the biosynthesis of lecithin (phosphatidylcholine). *Biochim. Biophys. Acta* 46: 205–216, 1961.
24. BROWN, E. S. Isolation and assay of dipalmityl lecithin in lung extracts. *Am. J. Physiol.* 207: 402–406, 1964.
25. BROWN, L. A. S., AND W. J. LONGMORE. Adrenergic and cholinergic regulation of lung surfactant secretion in the isolated perfused rat lung and in the alveolar type II cell in culture. *J. Biol. Chem.* 256: 66–72, 1981.
26. BRUMLEY, G. W., B. TUGGLE, L. LUXNER, AND J. D. CRAPO. Disaturated phosphatidylcholine in rat lungs with altered numbers of type II alveolar epithelial cells. *Am. Rev. Respir. Dis.* 119: 461–470, 1979.
27. BURNELL, J. M., E. C. KYRIAKIDES, R. H. EDMONDS, AND J. A. BALINT. The relationship of fatty acid composition and surface activity of lung extracts. *Respir. Physiol.* 32: 195–206, 1978.
28. BYGRAVE, F. L., AND R. M. C. DAWSON. Phosphatidylcholine biosynthesis and choline transport in the anaerobic protozoon *Entodinium caudatum*. *Biochem. J.* 160: 481–490, 1976.
29. CASOLA, P. G., A. YEUNG, G. F. FELLOWS, AND F. POSSMAYER. Pulmonary phosphatidic acid phosphatase: evidence for a membrane-bound phosphatidic acid-dependent activity associated with the high speed supernatant of rat lung. *Bio-

Chem. Biophys. Res. Commun. 82: 627–633, 1978.
30. CHAPMAN, D., R. M. WILLIAMS, AND B. D. LADBROOKE. Physical studies of phospholipid. VI. Thermotropic and lyotropic mesomorphism of some 1,2-diacylphosphatidylcholines (lecithins). *Chem. Phys. Lipids* 1: 445–475, 1967.
31. CHEVALIER, G., AND A. J. COLLET. In vivo incorporation of choline-^{3}H, leucine-^{3}H, and galactose-^{3}H in alveolar type II pneumonocytes in relation to surfactant synthesis. A quantitative radioautographic study in mouse by electron microscopy. *Anat. Rec.* 174: 289–310, 1972.
32. CHI, E. Y., J. L. PRUEITT, AND D. LAGUNOFF. Abnormal lamellar bodies in type II pneumocytes and increased lung surface active material in the beige mouse (Letter to the editor). *J. Histochem. Cytochem.* 23: 863–868, 1975.
33. CLEMENTS, J. A. Surface phenomena in relation to pulmonary function. *Physiologist* 5: 11–28, 1962.
34. CLEMENTS, J. A. The alveolar lining layer. In: *Development of the Lung*, edited by A. V. S. de Reuck and R. Porter. London: Churchill, 1967, p. 202–237.
35. CLEMENTS, J. A., R. F. HUSTEAD, R. P. JOHNSON, AND I. GRIBETZ. Pulmonary surface tension and alveolar stability. *J. Appl. Physiol.* 16: 444–450, 1961.
36. CLEMENTS, J. A., AND R. J. KING. Composition of surface active material. In: *Lung Biology in Health and Disease. The Biochemical Basis of Pulmonary Function*, edited by R. G. Crystal. New York: Dekker, vol. 2, 1976, p. 363–383.
37. CLEMENTS, J. A., J. NELLENBOGEN, AND H. J. TRAHAN. Pulmonary surfactant and evolution of the lungs. *Science* 169: 603–604, 1970.
38. COLACICCO, G., M. K. BASU, A. K. RAY, M. WITTNER, AND R. M. ROSENBAUM. Effects of prostaglandins E$_2$ and F$_{2\alpha}$ on lecithin biosynthesis by cultured lung cells. *Prostaglandins* 14: 283–294, 1977.
39. COLACICCO, G., A. R. BUCKELEW, JR., AND E. M. SCARPELLI. Protein and lipid-protein fractions of lung washings: chemical characterization. *J. Appl. Physiol.* 34: 743–749, 1973.
40. COLLET, A. J., AND G. CHEVALIER. Morphological aspects of type II alveolar pneumonocytes following treatment with puromycin in vivo. *Am. J. Anat.* 148: 275–294, 1977.
41. COLLINS, J. F., AND R. G. CRYSTAL. Protein synthesis. In: *Lung Biology in Health and Disease. The Biochemical Basis of Pulmonary Function*, edited by R. G. Crystal. New York: Dekker, vol. 2, 1976, p. 171–212.
42. CORBET, A. J. S., P. FLAX, AND A. J. RUDOLPH. Role of autonomic nervous system controlling surface tension in fetal rabbit lungs. *J. Appl. Physiol.: Respirat. Environ. Exercise Physiol.* 43: 1039–1045, 1977.
43. DAVIES, J. T., AND E. K. RIDEAL. *Interfacial Phenomena.* New York: Academic, 1961.
44. DERMER, G. B. The fixation of pulmonary surfactant for electron microscopy. II. Transport of surfactant through the air-blood barrier. *J. Ultrastruct. Res.* 31: 229–246, 1970.
45. DOBBS, L. G., AND R. J. MASON. Pulmonary alveolar type II cells isolated from rats: release of phosphatidylcholine in response to beta-adrenergic stimulation. *J. Clin. Invest.* 63: 378–387, 1978.
46. DUCK-CHONG, C. G. The isolation of lamellar bodies and their membranous content from rat lung, lamb tracheal fluid and human amniotic fluid. *Life Sci.* 22: 2025–2030, 1978.
47. ENGLE, M. J., R. L. SANDERS, AND W. J. LONGMORE. Phospholipid composition and acyl-transferase activity of lamellar bodies isolated from rat lung. *Arch. Biochem. Biophys.* 173: 586–594, 1976.
48. ERBLAND, J. F., AND G. V. MARINETTI. The enzymatic acylation and hydrolysis of lysolecithin. *Biochim. Biophys. Acta* 106: 128–138, 1965.
49. FARIDY, E. E. Effect of food and water deprivation on surface activity of lungs of rats. *J. Appl. Physiol.* 29: 493–498, 1970.
50. FARIDY, E. E. Effect of distension on release of surfactant in excised dogs' lungs. *Respir. Physiol.* 27: 99–114, 1976.
51. FARIDY, E. E., S. PERMUTT, AND R. L. RILEY. Effect of ventilation on surface forces in excised dogs' lungs. *J. Appl. Physiol.* 21: 1453–1462, 1966.
52. FARRELL, P. M. Fetal lung development and the influence of glucocorticoids on pulmonary surfactant. *J. Steroid Biochem.* 8: 463–470, 1977.
53. FARRELL, P. M., D. W. LUNDGREN, AND A. J. ADAMS. Choline kinease and choline phosphotransferase in developing fetal rat lung. *Biochem. Biophys. Res. Commun.* 57: 696–701, 1974.
54. FELDMAN, D. A., C. R. KOVAC, P. L. DRANGINIS, AND P. A. WEINHOLD. The role of phosphatidylglycerol in the activation of CTP:phosphocholine cytidylyltransferase from rat lung. *J. Biol. Chem.* 253: 4980–4986, 1978.
55. FERREIRA, S. H., AND J. R. VANE. Prostaglandins: their disappearance from and release into the circulation. *Nature London* 216: 868–873, 1967.
56. FINLEY, T. N., S. A. PRATT, A. J. LADMAN, L. BREWER, AND M. B. McKAY. Morphological and lipid analysis of the alveolar lining material in dog lung. *J. Lipid Res.* 9: 357–365, 1968.
57. FINLEY, T. N., W. H. TOOLEY, E. W. SWENSON, R. E. GARDNER, AND J. A. CLEMENTS. Pulmonary surface tension in experimental atelectasis. *Am. Rev. Respir. Dis.* 89: 372–378, 1964.
58. FISHER, H. K., M. H. HYMAN, AND S. J. ASHCRAFT. Alveolar surfactant phospholipids are not cleared via trachea (Abstract). *Federation Proc.* 38: 1373, 1979.
59. FORREST, J. B. The effect of hyperventilation on pulmonary surface activity. *Br. J. Anaesth.* 44: 313–320, 1972.
60. FROSOLONO, M. F., B. L. CHARMS, R. PAWLOWSKI, AND S. SLIVKA. Isolation, characterization and surface chemistry of a surface-active fraction from dog lung. *J. Lipid Res.* 11: 439–457, 1970.
61. FUJIWARA, T. Biochemical aspects of pulmonary alveolar surface lining layer. *Acta Pathol. Jpn.* 22: 805–810, 1972.
62. GAIL, D. B., G. D. MASSARO, AND D. MASSARO. Influence of cycloheximide on the lung. *J. Appl. Physiol.* 38: 623–629, 1975.
63. GAIL, D. B., G. D. MASSARO, AND D. MASSARO. Influence of fasting on the lung. *J. Appl. Physiol.: Respirat. Environ. Exercise Physiol.* 42: 88–92, 1977.
64. GALDSTON, M., D. O. SHAH, AND G. Y. SHINOWARA. Isolation and characterization of a lung lipoprotein surfactant. *J. Colloid Interface Sci.* 29: 319–334, 1969.
65. GASSENHEIMER, L. N., AND R. A. RHOADES. Influence of forced ventilation on substrate metabolism in the perfused rat lung. *J. Appl. Physiol.* 37: 224–227, 1974.
66. GASSENHEIMER, L. R., R. A. RHOADES, AND R. W. SCHOLZ. In vivo incorporation of ^{14}C-1-palmitate and ^{3}H-U-glucose into lung lecithin. *Respir. Physiol.* 15: 268–275, 1972.
67. GEIGER, K., M. L. GALLAGHER, AND J. HEDLEY-WHYTE. Cellular distribution and clearance of aerosolized dipalmitoyl lecithin. *J. Appl. Physiol.* 39: 759–766, 1975.
68. GIKAS, E. G., R. J. KING, E. J. MESCHER, A. C. G. PLATZKER, J. A. KITTERMAN, P. L. BALLARD, B. J. BENSON, W. H. TOOLEY, AND J. A. CLEMENTS. Radioimmunoassay of pulmonary surface active material in the tracheal fluid of fetal lamb. *Am. Rev. Respir. Dis.* 115: 587–594, 1977.
69. GIL, J., AND O. K. REISS. Isolation and characterization of lamellar bodies and tubular myelin from rat lung homogenates. *J. Cell Biol.* 58: 152–171, 1973.
70. GODINEZ, R. I., R. L. SANDERS, AND W. J. LONGMORE. Phosphatidylglycerol in rat lung. I. Identification as a metabolically active phospholipid in isolated perfused rat lung. *Biochemistry* 14: 830–834, 1975.
70a.GOERKE, J., AND J. A. CLEMENTS. Alveolar surface tension and lung surfactant. In: *Handbook of Physiology. The Respiratory System. Mechanics of Breathing*, edited by P. T. Macklem and J. Mead. Bethesda, MD: Am. Physiol. Soc., in press.
71. GOLDENBERG, V. E., S. BUCKINGHAM, AND S. C. SOMMERS. Pulmonary alveolar lesions in vagotomized rats. *Lab. Invest.* 16: 693–700, 1967.
72. GOLDENBERG, V. E., S. BUCKINGHAM, AND S. C. SOMMERS. Pilocarpine stimulation of granular pneumocyte secretion.

Lab. Invest. 20: 147–158, 1969.
73. GREENLEAF, R. D., R. J. MASON, AND M. C. WILLIAMS. Isolation of alveolar type II cells by centrifugal elutriation. *In Vitro* 15: 673–684, 1979.
74. GROSS, I. Nutritional and hormonal influences on lung phospholipid metabolism. *Federation Proc.* 36: 2665–2669, 1977.
75. GROSS, I., C. M. WILSON, L. D. INGLESON, A. BREHIER, AND S. A. ROONEY. The influence of hormones on the biochemical development of fetal rat lung in organ culture. I. Estrogen. *Biochim. Biophys. Acta* 575: 375–383, 1979.
76. HALLMAN, M., AND B. L. EPSTEIN. Role of myo-inositol in the synthesis of phosphatidylglycerol and phosphatidylinositol in the lung. *Biochem. Biophys. Res. Commun.* 92: 1151–1159, 1980.
77. HALLMAN, M., B. L. EPSTEIN, AND L. GLUCK. Analysis of labeling and clearance of lung surfactant phospholipids in rabbit. Evidence of bidirectional surfactant flux between lamellar bodies and alveolar lavage. *J. Clin. Invest.* 68: 742–751, 1981.
78. HALLMAN, M., AND L. GLUCK. Phosphatidylglycerol in lung surfactant. II. Subcellular distribution and mechanism of biosynthesis in vitro. *Biochim. Biophys. Acta* 409: 172–191, 1975.
79. HALLMAN, M., AND L. GLUCK. Phosphatidylglycerol in lung surfactant. III. Possible modifier of surfactant function. *J. Lipid Res.* 17: 257–262, 1976.
80. HAMOSH, M., AND P. HAMOSH. The effect of prolactin on the lecithin content of fetal rabbit lung. *J. Clin. Invest.* 59: 1001–1005, 1977.
81. HASS, M. A., AND W. J. LONGMORE. Surfactant cholesterol metabolism of the isolated perfused rat lung. *Biochim. Biophys. Acta* 573: 166–174, 1979.
82. HASSETT, R. J., R. L. SANDERS, A. E. VATTER, AND O. K. REISS. Lamellar bodies: isolation from rat lung, stability and conversion to tubular myelin figures (Abstract). *Federation Proc.* 36: 615, 1977.
83. HEATH, M. F., AND W. JACOBSON. Phospholipases A_1 and A_2 in lamellar inclusion bodies of the alveolar epithelium of rabbit lung. *Biochim. Biophys. Acta* 441: 443–452, 1976.
84. HEDQVIST, P. Basic mechanisms of prostaglandin action on autonomic neurotransmission. *Annu. Rev. Pharmacol. Toxicol.* 17: 259–279, 1977.
85. HEPPLESTON, A. G., K. FLETCHER, AND I. WYATT. Abnormalities of lung lipids following inhalation of quartz. *Experientia* 28: 938–939, 1972.
86. HILDEBRAN, J. N., J. GOERKE, AND J. A. CLEMENTS. Pulmonary surface film stability and composition. *J. Appl. Physiol.: Respirat. Environ. Exercise Physiol.* 47: 604–611, 1979.
87. HILDEBRAN, J. N., J. GOERKE, AND J. A. CLEMENTS. Surfactant release in excised rat lung is stimulated by air inflation. *J. Appl. Physiol.: Respirat. Environ. Exercise Physiol.* 51: 905–910, 1981.
88. HILL, P. Effect of a cholesterol-biosynthesis inhibitor on the fatty acid composition of phospholipids in the serum and tissue of rats. *Biochem. J.* 98: 696–701, 1966.
89. HILL, P., AND E. GRESELIN. Lung phospholipids: biochemical and histologic changes induced by the cholesterol-biosynthesis inhibitor AY-9944. *Toxicol. Appl. Pharmacol.* 11: 245–256, 1967.
90. HIRATA, F., AND J. AXELROD. Phospholipid methylation and biological signal transmission. *Science* 209: 1082–1090, 1980.
91. HOFFMAN, L. Isolation and inclusion bodies from rabbit lung parenchyma. *J. Cell Physiol.* 79: 65–72, 1972.
92. HOLDEN, K. R., W. R. HARLAN, JR., AND S. SAID. Failure of near-lethal inhibition of protein synthesis to alter pulmonary surfactant. *Johns Hopkins Med. J.* 126: 337–343, 1970.
93. HONG, S. C., R. POLSKY-CYNKIN, AND L. LEVINE. Stimulation of prostaglandin biosynthesis by vasoactive substances in methylcholanthrene-transformed mouse BALB/3T3. *J. Biol. Chem.* 251: 776–780, 1976.
94. HUNG, K. S., M. S. HERTWECK, J. D. HARDY, AND C. G. LOOSLI. Innervation of pulmonary alveoli of the mouse lung: an electron microscopic study. *Am. J. Anat.* 135: 477–496, 1972.
95. JACOBS, H., A. JOBE, M. IKEGAMI, AND S. JONES. Surfactant phosphatidylcholine source, fluxes, and turnover times in 3-day-old, 10-day-old, and adult rabbits. *J. Biol. Chem.* 257: 1805–1810, 1982.
96. JAIN, M. K. Role of cholesterol in biomembranes and related systems. *Curr. Top. Membr. Transp.* 6: 1–57, 1975.
97. JIMENEZ, J. M., AND J. M. JOHNSTON. Fetal lung maturation. IV. The release of phosphatidic acid phosphohydrolase and phospholipids into human amniotic fluid. *Pediatr. Res.* 10: 767–769, 1976.
98. JOBE, A. The labelling and biological half-life of phosphatidylcholine in subcellular fractions of rabbit lung. *Biochim. Biophys. Acta* 489: 440–453, 1977.
99. JOBE, A., E. KIRKPATRICK, AND L. GLUCK. Labelling of phospholipids in the surfactant and subcellular fractions of rabbit lung. *J. Biol. Chem.* 253: 3810–3816, 1978.
100. JOBE, A., A. KIRKPATRICK, AND L. GLUCK. Lecithin appearance and apparent biologic half-life in term newborn rabbit lung. *Pediatr. Res.* 12: 669–675, 1978.
101. KATYAL, S. L., AND B. LOMBARDI. Effects of dietary choline and N,N-dimethylaminoethanol on lung phospholipid and surfactant of newborn rats. *Pediatr. Res.* 12: 952–955, 1978.
102. KATYAL, S. L., AND G. SINGH. An immunological study of the apoproteins of rat lung surfactant. *Lab. Invest.* 40: 562–567, 1979.
103. KENNEDY, E. P. The metabolism and function of complex lipids. *Harvey Lect.* 57: 143–171, 1962.
104. KHOSLA, S. S., L. I. GOBRAN, AND S. A. ROONEY. Stimulation of phosphatidylcholine synthesis by 17β-estradiol in fetal rabbit lung. *Biochim. Biophys. Acta* 617: 282–290, 1980.
105. KIKKAWA, Y., AND E. MOTOYAMA. Effect of AY-9944, a cholesterol biosynthesis inhibitor, on fetal lung development and on the development of type II alveolar epithelial cells. *Lab. Invest.* 28: 48–54, 1973.
106. KIKKAWA, Y., AND K. YONEDA. The type II epithelial cell of the lung. I. Method of isolation. *Lab. Invest.* 30: 76–84, 1974.
107. KING, R. J. The surfactant system of the lung. *Federation Proc.* 33: 2238–2247, 1974.
108. KING, R. J. Metabolic fate of the apoproteins of pulmonary surfactant. *Am. Rev. Respir. Dis.* 115: 587–593, 1977.
109. KING, R. J. Utilization of alveolar epithelial type II cells for the study of pulmonary surfactant. *Federation Proc.* 38: 2637–2643, 1979.
110. KING, R. J., AND J. A. CLEMENTS. Surface active materials from dog lung. I. Method of isolation. *Am. J. Physiol.* 223: 707–714, 1972.
111. KING, R. J., AND J. A. CLEMENTS. Surface active materials from dog lung. II. Composition and physiological correlations. *Am. J. Physiol.* 223: 715–726, 1972.
112. KING, R. J., E. G. GIKAS, J. RUCH, AND J. A. CLEMENTS. The radioimmunoassay of pulmonary surface active material in sheep lung. *Am. Rev. Respir. Dis.* 110: 273–281, 1974.
113. KING, R. J., D. J. KLASS, E. G. GIKAS, AND J. A. CLEMENTS. Isolation of the apoproteins from canine surface active material. *Am. J. Physiol.* 224: 788–795, 1973.
114. KING, R. J., AND M. C. MACBETH. Physico-chemical properties of dipalmitoyl phosphatidylcholine after interaction with an apoprotein of pulmonary surfactant. *Biochim. Biophys. Acta* 557: 86–101, 1979.
115. KING, R. J., AND M. C. MACBETH. Interaction of the lipid and protein components of pulmonary surfactant. Role of phosphatidylglycerol and calcium. *Biochim. Biophys. Acta* 647: 159–168, 1981.
116. KING, R. J., AND H. MARTIN. Intracellular metabolism of the apoproteins of pulmonary surfactant in rat lung. *J. Appl. Physiol.: Respirat. Environ. Exercise Physiol.* 48: 812–820, 1980.
117. KING, R. J., AND H. MARTIN. Effects of inhibiting protein synthesis on the secretion of surfactant by type II cells in

primary culture. *Biochim. Biophys. Acta* 663: 289–301, 1981.
118. KING, R. J., H. MARTIN, D. MITTS, AND F. M. HOLMSTROM. Metabolism of the apoproteins in pulmonary surfactant. *J. Appl. Physiol.: Respirat. Environ. Exercise Physiol.* 42: 483–491, 1977.
119. KING, R. J., J. RUCH, E. G. GIKAS, A. C. G. PLATZKER, AND R. K. CREASY. Appearance of apoproteins of pulmonary surfactant in human amniotic fluid. *J. Appl. Physiol.* 39: 735–741, 1975.
120. KLEIN, R. M., AND S. MARGOLIS. Purification of pulmonary surfactant by ultracentrifugation. *J. Appl. Physiol.* 25: 654–658, 1968.
121. KOTAS, R. V., AND M. E. AVERY. Accelerated appearance of pulmonary surfactant in the fetal rabbit. *J. Appl. Physiol.* 30: 358–361, 1971.
122. KUHN, C. The cells of the lung and their organelles. In: *Lung Biology in Health and Disease. The Biochemical Basis of Pulmonary Functon*, edited by R. G. Crystal. New York: Dekker, vol. 2, 1976, p. 3–48.
123. KUHN, C., F. GYÖRKEY, B. E. LEVINE, AND J. RAMIREZ-R. Pulmonary alveolar proteinosis. A study using enzyme histochemistry, electron microscopy, and surface tension measurement. *Lab. Invest.* 15: 492–509, 1966.
124. KYRIAKIDES, E. C., D. A. BEELER, R. H. EDMONDS, AND J. A. BALINT. Alterations in phosphatidylcholine species and their reversal in pulmonary surfactant during essential fatty-acid deficiency. *Biochim. Biophys. Acta* 431: 399–407, 1976.
125. LANDS, W. E. M. Metabolism of glycerolipids. II. The enzymatic acylation of lysolecithin. *J. Biol. Chem.* 235: 2233–2237, 1960.
126. LAU, M.-J., AND K. M. W. KEOUGH. Lipid composition of lung and lung lavage fluid from map turtles (*Malaclemys geographica*) maintained at different environmental temperatures. *Can. J. Biochem.* 59: 208–219, 1981.
127. LAWSON, E. E., E. R. BROWN, J. S. TORDAY, H. W. MADANSKY, AND D. L. TAEUSCH, JR. The effect of epinephrine on tracheal fluid flow and surfactant efflux in fetal sheep. *Am. Rev. Respir. Dis.* 118: 1023–1026, 1978.
128. LIGGINS, G. C. Premature parturition after infusion of corticotrophin or cortisol into foetal lambs. *J. Endocrinol.* 42: 323–329, 1968.
129. LIGGINS, G. C., J. A. KITTERMAN, G. A. CAMPOS, J. A. CLEMENTS, C. S. FORSTER, C. H. LEE, AND R. K. CREASY. Pulmonary maturation in the hypophysectomised ovine fetus. Differential responses to adrenocorticotrophin and cortisol. *J. Dev. Physiol.* 3: 1–14, 1981.
130. LONGMORE, W. J., V. OLDENBORG, AND L. M. G. VAN GOLDE. Phospholipase A_2 in rat-lung microsomes: substrate specificity towards endogenous phosphatidylcholines. *Biochim. Biophys. Acta* 572: 452–460, 1979.
131. LYNN, W. S., S. C. SAHU, AND S. N. BHATTACHARYYA. Secretory alveolar glycoproteins (alveolyns). In: *Le lavage bronchoalvéolaire chez l'homme*, edited by G. Biserte, J. Chrétien, and C. Voisin. Paris: INSERM, 1979, p. 17–26.
132. MAGOON, M. W., A. G. BARITUSSIO, J. GOERKE, AND J. A. CLEMENTS. Precursor-product (PP) relationship between rabbit type II cell lamellar bodies (LB) and alveolar surface active material (SAM) and SAM turnover time (τ) (Abstract). *Federation Proc.* 40: 407, 1981.
133. MASON, R. J. Lipid metabolism. In: *Lung Biology in Health and Disease. The Biochemical Basis of Pulmonary Function*, edited by R. G. Crystal. New York: Dekker, vol. 2, 1976, p. 127–169.
134. MASON, R. J., AND L. G. DOBBS. Synthesis of phosphatidylcholine and phosphatidylglycerol by alveolar type II cells in primary culture. *J. Biol. Chem.* 255: 5101–5107, 1980.
135. MASON, R. J., G. HUBER, AND M. VAUGHAN. Synthesis of dipalmitoyl lecithin by alveolar macrophages. *J. Clin. Invest.* 51: 68–73, 1972.
136. MASON, R. J., M. C. WILLIAMS, R. D. GREENLEAF, AND J. A. CLEMENTS. Isolation and properties of type II alveolar cells from rat lung. *Am. Rev. Respir. Dis.* 115: 1015–1026, 1977.

137. MASSARO, D. In vivo protein secretion by lung. Evidence for active secretion and interspecies differences. *J. Clin. Invest.* 56: 263–271, 1975.
138. MASSARO, D., AND G. D. MASSARO. Synthesis, intracellular transport, and secretion of macromolecules by the lung. In: *Lung Biology in Health and Disease. The Biochemical Basis of Pulmonary Function*, edited by R. G. Crystal. New York: Dekker, vol. 2, 1976, p. 389–416.
139. MCCLENAHAN, J. B., AND A. URTNOWSKI. Effect of ventilation on surfactant, and its turnover rate. *J. Appl. Physiol.* 23: 215–220, 1967.
140. MEAD, J., AND C. COLLIER. Relation of volume history of lungs to respiratory mechanics in anesthetized dogs. *J. Appl. Physiol.* 14: 669–678, 1959.
141. MESCHER, E. J., A. C. G. PLATZKER, P. L. BALLARD, J. A. KITTERMAN, J. A. CLEMENTS, AND W. H. TOOLEY. Ontogeny of tracheal fluid, pulmonary surfactant, and plasma corticoids in the fetal lamb. *J. Appl. Physiol.* 39: 1017–1021, 1975.
142. METCALFE, I. L., G. ENHORNING, AND F. POSSMAYER. Pulmonary surfactant-associated proteins: their role in the expression of surface activity. *J. Appl. Physiol.: Respirat. Environ. Exercise Physiol.* 49: 34–41, 1980.
143. MEYRICK, B., AND L. REID. Nerves in rat intra-acinar alveoli: an electron microscopic study. *Respir. Physiol.* 11: 367–377, 1971.
144. MORGAN, T. E. Isolation and characterization of lipid N-methyl-transferase from dog lung. *Biochim. Biophys. Acta* 178: 21–34, 1969.
145. MORGAN, T. E., AND B. C. MORGAN. Surfactant synthesis, storage, and release by alveolar cells. In: *Respiratory Distress Syndrome*, edited by C. A. Villee, D. B. Villee, and J. Zuckerman. New York: Academic, 1973, p. 117–127.
146. MUNDER, P. G., M. MODOLLEL, E. FERBER, AND H. FISCHER. The relationship between macrophages and adjuvant activity. In: *Mononuclear Phagocytes*, edited by R. van Furth. Oxford, UK: Blackwell, 1970, p. 445–460.
147. NAIMARK, A. Pulmonary blood flow and the incorporation of palmitate-I-C^{14} by dog lung in vivo. *J. Appl. Physiol.* 21: 1292–1298, 1966.
148. NAIMARK, A. Cellular dynamics and lipid metabolism in the lung. *Federation Proc.* 32: 1967–1971, 1973.
149. NIELSEN, H. C., AND J. S. TORDAY. Sex differences in fetal rabbit pulmonary surfactant production. *Pediatr. Res.* 15: 1245–1247, 1981.
150. NIELSEN, H. C., H. M. ZINMAN, AND J. S. TORDAY. Dihydrotestosterone (DHT) inhibits fetal pulmonary surfactant production in vivo. *Pediatr. Res.* 15: 728, 1981.
151. OHNO, K., T. AKINO, AND T. FUJIWARA. Phospholipid metabolism in perinatal lung. In: *Reviews in Perinatal Medicine*, edited by E. M. Scarpelli and E. V. Cosmi. New York: Raven, 1978, p. 227–318.
152. OLDENBORG, V., AND L. M. G. VAN GOLDE. Activity of cholinephosphotransferase, lysolecithin:lysolecithin acyltransferase and lysolecithin acyltransferase in the developing mouse lung. *Biochim. Biophys. Acta* 441: 433–442, 1976.
153. OLDENBORG, V., AND L. M. G. VAN GOLDE. The enzymes of phosphatidylcholine biosynthesis in the fetal mouse lung. Effects of dexamethasone. *Biochim. Biophys. Acta* 489: 454–465, 1977.
154. OLSEN, D. B. Neurohumoral-hormonal secretory stimulation of pulmonary surfactant in the rat (Abstract). *Physiologist* 15: 230, 1972.
155. OP DEN KAMP, J. A. F., M. T. KAUERZ, AND L. L. M. VAN DEENEN. Action of pancreatic phospholipase A_2 on phosphatidylcholine bilayers in different physical states. *Biochim. Biophys. Acta* 406: 169–177, 1975.
156. OYARZÚN, M. J., AND J. A. CLEMENTS. Ventilatory and cholinergic control of pulmonary surfactant in the rabbit. *J. Appl. Physiol.: Respirat. Environ. Exercise Physiol.* 43: 39–45, 1977.
157. OYARZÚN, M. J., AND J. A. CLEMENTS. Control of lung surfactant by ventilation, adrenergic mediators, and prostaglandins in the rabbit. *Am. Rev. Respir. Dis.* 117: 879–891, 1978.

158. OYARZÚN, M. J., J. A. CLEMENTS, AND A. BARITUSSIO. Ventilation enhances pulmonary alveolar clearance of radioactive dipalmitoyl phosphatidylcholine in liposomes. *Am. Rev. Respir. Dis.* 121: 709–721, 1980.

159. PAGANO, R. E., AND J. N. WEINSTEIN. Interactions of liposomes with mammalian cells. *Annu. Rev. Biophys. Bioeng.* 7: 435–468, 1978.

160. PAGE-ROBERTS, B. A. Preparation and partial characterization of a lamellar body fraction from rat lung. *Biochim. Biophys. Acta* 260: 334–338, 1972.

161. PAPAHADJOPOULOS, D., G. POSTE, AND B. E. SCHAEFFER. Fusion of mammalian cells of unilamellar lipid vesicles: influence of lipid surface charge, fluidity and cholesterol. *Biochim. Biophys. Acta* 323: 23–42, 1973.

162. PASSERO, M. A., R. W. TYE, K. H. KILBURN, AND W. S. LYNN. Isolation and characterization of two glycoproteins from patients with alveolar proteinosis. *Proc. Natl. Acad. Sci. USA* 70: 973–976, 1973.

163. PFLEGER, R. C., AND H. G. THOMAS. Beagle dog pulmonary surfactant lipids. *Arch. Intern. Med.* 127: 863–872, 1971.

164. PLATZKER, A. C. G., J. A. KITTERMAN, E. J. MESCHER, J. A. CLEMENTS, AND W. H. TOOLEY. Surfactant in the lung and tracheal fluid of the fetal lamb and acceleration of its appearance by dexamethasone. *Pediatrics* 56: 554–561, 1975.

165. POSSMAYER, F., P. CASOLA, F. CHANG, S. HILL, I. L. METCALF, P. J. STEWART-DEHAAN, T. WONG, J. LAS HERAS, E. B. GAMMAL, AND P. G. HARDING. Glucocorticoid induction of pulmonary maturation in the rabbit fetus. The effect of maternal injection of betamethasone on the activity of enzymes in fetal lung. *Biochim. Biophys. Acta* 574: 197–211, 1979.

166. PRATT, S. A., T. N. FINLEY, M. H. SMITH, AND A. J. LADMAN. A comparison of alveolar macrophages and pulmonary surfactant(?) obtained from the lung of human smokers and nonsmokers by endobronchial lavage. *Anat. Rec.* 163: 497–508, 1969.

167. RAMIREZ-R, J., AND W. R. HARLAN, JR. Pulmonary alveolar proteinosis. Nature and origin of alveolar lipid. *Am. J. Med.* 45: 502–512, 1968.

168. RESCIGNO, A., AND G. SEGRE. *Drug and Tracer Kinetics*. Waltham, MA: Blaisdell, 1966.

169. RHOADES, R. A. Influence of starvation on the lung: effect on glucose and palmitate utilization. *J. Appl. Physiol.* 38: 513–516, 1975.

170. ROONEY, S. A., P. M. CANAVAN, AND E. K. MOTOYAMA. The identification of phosphatidylglycerol in the rat, rabbit, monkey, and human lung. *Biochim. Biophys. Acta* 360: 56–57, 1974.

171. ROONEY, S. A., L. GOBRAN, I. GROSS, T. S. WAI-LEE, L. L. NARDONE, AND E. S. MOTOYAMA. Studies on pulmonary surfactant. Effects of cortisol administration on lung phospholipid content, composition, and biosynthesis. *Biochim. Biophys. Acta* 450: 121–130, 1976.

172. ROONEY, S. A., P. A. MARINO, L. I. GOBRAN, I. GROSS, AND J. B. WARSHAW. Thyrotropin-releasing hormone increases the amount of surfactant in lung lavage from fetal rabbits. *Pediatr. Res.* 13: 623–625, 1979.

173. ROONEY, S. A., B. A. PAGE-ROBERTS, AND E. K. MOTOYAMA. Role of lamellar inclusions in surfactant production: studies on phospholipid composition and biosynthesis in rat and rabbit lung subcellular fractions. *J. Lipid Res.* 16: 418–425, 1975.

174. ROONEY, S. A., T. S. WAI-LEE, L. GOBRAN, AND E. K. MOTOYAMA. Phospholipid content, composition, and biosynthesis during fetal lung development in the rabbit. *Biochim. Biophys. Acta* 431: 447–458, 1976.

175. ROSEN, S. H., B. CASTLEMAN, AND A. A. LIEBOW. Pulmonary alveolar proteinosis. *N. Engl. J. Med.* 258: 1123–1142, 1958.

176. RYAN, J. W., R. S. NIEMEYER, AND U. RYAN. Metabolism of prostaglandin $F_{1\alpha}$ in the pulmonary circulation. *Prostaglandins* 10: 101–108, 1975.

177. SAHU, S., R. P. DIAUGUSTINE, AND W. S. LYNN. Lipids found in pulmonary lavage of patients with alveolar proteinosis and in rabbit lung lamellar organelles. *Am. Rev. Respir. Dis.* 114: 177–185, 1976.

178. SAID, S. I., W. R. HARLAN, JR., G. W. BURKE, AND C. M. ELLIOTT. Surface tension, metabolic activity, and lipid composition of alveolar cells in washings from normal dog lungs and after pulmonary artery ligation. *J. Clin. Invest.* 47: 336–343, 1968.

179. SAID, S. I., S. KITAMURA, AND C. VREIM. Prostaglandins: release from the lung during mechanical ventilation at large tidal volumes. *J. Clin. Invest.* 51: 83a–84a, 1972.

180. SAUNDERS, B. S., J. W. SHEPARD, JR., A. JOBE, K. MIYAI, K. M. MOSER, AND L. GLUCK. Alveolar CO_2 tension as a mediator of lamellar body release in experimental left pulmonary artery occlusion. *Chest* 72: 411–412, 1977.

181. SCARPELLI, E. M., S. CONDORELLI, G. COLACICCO, AND E. COSMI. Lamb fetal pulmonary fluid. II. Fate of phosphatidylcholine. *Pediatr. Res.* 9: 195–201, 1975.

182. SCHNEIDER, W. J., AND D. E. VANCE. Effect of choline deficiency on the enzymes that synthesize phosphatidylcholine and phosphatidylethanolamine in rat liver. *Eur. J. Biochem.* 85: 181–187, 1978.

183. SCHOLZ, R. W., B. M. WOODWARD, AND R. A. RHOADES. Utilization in vitro and in vivo of glucose and glycerol by rat lung. *Am. J. Physiol.* 223: 991–996, 1972.

184. SEARLE, G. L. The use of isotope turnover techniques in the study of carbohydrate metabolism in man. *Clin. Endocrinol. Metab.* 5: 783–804, 1976.

185. SEVERINGHAUS, J. W., E. W. SWENSON, T. N. FINLEY, M. T. LATEGOLA, AND J. WILLIAMS. Unilateral hypoventilation produced in dogs by occluding one pulmonary artery. *J. Appl. Physiol.* 16: 53–60, 1961.

186. SHELLEY, S. A., M. V. L'HEUREUX, AND J. U. BALIS. Characterization of lung surfactant factors promoting formation of artifactual lipid-protein complexes. *J. Lipid Res.* 16: 224–234, 1975.

187. SHEPARD, C. W. *Basic Principles of the Tracer Method*. New York: Wiley, 1962.

188. SHEPARD, J. W., JR., K. MIYAI, AND K. M. MOSER. Depletion and repletion of lamellar bodies from type II alveolar pneumocytes following unilateral pulmonary artery balloon occlusion (U.P.A.B.O.) and reperfusion (Abstract). *Federation Proc.* 36: 541, 1977.

189. SMITH, D. S., U. SMITH, AND J. W. RYAN. Freeze-fractured lamellar body membranes of the rat lung great alveolar cell. *Tissue Cell* 4: 457–468, 1972.

190. SMITH, F. B., AND Y. KIKKAWA. The type II epithelial cells of the lung. V. Synthesis of phosphatidylglycerol in isolated type II cells and pulmonary alveolar macrophages. *Lab. Invest.* 40: 172–177, 1980.

191. SMITH, F. B., Y. KIKKAWA, C. A. DIGLIO, AND R. C. DALEN. The type II epithelial cells of the lung. VI. Incorporation of ^3H-choline and ^3H-palmitate into lipids of cultured type II cells. *Lab. Invest.* 42: 296–301, 1980.

192. SMITH, R., AND C. TANFORD. The critical micelle concentration of L-α-dipalmitoylphosphatidylcholine in water and water-methanol solutions. *J. Mol. Biol.* 67: 75–83, 1972.

193. SPICER, S., A. SATO, R. VINCENT, M. EGUCHI, AND K. C. POON. Lysosome enlargement in the Chediak-Higashi syndrome. *Federation Proc.* 40: 1451–1455, 1981.

194. SPITZER, H. L., AND J. M. JOHNSTON. Characterization of phosphatidate phosphohydrolase activity associated with isolated lamellar bodies. *Biochim. Biophys. Acta* 531: 275–285, 1978.

195. SPITZER, H. L., AND J. R. NORMAN. The biosynthesis and turnover of surfactant lecithin and protein. *Arch. Intern. Med.* 127: 429–435, 1971.

196. STERN, W., C. KOVAC, AND P. A. WEINHOLD. Activity and properties of CTP:choline phosphate cytidylyltransferase in adult and fetal rat lung. *Biochim. Biophys. Acta* 441: 280–293, 1976.

197. STRATTON, C. J. The three-dimensional aspect of mammalian lung multi-lamellar bodies. *Tissue Cell* 8: 693–712, 1976.

198. SUEISHI, K., AND B. J. BENSON. Isolation of a major apoprotein of canine and murine pulmonary surfactant: biochemical

and immunochemical characteristics. *Biochim. Biophys. Acta* 665: 442–453, 1981.
199. THET, L. A., L. B. CLERCH, AND D. MASSARO. Relation of changes in sedimentation of surfactant(s) to volume history of lungs and changes in respiratory mechanics (Abstract). *Clin. Res.* 26: 455A, 1978.
200. THOMAS, T., JR., AND R. A. RHOADES. Incorporation of palmitate-1-^{14}C into lung tissue and "alveolar" lecithin. *Am. J. Physiol.* 219: 1535–1538, 1970.
201. TIERNEY, D. F., J. A. CLEMENTS, AND H. J. TRAHAN. Rates of replacement of lecithin and alveolar instability in rat lungs. *Am. J. Physiol.* 213: 671–676, 1967.
202. TOOLEY, W., R. GARDNER, N. THUNG, AND T. FINLEY. Factors affecting the surface tension of lung extracts (Abstract). *Federation Proc.* 20: 428, 1961.
203. TORDAY, J. S., H. C. NIELSEN, M. DE M. FENCL, AND M. E. AVERY. Sex differences in fetal lung maturation. *Am. Rev. Respir. Dis.* 123: 205–208, 1981.
204. TOSHIMA, N., T. AKINO, AND K. OHNO. Turnover time of lecithin in lung tissue and alveolar wash of rat. *Tohoku J. Exp. Med.* 108: 265–277, 1972.
205. VANCE, D. E., AND P. C. CHOY. How is phosphatidylcholine biosynthesis regulated? *Trends Biochem. Sci.* 4: 145–148, 1979.
206. VANCE, D. E., E. M. TRIP, AND H. B. PADDON. Poliovirus increases phosphatidylcholines biosynthesis in HeLa cells by stimulation of the rate-limiting reaction catalyzed by CTP:phosphocholine cytidylyltransferase. *J. Biol. Chem.* 255: 1064–1069, 1980.
207. VAN GOLDE, L. M. G. Metabolism of phospholipids in the lung. *Am. Rev. Respir. Dis.* 114: 977–1000, 1976.
208. WEBB, H. H., AND D. F. TIERNEY. Experimental pulmonary edema due to intermittent positive pressure ventilation with high inflation pressures. Protection by positive end-expiratory pressure. *Am. Rev. Respir. Dis.* 110: 556–565, 1974.
209. WEIBEL, E. R., P. GEHR, D. HAIES, J. GIL, AND M. BACHOFEN. The cell population of the normal lung. In: *Lung Cells in Disease*, edited by A. Bouhuys. Amsterdam: Elsevier, 1976, p. 3–16.
210. WILLIAMS, M. C. Conversion of lamellar body membranes into tubular myelin in alveoli of fetal rat lungs. *J. Cell Biol.* 72: 260–277, 1977.
211. WILLIAMS, M. C. Freeze-fracture studies of tubular myelin and lamellar bodies in fetal and adult rat lungs. *J. Ultrastruct. Res.* 44: 352–361, 1978.
212. WILLIAMS, M. C., AND B. J. BENSON. Immunocytochemical localization and identification of the major surfactant protein in adult rat lung. *J. Histochem. Cytochem.* 29: 291–305, 1981.
213. WYSZOGRODSKI, I., K. KYEI-ABOAGYE, H. W. TAEUSCH, JR., AND M. E. AVERY. Surfactant inactivation by hyperventilation: conservation by end-expiratory pressure. *J. Appl. Physiol.* 38: 461–466, 1975.
214. WYSZOGRODSKI, I., AND H. W. TAEUSCH, JR. Prolonged sympathetic activation and pulmonary surfactant: absence of effect in anesthetized cats. *Am. Rev. Respir. Dis.* 111: 619–622, 1975.
215. WYSZOGRODSKI, I., H. W. TAEUSCH, JR., AND M. E. AVERY. Isoxsuprine induced alterations of pulmonary pressure-volume relationships in premature rabbits. *Am. J. Obstet. Gynecol.* 119: 1107–1111, 1974.
216. YEAGLE, P. L., R. B. MARTIN, A. K. LALA, H. LIN, AND K. BLOCK. Differential effects of cholesterol and lanosterol on artificial membranes. *Proc. Natl. Acad. Sci. USA* 74: 4924–4926, 1977.
217. YOUNG, S. L., S. A. KREMERS, J. S. APPLE, J. D. CRAPO, AND G. W. BRUMLEY. Rat lung surfactant kinetics: biochemical and morphometric correlation. *J. Appl. Physiol.: Respirat. Environ. Exercise Physiol.* 51: 248–253, 1981.
218. YOUNG, S. L., AND D. F. TIERNEY. Dipalmitoyl lecithin secretion and metabolism by the rat lung. *Am. J. Physiol.* 222: 1539–1544, 1972.
219. ZILVERSMIT, D. B., C. ENTENMAN, AND M. FISHLER. On the calculation of "turnover time" and "turnover rate" from experiments involving the use of labeled agents. *J. Gen. Physiol.* 26: 325–331, 1942.

CHAPTER 9

5-Hydroxytryptamine and other amines in the lungs

ALAIN F. JUNOD | *Department of Medicine, University of Geneva, Hospital Cantonal, Geneva, Switzerland*

CHAPTER CONTENTS

5-Hydroxytryptamine Uptake
    Characterization of uptake process
    Localization of uptake process
    Monoamine oxidases of pulmonary endothelial cells
    Pharmacological inhibition of uptake process
    Efflux of accumulated 5-hydroxytryptamine
    Uptake in isolated and cultured endothelial cells
    Uptake and platelet-lung relationships
    Uptake by the lung and pharmacological action of
        5-hydroxytryptamine on pulmonary circulation
Norepinephrine Uptake
    Characterization of uptake process
    Localization of uptake process
    l-Norepinephrine uptake by isolated endothelial cells
    l-Norepinephrine uptake by the lung: uptake 1 (neuronal) or
        uptake 2 (extraneuronal)
Effects of Experimental and Clinical Conditions on
    5-Hydroxytryptamine and Norepinephrine Uptake
    Experimental conditions
        Anesthesia
        Monocrotaline
        Paraquat
        α-Naphthylthiourea
        Hyperoxia
        Cigarette smoke
        Spontaneous hypertension in rats
    Application to human clinical problems
Other Naturally Occurring Catecholamines
    β-Phenylethylamine
    Dopamine
    Epinephrine
    Octopamine
Sympathomimetic Drugs
    Metaraminol
    Isoprenaline
    Mescaline
Histamine
Uptake of Basic Amines by the Lung
Conclusion

INACTIVATION OF CIRCULATING vasoactive substances was first described by Eichholtz and Verney (34) in 1924. They found that the pressure rise in kidneys perfused with shed blood disappeared if a heart-lung preparation was included in the perfusion circuit. Hence they suggested that the lungs were able to remove a vasoconstrictor agent from the circulation, which years later turned out to be 5-hydroxytryptamine (5-HT), or serotonin. No further study ensued until Gaddum et al. (42) in 1953 demonstrated that perfused cat lungs inactivated circulating 5-HT. Axelrod and Inscoe (6) noted a decade later that 1 min after intravenous injection of labeled 5-HT the highest amount of radioactivity retained by various organs per gram of tissue was in the lung. From 1964 to 1967 several investigators, using different techniques and experimental protocols, independently reconsidered this problem. Eiseman et al. (35) perfused isolated dog lungs and observed a progressive decrease, over time, in the medium 5-HT concentration and the appearance of the deaminated product, 5-hydroxyindoleacetic acid (5-HIAA). Davis and Wang (32) injected boluses of radioactive 5-HT into living dogs and found that ~33% of the initial load was removed in one circulation; pretreatment with an inhibitor of monoamine oxidase (MAO), β-phenylisopropylhydrazine, had no significant effect on the amount of 5-HT removed. These results were challenged by Crawford (27), who found no arteriovenous (AV) difference in 5-HT levels of whole blood or plasma, and by Larmi and Heikkinen (71), who, in the absence of AV differences in humans infused with 5-HT (800 µg/min) concluded that thrombocytes were probably responsible for the disappearance of circulating 5-HT from plasma. Thomas and Vane (99) substantially settled this controversy by reporting that up to 98% of the injected 5-HT disappeared from the circulation after one passage through the lung. The platelets played a minor role in this process. By using a biological assay and the superfusion technique, Vane (101) showed that 5-HT, *l*-norepinephrine (*l*-NE), bradykinin, angiotensin I, and certain prostaglandins were hydrolyzed by or disappeared from the pulmonary circulation; this lung action could not be considered trivial because it affected up to 98% of the circulating substrate. These findings stimulated additional analytical investigations on how the lungs handle circulating 5-HT and other amines, biogenic or nonbiogenic (1, 11, 40, 46, 49, 53, 57, 66, 67, 90, 91, 101).

5-HYDROXYTRYPTAMINE UPTAKE

Characterization of Uptake Process

Most studies on 5-HT removal by the lungs have used the isolated perfused preparation. Cell-free perfusion medium generally was used to eliminate the problem of 5-HT uptake by platelets. Extraction rate or removal was usually analyzed with radiolabeled 5-HT, although Vane and co-workers (2, 3, 55, 99) derived useful information from biological assay. Catravas and Gillis (25) and Gillis et al. (48) recently gave a detailed account of various ways of determining 5-HT uptake with indicator-dilution techniques.

Disappearance of 5-HT from perfusion medium primarily results from its uptake by the lung and is independent from its subsequent intracellular oxidative deamination by MAO [Fig. 1; (65)]. The uptake is saturable and temperature dependent. The kinetic analysis of this process, determined by the transport rate of the amine, provided similar data to several authors despite differences in animal species and preparations: Michaelis constant (K_m) = 6.2 μM (65), 6.9 μM (7), 1.65 μM (80), and 5.2 μM (63); maximal velocity (V_{max}) = 19 nmol·g^{-1} lung·min^{-1} (65), 12.8 nmol·g^{-1} lung·min^{-1} (63), and 0.17 μmol·min^{-1} per rabbit lung (80).

TABLE 1. *5-Hydroxytryptamine Extraction by the Lung*

Species	Drug Administration*	Extraction, %	Ref.
Human	[^{14}C]5-HT: bolus injection of 0.45 μmol in vivo	65	50
	[^{14}C]5-HT: bolus injection of 0.6 μmol in vivo	62† 81‡	48
	5-HT: injection of 0.6–0.28 nmol into isolated perfused human lung, 8 ml/min for 10–15 g lung	71	4
Dog	[^{14}C]5-HT: bolus injection of 0.06–0.1 μmol/kg in vivo	18–45	32
	5-HT: infusion of 0.06–0.18 μmol/min in vivo	80–98	99
Rabbit	[^{14}C]5-HT: 30-min infusion 0.03 μmol/min (10 ml/min)	56	52
	[^{14}C]5-HT: 12-min infusion 0.4(?)–2.6 μmol/min (200 ml/min)	≤47	80
	[^{14}C]5-HT: bolus injection of 56 nmol in vivo	57–79	25
Guinea pig	5-HT: infusion of 0.12–1.14 nmol/min (20 ml/min)	30–82	56
	[^{14}C]5-HT: initial concn 0.25 μM in closed circuit (10 ml/min)	57	96
Rat	5-HT: 3- to 5-min infusion of 0.2–0.4 nmol/min (8 ml/min)	92	2
	[^{14}C]5-HT: 3-min infusion of 0.001–0.17 μmol/min (10 ml/min)	20–58.5	65
	[^{14}C]5-HT: initial concn 0.25 μM in closed circuit (14 ml/min)	77–81	17

* Doses used by investigators and expressed as micrograms were transformed into moles. It was assumed, when no mention was made, that authors took 5-HT as free base. † Arteriovenous difference. ‡ Extraction at peak of dextran dilution curve.

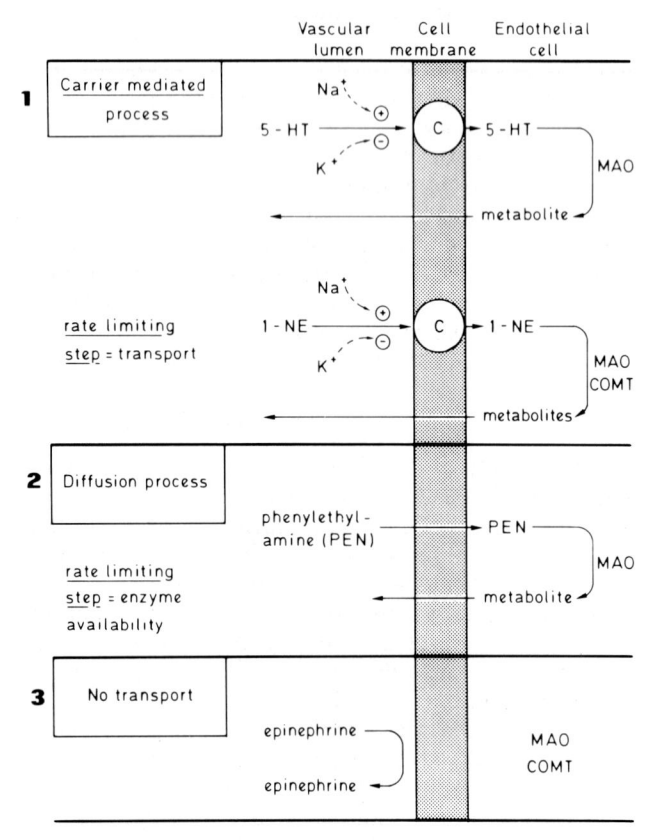

FIG. 1. Schematic illustration of 3 main processes involved in handling of amines by pulmonary circulation. C in process 1 (carrier-mediated process) represents carrier.

Other ways of expressing the extent of this process are by the percentage of extraction or by the percentage of removal when the outflow concentration of 5-HT is related to its inflow concentration. Pickett et al. (80) pointed out that results can be greatly influenced by the rate of supply, which depends on the concentration of substrate and the delivery of flow. Some of the reported data are listed in Table 1.

The changes in 5-HT uptake with alterations of the ionic composition of the medium and the presence of ouabain suggest a carrier-mediated and Na$^+$-dependent transport process: lack or decrease in [Na$^+$] and an increase in [K$^+$] or ouabain inhibit uptake.

Interestingly this type of uptake process, which is basically similar to that operating for *l*-NE in the lung, is also analogous to the mechanism of 5-HT and NE accumulation by nerve endings and synaptosomes (100). Platelets share the same mechanism to concentrate amines in their cytoplasm (94). This transport process utilizes the Na concentration gradient existing across the cell membrane and generated by the Na$^+$- and K$^+$-activated ATPase (Na$^+$ pump). Several groups have evaluated metabolic requirements for the transport process. Two studies reported a lack of effect of glucose-free medium and a small effect of hypoxia (63, 65). Steinberg et al. (96), however, reported that glucose-free medium had an inhibitory effect and that 2-deoxyglucose (a metabolic inhibitor that acts on the glycolytic pathway through competitive inhibition of the phosphoglucose isomerase and irreversible formation of 2-deoxyglucose 6-phosphate) also reduced 5-HT uptake. This inhibition was reversed by other substrates, e.g., pyruvate, lactate, acetate, alanine, β-hydroxybutyrate, palmitate, or glycerol (39). The lack of glucose effect in the initial studies may be attributed to a relatively short preincubation period.

Longitudinal studies performed on newborn rabbits for up to 4 wk after birth indicated that the uptake and metabolism of 5-HT were fully developed at birth and were not modified thereafter (45).

Localization of Uptake Process

Radioautographic studies performed in isolated perfused rat lungs with tritium-labeled 5-HT, in the presence of an MAO inhibitor, clearly demonstrated intense labeling of endothelial cells in large vessels and in capillaries (98). This was clearly a cell-specific phenomenon because 90% of the grains were found over endothelial cells. This finding was later confirmed by Cross et al. (29), who also used an isolated rat lung preparation. In the absence of MAO inhibition an examination by light microscope revealed labeling essentially in the cells outlining the alveolar wall. In the presence of mebanazine, an MAO inhibitor, all the endothelial cells, including those lining the lumen of arterioles and arteries, were labeled. This suggests the existence of different amounts or activities of MAO along the pulmonary vascular bed.

Fisher and Pietra (38), using vascular perfusion and endotracheal infusion of [³H]5-HT, also found that the major site for lung 5-HT accumulation was the pulmonary capillary endothelium.

Monoamine Oxidases of Pulmonary Endothelial Cells

Because various compounds had different inhibitory effects, Roth and Gillis (84) concluded that several types of MAO were responsible for the enzymatic degradation of the 5-HT taken up (Fig. 2). This view is based on the existence of two main forms of MAO in mitochondria (41, 105); they are defined in terms of either sensitivity to specific blockers or substrate specificity. The activity of MAO A is sensitive to chlorgyline and harmaline; its substrates are 5-HT, l-NE, epinephrine, and octopamine. The activity of MAO B is sensitive to deprenyl, imipramine, and pargyline and acts on benzylamine, tryptamine, and β-phenylethylamine. Other amines (e.g., tyramine, dopamine, and kynurenamine) are substrates for both types of mitochondrial MAO.

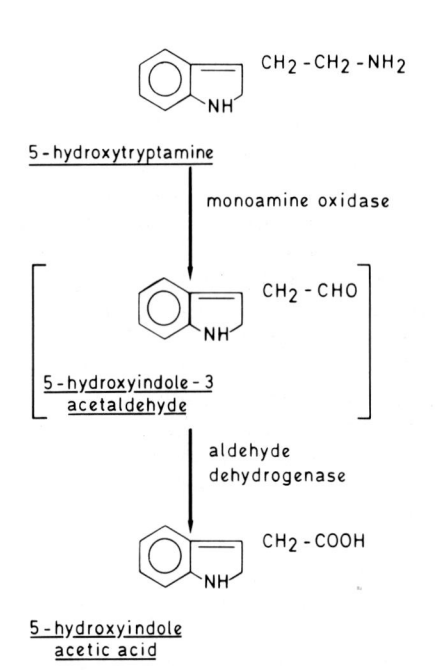

FIG. 2. Degradation of 5-hydroxytryptamine.

The lung also possesses a third type of MAO, similar to that described in plasma by McEwen et al. (73) and in arterial wall by Coquil et al. (26); its activity is best inhibited by semicarbazide hydrochloride (84). The use of preferential substrates and specific inhibitors has indicated that these different forms of MAO operate independently. Evidence proving the existence of these three MAO forms in endothelial cells is based on the use of these different substrates and inhibitors in isolated perfused lungs under the same conditions as those used in radioautographic studies. Experiments with lung homogenates only would have indicated the prevalence of various MAO forms in the lung but not in the endothelial cells in particular (12, 106). Bakhle and Ben-Harari (7) observed that the estrous cycle and the administration of 17β-estradiol could somewhat modulate the activity of lung MAO.

Pharmacological Inhibition of Uptake Process

Cocaine (10^{-5}–10^{-4} M), chlorpromazine, and tricyclic antidepressant drugs (imipramine, amitriptyline, desipramine) exerted a marked inhibitory effect on 5-HT uptake (2, 62, 63, 65). The inhibitory effect of imipramine appeared to be competitive.

According to Iwasawa and Gillis (62), other amines, such as phenoxybenzamine hydrochloride and normetanephrine, also decreased 5-HT uptake, whereas other investigators (3, 65) reported opposite results. Tryptamine also decreased 5-HT uptake, whereas reserpine, 6-hydroxydopamine, phentolamine hydrochloride, metaraminol bitartrate, and propranolol hydrochloride were without effect. Norepinephrine, which is also transported by endothelial cells, even at a concentration 100 times higher than that of 5-HT was only slightly inhibitory (62, 65).

Efflux of Accumulated 5-Hydroxytryptamine

Radioactivity accumulated in the lung during perfusion with labeled 5-HT was released more rapidly when lungs were treated with MAO inhibitors, presumably because diffusion of 5-HIAA out of the endothelium is faster than the efflux of 5-HT (65). In the presence of MAO inhibitors the efflux of 5-HT was accelerated by a higher concentration of 5-HT and by Na$^+$-free medium. These results are compatible with a carrier-mediated transport process and the presence of a counterflow phenomenon (efflux of substrate against an apparent concentration gradient). This explanation holds for the similar effect of imipramine and chlorpromazine, although these drugs could also displace 5-HT from intracellular binding sites, if they exist.

Uptake in Isolated and Cultured Endothelial Cells

Cultured endothelial cells have been used to study 5-HT uptake. Because they are generally isolated from large vessels, it was of primary importance to confirm that the endothelium of large vessels had the same properties as capillary endothelial cells when studied in isolated perfused lungs. This was demonstrated for cells freshly isolated from pig pulmonary arteries and in cells isolated from the aorta (69). Because of these results obtained with aortic endothelial cells, 5-HT uptake could not be considered to be a specific property of the endothelium of the pulmonary circulation. Shepro et al. (92), using fresh and cultured bovine aortic endothelial cells, detected evidence for an uptake process inhibited by temperature, metabolic inhibitors, and ouabain. Small et al. (93) found evidence for production of 5-HIAA by cultured endothelial cells derived from bovine aorta and human umbilical vein without MAO inhibitors. Finally, Pearson et al. (78) furnished experimental evidence of saturability for the uptake process by cultured aortic endothelial cells.

These in vitro experiments are important in several respects. *1*) They show that for 5-HT uptake the properties of lung capillary endothelial cells are also found in large pulmonary vessels, *2*) they extend the concept of 5-HT uptake to the endothelium of the systemic circulation, and *3*) they establish the validity of cell culture for in vitro experimental procedures related to in vivo processes. This last point should be accepted with caution, however, because the possibility of cell dedifferentiation with serial passage must be considered. Furthermore strict criteria for endothelial cell identification must be satisfied. However, though endothelial cells may retain markers, e.g., angiotensin-converting enzyme activity or production of factor VIII, other enzyme or membrane functions may still be modified during the culture process.

Uptake and Platelet-Lung Relationships

Thomas and Vane (99) concluded that the role played by platelets in 5-HT uptake could be negligible compared with the role played by the lung: the 10–80 ng/ml 5-HT half-life in whole blood varied between 60 and 120 s. Steinberg and Das (97) reexamined this problem and found that perfusion with platelet-rich plasma resulted in a decrease in the lung effect on the overall removal of 5-HT from the circulation, whereas the effect of platelets increased. These observations were made without measurable trapping of platelets inside the lungs. Few experiments have been performed to further characterize the possible interrelationship between lung endothelium and platelets. White et al. (103) have reported that normal lungs could take up a maximum of 72% of 5-HT stored in platelets during a single transit period, whereas abnormal lungs took up none. Obviously 5-HT loading in both lung and platelets with different isotopes could be used to study this problem in more detail. Endothelial cells metabolize 5-HT and release 5-HIAA, whereas platelets store 5-HT; this could be used to differentiate between platelet and lung uptake.

Uptake by the Lung and Pharmacological Action of 5-Hydroxytryptamine on Pulmonary Circulation

Rickaby et al. (81) concluded that the inactivation of 5-HT in the pulmonary circulation will not modulate its pharmacological action because they found that arterial vasoconstriction by 5-HT was uninfluenced by the inactivation processes occurring simultaneously. This is a logical conclusion in view of the limited amount of vascular endothelial surface available on the arterial side for 5-HT uptake. However, this explanation is questionable when other 5-HT actions elsewhere in the vascular bed (e.g., its effect on capillary permeability) are considered.

NOREPINEPHRINE UPTAKE

Norepinephrine uptake by the lung has received less attention probably because less NE than 5-HT disappears from the pulmonary circulation. In 1961 Whitby et al. (102) noticed the high concentration of [^{3}H]*l*-NE in the lung 2 min after injection. Eiseman et al. (35) reported that the NE half-life was considerably decreased when perfused through an isolated lung. In 1968 Ginn and Vane (55), using their superfusion technique, measured 0%–36% extraction of NE from the cat lung circulation and 7%–33% NE extraction in the dog lung circulation (infusion rates of 0.3–2 $\mu g \cdot kg^{-1} \cdot min^{-1}$; means of 18% and 19%, respectively). The biological activity of epinephrine, however, was not altered during its passage through the lungs of 13–14 animals.

Characterization of Uptake Process

Several groups of investigators have published more analytical studies since 1969 (3, 58, 62, 63, 76). Their main findings are summarized in Table 2. Like 5-HT

TABLE 2. *l-Norepinephrine Extraction by the Lung*

Species	Drug Administration*	Extraction, %	Ref.
Human	l-NE: bolus injection of 0.04 µmol in vivo	20–23	28, 47, 50
	AV difference in plasma NE concn	25	95
Dog	l-NE: infusion of 0.3–11.7 nmol· kg^{-1}·min^{-1} in vivo	19	55
	l-NE: 3- to 4-min infusion of 1.5–6 nmol/min in vivo	20	9
Cat	l-NE: infusion of 1.9–12 nmol· kg^{-1}·min^{-1} in vivo	18	55
Rabbit	l-NE: 30-min perfusion of 6–30 nmol/min (10 ml/min)	29–39	52
	[^{3}H]l-NE: bolus injection of 0.27 nmol in vivo	48–58	25
Rat	l-NE: 4-min infusion of 0.1–4.8 nmol/min (8 ml/min)	33–40	3
	[^{3}H]l-NE: 2-min infusion of 0.07–1.4 nmol/min (10 ml/min)	17–37	76
	[^{3}H]dl-NE: 2- to 40-min infusion of 0.27–32 nmol/min (9 µl/min)	16†	58

* Doses used by investigators and expressed as micrograms were transformed into moles. It was assumed, when no mention was made, that authors took NE as free base. † Per gram of lung.

uptake, NE uptake by the lung is determined by its rate of transport into endothelial cells (see Fig. 1). This saturable transport mechanism has been kinetically analyzed. The K_m values are between 1.1 and 2.4 µM, and those for V_{max} are between 2.2 and 5.6 nmol· g^{-1}·min^{-1}. Studies with d-NE and l-NE showed no stereospecificity for the transport step (63, 76). The uptake was temperature sensitive and was inhibited by ouabain and Na iodoacetic acid but not by glucose-free medium (63, 76). Transport also required the presence of Na$^+$ and was antagonized by the absence of K$^+$ and by increased concentrations of K$^+$. The efflux of accumulated NE was accelerated with Na$^+$-free perfusion medium (76).

Uptake was not markedly affected by the presence of inhibitors of MAO and catechol O-methyltransferase (COMT). However, Hughes et al. (58) and Nicholas et al. (76) found a slight increase in NE uptake in the presence of tropolone, iproniazid, or pargyline (which probably resulted from the slower efflux of NE than of NE metabolites). Without MAO and COMT inhibitors, lung extracts contained little NE (19%–23%) and higher amounts of deaminated and methylated metabolites, including normetanephrine, 3,4-dihydroxymandelic acid, and 3-methoxy-4-hydroxymandelic acid (Fig. 3). During a brief infusion period (2 min), metabolites had already appeared in the effluent.

Pharmacological inhibitors of 5-HT uptake (e.g., cocaine and imipramine) also markedly inhibited NE uptake. Normetanephrine, phentolamine hydrochloride, and phenoxybenzamine hydrochloride were found to inhibit this uptake mechanism by some investigators (62, 76) but not by others (3). Metaraminol had no effect (76).

Competition between the two biogenic amines 5-HT and l-NE has also been considered. Nicholas et al. (76) found a partial competitive inhibitory effect of 5-HT on NE uptake, but surprisingly 5-HT had no effect on NE efflux as expected if these amines shared the same carrier.

Although the effect of the estrous cycle on the lung uptake of l-NE was not tested, most steroid hormones (estradiol, corticosterone, hydrocortisone, deoxycorticosterone acetate) had a slightly negative effect except for progesterone, which had no effect (61). However, two anesthetic agents (halothane and N$_2$O) inhibited the clearance of l-NE from the pulmonary circulation (9, 75).

Localization of Uptake Process

Initial studies with radioautography done by Hughes et al. (58) suggested that endothelial cells were mainly responsible for the uptake of dl-NE from the pulmonary circulation. Nicholas et al. (76), using the same technique but employing l-NE and a higher magnification, confirmed this finding and added a new element, the heterogeneity of the site of uptake. Instead of an even spread along the pulmonary vascular bed, the uptake of [^{3}H]l-NE was preferentially local-

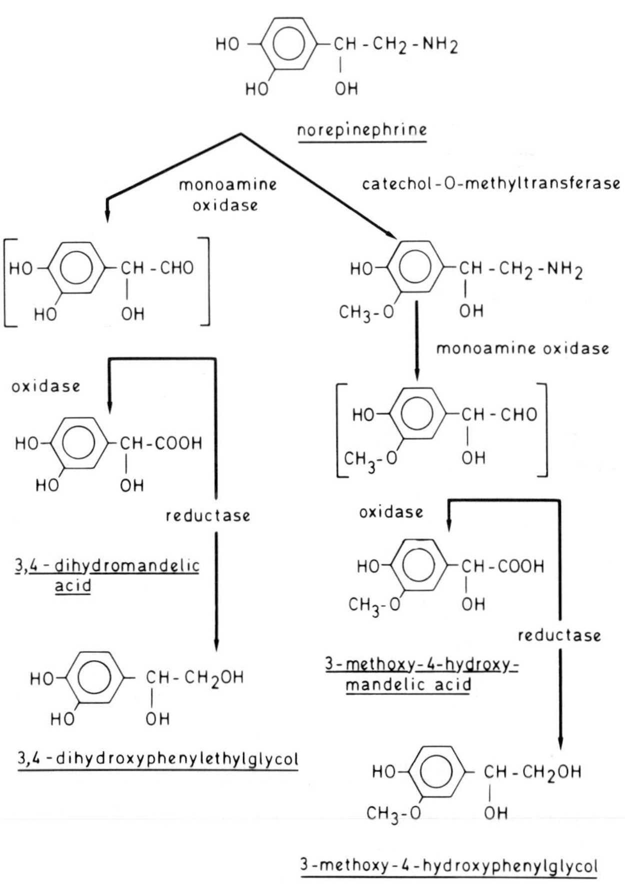

FIG. 3. Degradation of norepinephrine.

ized in pre- and postcapillaries. Only 31% of the capillaries and 12% of the arteries were labeled. Other studies by Iwasawa et al. (63), who used fluorescence microscopy, also showed that NE uptake was localized in endothelial cells only in the presence of MAO and COMT inhibitors.

l-Norepinephrine Uptake by Isolated Endothelial Cells

When isolated by the Häutchen technique or exposed to collagenase, endothelial cells from pulmonary arteries do not exhibit an uptake process identical to that operating in the perfused lung (69). The uptake of *l*-NE was insensitive to the effect of imipramine, not saturable, and not Na$^+$ dependent. However, evidence for intracellular metabolism of *l*-NE and for sensitivity to cold was obtained. These findings indicate that *l*-NE uptake in perfused lungs is different from that in large vessels. Radioautographic findings reported by Nicholas et al. (76) corroborate this difference by the relative inability of endothelial cells in large intrapulmonary arteries to accumulate *l*-NE. Similar results were obtained with isolated aortic endothelial cells, but no data are available on *l*-NE uptake by cultured endothelial cells.

l-Norepinephrine Uptake by the Lung: Uptake 1 (Neuronal) or Uptake 2 (Extraneuronal)

Iversen (60) has defined the characteristics of two types of uptake for *l*-NE: neuronal (uptake 1) and extraneuronal (uptake 2). The main criteria for the two types of uptake are listed in Table 3; the last column enumerates the properties of pulmonary endothelial cells. Although anatomically extraneuronal, pulmonary endothelial cells possess some of the characteristics of neuronal *l*-NE uptake: high affinity, Na$^+$ dependence, and sensitivity to imipramine and cocaine.

EFFECTS OF EXPERIMENTAL AND CLINICAL CONDITIONS ON 5-HYDROXYTRYPTAMINE AND NOREPINEPHRINE UPTAKE

Experimental Conditions

ANESTHESIA. As previously indicated, *l*-NE uptake was slightly reduced during exposure of rabbit lungs to nitrous oxide and halothane. There was additive inhibition when these two gases were combined (75). Bakhle and Block (9) also found that a halothane-air mixture decreased *l*-NE inactivation by dog lungs compared with control conditions (chloralose anesthesia).

MONOCROTALINE. Chronic ingestion of pyrrolizidine alkaloid isolated from the seeds of *Crotalaria spectabilis* produces pulmonary arterial hypertension that

TABLE 3. *Characteristics of Norepinephrine Uptake*

	Neuronal (Uptake 1)	Extraneuronal (Uptake 2)	Pulmonary Endothelial Cell
K_m	0.2–0.4 μM	250 μM	1.1–2.4 μM
Stereospecificity	+	−	−
Na$^+$ dependent	+	±	+
Inhibition by			
Cocaine	+	−	+
Imipramine	+	−	+
Normetanephrine	−	+	±
Phenoxybenzamine	−	+	±
Steroids	−	+	+
Uptake followed by			
Storage	+	−	−
Rapid degradation	−	+	+

leads to right ventricular hypertrophy and cor pulmonale. Gillis et al. (51) found that rats ingesting monocrotaline for 21 days removed and inactivated less 5-HT and NE (50%–60%), but their MAO activity was unaffected. Acute administration of monocrotaline had no pharmacological effect on 5-HT uptake. This suggests that the monocrotaline effect did not result from a direct pharmacological inhibition of uptake but from decreased pulmonary vascular surface and/or damage (unspecified) to endothelial cells. On the other hand, Huxtable et al. (59), despite similar protocol and use of the same species, found that chronic ingestion of monocrotaline affected only 5-HT uptake and not that of NE.

PARAQUAT. Ingestion of this herbicide results in the development of potentially fatal acute respiratory failure and subsequent pulmonary fibrosis. Although morphological evidence for a toxic damage to the pulmonary endothelium is contradictory, Roth et al. (88) were able to show that rat lungs became edematous and 5-HT extraction decreased significantly 3 days after exposure to paraquat. Uptake of 5-HT returned to normal values 10 days later. Decreased 5-HT extraction by the lung was not the result of a direct inhibitory effect of paraquat on 5-HT uptake. The MAO activity also decreased in the homogenates of paraquat-treated lungs. This study is of interest because it shows a clear distinction between the subacute and chronic effects of paraquat. It also established biochemical evidence of endothelial cell damage in the presence of still-disputed morphological alterations.

α-NAPHTHYLTHIOUREA. This compound, used to create acute pulmonary edema, reportedly provokes morphological changes affecting the pulmonary endothelium. Block and Schoen (20) showed that 5-HT uptake by rat lungs was significantly depressed 4 h after administration of this chemical, before any morphologic change and the development of pulmonary edema. The 5-HT uptake was further reduced after 24 h, when pulmonary edema was clearly present. This index returned to normal levels 10 days after initial administration of α-naphthylthiourea. This investigation demonstrates the value of 5-HT uptake measurement for early detection of endothelial damage.

HYPEROXIA. Block and Cannon (16) and Block and Fisher (17) found that uptake of 5-HT or l-NE by rat lung was significantly reduced after 18–24 h of exposure to 95% O_2 (1 ATA), before any histological alteration or change in the ratio of dry lung weight to wet lung weight could be demonstrated. Superoxide dismutase pretreatment partially prevented this reduction in 5-HT clearance (19). Exposure to hyperbaric oxygen accelerated the development of biochemical evidence of endothelial cell dysfunction; evidence of reversibility was shown under normal conditions after 4 h of breathing air (15, 18). Thus hyperoxia also turned out to be a good model to demonstrate early alteration in the function of the endothelium before changes in morphology or development of lung edema. Interestingly the pulmonary accumulation of imipramine was unaffected by hyperbaric oxygen (16).

CIGARETTE SMOKE. Short- and long-term exposure of rats to cigarette smoke did not affect 5-HT uptake by the lung (10).

SPONTANEOUS HYPERTENSION IN RATS. Spontaneously hypertensive rats can remove more NE and less 5-HT from the pulmonary circulation than control rats (87). The mechanisms of this differential behavior are unclear, and thus it is impossible to tell whether the response is adaptive or genetically determined.

It may be concluded from these recent applications to experimental pathology that the use of measurements of 5-HT or l-NE uptake represents major progress in understanding the involvement of pulmonary endothelial cells in various processes. The combined measurements of different indices of endothelial cell function (e.g., angiotensin-converting enzyme) may give a better assessment of the type of endothelial damage. The question still persists concerning distinguishing between a decreased pulmonary vascular surface and a real, qualitative dysfunction of the endothelium (or a combination of both). The simultaneous injection of two different markers, one dependent on endothelial function and the other dependent on endothelial surface, should help solve this problem, but presently no reliable marker for the endothelial cell surface is available. Nonetheless the use of endothelial cells in culture may represent a new and fruitful approach in evaluating endothelial responses to various pathological processes.

Application to Human Clinical Problems

Gillis et al. (48) recently described various ways of measuring 5-HT clearance by the lung using the indicator-dilution technique and two isotopes: [^{3}H]dextran (a marker of intravascular space) and [^{14}C]5-HT. Previously the same group measured extraction rates for 5-HT and l-NE using a bolus injection with only one isotope (l-NE and/or 5-HT) and no marker for intravascular space. They found that biogenic amine extraction by the lung increased after cardiopulmonary bypass (47, 50). In patients with postcapillary pulmonary hypertension undergoing valve replacement, however, the postbypass values for 5-HT and l-NE extraction rates decreased compared with their initial values (47). The return of pulmonary artery pressure toward normal values was thought to cause this decrease in the removal of amines from the pulmonary circulation.

Sole et al. (95) compared the AV difference for various catecholamines in normal subjects with results in patients having primary pulmonary hypertension. They observed a complete absence of AV difference for NE in patients with primary pulmonary hypertension, which suggests a marked reduction in the removal process of this amine by the lung. The reservations just expressed regarding the limitations of interpretation of these data are also valid for these clinical conditions. However, future research probably will bring about major advances in this field through use of multiple indicators of endothelial cell function as well as surface and intravascular space markers. The development of ^{11}C isotopes and the use of a γ-camera may allow visualization and quantification of endothelial cell function in the lung (43).

OTHER NATURALLY OCCURRING CATECHOLAMINES

Chemical structures of other naturally occurring catecholamines are shown in Figure 4.

β-Phenylethylamine

The compound β-phenylethylamine (PEN) is interesting not so much because of its importance as an endogenous product (89) but because it represents another model for the handling of amines by the lung.

Roth and Gillis (83) investigated this substance as an MAO substrate from rabbit lung mitochondrial preparation. They showed that imipramine (known to block amine uptake) also had MAO activity, primarily of the B type. Subsequently they analyzed the fate of perfused PEN in isolated rabbit lungs and found that it was 95% degraded in one passage (84). Even at high concentrations, removal was apparently linearly related to substrate concentration (54), a finding compatible with a single diffusion process (see Fig. 1).

Ben-Harari and Bakhle (13) reinvestigated this problem and found evidence for the presence of two components in the uptake process, one compatible with simple diffusion and the other compatible with a saturable transport mechanism. These results were

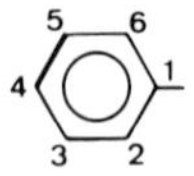

CATECHOLAMINES

Phenylethylamine			H	H	H
Epinephrine	3-OH	4-OH	OH	H	CH$_3$
Norepinephrine	3-OH	4-OH	OH	H	H
Dopamine	3-OH	4-OH	H	H	H
Octopamine		4-OH	OH	H	H
Isoproterenol	3-OH	4-OH	OH	H	CH(CH$_3$)$_2$
Metaraminol	3-OH		OH	CH$_3$	H
Amphetamine			H	CH$_3$	H
Mescaline	3-OCH$_3$ 5-OCH$_3$	4-OCH$_3$	H	H	H
Chlorphentermine		4-Cl	H	(CH$_3$)$_2$	H

FIG. 4. Chemical structure of major endogenous catecholamines and certain sympathomimetic drugs.

obtained without MAO inhibitors. However, with deprenyl present there was a marked reduction in uptake value. Unfortunately none of these studies achieved or demonstrated a complete blockade of MAO activity, thus some doubt exists about whether simple diffusion, facilitated diffusion, carrier-mediated transport, or a combination of these processes operates.

Because the kinetics for PEN metabolism were the same in subcellular preparations and perfused lungs, inactivation of circulating PEN appears to be determined by intracellular metabolism of the amine, not by the transport step. This conclusion is supported by observing that various drugs (desipramine, normetanephrine, amphetamine, benzylamine, propranolol hydrochloride) inhibit uptake and metabolism of PEN. Results of experiments performed with glucose-, Na$^+$-, and K$^+$-free media during anoxia and at 4°C varied, depending on PEN concentration.

Metabolism of PEN by MAO and degradation of 5-HT are under the same influence of the estrous cycle and exogenous estrogens (8). However, compared with 5-HT (a substrate for MAO A) PEN is preferentially metabolized by MAO B. This may explain the differential maturation rate of the degradative processes of postnatal rabbit lung: instead of the stable inactivation rate found for 5-HT in a 28-day period, the rate of PEN degradation increased with time (45).

Dopamine

No loss of dopamine (DA) biological activity was detected in humans, rats, or dogs by Boileau et al. (23) with DA injected into the pulmonary artery or into the aorta. Nicholas et al. (76) could not find retention of radioactivity when labeled DA was perfused through isolated rat lungs, but the nature of the radioactivity of the effluent was not analyzed. Sole et al. (95) did not find any AV difference for DA concentrations in normal subjects, whereas Gillis and Roth (54) reported that up to 32% of DA infused into isolated rabbit lung was recovered as deaminated metabolites.

Epinephrine

Ginn and Vane (55) did not find convincing evidence for a loss of epinephrine activity when injected into the pulmonary circulation of dogs and cats (see Fig. 1). Boileau et al. (22) in studies on dogs, cats, rats, and humans confirmed this lack of change. Sole et al. (95) also found no AV difference in their epinephrine determinations in plasma of normal subjects, whereas Hughes et al. (58) showed some accumulation of radioactivity in isolated rat lungs when epinephrine was injected together with pargyline and tropolone. Hughes and co-workers concluded that the uptake process for epinephrine was 4–5 times less important than for NE. Clearly a 5% loss in activity or a 5% difference in AV concentrations would hardly be detectable no matter which techniques, bioassay or isotopic studies, are used.

Octopamine

From the data reported by Gillis and Roth (54), octopamine apparently behaves similarly to NE.

SYMPATHOMIMETIC DRUGS

Chemical structures of sympathomimetic drugs are shown in Figure 4.

Metaraminol

The uptake of metaraminol in lung tissue slices (30, 31) was altered by changes in the ionic composition of the medium and ouabain, indicating that it was saturable and dependent on the temperature and integrity of Na$^+$- and K$^+$-activated ATPase.

Metaraminol uptake was also inhibited by cocaine, tyramine, imipramine, and desipramine. Because no experiment was done with perfused lungs, the site of uptake (likely found in endothelial cells) has not been established. Opposite results on the inhibitory effect of metaraminol on NE uptake were obtained by Alabaster and Bakhle (3) and Nicholas et al. (76), thus preventing an argument for identical carriers. Metaraminol's insensitivity to MAO and COMT action could prove potentially advantageous as a marker for endothelial cell function.

Isoprenaline

In an isolated dog lung perfused with plasma in a closed circuit, 3-O-methylisoprenaline formed by

COMT appears after injection of isoprenaline (24). Isoprenaline uptake was not measured directly. The new β_2-stimulants (e.g., terbutaline, a noncatechol compound), however, are generally not metabolized by the lung because they are not sensitive to the COMT effect.

Mescaline

Mescaline, a hallucinogenic compound, is also extensively metabolized during its passage through the lung. The degradative process, leading to the formation of trimethoxyphenylacetic acid, is blocked by semicarbazide but not by pargyline (86). This semicarbazide hydrochloride effect suggests that the enzyme involved is the plasma MAO and not the mitochondrial form. Mescaline also accumulated in the semicarbazide-treated lungs. This process, however, did not show strong evidence of saturability at concentrations of $2-8 \times 10^{-6}$ M and was insensitive to ouabain.

The efflux of mescaline from a lung previously loaded with this substance was slower than the efflux of its metabolites. Hyperventilation increased amine removal and degradation. Increased pH was thought to be primarily responsible for the increased removal (85). For mescaline and PEN, the lack of a detailed analysis of the removal process in the presence of enzyme inhibitors prevents its characterization. Removal thus appears to depend more on metabolism than on transport rate.

HISTAMINE

Despite observations by Lilja and Lindell (72) of a gradual histamine loss in their heart-lung preparation perfused with blood, histamine (Fig. 5) did not appear to be removed from circulation during its passage through the lung (21, 35, 37). Based on in vivo experiments in rats, Krell et al. (70) concluded that there was a small accumulation of unchanged histamine in the lung and a gradual increase in the proportion of metabolites. Inhibition of diamine oxidase by iproniazid and aminoguanidine prevented degradation of the histamine retained by the lung. This observation confirms that a small amount of histamine accumulates and is metabolized in the lung. The magnitude of this phenomenon is, however, much less impressive than it is for 5-HT and *l*-NE.

Previous experiments done with lung homogenates demonstrated the presence of enzymes capable of degrading histamine: diamine oxidase and imidazole-*N*-

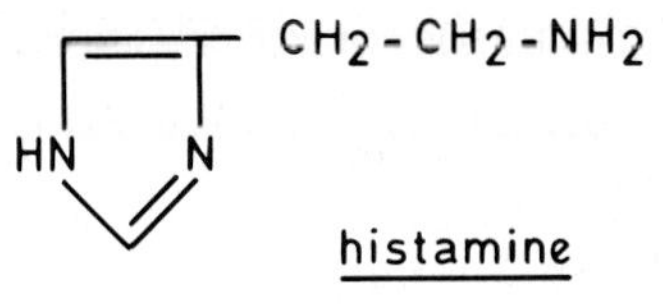

FIG. 5. Chemical structure of histamine.

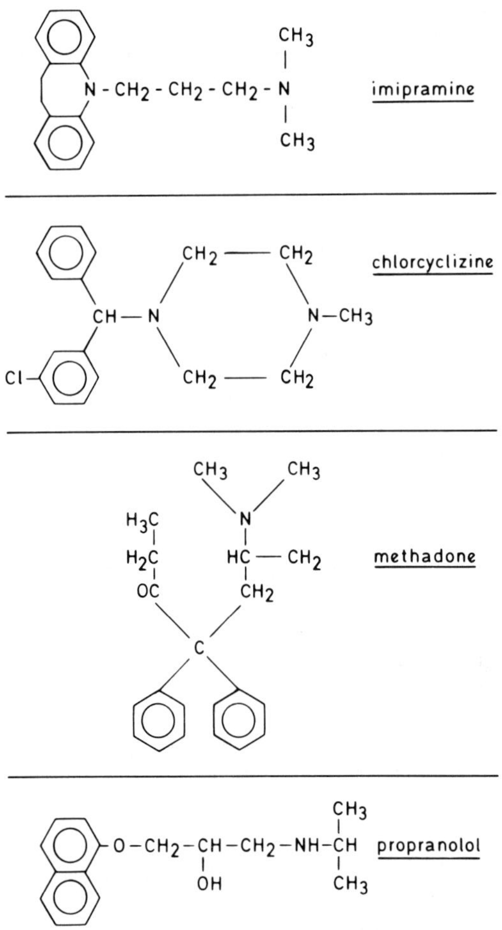

FIG. 6. Chemical structure of some basic amines taken up by the lung.

methyltransferase (14). Krell et al. (70) documented the presence and roles of these enzymes in the degradation of circulating histamine, although locally released histamine from mast cells, for example, can also be considered as an appropriate substrate. Histamine uptake, however, has not been precisely characterized.

UPTAKE OF BASIC AMINES BY THE LUNG

Several basic lipophilic amines accumulate in the lung (Fig. 6). These drugs share common characteristics of lung accumulation that are markedly different from the uptake of biogenic amines (68, 79).

Early studies on the general distribution of drugs in tissues revealed that certain compounds accumulated in the lung. Only after development of the isolated perfused lung preparation were investigations undertaken to specifically study drug uptake by the lung (82). One such study (64) showed a competitive inhibitory effect of imipramine on 5-HT uptake by the lung and concluded that imipramine (like 5-HT) was taken up by Na$^+$-dependent, carrier-mediated transport. Subsequent studies, however, showed that such transport for imipramine did not occur but attributed uptake to binding to receptor sites (64). Accumulation of imipramine was a saturable phenomenon during a 3-min perfusion in the lung but a plateau was seen only at concentrations above 10^{-3} M. There was little or no inhibition by cold, Na^+-free medium, 5-HT, or l-NE, and imipramine was not metabolized. Decreased uptake and increased efflux were observed in the presence of desipramine and chlorpromazine. Apparent K_m and V_{max} values were 200 μM and 2 μmol/g lung, respectively, compared with 6.2 μM and 19 nmol/g lung for 5-HT (64).

Orton et al. (77) reported similar findings and extended their investigations to other basic amines (amphetamine, chlorcyclizine, and methadone hydrochloride) (see Fig. 6). Uptake of nonbasic amines (aniline, imidazole, and propazine) resulted from simple diffusion, whereas uptake of basic amines, under steady-state conditions, was again found to be concentration dependent. Only methadone was partially metabolized. The same group (5), under steady-state conditions, examined the uptake of imipramine, chlorcyclizine, and amphetamine and determined, depending on the substrate concentration, that uptake of basic amines had a linear and a saturable (evident at low substrate concentration) component. Depending on the compounds tested, there were differences in the magnitude of the accumulation and in the mutual inhibitory effects of linear or saturable components. In some cases inhibition was competitive (imipramine vs. desipramine), whereas the interaction between imipramine and amphetamine was noncompetitive. The authors also confirmed previous observations concerning displacement of one previously accumulated drug by another.

Studies by Eling et al. (36) elaborated the kinetics of uptake and efflux of imipramine in an open, isolated perfused rabbit lung preparation. They concluded that the initial rate of imipramine removal from the circulation had two exponential components (rates 1 and 2). Their initial velocities were both linearly related to substrate concentration, and thus a diffusion-binding phenomenon (partitioning) could be considered. However, when calculated under steady-state conditions, if the imipramine amount accumulated over time by rate 1 was also linearly related to imipramine concentration, the other process related to rate 2 (saturable binding sites) was clearly nonlinear.

Efflux of previously accumulated imipramine was partitioned into four components: two with fast rates of efflux (half-lives of 18 and 58 s) resulting from rate 1 of accumulation, one with a slower rate of efflux (half-life of 8.25 min) corresponding to rate 2 of uptake, and an apparently noneffluxent pool of bound imipramine.

Similar data on methadone uptake by the lung were reported by the same group (104).

Dollery and Junod (33) also found evidence for the existence of at least two populations of binding sites in the lung with different affinities for propranolol. Minchin et al. (74) recently reported that the kinetics of chlorphentermine accumulation in isolated perfused rat lung had two components: one linearly related to substrate concentration, probably resulting from a partitioning process, and the other saturable, much larger, and probably caused by binding to cellular components. This saturable process was the only process to be influenced in a competitive inhibitory fashion by another drug (desipramine) known to accumulate in the lung. On the basis of pharmacokinetic data, these authors proposed that chlorphentermine accumulation could not be explained solely by diffusion-binding processes but also must involve a carrier-mediated uptake mechanism. This truly is the most important question that direct experimental evidence has not firmly answered.

What makes the accumulation process so spectacular in the lung? Is it partly related to the number of endothelial cells in this organ or does it have something to do with the somewhat organ-specific secretions of phospholipids? How could the two processes, partitioning and binding (a carrier-mediated process?), be visualized in morphological terms? In other words, are they cell specific, and if so which cell? Are different uptake and efflux rates related to different cellular and subcellular localizations? Answers to these questions are not only of academic interest, because use of these substances as markers of endothelial cell surface could also be considered. Block and Cannon (16) have already shown that imipramine accumulation in the lung, unlike l-NE or 5-HT uptake, is not influenced by hyperoxia. Geddes et al. (44) have also measured the extraction of propranolol across human lungs. Clearly more information on the nature of these processes is necessary before they can be of use in the assessment of pulmonary endothelial function and surface.

CONCLUSION

Some of the endogenous and exogenous amines appear to be suitable substrates for measurement and assessment of several functions of the pulmonary endothelium: transport, intracellular metabolism by various enzymes, and binding. Biogenic amine uptake and metabolism have been well characterized and localized, whereas the basic lipophilic drugs accumulated in the lung by processes involving several mechanisms, and possibly several sites, are not yet identified or precisely defined. The use of these metabolic properties of pulmonary endothelial cells has led to early detection of endothelial damage resulting from various causes (drugs and toxic gases). In this investigative field a distinction between a decreased pulmonary vascular surface and a real dysfunction of the endothelial cell or perhaps a combination of the two is needed.

General physiological considerations on the lung's handling of these amines remain somewhat vague. The only firmly established concepts are the lack of specificity of function of the pulmonary circulation (because aortic endothelial cells also take up 5-HT) and the existence of some heterogeneity of function of the endothelium depending on its localization [because the endothelium of the large branches of the pulmonary artery apparently do not take up l-NE (76)]. This latter finding was corroborated by studies on isolated endothelial cells derived from the main pulmonary artery (69). The unique role of the pulmonary circulation should be related to its strategic location and to its huge surface. Whether this function has a real physiological role is unsettled. There appears to be no mechanism for control or regulation of these uptake or extraction processes; in particular subtle changes in partial pressures of O_2 or CO_2 (likely to take place in the pulmonary circulation) have not been shown to significantly influence 5-HT uptake. The lung may, however, play a physiological role in controlling the plasma levels of some biogenic amines (49), but conclusive experimental evidence is necessary to confirm this assumption.

REFERENCES

1. ALABASTER, V. A. Inactivation of endogenous amines in the lungs. In: *Lung Biology in Health and Disease. Metabolic Functions of the Lung*, edited by Y. S. Bakhle and J. R. Vane. New York: Dekker, 1977, vol. 4, chapt. 1, p. 3–31.
2. ALABASTER, V. A., AND Y. S. BAKHLE. Removal of 5-hydroxytryptamine in the pulmonary circulation of rat isolated lungs. *Br. J. Pharmacol.* 40: 468–482, 1970.
3. ALABASTER, V. A., AND Y. S. BAKHLE. The removal of noradrenaline in the pulmonary circulation of rat isolated lungs. *Br. J. Pharmacol.* 47: 325–331, 1973.
4. AL-UBAIDI, F., AND Y. S. BAKHLE. Metabolism of vasoactive hormones in human isolated lung. *Clin. Sci.* 58: 45–51, 1980.
5. ANDERSON, M. W., T. C. ORTON, R. D. PICKETT, AND T. E. ELING. Accumulation of amines in the isolated perfused rabbit lung. *J. Pharmacol. Exp. Ther.* 189: 456–466, 1974.
6. AXELROD, J., AND J. K. INSCOE. The uptake and binding of circulating serotonin and the effect of drugs. *J. Pharmacol. Exp. Ther.* 141: 161–165, 1963.
7. BAKHLE, Y. S., AND R. R. BEN-HARARI. Effects of oestrous cycle and exogenous ovarian steroids on 5-hydroxytryptamine metabolism in rat lung. *J. Physiol. London* 291: 11–18, 1979.
8. BAKHLE, Y. S., AND R. R. BEN-HARARI. Effects of the oestrous cycle and exogenous ovarian steroids on metabolism of β-phenylethylamine in rat lung. *Br. J. Pharmacol.* 67: 109–114, 1979.
9. BAKHLE, Y. S., AND A. J. BLOCK. Effects of halothane on pulmonary inactivation of noradrenaline and prostaglandin E_2 in anaesthetized dogs. *Clin. Sci. Mol. Med.* 50: 87–90, 1976.
10. BAKHLE, Y. S., J. HARTIALA, H. TOIVONEN, AND P. UOTILA. Effects of cigarette smoke on the metabolism of vasoactive hormones in rat isolated lungs. *Br. J. Pharmacol.* 65: 495–499, 1979.
11. BAKHLE, Y. S., AND J. R. VANE. Pharmacokinetic function of the pulmonary circulation. *Physiol. Rev.* 54: 1007–1045, 1974.
12. BAKHLE, Y. S., AND M. B. H. YOUDIM. The metabolism of 5-hydroxytryptamine and β-phenylethylamine in perfused rat lung and in vitro. *Br. J. Pharmacol.* 65: 147–154, 1979.
13. BEN-HARARI, R. R., AND Y. S. BAKHLE. Uptake of β-phenylethylamine in rat isolated lung. *Biochem. Pharmacol.* 29: 489–494, 1980.
14. BENNETT, A. The metabolism of histamine by guinea-pig and rat lung in vitro. *Br. J. Pharmacol.* 24: 147–155, 1965.
15. BLOCK, E. R. Recovery from hyperoxic depression of pulmonary 5-hydroxytryptamine clearance: effect of inspired O_2 tension. *Lung* 155: 131–140, 1978.
16. BLOCK, E. R., AND J. K. CANNON. Effect of oxygen exposure on lung clearance of amines. *Lung* 155: 287–295, 1978.
17. BLOCK, E. R., AND A. B. FISHER. Depression of serotonin clearance by rat lungs during oxygen exposure. *J. Appl. Physiol.: Respirat. Environ. Exercise Physiol.* 42: 33–38, 1977.
18. BLOCK, E. R., AND A. B. FISHER. Effect of hyperbaric oxygen exposure on pulmonary clearance of 5-hydroxytryptamine. *J. Appl. Physiol.: Respirat. Environ. Exercise Physiol.* 43: 254–257, 1977.
19. BLOCK, E. R., AND A. B. FISHER. Prevention of hyperoxic-induced depression of pulmonary serotonin clearance by pretreatment with superoxide dismutase. *Am. Rev. Respir. Dis.* 116: 441–447, 1977.
20. BLOCK, E. R., AND F. J. SCHOEN. Effect of alpha naphthylthiourea on uptake of 5-hydroxytryptamine from the pulmonary circulation. *Am. Rev. Respir. Dis.* 123: 69–73, 1981.
21. BOILEAU, J. C., L. CAMPEAU, AND P. BIRON. Pulmonary fate of histamine, isoproterenol, physalaemin, and substance P. *Can. J. Physiol. Pharmacol.* 48: 681–684, 1970.
22. BOILEAU, J. C., L. CAMPEAU, AND P. BIRON. Comparative pulmonary fate of intravenous epinephrine. *Rev. Can. Biol.* 30: 281–286, 1971.
23. BOILEAU, J. C., C. CREXELLS, AND P. BIRON. Free pulmonary passage of dopamine. *Rev. Can. Biol.* 31: 69–72, 1972.
24. BRIANT, R. H., E. W. BLACKWELL, F. M. WILLIAMS, D. S. DAVIES, AND C. T. DOLLERY. The metabolism of sympathomimetic bronchodilator drugs by the isolated perfused dog lung. *Xenobiotica* 3: 787–799, 1973.
25. CATRAVAS, J. D., AND C. N. GILLIS. Pulmonary clearance of [^{14}C]5-hydroxytryptamine and [^{3}H]norepinephrine in vivo: effects of pretreatment with imipramine or cocaine. *J. Pharmacol. Exp. Ther.* 213: 120–127, 1980.
26. COQUIL, J. F., C. GORIDIS, G. MACK, AND N. H. NEFF. Monoamine oxidase in rat arteries: evidence for different forms and selective localization. *Br. J. Pharmacol.* 48: 590–599, 1973.
27. CRAWFORD, N. The lungs and serotonin metabolism: a study of the pulmonary arterio-venous levels of plasma free and platelet-bound serotonin in man. *Clin. Chim. Acta* 12: 264–273, 1965.
28. CRONAU, L. H., M. D. KERSTEIN, S. MANDEL, AND C. N. GILLIS. 5-Hydroxytryptamine extraction by the lung. *Surg. Gynecol. Obstet.* 143: 51–55, 1976.
29. CROSS, S. A. M., V. A. ALABASTER, Y. S. BAKHLE, AND J. R. VANE. Sites of uptake of ^{3}H-5-hydroxytryptamine in rat isolated lung. *Histochemistry* 39: 83–91, 1974.
30. DAVILA, D., AND T. DAVILA. Uptake and release of ^{3}H-metaraminol by rat lung. Basic aspects, ionic and energy requirements. *Arch. Int. Pharmacodyn. Ther.* 214: 53–61, 1975.
31. DAVILA, T., AND D. DAVILA. Uptake and release of ^{3}H-metaraminol by rat lung. The influence of various drugs. *Arch. Int. Pharmacodyn. Ther.* 215: 336–344, 1975.
32. DAVIS, R. B., AND Y. WANG. Rapid pulmonary removal of 5-hydroxytryptamine in the intact dog. *Proc. Soc. Exp. Biol. Med.* 118: 797–800, 1965.
33. DOLLERY, C. T., AND A. F. JUNOD. Concentration of (+/−)-propranolol in isolated perfused lungs of rat. *Br. J. Pharmacol.* 57: 67–71, 1976.
34. EICHHOLTZ, F., AND E. B. VERNEY. On some conditions af-

fecting the perfusion of isolated mammalian organs. *J. Physiol. London* 59: 340–344, 1924–1925.
35. EISEMAN, B., L. BRYANT, AND T. WALTUCH. Metabolism of vasomotor agents by the isolated perfused lung. *J. Thorac. Cardiovasc. Surg.* 48: 798–806, 1964.
36. ELING, T. E., R. D. PICKETT, T. C. ORTON, AND M. W. ANDERSON. A study of the dynamics of imipramine accumulation in the isolated perfused rabbit lung. *Drug Metab. Dispos.* 3: 389–399, 1975.
37. FERREIRA, S. H., K. K. NG, AND J. R. VANE. The continuous bioassay of the release and disappearance of histamine in the circulation. *Br. J. Pharmacol.* 49: 543–553, 1973.
38. FISHER, A. B., AND G. G. PIETRA. Comparison of serotonin uptake from the alveolar and capillary spaces of isolated rat lung. *Am. Rev. Respir. Dis.* 123: 74–78, 1981.
39. FISHER, A. B., H. STEINBERG, AND C. DODIA. Reversal of 2-deoxyglucose inhibition of serotonin uptake in isolated guinea pig lung. *J. Appl. Physiol.: Respirat. Environ. Exercise Physiol.* 46: 447–450, 1979.
40. FISHMAN, A. P., AND G. G. PIETRA. Handling of bioactive materials by the lung. Pt. 1. *N. Engl. J. Med.* 291: 884–890, 1974.
40a. FISHMAN, A. P., AND G. G. PIETRA. Handling of bioactive materials by the lung. Pt. 2. *N. Engl. J. Med.* 291: 953–959, 1974.
41. FOWLER, C. J., B. A. CALLINGHAM, T. J. MANTLE, AND K. F. TIPTON. Monoamine oxidase A and B: a useful concept? *Biochem. Pharmacol.* 27: 97–101, 1978.
42. GADDUM, J. H., C. O. HEBB, A. SILVER, AND A. A. B. SWAN. 5-Hydroxytryptamine. Pharmacological action and destruction in perfused lungs. *Q. J. Exp. Physiol.* 38: 255–262, 1953.
43. GALLAGHER, B., D. CHRISTMAN, J. FOWLER, R. MCGREGOR, A. P. WOLF, P. SOM, A. N. ANSARI, AND H. ATKINS. Radioisotope scintigraphy for the study of dynamics of amine regulation by the human lung. *Chest* 71, Suppl.: 282–284, 1977.
44. GEDDES, D. M., K. NESBITT, T. TRAILL, AND J. P. BLACKBURN. First pass uptake of ^{14}C-propranolol by the lung. *Thorax* 34: 810–813, 1979.
45. GEWITZ, M. H., AND C. N. GILLIS. Uptake and metabolism of biogenic amines in the developing rabbit lung. *J. Appl. Physiol.: Respirat. Environ. Exercise Physiol.* 50: 118–122, 1981.
46. GILLIS, C. N. Metabolism of vasoactive hormones by lung. *Anesthesiology* 39: 626–632, 1973.
47. GILLIS, C. N., L. H. CRONAU, N. M. GREENE, AND G. L. HAMMOND. Removal of 5-hydroxytryptamine and norepinephrine from the pulmonary vascular space of man: influence of cardiopulmonary bypass and pulmonary arterial pressure on these processes. *Surgery* 76: 608–616, 1974.
48. GILLIS, C. N., L. H. CRONAU, S. MANDEL, AND G. L. HAMMOND. Indicator dilution measurement of 5-hydroxytryptamine clearance by human lung. *J. Appl. Physiol.: Respirat. Environ. Exercise Physiol.* 46: 1178–1183, 1979.
49. GILLIS, C. N., AND N. M. GREENE. Possible clinical implications of metabolism of bloodborne substrates by the human lung. In: *Lung Biology in Health and Disease. Metabolic Functions of the Lung*, edited by Y. S. Bakhle and J. R. Vane. New York: Dekker, 1977, vol. 4, chapt. 6, p. 173–193.
50. GILLIS, C. N., N. M. GREENE, L. H. CRONAU, AND G. L. HAMMOND. Pulmonary extraction of 5-hydroxytryptamine and norepinephrine before and after cardiopulmonary bypass in man. *Circ. Res.* 30: 666–674, 1972.
51. GILLIS, C. N., R. J. HUXTABLE, AND R. A. ROTH. Effects of monocrotaline pretreatment of rats on removal of 5-hydroxytryptamine and noradrenaline by perfused lung. *Br. J. Pharmacol.* 63: 435–443, 1978.
52. GILLIS, C. N., AND Y. IWASAWA. Technique for measurement of norepinephrine and 5-hydroxytryptamine uptake by rabbit lung. *J. Appl. Physiol.* 33: 404–408, 1972.
53. GILLIS, C. N., AND J. A. ROTH. Pulmonary disposition of circulating vasoactive hormones. *Biochem. Pharmacol.* 25: 2547–2553, 1976.
54. GILLIS, C. N., AND J. A. ROTH. The fate of biogenic monoamines in perfused rabbit lung. *Br. J. Pharmacol.* 59: 585–590, 1977.
55. GINN, R., AND J. R. VANE. Disappearance of catecholamines from the circulation. *Nature London* 219: 740–742, 1968.
56. GRUBY, L. A., C. ROWLANDS, B. Q. VARLEY, AND J. H. WYLLIE. The fate of 5-hydroxytryptamine in the lungs. *Br. J. Surg.* 58: 525–532, 1971.
57. HEINEMANN, H. O., AND A. P. FISHMAN. Nonrespiratory functions of mammalian lung. *Physiol. Rev.* 49: 1–47, 1969.
58. HUGHES, J., C. N. GILLIS, AND F. E. BLOOM. The uptake and disposition of dl-norepinephrine in perfused rat lung. *J. Pharmacol. Exp. Ther.* 169: 237–248, 1969.
59. HUXTABLE, R., D. CIARAMITARO, AND D. EISENSTEIN. The effect of a pyrrolizidine alkaloid, monocrotaline, and a pyrrole, dehydroretronecine, on the biochemical functions of the pulmonary endothelium. *Mol. Pharmacol.* 14: 1189–1203, 1978.
60. IVERSEN, L. L. Uptake mechanisms for neurotransmitter amines. *Biochem. Pharmacol.* 23: 1927–1935, 1974.
61. IWASAWA, Y., AND C. N. GILLIS. Effect of steroid and other hormones on lung removal of noradrenaline. *Eur. J. Pharmacol.* 22: 367–370, 1973.
62. IWASAWA, Y., AND C. N. GILLIS. Pharmacological analysis of norepinephrine and 5-hydroxytryptamine removal from the pulmonary circulation: differentiation of uptake sites for each amine. *J. Pharmacol. Exp. Ther.* 188: 386–393, 1974.
63. IWASAWA, Y., C. N. GILLIS, AND G. AGHAJANIAN. Hypothermic inhibition of 5-hydroxytryptamine and norepinephrine uptake by lung: cellular location of amines after uptake. *J. Pharmacol. Exp. Ther.* 186: 498–507, 1973.
64. JUNOD, A. F. Accumulation of ^{14}C-imipramine in isolated perfused rat lungs. *J. Pharmacol. Exp. Ther.* 183: 182–187, 1972.
65. JUNOD, A. F. Uptake, metabolism and efflux of ^{14}C-5-hydroxytryptamine in isolated, perfused rat lungs. *J. Pharmacol. Exp. Ther.* 183: 341–355, 1972.
66. JUNOD, A. F. Mechanism of uptake of biogenic amines in the pulmonary circulation. In: *Lung Metabolism*, edited by A. F. Junod and R. de Haller. London: Academic, 1975, p. 387–398.
67. JUNOD, A. F. Metabolism, production, and release of hormones and mediators in the lung. *Am. Rev. Respir. Dis.* 112: 93–108, 1975.
68. JUNOD, A. F. Uptake, release and metabolism of drugs in the lungs. In: *International Encyclopedia of Pharmacology and Therapeutics. Respiratory Pharmacology*, edited by J. G. Widdicombe. Oxford, UK: Pergamon, 1981, p. 733–745.
69. JUNOD, A. F., AND C. ODY. Amine uptake and metabolism by endothelium of pig pulmonary artery and aorta. *Am. J. Physiol.* 232 (*Cell Physiol.* 1): C88–C94, 1977.
70. KRELL, R. D., J. MCCOY, AND P. CHRISTIAN. Accumulation and metabolism of [^{14}C]histamine by rat lung in vivo. *Biochem. Pharmacol.* 27: 820–821, 1978.
71. LARMI, T. K. I., AND E. HEIKKINEN. Pulmonary degradation and cardiovascular effects of intracavally infused 5-hydroxytryptamine in man. *Scand. J. Thorac. Cardiovasc. Surg.* 1: 123–126, 1967.
72. LILJA, B., AND S. E. LINDELL. Metabolism of [^{14}C]histamine in heart-lung-liver preparations of cats. *Br. J. Pharmacol.* 16: 203–208, 1961.
73. MCEWEN, C. M., JR., K. T. CULLEN, AND A. J. SOBER. Rabbit serum monoamine oxidase. Purification and characterization. *J. Biol. Chem.* 241: 4544–4556, 1966.
74. MINCHIN, R. F., B. W. MADSEN, AND K. F. ILETT. Effect of desmethylimipramine on the kinetics of chlorphentermine accumulation in isolated perfused rat lung. *J. Pharmacol. Exp. Ther.* 211: 514–518, 1979.
75. NAITO, H., AND C. N. GILLIS. Effects of halothane and nitrous oxide on removal of norepinephrine from the pulmonary circulation. *Anesthesiology* 39: 575–580, 1973.
76. NICHOLAS, T. E., J. M. STRUM, L. S. ANGELO, AND A. F. JUNOD. Site and mechanism of uptake of ^{3}H-*l*-norepinephrine

by isolated perfused rat lungs. *Circ. Res.* 35: 670–680, 1974.
77. ORTON, T. C., M. W. ANDERSON, R. D. PICKETT, T. E. ELING, AND J. R. FOUTS. Xenobiotic accumulation and metabolism by isolated perfused rabbit lungs. *J. Pharmacol. Exp. Ther.* 186: 482–497, 1973.
78. PEARSON, J. D., H. J. OLVERMAN, AND J. L. GORDON. Transport of 5-hydroxytryptamine by endothelial cells. *Biochem. Soc. Trans.* 5: 1181–1183, 1977.
79. PHILPOT, R. M., M. W. ANDERSON, AND T. E. ELING. Uptake, accumulation and metabolism of chemicals by the lung. In: *Lung Biology in Health and Disease. Metabolic Functions of the Lung*, edited by Y. S. Bakhle and J. R. Vane. New York: Dekker, 1977, vol. 4, chapt. 5, p. 123–171.
80. PICKETT, R. D., M. W. ANDERSON, T. C. ORTON, AND T. E. ELING. The pharmacodynamics of 5-hydroxytryptamine uptake and metabolism by the isolated perfused rabbit lung. *J. Pharmacol. Exp. Ther.* 194: 545–553, 1975.
81. RICKABY, D. A., C. A. DAWSON, AND M. B. MARON. Pulmonary inactivation of serotonin and site of serotonin pulmonary vasoconstriction. *J. Appl. Physiol.: Respirat. Environ. Exercise Physiol.* 48: 606–612, 1980.
82. ROSENBLOOM, P. M., AND A. D. BASS. A lung perfusion preparation for the study of drug metabolism. *J. Appl. Physiol.* 29: 138–144, 1970.
83. ROTH, J. A., AND C. N. GILLIS. Deamination of β-phenylethylamine by monoamine oxidase-inhibition by imipramine. *Biochem. Pharmacol.* 23: 2537–2545, 1974.
84. ROTH, J. A., AND C. N. GILLIS. Multiple forms of amine oxidase in perfused rabbit lung. *J. Pharmacol. Exp. Ther.* 194: 537–544, 1975.
85. ROTH, R. A., AND C. N. GILLIS. Effect of ventilation and pH on removal of mescaline and biogenic amines by rabbit lung. *J. Appl. Physiol.: Respirat. Environ. Exercise Physiol.* 44: 553–558, 1978.
86. ROTH, R. A., JR., J. A. ROTH, AND C. N. GILLIS. Disposition of ^{14}C-mescaline by rabbit lung. *J. Pharmacol. Exp. Ther.* 200: 394–401, 1977.
87. ROTH, R. A., AND K. B. WALLACE. Disposition of biogenic amines and angiotensin I by lungs of spontaneously hypertensive rats. *Am. J. Physiol.* 239 (*Heart Circ. Physiol.* 8): H736–H741, 1980.
88. ROTH, R. A., K. B. WALLACE, R. H. ALPER, AND M. D. BAILIE. Effect of paraquat treatment of rats on disposition of 5-hydroxytryptamine and angiotensin I by perfused lung. *Biochem. Pharmacol.* 28: 2349–2355, 1979.
89. SABELLI, H. C., R. L. BORISON, B. I. DIAMOND, H. S. HAVDALA, AND N. NARASIMHACHARI. Phenylethylamine and brain function. *Biochem. Pharmacol.* 27: 1729–1730, 1978.
90. SAID, S. I. The lung as a metabolic organ. *N. Engl. J. Med.* 279: 1330–1334, 1969.
91. SAID, S. I. The lung in relation to vasoactive hormones. *Federation Proc.* 32: 1972–1975, 1973.
92. SHEPRO, D., J. C. BATBOUTA, L. S. ROBBLEE, M. P. CARSON, AND F. A. BELAMARICH. Serotonin transport by cultured bovine aortic endothelium. *Circ. Res.* 36: 799–805, 1975.
93. SMALL, R., E. MACARAK, AND A. B. FISHER. Production of 5-hydroxyindoleacetic acid from serotonin by cultured endothelial cells. *J. Cell. Physiol.* 90: 225–232, 1976.
94. SNEDDON, J. M. Sodium-dependent accumulation of 5-hydroxytryptamine by rat blood platelets. *Br. J. Pharmacol.* 37: 680–688, 1969.
95. SOLE, M. J., M. DROBAC, L. SCHWARTZ, M. N. HUSSAIN, AND E. F. VAUGHAN-NEIL. The extraction of circulating catecholamines by the lungs in normal man and in patients with pulmonary hypertension. *Circulation* 60: 160–163, 1979.
96. STEINBERG, H., D. J. P. BASSETT, AND A. B. FISHER. Depression of pulmonary 5-hydroxytryptamine uptake by metabolic inhibitors. *Am. J. Physiol.* 228: 1298–1303, 1975.
97. STEINBERG, H., AND D. K. DAS. Competition between platelets and lung for 5-hydroxytryptamine uptake. *Exp. Lung Res.* 1: 121–130, 1980.
98. STRUM, J. M., AND A. F. JUNOD. Radioautographic demonstration of 5-hydroxytryptamine-^{3}H uptake by pulmonary endothelial cells. *J. Cell Biol.* 54: 456–467, 1972.
99. THOMAS, D. P., AND J. R. VANE. 5-Hydroxytryptamine in the circulation of the dog. *Nature London* 216: 335–338, 1967.
100. TISSARI, A. H., AND D. F. BOGDANSKI. Biogenic amine transport. IV. Comparison of effects of ouabain and K$^+$ deficiency on the transport of 5-hydroxytryptamine and norepinephrine by synaptosomes. *Pharmacology* 5: 225–234, 1977.
101. VANE, J. R. The release and fate of vaso-active hormones in the circulation. *Br. J. Pharmacol.* 35: 209–242, 1969.
102. WHITBY, L. G., J. AXELROD, AND H. WEIL-MALHERBE. The fate of H^3-norepinephrine in animals. *J. Pharmacol. Exp. Ther.* 132: 193–201, 1961.
103. WHITE, M. K., H. B. HECHTMAN, AND D. SHEPRO. Canine lung uptake of plasma and platelet serotonin. *Microvasc. Res.* 9: 230–241, 1975.
104. WILSON, A. G. E., F. C. P. LAW, T. E. ELING, AND M. W. ANDERSON. Uptake, metabolism and efflux of methadone in "single pass" isolated perfused rabbit lungs. *J. Pharmacol. Exp. Ther.* 199: 360–367, 1976.
105. YANG, H.-Y. T., AND N. H. NEFF. The monoamine oxidases of brain: selective inhibition with drugs and the consequences for the metabolism of the biogenic amines. *J. Pharmacol. Exp. Ther.* 189: 733–740, 1974.
106. YOUDIM, M. B. H., Y. S. BAKHLE, AND R. R. BEN-HARARI. Inactivation of monoamines by the lung. In: *Metabolic Functions of the Lung.* Amsterdam: Excerpta Med., 1980, p. 105–128. (Ciba Found. Symp. 78.)

CHAPTER 10

Processing of angiotensin and other peptides by the lungs

UNA S. RYAN | *Department of Medicine, University of Miami School of Medicine, Miami, Florida*

CHAPTER CONTENTS

Historical Background
Pulmonary Metabolism
   Angiotensin I
   Bradykinin
   Angiotensin II
   Angiotensin III
   Angiotensin-converting enzyme: kininase II
   Cellular and subcellular sites of relevant pulmonary enzymes
   Immunocytochemistry
   Pulmonary endothelial cells as a model system
      Cell culture methods
      Scale-up methods
      Do endothelial cells synthesize angiotensin-converting enzyme?
   Clinical implications
   Actions of peptide hormones on lungs
      Interdependence of endothelial cells and smooth muscle cells
      Interactions among vasoactive agents and their target cells
   Other peptides
Discussion and Future Directions

NOTING THAT LUNGS evolved from gills, Comroe (23) points out that the gill circulation represents a huge absorbing surface through which chemical materials in the water, in addition to O_2, might enter the circulating blood. A detoxifying station in the gills would serve as a useful defense mechanism for the rest of the body. Perhaps as the respiratory surfaces become internalized the detoxifying function could still serve a useful purpose. Vane (138) proposed that the pulmonary circulation can be biologically useful in removing from the blood substances never intended to enter the systemic circulation (local hormones), whereas those intended for wide distribution to tissues are not removed from blood in the lungs. The hypotheses seem to hold reasonably well for peptide hormones. For example, bradykinin is inactivated and angiotensin I (ANG I) is converted to ANG II, but eledoisin, substance P, physalaemin, vasopressin, and oxytocin pass through unchanged.

The pulmonary vascular bed can be considered as a sluice gate for controlling the quality of biologically active peptides allowed to enter the systemic circulation. Whether the selective control exercised by the lungs should be envisaged more as a fail-safe mechanism or as a prefilter for final adjustments to be made by cells of the target organs themselves is worth examination. The remarkable feature of the lungs is the selectivity of the processing, especially when one considers that most peptides are indiscriminately degraded by blood enzymes, tissue homogenates, and many enzymes familiar on laboratory shelves. What is unique about the pulmonary circulation? Important features must be in part anatomical (e.g., the position of the lungs in the circulation and the extensiveness of the pulmonary vasculature) and in part chemical (e.g., which of the circulating peptides are substrates for pulmonary enzymes). Nevertheless one of the most critical determinants of the selectivity of metabolism of peptides is the location of their inactivating enzymes. Thus it is the cell biology that to a great extent determines the access of peptides to their metabolizing enzymes.

The mechanisms of formation and inactivation of the kinins and angiotensins are probably directly related to the onset and duration of actions of these substances. It is no longer a surprise to find that a substance entering the lungs may not emerge unscathed; however, a full understanding of the selectivity of the pulmonary metabolism of peptides must take into account not only the circulating levels of peptide hormones but where, when, and how they are produced, released, modified, or inactivated and when, how, and where they act.

This chapter is devoted to the processing of polypeptide hormones by the lungs. Previous reviews cover certain aspects with a broader scope (8, 47–49, 51, 59, 68, 108–110, 120, 133, 135) or with a finer focus (38, 98, 115, 134).

HISTORICAL BACKGROUND

Bradykinin and angiotensin are the most studied of the physiologically important peptide hormones pro-

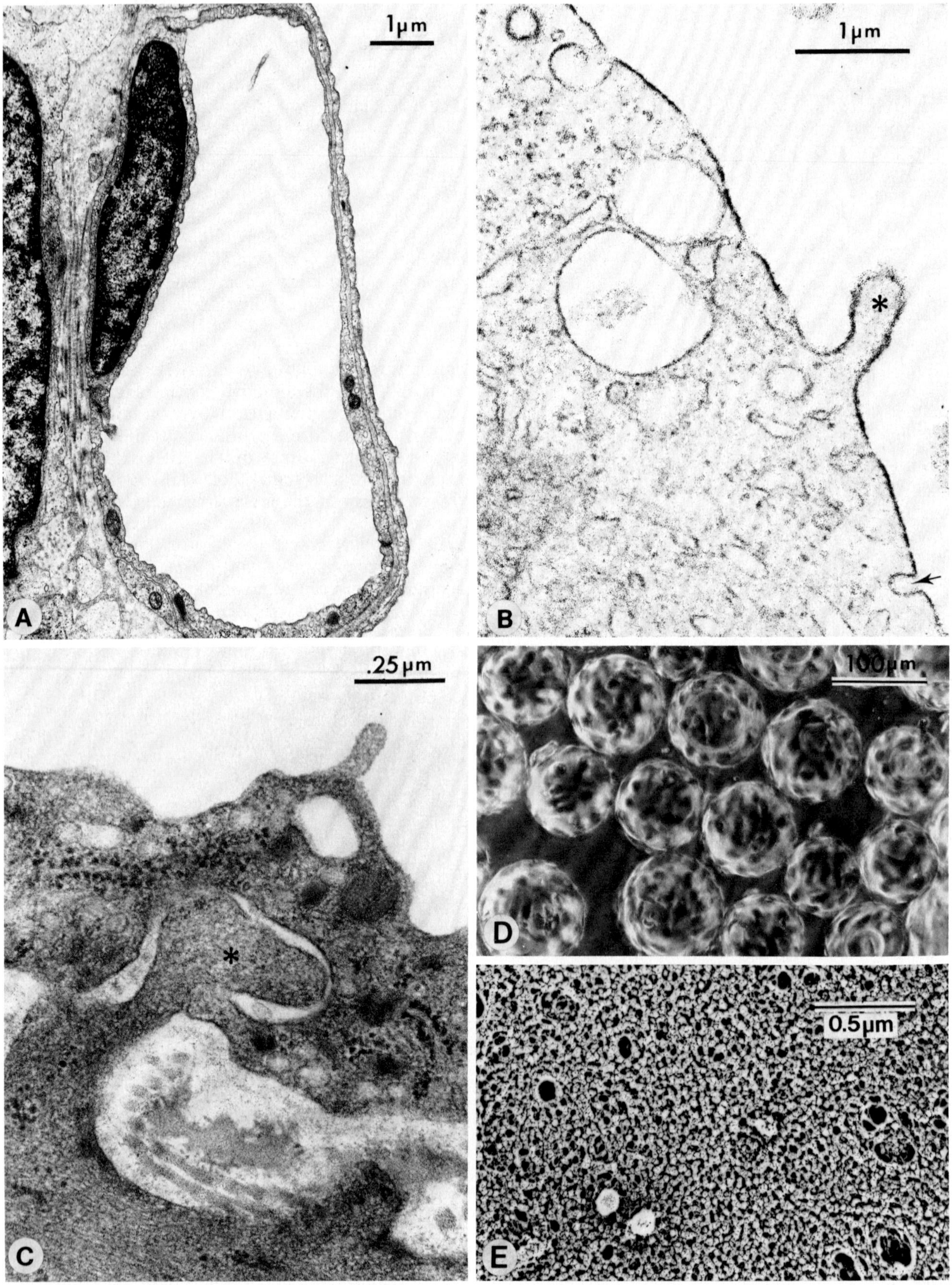
1μm
A
1μm
*
B
.25μm
*
C
100μm
D
0.5μm
E

TABLE 1. *Structures of Angiotensins and Bradykinin*

1	2	3	4	5	6	7	8	9	10

Asp-Arg-Val-Tyr-Ile-His-Pro-Phe-His-Leu
ANG I

Arg-Val-Tyr-Ile-His-Pro-Phe-His-Leu
[des-Asp^1]ANG I

Asp-Arg-Val-Tyr-Ile-His-Pro-Phe
ANG II

Arg-Val-Tyr-Ile-His-Pro-Phe
ANG III

Arg-Pro-Pro-Gly-Phe-Ser-Pro-Phe-Arg
Bradykinin

cessed by the lungs. Since the discoveries of angiotensin (15, 86) and bradykinin (94) it has been known that blood and tissues contain enzymes capable of terminating their biological activities (42, 94). Initially it was thought that the enzymes were specific for angiotensin and bradykinin. However, when the primary structures of the angiotensins (37, 74, 130) and bradykinin (36) were established (see Table 1 for chemical structures), it became apparent that enzymes having specificities like those of trypsin, chymotrypsin, pepsin, aminopeptidases, and carboxypeptidases could reduce or eliminate biological activities. Studies indicate that hydrolysis of any peptide bond of bradykinin eliminates biological activity (for review see ref. 128). Similarly hydrolysis of any of the peptide bonds from Arg^2 to Phe^8 of ANG II either eliminates or reduces biological activity. Hydrolysis of the Asp^1-Arg^2 bond reduces activity on vascular smooth muscle by at least 50% (87) but increases activity on adrenal cortex (20). Only one peptide cleavage site in ANG I is compatible with preservation and enhancement of biological activity, the hydrolysis of the Phe^8-His^9 bond (74) that forms ANG II.

Virtually every tissue studied contains an abundance of enzymes capable of inactivating ANG II and bradykinin (16, 39, 42, 65). However, which of these enzymes has access to angiotensin or bradykinin in vivo is a central question in studies of the fates of these polypeptides (67, 103, 104, 110, 126). Many tissue enzymes do not have access. For example, bradykinin is degraded to a series of characteristic peptides during circulation through the lungs but is reduced to free amino acids by lung homogenates (102, 103). Similarly ANG I is converted to ANG II during circulation through the lungs (78, 79, 101, 102, 114) but is inactivated by lung homogenates (6). Homogenates of the lung also rapidly inactivate ANG II (65), yet only a small proportion of ANG II entering the pulmonary artery fails to emerge in the pulmonary vein (11, 12, 54, 61, 73).

Red cells, white cells, and plasma contain enzymes capable of degrading the angiotensins and the kinins (39, 42, 55), but the importance of blood enzymes in terminating the activities of these polypeptides is in doubt. When cell damage (e.g., evident by hemolysis) is avoided, inactivation of ANG II and bradykinin is slow (30, 39, 45, 61, 78, 79). The brief durations of action of bradykinin and ANG II cannot be explained in terms of blood enzymes (34, 45). Furthermore tissues perfused with artificial salt solutions degrade bradykinin (103, 104) and ANG II (73) at rates comparable to those of tissues perfused with blood.

PULMONARY METABOLISM

Bradykinin and ANG I are almost completely eliminated during the few seconds required for blood to pass through the pulmonary vascular bed (110). Elimination is accomplished by the hydrolysis of peptide bonds. Hydrolysis of bradykinin, a substance that lowers blood pressure, yields biologically inactive products. Hydrolysis of ANG I yields, among other products, the potent vasopressor hormone ANG II. Angiotensin II is released into the systemic arterial circulation. Thus as central venous blood is converted into arterial blood a blood pressure–raising substance is formed and a blood pressure–lowering substance is inactivated with concomitant implications for blood pressure homeostasis. In the metabolism of bradykinin and ANG I the reactions are catalyzed by peptidase enzymes situated along the luminal surface (Fig. 1*A, B*) of pulmonary endothelial cells, with no require-

FIG. 1. *A*: transverse section of a pulmonary capillary endothelial cell. At the level of the alveolar capillary unit, processing of vasoactive substances is likely to be maximal. Cells are extremely thin but present a vast surface area that is further enhanced by caveolae and surface projections. *B*: immunocytochemical localization of angiotensin-converting enzyme on plasma membrane of a pulmonary endothelial cell in culture including caveolae (*arrow*) and projection (***). The endothelial surface is not only extensive but contains specific enzymes accessible to circulating substrates. *C*: vasoactive peptides are not only inactivated during circulation through the lungs but also exert effects on pulmonary vascular tone. The mechanism is not fully understood; however, some pulmonary vessels, in this case a small pulmonary artery ~200 μm in diameter, exhibit structural interactions known as myoendothelial junctions (***) between endothelial and smooth muscle layers. *D*: with current technology for large-scale, long-term culture, pulmonary endothelial cells are propagated on microcarrier beads in roller bottles. *E*: surface replicas of plasma membrane of endothelial cells illustrate the true unfractured face normally exposed to circulating substrates. Particles of various sizes are evident, but identification of specific enzymatic or receptor sites awaits future studies. [From Ryan (116a).]

ment for enzymes of blood nor access to intracellular enzymes of lung cells (120).

Angiotensin I

During one passage through the pulmonary circulation (114) up to 20% of ANG I is converted to ANG II, its more potent lower-molecular-weight homologue. Initial studies showed that [^{14}C-Leu^{10}]ANG I is metabolized to yield radioactive His-Leu and a biologically active nonradioactive peptide. With [^{14}C-Phe^{8}]-ANG I, chemical and biological identification techniques subsequently confirmed that ANG II is the major large polypeptide metabolite (102).

There are several striking features of the metabolism of ANG I during passage through the lungs (114, 133). 1) Metabolism is not due to enzymes present in the blood. 2) The hydrolase enzymes required to degrade ANG I are not secreted by the lungs. 3) Lungs perfused with radioactive ANG I do not retain radioactivity. These features suggest that the requisite hydrolase enzymes exist on or very near the luminal surface of pulmonary endothelial cells. This concept is supported by the kinetics of disappearance of [^{14}C-Phe^{8}]ANG I during circulation through isolated rat lungs washed free of blood (102). The mean transit time and the volume of distribution of radioactivity are no greater than those of blue dextran (M_r > 2,000,000), a compound unlikely to leave the vascular space. There is a quantitative recovery of radioactivity in the venous effluent, yet little if any of the radioactivity remains in the form of ANG I.

Plasma contains a carboxypeptidase capable of hydrolyzing ANG I to yield ANG II and His-Leu (31, 74), yet the physiological role of the plasma enzyme is still in question (79, 101, 102, 113, 114). During circulation through the lungs the conversion rate of ANG I is greater than can be accounted for by blood enzymes. Similarly the apparent concentration of the dipeptidyl carboxypeptidase enzyme in lung homogenates is greater than that in plasma (31). The role of nonpulmonary vascular beds in the metabolism of ANG I is less clear. However, homogenates of a variety of tissues (notably the liver, diaphragm, lung, and ileum) contain enzymes capable of metabolizing ANG I or alternative substrates of the ANG I–converting enzyme (25, 26, 62). Evidence indicates that substances known to inhibit the ANG I–converting enzyme, e.g., the bradykinin-potentiating peptide BPP$_{5a}$ (Pyroglutamyl-Lys-Trp-Ala-Pro), can reduce or abolish biological effects (e.g., increased renovascular resistance) ordinarily considered a consequence of infusing ANG I (2).

Methot et al. (77) assumed that the disappearance of ANG I in the liver was accounted for by enzymatic degradation. Hodge et al. (61) considered removal of the hormone from the vascular space followed by either degradation or subsequent release back into the bloodstream. Ferreira and Vane (45) thought that bradykinin might be degraded by enzymes of the interstitial space, cell surfaces, or intracellular organelles. The apparent activation of ANG I during passage through the lungs (78) implied an enzymatic mechanism that Ng and Vane (80) sought to clarify by studying the biological effects of [His^{10}]ANG I, the synthetic analogue of ANG I, before and after perfusion through the pulmonary circulation of the dog. They found that the activity (effects on rat colon) of the analogue is <1% of that of ANG I itself and that its apparent activity decreases during passage through the lungs. From their findings they concluded that [His^{10}]ANG I was not a substrate for the postulated pulmonary converting enzyme. They further stated that the enzyme responsible for degrading ANG I must be an endopeptidase. Bakhle (5) provided additional evidence implicating an enzymatic mechanism by showing that the effects of ANG I (stimulation of isolated rat colon) are increased by a factor of 2 during incubation with a high-speed pellet (20,000–105,000 g) of homogenized dog lung. Cushman and Cheung (25) reported shortly thereafter that an enzyme capable of hydrolyzing Hip-His-Leu to yield His-Leu could be purified from a particulate fraction of whole-lung homogenate.

Early studies (11, 12, 19, 45, 73, 77–79) illustrate that the elimination of the angiotensins and kinins, as they occur in the circulation, is more closely related to activities of a given vascular bed than to blood enzymes. However, these studies were based on the results obtained from bioassay techniques (7, 45, 61, 78–80). The technique is dynamic (138), and there is little doubt that the data would have been difficult or impossible to obtain by other methods available at the time. However, the bioassay method provides no information on the subcellular or molecular mechanisms by which some compounds are removed and some are activated within the circulation. With hindsight it is now possible to understand the processing of ANG I to ANG II in terms of endothelial cell–bound angiotensin-converting enzyme (ACE).

Bradykinin

Ferreira and Vane (45) found that bradykinin disappears during circulation through the head, hindquarters, and kidney and is not spared during circulation through the lungs, as is ANG II. Its half-life in blood alone was ~17 s, whereas its half-life in the various vascular beds could not exceed 3–4 s. Bradykinin is not removed by cellular uptake during passage through the lungs but is metabolized by hydrolytic degradation (100, 102, 103). When [^{14}C-Pro^{2}]bradykinin is perfused through blood-free lungs, the major radioactive metabolites are Pro-Pro (60%) and Arg-Pro-Pro-Gly (40%). When [^{3}H-Phe^{8}]bradykinin is used, the major radioactive metabolite is Phe-Arg. The metabolites can be varied by the use of substances that potentiate the biological actions of bradykinin.

For example, when 2-mercaptoethanol and bradykinin-potentiating factor (44) are included in the perfusion system containing [^{3}H-Phe^8]bradykinin, the sole radioactive metabolite is Pro-Phe-Arg (103). The findings imply that bradykinin is metabolized in at least five peptide bonds during the few seconds required to pass from the pulmonary artery to the pulmonary vein.

The pulmonary metabolism of bradykinin has several distinguishing features. *1*) With either [^{14}C-Pro^2]-bradykinin or [^{3}H-Phe^8]bradykinin virtually all the radioactivity entering the pulmonary artery emerges in the pulmonary vein. Less than 1% of the radioactivity remains in the lungs. None of the radioactivity of the venous effluent remains in the form of bradykinin. *2*) Even though the degradation of bradykinin is extensive, the associated radioactivity is not delayed in transit, its mean transit time and volume of distribution being precisely that of blue dextran (M_r 2,000,000), a compound unlikely to leave the vascular space during one circulation. *3*) Metabolism of bradykinin does not depend on blood enzymes, because degradation is not impaired during passage through lungs free of blood. *4*) Metabolites produced by intact lungs are specific and different from those produced by lung homogenates; enzymes of the latter cause complete degradation of bradykinin to its component amino acids (104). Thus the lungs contain a variety of peptide hydrolase enzymes that do not have access to circulating bradykinin.

The characteristics of the pulmonary metabolism of bradykinin are strikingly similar to those of ANG I. Accordingly it was postulated that bradykinin is also metabolized by enzymes on or close to the pulmonary endothelium (103). Metabolism of bradykinin is highly specific. All higher homologues of bradykinin are metabolized at rates slower than that of bradykinin itself (93, 104). For example, Lys-bradykinin is metabolized at about one-half the rate, and Met-Lys-bradykinin and phyllokinin are metabolized at about one-tenth the rate. Polistes kinin, an 18-residue kinin, is not metabolized at all during passage through the lungs. All these peptides contain the same five peptide bonds of bradykinin, suggesting that the relevant lung enzymes are either highly specific or are sequestered in an exclusive microenvironment so that some substrates have access to the enzymes but others do not (131). In fact the specificity appears to reside with the enzyme (33).

Angiotensin II

The selectivity of the lungs in processing vasoactive polypeptides is illustrated by the apparent fates of ANG I and II. Goffinet and Mulrow (54) found that ANG II infused via the portal vein or the common iliac artery had reduced blood pressure effects compared with angiotensin infused via the jugular vein or the aortic arch. They found little difference between effects of angiotensin infused via the jugular vein or aortic arch and concluded that ANG II is cleared by the liver and hindlimb but not by the lungs. Their results were confirmed (12, 19, 73). Hodge et al. (61) and Leary and Ledingham (73) extended previous findings to show that ANG II also disappears during circulation through the head and kidneys. The apparent half-life of ANG II in blood circulated through silicone tubing, but not through a vascular bed, was ~3 min. For undetermined reasons [Asp^1, Val^5]ANG II had a longer half-life (282 s) than [Asp^1, Ile^5]ANG II (183 s) and [Asn^1, Val^5]ANG II (146 s). In contrast the half-lives of these angiotensins in vivo were estimated to be no more than one circulation time (~15 s). Thus compared with ANG I (78, 79), its higher homologue, little or no ANG II–like activity disappears during passage through the pulmonary vascular bed.

Osborne et al. (85) provided the first direct evidence on the mechanisms of disappearance of ANG II in other vascular beds. Using [^{3}H-Tyr^4]ANG II, they found that 30%–80% of the biological activity disappears during passage through the renal or coronary circulation. More than 80% of the radioactivity was recovered in the venous effluent simultaneously with the emergence of biological activity; <2% of the radioactivity was retained by the heart and <3% was retained by the kidneys; the remaining radioactivity was not recovered. On gel chromatography, most of the radioactivity was retarded in elution compared with angiotensin, occurring as a complex mixture of lower homologues. The data indicate that ANG II is eliminated by enzymatic hydrolysis, possibly by enzymes on or near the endothelium (for review see ref. 97).

Angiotensin III

The peptide [des-Asp^1]ANG II is a normal constituent of blood and is believed to be formed from ANG II through the action of an aminopeptidase A–like enzyme (see ref. 129). Similarly Lys-bradykinin (kallidin 10) is rapidly converted into bradykinin after its entry into venous blood (81), presumably through the action of a selective lysine aminopeptidase. Given the differences in pharmacological activities between ANG II and ANG III and those between Lys-bradykinin and bradykinin, perhaps aminopeptidase enzymes are important in the overall control of blood pressure hemostasis, but little is known about the distribution of these enzymes among blood and tissues.

In any event [des-Asp^1]ANG I is among the major products formed by rat lungs perfused with ANG I (1, 114) and can be converted to ANG III by ACE (22, 136). Under similar conditions the NH$_2$-terminal amino acid residue of bradykinin is removed, a finding that implies the action of an aminopeptidase enzyme (110).

Capillaries of the adrenal cortex possess both ACE

and aminopeptidase A activity (27). Aminopeptidase A is of interest in terms of blood pressure control, because it converts ANG II into ANG III, a possible aldosterone secretagogue (13). Thus endothelial cells of the adrenal cortex and probably other arterial and microvascular beds are capable of making fine adjustments to the concentrations of kinins and angiotensins.

Angiotensin-Converting Enzyme: Kininase II

Shortly after the discoveries that bradykinin and ANG I are eliminated during passage through the lungs, several investigators began to consider that the two polypeptides might be eliminated by a common mechanism (5, 79). Bakhle (5) reported that a crude particulate fraction of lung homogenate was capable of converting ANG I and of inactivating bradykinin. Both activities were inhibited by ethylenediaminetetraacetic acid (EDTA) and bradykinin-potentiating factor. However, the bradykininase activity was inhibited by 2-mercaptoethanol and 8-hydroxyquinoline, whereas the converting enzyme was not. In an analogous study, Sander and Huggins (125) showed that bradykinin acts as a competitive inhibitor of the metabolism of ANG I, a result subsequently confirmed by Cushman and Cheung (26). Igic et al. (64) reported that purified fractions of lung, kidney, and plasma were capable of cleaving dipeptides from the COOH-terminal ends of ANG I, bradykinin, the B chain of insulin, and Dns-Gly-Gly-Gly.

Dorer et al. (32) isolated a homogeneous preparation of hog lung converting enzyme that hydrolyzes ANG I to yield ANG II plus His-Leu. This enzyme has also been found to hydrolyze bradykinin through at least two steps (33), thus establishing the two activities as one enzyme.

Cellular and Subcellular Sites of Relevant Pulmonary Enzymes

Angiotensin I and bradykinin are metabolized by several different enzymes during a single passage through the pulmonary bed (110). Only one of these enzymes (ACE, kininase II) has been characterized in detail (for review see refs. 98, 115, 134). Nonetheless there is considerable indirect evidence indicating that all the relevant enzymes must exist on or near the luminal surface of pulmonary endothelial cells.

According to this concept the plasma membrane fraction of whole-lung homogenates should contain the enzyme(s) capable of converting ANG I to ANG II plus the dipeptide His-Leu. Therefore a technique based on the localization of 5'-nucleotidase on plasma membrane, specifically within the caveolae intracellulares, was developed (112). Plasma membrane collected by this method is capable of degrading bradykinin and of converting ANG I to ANG II at rates comparable to those of intact lungs (105, 112, 113).

However, it is not known what proportion of the plasma membrane preparation is derived from endothelium and what proportion comes from other cell types. Therefore to study the problem more directly, endothelial cells were isolated from the main stem pulmonary artery. By means of a Häutchen preparation (90), monolayers of endothelial cells were obtained on a cellulose acetate support (132) and shown to convert ANG I to ANG II and to degrade bradykinin to yield characteristic products (133).

Techniques modified from those used to obtain endothelium from human umbilical vein (63, 66) were used to harvest larger numbers of pulmonary artery endothelial cells. These techniques made it possible to maintain cells in culture and to confirm our previous work (117, 124). The cells degrade ^{125}I-labeled Tyr^8-bradykinin to yield ^{125}I-Tyr-Arg, the product formed by ACE (21). Simpler substrates are now available for the assay of ACE as it occurs in association with endothelial cells in culture (99, 117), and it now appears that ACE activity is a property of all endothelial cells.

Immunocytochemistry

When Dorer et al. (32) purified ACE to apparent homogeneity, we began collaborative studies. Antibodies were prepared against the enzyme (from hog lung) to localize by immunocytochemistry the cellular and subcellular site of ACE at the level of electron microscopy. Antibodies (from goat) coupled to 11-microperoxidase (11-MP) with glutaraldehyde (111, 122) localized the enzyme to endothelial cells of rat lung as well as porcine and bovine pulmonary endothelial cells. To increase the resolution of the immunocytochemical reaction and to minimize possible nonspecific adherence of aldehyde conjugates to cells, we used a technique that coupled the partially purified antibody via a bifunctional active ester to 8-microperoxidase (8-MP), a lower homologue of 11-MP (100). Results obtained with the improved conjugate were precisely the same as those obtained previously: ACE is distributed along the luminal surface of pulmonary and aortic endothelial cells [Fig. 1B; (124)].

Caldwell et al. (18) independently showed that fluorescein-labeled goat antibodies to pure rabbit lung ACE react with rabbit tissues to bind to the luminal surface of blood vessels of lungs, spleen, adrenal gland, pancreas, and liver. However, the most prominent site of labeling in the kidney is on the brush border of the proximal tubules.

Pulmonary Endothelial Cells as a Model System

Because circulating kinins and angiotensins are processed almost exclusively by enzymes on or near the luminal surface of pulmonary endothelial cells (see ref. 124), much current work has focused on the activities of pulmonary endothelial cells in culture. However, recognizing that under these conditions endothelial cells serve as a model system and are thus subject to the disadvantages inherent in any model system, it is prudent to validate the cultures in terms of metabolic properties expected of the cells in vivo (121) and to compare data with those obtained with isolated perfused rat lungs.

The fate of [^{3}H-Phe^8]bradykinin (10 ng/ml at 37°C) was examined. The lungs were perfused at 10 ml/min at pressures between 4 and 20 mmHg. In some experiments SQ 14225 was used at 10^{-6} M, a concentration sufficient to inhibit ACE completely. In the absence of SQ 14225, [^{3}H-Phe^8]bradykinin is converted quantitatively into [^{3}H]Phe-Arg, the product expected from the action of ACE. Under these conditions the mean transit time across the lungs was ~3 s. By taking the quantitative recovery of Phe-Arg to represent no fewer than four half-lives (93% degradation), the half-life of [^{3}H-Phe^8]bradykinin within the pulmonary vascular bed thus could not have been >0.75 s. When SQ 14225 was added to the perfusion solution, the formation of [^{3}H]Phe-Arg was completely inhibited. Radioactivity was recovered quantitatively in the venous effluent in the form of Pro-Phe-Arg (40%), Ser-Pro-Phe-Arg (22%), [des-Arg^1]bradykinin (18%), and Gly^4-Arg^9 (20%). None of the radioactivity was recovered in the form of bradykinin itself (110).

Within the limits examined, pulmonary endothelial cells in culture appear to account for most, if not all, of the metabolic events. In our laboratory we have routinely used bovine pulmonary endothelial cells (116). Confluent monolayers of endothelial cells in the 25-cm^2 growing area of T25 flasks (3.5 × 10^6) are washed six times with medium 199 and then incubated at 37°C in fresh medium 199 containing [^{3}H-Phe^8]-bradykinin at 10–40 ng/ml. To inhibit ACE, SQ 14225 (10^{-6} M) or the bradykinin-potentiating peptide BPP$_{9a}$ (10^{-6} M) is included in some reactions. When ACE is not inhibited, [^{3}H]Phe-Arg accumulates 72%–80% of the total radioactivity over a period of 120 min. As much as 15% of the starting amount of radioactivity remains in the form of bradykinin, and 5%–10% accumulates in the form of Ser-Pro-Phe-Arg and Pro-Phe-Arg. Either of the ACE inhibitors prevents the formation of [^{3}H]Phe-Arg. However, the formation of Ser-Pro-Phe-Arg and Pro-Phe-Arg is not inhibited. As much as 30% of the starting quantity of bradykinin may remain intact after 120 min of incubation. Thus bovine endothelial cells in culture replicate part, but not all, of the reactions conducted by isolated rat lungs (110). These reactions may appear to be relatively slow, but it should be kept in mind that intact bovine lungs contain 10^{14} endothelial cells.

CELL CULTURE METHODS. Pure lines of endothelial cells have been isolated from the pulmonary artery, inferior vena cava, and aorta of the cow, pig, rat, and rabbit (117). The technique is based on methods for isolating endothelial cells from human umbilical veins (53, 66). The vessels are washed with 0.2% collagenase in a balanced salt solution (e.g., Puck's phosphate-buffered saline), and the cells are maintained in medium 199 containing 20% fetal calf serum and antibiotics. The endothelial cells have been characterized by light and electron microscopy and by the presence of ACE activity (117). Endothelial cells obtained from the microvasculature of the lungs have the same growth characteristics (doubling time 24 h) as cells obtained from the large pulmonary vessels, and ACE activity on the plasma membrane and caveolae has been demonstrated by immunocytochemistry (56, 116, 124a).

SCALE-UP METHODS. Metabolism of some blood-borne substrates may be accomplished through the action of enzymes on the luminal surface of the endothelial cells. Definitive testing of this hypothesis has depended on cultivating endothelial cells free of artifacts that may arise when cells are harvested and passaged with exogenous enzymes (e.g., trypsin and collagenase). Functional activities of endothelial cells, such as those conducted by ACE, can be heavily damaged by the methods used commonly for cell culture. Isolation and passaging of endothelial cells by the use of protease enzymes commonly yields cells in culture that do not have all the surface enzymes and proteins believed to exist on endothelial cells in situ. To overcome this problem techniques have been developed for the culture of pulmonary endothelial cells that avoid exposure to exogenous proteolytic enzymes at both the isolation step and during successive passages (116, 119, 124a).

The cells are harvested by scraping the luminal surface of the pulmonary artery of a newborn calf with a scalpel. The sheet of cells thus removed can be seeded into flasks or directly onto microcarriers. The cells on microcarriers (Fig. 1D) are grown in roller bottles, a system with numerous advantages. The surface area for attachment is enormous. The cells on each bead form a confluent monolayer, a feature important for assay of surface enzymes (121), while retaining the advantages of a suspension culture for adequate mixing and utilization of nutrients. Perhaps the most important advantage is that the system allows the cells to be passaged without exposure to trypsin. The cell-covered bead suspension can be split into new flasks to which fresh medium and new beads are also added. The cells colonize the new beads, and the process can be repeated to provide long-term, large-scale cultures of pulmonary endothelial cells that retain the structural and functional properties of primary or early-passage cultures and are responsive to hormones.

DO ENDOTHELIAL CELLS SYNTHESIZE ANGIOTENSIN-CONVERTING ENZYME? Pulmonary endothelial cells can be propagated in medium 199 containing 20% fetal bovine serum previously inactivated by heat

(61°C for 30 min). Under these conditions the ACE of fetal bovine serum is completely inactivated and therefore cannot contribute to the ACE activity of the cell monolayers. For example, endothelial cells were seeded, grown to confluence, passaged 1:2 (i.e., contents of one flask were distributed between two new flasks), and the procedure was continued through four passages. The cell seed and cells of each subsequent passage were assayed for ACE with [^{3}H]benzoyl-Phe-Ala-Pro as substrate. The progeny of each original seed cell was estimated to be ~6,400 cells in the fourth passage at confluence. The cells possessed 12,000 times more ACE activity than could have been contributed by the original seed cells. Thus bovine pulmonary endothelial cells clearly have the ability to synthesize ACE (117).

Hayes et al. (58) independently showed that pig aortic endothelial cells are capable of synthesizing ACE. They further adduced evidence that the enzyme is secreted into the cell culture medium and have postulated that plasma ACE is contributed by the endothelial cell lining.

Clinical Implications

Several types of injury to the lungs affect the quantities of vasoactive substances entering the systemic circulation, suggesting that damage to pulmonary endothelial cells may alter their capacity to process circulating substances.

Although the exact mechanism has not yet been determined, acute hypoxia appears to influence the metabolism of ANG I and bradykinin by the lungs. In anesthetized dogs, acute hypoxia has been reported to inhibit ACE activity, rapidly and reversibly, as assessed by extraction of bradykinin (134b) and conversion of ANG I (134d). Studies with cultured endothelial cells suggest that acute hypoxia has similar inhibitory effects on the converting enzyme in vitro (134c). Other studies indicate that the hypoxia-induced inhibition of the metabolism of ANG I and bradykinin may be secondary to hemodynamic alterations induced by hypoxia (18a, 84a). Chronic hypoxic lung diseases in humans are associated with abnormal blood pressure regulation, suggesting that the activity of ACE may be altered. Whereas the function of the converting enzyme may be impaired in experimental emphysema in dogs (134a), chronic hypoxia has been reported to have no effect on ACE activity in cultured endothelial cells (24a).

Neither the physiological nor pathophysiological implications of metabolic functions of the lungs are known (13a). Consequently it is premature to assess the usefulness of alterations in endothelial cell functions for the early detection of pulmonary vascular injury. However, an exciting new area has opened up in the therapeutic use of inhibitors of the pulmonary metabolism of peptides.

Enzymes that interconvert and inactivate kinins and angiotensins must play an important role in determining the overall expression of the activities of the kallikrein-kinin and renin-angiotensin systems. The snake venom peptide BPP$_{5a}$ (SQ 20475), given intravenously, reduces the blood pressure of rats with two-kidney Goldblatt hypertension (71); BPP$_{9a}$ is a potent but short-lasting inhibitor of ACE. Gavras et al. (50) have shown that BPP$_{9a}$ (SQ 20881; teprotide) can be used to reduce blood pressures of ~60% of the hypertensive population, sometimes to levels within the normal range. Neither BPP$_{9a}$ nor BPP$_{5a}$ can be administered orally. However, orally effective inhibitors of ACE have now been developed (3a, 83, 98a, 133a).

Although the use of ACE inhibitors has been associated with side effects (cf. ref. 35a), the side effects are unlikely to be caused by inhibition of ACE per se. Inhibition of ACE provides a mild means of controlling blood pressure for most hypertensive patients. Furthermore, inhibition of ACE can provide rapid and dramatic relief to patients with congestive heart failure (35, 50). Because the successful clinical use of inhibitors of ACE implies that a large number of patients may live periods of their lives without the benefits of ACE activity, it becomes important to define the alternative fates of kinins and ANG I (and [des-Asp^1]ANG I) under conditions in which ACE cannot function.

Actions of Peptide Hormones on Lungs

Historically the pulmonary circulation has been thought to be privileged compared with other vascular beds (e.g., kidney, skin, skeletal muscle, and intestinal tract). The tone and resistance of pulmonary blood vessels do not undergo striking changes in response to nerve impulses, chemical agents, changes in temperature, moderate blood loss, and other stimuli. Presumably the pulmonary circulation, a high-flow, low-pressure system having as its primary function the exchange of gases, should not undergo great changes in pressure and resistance to facilitate transfer of blood from resting to active organs. In fact pulmonary arterioles do not have the same investment of smooth muscle as do arterioles in the systemic circulation. Although the pulmonary circulation responds to agonists such as ANG II and norepinephrine, the responses in absolute terms are not dramatic (e.g., compared with the renal circulation) and are in some respects atypical. Thus ANG II increases pulmonary vascular resistance largely by its effect on large vessels (9, 60). In the systemic circulation, ANG II affects primarily small arteries and arterioles. Similarly bradykinin has relatively weak effects on pressure within the pulmonary artery but reduces total pulmonary resistance (in percent change) as much as it reduces total systemic resistance (95).

Reasons such as these suggest that pulmonary vascular smooth muscle may differ from smooth muscle of other vascular beds. It may be pertinent to add that other cell types of the pulmonary vascular bed differ qualitatively. Pulmonary endothelial cells do not appear to possess angiotensinase enzymes, a class of enzymes occurring abundantly in liver, spleen, and kidney (54, 61), presumably in association with endothelial cells.

INTERDEPENDENCE OF ENDOTHELIAL CELLS AND SMOOTH MUSCLE CELLS. Evidence indicates that the functions of endothelial cells and those of smooth muscle cells are interdependent. *1)* There is no apparent means by which intravascular bradykinin can gain direct access to smooth muscle other than by way of the endothelium. *2)* There is a morphological basis for these intercellular interactions in that junctions between the two cell types exist that have been called "myoendothelial junctions" [Fig. 1C; (91, 123)]. *3)* The mechanics of the vessel wall contractions make it likely that the endothelium and smooth muscle act as a unit.

Precisely how circulating vasoactive agents gain access to smooth muscle is not clear. It has been shown that bradykinin is rapidly metabolized during a single passage through the pulmonary circulation and that the metabolic reactions occur while the kinin is confined to the vascular space (103, 104). The major kininase enzyme [dipeptidyl carboxypeptidase (kininase II, also known as ACE)] is situated on the luminal surface of pulmonary endothelial cells (111, 124). Nonetheless bradykinin administered intravenously (or presumably that generated on the venous side of the systemic circulation) decreases pulmonary vascular resistance (95).

Angiotensin II can raise pulmonary artery blood pressure and increase pulmonary vascular resistance (60). Richardson and Beaulnes (92) have shown that ANG II conjugated to horseradish peroxidase exerted typical hypertensive effects under conditions in which the conjugate was found (by electron microscopy) to be confined to the vascular space. Thus bradykinin and ANG II appear to be capable of affecting pulmonary vascular tone under conditions in which they are unlikely to have direct access to vascular smooth muscle. Whether small polypeptides such as ANG II and bradykinin can be taken up and transported within cells, as suggested for insulin (127), has not been adequately examined.

Myoendothelial junctions provide a morphological basis for interactions between endothelial cells and adjacent smooth muscle cells (Fig. 1C). Furthermore there is reason to believe that endothelial cells possess specific receptors for angiotensins, kinins, and other polypeptide hormones (118, 121). Buonassisi and Venter (17) have shown that rabbit aorta endothelial cells in culture have a high affinity (specific binding sites) for ANG II, among other vasoactive agents. Gimbrone and Alexander (52) have shown high-affinity binding sites for insulin on human umbilical vein endothelial cells in culture.

INTERACTIONS AMONG VASOACTIVE AGENTS AND THEIR TARGET CELLS. Evidence indicates that some of the effects of ANG II and bradykinin on blood vessels are modulated and/or mediated by prostaglandins and related substances (14, 142). Data obtained by Blumberg et al. (14) imply possible qualitative differences among blood vessels. Thus release of a PGE-like prostaglandin from the kidney is most sensitive to ANG II, whereas release of a similar substance by mesenteric vasculature is most sensitive to ANG III.

Wong et al. (142) have argued that venous tissue can be distinguished from arterial tissue by the prostaglandins released in response to bradykinin. The mesenteric artery releases primarily a PGE_2-like substance, whereas the mesenteric vein releases primarily $PGF_{2\alpha}$ (142). If the vein is treated with indomethacin, the venoconstrictor effect of bradykinin is lost. Higher levels of complexity are evident when one considers that bradykinin acts on the mesenteric vein to release PGE_2, which is converted via PGE 9-ketoreductase to $PGF_{2\alpha}$. Arterial tissue contains the same enzyme but does not convert PGE_2 to $PGE_{2\alpha}$ unless pretreated with BPP_{9a}, an inhibitor of kininase II. Thus interactions among angiotensins, kinins, and prostaglandins occur within the pulmonary circulation. It may be pertinent that ANG II can exaggerate the hypertensive response to hypoxia (3) and that prostaglandin synthetase inhibitors also enhance the response to hypoxia (141). Piper and Vane (89) have shown that the venous effluent of lungs perfused with bradykinin contains prostaglandins and labile vasoactive substances (probably thromboxane A_2). However, the bradykinin effect is not sustained.

Endothelial cells isolated and cultured without exposure to proteolytic enzymes are in fact responsive to angiotensins and kinins as hormones (121). *1)* It is evident that both bradykinin and angiotensin stimulate synthesis of cyclic nucleotides of endothelial cells in culture (118). *2)* Bradykinin (in physiological doses) stimulates prostacyclin (PGI_2) release (24). Curiously, thromboxane A_2 (measured as thromboxane B_2) is also released in readily measurable quantities (~5% of total radioactivity). Prostacyclin is a potent vasodilator in its own right. Furthermore, unlike prostaglandins of the E and F series, PGI_2 is not degraded during passage through the lungs (4) and may be capable of reaching pulmonary vascular smooth muscle (i.e., bradykinin could exert some of its effects on pulmonary vascular tone by stimulating endothelial cells to release the vasodilator PGI_2).

Note that PGI_2 is among the most potent of the known inhibitors of platelet aggregation (4, 139) and may represent a means by which bradykinin could indirectly affect fluidity of blood (24, 121).

Other Peptides

The selectivity of the pulmonary inactivation mechanism is strikingly illustrated by the way the lungs inactivate bradykinin but allow three other vasodepressor peptides (eledoisin, substance P, and physalaemin) to pass through. Vasopressin and oxytocin also survive passage through the pulmonary circulation of the species tested (140).

Little is known of how the lung treats fibrinopeptides, although the lung may be an active site for fibrinopeptide metabolism (10). It is not known whether the lungs have any effects on the activity of cholecystokinin, pancreozymin, glucagon, and other peptide hormones of gastrointestinal origin.

There have been reports that insulin may be metabolized during circulation through the lungs (96) and that pulmonary ACE can metabolize the B chain of insulin (64). Such reports remain unconfirmed, however, and it is still not clear whether insulin is metabolized by the lungs (120). When lung slices are incubated with insulin and proinsulin, the rate of degradation appears to be insignificant compared with that of liver and muscle (69).

The physiological actions of exogenously administered gastrin are short-lived (75), the sites of catabolism are not fully known, and the role of the lungs is not agreed on. Korman et al. (70) have reported that the lung inactivates gastrin and may well be the major site for this catabolism. Inactivation of synthetic human gastrin I and its analogue pentagastrin has also been studied in slices of several mammalian tissues. Both gastrin and pentagastrin are inactivated in vitro, as determined by radioimmunoassay and bioassay in all tissue homogenates tested, including lung (41). However, studies of isolated perfused dog lungs have indicated that the normal, edema-free lung does not catabolize gastrin and that there is no physiological role for the lung in the degradation of gastrin (28, 29).

DISCUSSION AND FUTURE DIRECTIONS

The biological activities of the kinins and ANG II disappear, whereas the activity of ANG I is enhanced during circulation through various vascular beds. To a large degree the changes in activities of the vasoactive polypeptides are independent of enzymes and cellular elements of blood but are closely related to peptidase activities of the vascular bed itself. There are also qualitative differences among different vascular beds in the processing of the substances. *1*) Angiotensin II is not inactivated in all vascular beds; most notably it is not inactivated in the pulmonary circulation. Similarly ANG I may not be activated in all vascular beds. *2*) The apparent biological half-lives of the angiotensins and kinins differ among vascular beds.

Our aim is to understand interactions of soluble or circulating components of the renin-angiotensin system and the kallikrein-kinin system with cellular components. This approach is important because both systems function, at least in some respects, as local hormones. However, even their systemic actions may presume critically important reactions with cellular components that are not uniformly distributed within organs or within particular cell types of a given organ or tissue.

Over the past several years aspects of the metabolism of kinins and ANG I by pulmonary endothelium have been defined. Our focus has been on a cell not previously known to exist until the advent of electron microscopy (Fig. 1). Endothelial cells selectively process a series of vasoactive substances, including ANG I and bradykinin. Studies show that endothelial cells of the lung can be considered a very complex solid-phase reactor capable of extremely fast reactions of high selectivity, perhaps even specificity. A number of other enzymes participate, and what little is known about them suggests that a fuller understanding of these systems will lend itself to a cell biology approach. Thus the concentration of ANG II in systemic arterial blood, and possibly that of ANG III and bradykinin, depends greatly on what happens as they or their precursors pass through the pulmonary circulation.

The critical disposition of an enzyme on one cell type or another, or of the same cell type within different organs, bespeaks important control. A point has been reached where it is not highly informative to know, for example, the angiotensinase activity of tissue homogenates or to seek receptors in tissue homogenates. We are now in a position to look for receptors, converting enzymes, and degradative enzymes in terms of specific cell types and their subcellular organelles.

Figure 1*E* shows a surface replica of the true outer membrane face of an endothelial cell in culture and presumably is representative of the cell surface normally exposed to the circulation. Studies of the pulmonary processing of angiotensins and related peptides clearly show that the critical, initial reactions occur at the cell surface—this is true of metabolic enzymes, receptors, and the release of products. A challenge for the future is to begin to chart the geography of the pulmonary endothelial cell surface.

It is a pleasure to acknowledge the support of Dr. J. W. Ryan and many collaborators (Drs. D. S. Smith, D. R. Schultz, F. E. Dorer, and D. J. Crutchley) and the assistance of L. A. White and C. M. Oberto in the preparation of the manuscript.

This work was supported by grants from the National Institutes of Health (HL-22087, HL-21568) and the Council of Tobacco Research, Inc.

REFERENCES

1. ACKERLY, J. A., M. J. PEACH, E. D. VAUGHAN, JR., AND A. W. GLENN. Formation of [Des-Asp¹]angiotensin I by the perfused rat lung. *Endocrinology* 107: 1699–1704, 1980.

2. AIKEN, J. W., AND J. R. VANE. Intrarenal prostaglandin release attenuates the renal vasoconstrictor activity of angiotensin. *J. Pharmacol. Exp. Ther.* 184: 678–687, 1972.

3. ALEXANDER, J. M., M. D. NYBY, AND K. A. JASBERG. Effect of angiotensin on hypoxic pulmonary vasoconstriction in isolated dog lung. *J. Appl. Physiol.* 41: 84–88, 1976.

3a. ANTONACCIO, M. J. Angiotensin converting enzyme (ACE) inhibitors. *Annu. Rev. Pharmacol. Toxicol.* 22: 57–87, 1982.

4. ARMSTRONG, J. M., N. LATTIMER, S. MONCADA, AND J. R. VANE. Comparison of the vasodepressor effects of prostacyclin and 6-oxo-prostaglandin $F_{1\alpha}$ with those of prostaglandin E_2 in rats and rabbits. *Br. J. Pharmacol.* 62: 125–130, 1978.

5. BAKHLE, Y. S. Conversion of angiotensin I to angiotensin II by cell-free extracts of dog lung. *Nature London* 220: 919–921, 1968.

6. BAKHLE, Y. S. Converting enzyme: in vitro measurement and properties. In: *Handbook of Experimental Pharmacology. Angiotensin*, edited by I. H. Page and F. M. Bumpus. Berlin: Springer-Verlag, 1974, vol. 37, p. 41–80.

7. BAKHLE, Y. S., A. M. REYNARD, AND J. R. VANE. Metabolism of the angiotensins in isolated perfused tissues. *Nature London* 222: 956–959, 1969.

8. BAKHLE, Y. S., AND J. R. VANE. Pharmacokinetic function of the pulmonary circulation. *Physiol. Rev.* 54: 1007–1045, 1974.

9. BAUM, M. D., AND P. A. KOT. Response of pulmonary vascular segments to angiotensin and norepinephrine. *J. Thorac. Cardiovasc. Surg.* 63: 322–328, 1972.

10. BAYLEY, T., J. A. CLEMENTS, AND A. J. OSBAHR. Pulmonary and circulatory effects of fibrinopeptides. *Circ. Res.* 21: 469–485, 1967.

11. BIRON, P., L. CAMPEAU, AND P. DAVID. Fate of angiotensin I and II in the human pulmonary circulation. *Am. J. Cardiol.* 24: 544–547, 1969.

12. BIRON, P., AND C. G. HUGGINS. Pulmonary activation of synthetic angiotensin I. *Life Sci.* 7: 965–970, 1968.

13. BLAIR-WEST, J. R., J. P. COGHLAN, D. A. DENTON, J. W. FUNDER, B. A. SCOGGINS, AND R. D. WRIGHT. The effect of the heptapeptide (2-8) and hexapeptide (3-8) fragments of angiotensin II on aldosterone secretion. *J. Clin. Endocrinol. Metab.* 32: 575–578, 1971.

13a. BLOCK, E. R., AND S. A. STALCUP. Metabolic functions of the lung. Of what clinical relevance? *Chest* 2: 215–223, 1982.

14. BLUMBERG, A. L., S. E. DENNY, G. R. MARSHALL, AND P. NEEDLEMAN. Blood vessel-hormone interactions: angiotensin, bradykinin, and prostaglandins. *Am. J. Physiol.* 232 (*Heart Circ. Physiol.* 1): H305–H310, 1977.

15. BRAUN-MENENDEZ, E., J. C. FASCIOLO, L. F. LELOIR, AND J. M. MUNOZ. La substancia hipertensora de la sagre del rinon isquemiado. *Rev. Soc. Argent. Biol.* 15: 420, 1939.

16. BUMPUS, F. M., R. SMEBY, I. H. PAGE, AND P. A. KHAIRALLAH. Distribution and metabolic fate of angiotensin II and various derivatives. *Can. Med. Assoc. J.* 90: 190–193, 1964.

17. BUONASSISI, V., AND J. C. VENTER. Hormone and neurotransmitter receptors in an established vascular endothelial cell line. *Proc. Natl. Acad. Sci. USA* 73: 1612–1616, 1976.

18. CALDWELL, P. R. B., H. J. WIGGER, M. DAS, AND R. L. SOFFER. Angiotensin-converting enzyme: effect of antienzyme antibody in vivo. *FEBS Lett.* 63: 82–84, 1976.

18a. CATRAVAS, J. D., AND C. N. GILLIS. Metabolism of [^{3}H]-benzoyl-phenylalanyl-alanyl-proline by pulmonary angiotensin converting enzyme in vivo: effects of bradykinin, SQ14225 or acute hypoxia. *J. Pharmacol. Exp. Ther.* 217: 263–270, 1981.

19. CHAMBERLAIN, J., N. L. BROWSE, D. G. GIBSON, AND J. A. GLEESON. Angiotensin and reno-portal anastomosis. *Br. Med. J.* 2: 1507–1508, 1964.

20. CHIU, A. T., AND M. J. PEACH. Stimulation of aldosterone biosynthesis by angiotensin heptapeptide (Abstract). *Federation Proc.* 32: 765, 1973.

21. CHIU, A. T., J. W. RYAN, U. S. RYAN, AND F. E. DORER. A sensitive radiochemical assay for angiotensin-converting enzyme (kininase II). *Biochem. J.* 149: 297–300, 1975.

22. CHIU, A. T., J. W. RYAN, J. M. STEWART, AND F. E. DORER. Formation of angiotensin III by angiotensin-converting enzyme. *Biochem. J.* 155: 189–192, 1976.

23. COMROE, J. H. *Physiology of Respiration*. Chicago, IL: Year Book, 1974.

24. CRUTCHLEY, D. J., J. W. RYAN, U. S. RYAN, G. H. FISHER, AND S. M. PAUL. Effects of bradykinin and its homologs on the metabolism of arachidonate of endothelial cells. *Adv. Exp. Med. Biol.* 156: 527–532, 1983.

24a. CUMMISKEY, J., N. PETIT, AND G. YU. Effects of chronic hypoxia on pulmonary artery endothelial cells in vitro (Abstract). *Am. Rev. Respir. Dis.* 125: 266, 1982.

25. CUSHMAN, D. W., AND H. S. CHEUNG. A simple substrate for assay of dog lung angiotensin converting enzyme (Abstract). *Federation Proc.* 28: 799, 1969.

26. CUSHMAN, D. W., AND H. S. CHEUNG. Spectrophotometric assay and properties of the angiotensin-converting enzyme of rabbit lung. *Biochem. Pharmacol.* 20: 1637–1648, 1971.

27. DEL VECCHIO, P. J., J. W. RYAN, A. CHUNG, AND U. S. RYAN. Capillaries of adrenal cortex possess aminopeptidase A and angiotensin converting enzyme. *Biochem. J.* 186: 605–608, 1980.

28. DENT, R. I., B. LEVINE, H. HIRSCH, H. JAMES, AND J. E. FISCHER. Changes in plasma gastrin levels during isolated perfusions of canine lung and kidney. *J. Surg. Res.* 14: 353–358, 1973.

29. DENT, R. I., B. LEVINE, J. H. JAMES, H. HIRSCH, AND J. E. FISCHER. Effects of isolated perfused canine lung and kidney on gastrin heptadecapeptide. *Am. J. Physiol.* 225: 1038–1044, 1973.

30. DEXTER, L. The hypertensinase content of plasma of normal, hypertensive and nephrectomized dogs. *Ann. Intern. Med.* 17: 447–450, 1942.

31. DORER, F. E., J. R. KAHN, K. E. LENTZ, M. LEVINE, AND L. T. SKEGGS. Angiotensin converting enzyme: method of assay and partial purification. *Anal. Biochem.* 33: 102–103, 1970.

32. DORER, F. E., J. R. KAHN, K. E. LENTZ, M. LEVINE, AND L. T. SKEGGS. Purification and properties of angiotensin-converting enzyme from hog lung. *Circ. Res.* 31: 356–366, 1972.

33. DORER, F. E., J. R. KAHN, K. E. LENTZ, M. LEVINE, AND L. T. SKEGGS. Hydrolysis of bradykinin by angiotensin converting enzyme. *Circ. Res.* 34: 823–827, 1974.

34. DOYLE, A. E. Studies on the metabolism of angiotensin. *Postgrad. Med. J.* 44: 31–35, 1968.

35. DZAU, V. J., W. S. COLUCCI, G. H. WILLIAMS, G. CURFMAN, L. MEGGS, AND N. K. HOLLENBERG. Sustained effectiveness of converting-enzyme inhibition in patients with severe congestive heart failure. *N. Engl. J. Med.* 302: 1373–1379, 1980.

35a. Editorial. Inhibitors of angiotensin 1 converting enzyme for treating hypertension. *Brit. Med. J.* 281: 630–631, 1980.

36. ELLIOTT, D. F., G. P. LEWIS, AND E. W. HORTON. The structure of bradykinin—a plasma kinin from blood. *Biochem. Biophys. Res. Commun.* 3: 87–91, 1960.

37. ELLIOTT, D. F., AND W. S. PEART. The amino acid sequence in a hypertensin. *Biochem. J.* 65: 246, 1957.

38. ERDÖS, E. G. Conversion of angiotensin I to angiotensin II. *Am. J. Med.* 60: 749–759, 1976.

39. ERDÖS, E. G., A. G. RENFEW, E. M. SLOANE, AND J. R. WOHLER. Enzymatic studies on bradykinin and similar peptides. *Ann. NY Acad. Sci.* 104: 222–235, 1963.

40. ERDÖS, E. G., AND H. Y. T. YANG. Bradykinin, kallidin and kallikrein. In: *Handbook of Experimental Pharmacology. Bradykinin, Kallidin and Kallikrein*, edited by E. G. Erdös. Berlin: Springer-Verlag, 1970, vol. 25, p. 289–323.

41. EVANS, J. C., D. D. REEDER, AND J. C. THOMPSON. Inactivation of gastrin and pentagastrin by tissue slices. *Proc. Soc. Exp. Biol. Med.* 143: 168–170, 1973.

42. FASCIOLO, J. C., L. F. LELOIR, J. M. MUNOZ, AND E. BRAUN-MENENDEZ. La hipertensinasa, su dosaje y dostribucion. *Rev. Soc. Argent. Biol.* 16: 643, 1940.

43. FELDBERG, W., AND G. P. LEWIS. Further studies on the effects of peptides on the suprarenal medulla of cats. *J. Physiol. London* 178: 239–251, 1965.

44. FERREIRA, S. H. A bradykinin-potentiating factor (BPF) present in the venom of *Bothrops jararaca*. *Br. J. Pharmacol. Chemother.* 24: 163–169, 1965.

45. FERREIRA, S. H., AND J. R. VANE. Half-lives of peptides and a-

mines in the circulation. *Nature London* 215: 1237–1240, 1967.
46. FERREIRA, S. H., AND J. R. VANE. Prostaglandins. Their disappearance from and release into the circulation. *Nature London* 216: 868–873, 1967.
47. FISHMAN, A. P. Nonrespiratory functions of the lungs. *Chest* 72: 84–89, 1977.
48. FISHMAN, A. P., AND G. G. PIETRA. Handling of bioactive materials by the lung. Pt. 1. *N. Engl. J. Med.* 291: 884–890, 1974.
49. FISHMAN, A. P., AND G. G. PIETRA. Handling of bioactive materials by the lung. Pt. 2. *N. Engl. J. Med.* 291: 953–959, 1974.
50. GAVRAS, H., H. R. BRUNNER, J. H. LARAGH, J. E. SEALEY, I. GAVRAS, AND R. A. VUKOVICH. An angiotensin converting-enzyme inhibitor to identify and treat vasoconstrictor and volume factors in hypertensive patients. *N. Engl. J. Med.* 291: 817–821, 1974.
51. GILLIS, C. N., AND J. A. ROTH. Pulmonary disposition of circulating vasoactive hormones. *Biochem. Pharmacol.* 25: 2547–2553, 1976.
52. GIMBRONE, M. A., AND R. ALEXANDER. Insulin receptors in cultured human vascular endothelial cells (Abstract). *Circulation* 56: 809, 1977.
53. GIMBRONE, M. A., R. S. COTRAN, AND J. FOLKMAN. Human vascular endothelial cells in culture. *J. Cell Biol.* 60: 673–684, 1974.
54. GOFFINET, J. A., AND P. J. MULROW. Estimation of angiotensin clearance by an in vivo assay (Abstract). *Clin. Res.* 11: 408, 1963.
55. GREENBAUM, L. M., AND K. S. KIM. The kinin forming and kininase activities of rabbit polymorphonuclear leucocytes. *Br. J. Pharmacol. Chemother.* 27: 230–238, 1967.
56. HABLISTON, D. L., C. WHITAKER, M. A. HART, U. S. RYAN, AND J. W. RYAN. Isolation and culture of endothelial cells from the lungs of small animals. *Am. Rev. Respir. Dis.* 119: 853–868, 1979.
57. HART, M. A., AND U. S. RYAN. Surface replicas of pulmonary endothelial cells in culture. *Tissue Cell* 10: 441–449, 1978.
58. HAYES, L. W., C. A. GOGUEN, S. F. CHING, AND L. L. SLAKEY. Angiotensin-converting enzyme: accumulation in medium from cultured endothelial cells. *Biochem. Biophys. Res. Commun.* 82: 1147–1153, 1978.
59. HEINEMANN, H. O., AND A. P. FISHMAN. Nonrespiratory functions of mammalian lung. *Physiol. Rev.* 49: 1–47, 1969.
60. HIRSCHMAN, J., AND R. BOUCEK. Angiographic evidence of pulmonary vasomotion in the dog. *Br. Heart J.* 25: 375–381, 1963.
61. HODGE, R. L., K. K. F. NG, AND J. R. VANE. Disappearance of angiotensin from the circulation of the dog. *Nature London* 215: 138–141, 1967.
62. HUGGINS, C. G., AND N. S. THAMPI. A simple method for the determination of angiotensin I converting enzyme. *Life Sci.* 7: 633–639, 1968.
63. IGIC, R., E. G. ERDÖS, H. S. YEH, K. SORRELS, AND T. NAKAJIMA. Angiotensin I converting enzyme of the lung. *Circ. Res.* 31, Suppl. 2: 51–61, 1972.
64. IGIC, R., H. S. YEH, K. SORRELS, AND E. G. ERDÖS. Cleavage of active peptides by a lung enzyme. *Experientia* 28: 135–136, 1972.
65. ITSKOVITZ, H. D., AND L. MILLER. Differential studies of angiotensinase activities from several tissue sources. *Am. J. Med. Sci.* 254: 659–666, 1967.
66. JAFFE, E. A., R. L. NACHMAN, C. G. BECKER, AND C. R. MINICK. Culture of human endothelial cells derived from umbilical veins. *J. Clin. Invest.* 52: 2745–2756, 1973.
67. JOHNSON, D. C., AND J. W. RYAN. Degradation of angiotensin II by a carboxypeptidase of rabbit liver. *Biochim. Biophys. Acta* 160: 196–203, 1968.
68. JUNOD, A. F. Metabolism, production, and release of hormones and mediators in the lungs. *Am. Rev. Respir. Dis.* 112: 93–108, 1975.
69. KITABCHI, A. E., AND F. B. STENTZ. Degradation of insulin and proinsulin by various organ homogenates of rat. *Diabetes* 21: 1091–1101, 1972.
70. KORMAN, M. G., J. HANSKY, B. C. RITCHIE, J. M. WATTS, AND J. E. MALONEY. Disappearance of gastrin across the lung. *Aust. J. Exp. Biol. Med. Sci.* 51: 679–687, 1973.
71. KRIEGER, E. M., H. C. SALGADO, C. J. ASSAN, L. L. J. GREENE, AND S. H. FERREIRA. Potential screening test for detection of over-activity of renin-angiotensin system. *Lancet* 1: 269–271, 1971.
72. LARAGH, J. H., M. ANGERS, W. G. KELLY, AND S. LIEBERMAN. Hypotensive agents and pressor substances: the effects of epinephrine, norepinephrine, angiotensin II and others on the secretory rate of aldosterone in man. *J. Am. Med. Assoc.* 174: 234–240, 1960.
73. LEARY, W. P., AND J. G. LEDINGHAM. Removal of angiotensin by isolated perfused organs of the rat. *Nature London* 222: 959–960, 1969.
74. LENTZ, K. E., L. T. SKEGGS, K. R. WOODS, J. R. KAHN, AND N. P. SHUMWAY. The amino acid composition of hypertensin II and its biochemical relationship to hypertensin I. *J. Exp. Med.* 104: 183–191, 1956.
75. MAKHLOUF, G. M., J. P. MCMANUS, AND W. I. CARD. Action of gastrin II on gastric secretion in man. In: *Gastrin*, edited by M. I. Grossman. Berkeley: Univ. of California Press, 1966, p. 139–169.
76. MCCAA, R. E., J. E. HALL, AND C. S. MCCAA. The effects of angiotensin I converting enzyme inhibitors on arterial blood pressure and urinary sodium excretion: role of the renal renin-angiotensin and kallikrein-kinin systems. *Circ. Res.* 43: I32–I39, 1978.
77. METHOT, A. L., P. MEYER, P. BIRON, M. F. LORAIN, G. LAGRUE, AND P. MILLIEZ. Hepatic inactivation of angiotensin. *Nature London* 203: 531–532, 1964.
78. NG, K. K. F., AND J. R. VANE. Conversion of angiotensin I to angiotensin II. *Nature London* 216: 762–766, 1967.
79. NG, K. K. F., AND J. R. VANE. Fate of angiotensin I in the circulation. *Nature London* 218: 144–150, 1968.
80. NG, K. K. F., AND J. R. VANE. Some properties of angiotensin converting enzyme in the lung in vivo. *Nature London* 225: 1142–1144, 1970.
81. OATES, J. A., W. A. PETTINGER, AND R. B. DOCTOR. Evidence for the release of bradykinin in carcinoid syndrome. *J. Clin. Invest.* 45: 173–179, 1966.
82. OEHME, P., S. KATZWINKEL, W. E. VOGT, AND H. NIEDRICH. Retarded enzymatic degradation of heterologous eledoisin sequences. *Experientia* 29: 947–948, 1973.
83. ONDETTI, M. A., B. RUBIN, AND D. W. CUSHMAN. Design of specific inhibitors of angiotensin converting enzyme: a new class of orally active hypertensive agents. *Science* 196: 441–444, 1977.
84. OPARIL, S., C. A. SANDERS, AND E. HABER. In-vivo and in-vitro conversion of angiotensin I to angiotensin II in dog blood. *Circ. Res.* 26: 591–599, 1970.
84a. OPARIL, S., S. WINTERNITZ, V. GOULD, M. BAERWALD, AND P. SZIDON. Effect of hypoxia on the conversion of angiotensin I to II in the isolated perfused rat lung. *Biochem. Pharmacol.* 31: 1375–1379, 1982.
85. OSBORNE, M. J., A. D'AURIAC, P. MEYER, AND M. WORCEL. Mechanism of extraction of angiotensin II in coronary and renal circulations. *Life Sci.* 9: 859–867, 1970.
86. PAGE, I. H., AND O. M. HELMER. A crystalline pressor substance (angiotonin) resulting from the reaction between renin and renin-activator. *J. Exp. Med.* 71: 29–42, 1940.
87. PAGE, I. H., AND J. W. MCCUBBIN. *Renal Hypertension.* Chicago, IL: Year Book, 1968, chapt. 2.
88. PEART, W. S. The renin-angiotensin system. *Pharmacol. Rev.* 17: 143–182, 1965.
89. PIPER, P. J., AND J. R. VANE. The release of prostaglandins from the lung and other tissues. *Ann. NY Acad. Sci.* 180: 363–385, 1971.

90. Pugatch, E. M. J., and A. M. Saunders. A new technique for making Häutchen preparations of unfixed aortic endothelium. *J. Atheroscler. Res.* 8: 735–738, 1968.
91. Rhodin, J. A. G. The ultrastructure of mammalian arterioles and precapillary sphincters. *J. Ultrastruct. Res.* 18: 181–223, 1967.
92. Richardson, J. B., and A. Beaulnes. The cellular site of action of angiotensin. *J. Cell Biol.* 51: 419–432, 1971.
93. Roblero, J., J. W. Ryan, and J. M. Stewart. Assay of kinins by their effects on blood pressure. *Res. Commun. Chem. Pathol. Pharmacol.* 6: 207–212, 1973.
94. Rocha e Silva, M., W. T. Beraldo, and G. Rosenfeld. Bradykinin, a hypotensive and smooth muscle stimulating factor released from plasma globulin by snake venoms and by trypsin. *Am. J. Physiol.* 156: 261–273, 1949.
95. Rowe, G. G., S. Afonson, C. A. Castillo, F. Lioy, J. E. Lugo, and C. W. Crumpton. The systemic and coronary hemodynamic effects of synthetic bradykinin. *Am. Heart J.* 65: 656–663, 1963.
96. Rubenstein, A. H., S. Zwi, and K. Miller. Insulin and the lung. *Diabetologia* 4: 236–238, 1968.
97. Ryan, J. W. The fate of angiotensin II. In: *Handbook of Experimental Pharmacology. Angiotensin*, edited by I. H. Page and F. M. Bumpus. New York: Springer-Verlag, 1974, vol. 37, p. 81–110.
98. Ryan, J. W. Processing of endogenous polypeptides by the lungs. *Annu. Rev. Physiol.* 44: 241–255, 1982.
98a. Ryan, J. W., and A. Chung. A new class of inhibitors of angiotensin converting enzyme. *Adv. Exp. Med. Biol.* 156: 1138–1139, 1983.
99. Ryan, J. W., A. Chung, L. C. Martin, and U. S. Ryan. New substrates for the radioassay of angiotensin converting enzyme of endothelial cells in culture. *Tissue Cell* 10: 555–562, 1978.
100. Ryan, J. W., A. R. Day, D. R. Schultz, U. S. Ryan, A. Chung, D. I. Marlborough, and F. E. Dorer. Localization of angiotensin converting enzyme (kininase II). I. Preparation of antibody-heme-octapeptide conjugates. *Tissue Cell* 8: 111–124, 1976.
101. Ryan, J. W., R. S. Niemeyer, and D. W. Goodwin. Metabolic fates of bradykinin, angiotensin I, adenine nucleotides and prostaglandins E_1 and $F_{1\alpha}$ in the pulmonary circulation. *Adv. Exp. Med. Biol.* 21: 259–266, 1972.
102. Ryan, J. W., R. S. Niemeyer, D. W. Goodwin, U. Smith, and J. M. Stewart. Metabolism of (8-L-[^{14}C]phenylalanine)-angiotensin I in the pulmonary circulation. *Biochem. J.* 125: 921–923, 1971.
103. Ryan, J. W., J. Roblero, and J. M. Stewart. Inactivation of bradykinin in the pulmonary circulation. *Biochem. J.* 110: 795–797, 1968.
104. Ryan, J. W., J. Roblero, and J. M. Stewart. Inactivation of bradykinin in the rat lung. *Adv. Exp. Med. Biol.* 8: 263–272, 1970.
105. Ryan, J. W., and U. S. Ryan. Metabolic activities of plasma membrane and caveolae of pulmonary endothelial cells with a note on pulmonary prostaglandin synthetase. In: *Lung Metabolism*, edited by A. F. Junod and R. de Haller. New York: Academic, 1975, p. 399–424.
106. Ryan, J. W., and U. S. Ryan. Biochemical and morphological aspects of the actions and metabolism of kinins. In: *Chemistry and Biology of the Kallikrein-Kinin System in Health and Disease*, edited by J. J. Pisano and K. F. Austen. Washington, DC: US Govt. Printing Office, 1976, chapt. 41, p. 315–333. (Fogarty Int. Proc. 27.)
107. Ryan, J. W., and U. S. Ryan. Is the lung a para-endocrine organ? *Am. J. Med.* 63: 595–603, 1977.
108. Ryan, J. W., and U. S. Ryan. Pulmonary endothelial cells. *Federation Proc.* 36: 2683–2691, 1977.
109. Ryan, J. W., and U. S. Ryan. Metabolic functions of the pulmonary vascular endothelium. *Adv. Vet. Sci. Comp. Med.* 26: 79–98, 1982.
110. Ryan, J. W., and U. S. Ryan. Endothelial surface enzymes and the dynamic processing of plasma substrates. *Int. Rev. Exp. Pathol.* 26: 1–43, 1983.
111. Ryan, J. W., U. S. Ryan, D. R. Schultz, C. Whitaker, A. Chung, and F. E. Dorer. Subcellular localization of pulmonary angiotensin converting enzyme (kininase II). *Biochem. J.* 146: 497–499, 1975.
112. Ryan, J. W., and U. Smith. A rapid, simple method for isolating pinocytotic vesicles and plasma membrane of lung. *Biochim. Biophys. Acta* 249: 177–180, 1971.
113. Ryan, J. W., U. Smith, and R. S. Niemeyer. Angiotensin I: metabolism by plasma membrane of lung. *Science* 176: 64–66, 1972.
114. Ryan, J. W., J. M. Stewart, W. P. Leary, and J. G. Ledingham. Metabolism of angiotensin I in the pulmonary circulation. *Biochem. J.* 120: 221–223, 1970.
115. Ryan, U. S. Structural bases for metabolic activity. *Annu. Rev. Physiol.* 44: 223–239, 1982.
116. Ryan, U. S. Culture of pulmonary endothelial cells on microcarriers. In: *Biology of the Endothelial Cell*, edited by E. A. Jaffe. The Hague, The Netherlands: Nijhoff, 1983, chapt. 4, p. 34–50.
116a. Ryan, U. S. New uses for endothelial cell culture. *BioEssays* 1: 114–116, 1984.
117. Ryan, U. S., E. Clements, D. Habliston, and J. W. Ryan. Isolation and culture of pulmonary endothelial cells. *Tissue Cell* 10: 535–554, 1978.
118. Ryan, U. S., D. C. Lehotay, and J. W. Ryan. Effects of bradykinin and angiotensin II on pulmonary endothelial cells in culture. *Adv. Exp. Med. Biol.* 156: 767–774, 1983.
119. Ryan, U. S., M. Mortara, and C. Whitaker. Methods for microcarrier culture of bovine pulmonary artery endothelial cells avoiding the use of enzymes. *Tissue Cell* 12: 619–635, 1980.
120. Ryan, U. S., and J. W. Ryan. Correlations between the fine structure of the alveolar-capillary unit and its metabolic activities. In: *Lung Biology in Health and Disease. Metabolic Functions of the Lung*, edited by Y. S. Bakhle and J. R. Vane. New York: Dekker, 1977, vol. 4, chapt. 7, p. 197–232.
121. Ryan, U. S., and J. W. Ryan. Vital and functional activities of endothelial cells. In: *Pathobiology of the Endothelial Cell*, edited by H. L. Nossel and H. J. Vogel. New York: Academic, 1982, p. 455–469.
122. Ryan, U. S., J. W. Ryan, D. R. Schultz, and F. E. Dorer. Localization of pulmonary angiotensin converting enzyme (Abstract). *J. Cell Biol.* 63: 294a, 1974.
123. Ryan, U. S., J. W. Ryan, and C. Whitaker. How do kinins affect vascular tone? In: *Kinins—II. Biochemistry, Pathobiology and Clinical Aspects*, edited by S. Fujii, H. Moriya, and T. Suzuki. New York: Plenum, 1979, p. 375–391.
124. Ryan, U. S., J. W. Ryan, C. Whitaker, and A. Chiu. Localization of angiotensin converting enzyme (kininase II). II. Immunocytochemistry and immunofluorescence. *Tissue Cell* 8: 125–145, 1976.
124a. Ryan, U. S., L. A. White, M. Lopez, and J. W. Ryan. Use of microcarriers to isolate and culture pulmonary microvascular endothelium. *Tissue Cell* 14: 597–606, 1982.
125. Sander, G. E., and C. G. Huggins. Subcellular enzyme in rabbit lung. *Nature London New Biol.* 230: 27–29, 1971.
126. Saperstein, L. A., R. K. Reed, and E. W. Page. The site of angiotonin destruction. *J. Exp. Med.* 83: 425–439, 1946.
127. Schlessinger, J., Y. Shechter, M. C. Willingham, and I. Pastan. Direct visualization of binding, aggregation and internalization of insulin and epidermal growth factor on living fibroblastic cells. *Proc. Natl. Acad. Sci. USA* 75: 2659–2663, 1978.
128. Schroder, E., and K. Lubke. Linear peptides. A. Tissue hormones (kinin hormones). In: *The Peptides*, translated by E. Gross. New York: Academic, 1966, vol. 2, chapt. 1, p. 109–120.
129. Semple, P. F., and J. J. Morton. Angiotensin II and angiotensin III in rat blood. *Circ. Res.* 38, Suppl. II: 122–126, 1976.

130. SKEGGS, L. T., J. R. KAHN, AND N. P. SHUMWAY. The preparation and function of the hypertensin-converting enzyme. *J. Exp. Med.* 103: 295-299, 1956.
131. SMITH, U., AND J. W. RYAN. An electron microscopic study of the vascular endothelium as a site for bradykinin and adenosine-5'-triphosphate inactivation in rat lung. *Adv. Exp. Med. Biol.* 8: 249-262, 1970.
132. SMITH, U., AND J. W. RYAN. Pinocytotic vesicles of the pulmonary endothelial cell. *Chest* 59: 12S-15S, 1971.
133. SMITH, U., AND J. W. RYAN. Electron microscopy of endothelial and epithelial components of the lungs: correlations of structure and function. *Federation Proc.* 32: 1957-1966, 1973.
133a. SOFFER, R. L. Angiotensin-converting enzyme and the regulation of vasoactive peptides. *Annu. Rev. Biochem.* 45: 73-94, 1976.
134. SOFFER, R. L. Angiotensin converting enzyme. In: *Biochemical Regulation of Blood Pressure*, edited by R. L. Soffer. New York: Wiley, 1981, p. 123-164.
134a. STALCUP, S. A., P. J. LEUENBERGER, J. S. LIPSET, M. M. OSMAN, J. M. CERRETA, R. B. MELLINS, AND G. M. TURINO. Impaired angiotensin conversion and bradykinin clearance in experimental canine pulmonary emphysema. *J. Clin. Invest.* 67: 201-209, 1981.
134b. STALCUP, S. A., J. S. LIPSET, P. M. LEGANT, P. J. LEUENBERGER, AND R. B. MELLINS. Inhibition of converting enzyme activity by acute hypoxia in dogs. *J. Appl. Physiol.: Respirat. Environ. Exercise Physiol.* 46: 227-234, 1979.
134c. STALCUP, S. A., J. S. LIPSET, J. M. WOAN, P. LEUENBERGER, AND R. B. MELLINS. Inhibition of angiotensin converting enzyme activity in cultured endothelial cells by hypoxia. *J. Clin. Invest.* 63: 966-976, 1979.
134d. SZIDON, P., N. BAIREY, AND S. OPARIL. Effect of acute hypoxia on the pulmonary conversion of angiotensin I to angiotensin II in dogs. *Circ. Res.* 46: 221-226, 1980.
135. TIERNEY, D. F. Lung metabolism and biochemistry. *Annu. Rev. Physiol.* 36: 209-231, 1974.
136. TSAI, B. S., M. J. PEACH, M. C. KHOSLA, AND F. M. BUMPUS. Synthesis and evaluation of [Des-Asp^1] angiotensin I as a precursor for [Des-Asp^1]angiotensin II (angiotensin III). *J. Med. Chem.* 18: 1180-1183, 1975.
137. TURKER, R. K., M. YAMAMOTO, F. M. BUMPUS, AND P. A. KHAIRALLAH. Lung perfusion with angiotensin I and II. Evidence of release myotropic and inhibitory substances. *Circ. Res.* 28: 559-597, 1971.
138. VANE, J. R. The release and fate of vaso-active hormones in the circulation. *Br. J. Pharmacol.* 35: 209-242, 1969.
139. VANE, J. R. Inhibition of prostaglandin synthesis as a mechanism of action for aspirin-like drugs. *Nature London New Biol.* 231: 232-235, 1971.
140. VANE, J. R. Introduction. In: *Metabolic Activities of the Lung.* Amsterdam: Excerpta Med., 1980, p. 1-10. (Ciba Found. Symp. 78.)
141. VOELKEL, N. F., J. G. GERBER, I. F. MCMURTY, A. S. NIES, AND J. T. REEVES. Release of vasodilator prostaglandin, PGI_2, from isolated rat lung during vasoconstriction. *Circ. Res.* 48: 207-213, 1981.
142. WONG, P. Y. K., N. A. TERRAGNO, AND J. C. MCGIFF. Dual effects of bradykinin on prostaglandin metabolism: relationship to the dissimilar vascular actions of kinins. *Prostaglandins* 13: 1113-1125, 1977.

CHAPTER 11

Lung metabolism of eicosanoids: prostaglandins, prostacyclin, thromboxane, and leukotrienes

Y. S. BAKHLE | Department of Pharmacology, Royal College of Surgeons of England, London, England

SERGIO H. FERREIRA | Department of Pharmacology, Medical School of Ribeirao Preto, Sao Paulo, Brazil

CHAPTER CONTENTS

History of Eicosanoids
Overview of Eicosanoid Biosynthesis
Antagonists of Eicosanoids and Inhibitors of Their Synthesis
Lung Pharmacology of Eicosanoids
Inactivation of Eicosanoids in Lung
Synthesis of Eicosanoids by Lung
   Synthesis from exogenous arachidonic acid
   Synthesis from endogenous arachidonic acid
      Release of eicosanoids after anaphylactic reactions
      Release of eicosanoids by mechanical stimulation
      Release of eicosanoids by endogenous mediators
Summary

SINCE THE RENAISSANCE of interest in metabolic functions of the lung in the late 1960s, our knowledge of these functions has grown at an exponential rate common to many fields of research. Within this rapidly growing field, however, one area has expanded in an almost explosive manner: the study of the metabolism of arachidonic acid (AA) and its oxygenated metabolites in the lung. These metabolites [prostaglandins (PGs), prostacyclin, thromboxanes, and leukotrienes] are all, like AA, basically molecules containing 20 carbon atoms. Because the chemical name for AA is eicosatrienoic acid, these metabolites and their precursors are often called eicosanoids.

An early paper on PG biosynthesis demonstrated a highly active enzyme in guinea pig lung extracts (16), and the most recent advance in eicosanoid biochemistry was the identification of leukotrienes generated by lung tissue during anaphylaxis (195). These developments increased our knowledge of the lung and are important and sometimes essential elements in the development of our understanding of the eicosanoids in general.

HISTORY OF EICOSANOIDS

Over the last 20 years the advances in our understanding of PGs and allied AA metabolites have surprised biologists. Primary PGs were first isolated, characterized, and synthesized in the 1960s. The availability of these pure PGs strongly stimulated the investigation of their pharmacological properties, and they were soon shown to have wide-ranging effects. These investigations resulted in the use of PGs and their analogues in humans to induce midtrimester abortion (163); they were also used to synchronize the sexual cycle of cattle, thus improving the efficiency of artificial insemination (236). The intensive search for potent and specific antagonists of PG action has been less successful, and this important breakthrough has not been made.

In the 1970s Vane (279) discovered that PG synthesis was inhibited by the anti-inflammatory drugs (e.g., aspirin) referred to as nonsteroid, anti-inflammatory drugs (NSAIDs). This discovery had several important effects. For basic research it provided a conceptual substitute for a potent and specific PG antagonist. If a process is altered by aspirin or indomethacin, that finding is commonly accepted as evidence for the involvement of PGs. Furthermore sensitivity to NSAIDs is one of the criteria suggested for establishing PG biosynthesis as a causal factor in biological events (204).

The discovery of NSAIDs demonstrated clearly that PGs were important participants in inflammation and added several more possible substances to the list of the mediators of inflammation. This discovery also provided a logical explanation for the efficacy of aspirinlike drugs in the treatment of inflammatory diseases.

An important extension of the therapeutic use of

inhibitors of PG biosynthesis came in treating disorders that were thought unsuitable for such therapy until the connection between PGs and NSAIDs was made. These disorders (e.g., Bartter's syndrome, Crohn's disease, and refractory diarrhea accompanying medullary carcinoma of the thyroid) are all associated with supranormal levels of PGs; clinical improvement follows inhibition of their biosynthesis. Aspirinlike drugs are also being tested to prevent premature labor or abortion, to aid the closure of patent ductus arteriosus, to treat malignant osteolytic metastases, and to prevent subsequent heart attacks in patients who have already suffered one (and who are therefore at greater risk for additional attacks). Although these considerations are not strictly physiological, they show that one aim of physiological research is the improved therapy of disease.

It was clear from the earliest studies on PGs that these endogenous agents are not stored preformed in vesicles or granules like biogenic amines or many peptide hormones but are instead synthesized on demand in response to a multitude of different stimuli. One such stimulus was tissue homogenization. This procedure yielded basal PG levels that were more related to homogenization itself than to any previous experimental manipulation of the tissue. With the discovery of the inhibitory effects of aspirin and indomethacin on PG biosynthesis, it was possible to minimize the homogenization artifact and measure real changes in tissue PG content.

The ability of nearly every tissue to generate PGs was compatible with the early discovery that the precursor for PGs was AA, a 20-carbon unsaturated fatty acid that is ubiquitously distributed in the body, chiefly as a component of membrane phospholipid. Free AA is rapidly oxidized by a series of enzymes, the first of which is a cyclooxygenase. Its products are the PG endoperoxides, which are themselves substrates for a variety of further enzymatic transformations into the different PGs. Aspirinlike drugs block cyclooxygenase activity in vitro, and most of the relevant actions of these drugs in vivo are thought to be due to the inhibition of this enzyme.

Studies of AA metabolism in isolated perfused lung preparations showed that other highly active products distinct from the known PGs were formed from the endoperoxides produced by cyclooxygenase (230). These new metabolites had not been previously detected by the traditional chemical methods of isolation because they were unstable in aqueous media, with half-lives of just a few minutes. The first new metabolite identified was thromboxane A_2 (TXA_2) (122); it exhibited bronchoconstrictor and vasoconstrictor activities and was a highly potent platelet-aggregating agent. Both lung tissue and platelets formed TXA_2 under appropriate stimulation.

The next endoperoxide metabolite discovered was prostacyclin (PGI_2) (144, 188). In contrast to TXA_2, PGI_2 is an antiaggregatory agent and a potent vasodilator. Prostacyclin may be continuously generated by endothelial cells, most probably to counteract the normal tendency of platelets to adhere to vessels and thus cause thrombus formation (190). It is proposed (68, 249) that atheromatous plaques decrease PGI_2 synthesis by vascular endothelium, thus allowing accumulation of platelets and thrombus formation. The therapeutic use of PGI_2 as a partial substitute for heparin (based on its antiaggregating activity) has been assessed in studies of cardiopulmonary bypass and kidney dialysis (51, 174, 295). The antiaggregatory effect, coupled with potent vasodilation, is probably the reason for the long-term improvement of patients with severe peripheral vascular disease after infusions of PGE_1 and PGI_2 (269, 271).

The 1980s opened with the demonstration of another important oxidative metabolic pathway for AA, i.e., through 5-lipoxygenase and leading to leukotriene formation (245). These metabolites are particularly synthesized by the lung during anaphylaxis (195, 228) and are the major constituents of what was called the slow-reacting substance of anaphylaxis (SRS-A). Some leukotrienes have potent chemotactic activities (99, 226) and increase vascular permeability (226) and therefore may be important during inflammation; others are bronchoconstrictors and vasoconstrictors and thus may be involved in asthma (228, 245).

During the last 20 years the study of eicosanoids has progressed because of interactions among pharmacologists, biochemists, and chemists. Although the chemical identification and quantification of AA metabolites is highly sophisticated, substances detected by bioassay have always stimulated the main direction of research.

The lung is one of the most important tissues in which the metabolism of AA can be demonstrated. Early work showed PG biosynthesis in guinea pig lung homogenates (16). This was followed by demonstrations in lung preparations of the formation of rabbit aorta contracting substance (RCS) in anaphylaxis (229), the inhibition of PG biosynthesis by indomethacin and its congeners (279), the identification of TXA_2 (122), the production of PGI_2 (114), and the identification of leukotrienes in SRS-A from guinea pig (195) and human lung (170). It seems that progress in our understanding of both AA and pulmonary metabolism shall always be linked.

Other detailed reviews of the topics discussed here are available (82, 87, 94, 95, 193, 224, 243, 255).

OVERVIEW OF EICOSANOID BIOSYNTHESIS

Although at least three naturally occurring 20-carbon acids (dihomo-γ-linolenic, arachidonic, and eicosapentaenoic), are all substrates for cyclooxygenase, the metabolites of AA (5,8,11,14-eicosatetraenoic acid) are believed to be the major physiologically relevant eicosanoids because of the relative abundance of this precursor in humans. Two major routes of eicosanoid formation are known (Figs. 1 and 2). The first stable compounds to be described that were active on both smooth muscle preparations and blood pressure were the primary PGs (PGE and PGF). At least 20 years elapsed between their initial biological characterization and the availability of the synthetic material (35, 107, 282a). Prostaglandins of the "2 series" (2 double bonds, e.g., PGE$_2$) are synthesized via oxidation and cyclization of AA by cyclooxygenase (35, 278), a microsomal enzyme that is present in most cells. In this process two unstable cyclic endoperoxides, PGG$_2$ and PGH$_2$, are formed (119, 210). The conversion of PGG$_2$ to PGH$_2$ is catalyzed by a relatively nonspecific peroxidase. The activity of cyclooxygenase is critically dependent on the concentration of hydroperoxy free radicals (134). The fatty acid hydroperoxides from which these radicals are derived may accumulate during cyclooxygenase action, causing the delay followed by accelerating formation of product characteristic of this enzyme. Another corollary of this dependence is termination of cyclooxygenase action if the hydroperoxides are removed by tissue peroxidases; this is probably one of the normal controls of PG biosynthesis. The conversion of PGH$_2$ to PGF$_{2\alpha}$ seems to be mainly nonenzymatic and directed by cofactors, whereas the conversion of PGH$_2$ to PGE$_2$ or PGD$_2$ is enzymatically catalyzed (272).

Depending on the tissue in which the endoperoxides are generated, they are enzymatically transformed into two nonprostanoid substances: TXA$_2$ (122) and PGI$_2$ (188). Both TXA$_2$ and PGI$_2$ are unstable in biological fluids and break down to TXB$_2$ (122) and 6-oxo-PGF$_{1\alpha}$, respectively (144). Both of these breakdown products have very little biological activity. Malondialdehyde and 12-hydroxy-5,8,10-heptadecatrienoic acid (a 17-carbon hydroxy acid), substances with no biological activity, can be formed either by spontaneous degradation of PGH$_2$ or by the enzyme that synthesizes TXA$_2$. The further metabolism of primary PGs is discussed in a later section (see INACTIVATION OF EICOSANOIDS IN LUNG, p. 370).

Incomplete cyclooxygenase reactions may lead to noncyclized hydroxy acids, i.e., 11- or 15-hydroxyeicosatetraenoic acid (11- or 15-HETE). The major route of formation for linear eicosanoids, however, is via lipoxygenases found in platelets, leukocytes, and the lung. Platelets synthesize 12-hydroperoxyeicosatetraenoic acid (12-HPETE), which spontaneously degrades to 12-HETE (120, 209). The lipoxygenase in leukocytes, besides catalyzing the formation of 5-HPETE, also gives rise to an unstable compound (Fig. 2) containing a conjugate triene structure (195, 200), leukotriene A$_4$ (LTA$_4$, subscript indicating 4 double bonds). The LTA$_4$ (5,6 epoxide of AA) can then be converted into either LTB$_4$ or LTC$_4$. The LTC$_4$ is generated by a glutathione S-transferase and metabolized to LTD$_4$ by γ-glutamyl transpeptidase. In all probability the family of leukotrienes will increase as additional biologically active substances with minor structural modifications are discovered (213). The slow reacting substances generated either during anaphylaxis or by calcium ionophore stimulation are mixtures of leukotrienes formed via this pathway.

ANTAGONISTS OF EICOSANOIDS AND INHIBITORS OF THEIR SYNTHESIS

The eicosanoid antagonists now known cannot in-

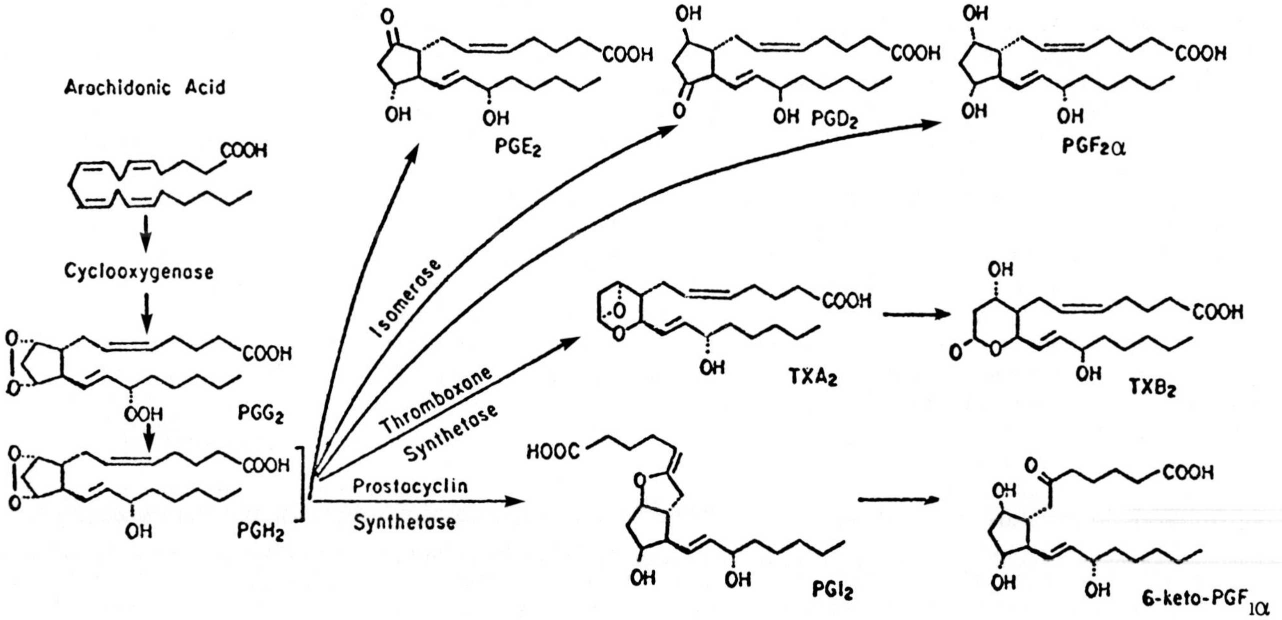

FIG. 1. Synthetic pathway of cyclooxygenase products.

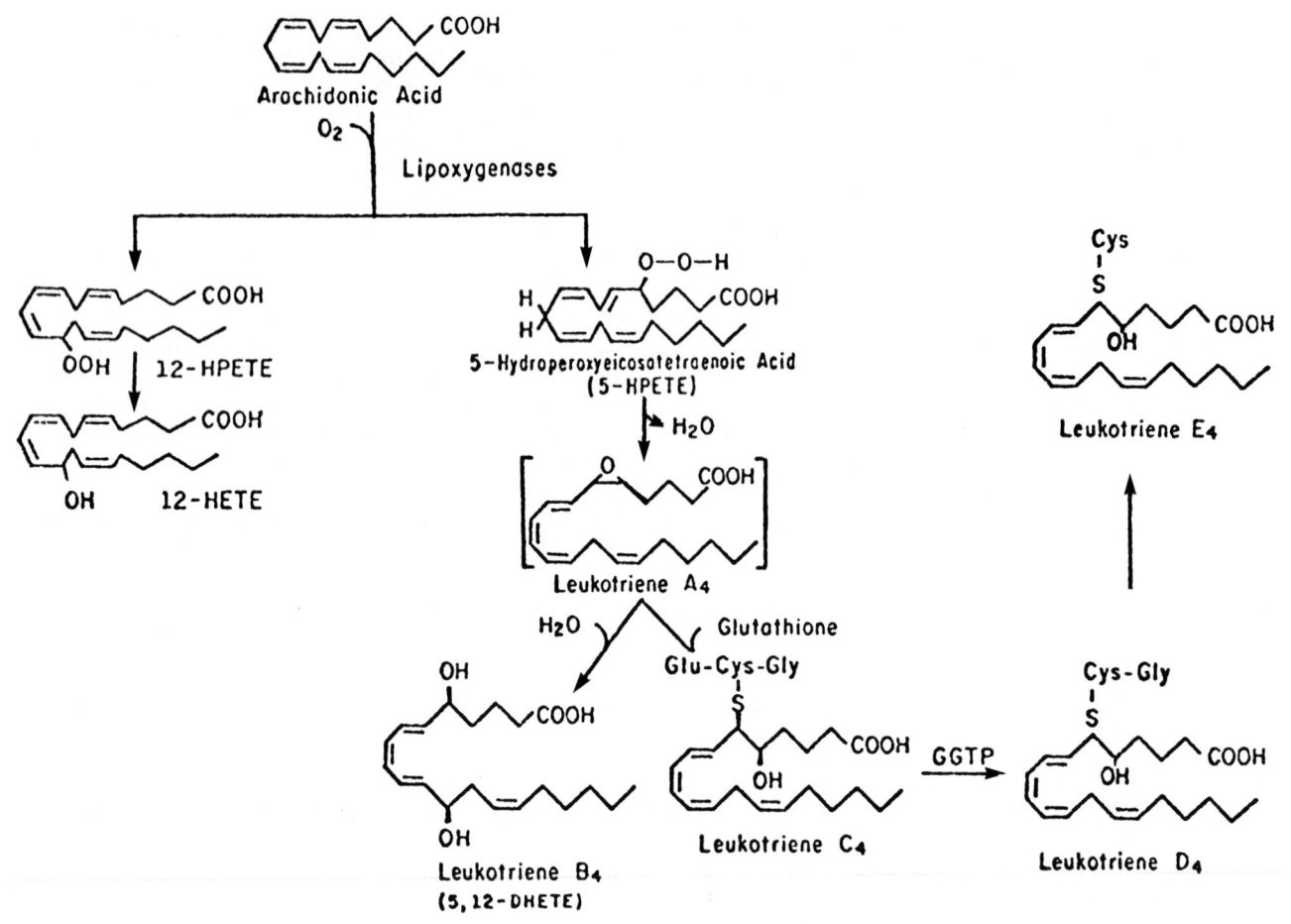

FIG. 2. Synthetic pathway of lipoxygenase products.

hibit all of the pharmacological effects of PGs, although they are quite effective antagonists of the spasmogenic effect of primary PGs in smooth muscle preparations. Those antagonists derived from dibenzoxozine (SC 19220) seem to be more reliable than analogues of PGs or the polymers of phloretin phosphate (246). Meclofenamate, flufenamate, and phenylbutazone antagonize the contraction of human isolated bronchial muscle caused by $PGF_{2\alpha}$ (63). In such instances the fenamates are at least 100 times more active against $PGF_{2\alpha}$ than they are against SRS-A.

Contractions of the guinea pig ileum caused by SRS-A are strongly inhibited by FPL 55712, whereas those due to histamine are unaffected (20). Flurbiprofen also antagonizes SRS-A (110). It differs from FPL 55712 (the most specific antagonist) in that it has a powerful inhibitory action in tracheal preparations but only minor effects on guinea pig ileum contractions induced by SRS-A. The bronchoconstrictor and contractile effects of LTC_4 and LTD_4 on isolated tissues are antagonized by FPL 55712.

In 1971 the generation of PGs was shown to be inhibited by aspirinlike drugs in three different systems and species. Vane (279) worked with a cell-free preparation of PG synthetase obtained from lung homogenates, whereas Smith and Willis (253) demonstrated aspirin's inhibition of PG synthesis in human platelets, and Ferreira et al. (85) studied PG synthesis in a dog spleen preparation stimulated by catecholamines. This inhibition of PG synthesis has been confirmed in a large number of species and systems and was extended to a great variety of NSAIDs. The concentration of the various NSAIDs necessary to inhibit the cyclooxygenase activity of isolated tissues or homogenates (0.1–10 µg/ml) is comparable to their therapeutic levels in human and animal models (87, 94).

Most of the aspirinlike drugs block the initial stage of AA metabolism in cell-free enzyme preparations through a time-dependent, competitive-irreversible mechanism (94, 157). They probably combine slowly with an allosteric site that reduces the catalytic activity of cyclooxygenase. Although acetylation of the cyclooxygenase protein by aspirin has been demonstrated (239) and correlated with inhibition of catalytic function, this cannot be the only mechanism of inhibition, because salicylate and indomethacin, which are not acetyl donors, also show the same kinetics of inhibition (160, 277).

In vivo, however, there are important differences in

efficacy and duration between the different NSAIDs. First, cyclooxygenase sensitivity to the inhibitory action of NSAIDs varies from tissue to tissue. This fact is not yet well explained and may be due to isoenzymes of cyclooxygenase or to differing tissue contents of cofactors. The strong antipyretic and analgesic action of p-acetaminophenol contrasts with its weak anti-inflammatory activity and has been correlated with its greater inhibition of cyclooxygenase from the central nervous system (97).

Second, the duration of inhibition may depend on the type of cell in which cyclooxygenase is inhibited. Inhibition by aspirin is irreversible; thus the recovery of cyclooxygenase activity depends on the synthesis of more new enzyme. This effect is best illustrated by contrasting the duration of inhibition of cyclooxygenase in platelets, which lack protein synthesis enzymes (261), with that in endothelial cells, which are fully equipped for protein synthesis. After a single dose of aspirin, PG biosynthesis in the platelet is blocked for 2–3 days, whereas the endothelial cell cyclooxygenase activity returns to normal within a few hours. Generally, however, the de novo synthesis of cyclooxygenase is a slow process because the whole body synthesis of PGs in humans is depressed for >24 h after therapeutic doses of aspirin, salicylate, or indomethacin (160). This certainly is not the case when there is an overproduction of PGs by local or migrating cells (e.g., in inflammation) and when a regimen of dosage lasting <6 h ensures an effective anti-inflammatory result.

Several polyunsaturated fatty acids were shown to be competitive inhibitors of cyclooxygenase, possessing an inhibition binding constant similar to the affinity of the substrate AA (160, 208, 277). The most used substrate antagonist is 5,8,11,14-eicosatetraynoic acid (TYA), an acetylenic analogue of AA. This acid exhibits two distinct types of cyclooxygenase inhibition: an instantaneous, concentration-dependent inhibition and an irreversible, time-dependent inhibition. In contrast to most of the NSAIDs, TYA also inhibits the lipoxygenase pathway. A third type of anticyclooxygenase agent has been proposed, causing a rapidly reversible, noncompetitive inhibition by free-radical trapping (277). The inflammatory activity of the experimental drug MK-447 has been explained by its free radical–scavenger property (158), and the analgesic effect of acetaminophen was recently related to its antioxidant activity (134).

The transformation of endoperoxides into primary PGs can be nonenzymatic, and there are no known inhibitors of this transformation. However, inhibitors of the enzymes synthesizing TXA_2 or PGI_2 are known. Synthesis of TXA_2 is blocked by a number of imidazole compounds (45, 187) and analogues of PGH_2 (108); one imidazole derivative is undergoing clinical evaluation (169a). Prostacyclin synthetase is inhibited by fatty acid hydroperoxides [e.g., 15-hydroperoxy-AA; (189)] and by tranylcypromine (113).

Most NSAIDs have little effect on the lipoxygenase pathways. The experimental anti-inflammatory compound BW 755C equally inhibits both cyclooxygenase and lipoxygenase activities in vitro and probably in vivo as well (136). Benoxaprofen is also thought to inhibit both enzymes (72, 285).

Cyclooxygenase acts only on free AA. Most of this substrate is esterified in phospholipids, and therefore an essential step in eicosanoid biosynthesis is the hydrolysis of arachidonate-containing phospholipids by phospholipase A_2. Inhibitors of this enzyme (e.g., mepacrine and p-bromophenacetyl bromide) prevent eicosanoid synthesis in perfused lung and platelets (280). Glucocorticoids also prevent eicosanoid formation, but only in leukocytes and other intact cell preparations (73), in inflamed synovial tissue (93), and in guinea pig lungs. At present this inhibitory effect of glucocorticoids is attributed to the synthesis of a peptide inhibitor of phospholipase A_2 (44, 69, 96). This peptide blocks the release of AA and consequently also blocks the synthesis of cyclooxygenase and lipoxygenase products (43).

LUNG PHARMACOLOGY OF EICOSANOIDS

The effects of the various AA metabolites on isolated preparations of bronchial and tracheal muscle vary depending both on the species used and the basal tone of the preparation (159). These effects have been attributed to the presence of both contractor and relaxant receptors on tracheobronchial muscle that are stimulated to different extents by the eicosanoids (61).

The contraction of bronchial and tracheal preparations has been described for $PGF_{2\alpha}$ (63, 103), PGD_2 (139), TXA_2 (122), PGI_2 (61), LTC_4 or LTD_4 (37, 245), and PGG_2 or PGH_2 (118). The TXA_2 was generally more potent in causing contractions in vascular and airway smooth muscle in vitro than the parent endoperoxides (192). In guinea pig tracheal muscle the endoperoxides were several times more active than $PGF_{2\alpha}$ (118). Surprisingly, in view of its vasodilator effect (19), PGI_2 was as active as $PGF_{2\alpha}$ in stimulating contractions in isolated strips of guinea pig lung (281). On isolated human bronchial smooth muscle, LTC_4 was at least 500 times more potent than $PGF_{2\alpha}$ and 1,000 times more active than histamine (67). Both LTC_4 and LTA_4 were equipotent on isolated human and guinea pig tracheobronchial preparations, whereas LTA_4 showed a potency similar to that of histamine (67, 131).

Most AA metabolites with bronchoconstrictor activity in vitro also retain their activity in vivo. Bronchoconstriction can be induced by doses of 2–10 µg of $PGF_{2\alpha}$. Two of the most potent AA metabolites are LTC_4 and LTD_4 (131). The order of potency relative to $PGF_{2\alpha}$ in the guinea pig lung (Konzett-Rössler preparation) is LTC$_4$ or LTD$_4$ (500), TXA$_2$ (60), PGH$_2$ (5), PGF$_{2\alpha}$ (1), and PGD$_2$ (0.5). When given by aerosol the endoperoxides cause a smaller increase in airflow resistance than PGF$_{2\alpha}$ (281). These ratios should be interpreted with caution because some of these substances can be transformed to other active metabolites by the lung tissue or may stimulate some additional synthesis from endogenous AA. Indeed the bronchoconstrictor effects of SRS-A and the leukotrienes are inhibited by treating the animal with NSAIDs; in the guinea pig their bronchoconstrictor activity is mainly mediated by the release of thromboxanes (39, 225, 226, 281). Furthermore, although isolated animal preparations are useful for comparing the actions of PGs, in many instances they do not predict the effects of PGs on humans. For example, PGA$_2$, PGB$_1$, PGF$_{1\alpha}$, and 15-methyl PGE$_2$ all produce bronchodilation in the guinea pig but bronchoconstriction in humans (152). Cats and dogs are also responsive to the bronchoconstrictor activities of these AA metabolites (256–258, 286). Furthermore stable analogues of the endoperoxides increase bronchomotor tone and decrease lung compliance and lung volume in the dog. These effects are probably directly on the lung, as opposed to on the pulmonary vasculature, because mechanically induced increases in pulmonary vascular pressure have little effect on lung compliance (150, 257).

In humans, PGF$_{2\alpha}$ (given by aerosol to healthy subjects) is a short-lasting but very potent bronchoconstrictor (132, 182). Asthmatics are 8,000 times more sensitive to PGF$_{2\alpha}$ inhalation than healthy subjects (182, 251); for example, an asthma patient developed bronchospasm when treated with PGF$_{2\alpha}$ for therapeutic abortion (88). Flufenamate antagonized the contractions of human isolated bronchial muscle caused by PGF$_{2\alpha}$ (63) but failed to modify its bronchoconstrictor effects when inhaled (251).

Several studies with isolated human bronchial muscle preparations showed that PGE$_1$ and PGE$_2$ cause relaxation, with the bronchodilator potency of PGE$_1$ aerosols being 10–100 times greater than that of isoproterenol (161). In vivo PGE$_1$ and PGE$_2$ antagonized increases in bronchial resistance induced by either histamine or vagal stimulation (161, 178, 238).

In general the bronchodilator activity of either PGE$_1$ or PGE$_2$ is greater when they are administered by aerosol rather than by infusions. This might reflect the rapid removal and inactivation of PGE$_1$ or PGE$_2$ in the pulmonary circulation (86). The PGE$_1$ and PGE$_2$ had equipotent effects on bronchial muscle tone in healthy and asthmatic subjects and were 100 times as potent as isoprenaline (250). Prostaglandins and their analogues have not been therapeutically useful bronchodilators because of their tendency to irritate the upper respiratory tract (66). However, the receptors involved in coughing and bronchodilation are apparently different (61), and some PG derivatives with little or no irritant activity but potent bronchial relaxant activity have recently been described (104, 199).

Arachidonic acid and its metabolites also affect the smooth muscle of pulmonary blood vessels (151). Changes in pulmonary vascular pressure or flow in vivo may reflect the combination of a direct effect on vascular smooth muscle and a secondary effect due to increased platelet aggregation. It has been possible to demonstrate a direct effect of many eicosanoids on the pulmonary vasculature, however. Thus infusions of AA probably increase pulmonary arterial pressure by conversion to more active metabolites. The endoperoxides PGH$_2$ (149) and PGF$_{2\alpha}$ (76, 141) are also vasoconstrictors in the pulmonary vascular bed.

Vasodilation is produced consistently by PGE$_1$ (129, 141) and in some species also by PGE$_2$ (143). Prostacyclin is a potent vasodilator of the pulmonary circulation in humans (270) and in dogs (148, 198). In the fetal lamb PGE$_2$, PGF$_{2\alpha}$, and PGI$_2$ all dilated the pulmonary vascular bed (166).

INACTIVATION OF EICOSANOIDS IN LUNG

Lung homogenates contain a great variety of enzymes that can inactivate many endogenous mediators. However, the presence of inactivating enzymes in intracellular compartments or in tissue homogenates does not mean that the biologically active substrate is removed and inactivated during passage through the pulmonary circulation (83). The presence of membrane-bound enzymes in direct contact with blood allows some peptides (e.g., bradykinin and angiotensin I) to be hydrolyzed during passage through the lungs (see the chapter by Ryan in this *Handbook*). Despite the presence of endopeptidases, aminopeptidases, and carboxypeptidases within the lung cells, the absence of an uptake transport system for some peptides (e.g., oxytocin, vasopressin, substance P, angiotensin II) ensures that they pass through the pulmonary circulation intact (83, 84). Lack of transport to the intracellular enzyme site also seems to be why dopamine and epinephrine pass through the pulmonary circulation unchanged, whereas 5-hydroxytryptamine (5-HT) and norepinephrine are metabolized during the passage [(2, 296); see also the chapter by Junod in this *Handbook*].

Although the metabolic activity of the lung toward endogenous substrates is not due to a cell that is specific to the lung, the precise substrate specificity exhibited by the lung is not shared by other vascular beds. For instance, the hepatic portal circulation not only inactivated norepinephrine and 5-HT but also inactivated epinephrine and dopamine (296). In addition the majority of peptides are also metabolized during their passage through the portal circulation. Thus it seems that discriminating between different substrates may be a special feature of the pulmonary circulation.

The metabolism of PGs was first demonstrated with homogenates of the lung; subsequent investigation has disclosed that several enzymes are involved in this overall metabolic scheme.

Two closely associated enzymes are responsible for the inactivation of primary PGs by the lungs: 15-hydroxy-PG dehydrogenase (PGDH) and PG Δ^{13}-reductase (PGR). The PGDH oxidizes the 15-hydroxyl group to form 15-oxo-PGs with either NAD (type I PGDH) or NADP (type II PGDH) as a cofactor (17); PGDH is a soluble, ubiquitous enzyme and is found in high concentrations in the lung (125, 162). Most natural PGs are substrates (PGE$_2$, PGF$_{2\alpha}$, and PGI$_2$) (185, 263). Although PGA$_2$ is a substrate, PGB$_2$ (263) and TXB$_2$ (269) are not. The formation of 15-oxo-TXB$_2$ (58) was thus thought to represent metabolism of TXA$_2$ itself. Recently, however, the metabolism of TXB$_2$ to the 13,14-dihydro-15-oxo- derivative has been demonstrated in perfused lung (219a, 237a); this paradoxical finding has yet to be resolved. Although there are reports that the reaction catalyzed by PGDH is reversible in vitro (180, 272), in perfused lungs and in vivo the formation of the 15-oxo- derivative is favored. Because 15-oxo-PGs exhibit only weak biological activity relative to the parent 15-OH-PGs, the action of PGDH leads to inactivation.

The second enzyme, PGR, is also soluble and present in lung tissue in high concentrations (14); it uses NADH to reduce the 13,14 double bond of the 15-oxo- product of PGDH. This enzyme does not accept the 15-hydroxy-PGs as substrates (126, 165). Thus PGDH and PGR act sequentially, with PGDH catalyzing the rate-limiting step. Reduction of the 13,14 double bond does not change markedly the biological activity of the 15-oxo- derivative and the "double" metabolites (13,14-dihydro-PGs and 15-oxo-PGs) remain relatively inactive.

Other enzymes metabolizing PGs, i.e., those catalyzing β- and ω-oxidation (203, 235), and the PG-9 keto reductase (169) have been found in lung homogenates. However, in both perfused lung and in vivo, the PGDH action is so rapid that these other enzymes cannot contribute significantly to the inactivation of blood-borne PGs in the pulmonary circulation.

Although PGDH seems to be responsible for the inactivation of PGs, the broad substrate specificity of this enzyme in the intact lung is limited. Thus PGE$_2$, PGE$_1$, and PGF$_{2\alpha}$ are extensively metabolized and inactivated (70, 86, 231), but PGA$_2$ (124, 138, 184) and PGI$_2$ pass through the pulmonary circulation unchanged (76, 130). This is because both PGDH and PGR are intracellular enzymes requiring the transfer of substrates across the cell membrane. This carrier-mediated transport process is unable to transfer PGA$_2$, PGI$_2$, and 6-oxo-PGF$_{1\alpha}$ into the lung from the pulmonary circulation (13, 40, 78, 130). It is important to note that the liver does not exhibit a similar specificity, because both PGA$_2$ and PGI$_2$ are metabolized, together with PGE$_2$ and PGF$_{2\alpha}$, on passing through the portal circulation (76, 184).

Another divergence between the substrate specificity of the pulmonary transport system and PGDH is illustrated by the fate of the methylated PG analogues, 16,16-dimethyl- and 15-methyl-PGE$_2$. These compounds are not substrates for PGDH, presumably because of steric hindrance to the 15-hydroxyl group (176), but they are substrates for the pulmonary transport system (28). Thus they are not inactivated on transit through the pulmonary circulation; their appearance in the pulmonary venous effluent is delayed, however.

In vitro inhibitors of PGDH, e.g., furosemide (125), sulfasalazine (140), and diphloretin phosphate (65), also inhibit PG inactivation in the perfused lung; apparently they do so by inhibiting the carrier-mediated transport step (23–25). Other compounds that only act on the transport step, e.g., probenecid (40) and some organic dye molecules (27), also inhibit PG metabolism and inactivation. Clinically used dyes like indocyanine green can potently protect PGE$_2$ from inactivation (25), presumably by blocking its transport.

The cellular site of the PG-inactivating system in the lung is still unknown. Although many different substrates (5-HT, bradykinin, ADP, and even AA itself) are metabolized by endothelial cells of the pulmonary circulation, studies with cultured endothelial cells clearly show that these cells do not exhibit PGDH activity or inactivate PGs (6, 211). Furthermore smooth muscle cells, pulmonary fibroblasts (211), and several cultured fibroblast cell lines also lack PGDH activity (6). Endothelial cells in culture may somehow lose their normal PGDH activity; it must be remembered, however, that other enzymatic activities, e.g., those of monoamine oxidase [MAO; amine oxidase (flavin-containing)] (147, 240) and the membrane-bound, angiotensin-converting enzyme are retained (241). Whichever cell types are involved in pulmonary inactivation, they must be reasonably numerous to effect the extensive and rapid metabolism of PGs. In addition, inhibition by large ionized, nondiffusing molecules like diphloretin phosphate or bromocresol green indicates that they must be near the capillary lumen.

Although the metabolism of PGI$_2$ by PGDH has been thoroughly investigated (185), the metabolism of other short-lived AA metabolites has not received equal attention. Of the endoperoxides, PGG$_2$ cannot be a substrate, because it has a 15-hydroperoxy group; PGH$_2$, on the other hand, has a 15-hydroxy group and is a good substrate (262). The great instability of TXA$_2$ creates difficulties in studies of metabolism, but the presence of 15-oxo-TXB$_2$ in effluent from guinea pig lungs after anaphylaxis (58, 71), coupled with the inability of PGDH to oxidize TXB$_2$ in vitro (265), implies that TXA$_2$ may indeed survive long enough in vivo to be metabolized by PGDH. Crutchley et al. (64) demonstrated a potentially important corollary of this possibility when they showed a greater output of TXA_2 from guinea pig lungs after the PGDH levels had been decreasd by in vivo exposure to 100% O_2. Increases in TXA_2 levels and its effects may thus reflect decreased metabolism rather than increased synthesis. The more stable TXB_2 has been shown to decrease PGE_2 metabolism in dog lung in vivo, even though it is not itself metabolized (102). This effect was observed with high doses of TXB_2 and has been attributed to TXB_2 blocking the transport of PGE_2. This possibility is supported by the paradoxical ability of perfused lung to take up and metabolize TXB_2 (219a, 237a).

Before considering how the pulmonary inactivation of PGs can be modulated, it is worth emphasizing that the inactivation processes apply both to substrate in the pulmonary vascular bed (i.e., extrapulmonary PG) and to substrate generated in situ (i.e., intrapulmonary PG). Because the lung can produce nearly all the known eicosanoids, this ability to inactivate highly potent eicosanoids before they enter the vascular space is clearly a very important protective mechanism. Thus in guinea pig lung during anaphylaxis most of the eicosanoids present in the perfusate leaving the lung are inactive metabolites of the TXA_2 originally formed (71, 172).

Pulmonary inactivation of the primary PGs is susceptible to modulation by both physiological and pathological factors, apart from any pharmacological means of inhibition. The first physiological factor to be considered is the animal's development. In the immediate postnatal days, PGDH levels are equal to or slightly higher than levels in the adult (215, 216); in addition, inactivation of PGE_1 in the pulmonary circulation of fetal lambs equals that in newborn (11–12 days) or 6-mo-old lambs (212). These results were essentially confirmed in a more recent study with fetal and neonatal isolated rabbit lungs (248). Here PGE_2 inactivation was extensive by 28 days of gestation, increased up to birth, and remained on this higher level for up to 1 wk after birth. This pattern of early development of PG inactivation contrasts with the finding that the limited fetal metabolism of angiotensin I and bradykinin increases dramatically postnatally (156, 260), accompanied by a comparable postnatal development of monoamine oxidase (33). Pulmonary PG inactivation is apparently also important in utero as well as after birth.

Prostaglandin metabolism is affected by the progress of the estrous cycle (31) but a greater effect is seen during the later stages of pregnancy. The metabolism of PGs in the maternal lung increased sharply at term, when measured as enzyme levels either in vitro or in vivo in rabbits but not in rats (32, 77, 262). However, changes in PGDH and the inactivation of PGE_2 in isolated rat lungs have also been reported during late pregnancy (42, 49). The 20-hydroxylation of PGs by a particulate fraction of rabbit lung is markedly stimulated in pregnant animals (235). The purpose of these increases may be to protect the increasingly sensitive uterine smooth muscle from stimulation by PGs liberated from extrauterine sources. Treatment with progesterone also causes some similar changes (32, 234).

Pathological factors influencing pulmonary PG inactivation have been investigated for a limited number of alterations in the ventilating gases. Exposure to anesthetic mixtures of halothane did not affect PGE_2 inactivation but did decrease norepinephrine inactivation in dogs (26). Cardiopulmonary bypass is associated with increases in arterial levels of PGs because pulmonary inactivation cannot take place (53, 232, 247). When pulmonary circulation is restored, however, the full metabolic potential of the lung is not immediately exhibited; less PGE_1 is removed postbypass in humans (124, 232). These changes in PG metabolism clearly affect the cardiovascular system both during and after bypass procedures.

The toxic effects of hyperoxia (exposure to 90%–100% O_2) are associated with damage to the alveolar septum and consequent defects in gas exchange. These morphological changes are accompanied by enzymatic changes. The PGDH activity in homogenates of the lungs from guinea pigs exposed in vivo to 100% O_2 was decreased (54, 219), and with perfused rat lungs, a decrease in PG inactivation has been correlated with the duration of exposure to high O_2 concentrations (155, 274). Direct measurement of PG oxidation in rat lung homogenates showed a fall to 13% of normal levels after a 48-h exposure (276). The mechanism of the decrease in PGDH activity has not been elucidated but may be related to the susceptibility of protein sulfhydryl groups in the enzyme (125) to oxidation. Prostaglandin inactivation may be affected earlier than either 5-HT metabolism or angiotensin I–converting enzyme activity; this suggests that a nonendothelial cell type is responding earlier than the endothelial cell, the site of early morphological changes (154).

Tobacco smoke is another common pulmonary insult that is delivered via the airways. Inhaled cigarette smoke had no effect on the metabolism of $PGF_{2\alpha}$ in isolated rabbit lung (117) when the ventilating gas (room air) was replaced by cigarette smoke for four 2-s puffs. However, more prolonged smoke exposure (up to 10 days) is known to increase the metabolism and binding of benzo[a]pyrene (59), to affect testosterone metabolism in rat lung (127), and to decrease the inactivation of PGE_2 in isolated perfused lungs (27). The ventilation of isolated rat lungs with cigarette smoke decreased the formation of 15-oxo-PGE_2 after the infusion of [^{14}C]PGE_2 through the pulmonary circulation (179). Decreases in PG metabolism are not accompanied by decreases in the metabolism of other substrates (27), arguing against a nonspecific "poisoning" of the lung cells. Furthermore these experiments suggest that the normal control function of the pulmonary circulation is altered by exposure to smoke, and this may be a mechanism for initiating the cardiovascular changes associated with cigarette smoking.

Systemic hypertension as a factor affecting pulmonary metabolism has not been extensively studied. There is some disagreement between those who find decreases in pulmonary inactivation (49, 164) and increases in pulmonary PGDH activity (273) in genetically hypertensive rats. Systemic hypotension resulting from endotoxin or hemorrhagic shock also affects PG metabolism in the lung. Thus after endotoxin injection, PG metabolizing activity in rat lung homogenates was decreased (203). However, in baboons the in vivo pulmonary metabolism of $PGF_{2\alpha}$ increased after endotoxin injection (91), but metabolism of PGE_2 and $PGF_{2\alpha}$ decreased with hemorrhagic shock (92). This decrease may reflect the increased venous levels of PGs saturating the pulmonary removal processes rather than a real decrease in PG inactivation.

Modulation of PG inactivation by clinically used drugs is not very likely because the agents affecting inactivation are either not used clinically (e.g., N-ethylmaleimide and p-chloromercuribenzoic acid) or are not very potent. The latter class includes diuretics like furosemide and ethacrynic acid that inhibit PGDH (125); the concentrations of ~1 mM needed to modulate such inhibition in the perfused lung are much higher than are required to cause diuretic activity in vivo. The most potent uptake inhibitors (bromocresol green and diphloretin phosphate) are not used therapeutically (27). Several clinically used dyes (e.g., indocyanine green and bromsulfophthalein sodium) have been shown to inhibit PG inactivation in isolated lungs (25), and these compounds may indeed affect pulmonary PG inactivation in vivo after clinical use.

SYNTHESIS OF EICOSANOIDS BY LUNG

Eicosanoids are not stored preformed but are instead synthesized by the lung as needed. Much effort has been spent in analyzing the stimuli for eicosanoid production, identifying pathways and rate-limiting steps, and characterizing the actual mixture of eicosanoids formed in response to each stimulus.

Eicosanoid production is discussed in two general subdivisions: synthesis from exogenous AA (i.e., extrapulmonary AA, present as a component of plasma free fatty acids) and synthesis from endogenous AA (i.e., intrapulmonary AA, usually esterified and present in phospholipids or neutral lipids).

The crucial difference between these pathways is that synthesis from exogenous AA depends solely on the activity of cyclooxygenase, whereas synthesis from endogenous AA supplies appears to be controlled at the earlier stage of lipid hydrolysis, probably by a phospholipase or a glyceride lipase. Thus the maximum potential of the lungs to synthesize eicosanoids may be estimated by providing exogenous AA; synthesis from endogenous supplies may be a more realistic estimate of potential synthesis after a given stimulus, however. Both estimates are useful and, although they may coincide in magnitude or type of eicosanoid formed, this coincidence must not be assumed.

One reason for this caution is the multiplicity of cell types in the lung. Endothelial cells, for example, have a profile of eicosanoid formation that differs from platelets (193), but we know comparatively little about the synthetic potential of other lung cells. Thus two stimuli for endogenous synthesis (e.g., anaphylaxis and pulmonary embolism) may stimulate different populations of cells, including cells that differ from those that synthesize eicosanoids from exogenous AA. The presence of highly active PG inactivating systems in the lung introduces a further complication. This means that eicosanoid synthesis and activation could occur locally, with the precise cellular environment in which synthesis occurred influencing the mixture of eicosanoids present in pulmonary vascular effluent.

Synthesis From Exogenous Arachidonic Acid

In vivo infusion of AA into the pulmonary circulation affects both bronchial and vascular smooth muscle (151, 258); these effects are blocked by indomethacin and other NSAIDs and have thus been attributed to the synthesis of cyclooxygenase products (COPs), i.e., PGs and TXA_2. Because AA also causes platelet aggregation, the synthesis of COP by the lungs must be dissociated from COP synthesis resulting from the platelet aggregates in the pulmonary vascular bed. Dog platelets, however, are resistant to the aggregatory effects of AA and its metabolites (56), and Hyman and his colleagues (142) showed that AA had both vasoconstrictor and vasodilator effects on the canine pulmonary circulation in vivo. With bolus injections or infusions of high concentrations of AA, broncho- and vasoconstriction were observed both in vivo and in lungs perfused with a salt solution (142, 290). Infusions of low concentrations of AA in vivo did not change airway tone but did decrease the pulmonary vascular resistance. Increasing the concentration of infused AA changed pulmonary vasodilation to vasoconstriction (256). There is now evidence in other systems that, at low concentrations of AA, mainly PGI_2 is formed, whereas at high AA concentrations the proportion of vasoconstrictor TXA_2 is much increased (259, 264).

The bronchoconstriction induced in vivo by intravenous administration of AA in the dog (256), cat (101), and guinea pig (60, 168) was abolished by NSAIDs. In the guinea pig, bronchoconstriction induced by AA infusion apparently is not caused by the formation of TXA_2 resulting from platelet aggregates, because thrombocytopenia induced by antiplatelet serum does not modify this effect (168). This bronchoconstriction is also resistant to blockade by imidazole (55, 237), an inhibitor of TXA_2 synthetase in vitro, suggesting that TXA_2 produced by the lung is not involved. However, this drug is probably not effective in vivo because it did not affect the thrombocytopenia caused by AA as effectively as cyclooxygenase inhibitors (281).

The ability of the airways to generate a constrictor COP concurrent with the vasculature's generation of a dilator metabolite exemplifies the different profiles of the COPs generated by different cell types. In the guinea pig lung the following compartmentalization of COP synthesis has been proposed: PGs, in the smooth muscle of large airways; TXA_2, in the interstitial cells of lung parenchyma; and PGI_2, in the pulmonary endothelium (113). This proposal was based on the observations that contracting guinea pig trachea releases PGE_2, that parenchymal lung strips synthesize mainly TXA_2, and that isolated perfused lungs synthesize PGI_2 from exogenous AA.

The fate of exogenous AA has been analyzed in some detail with isolated lungs perfused with Krebs solution. A mixture of endoperoxides and TXA_2 (originally referred to as RCS) forms after the perfusion of AA through isolated guinea pig lungs (121, 266, 282). Imidazole effectively blocks TXA_2 production in this preparation (206). The inhibition of RCS formation by NSAIDs after AA infusion was demonstrated previously (282). In a comparative analysis of the fate of exogenous AA in isolated lungs from the guinea pig, rat, and human, 80%–90% of the radioactivity derived from [^{14}C]AA was taken up and retained in the lungs of all species after a single passage through the pulmonary circulation (8–10, 146). The retained radioactivity was rapidly esterified (within 10 min), chiefly into phospholipids, with lesser amounts in neutral lipids.

The major difference between species was the amount and type of COPs produced by the lung; guinea pig lung produced the most COPs (including TXA_2), whereas in both rat and human lung effluent fivefold less COP was formed and activity similar to that of TXA_2 was undetectable. This apparent inability to synthesize TXA_2 in human lung was also seen after stimulation by the calcium ionophore A23187 (11). These results suggest strongly that TXA_2 formation may be particularly prevalent in guinea pig lungs and that other species may not produce as much of this vasoconstrictor and bronchoconstrictor COP. They also suggest that species differences are extremely important at least in terms of the metabolism of AA and that rat lung may be a better analogue of human lung than the more commonly used guinea pig lung (10, 11).

The metabolism of the intermediate endoperoxides PGG_2 and PGH_2 was studied in vivo by comparing their hypotensive effects after intravenous or intra-arterial administration in rats (18). Both endoperoxides were more potent in lowering the systemic arterial blood pressure when given intravenously, suggesting that they are transformed in the lung into a more potent vasodilator, possibly PGI_2. These results are at variance with experiments with isolated lungs perfused with Krebs solution, which show the inactivation of exogenous PGH_2. In guinea pig lungs, only a 10%–12% conversion of intermediate endoperoxides to TXA_2 and <5% conversion to PGE_2 was observed by bioassay. Even less metabolism to TXA_2, PGI_2 or PGE_2, and $PGF_{2\alpha}$ was seen in rabbit lungs (3, 4). A parallel study (7) with guinea pig and rat lungs concluded that exogenous PGH_2 did not follow the same metabolic pathway as endoperoxide formed in situ from exogenous AA; i.e., it was mostly inactivated and not converted to the same mixture of COPs as was its precursor, AA.

A number of factors influence the formation of COPs by the lungs from exogenous AA. Two studies of gender differences in AA metabolism are available (30, 177). In both studies the metabolism of exogenous AA in perfused lungs was assayed radiochemically and showed that the formation of COP was greater in males than in females. The metabolism of AA in females also changed during the estrous cycle with the most marked changes occurring between proestrous and estrous (30). It seems therefore that naturally induced changes in the levels of sex hormones could affect the normal synthesis of COP, a finding with important physiological and pharmacological implications.

An important factor in relating experiments in perfused lungs to those in vivo is the effect of albumin on COP formation. In guinea pig lungs perfused with Krebs solution, the synthesis of myotropic COPs from exogenous AA was decreased markedly by the addition of albumin (1% bovine serum albumin) to the perfusing solution (7). The replacement of blood in dog lungs with a saline perfusate led to an increased vascular response to AA and increased PGE- and PGF-like products in lung effluent (measured by radioimmunoassay); perfusion with 1% albumin in saline gave results equivalent to blood perfusion (142, 143). Apparently the presence of albumin in vivo may inhibit total COP formation. Whether it also changes the composition of the mixture of COPs is not known.

A diminished vascular response to AA despite an increased sensitivity to PGE_2 and $PGF_{2\alpha}$ during hypoxia [partial pressure of O_2 in arterial blood (Pa_{O_2}) = 46 mmHg] implies a diminished synthesis of COPs (142). Changes in blood pH from 7.1 to 7.6 did not affect responses to AA, although responses to PGs were altered; in addition it seems that small compensatory alterations in COP synthesis may have occurred (142). The effects of these variables (Pa_{O_2}, pH) on the activity of systems inactivating PG must be considered before any firm conclusions can be drawn.

Synthesis From Endogenous Arachidonic Acid

As mentioned earlier (see ANTAGONISTS OF EICOSANOIDS AND INHIBITORS OF THEIR SYNTHESIS, p. 367) the synthesis of eicosanoids from endogenous substrate requires the activation of lipases to liberate AA from its esterified lipid forms. Eicosanoids are probably continuously produced at a low level; this is because the lipids are turned over under normal basal metabolic conditions. However, in other, pathological, conditions this production is greatly increased, with clear pharmacological effects on the lung and extrapulmonary systems.

RELEASE OF EICOSANOIDS AFTER ANAPHYLACTIC REACTIONS. The first evidence for eicosanoid production in guinea pig lungs during anaphylaxis was provided by Piper and Vane (229). They found that PG-like material in lung effluent was also accompanied by RCS (subsequently shown to be TXA_2). Several PGs and their metabolites have been clearly identified in this system (71, 172, 183). Steroids or NSAIDs prevented the release of these COPs after immunological stimulation, a reaction that was consistent with the liberation of endogenous AA as a substrate for cyclooxygenase. However, although the COPs formed have potent broncho- and vasoconstrictor activities, the in vivo pharmacological effects of anaphylaxis were already known to be only partially inhibited by NSAIDs (62). Furthermore indomethacin did not decrease the pulmonary effects of allergic asthma (252); indeed aspirin can induce asthma (268). Apparently the COPs so far identified were not the major mediators of the effects of anaphylaxis, although they were somehow associated with it.

This association can be demonstrated in immunologically sensitized animals even without anaphylaxis. Dawson and co-workers (34, 47) showed that in guinea pig lungs, sensitization increased both the total COP formation from exogenous AA and the proportion of COPs present as TXB_2. In lungs from animals sensitized and repeatedly challenged, over 80% of the COPs corresponded to TXB_2 and its metabolites. If a similar situation exists in humans, it is possible that the apparent inability to form TXA_2 in the normal lung may be markedly altered by sensitization and continuous exposure to low levels of antigen (11).

Another myotropic agent associated with anaphylaxis is SRS-A, and this agent has recently been shown to be a metabolite of AA that is synthesized via lipoxygenase and not via cyclooxygenase. It was first described as a potent myotropic agent, pharmacologically distinguishable from histamine and released from guinea pig lungs during anaphylaxis (153). It showed the same pharmacological profile (50) as other poorly defined materials released from dog and monkey lungs after perfusion with cobra venom (81). Like the PGs, SRS-A is not stored preformed but is synthesized after immunological stimulation.

The generation of SRS-A by immunological activation was increased by the concomitant infusion of AA (196) and was further increased by administration of cyclooxygenase inhibitors (79, 283). These observations strongly suggested that PGs and SRS-A shared the same precursor, AA, for their synthesis. The structures of the components of SRS-A were established and given the name leukotrienes [Fig. 2; (48, 195, 200)]. It is now clear that AA is the common precursor, through two different pathways, both of PGs and the mixtures of leukotrienes referred to as SRS-A.

The most potent leukotrienes presently known in terms of causing contractions in smooth muscle are LTC_4 and LTD_4 (22, 74, 226). Another leukotriene, LTB_4, has much less potent effects on smooth muscle but is a powerful chemotactic agent for leukocytes (254). Although the leukotrienes can be synthesized chemically, the many possible isomers (*cis* or *trans* configurations) resulting from the four double bonds in the molecule introduce an additional difficulty into the structure-activity analysis of these compounds (171). Separation and unequivocal identification of each isomer present problems, and the possibility of different mixtures of isomers makes it difficult to know which leukotriene is being assessed biologically. Apparently only one configuration of double bonds possesses the potency of naturally synthesized SRS-A (98). Further complications arise from the conversion of LTC_4 to LTD_4 by the loss of a glutamic acid residue catalyzed by γ-glutamyl transpeptidase, an enzyme widely distributed in animal tissue (111). Thus in isolated tissue and even in vivo, the effects of LTC_4 might be due to its partial or total transformation to LTD_4. For this reason the biological activities associated with SRS-A are usually attributed to a mixture (of variable proportions) of LTC_4, LTD_4, and LTE_4 [Fig. 2; (170)].

The biological activities of particular interest here are the contraction of bronchial and tracheal smooth muscle and of lung parenchymal strips. This lung parenchyma preparation (175, 186) has been a model of the peripheral airway smooth muscle, at least in the guinea pig and cat, and it is at this level that reduced air flow in asthmatics is said to occur, not in the larger airways from which bronchial or tracheal smooth muscle strips may be taken. Both SRS-A and LTC_4 and LTD_4 are very powerful contractors of the guinea pig lung parenchymal strip (10^{-11} mol of LTC_4 causes a large response). On parenchymal strips from rat lung, however, LTC_4 and LTD_4 are 100- to 200-fold less effective (225).

An important property of SRS-A, LTC_4, and LTD_4 is the ability to release TXA_2 and other COPs from guinea pig lung, perfused either in isolation or in strips

(225). This can be inhibited by cyclooxygenase inhibitors (aspirin, indomethacin) or by thromboxane synthetase inhibitors (imidazole), and in the presence of these compounds, the effects of LTC_4 and LTD_4 on guinea pig lung strip are markedly decreased (225). Neither purified SRS-A nor LTC_4 releases TXA_2 from perfused rat or human lung (9), and on strips from rat and rabbit lung the effects of LTC_4 and LTD_4 are resistant to indomethacin (225). The high potency of LTC_4 and LTD_4 on guinea pig lung is therefore not a direct effect but occurs via TXA_2 synthesis. This indirect effect (and thus potency) is lacking in the lungs of other animals and in humans.

The synthesis of the leukotrienes proceeds via a lipoxygenase-catalyzed oxidation of AA and not via cyclooxygenase. Thus the NSAID inhibitors of cyclooxygenase actually increase leukotriene synthesis (79, 283), probably by decreasing competition for the substrate AA. Steroids decrease the amount of AA available and are therefore effective inhibitors of both SRS-A and COP formation (44, 52, 115). Also analogues of AA, e.g., TYA (an acetylenic derivative of AA), and an unrelated group of compounds (phenylpyrazolidone, BW 775C, and benoxaprofen) inhibit both AA oxygenases and decrease leukotriene formation (52, 137, 227, 284). A specific inhibitor of the 5-lipoxygenase has not been synthesized, however.

One of the most important incentives for the study of leukotrienes and COP in the lung was the search for the primary mediator(s) of allergic asthma. At present two possible mediators have been eliminated: histamine and COPs. Histamine antagonists, although active in many other systems, were ineffective in allergic asthma, as were inhibitors of COP formation like aspirin or indomethacin (252). The formation of SRS-A was not inhibited by NSAIDs, and the increased synthesis observed in the presence of indomethacin could explain aspirin-induced asthma. Some of the leukotrienes in SRS-A were potent myotropic agents and stimulated the synthesis of TXA_2, another potent myotropic agent. In addition, LTB_4 also increased vascular permeability and could be involved in the bronchial edema often associated with asthma. Experimental studies with TYA and BW 755C, inhibitors of lipoxygenase and cyclooxygenase both in vitro and in vivo, showed a decreased production of SRS-A (220, 284) and a decreased airways response to immunological stimuli (207, 221, 222).

Less supportive evidence of leukotriene mediation of asthma includes the following points: LTC_4 and LTD_4 were much less potent on rat and rabbit lung strips than on guinea pig strips and did not stimulate TXA_2 release in human lung; indomethacin blocked the bronchoconstriction caused by injection of LTC_4 in guinea pigs, showing that this is an indirect effect.

Whether leukotrienes are the "missing mediators" in asthma is not known. However, the efficacy of steroids in this disorder, coupled with their indirect inhibition of phospholipase A_2 (41), does suggest strongly the involvement of some metabolite of AA. Leukotrienes and COPs might interact to sensitize airway smooth muscle to another unknown mediator, other lipoxygenase products besides LTC_4 potentiate the action of histamine on bronchial smooth muscle (1), and PGs are known to sensitize uterine smooth muscle to other agonists (57, 291).

Mast cells in the lung are thought to be the major source of SRS-A, because its release is associated with an IgE-dependent reaction (214). Other cells can also form a mixture of leukotrienes, however. In rats SRS-A can be formed from an IgG complement-dependent reaction involving neutrophils (197), and the calcium ionophore A23187 causes leukocytes to synthesize leukotrienes without any immunological involvement (21).

Activation of the complement system can induce COP synthesis, probably via the formation of anaphylatoxin or C5a. Injections of purified hog C5a in dogs (223) produced pulmonary hypertension, tachypnea, and systemic hypotension accompanied by an output of PG-like substances in the arterial blood; pretreatment with indomethacin prevented the systemic hypotension. In isolated lungs from guinea pigs, crude rat anaphylatoxin (242) and purified hog C5a (223) released both COPs and histamine. Furthermore, TXA_2-, PGE-, and PGF-like activity were identified as components of the released COP and release was blocked by indomethacin. In this preparation, however, no evidence for SRS formation was found.

There is therefore reason to believe that some of the effects of C5a in vivo are related to a release of COP from the lung. Although Pavek and colleagues (223) compared C5a with anaphylaxis, complement activation can be brought about by contact between complement precursors and the bacterial cell walls. Thus in patients with sepsis, the development of shock lung or the adult respiratory distress syndrome (characterized by hypoxemia, interstitial infiltrates, and reduced compliance) correlated strongly with plasma levels of C5a (123). The role of complement in endotoxin shock in animals is still unclear, but COP seems to be involved because endotoxin releases primary PGs (13) and aspirinlike drugs partially reverse the hemodynamic changes observed in shock (90). A further link between C5a and the lung is the fact that C5a causes leukocyte aggregation. These leukocyte aggregates accumulated in the lung and were associated with pulmonary dysfunction (i.e., hypertension and fall in Pa_{O_2}). Sulfinpyrazone, which is known to inhibit PG synthesis, inhibited pulmonary dysfunction but not leukocyte aggregation (100). When complement is activated, leukocytes aggregate and form leukoemboli in the pulmonary microvasculature. They then generate COP, probably by interacting with the endothelium, and these COP can affect pulmonary smooth muscle in the blood vessels or airways.

RELEASE OF EICOSANOIDS BY MECHANICAL STIMULATION. Simple manipulation of isolated perfused organs, such as the spleen (86, 105, 106, 116) or the lungs (217), causes PG release. Chopped guinea pig lung also releases PGs when agitated by stirring. Infusion of particles (Sephadex or polystyrene spheres) or emulsions of fats through the pulmonary circulation of guinea pigs or rats (173, 230) leads to the release of PGE$_2$- and TXA$_2$-like activity.

The effects of pulmonary emboli in vivo, from whatever cause, are diminished after administering indomethacin and steroids. Thus the bronchoconstriction occurring after BaSO$_4$ microembolization (201) and the pulmonary hypertension caused by endotoxin-induced embolization were both blocked by either aspirin (109) or methyl prednisolone (181). This, together with increased arterial levels of PGs (12, 91) after embolization, could be taken as evidence for the synthesis of COP in the lung in these situations. However, the aggregation of platelets and leukocytes in the lung provides an alternate source of COP. Indeed there is evidence that in thrombocytopenic animals, infusion of BaSO$_4$ no longer causes contraction of pulmonary vascular muscle (46). The relative contribution of pulmonary and nonpulmonary cells to COP formation during pulmonary embolus formation in vivo is therefore uncertain, and in this case it seems that whichever cells are responsible, the balance of COP formation is toward the constrictor species, TXA$_2$ and PGF$_{2\alpha}$.

In anesthetized cat, dog, and rabbit the lungs seem to generate PGI$_2$ continuously (112, 114, 191). This spontaneous release of PGI$_2$ is also detectable in isolated perfused lung of the guinea pig, rat, and cat and is increased by mechanical stimulation, AA, or vasoactive substances (259). Generation of PGI$_2$ is increased by artificial ventilation of anesthetized patients (76a). In animals, respiratory stimulants such as lobeline are as effective as mechanical hyperventilation in increasing PGI$_2$ production by lung (259). This increased production is secondary to the increased ventilatory movement, because the respiratory stimulants do not increase PGI$_2$ in isolated lung or after bilateral vagotomy in vivo, conditions in which they also do not increase ventilatory movements.

It has been proposed that PGI$_2$ continuously released by the lungs into the arterial circulation would act in peripheral vascular beds, supplementing the antiaggregatory and vasodilatory actions of locally released PGI$_2$ (112). Too little PGI$_2$ is released by the lungs (100–200 pg/ml) (114, 135) to affect blood pressure and platelet aggregation; recent measurements suggest that the circulating levels in conscious resting subjects are even lower (<3 pg/ml) (45a). Additional PGI$_2$ release induced by mechanical stimulation, i.e., ventilatory movements of lung, might protect against the formation of microthrombi in lung vasculature and also serve as a local vasodilator, ensuring maximal matching of ventilation with perfusion within the pulmonary circulation. Artificial ventilation of anesthetized patients increased blood levels of 6-oxo-PGF$_{1\alpha}$ from ~20 pg/ml to 190 pg/ml (76a). The synthesis of COP induced by respiratory movements may also be important in the rapid fall in pulmonary vascular resistance immediately after birth. In fetal goats indomethacin blocked a part of the decrease in pulmonary vascular resistance after ventilation (167); this could be due to COP synthesis by lung tissue comparable with that seen in adult lungs during hyperventilation (36).

The release of COP during hyperventilation does not seem to be related to either increased oxygen tension or pH changes in the pulmonary blood. On the contrary, pulmonary events occurring during hypoxia might be associated with the formation of COP products. The mediators of hypoxic vasoconstriction in the lung are still unknown. As Fishman (89) pointed out, almost every known mediator has had its proponents and none have been convincing. The demonstration that Ca^{2+} antagonists (e.g., verapamil) are inhibitors of this response does not identify the agent causing the increased Ca^{2+} flux in vascular smooth muscle. Prostaglandin-like compounds were thought to be involved as mediators of hypoxic vasoconstriction (244) until indomethacin was found to be ineffective as an inhibitor of the hypoxic response (275, 289). Indeed most workers agree that COP formation increases during hypoxia and the effect of this increased synthesis may be to diminish rather than to cause hypoxic vasoconstriction, because indomethacin or aspirin treatment potentiated hypoxic pulmonary hypertension (275, 289). However, because hypoxia alone potentiated the responses to the constrictor PGF$_{2\alpha}$ and because COP formation was deduced from smooth muscle responses, further analysis of these results is needed to differentiate between increased synthesis and increased muscle sensitivity before they can be adequately interpreted.

RELEASE OF EICOSANOIDS BY ENDOGENOUS MEDIATORS. A variety of myotropic agents also induce the synthesis of COP from endogenous AA. Bradykinin, histamine, 5-HT, and angiotensin II infused through the pulmonary circulation all cause COP release as identified either by bioassay (5, 29, 230) or by radioimmunoassay (37, 38). Interesting features of this release included tachyphylaxis; i.e., repeated doses of the agonist produced a diminishing release of COP and the release was mediated via specific receptors. For example, 5-HT–induced release was blocked by methysergide, whereas histamine-induced release in the same lung was unaffected. The release of TXA$_2$ from guinea pig isolated lung and of PGF$_{2\alpha}$ from human lung fragments (both induced by histamine) were blocked by H$_1$ antagonists. The H$_2$ agonists could not induce release and H$_2$ antagonists were unable to block the release caused by histamine (38, 233). Indomethacin, however, was able to block the COP release induced by any agonist. Another important characteristic of this type of induced COP formation is its species variation (5, 29): histamine caused COP release from guinea pig, dog, or rat lung, but 5-HT and tryptamine were effective only in rat lung. Superimposed on this is the species variation in the type of COP formed (see *Synthesis From Exogenous Arachidonic Acid*, p. 373). It is thus difficult to relate this phenomenon directly to either the human lung or human pathology.

Both ATP and ADP provide a rather unusual stimulus for COP biosynthesis. In isolated rat lungs, ATP infused through the pulmonary circulation stimulated the release of a PGE_2-like substance, which was not further characterized (205). In dogs the intravenous infusion of ADP and ATP produced a substance described as PGI_2-like on the basis of its antiaggregatory and myotropic activities, its short half-life, and its inhibition by indomethacin (133). The ADP undoubtedly caused platelet aggregation in the in vivo pulmonary circulation, and this generation of COP could therefore be classified as embolus induced. Needleman et al. (205) used blood-free perfusate to show that lung tissue can be stimulated directly by ADP and ATP to produce COP from endogenous AA. This stimulus for COP formation is probably of little importance under physiological conditions, when the adenine nucleotides would normally be retained inside cells. Where the blood levels of these nucleotides are raised by leakage from injured tissues and platelet aggregation this mechanism may be more important.

Bradykinin or angiotensin II (but not other biologically active peptides, amines, and nucleotides) increased the release of PGI_2 from perfused guinea pig lungs (259). The effect mediated by angiotensin II was blocked by saralasin, an antagonist of angiotensin II, and bradykinin's effect was enhanced by captopril, an inhibitor of bradykinin breakdown in the lung. These results again are probably indications of the potential for modulating pulmonary COP synthesis in pathological conditions rather than demonstrations of a physiological mechanism.

Edema is a cardinal sign of inflammation. For over 10 years, PGs have been identified as one of the mediators of inflammation (294). It is therefore not surprising that AA metabolites have been investigated in states of pulmonary edema, both as mediators of the increased lung permeability and as products of the edematous lung.

Infusions of AA or a number of COPs into the pulmonary artery of sheep did not directly increase vascular permeability, but the vasoconstrictor COP increased lung lymph flow by increasing microvascular pressure. In agreement with this, cyclooxygenase inhibitors (indomethacin and meclofenamate) did not block the phase of increased permeability in the lung's response to endotoxin, although the earlier pulmonary hypertension was reduced. Either treatment with steroids or the depletion of granulocytes blocked the increased permeability responses, however (49a). These results parallel those obtained in skin microvasculature of rabbits (288), where LTB_4, a lipoxygenase metabolite of AA, was shown to increase vascular permeability via a leukocyte-dependent mechanism. The formation of LTB_4 would be unaffected by cyclooxygenase inhibitors, but sensitive to inhibition by steroids, at an earlier stage in its synthesis. It is interesting to note in this context that PGs did not affect permeability in the skin microvasculature but the vasodilator PGs synergized powerfully with agents causing increased permeability (e.g., histamine or C5a) to produce marked edema (292, 293). Therefore it is possible that cyclooxygenase metabolites mediate changes in vascular resistance, whereas lipoxygenase metabolites mediate changes in permeability in pulmonary edema.

SUMMARY

The lungs, like most other organs of the body, can both synthesize and inactivate biologically active, oxygenated metabolites of AA. This ability is obviously important in studies of the intrapulmonary effects of these metabolites.

This metabolic activity is also potentially important in terms of extrapulmonary effects because of the lung's unique position in the vascular system. The pulmonary circulation receives the total cardiac output and is placed at the point of division between systemic venous and arterial circulations. Thus the composition and amount of AA metabolites entering the systemic arterial circulation for distribution to the peripheral tissues is crucially dependent on events in the lung.

The control exercised by the lung is supplemented by the selectivity of lung metabolism. For AA metabolites this is most obvious in the selective inactivation of PGE_2 and $PGF_{2\alpha}$ and the free passage of PGI_2. If the lung's inactivating mechanisms are deficient, the PGs formed in peripheral tissues and drained into the venous blood are carried over into the systemic arterial circulation; if the inactivating mechanisms are more effective than usual, as in the last days of pregnancy, then a greater protection against recirculating PGs is possible. Similarly, if the lung suffers some insult and is synthesizing TXA_2 or leukotrienes, then the arterial blood is contaminated with these highly active agents. Although TXA_2 has a short half-life (30 s), there is more than enough time for it to reach the most peripheral parts of the systemic arterial bed.

A variety of physiological and pathological factors modify the metabolic activities of the lung. Although there are presently no clear examples of disturbed lung metabolism leading directly to disturbances in systemic homeostasis, the potential for such correlations clearly exists.

The intrapulmonary effects of AA metabolites probably depend more on the availability of endogenous intrapulmonary AA than on its coming from blood-borne extrapulmonary sources. This is certainly true in anaphylaxis, where the immunological reactions provide free AA from endogenous lipids and where the synthesis of all AA metabolites depends on its liberation by lipases from esterified pools. Whether TXA_2 or leukotrienes are responsible for this bronchoconstriction, their synthesis and their effects are reduced by steroids (probably via inhibition of phospholipase A_2). Although steroids given as aerosols are much more therapeutically effective than those given systemically, the inhibition of phospholipase A_2 (even in lung) could have serious side effects on surfactant synthesis. From the direction of current research it seems that a specific inhibitor of 5-lipoxygenase would have a better therapeutic index than the steroids and finally settle the question of the involvement of leukotrienes in asthma.

Two of the most important aspects of intrapulmonary AA metabolism may be the synthesis of PGI_2 and the inactivation of PGH_2 in the pulmonary circulation. The synthesis of a potent antiaggregatory agent and the degradation of a proaggregatory agent, together with the degradation of two other proaggregatory substances, ADP and 5-HT, mean that the pulmonary circulation is well equipped to maintain the patency of the pulmonary capillaries. In a vascular bed where the capillaries physically filter out microthrombi, cellular aggregates, and debris in mixed venous blood, it is important to ensure that occlusion is not transformed into a focus for platelet aggregation.

The increased synthesis of PGI_2 stimulated by bradykinin could also serve as a protective mechanism, because kinin formation may be increased after either tissue damage or after the activation of the Hagemann factor by bacterial cell walls; both of these are conditions in which aggregates of disrupted tissue or leukocytes might accumulate in lung capillaries.

To some extent, the metabolism of AA in the lung is a phenomenon looking for a function. An understanding of this phenomenon is necessary to elucidate its function. The relationship of PGs, TXA_2 and TXB_2, and leukotrienes to the lung is still incompletely understood, but their effects are known too well to be disregarded in any future investigation of lung function.

REFERENCES

1. ADCOCK, J. J., AND L. G. GARLAND. A possible role for lipoxygenase products as regulators of airway smooth muscle reactivity. *Br. J. Pharmacol.* 69: 167–169, 1980.
2. ALABASTER, V. A. Inactivation of endogenous amines in the lungs. In: *Lung Biology in Health and Disease. Metabolic Functions of the Lung*, edited by Y. S. Bakhle and J. R. Vane. New York: Dekker, 1977, vol. 4, p. 3–31.
3. ALABASTER, V. A. Metabolism of arachidonic acid and its endoperoxide prostaglandin H_2 in isolated lungs from guinea pigs and rabbits (Abstract). *J. Physiol. London* 293: 28P, 1979.
4. ALABASTER, V. A. Metabolism of arachidonic acid and its endoperoxide (PGH_2) to myotropic products in guinea-pig and rabbit isolated lungs. *Br. J. Pharmacol.* 69: 479–489, 1980.
5. ALABASTER, V. A., AND Y. S. BAKHLE. Release of smooth muscle contracting substances from isolated perfused lungs. *Eur. J. Pharmacol.* 35: 349–360, 1976.
6. ALI, A. E., J. C. BARRETT, AND T. E. ELING. Prostaglandin and thromboxane production by fibroblasts and vascular endothelial cells. *Prostaglandins* 20: 667–688, 1980.
7. AL-UBAIDI, F., AND Y. S. BAKHLE. What is the fate of exogenous prostaglandin endoperoxide, PGH_2, in isolated lung (Abstract)? *J. Physiol. London* 293: 20P, 1979.
8. AL-UBAIDI, F., AND Y. S. BAKHLE. The fate of exogenous arachidonic acid in guinea-pig isolated lungs. *J. Physiol London* 295: 445–455, 1979.
9. AL-UBAIDI, F., AND Y. S. BAKHLE. Differences in biological activation of arachidonic acid in perfused lungs from guinea pig, rat and man. *Eur. J. Pharmacol.* 62: 89–96, 1980.
10. AL-UBAIDI, F., AND Y. S. BAKHLE. Metabolism of ^{14}C-arachidonate in rat isolated lung. *Prostaglandins* 19: 747–759, 1980.
11. AL-UBAIDI, F., AND Y. S. BAKHLE. Metabolism of vasoactive hormones in human isolated lung. *Clin. Sci.* 58: 45–51, 1980.
12. ANDERSON, F. L., W. JUBIZ, T. J. TSAGARIS, AND H. KUIDA. Endotoxin-induced prostaglandin E and F release in dogs. *Am. J. Physiol.* 228: 410–414, 1975.
13. ANDERSON, M. W., AND T. E. ELING. Prostaglandin removal and metabolism by isolated perfused rat lung. *Prostaglandins* 11: 645–677, 1976.
14. ÄNGGÅRD, E., C. LARSSON, AND B. SAMUELSSON. The distribution of 15-hydroxy prostaglandin dehydrogenase and prostaglandin-Δ13-reductase in tissues of the swine. *Acta Physiol. Scand.* 81: 396–404, 1971.
15. ÄNGGÅRD, E., AND B. SAMUELSSON. Prostaglandins and related factors. 28. Metabolism of prostaglandin E_1 in guinea pig lung: the structures of two metabolites. *J. Biol. Chem.* 239: 4097–4102, 1964.
16. ÄNGGÅRD, E., AND B. SAMUELSSON. Prostaglandins and related factors. 38. Biosynthesis of prostaglandins from arachidonic acid in guinea pig lung. *J. Biol. Chem.* 240: 3518–3521, 1965.
17. ÄNGGÅRD, E., AND B. SAMUELSSON. Purification and properties of a 15-hydroxyprostaglandin dehydrogenase from swine lung. *Ark. Kemi.* 25: 293–300, 1966.
18. ARMSTRONG, J. M., A. L. A. BOURA, M. HAMBERG, AND B. SAMUELSSON. A comparison of the vasodepressor effects of the cyclic endoperoxides PGG_2 and PGH_2 with those of PGD_2 and PGE_2 in hypertensive and normotensive rats. *Eur. J. Pharmacol.* 39: 251–258, 1976.
19. ARMSTRONG, J. M., N. LATTIMER, S. MONCADA, AND J. R. VANE. Comparison of the vasodepressor effects of prostacyclin and 6-oxo-prostaglandin $F_{1\alpha}$ with those of prostaglandin E_2 in rats and rabbits. *Br. J. Pharmacol.* 62: 125–130, 1978.
20. AUGSTEIN, J., J. B. FARMER, T. B. LEE, P. SHEARD, AND M. L. TATTERSALL. Selective inhibitor of slow reacting substance of anaphylaxis. *Nature London New Biol.* 245: 215–217, 1973.
21. BACH, M. K., AND J. R. BRASHLER. In vivo and in vitro production of a slow reacting substance in the rat upon treatment with calcium ionophores. *J. Immunol.* 113: 2040–2044, 1974.
22. BACH, M. K., J. R. BRASHLER, M. A. JOHNSON, AND J. M. DRAZEN. Two rat mononuclear cell-derived slow reacting substances: kinetic evidence that the peripheral airways-selective spasmogen is derived from a nonselectively acting precursor. *Immunopharmacology* 2: 361–373, 1980.
23. BAKHLE, Y. S. Action of prostaglandin dehydrogenase inhibitors on prostaglandin uptake in rat isolated lung. *Br. J. Phar-*

macol. 65: 635–639, 1979.
24. BAKHLE, Y. S. Biosynthesis of prostaglandins and thromboxanes in lung. *Bull. Eur. Physiopathol. Respir.* 17: 491–508, 1981.
25. BAKHLE, Y. S. Inhibition by clinically used dyes of prostaglandin inactivation in rat and human lung. *Br. J. Pharmacol.* 72: 715–722, 1981.
26. BAKHLE, Y. S., AND A. J. BLOCK. Effects of halothane on pulmonary inactivation of noradrenaline and prostaglandin E_2 in anaesthetized dogs. *Clin. Sci. Mol. Med.* 50: 87–90, 1976.
27. BAKHLE, Y. S., J. HARTIALA, H. TOIVONEN, AND P. UOTILA. Effects of cigarette smoke on the metabolism of vasoactive hormones in rat isolated lungs. *Br. J. Pharmacol.* 65: 495–500, 1979.
28. BAKHLE, Y. S., S. JANCAR, AND B. J. R. WHITTLE. Uptake and inactivation of prostaglandin E_2 methyl analogues in the rat pulmonary circulation. *Br. J. Pharmacol.* 62: 275–280, 1978.
29. BAKHLE, Y. S., AND T. W. SMITH. Release of spasmogens from rat isolated lungs by tryptamines. *Eur. J. Pharmacol.* 46: 31–39, 1977.
30. BAKHLE, Y. S., AND J. T. ZAKRZEWSKI. Effects of the oestrous cycle on the metabolism of arachidonic acid in rat isolated lung. *J. Physiol. London* 326: 411–423, 1982.
31. BAKHLE, Y. S., AND J. T. ZAKRZEWSKI. Inactivation of prostaglandin E_2 by rat isolated lung during the oestrous cycle. *J. Endocrinol.* 98: 47–53, 1983.
32. BEDWANI, J. R., AND P. B. MARLEY. Enhanced inactivation of prostaglandin E_2 by the rabbit during pregnancy or progesterone treatment. *Br. J. Pharmacol.* 53: 547–554, 1979.
33. BEN-HARARI, R. R., AND M. B. H. YOUDIM. Ontogenesis of uptake and deamination of 5-hydroxytryptamine, dopamine and β-phenylethylamine in isolated perfused lung and lung homogenates from rats. *Br. J. Pharmacol.* 72: 731–737, 1981.
34. BENZIE, R., J. R. BOOT, AND W. DAWSON. A preliminary investigation of prostaglandin synthetase activity in normal, sensitized and challenged sensitized guinea-pig lung (Abstract). *J. Physiol. London* 246: 80P–81P, 1975.
35. BERGSTRÖM, S., AND B. SAMUELSSON. The prostaglandins. *Endeavour* 23: 109–113, 1968.
36. BERRY, E. M., J. F. EDMONDS, AND J. H. WYLLIE. Release of prostaglandin E_2 and unidentified factors from ventilated lungs. *Br. J. Surg.* 58: 189–192, 1971.
37. BERTI, F., G. C. FOLCO, A. GIACHETTI, S. MALANDRINO, C. OMINI, AND T. VIGANO. Atropine inhibits thromboxane A_2 generation in isolated lungs of the guinea pig. *Br. J. Pharmacol.* 68: 467–472, 1980.
38. BERTI, F., G. C. FOLCO, S. NICOSIA, C. OMINI, AND R. PASARGIKLIAN. The role of histamine H_1- and H_2-receptors in the generation of thromboxane A_2 in perfused guinea-pig lungs. *Br. J. Pharmacol.* 65: 629–633, 1979.
39. BERTI, F., G. C. FOLCO, AND C. OMINI. Pharmacological control of thromboxane A_2 in lung. *Bull. Eur. Physiopathol. Respir.* 17: 509–552, 1981.
40. BITO, L. Z., R. A. BAROODY, AND M. E. REITZ. Dependence of pulmonary prostaglandin metabolism on carrier-mediated transport processes. *Am. J. Physiol.* 232 (*Endocrinol. Metab. Gastrointest. Physiol.* 1): E382–E387, 1977.
41. BLACKWELL, G. J., R. CARNUCCIO, M. DI ROSA, R. J. FLOWER, L. PARENTE, AND P. PERSICO. Macrocortin: a polypeptide causing the anti-phospholipase effect of glucocorticoids. *Nature London* 287: 147–149, 1980.
42. BLACKWELL, G. J., AND R. J. FLOWER. Effects of steroid hormones on tissue levels of prostaglandin 15-hydroxydehydrogenase in the rat (Abstract). *Br. J. Pharmacol.* 56: 343P–344P, 1976.
43. BLACKWELL, G. J., AND R. J. FLOWER. Glucocorticoids, lungs and prostaglandins. *Bull. Eur. Physiopathol. Respir.* 17: 595–607, 1981.
44. BLACKWELL, G. J., R. J. FLOWER, F. P. NIJKAMP, AND J. R. VANE. Phospholipase A_2 activity of guinea-pig isolated perfused lungs: stimulation, and inhibition by anti-inflammatory steroids. *Br. J. Pharmacol.* 62: 79–89, 1978.
45. BLACKWELL, G. J., R. J. FLOWER, N. RUSSELL-SMITH, J. A. SALMON, P. B. THOROGOOD, AND J. R. VANE. 1-n-Butylimidazole: a potent and selective inhibitor of "thromboxane synthetase" (Abstract). *Br. J. Pharmacol.* 64: 435P, 1978.
45a. BLAIR, I. A., S. E. BARROW, K. A. WADDELL, P. J. LEWIS, AND C. T. DOLLERY. Prostacyclin is not a circulating hormone in man. *Prostaglandins* 23: 579–589, 1982.
46. BØ, G., J. HOGNESTAD, AND J. VAAGE. The role of blood platelets in pulmonary responses to microembolization with barium sulphate. *Acta Physiol. Scand.* 90: 244–251, 1974.
47. BOOT, J. R., A. F. COCKERILL, W. DAWSON, D. N. MALLEN, AND D. J. OSBORNE. Modification of prostaglandin and thromboxane release by immunological sensitization and successive immunological challenges from guinea-pig lungs. *Int. Arch. Allergy Appl. Immunol.* 57: 159–164, 1978.
48. BORGEAT, P., AND B. SAMUELSSON. Arachidonic acid metabolism in polymorphonuclear leukocytes: unstable intermediate in formation of dihydroxy acids. *Proc. Natl. Acad. Sci. USA* 76: 3213–3217, 1979.
49. BOURA, A. L. A., AND R. D. MURPHY. Some factors affecting inactivation of prostaglandin E_2 (PGE_2) by the rat isolated perfused lung (Abstract). *Br. J. Pharmacol.* 62: 411P, 1978.
49a. BRIGHAM, K. L., AND M. L. OGLETREE. Effects of prostaglandins and related compounds on lung vascular permeability. *Bull. Eur. Physiopathol. Respir.* 17: 703–722, 1981.
50. BROCKLEHURST, W. E. The release of histamine and formation of a slow-reacting substance (SRS-A) during anaphylactic shock. *J. Physiol. London* 151: 416–435, 1960.
51. BUNTING, S., S. MONCADA, J. R. VANE, H. F. WOODS, AND M. J. WESTON. Prostacyclin improves hemocompatibility during charcoal hemoperfusion. In: *Prostacyclin*, edited by S. Bergström and J. R. Vane. New York: Raven, 1979, p. 361–369.
52. BURKA, J. F., AND R. J. FLOWER. Effects of modulators of arachidonic acid metabolism on the synthesis and release of slow-reacting substance of anaphylaxis. *Br. J. Pharmacol.* 65: 35–41, 1979.
53. CEDRO, A., AND K. HERBACZYŃSKA-CEDRO. Increased blood level of prostaglandin-like substances during cardiopulmonary bypass in the dog. *Cardiovasc. Res.* 12: 516–522, 1978.
54. CHAUDHARI, A., K. SIVARAJAH, R. WARWICK, T. E. ELING, AND M. W. ANDERSON. Inhibition of pulmonary prostaglandin metabolism by exposure of animals to oxygen or nitrogen dioxide. *Biochem. J.* 184: 51–57, 1979.
55. CHIGNARD, M., A. PRANCAN, J. LEFORT, F. DRAY, AND B. B. VARGAFTIG. Arachidonate-mediated bronchoconstriction and platelet activation are inhibited by microgram doses of compound L8027 which are not selective for thromboxane synthetase. *Agents Actions* 4, Suppl.: 184–187, 1979.
56. CHIGNARD, M., AND B. B. VARGAFTIG. Dog platelets fail to aggregate when they form aggregating substances upon stimulation with arachidonic acid. *Eur. J. Pharmacol.* 38: 7–18, 1976.
57. CLEGG, P. C., W. J. HALL, AND V. R. PICKLES. The action of ketonic prostaglandins on the guinea-pig myometrium. *J. Physiol. London* 183: 123–144, 1966.
58. COCKERILL, A. F., D. N. B. MALLEN, D. J. OSBORNE, J. R. BOOT, AND W. DAWSON. The identification of two novel prostaglandins and a thromboxane. *Prostaglandins* 13: 1033–1042, 1977.
59. COHEN, G. M., P. UOTILA, J. HARTIALA, E. M. SUOLINNA, N. SIMBERG, AND O. PELKONEN. Metabolism and covalent binding of [³H]benzo(a)pyrene by isolated perfused lungs and short-term tracheal organ culture of cigarette smoke-exposed rats. *Cancer Res.* 37: 2147–2155, 1977.
60. COLLIER, H. O. J. New light on how aspirin works. *Nature London* 223: 35–37, 1969.
61. COLLIER, H. O. J., AND P. J. GARDINER. Prostaglandin receptors in the airways. In: *Metabolic Activities of the Lung*, edited by R. Porter and J. Whelan. Amsterdam: Excerpta Med., 1980,

p. 333–350. (Ciba Found. Symp. 78.)
62. COLLIER, H. O. J., AND G. W. L. JAMES. Humoral factors affecting pulmonary inflation during acute anaphylaxis in the guinea-pig in vivo. *Br. J. Pharmacol.* 30: 283–301, 1967.
63. COLLIER, H. O. J., AND W. J. F. SWEATMAN. Antagonism by fenamates of prostaglandin F$_{2\alpha}$ and of slow reacting substance on human bronchial muscle. *Nature London* 219: 864–865, 1968.
64. CRUTCHLEY, D. J., J. A. BOYD, AND T. E. ELING. Enhanced thromboxane B$_2$ release from challenged guinea pig lung after oxygen exposure. *Am. Rev. Respir. Dis.* 121: 695–699, 1980.
65. CRUTCHLEY, D. J., AND P. J. PIPER. Inhibition of the pulmonary inactivation of prostaglandins in vivo by di-4-phloretin phosphate. *Br. J. Pharmacol.* 54: 301–307, 1975.
66. CUTHBERT, M. F. Prostaglandins and asthma. *Br. J. Clin. Pharmacol.* 2: 293–295, 1975.
67. DAHLÉN, S. E., P. HEDQVIST, S. HAMMARSTRÖM, AND B. SAMUELSSON. Leukotrienes are potent constrictors of human bronchi. *Nature London* 288: 484–486, 1980.
68. D'ANGELO, V., S. VILLA, M. MYSLIWIEC, M. B. DONATI, AND G. DE GAETANO. Defective fibrinolytic and prostacyclin-like activity in human atheromatous plaques. *Thromb. Diath. Haemorrh.* 39: 535–536, 1978.
69. DANON, A., AND G. ASSOULINE. Inhibition of prostaglandin biosynthesis by corticosteroids requires RNA and protein synthesis. *Nature London* 273: 552–554, 1978.
70. DAWSON, C. A., B. O. COZZINI, AND A. J. LONIGRO. Metabolism of [2-^{14}C]prostaglandin E$_1$ on passage through the pulmonary circulation. *Can. J. Physiol. Pharmacol.* 53: 610–615, 1975.
71. DAWSON, W., J. R. BOOT, A. F. COCKERILL, D. N. B. MALLEN, AND D. J. OSBORNE. Release of novel prostaglandins and thromboxanes after immunological challenge of guinea pig lung. *Nature London* 262: 699–702, 1976.
72. DAWSON, W., J. R. BOOT, E. A. KITCHEN, AND J. R. WALKER. Inhibition of lipoxygenase related effector systems. In: *SRS-A and Leukotrienes*, edited by P. J. Piper. New York: Wiley, 1981, p. 219–226.
73. DI ROSA, M., AND P. PERSICO. Latency and reversion of hydrocortisone inhibition of prostaglandin biosynthesis in rat leucocytes. In: *Arachidonic Acid Metabolism: Proc. Eur. Workshop on Inflammation, 1st, Basel*, edited by K. Brune and M. Baggiolini. Basel: Springer-Verlag, 1979, p. 63–68.
74. DRAZEN, J. M., R. A. LEWIS, S. I. WASSERMAN, R. P. ORANGE, AND K. F. AUSTEN. Differential effects of a partially purified preparation of slow-reacting substance of anaphylaxis on guinea pig tracheal spirals and parenchymal strips. *J. Clin. Invest.* 63: 1–5, 1979.
75. DUCHARME, D. W., J. R. WEEKS, AND R. G. MONTGOMERY. Studies on the mechanism of the hypertensive effect of prostaglandin F$_{2\alpha}$. *J. Pharmacol. Exp. Ther.* 160: 1–10, 1968.
76. DUSTING, G. J., S. MONCADA, AND J. R. VANE. Recirculation of prostacyclin PGI$_2$ in the dog. *Br. J. Pharmacol.* 64: 315–320, 1978.
76a. EDLUND, A., W. BONFIM, L. KAIJSER, C. OLIN, C. PATRONO, E. PINCA, AND W. WENNMALM. Pulmonary formation of prostacyclin in man. *Prostaglandins* 22: 323–332, 1981.
77. EGERTON-VERNON, J. M., AND J. R. BEDWANI. Prostaglandin 15-hydroxydehydrogenase activity during pregnancy in rabbits and rats. *Eur. J. Pharmacol.* 33: 405–408, 1975.
78. ELING, T. E., H. J. HAWKINS, AND M. W. ANDERSON. Structural requirements for, and the effects of chemicals on, the rat pulmonary inactivation of prostaglandins. *Prostaglandins* 14: 51–60, 1977.
79. ENGINEER, D. M., U. NIEDERHAUSER, P. J. PIPER, AND P. SIROIS. Release of mediators of anaphylaxis: inhibition of prostaglandin synthesis and the modification of the release of slow-reacting substance of anaphylaxis and histamine. *Br. J. Pharmacol.* 62: 61–66, 1978.
81. FELDBERG, W., AND C. H. KELLAWAY. Liberation of histamine and formation of lysolecithin-like substances by cobra venom. *J. Physiol. London* 94: 187–226, 1938.
82. FERREIRA, S. H. Prostaglandins. In: *Chemical Messengers of the Inflammatory Process*, edited by J. C. Houck. Amsterdam: North-Holland, 1979, p. 113–151.
83. FERREIRA, S. H., AND Y. S. BAKHLE. Inactivation of bradykinin and related peptides in the lungs. In: *Lung Biology in Health and Disease. Metabolic Functions of the Lung*, edited by Y. S. Bakhle and J. R. Vane. New York: Dekker, 1977, vol. 4, p. 35–53.
84. FERREIRA, S. H., L. J. GREENE, M. C. O. SALGADO, AND E. M. KRIEGER. The fate of circulating biologically active peptides in the lungs. In: *Metabolic Activities of the Lungs*, edited by R. Porter and J. Whelan. Amsterdam: Excerpta Med., 1980, p. 129–140. (Ciba Found. Symp. 78.)
85. FERREIRA, S. H., S. MONCADA, AND J. R. VANE. Indomethacin and aspirin abolish prostaglandin release from the spleen. *Nature London New Biol.* 231: 237–239, 1971.
86. FERREIRA, S. H., AND J. R. VANE. Prostaglandins: their disappearance from and release into the circulation. *Nature London* 216: 868–873, 1967.
87. FERREIRA, S. H., AND J. R. VANE. Mode of action of anti-inflammatory agents which are prostaglandin synthetase inhibitors. In: *Handbook of Experimental Pharmacology. Anti-Inflammatory Drugs*, edited by J. R. Vane and S. H. Ferreira. Berlin: Springer-Verlag, 1979, vol. 50, pt. 2, p. 348–398.
88. FISHBURNE, J. T., W. F. BRENNER, J. T. BRAKSMA, AND C. H. HENDRICKS. Bronchospasm complicating intravenous prostaglandin F$_{2\alpha}$ for therapeutic abortion. *Obstet. Gynecol.* 39: 892–898, 1972.
89. FISHMAN, A. P. Hypoxia on the pulmonary circulation. *Circ. Res.* 38: 221–231, 1976.
90. FLETCHER, J. R., AND P. W. RAMWELL. Altered lung metabolism of prostaglandins during hemorrhagic and endotoxin shock. *Surg. Forum* 28: 184–186, 1977.
91. FLETCHER, J. R., AND P. W. RAMWELL. Modification by aspirin and indomethacin of the haemodynamic and prostaglandin releasing effects of E. coli endotoxin in the dog. *Br. J. Pharmacol.* 61: 175–181, 1977.
92. FLETCHER, J. R., AND P. W. RAMWELL. Modulation of prostaglandins E and F by the lung in baboon hemorrhagic shock. *J. Surg. Res.* 26: 465–472, 1979.
93. FLOMAN, Y., N. FLOMAN, AND U. ZOR. Inhibition of prostaglandin E release by anti-inflammatory steroids. *Prostaglandins* 11: 591–594, 1976.
94. FLOWER, R. J. Drugs which inhibit prostaglandin biosynthesis. *Pharmacol. Rev.* 26: 33–67, 1974.
95. FLOWER, R. J. Prostaglandins and related compounds. In: *Handbook of Experimental Pharmacology. Anti-Inflammatory Drugs*, edited by J. R. Vane and S. H. Ferreira. Berlin: Springer-Verlag, 1979, vol. 50, pt. 2, p. 373–415.
96. FLOWER, R. J. Steroidal anti-inflammatory drugs as inhibitors of phospholipase A$_2$. *Adv. Prostaglandin Thromboxane Res.* 3: 105–112, 1978.
97. FLOWER, R. J., AND J. R. VANE. Inhibition of prostaglandin synthetase in brain explains the anti-pyretic activity of paracetamol (4-acetamidophenol). *Nature London* 240: 410–411, 1972.
98. FORD-HUTCHINSON, A. W., M. A. BRAY, F. M. CUNNINGHAM, E. M. DAVIDSON, AND M. J. H. SMITH. Isomers of leukotriene B$_4$ possess different biological potencies. *Prostaglandins* 21: 143–152, 1981.
99. FORD-HUTCHINSON, A. W., M. A. BRAY, M. V. DOIG, M. E. SHIPLEY, AND M. J. H. SMITH. Leukotriene B, a potent chemokinetic and aggregating substance released from polymorphonuclear leukocytes. *Nature London* 286: 264–265, 1980.
100. FOUNTAIN, S. W., B. A. MARTIN, C. E. MUSCLOW, AND J. D. COOPER. Pulmonary leukostasis and its relationship to pulmonary dysfunction in sheep and rabbits. *Circ. Res.* 46: 175–180, 1980.
101. FREY, H.-H., AND C. DENGJEL. Antagonism of arachidonic acid-induced bronchoconstriction in cats by aspirin-like anal-

gesics. *Eur. J. Pharmacol.* 40: 345–348, 1976.
102. FRIEDMAN, L. S., T. M. FITZPATRICK, P. W. RAMWELL, AND P. A. KOT. Thromboxane B$_2$ inhibits the pulmonary metabolism of PGE$_2$ in the anesthetized dog. *Adv. Prostaglandin Thromboxane Res.* 7: 981–983, 1980.
103. GARDINER, P. J., AND H. O. J. COLLIER. Specific receptors for prostaglandins in airways. *Prostaglandins* 19: 819–841, 1980.
104. GARDINER, P. J., J. L. COPAS, C. SCHNEIDER, AND H. O. J. COLLIER. 2-Decarboxy-2-hydroxymethyl prostaglandin E$_1$ (TR4161), a prostaglandin bronchodilator of low tracheobronchial irritancy. *Prostaglandins* 19: 349–370, 1980.
105. GILMORE, N., J. R. VANE, AND J. H. WYLLIE. Prostaglandins released by the spleen. *Nature London* 218: 1135–1140, 1968.
106. GILMORE, N., J. R. VANE, AND J. H. WYLLIE. Prostaglandin release by the spleen in response to an infusion of particles. In: *Prostaglandins, Peptides and Amines*, edited by P. Mantegazza and E. W. Horton. London: Academic, 1969, p. 21–29.
107. GOLDBLATT, M. W. Properties of human seminal fluid. *J. Physiol London* 84: 208–218, 1935.
108. GORMAN, R. R., G. L. BUNDY, D. C. PETERSON, F. F. SUN, O. V. MILLER, AND F. A. FITZPATRICK. Inhibition of human platelet thromboxane synthetase by 9,11-azoprosta-5,13-dienoic acid. *Proc. Natl. Acad. Sci. USA* 74: 4007–4011, 1977.
109. GREENWAY, C. V., AND V. S. MURTHY. Mesenteric vasoconstriction after endotoxin administration in cats pretreated with aspirin. *Br. J. Pharmacol.* 43: 259–269, 1971.
110. GREIG, M. E., AND R. L. GRIFFIN. Antagonism of slow reacting substance in anaphylaxis (SRS-A) and other spasmogens on the guinea pig tracheal chain by hydrotropic acids and their effects on anaphylaxis. *J. Med. Chem.* 18: 112–116, 1975.
111. GRIFFITH, O. W., AND A. MEISTER. Translocation of intracellular glutathione to membrane-bound γ-glutamyl transpeptidase as a discrete step in the γ-glutamyl cycle: glutathionuria after inhibition of transpeptidase. *Proc. Natl. Acad. Sci. USA* 76: 268–272, 1979.
112. GRYGLEWSKI, R. J. Prostacyclin as a circulating hormone. *Biochem. Pharmacol.* 28: 2161–2166, 1979.
113. GRYGLEWSKI, R. J., A. DEMBINSKA-KIEC, L. GRODZINSKA, AND B. PANCZENKO. Differential generation of substances with prostaglandin-like and thromboxane-like activities by guinea pig trachea and lung strips. In: *Lung Cells in Disease*, edited by A. Bouhuys. Amsterdam: North-Holland, 1976, p. 289–307.
114. GRYGLEWSKI, R. J., R. KORBUT, AND A. C. OCETKIEWICZ. Generation of prostacyclin by lungs in vivo and its release into the arterial circulation. *Nature London* 273: 765–767, 1978.
115. GRYGLEWSKI, R. J., B. PANCZENKO, R. KORBUT, L. GRODZINSKA, AND A. OCETKIEWICZ. Corticosteroids inhibit prostaglandin release from perfused mesenteric blood vessels of rabbit and from perfused lungs of sensitized guinea pig. *Prostaglandins* 10: 343–355, 1975.
116. GRYGLEWSKI, R. J., AND J. R. VANE. The release of prostaglandins and rabbit aorta contracting substance (RCS) from rabbit spleen and its antagonism by anti-inflammatory drugs. *Br. J. Pharmacol.* 45: 37–47, 1972.
117. HAGEDORN, B., AND H. B. KOSTENBAUDER. Studies on the effect of tobacco smoke on the biotransformation of vasoactive substances in the isolated perfused rabbit lung. I. Prostaglandin F$_{2\alpha}$. *Res. Commun. Chem. Pathol. Pharmacol.* 18: 495–506, 1977.
118. HAMBERG, M., P. HEDQVIST, K. STRANDBERG, J. SVENSSON, AND B. SAMUELSSON. Prostaglandin endoperoxides. IV. Effects on smooth muscle. *Life Sci.* 16: 451–462, 1975.
119. HAMBERG, M., AND B. SAMUELSSON. Detection and isolation of an endoperoxide intermediate in prostaglandin biosynthesis. *Proc. Natl. Acad. Sci. USA* 70: 899–903, 1973.
120. HAMBERG, M., AND B. SAMUELSSON. Prostaglandin endoperoxides. Novel transformations of arachidonic acid in human platelets. *Proc. Natl. Acad. Sci. USA* 71: 3400–3404, 1974.
121. HAMBERG, M., J. SVENSSON, P. HEDQVIST, K. STRANDBERG, AND B. SAMUELSSON. Involvement of endoperoxides and thromboxanes in anaphylactic reactions. *Adv. Prostaglandin Thromboxane Res.* 1: 495–501, 1976.
122. HAMBERG, M., J. SVENSSON, AND B. SAMUELSSON. Thromboxanes, a new group of biologically active compounds derived from prostaglandin endoperoxides. *Proc. Natl. Acad. Sci. USA* 71: 345–349, 1975.
123. HAMMERSCHMIDT, D. E., L. J. WEAVER, L. D. HUDSON, P. R. CRADDOCK, AND H. S. JACOB. Association of complement activation and elevated plasma C5a with adult respiratory distress syndrome. *Lancet* 1: 947–949, 1980.
124. HAMMOND, G. L., L. CRONAU, D. WHITTAKER, AND C. N. GILLIS. Fate of prostaglandins E$_1$ and A$_1$ in the human pulmonary circulation. *Surgery* 81: 716–722, 1977.
125. HANSEN, H. S. 15-Hydroxyprostaglandin dehydrogenase. A review. *Prostaglandins* 12: 647–679, 1976.
126. HANSEN, H. S. Purification and characterization of a 15-ketoprostaglandin Δ13-reductase from bovine lung. *Biochim. Biophys. Acta* 574: 136–145, 1979.
127. HARTIALA, J., P. UOTILA, AND T. W. NIENSTEDT. The effects of cigarette smoke exposure on testosterone metabolism in the isolated perfused rat lung. *J. Steroid Biochem.* 9: 365–368, 1978.
128. HASLAM, R. J., AND M. D. MCCLENAGHAN. Measurement of circulating prostacyclin. *Nature London* 292: 364–366, 1981.
129. HAUGE, A., P. K. M. LUNDE, AND B. A. WAALER. Effects of prostaglandin E$_1$ and adrenaline on the pulmonary vascular resistance (PVR) in isolated rabbit lungs. *Life Sci.* 6: 673–680, 1967.
130. HAWKINS, H. J., J. B. SMITH, K. C. NICOLAOU, AND T. E. ELING. Studies of the mechanism involved in the fate of prostacyclin (PGI$_2$) and 6-keto-PGF$_{1\alpha}$ in the pulmonary circulation. *Prostaglandins* 16: 871–884, 1978.
131. HEDQVIST, P., S. E. DAHLEN, L. GUSTAFSSON, S. HAMMARSTRÖM, AND B. SAMUELSSON. Biological profile of leukotrienes C$_4$ and D$_4$. *Acta Physiol. Scand.* 110: 331–333, 1980.
132. HEDQVIST, P., A. HOLMGREN, AND A. A. MATHÉ. Effect of prostaglandin F$_{2\alpha}$ on airway resistance in man (Abstract). *Acta Physiol. Scand.* 82: 29A, 1971.
133. HEMKER, D. P., R. J. SHEBUSKI, AND J. W. AIKEN. Release of a prostacyclin-like substance into the circulation of dogs by intravenous adenosine diphosphate. *J. Pharmacol. Exp. Ther.* 212: 246–252, 1980.
134. HEMLER, M. E., AND W. E. M. LANDS. Evidence for a peroxide-initiated free radical mechanism of prostaglandin biosynthesis. *J. Biol. Chem.* 255: 6253–6261, 1980.
135. HENSBY, C. N., P. J. BARNES, C. T. DOLLERY, AND H. DARGIE. Production of 6-oxo-PGF$_{1\alpha}$ by human lung in vivo. *Lancet* 2: 1162–1163, 1979.
136. HIGGS, G. A., AND R. J. FLOWER. Anti-inflammatory drugs and the inhibition of arachidonate lipoxygenase. In: *SRS-A and Leukotrienes*, edited by P. J. Piper. New York: Wiley, 1981, p. 197–207.
137. HITCHCOCK, M. Effect of inhibitors of prostaglandin synthesis and prostaglandins E$_2$ and F$_{2\alpha}$ on the immunologic release of mediators of inflammation from actively sensitized guinea-pig lung. *J. Pharmacol. Exp. Ther.* 207: 630–640, 1978.
138. HORTON, E. W., AND R. L. JONES. Prostaglandins A$_1$, A$_2$ and 19-hydroxy A$_1$; their actions on smooth muscle and their inactivation on passage through the pulmonary and hepatic portal vascular beds. *Br. J. Pharmacol.* 37: 705–722, 1969.
139. HORTON, E. W., AND R. L. JONES. Biological activity of prostaglandin D$_2$ on smooth muscle (Abstract). *Br. J. Pharmacol.* 52: 110P–111P, 1974.
140. HOULT, J. R. S., AND P. K. MOORE. Effects of sulphasalazine and its metabolites on prostaglandin synthesis, inactivation and actions on smooth muscle. *Br. J. Pharmacol.* 68: 719–730, 1980.
141. HYMAN, A. L. The active responses of pulmonary veins in intact dogs to prostaglandins F$_{2\alpha}$ and E$_1$. *J. Pharmacol. Exp. Ther.* 165: 267–273, 1969.
142. HYMAN, A. L., A. A. MATHÉ, C. A. LESLIE, C. C. MATTHEWS,

J. T. Bennett, E. W. Spannhake, and P. J. Kadowitz. Modification of pulmonary vascular responses to arachidonic acid by alterations in physiologic state. *J. Pharmacol. Exp. Ther.* 207: 388–401, 1978.
143. Hyman, A. L., E. W. Spannhake, and P. J. Kadowitz. Prostaglandins and the lung. *Am. Rev. Respir. Dis.* 117: 111–136, 1978.
144. Johnson, R. A., D. R. Morton, J. H. Vinner, R. R. Gorman, J. C. McGuire, F. F. Sun, N. Whittaker, S. Bunting, J. A. Salmon, S. Moncada, and J. R. Vane. The chemical structure of prostaglandin X (prostacyclin). *Prostaglandins* 12: 915–928, 1976.
145. Jose, P. J., U. Niederhauser, P. J. Piper, C. Robinson, and A. P. Smith. Degradation of prostaglandin $F_{2\alpha}$ in the human pulmonary circulation. *Thorax* 31: 713–719, 1976.
146. Jose, P. J., and J. P. Seale. Incorporation and metabolism of [^{14}C]-arachidonic acid in guinea-pig lungs. *Br. J. Pharmacol.* 67: 519–526, 1979.
147. Junod, A. F., and C. Ody. Amine uptake and metabolism by endothelium of pig pulmonary artery and aorta. *Am. J. Physiol.* 232 (*Cell Physiol.* 1): C88–C94, 1977.
148. Kadowitz, P. J., B. M. Chapnick, L. P. Feigen, A. L. Hyman, P. K. Nelson, and E. W. Spannhake. Pulmonary and systemic vasodilator effects of the newly discovered prostaglandin, PGI_2. *J. Appl. Physiol.: Respirat. Environ. Exercise Physiol.* 45: 408–413, 1978.
149. Kadowitz, P. J., C. A. Gruetter, D. B. McNamara, R. R. Gorman, E. W. Spannhake, and A. L. Hyman. Comparative effects of endoperoxide PGH_2 and an analog on the pulmonary vascular bed. *J. Appl. Physiol.: Respirat. Environ. Exercise Physiol.* 42: 953–958, 1977.
150. Kadowitz, P. J., and A. L. Hyman. Influence of a prostaglandin endoperoxide analogue on the canine pulmonary vascular bed. *Circ. Res.* 40: 282–287, 1977.
151. Kadowitz, P. J., D. B. McNamara, H. S. She, E. W. Spannhake, and A. L. Hyman. Arachidonic acid responses in the lung. *Bull. Eur. Physiopathol. Respir.* 17: 659–674, 1981.
152. Karim, S. M. M., P. G. Adaikan, and S. R. Kottegoda. Prostaglandins and human respiratory tract smooth muscle: structure activity relationship. *Adv. Prostaglandin Thromboxane Res.* 7: 969–980, 1980.
153. Kellaway, C. H., and E. R. Trethewie. The liberation of a slow reacting smooth muscle-stimulating substance in anaphylaxis. *Q. J. Exp. Physiol.* 30: 121–145, 1940.
154. Kistler, G. S., P. R. B. Caldwell, and E. R. Weibel. Development of fine structural damage to alveolar and capillary lining cells in oxygen-poisoned rat lungs. *J. Cell Biol.* 32: 605–628, 1967.
155. Klein, L. S., A. B. Fisher, S. Soltoff, and R. F. Colburn. Effect of oxygen exposure on pulmonary metabolism of prostaglandin E_2. *Am. Rev. Respir. Dis.* 118: 622–625, 1978.
156. Kokobu, T., E. Ueda, K. Nishimura, and N. Yoshida. Angiotensin I converting enzyme activity in pulmonary tissue of fetal and newborn rabbits. *Experientia* 33: 1137–1138, 1977.
157. Ku, E. C., and J. M. Wasvary. Inhibition of prostaglandin synthetase by Su-21524 (Abstract). *Federation Proc.* 32: 3302, 1973.
158. Kuehl, F. A., Jr., J. L. Humes, E. A. Ham, R. W. Egan, and H. W. Dougherty. Inflammation: the role of peroxidase-derived products. *Adv. Prostaglandin Thromboxane Res.* 6: 77–86, 1980.
159. Lambley, J. E., and A. P. Smith. The effects of arachidonic acid, indomethacin and SC-19220 on guinea-pig tracheal muscle tone. *Eur. J. Pharmacol.* 30: 148–153, 1975.
160. Lands, W. E. M., P. R. Letellier, L. H. Rome, and J. Y. Vanderhoek. Modes of inhibiting the prostaglandin biosynthesis. In: *Advances in the Biosciences*, edited by S. Bergström and S. Bernhard. New York: Pergamon, 1973, vol. 9, p. 15–28.
161. Large, B. J., P. F. Leswell, and P. R. Maxwell. Bronchodilator activity of prostaglandin E_1 in experimental animals. *Nature London* 224: 78–80, 1969.

162. Larsson, C., and E. Änggård. Distribution of prostaglandin metabolizing enzymes in tissues of the swine. *Acta Pharmacol. Toxicol. Suppl.* 28: 61, 1970.
163. Lauersen, N. H., and K. H. Wilson. The role of a long-acting vaginal suppository of 15-ME-$PGB_{2\alpha}$ in first and second trimester abortion. *Adv. Prostaglandin Thromboxane Res.* 8: 1435–1441, 1980.
164. Leary, W. P., A. C. Asmal, and J. Botha. Pulmonary inactivation of prostaglandins by hypertensive rats. *Prostaglandins* 13: 697–700, 1977.
165. Lee, S. C., and L. Levine. Purification and properties of chicken heart prostaglandin Δ^{13}-reductase. *Biochem. Biophys. Res. Commun.* 61: 14–21, 1974.
166. Leffler, C.W., and J. R. Hessler. Pulmonary and systemic vascular effect of exogenous prostaglandin I_2 in fetal lambs. *Eur. J. Pharmacol.* 54: 37–42, 1979.
167. Leffler, C. W., T. L. Tyler, and S. Cassin. Effect of indomethacin on pulmonary vascular response to ventilation of fetal goats. *Am. J. Physiol.* 234 (*Heart Circ. Physiol.* 3): H346–H351, 1978.
168. Lefort, J., and B. B. Vargaftig. Role of platelets in aspirin-sensitive bronchoconstriction in the guinea-pig; interactions with salicylic acid. *Br. J. Pharmacol.* 63: 35–42, 1978.
169. Leslie, C. A., and L. Levine. Evidence for the presence of a prostaglandin E_2-9-keto reductase in rat organs. *Biochem. Biophys. Res. Commun.* 52: 717–724, 1973.
169a. Lewis, P., and H. M. Tyler (editors). Clinical prospects for a thromboxane synthetase inhibitor. *Br. J. Clin. Pharmacol.* 15, Suppl. 1: 5S–139S, 1983.
170. Lewis, R. A., K. F. Austen, J. M. Drazen, D. A. Clark, A. Marfat, and E. J. Corey. Slow reacting substances of anaphylaxis: identification of leukotrienes C-1 and D from human and rat sources. *Proc. Natl. Acad. Sci. USA* 77: 3710–3714, 1980.
171. Lewis, R. A., J. M. Drazen, K. F. Austen, D. A. Clark, and E. J. Corey. Identification of the C(6)-S conjugate to leukotriene A with cysteine as a naturally occurring slow reacting substance of anaphylaxis (SRS-A). Importance of the 11-*cis*-geometry for biological activity. *Biochem. Biophys. Res. Commun.* 96: 271–277, 1980.
172. Liebig, R., W. Bernauer, and B. A. Peskar. Release of prostaglandins, a prostaglandin metabolite, slow reacting substance and histamine from anaphylactic lungs and its modification by catecholamines. *Naunyn-Schmiedebergs Arch. Pharmakol.* 284: 279–293, 1974.
173. Lindsey, H. E., and J. H. Wyllie. Release of prostaglandins from embolized lungs. *Br. J. Surg.* 57: 738–741, 1970.
174. Longmore, D. B., G. Bennett, D. Gueirrara, M. Smith, S. Bunting, S. Moncada, P. Reed, N. G. Read, and J. R. Vane. Prostacyclin: a solution to some problems of extracorporeal circulation. Experiments in greyhounds. *Lancet* 1: 1002–1005, 1979.
175. Lulich, K. M., H. W. Mitchell, and M. P. Sparrow. The cat lung strip as an in vitro preparation of peripheral airways: a comparison of β-adrenoceptor agonists, autacoids and anaphylactic challenge on the lung strip and trachea. *Br. J. Pharmacol.* 58: 71–79, 1976.
176. Magerlein, B. J., D. W. Ducharme, W. E. Magee, W. L. Miller, A. Robert, and J. R. Weeks. Synthesis and biological properties of 16-alkylprostaglandins. *Prostaglandins* 4: 143–145, 1973.
177. Maggi, F. M., N. Tyrrell, Y. Maddox, W. Watkins, E. R. Ramey, and P. W. Ramwell. Prostaglandin synthetase activity in vascular tissue of male and female rats. *Prostaglandins* 19: 985–993, 1980.
178. Main, I. H. M. The inhibitory actions of prostaglandins on respiratory smooth muscle. *Br. J. Pharmacol.* 22: 511–519, 1964.
179. Männistö, J., and P. Uotila. Cigarette smoke ventilation decreases prostaglandin inactivation in rat and hamster lungs. *Prostaglandins* 23: 833–839, 1982.

180. MARRAZZI, M. A., J. E. SHAW, F. T. TAO, AND F. M. MATCHINSKY. Reversibility of 15-hydroxyprostaglandin dehydrogenase from swine lung. *Prostaglandins* 1: 389–395, 1972.
181. MASSION, W. H., B. ROSENBLUTH, AND M. KUX. Protective effect of methyl prednisolone against lung complications in endotoxin shock. *South. Med. J.* 65: 941–944, 1972.
182. MATHÉ, A. A., P. HEDQVIST, A. HOLMGREN, AND N. SVANBORG. Bronchial hyperreactivity to prostaglandin $F_{2\alpha}$ and histamine in patients with asthma. *Br. Med. J.* 1: 193–196, 1973.
183. MATHÉ, A. A., AND L. LEVINE. Release of prostaglandins and metabolites from guinea-pig lung: inhibition by catecholamines. *Prostaglandins* 4: 877–890, 1973.
184. MCGIFF, J. C., N. A. TERRAGNO, J. C. STRAND, J. B. LEE, AND A. J. LONIGRO. Selective passage of prostaglandins across the lung. *Nature London* 223: 742–745, 1969.
185. MCGUIRE, J. C., AND F. F. SUN. Metabolism of prostacyclin. Oxidation by rhesus monkey lung 15-hydroxyl prostaglandin dehydrogenase. *Arch. Biochem. Biophys.* 189: 92–96, 1978.
186. MITCHELL, H. W., AND M. A. DENBOROUGH. Anaphylaxis in guinea-pig peripheral airways in vitro. *Eur. J. Pharmacol.* 54: 69–78, 1979.
187. MONCADA, S., S. BUNTING, K. M. MULLANE, P. THOROGOOD, J. R. VANE, A. RAZ, AND P. NEEDLEMAN. A selective potent antagonist of thromboxane synthetase. *Prostaglandins* 13: 611–618, 1977.
188. MONCADA, S., R. J. GRYGLEWSKI, S. BUNTING, AND J. R. VANE. An enzyme isolated from arteries transforms prostaglandin endoperoxides to an unstable substance that inhibits platelet aggregation. *Nature London* 263: 663–665, 1976.
189. MONCADA, S., R. J. GRYGLEWSKI, S. BUNTING, AND J. R. VANE. A lipid peroxide inhibits the enzyme in blood vessel microsomes that generates from prostaglandin endoperoxides the substance (prostaglandin X) which prevents platelet aggregation. *Prostaglandins* 12: 715–737, 1976.
190. MONCADA, S., A. G. HERMAN, E. A. HIGGS, AND J. R. VANE. Differential formation of prostacyclin (PGX or PGI_2) by layers of the arterial wall. An explanation for the anti-thrombotic properties of vascular endothelium. *Thromb. Res.* 11: 323–344, 1977.
191. MONCADA, S., R. KORBUT, S. BUNTING, AND J. R. VANE. Prostacyclin is a circulating hormone. *Nature London* 273: 767–768, 1978.
192. MONCADA, S., P. NEEDLEMAN, S. BUNTING, AND J. R. VANE. Prostaglandin endoperoxide and thromboxane generating systems and their selective inhibition. *Prostaglandins* 12: 323–325, 1976.
193. MONCADA, S., AND J. R. VANE. Pharmacology and endogenous roles of prostaglandin endoperoxides, thromboxane A_2 and prostacyclin. *Pharmacol. Rev.* 30: 293–331, 1979.
194. MORRIS, H. R., P. J. PIPER, G. W. TAYLOR, AND J. R. TIPPINS. The role of arachidonate lipoxygenase in the release of SRS-A from guinea-pig chopped lung. *Prostaglandins* 19: 371–383, 1980.
195. MORRIS, H. R., G. W. TAYLOR, P. J. PIPER, M. N. SAMHOUN, AND J. R. TIPPINS. Slow reacting substances (SRSs): the structure identification of SRSs from rat basophil leukaemia (RBL-1) cells. *Prostaglandins* 19: 185–201, 1980.
196. MORRIS, H. R., G. W. TAYLOR, P. J. PIPER, AND J. R. TIPPINS. Structure of slow reacting substance of anaphylaxis from guinea-pig lung. *Nature London* 285: 104–106, 1980.
197. MORSE, H. C., III, K. J. BLOCH, AND K. F. AUSTEN. Biologic properties of rat antibodies. II. Time-course of appearance of antibodies involved in antigen-induced release of slow reacting substance of anaphylaxis (SRS-A rat); association of the activity with rat IgGa. *J. Immunol.* 101: 658–663, 1968.
198. MULLANE, K. M., G. J. DUSTING, J. A. SALMON, S. MONCADA, AND J. R. VANE. Biotransformation and cardiovascular effects of arachidonic acid in the dog. *Eur. J. Pharmacol.* 54: 217–228, 1979.
199. MURAO, M., K. UCHIYAMA, A. SHIDA, K. SAKAI, T. YUSA, AND T. YAMOGUCHI. Studies on 20-isopropylidene PGE_2 as a new aerosol bronchodilator. *Adv. Prostaglandin Thromboxane Res.* 7: 985–988, 1980.
200. MURPHY, R. C., S. HAMMARSTRÖM, AND B. SAMUELSSON. Leukotriene C: a slow reacting substance from murine mastocytoma cells. *Proc. Natl. Acad. Sci. USA* 76: 4275–4279, 1979.
201. NAKANO, J., AND R. B. MCCLOY, JR. Effects of indomethacin on the pulmonary vascular and airway resistance responses to pulmonary microembolization. *Proc. Soc. Exp. Biol. Med.* 143: 218–221, 1973.
202. NAKANO, J., AND N. Y. MORSY. Beta oxidation of prostaglandins E_1 and E_2 in rat lung and kidney homogenates (Abstract). *Clin. Res.* 19: 142, 1971.
203. NAKANO, J., AND A. V. PRANCAN. Metabolic degradation of prostaglandin E_1 in lung and kidney of rats in endotoxin shock. *Proc. Soc. Exp. Biol. Med.* 144: 506–508, 1973.
204. NEEDLEMAN, P. Experimental criteria for evaluating prostaglandin biosynthesis and intrinsic function. *Biochem. Pharmacol.* 27: 1515–1518, 1978.
205. NEEDLEMAN, P., M. S. MINKES, AND J. R. DOUGLAS. Stimulation of prostaglandin biosynthesis by adenine nucleotides. Profile of prostaglandin release by perfused organs. *Circ. Res.* 34: 455–460, 1974.
206. NIJKAMP, F. P., S. MONCADA, H. L. WHITE, AND J. R. VANE. Diversion of prostaglandin endoperoxide metabolism by selective inhibition of thromboxane A_2 biosynthesis in lung, spleen or platelets. *Eur. J. Pharmacol.* 44: 179–187, 1977.
207. NIJKAMP, F. P., AND A. G. M. RAMAKERS. Prevention of anaphylactic bronchoconstriction by a lipoxygenase inhibitor. *Eur. J. Pharmacol.* 62: 121–122, 1980.
208. NUGTEREN, D. H. Inhibition of prostaglandin biosynthesis by 8cis, 12trans, 14cis-eicosatrienoic acid and 5cis, 8cis, 12trans, 14cis-eicosatetraenoic acid. *Biochim. Biophys. Acta* 210: 171–176, 1970.
209. NUGTEREN, D. H. Arachidonate lipoxygenase in blood platelets. *Biochim. Biophys. Acta* 380: 299–307, 1975.
210. NUGTEREN, D. H., AND E. HAZELHOF. Isolation and properties of intermediates in prostaglandin biosynthesis. *Biochim. Biophys. Acta* 326: 448–461, 1973.
211. ODY, C., Y. DIETERLE, I. WAND, H. STALDER, AND A. F. JUNOD. PGA_1 and $PGF_{2\alpha}$ metabolism by pig pulmonary endothelium, smooth muscle, and fibroblasts. *J. Appl. Physiol.: Respirat. Environ. Exercise Physiol.* 46: 211–216, 1979.
212. OLLEY, P. M., F. COCEANI, AND G. KENT. Inactivation of prostaglandin E_1 by lungs of the foetal lamb. *Experientia* 30: 58–59, 1974.
213. ONISHI, H., H. KOSUZUME, Y. KITAMURA, K. YAMAGUCHI, M. NOBUHARA, Y. SUZUKI, S. YOSHIDA, H. TOMIOKA, AND A. KUMAGAI. Structure of slow-reacting substance of anaphylaxis (SRS-A). *Prostaglandins* 20: 655–667, 1980.
214. ORANGE, R. P., D. J. STECHSCHULTE, AND K. F. AUSTEN. Immunochemical and biologic properties of rat IgE. II. Capacity to mediate the immunologic release of histamine and slow reacting substance of anaphylaxis (SRS-A). *J. Immunol.* 105: 1087–1095, 1970.
215. PACE-ASCIAK, C. R. Biosynthesis and metabolism of prostaglandin during animal development. *Adv. Prostaglandin Thromboxane Res.* 1: 35–46, 1976.
216. PACE-ASCIAK, C., AND D. MILLER. Prostaglandins during development. Age-dependent activity profiles of prostaglandin 15-hydroxydehydrogenase and 13, 14-reductase in lung tissue from late prenatal, early postnatal and adult rats. *Prostaglandins* 4: 351–362, 1973.
217. PALMER, M. A., P. J. PIPER, AND J. R. VANE. Release of rabbit aorta contracting substance (RCS) and prostaglandins induced by chemical or mechanical stimulation of guinea-pig lungs. *Br. J. Pharmacol.* 49: 226–242, 1973.
218. PALMER, R. J., R. STEPNEY, G. A. HIGGS, AND K. E. EAKINS. Chemokinetic activity of arachidonic acid lipoxygenase products on leukocytes from different species. *Prostaglandins* 20: 411–418, 1980.

219. PARKES, D. P., AND T. E. ELING. The influence of environmental agents on prostaglandin biosynthesis and metabolism by the lung. *Biochem. J.* 146: 549–556, 1975.
219a.PATEL, K., AND Y. S. BAKHLE. Thromboxane B_2 (TxB_2) metabolism in rat isolated lung and its inhibition by drugs. *Prostaglandins Med.* 10: 221–229, 1983.
220. PATERSON, N. A. M., J. F. BURKA, AND I. D. CRAIG. Release of slow-reacting substance of anaphylaxis from dispersed pig lung cells: effects of cyclooxygenase and lipoxygenase inhibitors. *J. Allergy Clin. Immunol.* 67: 426–434, 1981.
221. PATTERSON, R., AND K. E. HARRIS. Inhibition of immunoglobulin E-mediated, antigen-induced monkey asthma and skin reactions by 5, 8, 11, 14-eicosatetraynoic acid. *J. Allergy Clin. Immunol.* 67: 146–152, 1981.
222. PATTERSON, R., J. J. PRUZANSKY, AND K. E. HARRIS. An agent that releases basophil and mast cell histamine but blocks cyclooxygenase and lipoxygenase metabolism of arachidonic acid inhibits immunoglobulin E-mediated asthma in rhesus monkeys. *J. Allergy Clin. Immunol.* 67: 444–449, 1981.
223. PAVEK, K., P. J. PIPER, AND G. SMEDEGÅRD. Anaphylatoxin-induced shock and two patterns of anaphylactic shock: hemodynamics and mediators. *Acta Physiol. Scand.* 105: 393–403, 1979.
224. PIPER, P. J. (editor). *SRS-A and the Leukotrienes.* New York: Wiley, 1981.
225. PIPER, P. J., AND M. N. SAMHOUN. The mechanism of action of leukotrienes C_4 and D_4 in guinea-pig isolated perfused lung and parenchymal strips of guinea pig, rabbit and rat. *Prostaglandins* 21: 793–803, 1981.
226. PIPER, P. J., M. N. SAMHOUN, J. R. TIPPINS, T. J. WILLIAMS, M. A. PALMER, AND M. J. PECK. Pharmacological studies on pure SRS-A and synthetic leukotrienes C_4 and D_4. In: *SRS-A and Leukotrienes*, edited by P. J. Piper. New York: Wiley, 1981, p. 81–99.
227. PIPER, P. J., AND D. M. TEMPLE. The effect of lipoxygenase inhibitors and diethylcarbamazine on the immunological release of slow reacting substance of anaphylaxis (SRS-A) from guinea-pig chopped lung. *J. Pharm. Pharmacol.* 33: 384–386, 1981.
228. PIPER, P. J., J. R. TIPPINS, M. N. SAMHOUN, H. R. MORRIS, G. W. TAYLOR, AND C. M. JONES. SRS-A and its formation by the lung. *Bull. Eur. Physiopathol. Respir.* 17: 571–586, 1981.
229. PIPER, P. J., AND J. R. VANE. Release of additional factors in anaphylaxis and its antagonism by anti-inflammatory drugs. *Nature London* 223: 29–35, 1969.
230. PIPER, P. J., AND J. R. VANE. The release of prostaglandin from lung and other tissues. *Ann. NY Acad. Sci.* 180: 363–385, 1971.
231. PIPER, P. J., J. R. VANE, AND J. H. WYLLIE. Inactivation of prostaglandins by the lungs. *Nature London* 225: 600–604, 1970.
232. PITT, B. R., C. N. GILLIS, AND G. L. HAMMOND. Influence of the lung on arterial levels of endogenous prostaglandins E and F. *J. Appl. Physiol.: Respirat. Environ. Exercise Physiol.* 50: 1161–1167, 1981.
233. PLATSHON, L. F., AND M. KALINER. The effects of the immunological release of histamine upon human lung cyclic nucleotide levels and prostaglandin generation. *J. Clin. Invest.* 62: 1113–1121, 1978.
234. POWELL, W. S. Omega-oxidation of prostaglandins by lung and liver microsomes. Changes in enzyme activity induced by pregnancy, pseudopregnancy, and progesterone. *J. Biol. Chem.* 253: 6711–6716, 1978.
235. POWELL, W. S., AND S. SOLOMON. Formation of 20-hydroxyprostaglandins by lungs of pregnant rabbits. *J. Biol. Chem.* 253: 4609–4616, 1978.
236. POYSER, N. L. *Prostaglandins in Reproduction.* New York: Wiley, 1981, chapt. 9, p. 238–242.
237. PRANCAN, A. V., J. LEFORT, M. CHIGNARD, K. GEROZISSIS, F. DRAY, AND B. B. VARGAFTIG. L8027 and 1-nonyl-imidazole as non-selective inhibitors of thromboxane synthesis. *Eur. J. Pharmacol.* 60: 287–297, 1979.
237a.ROBINSON, C., S. H. PEERS, K. A. WADDELL, I. A. BLAIR, AND J. R. S. HOULT. Thromboxane B_2 uptake and metabolism in isolated perfused lung: identification and comparison with prostaglandin $F_{2\alpha}$. *Biochim. Biophys. Acta* 712: 315–325, 1982.
238. ROSENTHALE, M. E., A. DERVINIS, AND J. KASSARICH. Bronchodilator activity of prostaglandins E_1 and E_2. *J. Pharmacol. Exp. Ther.* 178: 541–548, 1971.
239. ROTH, G. J., AND P. W. MAJERUS. The mechanism of the effect of aspirin on human platelets. I. Acetylation of a particulate fraction protein. *J. Clin. Invest.* 56: 624–628, 1975.
240. ROTH, J. A., AND J. C. VENTER. Predominance of the B form of monoamine oxidase in cultured vascular intimal endothelial cells. *Biochem. Pharmacol.* 27: 2371–2372, 1978.
241. RYAN, J. W., AND U. S. RYAN. Pulmonary endothelial cells. *Federation Proc.* 36: 2683–2691, 1977.
242. SACKEYFIO, A. C. Anaphylatoxin-induced release of a substance with prostaglandin-like activity in isolated perfused guinea-pig lungs (Abstract). *Br. J. Pharmacol.* 46: 544P–545P, 1972.
243. SAID, S. I. (editor). Prostaglandins and the lung. *Bull. Eur. Physiopathol. Respir.* 17: 487–736, 1981.
244. SAID, S. I., T. YOSHIDA, S. KITAMURA, AND C. VREIM. Pulmonary alveolar hypoxia: release of prostaglandins and other humoral mediators. *Science* 185: 1181–1183, 1974.
245. SAMUELSSON, B., S. HAMMARSTRÖM, R. C. MURPHY, AND P. BORGEAT. Leukotrienes and slow reacting substance of anaphylaxis (SRS-A). *Allergy* 35: 375–381, 1980.
246. SANNER, J. H. Substances that inhibit the actions of prostaglandins. *Arch. Intern. Med.* 133: 133–146, 1974.
247. SAUNDERS, C. R., E. R. RITTENHOUSE, B. M. JAFFE, AND D. B. DOTY. Prostaglandin E biosynthesis during cardiopulmonary bypass. *J. Surg. Res.* 24: 188–192, 1978.
248. SIMBERG, N., H. TOIVONEN, J. HARTIALA, AND Y. S. BAKHLE. The inactivation of prostaglandin E_2 and 5-hydroxytryptamine in isolated perfused fetal and neonatal rabbit lungs. *Acta Physiol. Scand.* 113: 291–295, 1982.
249. SINZINGER, H., W. FEIGH, AND K. SILBERBAUER. Prostacyclin generation in atherosclerotic arteries. *Lancet* 2: 469, 1979.
250. SMITH, A. P., AND M. F. CUTHBERT. The antagonistic action of prostaglandin $F_{2\alpha}$ and E_2 aerosols on bronchial tone in man. *Br. Med. J.* 3: 212–213, 1972.
251. SMITH, A. P., M. F. CUTHBERT, AND L. S. DUNLOP. Effects of inhaled prostaglandins E_1, E_2 and $F_{2\alpha}$ on the airway resistance of healthy and asthmatic man. *Clin. Sci. Mol. Med.* 48: 421–430, 1975.
252. SMITH, A. P., AND L. S. DUNLOP. Prostaglandins and asthma (Letter). *Lancet* 1: 39, 1975.
253. SMITH, J. B., AND A. L. WILLIS. Aspirin selectively inhibits prostaglandin production in human platelets. *Nature London New Biol.* 231: 235–237, 1971.
254. SMITH, M. J. H., A. W. FORD-HUTCHINSON, AND M. A. BRAY. Leukotriene B: a potent mediator of inflammation. *J. Pharm. Pharmacol.* 32: 517–518, 1980.
255. SORS, H., AND P. EVEN. Biosynthesis and metabolism of prostaglandins and related compounds by the lung. In: *Scientific Foundations of Respiratory Medicine*, edited by J. G. Scadding, G. Cumming, and W. M. Thurlbeck. London: Heinemann, 1981, p. 297–315.
256. SPANNHAKE, E. W., A. L. HYMAN, AND P. J. KADOWITZ. Dependence of the airway and pulmonary vascular effects of arachidonic acid upon route and rate of administration. *J. Pharmacol. Exp. Ther.* 212: 584–590, 1980.
257. SPANNHAKE, E. W., R. J. LEMEN, M. J. WEGMANN, A. L. HYMAN, AND P. J. KADOWITZ. Analysis of airway effects of a PGH_2 analog in the anesthetized dog. *J. Appl. Physiol.: Respirat. Environ. Exercise Physiol.* 44: 406–415, 1978.
258. SPANNHAKE, E. W., J. L. LEVIN, D. B. MCNAMARA, A. L. HYMAN, AND P. KADOWITZ. In vivo synthesis of airway-active agents from arachidonic acid. *Bull. Eur. Physiopathol. Respir.* 17: 523–530, 1981.

259. SPLAWINSKI, J., AND R. J. GRYGLEWSKI. Release of prostacyclin by the lung. *Bull. Eur. Physiopathol. Respir.* 17: 553–570, 1981.
260. STALCUP, S. A., L. M. PANG, J. S. LIPSET, C. E. ODYA, T. L. GOODFRIEND, AND R. B. MELLINS. Gestational changes in pulmonary converting enzyme activity in the fetal rabbit. *Circ. Res.* 43: 705–711, 1978.
261. STEINER, M. Platelet protein synthesis studied in a cell-free system. *Experientia* 26: 786–789, 1970.
262. SUN, F. F., AND S. B. ARMOUR. Prostaglandin 15-hydroxydehydrogenase and Δ^{13} reductase levels in the lungs of maternal, fetal and neonatal rabbits. *Prostaglandins* 7: 327–338, 1974.
263. SUN, F. F., S. B. ARMOUR, V. R. BOCKSTANZ, AND J. C. MCGUIRE. Studies on 15-hydroxyprostaglandin dehydrogenase from monkey lung. *Adv. Prostaglandin Thromboxane Res.* 1: 163–169, 1976.
264. SUN, F. F., J. P. CHAPMAN, AND J. C. MCGUIRE. Metabolism of prostaglandin endoperoxide in animal tissues. *Prostaglandins* 14: 1055–1074, 1977.
265. SVENSSON, J. Structure and quantitative determination of the major urinary metabolite of thromboxane B_2 in the guinea pig. *Prostaglandins* 17: 351–365, 1979.
266. SVENSSON, J., M. HAMBERG, AND B. SAMUELSSON. Prostaglandin endoperoxides IX. Characterization of rabbit aorta contracting substance (RCS) from guinea pig lung and human platelets. *Acta Physiol. Scand.* 94: 222–228, 1975.
267. SWEATMAN, W. O. J., AND H. O. J. COLLIER. Effects of prostaglandins on human bronchial muscle. *Nature London* 217: 69, 1968.
268. SZCZEKLIK, A., AND R. J. GRYGLEWSKI. Prostaglandins and aspirin-sensitive asthma. *Am. Rev. Respir. Dis.* 118: 799–800, 1978.
269. SZCZEKLIK, A., AND R. J. GRYGLEWSKI. Treatment of vascular disease with prostacyclin. In: *Clinical Pharmacology of Prostacyclin*, edited by P. J. Lewis and J. O'Grady. New York: Raven, 1981, p. 159–167.
270. SZCZEKLIK, A., R. J. GRYGLEWSKI, E. NIZANKOWSKA, R. NIZANKOWSKA, AND J. MUSIAL. Pulmonary and anti-platelet effects of intravenous and inhaled prostacyclin in man. *Prostaglandins* 16: 654–660, 1978.
271. SZCZEKLIK, A., R. NIZANKOWSKI, S. SKAWINSKI, J. SZCZEKLIK, P. GLUSZKO, AND R. J. GRYGLEWSKI. Successful therapy of advanced arteriosclerosis obliterans with prostacyclin. *Lancet* 1: 1111–1114, 1979.
272. TAI, H. H. Biosynthesis and metabolism of pulmonary prostaglandins, thromboxanes and prostacyclin. *Bull. Eur. Physiopathol. Respir.* 17: 627–646, 1981.
273. TAI, H. H., B. YUAN, AND M. SUN. Metabolism of prostaglandins in spontaneously hypertensive rats: NAD^+-dependent 15-hydroxyprostaglandin dehydrogenase activity is decreased in kidney and increased in lung. *Life Sci.* 24: 1275–1280, 1979.
274. TOIVONEN, H., J. HARTIALA, AND Y. S. BAKHLE. Effects of high oxygen tension on the metabolism of vasoactive hormones in isolated perfused rat lung. *Acta Physiol. Scand.* 111: 185–192, 1981.
275. VAAGE, J., L. BJERTNAES, AND A. HAUGE. The pulmonary vasoconstrictor response to hypoxia: effects of inhibitors of prostaglandin biosynthesis. *Acta Physiol. Scand.* 95: 95–101, 1975.
276. VADER, C. R., M. M. MATHIAS, AND C. L. SCHATTE. Pulmonary prostaglandin metabolism during normobaric hyperoxia. *Prostaglandins Med.* 6: 101–110, 1981.
277. VANDERHOEK, J. Y., AND W. E. M. LANDS. Acetylenic inhibitors of sheep vesicular gland oxygenase. *Biochim. Biophys. Acta* 296: 274–281, 1973.
278. VAN DORP, D. A. Aspects of the biosynthesis of prostaglandins. *Prog. Biochem. Pharmacol.* 3: 171–182, 1967.
279. VANE, J. R. Inhibition of prostaglandin synthesis as a mechanism of action for aspirin-like drugs. *Nature London New Biol.* 231: 232–235, 1971.
280. VARGAFTIG, B. B. Carrageenan and thrombin trigger prostaglandin synthetase-independent aggregation of rabbit platelets: inhibition by phospholipase A_2 inhibitors. *J. Pharm. Pharmacol.* 29: 222–228, 1977.
281. VARGAFTIG, B. B., M. CHIGNARD, J. M. MERCIA-HUERTA, B. ARNOUX, AND J. BENEVISTE. Pharmacology of arachidonate metabolites and of platelet-activating factor (PAF-acether). In: *Platelets in Biology and Pathology*, edited by J. L. Gordon. Amsterdam: Elsevier/North-Holland, 1981, vol. 2, p. 373–408.
282. VARGAFTIG, B. B., AND N. DAO-HAI. Release of vasoactive substances from guinea-pig lungs by slow reacting substance C and arachidonic acid. *Pharmacology* 6: 99–108, 1971.
282a. VON EULER, U. S. On the specific vasodilating and plain muscle stimulating substance from accessory genital glands in man and certain animals (prostaglandin and vesiglandin). *J. Physiol. London* 94: 187–226, 1938.
283. WALKER, J. L. The regulatory role of prostaglandins in the release of histamine and SRS-A from passively sensitized human lung tissue. In: *Advances in the Biosciences*, edited by S. Bergström and S. Bernhard. New York: Pergamon, 1973, vol. 9, p. 235–239.
284. WALKER, J. R., J. R. BOOT, B. COX, AND W. DAWSON. Inhibition of the release of slow reacting substance of anaphylaxis by inhibitors of lipoxygenase activity. *J. Pharm. Pharmacol.* 32: 866–867, 1980.
285. WALKER, J. R., AND W. DAWSON. Inhibition of rabbit PMN lipoxygenase activity by benoxaprofen. *J. Pharm. Pharmacol.* 31: 778–780, 1979.
286. WASSERMAN, M. A. Bronchopulmonary pharmacology of some prostaglandin endoperoxide analogs in the dog. *Eur. J. Pharmacol.* 36: 103–114, 1976.
287. WASSERMAN, M. A., D. W. DUCHARME, M. G. WENDELING, R. L. GRIFFIN, AND G. L. GRAAF. Bronchodilator effects of prostacyclin (PGI_2) in dogs and guinea pigs. *Eur. J. Pharmacol.* 66: 53–58, 1980.
288. WEDMORE, C. V., AND T. J. WILLIAMS. Control of vascular permeability by polymorphonuclear leukocytes in inflammation. *Nature London* 284: 646–650, 1981.
289. WEIR, E. K., I. F. MCMURTRY, A. TUCKER, J. T. REEVES, AND R. F. GROVER. Prostaglandin synthetase inhibitors do not decrease hypoxic pulmonary vasoconstriction. *J. Appl. Physiol.* 41: 714–718, 1976.
290. WICKS, T. C., J. C. ROSE, M. JOHNSON, P. W. RAMWELL, AND P. A. KOT. Vascular responses to arachidonic acid in the perfused canine lung. *Circ. Res.* 38: 167–171, 1976.
291. WILLIAMS, K. I., K. E. H. EL-TAHIR, AND E. MARCINKIEWICZ. Dual actions of prostacyclin (PGI_2) on the rat pregnant uterus. *Prostaglandins* 17: 667–672, 1979.
292. WILLIAMS, T. J., AND P. J. JOSE. Mediation of increased vascular permeability after complement activation. *J. Exp. Med.* 153: 136–153, 1981.
293. WILLIAMS, T. J., AND M. J. PECK. Role of prostaglandin-mediated vasodilation in inflammation. *Nature London* 270: 530–532, 1977.
294. WILLIS, A. L. Parallel assay of prostaglandin-like activities in rat inflammatory exudate by means of cascade superfusion. *J. Pharm. Pharmacol.* 21: 126–128, 1969.
295. WOODS, H. F., G. ASH, M. J. WESTON, S. BUNTING, S. MONCADA, AND J. R. VANE. Prostacyclin can replace heparin in haemodialysis in dogs. *Lancet* 2: 1075–1077, 1978.
296. YOUDIM, M. B. H., Y. S. BAKHLE, AND R. R. BEN-HARARI. Inactivation of monoamines by the lung. In: *Metabolic Activities of the Lung*, edited by R. Porter and J. Whelan. Amsterdam: Excerpta Med., 1980, p. 105–128. (Ciba Found. Symp. 78.)

CHAPTER 12

Lipoproteins and lipoprotein lipase

MARGIT HAMOSH | Department of Pediatrics and Department of Physiology and Biophysics,
PAUL HAMOSH | Georgetown University Medical School, Washington, DC

CHAPTER CONTENTS

History
Lipoproteins
   Chylomicrons
   Very-low-density lipoproteins
   Low-density lipoproteins
   High-density lipoproteins
Lipoprotein Lipase
   History of lipoprotein lipase
   Distribution of lipoprotein lipase
   Regulation of lipoprotein lipase activity
      Nutritional and hormonal effects
      Substrate affinity
      Cellular regulation
   Ontogeny of lipoprotein lipase
   Characteristics of lipoprotein lipase
   Mechanisms of hydrolysis of circulating triglycerides
      Endothelial lipoprotein lipase
      Origin of endothelial lipoprotein lipase
      Mechanism of binding to endothelium
      Role of apoprotein C-II
      Role of apoprotein E
   Characteristics of lipolytic activity of lipoprotein lipase
Lipoprotein Lipase in Lung
   Tissue distribution and regulation of activity
   Lung lipoprotein lipase in disease
      Diabetes
      Trauma
      Severe lipemia
   Origin
   Functions
      Lipid metabolism
      Apoprotein metabolism

THIS CHAPTER PRESENTS a brief review of the major classes of lipoproteins and an extensive discussion of lipoprotein lipase, the enzyme that regulates the uptake of circulating triglycerides by extrahepatic tissues. More information on lipoproteins can be found in several excellent recent reviews specifically on lipoprotein synthesis, structure, function, and catabolism (20, 60, 105, 107, 146, 185, 206, 244, 277, 342, 343, 345, 369, 370, 379–381).

HISTORY

Chyle, the fat-rich fluid that leaves the intestine after a meal, was first described by Claude Bernard (36), who reported that the lymphatics, distal to the pancreatic duct, became cloudy after the ingestion of fat. Virchow (401) first showed that the milky appearance of sera was due to the presence of fat. The first lipoproteins to be described were the chylomicrons, identified in 1920 with dark-field microscopy by Gage and Fish (144, 145). The other (less-lipid-filled) lipoproteins were not identified until the discovery of the ultracentrifuge (389). Lindgren (248), one of the pioneers in the field, cites Claude Bernard, who said, "Every advance in science is first preceded by an advance in technique." Originally the inventors of the ultracentrifuge, Svedberg and Rinde (389), used it to study the particle size of gold colloids. A higher speed ultracentrifuge developed a few years later was used for protein analysis (268, 389). At the same time Macheboeuf (257, 258) described a protein fraction from horse serum that contained lipid. This protein, isolated by precipitation with ammonium sulfate and labeled "coenapse precipitated by acid," was later found to be an α-globulin and thus a high-density lipoprotein (248). The era of lipoprotein research began when Gofman et al. (152) introduced the concept of lipoprotein flotation by raising the serum density above 1.03 g/ml. The marked advances in methodology of protein and lipid chemistry during the last 30 years have clarified many aspects of lipoprotein structure, function, and metabolism (158, 249–251, 285, 311, 395).

LIPOPROTEINS

Lipids are nonpolar or amphipathic substances (Fig. 1) insoluble in aqueous media. They can be transported in the circulation only in association with specific proteins. Polar lipids [e.g., free fatty acids (140) and lysolecithin (12)] bind to plasma albumin, whereas nonpolar lipids are transported in association with much larger particles, the lipoproteins. The nonpolar lipids (triglyceride and cholesteryl ester) form the hydrophobic core of the lipoproteins, whereas amphipathic lipids, phospholipids, cholesterol, small amounts of free fatty acids, and partial glycerides combine with apoproteins to form the surface film.

The lipoproteins are generally divided into four categories: chylomicrons, very-low-density lipoproteins (VLDL), low-density lipoproteins (LDL), and high-density lipoproteins (HDL). The classification of the major lipoprotein classes (Table 1) is based on the initial techniques employed for their isolation from plasma: ultracentrifugal flotation and electrophoretic mobility. The most widely used classification of lipoproteins, based on their flotation at densities of 1.063–1.21 g/ml, was introduced by Gofman et al. (152). It takes advantage of the high lipid content, which gives these particles a lower density than other proteins in the circulation.

The primary function of the lipoproteins is to transport lipids, chiefly cholesterol and triglyceride. Studies during the last several years show that in addition to their transport function (solubilizing hydrophobic lipid in the aqueous environment of blood) the protein component of lipoproteins, the apolipoproteins, has important metabolic functions (60, 113, 343, 380). Although there is not yet consensus on the nomenclature of lipoprotein apoproteins, the classification introduced by Alaupovic et al. (3) is most widely used. There are at least seven different lipoprotein apoproteins (343); five (apoproteins A–E) have been investigated extensively [Table 2; (343)]. The apoproteins differ in their structure, function, and distribution among the lipoprotein classes (Table 2). Some (apoB and apoA-II) have primary roles in lipid transport, whereas others (apoC-II and apoA-I) specifically activate enzymes involved in lipolysis (lipoprotein lipase) and interconversion of lipoproteins [lecithin:cholesterol acyltransferase (LCAT)] (107, 206, 277, 343, 380).

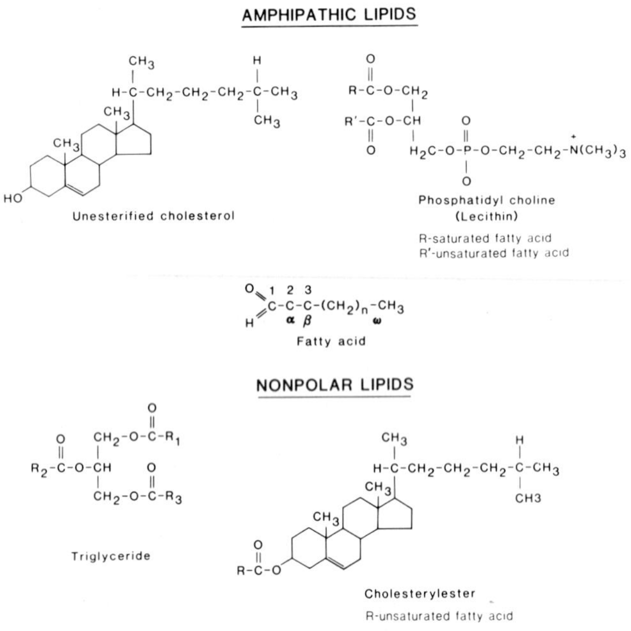

Chylomicrons

Dietary triglyceride and cholesterol enter the circulation in the form of chylomicrons formed exclusively in the intestine. After hydrolysis of dietary fat in the stomach (175) and intestine (50), the products of lipolysis are taken up by intestinal mucosal cells. There the free fatty acids are reesterified to triglyceride in the smooth endoplasmic reticulum (66, 143) and combine with cholesterol, cholesteryl ester, phospholipids (325, 326), and apoproteins to form the largest of the lipoprotein particles (80–500 nm)—the chylomicrons [Tables 1 and 3; (385)]. Chylomicrons have a core of triglyceride surrounded by an outer monomolecular layer of phosphatidylcholine, cholesterol, and apolipoproteins on the surface of the particles (139). The apoproteins in chylomicrons consist of ~66% C apolipoproteins (apoC-I, apoC-II, and apoC-III), 22% apoB, and 12% apoA (231). The large size of chylomicrons is probably related to a need to conserve apoB, which is essential for their secretion from the intestinal mucosa into the lymphatics (157).

Intestinal secretion of triglyceride-rich particles differs from hepatic secretion of VLDL in three major aspects (380): the much larger size of chylomicrons, the lack of synthesis of the C apoproteins, and the intermediary phase of transport in lymph. Chylomicrons emerge into the lymph with a full complement of cholesteryl ester (201), apoA (202, 321), and apoB (320) but are deficient in C apoproteins (149). The

FIG. 1. Principal lipid components of plasma. Amphipathic lipids: unesterified cholesterol and phosphatidylcholine. Nonpolar lipids: triglyceride and cholesteryl ester. Free fatty acids are present in plasma as a complex with albumin.

TABLE 1. *Properties of Human Serum Lipoproteins*

Lipoprotein	Density, g/ml	Diameter, nm	Molecular Weight × 10^5	Flotation Coefficient $S_f = 1.063$	Flotation Coefficient $S_f = 1.21$	Electrophoresis
Chylomicrons	0.93	80–500	10^4–10^5	400		Origin
Very-low-density lipoprotein	0.95–1.006	30–80	50–270	20–400		Pre-β
Intermediate-density lipoprotein	1.006–1.019	25–35	27–35	12–20		Slow pre-β
Low-density lipoprotein	1.019–1.063	21.6	22–27	0–12		β
High-density lipoprotein						
Type 2	1.063–1.125	8.5–10	1.75–2.6		3.6	α_1
Type 3	1.125–1.210	7.5–8.5	1.5–1.75		0.35	α_1

S_f, Svedberg flotation unit. (Data from refs. 146, 184, 206, 342, 343.)

TABLE 2. *Properties and Functions of Apoproteins of Plasma Lipoproteins*

Apo-protein	Peptide Structure	No. of Amino Acids per Chain	Molecular Weight × 10³	Function	Site of Synthesis
ApoA-I	Single chain	245	28.000	Activates LCAT	Intestine, liver
ApoA-II	2 Identical chains		17.000		Intestine, liver
ApoB			*	Transports triglyceride	Intestine, liver
ApoC-I	Single chain	57	6.331	Activates LCAT	Liver
ApoC-II	Single chain	78	8.837	Activates lipoprotein lipase	Liver
ApoC-III	Single chain	79	8.764	Inhibits lipoprotein lipase	Liver
ApoD			22.000	Transfer protein	
ApoE			33.000	Binds to specific liver and endothelial receptors	Intestine†

LCAT, lecithin-cholesterol acyltransferase. * Reported to be between 8 and 275 × 10³ (107). † Possibly liver also. (Data from refs. 60, 146, 184, 206, 303, 342, 343, 380.)

TABLE 3. *Composition of Human Serum Lipoproteins*

Lipoprotein	Protein*	Triglyceride	Cholesteryl ester	Cholesterol	Phospholipids	Major	Minor
Chylomicrons	2.0	84	5.0	2.0	8.0	C	A, B, E
Very-low-density lipoprotein	8–10	56	13.0	8.0	20.0	B, C	E
Low-density lipoprotein	25	10	50.0	10.0	30.0	B	C, E
High-density lipoprotein							
Type 2	41	7.6	28.0	9.0	50.0	A	C, D, E
Type 3	55	6.6	28.0	6.5	50.0	A	C, D, E

* Weight percent per particle. † Weight percent of total lipid. (Data from refs. 146, 184, 206, 342, 343.)

rapid transfer of apoC from HDL to chylomicrons in the circulation [Fig. 2; (186)] increases the apoC content of rat chylomicrons sixfold (201) and the human chylomicron content three- to fourfold (160). With the enrichment in protein, phospholipids are lost from the surface layer of chylomicrons (273). There are therefore marked differences in the composition and size of chylomicrons isolated from lymph or plasma.

Chylomicrons are the most rapidly catabolized of all lipoproteins, with a half-life of less than 5 min in the human (166). The catabolism of chylomicrons proceeds in two main phases. In the first phase the triglyceride core is markedly reduced by the action of lipoprotein lipase, an enzyme that hydrolyzes lipoprotein triglyceride at the luminal surface of the capillary endothelium (45, 294, 333, 355). Hydrolysis in extrahepatic tissues reduces the particles to cholesterol-enriched remnants that are removed by the liver [Fig. 2; (324)]. Remnant recognition by the liver does not depend on particle size or triglyceride composition (362). Recent evidence suggests that changes in the composition of the apoproteins on the surface of chylomicron remnants are the main determinant; a reduction in apoC (413) and an increase in apoE content (184) are prerequisites for efficient remnant uptake by the liver.

Very-Low-Density Lipoproteins

Very-low-density lipoproteins transport endogenously synthesized triglyceride. These particles are formed in the liver (78, 242, 377, 414) and to a lesser extent in the intestinal mucosa (297, 338, 414). At the two extremes of the density range, VLDL overlap with chylomicrons and with LDL. They are isolated from chylomicron-free plasma at densities less than 1.006 g/ml. The VLDL form a continuum of various sizes (30–88 nm diam) and molecular weights (5–30 × 10⁶) that reflects the extensive changes in composition occurring in the circulation (Table 1). In addition the metabolism of VLDL in various species differs markedly.

Long-chain fatty acids are diverted to triglyceride synthesis when their concentration exceeds the transmitochondrial transfer capacity of fatty acyl-CoA: carnitine transferase, the key enzyme in fatty acid oxidation (268). The intracellular sites of synthesis of various components of VLDL have been studied in detail in the rat (377) and other species (78, 242). One may assume that in general the mechanisms are similar in human liver. A major difference between the human and the rat is the content of cholesteryl ester in the nascent VLDL particle: human VLDL acquires most of its cholesteryl ester in the circulation [Fig. 2; (151)], whereas rat VLDL is secreted with a full complement of cholesteryl ester (380). In humans the major difference between VLDL synthesized in the liver and VLDL synthesized in the intestine is the full complement of cholesteryl ester and very low levels of apoC in intestinal VLDL. The size of the VLDL particles is directly related to the triglyceride content and inversely to the phospholipid and protein content;

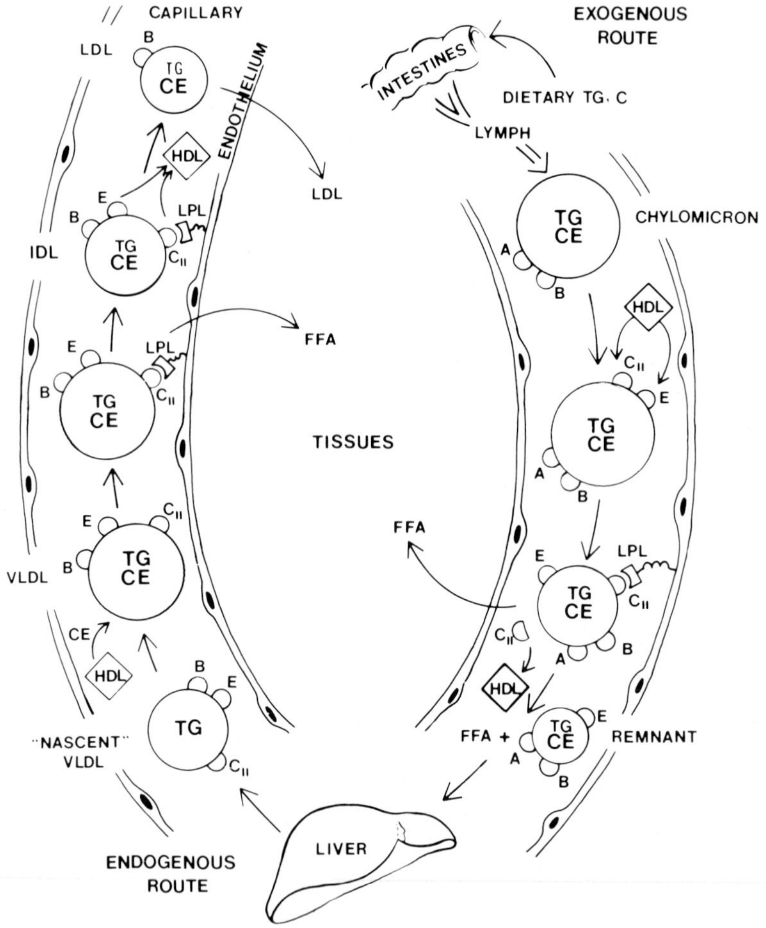

FIG. 2. Metabolism of triglyceride-rich lipoproteins. TG, triglyceride; CE, cholesteryl ester; LPL, lipoprotein lipase; FFA, free fatty acids; VLDL, very-low-density lipoprotein; IDL, intermediate-density lipoprotein; LDL, low-density lipoprotein; HDL, high-density lipoprotein; A, B, C, and E, apoproteins.

apoB accounts for 20%–40% of total VLDL protein (62, 343, 347), apoC for 50%, and apoE for 13% (343).

The organization of the components of VLDL resembles that of chylomicrons, with a neutral lipid core (composed of triglycerides and cholesteryl esters) and a surface film of phospholipids (phosphatidylcholine, sphingomyelin), cholesterol, and apoproteins (360). The triglyceride component is present in its entirety in nascent human VLDL, whereas most other constituents change when they enter the circulation: apoC, apoE (151), and cholesteryl ester are transferred from HDL to VLDL [Fig. 2; (2, 72, 150, 310, 421)]. In the latter the esterified cholesterol is accumulated in nascent HDL by the LCAT reaction (2, 150) and then is transferred to nascent VLDL. A specific transfer protein (421), recently identified as apoD, aids the transfer of cholesteryl ester (72). The phosphate groups of HDL phospholipids might also be involved in the cholesteryl ester transfer reaction (310). No such transfer occurs in the rat (339), a species that probably lacks this specific transfer protein (22).

The VLDL are catabolized by a stepwise reduction of the triglyceride core through the action of lipoprotein lipase, a process that in humans leads to the formation first of intermediate-density lipoproteins (IDL) (245) and ultimately of LDL. The first step occurs at the endothelium of extrahepatic tissues. It is not clear whether IDL are delipidated at the peripheral capillary endothelium or whether hepatic lipase hydrolyzes the triglyceride in the liver endothelium.

Although IDL contain only 1%–5% of the triglyceride originally present in VLDL, they are still regarded as triglyceride-rich lipoproteins. A precursor-product relationship has consistently been reported for the apoB moiety of VLDL, IDL, and LDL (35, 323, 366), indicating that LDL are the end product of a series of delipidation steps of VLDL (105). Because VLDL and LDL particles contain approximately the same number of apoB molecules in single lipoproteins (106), Eisenberg (105) concluded that only one product particle is formed from each precursor VLDL particle and that fission or fusion of the IDL core does not take place during the delipidation process. The formation of LDL is the result of removal of triglycerides, while cholesteryl ester, apoB, and surface lipids are left behind (105). However, apoC molecules are removed from VLDL as lipolysis progresses (111) and are transferred to HDL in the circulation, the latter acting as a reservoir for apoC molecules. However, in vitro studies have recently shown that HDL are not necessary for the removal of apoC molecules from VLDL (147). Along with triglyceride hydrolysis, the surplus surface constituents apoC, apoE, and lipids (60% of free cholesterol, 90% of phosphatidylcholine, and 100% of sphingomyelin) are removed from VLDL (111). During in vitro hydrolysis of VLDL triglyceride in the absence of plasma, the surface constituents are released in particulate form and associate into disk-shaped structures similar to HDL precursors isolated from intestinal lymph (161) or from rat liver perfusate (174).

Unlike the pathway in humans, in the rat the liver rapidly removes VLDL after partial lipolysis (109, 110, 117, 274); VLDL-apoB and cholesteryl ester are cleared from the circulation with a half-life of 5–10 min (109, 110, 117, 274). However, the apoC moiety of rat VLDL equilibrates rapidly with HDL, as it does in humans. The low levels of LDL in rat could therefore be the result of efficient clearing of VLDL from the circulation (105).

Low-Density Lipoproteins

Whereas the chylomicrons and VLDL transport exogenous and endogenous triglycerides from intestine and liver to tissues, the LDL and HDL transport cholesterol. Cholesterol is needed by all cells for plasma membrane synthesis, by specialized organs for the synthesis of steroid hormones, and by the liver for bile salt synthesis. The LDL contain 70% of the plasma cholesterol in humans (avg 200 mg/dl plasma). Lipids comprise 75% of the mass of the LDL particles and, as in the triglyceride-rich lipoproteins, form the core of the LDL particle (Table 3). Cholesterol amounts to 60% of the lipid content; the main part (50%) is cholesteryl ester. Free cholesterol (10%) and phospholipids (phosphatidylcholine and sphingomyelin) form a lipid coat that surrounds the nonpolar core. Only 10% of the lipid in LDL is triglyceride. The main protein of LDL is apoB, the least well characterized of the plasma apolipoproteins (Table 2). It is assumed that this protein, which contains 5%–9% carbohydrate (390), consists of several subunits, one part buried in the lipid core and another part exposed to the water surface (206).

As discussed in *Very-Low-Density Lipoproteins*, p. 389, LDL are the remnants of VLDL catabolism (Fig. 2). In normal humans and in the rat, the liver does not secrete LDL directly into the blood. Studies with ^{125}I-labeled apoB-LDL show that virtually all plasma LDL is derived from VLDL (366). Indeed, when most of the triglycerides have been removed and the content of cholesteryl ester has increased markedly [a result of the activity of the cholesteryl ester transfer complex of human plasma (132)] and after most apoC and apoE have left the particle, VLDL become LDL (238).

The main function of LDL is to transfer cholesteryl ester to nonhepatic tissues. The interaction of plasma LDL with specific cell surface receptors initiates this (55–57, 60, 155). During cholesterol delivery the protein component of LDL is hydrolyzed to amino acids; thus the entire LDL particle is catabolized. The complete hydrolysis of apoB during the transfer of cholesterol to various tissues indicates that this is the only apoprotein that does not shuttle back and forth between lipoprotein particles of various classes. ApoB enters the circulation in chylomicrons and VLDL [recent reports suggest structural differences between apoB synthesized in the intestine (chylomicrons, VLDL) and that formed in the liver (VLDL) (216, 236)]. After delipidation of chylomicrons, apoB is catabolized in the liver as part of the chylomicron remnant, whereas the apoB of VLDL remains with the same particle throughout its transformation into LDL and until its degradation in nonhepatic tissues (105). The hypothesis that most LDL are degraded in extrahepatic tissues is supported by the observation that removing the liver does not lower the rate of LDL catabolism (372). Futhermore a variety of human cells in culture [fibroblasts (153), arterial smooth muscle cells (4, 154), lymphoid cells (197), and endothelial cells (112)] can degrade LDL through the LDL pathway (155). In the cow the LDL receptors have been detected in cell membranes (23) prepared from many tissues (233). The number of receptors was highest in the adrenal cortex and in the ovarian corpus luteum, the two tissues that secrete steroids and therefore have the highest requirement for cholesterol. A detailed description of the regulation of cholesterol metabolism is outside the scope of this review. However, several recent excellent reviews (57–61, 155) can supplement the brief outline of LDL catabolism that follows.

The "LDL pathway" (58–61, 155) has three steps: *1*) binding of LDL to a cell surface receptor, *2*) endocytosis, and *3*) lysosomal degradation [Fig. 3; (7)]. The LDL receptor, a glycoprotein located within "coated" regions on the cell surface (7), binds only lipoproteins that contain apoB (LDL and VLDL). Although binding of LDL is competitively inhibited by VLDL but not by HDL (which lacks apoB) (153), recent studies

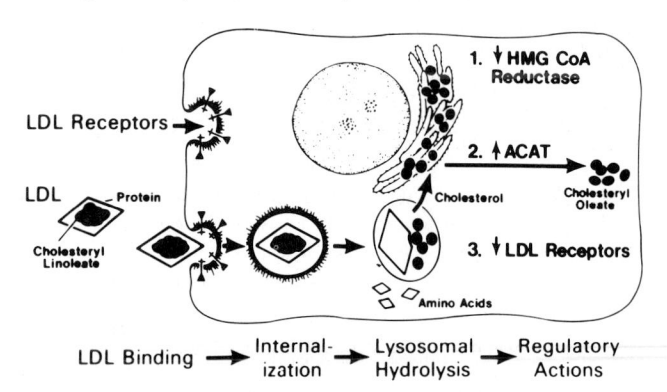

FIG. 3. Low-density lipoprotein (LDL) pathway. Sequential steps in catabolism of LDL. HMG CoA reductase, 3 hydroxy-3-methylglutaryl-CoA reductase; ACAT, acyl-CoA:cholesterol *O*-acyltransferase. [From Brown et al. (59).]

show that binding of VLDL occurs only after the latter has been acted on by lipoprotein lipase (69), suggesting that lipolysis-associated rearrangement of lipoprotein components is a prerequisite for the interaction of the lipoprotein with the cell surface receptor. Another lipoprotein that binds to the LDL receptor is HDL$_c$, a cholesterol-rich lipoprotein high in apoE, which is present in the plasma of swine fed high-cholesterol diets (260). After binding, LDL are incorporated into endocytotic vesicles, but breakdown of the lipoproteins starts only after fusion with lysosomes. Within the lysosomes the protein is hydrolyzed to a mixture of amino acids and small peptides (153) and the cholesteryl ester is hydrolyzed by an "acid" lipase (156). Release of free cholesterol is the key step in the regulation of the several cellular receptors for LDL, as well as in cellular cholesterol synthesis (57). The latter is accomplished by the regulation of two microsomal enzymes: suppression of the activity of 3-hydroxy-3-methylglutaryl-CoA reductase (the rate-limiting step in cholesterol synthesis) and activation of acyl-CoA:cholesterol O-acyltransferase. The net effect is a reduction in cellular cholesterol synthesis and storage of the LDL cholesterol as cholesteryl ester within the cell. During this process the fatty acid esterified to cholesterol is changed from linoleate in LDL cholesteryl ester to oleate in cellular cholesteryl ester (156). The elegant studies of Goldstein, Brown, and co-workers (7, 23, 55, 56, 153, 156; reviewed in refs. 57–61, 154, 155) show that several metabolic disorders associated with hypercholesterolemia are the result of genetic defects in several steps of the receptor-linked LDL catabolism.

About one-third of the circulating LDL are catabolized by an additional nonspecific process—bulk-phase phagocytosis—that does not require prior binding of the LDL to the cell surface (153, 155). In this process LDL particles are taken up at a rate proportional to their concentration in the medium. This process, however, does not regulate the rate of intracellular synthesis of cholesterol.

High-Density Lipoproteins

High-density lipoproteins, isolated in the density range of 1.063–1.21 g/ml, contain ~50% protein, ~25% phospholipid, ~20% cholesterol, and ~5% triglyceride [Tables 1 and 3; (185, 206, 277, 342, 345, 379, 391)]. They are composed of two density groups: HDL$_2$ (~40% protein, ~60% lipid) and HDL$_3$ (55% protein, 45% lipid). The principal apoproteins of HDL, apoA-I and apoA-II, constitute 90% of total HDL protein. The remaining 10% is apoC, apoD, apoE (Tables 2 and 3), and a recently described apolipoprotein, apoF (303).

In the circulation, HDL has a half-life of 3–6 days in the normal human; the apoprotein has a similar half-life (343). Several different lipoprotein species containing different apoproteins have been reported within the HDL group (345). A significant amount of apoA is synthesized in the intestine [56% of total plasma apoA-I in rats (415) and a similar amount in humans (160)] and is released into the circulation in chylomicrons. Rapid transfer of these apoproteins from chylomicrons to HDL has been reported in the human (344) and the rat (327). The other apoproteins of HDL originate in the liver.

Recently the interest in HDL has increased greatly because of the strong inverse relationship between plasma levels of HDL and morbidity or mortality from cardiovascular disease (19, 371). This relationship may be the result of the special function of HDL in transport of cholesterol from peripheral tissues to the liver for final catabolism (151), which reduces the amount of lipid deposited in the arterial wall (67, 370). The HDL are synthesized in the liver (264, 295) and intestine (266). The fraction produced by the intestine acquires its apoC complement in the circulation from HDL of hepatic origin; the HDL are released from the liver with a full complement of apoC. Nascent HDL produced by the liver have a higher proportion of apoE than do plasma HDL (146) and appear as disks of ~450 nm (172). These particles are rich in protein, phospholipid, and cholesterol, but they are deficient in cholesteryl ester (296). The maturation of disk-shaped HDL requires cholesterol esterification, which is mediated by the LCAT reaction. An enzyme released from the liver into the circulation, LCAT acts specifically on plasma HDL by converting the phosphatidylcholine (lecithin) and unesterified cholesterol of HDL to cholesteryl ester and lysolecithin (150, 151). Once esterified the free cholesterol leaves the surface coat and moves into the nonpolar lipid core in the center of the particle, transforming disk-shaped HDL into spherical (mature) HDL. ApoA-I, the principal apoprotein of HDL, is an activator of this reaction (343). As mentioned in *Very-Low-Density Lipoproteins*, p. 389, nascent HDL–like particles are formed during the in vitro hydrolysis of VLDL triglyceride by lipoprotein lipase (111). These observations suggest that, in addition to sites of synthesis within tissues (liver, intestine), many HDL particles could be formed in the circulation during lipolysis of triglyceride-rich lipoproteins (chylomicrons and VLDL) (Fig. 2). A mechanism whereby the triglyceride-rich core is reduced by lipoprotein lipase at the capillary endothelium, which leaves excess surface constituents (containing mainly apoproteins, cholesterol, and phospholipid) (421) to form bilayer folds resembling nascent HDL, has recently been proposed (391). These nascent HDL disks would then acquire cholesteryl ester through the LCAT reaction and become spherical HDL particles.

Formation of HDL particles would thus be increased during the catabolism of triglyceride-rich lipoproteins and would be directly proportional to the level of lipoprotein lipase activity (391). Indeed such a relationship has been reported (218, 289) during exercise

(287, 288) and after alcohol consumption (412). An important function of HDL is to act as a reservoir of both apoproteins and cholesteryl ester for other circulating lipoproteins (Table 4; Fig. 2). Because the intestine does not synthesize apoC, all the lipoproteins originating there (chylomicrons, VLDL, HDL) acquire apoC in the circulation from HDL. Nascent VLDL particles synthesized in the liver also do not contain cholesteryl ester and depend on HDL for this component. This transfer reaction occurs in two steps: *1)* cholesteryl ester is generated by interaction of HDL with LCAT in plasma, and *2)* the newly generated cholesteryl ester is transferred nonenzymatically to VLDL and LDL. The transfer reaction is mediated by a transfer protein similar to apoD (72). Recent evidence suggests a close link between LCAT, apoD, apoA-I, and the transfer of cholesteryl ester from HDL to VLDL (132). The complex between LCAT, apoA-I (cofactor of reaction), and apoD (carrier of product) has recently been named the cholesteryl ester transfer complex (132).

Very little is known about the catabolism of HDL. Receptor-mediated uptake by peripheral tissues and liver does not seem to occur, except in special conditions (260, 363) when HDL contain apoE, the specific recognition factor for lipoprotein remnant receptors (184, 363). Several tissues can take up and degrade HDL [e.g., hepatocytes (284), Kupfer cells (400), smooth muscle cells (38), and fibroblasts (373)]. Nonhepatic tissues probably take up the most HDL (68) by bulk-phase adsorptive endocytosis. Uptake and catabolism of the particle involve the concomitant breakdown of lipid, apoA-I, and apoA-II (185, 343).

An attempt to unify different aspects of lipoprotein catabolism and to further elucidate some of the interactions between the various lipoprotein particles has recently been made (105, 391). According to Eisenberg (105) all plasma lipoproteins are integral components of one process, the transport of triglycerides. Thus VLDL (the major transport vehicle for endogenously synthesized triglycerides) are the direct precursors of both LDL and HDL. Indeed there is good evidence of a precursor-product relationship between VLDL and LDL. Furthermore concomitant with the delipidation process, which leads to a loss of core triglycerides through the action of lipoprotein lipase, there is a continuous transfer of apoproteins, phospholipids, and cholesterol to HDL. Therefore LDL and HDL can be viewed as the end products of intravascular VLDL catabolism (391): LDL are thus the final form of the core remnant, whereas nascent HDL particles (138, 173, 296), which are similar to surface fragments (71, 94) formed during lipolysis, can be viewed as the final form of the surface coat remnant.

Lipoprotein lipase, the key enzyme in removal of lipoprotein triglyceride, is thus important in the formation of both LDL and HDL lipoprotein; LCAT catalyzes the synthesis of almost the entire cholesteryl ester of circulating lipoproteins. These two key enzymes differ in one important aspect: lipoprotein lipase is active at the capillary wall (Fig. 4) and under normal conditions is completely absent from the circulation. This specific location probably facilitates the uptake of lipolytic products (free fatty acid and monoglyceride) into tissues. On the other hand LCAT acts exclusively in plasma, where it continuously modulates the cholesteryl ester content of circulating lipoproteins.

LIPOPROTEIN LIPASE

Long-chain fatty acids are essential to all mammalian tissues, both as constituents of complex lipids necessary for the structural and functional integrity of cells and as an important energy source (140, 352).

Long-chain fatty acids are carried in the circulation in two forms—as free fatty acids bound to albumin (374) and as triglyceride fatty acids within chylomicrons and VLDL. The uptake of free fatty acids by individual tissues is largely a function of their concentration in the blood and of the rate of blood flow through the tissue (140, 352). Triglyceride fatty acids, however, are contained in the core of large particles that cannot cross the capillary endothelium; therefore their removal from the blood depends on prior hydrolysis at the capillary lumen, a reaction catalyzed by the enzyme lipoprotein lipase (45, 86, 333, 355, 394). The extent to which circulating lipoprotein triglyceride fatty acids are taken up by individual tissues

TABLE 4. *Functions of Plasma Lipoproteins*

Lipoprotein	Origin	Composition Change in Circulation	Half-Life	Function
Chylomicrons	Intestine*	Acquire apoC-II	<5 min	Transports triglyceride
Very-low-density lipoprotein	Intestine†	Acquire apoC-II and cholesteryl ester	Hours	Transports triglyceride
	Liver	Acquire cholesteryl ester		
Low-density lipoprotein	Circulation	From very-low-density lipoprotein through loss of triglyceride	Hours	Transports cholesterol to tissues (anabolic)
High-density lipoprotein	Intestine, liver	Acquire cholesteryl ester	Days	Transports cholesterol from tissues to liver (catabolic)
	Circulation‡			Reservoir of cholesteryl ester and apoC-II

* Dietary fat.   † Endogenous fat.   ‡ From surface coat of chylomicrons and very-low-density lipoproteins during lipolysis.

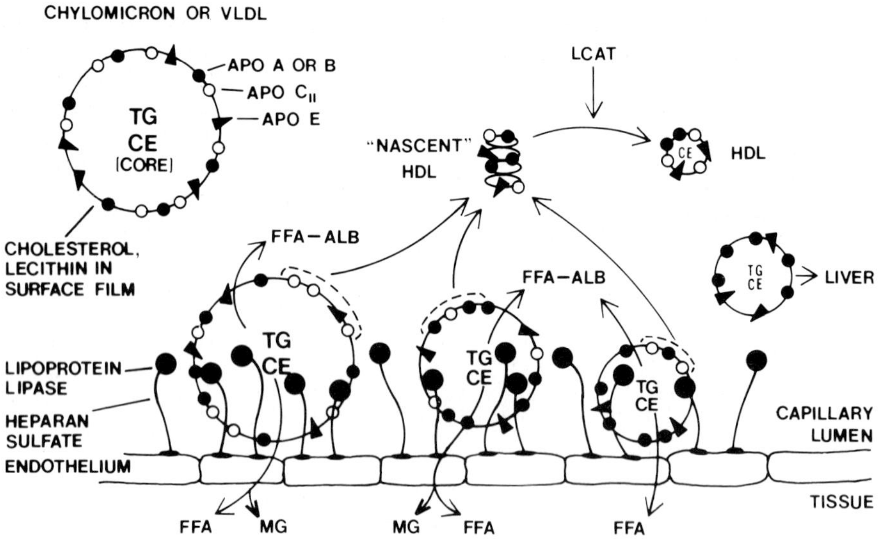

FIG. 4. Scheme for hydrolysis of triglyceride (TG) in chylomicrons and very-low-density lipoproteins (VLDL) by endothelial lipoprotein lipase. Triglyceride-rich lipoproteins are represented as large particles with a neutral lipid core and a surface film composed of lecithin (phosphatidylcholine), cholesterol, and apoproteins (apoA, apoB, etc.). VLDL, smaller than chylomicrons, contain different amounts of apoproteins. Lipoprotein lipase bound to endothelial surface through heparan sulfate hydrolyzes lipoprotein triglyceride to monoglyceride (MG) and free fatty acids (FFA); FFA are taken up by tissue or released into circulation where they bind to albumin (ALB). Shrinking particle core by lipolysis leaves excess surface constituents (*broken line*), which break off as disks similar to "nascent" high-density lipoprotein (HDL). These newly formed particles acquire cholesteryl ester (CE) via lecithin-cholesterol acyltransferase (LCAT) reaction, becoming spherical HDL particles.

thus depends on the relative lipoprotein lipase activity of each tissue (333). Because the activity of lipoprotein lipase in various tissues can change rapidly under different physiological conditions, the enzyme directs the distribution of the plasma triglycerides. Thus lipoprotein lipase is important in determining, not only the rate, but the pattern of uptake of triglyceride fatty acids from the blood. The ability to change the supply of triglyceride fatty acids according to the specific demands of each tissue is particularly important because there is no other mechanism for controlling the tissue distribution of circulating free fatty acids (140, 333, 352, 355). Lipoprotein lipase is thus not only the key enzyme in removing triglyceride from the circulation (the first step in the catabolism of triglyceride-rich lipoproteins); it provides the only way to channel long-chain fatty acids to the tissues where they are needed.

Lipoprotein lipase differs from other tissue lipases in the following ways: it has an alkaline pH optimum (8.0–9.0), is activated by low concentrations of heparin, depends on apoC-II for optimal activity, and is inhibited by high ionic strength (usually 1 M NaCl) and by protamine sulfate. Lipoprotein lipase from various tissues (liver is an exception) shows the same characteristics.

History of Lipoprotein Lipase

Hahn (169) in 1943 first reported the clearing of severe alimentary lipemia in dogs after transfusion of heparin-containing blood. He then injected only heparin and again obtained rapid clearing of lipemic plasma. The in vivo observations (169, 409) were followed by in vitro studies that established that mixing lipemic plasma with plasma obtained after injecting heparin (postheparin plasma) rapidly cleared the lipemia (6). These studies suggested that a factor, released into the circulation after heparin administration, can clear alimentary lipemia under in vivo or in vitro conditions. This lipase, initially called clearing-factor lipase, was named lipoprotein lipase by Korn (227), who showed that the enzyme hydrolyzes chylomicron triglycerides. Early studies by Korn and Quigley (227, 229, 230), Robinson and French (332, 334), and several other groups established that the enzyme is present in various tissues, that it probably is located close to the capillary wall [it appeared in the femoral vein 20 s after heparin injection into the femoral artery of rabbits (335)], and that the level of tissue lipoprotein lipase activity and the rate of lipoprotein triglyceride uptake are directly related (37). The early studies are discussed in excellent reviews by Robinson and French (332–334). Within the last 20 years lipoprotein lipase has been extensively researched, particularly the mechanism of hydrolysis of triglyceride-rich lipoproteins, the regulation of enzyme activity, and the relationship between the enzymes in parenchymal cells (the site of synthesis) and at the endothelial surface (the site of triglyceride hydrolysis). The availability of purified enzyme preparations from various sources has markedly advanced our understanding of the mechanism of lipoprotein lipase activity.

Distribution of Lipoprotein Lipase

The earliest and most extensive studies were carried out with adipose tissue, which takes up and stores most of the circulating triglyceride fatty acids (37, 230, 332, 333, 335, 355). Lipoprotein lipase activity is present in the adipose tissue of many species (32, 80, 88, 91, 95, 96, 115, 116, 176, 178, 305, 316, 340), including humans (182, 291, 313, 314, 318, 352). The highest levels of lipoprotein lipase activity are found in heart (5, 47, 48, 74, 82, 95, 96, 103, 210, 217, 322, 337), in lactating mammary gland (176, 265, 305, 331, 422), and in milk (102, 179, 193, 331). Other tissues in which lipoprotein lipase has recently been described are lung (1, 88, 177, 181, 188), skeletal muscle (24, 90, 115, 247, 253, 292), aorta (85, 98, 190, 306), corpus luteum (34, 359), and brain (53, 75). Lipoprotein lipase in placenta (114, 263) may facilitate the transfer of maternal triglyceride fatty acids to the fetus.

Regulation of Lipoprotein Lipase Activity

NUTRITIONAL AND HORMONAL EFFECTS. To effectively channel circulating triglyceride fatty acids to various organs according to their specific needs, the enzyme must fulfill two demands: *1*) its level must adjust rapidly and specifically to the temporary needs of each organ, and *2*) its location in the tissues must maximize the contact between circulating lipoproteins and enzyme. Indeed the location of the enzyme at the luminal surface of the capillary endothelium (from which it can be rapidly released by heparin) was one of the first reported characteristics of lipoprotein lipase (335). Studies during the last 20 years have shown that lipoprotein lipase activity levels change rapidly under a variety of physiological conditions. Table 5 summarizes the major findings.

In the fed animal a large amount of the circulating triglyceride fatty acids is taken up by adipose tissue, reesterified, and stored in adipocytes. The activity of lipoprotein lipase is therefore high in this tissue after feeding. Lipoprotein lipase activity during fasting decreases sharply, and a second lipase that hydrolyzes intracellular, stored triglyceride becomes active in the tissue, leading to the release of free fatty acids into the blood (220). Another tissue that takes up a major part of the circulating triglycerides is skeletal muscle (52, 213, 333). There fatty acids are an important energy source, especially in muscles containing a large proportion of slow-twitch red fibers (e.g., soleus). Indeed lipoprotein lipase activity is much higher in red than in white skeletal muscle (49, 247, 353, 392). Furthermore, whereas lipoprotein lipase activity does not change in white muscle during fasting, it increases in red muscle, enabling the red muscles to use VLDL triglyceride during this period. At comparable wet weights the lipoprotein lipase activity in cardiac muscle is much higher than in skeletal muscle; the activity

TABLE 5. *Factors That Regulate Level of Lipoprotein Lipase Activity in Various Tissues*

	Activity Under Optimal Conditions, μmol FFA· g^{-1}·h^{-1}	Feeding	Fasting	Exercise	Lactation	Ref.	Endocrine				
							Insulin	Corticosteroids	Prolactin	Estrogen	Thyroxine
Lung	15–30	0	↑, 0	↑	0	88, 171, 181		↑		0	0
Heart	60–140	↓↓	↑↑	↑	0	47–49, 74, 88, 210, 217, 290, 333	0	↑		0	↑
Adipose tissue	15–30	↑↑	↓↓	↑	↓↓	88, 90, 176, 288, 290, 305, 333, 340, 422	↑↑	↑	↓↓	↓	↓
Skeletal muscle											
Red	20–45	↓	↑	↑		24, 49, 88, 90, 247, 288, 290, 292	↑			0	
White	3–6	0	0	↑						0	
Lactating mammary gland	150–200	0	0		↑↑	176, 265, 305, 331, 382, 422		↑	↑↑		
Ref.							14, 198, 247, 333, 340	14, 96, 181	422	178, 411	5, 294

Data mainly from studies with rat tissues. Activity was measured in fresh tissue homogenate or acetone ether preparations of whole tissue. FFA, free fatty acid.

rises markedly after fasting, indicating that the utilization efficiency of plasma triglyceride fatty acids (mainly from VLDL) increases under fasting conditions. The lung lipoprotein lipase activity seems independent of nutritional status in the rat (88, 177), whereas in some other species (e.g., the mouse) an increase in activity occurs after a 24-h fast (88). The normal or higher-than-normal activity of lipoprotein lipase in lung, heart, and red skeletal muscle during fasting, coupled with the almost complete lack of activity in adipose tissue, effectively channels circulating VLDL triglyceride to tissues that have to be supplied with long-chain fatty acids for their normal metabolic function. Because all tissues compete equally for circulating free fatty acids, the tissues that maintain or increase their lipoprotein lipase activity have the additional advantage of access to circulating triglyceride fatty acids during fasting.

The most striking example of the role of lipoprotein lipase in diverting plasma triglycerides from one tissue to another occurs during lactation. The nonlactating mammary gland is completely devoid of lipoprotein lipase; shortly before parturition, however, enzyme activity rises dramatically while the enzyme from adipose tissue is almost completely lost (176). These dramatic changes in enzyme activity are regulated by pituitary prolactin (422), which throughout lactation completely depresses lipoprotein lipase activity in adipose tissue while maintaining a high level of activity in the mammary gland. As a result more than 50% of the dietary fat is diverted to the mammary gland for milk production (39, 148). Indeed, immediately prior to parturition and throughout lactation, the concentration of blood triglyceride is inversely related to the activity of mammary gland lipoprotein lipase (176). Furthermore, because of the extremely high level of lipoprotein lipase activity, which probably leads to rapid depletion of the chylomicron triglyceride core (with the formation of surplus surface film), the mammary gland can take up considerable amounts of chylomicron cholesterol (423).

In addition to parturition and lactation, other aspects of hormonal control of lipoprotein lipase have been investigated in several tissues. These studies show that administering insulin raises enzyme levels in adipose tissue (141, 198, 333, 340), that fluctuations in enzyme activity in adipose tissue parallel diurnal variations in plasma insulin levels (90, 318) in meal-fed rats (328), and that insulin regulates the synthesis and release of lipoprotein lipase from adipocytes in tissue culture (375, 376). Recent evidence suggests that glucocorticoids enhance the insulin effect (14). Administering glucocorticoids independently of insulin also increases enzyme activity in adipose tissue (96).

Estrogen administration markedly inhibits adipose tissue lipoprotein lipase (178, 411) and hepatic lipase activity (10), suggesting that the lipemia accompanying high plasma estrogen levels is associated with decreased triglyceride clearing (416, 424). In general, adipose tissue lipoprotein lipase, an enzyme that regulates the uptake of triglyceride fatty acids into tissues, is inhibited by most agents that stimulate fat mobilization by activating the hormone-sensitive lipase of this tissue (220, 309).

Much less is known about the hormonal regulation of lipoprotein lipase activity in other tissues. Insulin does not seem to affect enzyme activity in cardiac muscle (247, 333). Reports on the effect of glucagon on heart lipoprotein lipase activity conflict (46, 96, 232), perhaps because glucagon has different effects on endothelial and interstitial enzymes (210). Several reports indicate that enzyme activity increases in the heart after thyroid hormones, corticosteroids, and catecholamines are administered (5, 86, 394). With few exceptions (247) skeletal muscle responds much like the heart, including a marked rise in activity during exposure to cold or during fasting (217, 332, 337). Lipoprotein lipase activity in lung increases after glucocorticoid administration (181), but like the enzyme in heart it seems unaffected by insulin levels, because there were no changes in activity in diabetic animals (181).

SUBSTRATE AFFINITY. The delivery of circulating triglyceride fatty acids to specific tissues could also be regulated by differences in affinity between lipoprotein lipase and lipoproteins. Comparing the kinetics of triglyceride removal by isolated perfused rat heart and adipose tissue shows that lipoprotein lipase in heart endothelium has a high substrate affinity [K_m (Michaelis constant) 0.07 mM triglyceride], whereas the enzyme in the endothelium of adipose tissue has a low substrate affinity (K_m 0.70 mM triglyceride) (124, 134). These tissue-specific lipoprotein lipases differ not only kinetically but also structurally (133, 134). It has been proposed (129) therefore that the activity of high- and low-affinity lipoprotein lipase in heart and adipose tissue, respectively, may be important in the regulation of triglyceride clearance. At physiological levels of plasma triglyceride, adipose tissue lipoprotein lipase is not fully saturated and the rate of triglyceride removal is a function of plasma triglyceride concentration. Because of the high affinity of the heart enzyme for lipoprotein triglyceride, uptake of lipid remains constant even at low plasma triglyceride concentrations (e.g., during fasting). This mechanism provides a constant supply of circulating triglyceride fatty acids to the heart, regardless of nutritional state, while permitting storage in adipose tissue only at high plasma triglyceride concentrations.

CELLULAR REGULATION. Present evidence indicates that lipoprotein lipase is synthesized within parenchymal cells, released from these cells, and transported to the luminal surface of the capillary endothelium. Little is known about the regulation of enzyme synthesis within parenchymal cells, the mechanism of release from the cells, its transport through interstitium and basement membrane to the endothelial cell, or the mechanism by which it reaches the luminal surface of the endothelium.

Earlier studies proposed that lipoprotein lipase in adipose tissue exists in two forms—an intracellular, precursor form (LPL-b) and an extracellular form (LPL-a), representing ~5%-10% of total tissue enzyme (293). Accordingly the transformation of LPL-b to LPL-a is independent of protein synthesis, occurs just prior to its release from the cell, and therefore could represent activation of the precursor enzyme (293). These investigators suggested that the high activity of lipoprotein lipase in adipose tissue of fed rats results from an increase in enzyme protein (209). Ashby et al. (13) have recently proposed a scheme for the synthesis and release of the enzyme from adipocytes that probably applies equally to the release of the enzyme from parenchymal cells of other tissues [Table 6; (14)]. The synthesis of a proenzyme is regulated by insulin and corticosteroids (14). The next step is hormone and energy independent but requires glucose and probably involves the glycosylation of the proenzyme (307, 376). Inhibiting glycosylation with tunicamycin completely inhibits enzyme secretion (86, 211). The complete, active enzyme is released from the cell by microtubular transport, a mechanism suggested by the inhibition of enzyme secretion by colchicine (73, 89).

Ashby et al. (13, 14) suggested that catecholamine

TABLE 6. *Intracellular Regulation of Lipoprotein Lipase Synthesis*

Stimulation		Inhibition
	Amino Acids	
Insulin, glucocorticoids	→ (Synthesis) ←	Cycloheximide
	Proenzyme	
Glucose	→ Glycosylation ←	Tunicamycin
	↓ (Activation)	
	*Active Enzyme**	
	Microtubular transport ←	Colchicine
	↓ (Secretion)	
	Interstitial transport	
	↓ (Mechanism unknown)	
	Endothelial transport	
	↓ (Mechanism unknown)	
	Capillary lumen (Active site)	

* Catecholamines and theophylline inactivate enzyme.

TABLE 7. *Characteristics of Purified Lipoprotein Lipase Isolated From Various Tissues*

Source	Molecular Weight × 10³	Carbohydrate Content, %	Ref.
Postheparin plasma			
Human	75	a	104
Human[b]	69	8	15
Human[c]	67	8	15
Rat	72		133
Rat[d]	37.5	6.9	132
Rat[e]	69.25	10	133
Heart			
Rat	34	3.3	82
Rat	60		396
Pig	73		103
Adipose tissue			
Pig	60–62	a	32
Chicken	60		79
Milk			
Human	63		193
Bovine	62–66	a	102
Bovine	55	2.7	222

[a] Carbohydrate present but not quantitated. [b] Enzyme of hepatic origin. [c] Enzyme of extrahepatic origin, i.e., true lipoprotein lipase. [d] High-affinity lipoprotein lipase probably released from heart. [e] Low-affinity lipoprotein lipase probably released from adipose tissue.

inactivation of the enzyme just prior to its secretion from the parenchymal cell also controls enzyme activity. In the first step, hormonal regulation of proenzyme synthesis, glucocorticoids probably enhance lipoprotein lipase activity (14, 43, 44, 96, 181) at the level of RNA synthesis (14), whereas insulin probably stimulates protein synthesis generally (14, 376). Recent studies (225) suggest that fluctuations in hormone concentrations are great enough to account for the nutrition-associated changes in adipose tissue lipoprotein lipase activity (14). The second step, conversion of proenzyme to complete enzyme, is essential for enzyme secretion and probably involves glycosylation of the proenzyme protein (86, 211). Evidence that tunicamycin (a specific inhibitor of glycosylation) inhibits enzyme secretion (86, 211), that purified lipoprotein lipase is a glycosylated protein (Table 7), and that glycosylation of proteins is usually necessary for their secretion from cells (100) supports this assumption. The possible additional step of regulation of enzyme activity (inactivating the complete enzyme just before its release from the cell) by catecholamines (13, 14) could rapidly alter the functional activity at the endothelial surface. Ashby et al. (13) suggested that such a rapid change effected by adrenergic stimuli would stop triglyceride uptake more rapidly than changing the rate of enzyme synthesis.

Ontogeny of Lipoprotein Lipase

The main supply of calories changes suddenly at birth from primarily carbohydrate and fatty acids to the fetus to primarily milk triglyceride to the newborn.

Well-developed mechanisms of triglyceride clearing are therefore essential for the normal development of newborn mammals. Because it controls the supply of fatty acids at the tissue level, lipoprotein lipase is probably important in the growth and maturation of individual organs. Studies during the last several years suggest that local factors specific for each tissue regulate the development of lipoprotein lipase activity (75, 87, 180, 194, 195, 312, 317). Lipoprotein lipase activity in the heart is very low in the fetus and increases during the first 3 wk after birth (75, 180, 317); thus it is closely related to the developmental pattern of the heart, which in the rat differentiates only after birth (350). In the lung, contrary to the heart, lipoprotein lipase activity is detectable 5 days before birth, reaches its highest level 1 day before birth, and remains at ~50% of the adult activity level until weaning (75, 180, 195, 317). These studies show that enzyme activity is high during rapid surfactant synthesis characteristic of prenatal differentiation and maturation of the lung (119). Because VLDL are present in the fetal circulation at 21 days of gestation (11) (rat gestation period is 22 days), the lung could utilize triglyceride fatty acids in addition to free fatty acids for surfactant synthesis. Enzyme activity increases precociously after administration of dexamethasone (279), suggesting that the control mechanisms for lipoprotein lipase activity are similar in the fetal and adult lung (181).

Lipoprotein lipase might also play a special role during development in the brain (75). Lipoprotein lipase activity is low in brain except during the first 10 days after birth, when brain weight and cholesterol content increase dramatically (92). Because of the concomitant eightfold increase in 3-hydroxy-3-methylglutaryl-CoA reductase activity (386), Chajek et al. (75) suggested that lipoprotein lipase might be involved in the delivery of fatty acids necessary for the synthesis of phospholipids, which together with free cholesterol are necessary for cell membrane synthesis.

Lipoprotein lipase activity and the developmental pattern in adipose tissue differ according to location (75). Lipoprotein lipase activity in preadipocytes probably has a regulatory role in the lipid filling of this tissue during the early postnatal period (194). Lipoprotein lipase activity thus exhibits a triphasic pattern of activity: high during a period of active cell proliferation, declining toward the end of suckling, and high again when fat storage occurs. The mature control mechanisms are operative from birth in adipose tissue. Low levels of plasma insulin within the first 6 h after birth (43, 44) probably cause the decrease in lipoprotein lipase activity during this period (312); the reciprocity between lipoprotein lipase and hormone-sensitive lipase that normally exists in adipose tissue of adult rats (220, 309) is evident also in suckling pups (170). Skeletal muscle lipoprotein lipase probably contributes 60%–85% of the total triglyceride-clearing ability in suckling animals. Although enzyme activity develops in the early postnatal period in muscle, the mature control mechanisms are absent until 2 wk after birth in the rat. Thus fasting does not affect muscle lipoprotein lipase until the age of 14 days, when activity increases (317).

The liver is another organ where the lipase has high activity levels in the fetus and newborn but lacks the adult characteristics. Here resistance to 1 M NaCl (characteristic of hepatic lipase) develops only at weaning (75, 254).

The lipemia that develops at birth and persists for 1–3 days postnatally in the rat (180, 317) is probably related to low lipolytic activity in skeletal muscle (317). Inadequate clearing of circulating triglyceride is evident also during human development. If unable to feed orally after birth, premature infants may be maintained for weeks on parenteral nutrition (255). A major source of calories in parenteral feeding is Intralipid, a 10% triglyceride emulsion. Fat particles of Intralipid emulsion are similar in size to chylomicrons and, like the latter, are cleared from the circulation by lipoprotein lipase (167, 171, 298). Premature infants of gestational ages less than 32 wk clear this lipid emulsion less efficiently than infants at more than 32 wk of gestation or than term infants (8, 97, 361). Recent studies show that the impaired triglyceride clearing is directly related to low levels of postheparin lipolytic activity (97). This study indicates that lipoprotein lipase reserves are low in premature infants of 25–26 wk of gestation and suggests that in the human the lipid-clearing mechanisms are not well developed before 28 wk of gestation.

Characteristics of Lipoprotein Lipase

Lipoprotein lipase has been purified from several sources. Because of its high activity in bovine milk, this was one of the first sources from which a well-purified preparation of lipoprotein lipase was obtained (79, 102, 193). Another early source of enzyme was human postheparin plasma (104, 123, 133, 134). Purified preparations have been obtained from adipose tissue and heart of several species. The enzyme, isolated from different sources, is a glycoprotein with a molecular weight of 55,000–73,000 and a carbohydrate content of 3%–10%. The only exception seems to be a smaller-molecular-weight species isolated from heart (82) and from postheparin plasma (133) into which the enzyme is probably released from the heart (Table 7). Because postheparin plasma contains both lipoprotein lipase and hepatic lipase, the characteristics of both are listed in Table 7.

The amino acid composition of several of the lipoprotein lipase preparations (listed in Table 7) has recently been reported [Table 8; (15, 79, 82, 134, 304)]. Although the various preparations have general similarities, they probably represent different proteins. The two low-molecular-weight preparations [from pig heart (82) and postheparin plasma (134)] differ in both their amino acid composition and their carbohydrate content: 3.0% and 6.9%, respectively. Although the low-molecular-weight lipoprotein lipase isolated from postheparin plasma has the same high substrate affinity as the enzyme functioning at the vascular surface of the perfused heart (124, 130), this preparation probably also contains endothelial enzyme released from other tissues. The three lipoprotein lipase preparations from milk are very similar to each other. Hepatic lipase, i.e., heparin-released enzyme from liver (16, 235), which hydrolyzes triglycerides in the absence of the apoC-II cofactor and is not inhibited by high salt concentration or protamine sulfate (the two criteria used to identify lipoprotein lipase), has recently been purified from rat liver (237). This lipase was purified previously from postheparin plasma, and its amino acid composition has been determined (123, 304). There are marked differences in molecular weight between preparations of hepatic lipase isolated from liver perfusate and from postheparin plasma (237). The difference in amino acid composition between hepatic and extrahepatic lipases is greater in one study (304) than in another (15) probably because of differences in the purity of the preparations (304). Immunological studies indicate similarities and differences between different lipoprotein lipase preparations that are difficult to interpret. Thus antisera prepared against lipoprotein lipase isolated from chicken adipose tissue (226) or from rat heart (348) inhibit enzyme activity in other tissues of the same species. However, no antigenic determinant for milk lipoprotein lipase seems to be species specific; antibodies prepared against bovine milk lipoprotein lipase cross-react with lipoprotein lipase in human milk or with lipases in human postheparin plasma (192). There is no cross-reaction between hepatic lipase and extrahepatic lipoprotein lipase, which Augustin and Greten (16) attributed to differences in the carbohydrate moiety of the two enzymes. These investigators suggest that the main differences between these two enzymes, such as sensitivity to high ionic strength and the requirement of apoC-II for esterolytic activity, could be related to the differences in carbohydrate composition (16).

Mechanisms of Hydrolysis of Circulating Triglycerides

It is now well established that hydrolysis of lipoprotein triglycerides occurs at the luminal surface of the capillary endothelium (333, 355, 370, 379). Several questions therefore have to be answered: *1*) What is the distribution of lipoprotein lipase within tissues, i.e., how much of it is present at the capillary endothelium? *2*) To what extent does loss of endothelial enzyme interfere with the catabolism of lipoprotein triglyceride? *3*) Is the enzyme synthesized within the endothelium, or is it synthesized deeper in the tissue and transported later to the endothelium? *4*) What mechanism anchors the enzyme to the luminal side of the capillaries? Some of these questions have been

TABLE 8. *Amino Acid Composition of Lipoprotein Lipase and Hepatic Lipase*

Amino Acid	Rat LPL, Heart	Rat Postheparin Plasma "Heart" LPL*	Rat Postheparin Plasma "Adipose tissue" LPL†	Human Postheparin Plasma LPL	Human Postheparin Plasma HL	Human Postheparin Plasma LPL	Human Postheparin Plasma HL	Bovine Milk Lipase		
Valine, mol/10³ mol amino acid‡	50.2	62.0	63.3	§	§	52.8	53.4	63.8	§	§
Lysine	1.36	0.94	1.29			1.84	1.78	1.00		1.07
Histidine	0.43	0.22	0.34			0.45	0.45	0.36		0.43
Arginine	0.84	1.01	0.76			0.85	0.85	0.47		0.68
Aspartic acid	1.51	1.31	1.63	1.51	1.34	1.59	1.54	1.30	1.51	1.43
Threonine	1.10	0.94	0.79	0.84	1.27	1.20	1.17	0.87	0.80	0.78
Serine	1.68	1.23	1.33	1.40	1.25	1.44	1.16	1.20	1.19	1.21
Glutamic acid	2.66	2.55	1.61	1.63	2.02	2.21	2.12	1.77	1.28	1.21
Proline	0.88	0.76	0.94	0.77	0.86	0.85	0.85	0.87	0.71	0.64
Glycine	1.65	1.25	0.99	1.15	1.33	1.78	1.76	1.53	1.11	1.07
Alanine	1.44	1.21	1.03	1.05	0.96	1.21	1.30	1.30	0.82	0.82
Half-cystine	0.18	0.33	0.43			0.20	0.22	0.20		0.28
Methionine	0.18	0.33	0.24	0.18	0.33	0.14	0.15	0.20	0.24	0.25
Isoleucine	0.59	0.52	0.63	0.71	1.11	0.83	0.79	0.63	0.69	0.68
Leucine	1.57	1.40	1.35	0.99	1.58	1.51	1.51	1.20	1.14	1.00
Tyrosine	0.44	0.44	0.49	0.55	0.40	0.46	0.47	0.40	0.63	0.61
Phenylalanine	0.53	0.44	0.72	0.67	0.81	0.84	0.82	0.43	0.69	0.71
Tryptophan	0.12	0.21	0.22			0.47	0.46			0.28
Ref.	82	133	133	304	304	15	13	222	304	205

LPL, lipoprotein lipase; HL, hepatic lipase, with resistance to high salt concentration (1.0 M NaCl). * High-affinity LPL similar to that described in heart. † Low-affinity LPL similar to that described in adipose tissue. ‡ All other values are relative to valine measurements. § No absolute values were given.

answered; others are at present the subject of extensive investigation.

ENDOTHELIAL LIPOPROTEIN LIPASE. This section discusses the quantitative relationship of endothelial lipoprotein lipase to total tissue enzyme and to the hydrolysis of circulating triglyceride. Infusion of heparin into isolated perfused organs such as heart (48, 129, 130, 337), lung (177, 181), or adipose tissue (129, 130, 355) leads to the rapid release of lipoprotein lipase into the venous effluent. The amount of enzyme released varies with the tissue: 10%–15% of total tissue lipoprotein lipase is released from lung and adipose tissue and 25% or more from heart. Loss of endothelial enzyme dramatically decreases the ability of the tissue to hydrolyze infused lipoprotein triglyceride (48, 84, 129, 130, 355). Additional evidence that the easily accessible endothelial enzyme is directly related to triglyceride hydrolysis comes from recent studies in which specific antibodies have been prepared against rat (348) and bird lipoprotein lipase (226). These studies show that within 6 min after infusion of antibody to heart lipoprotein lipase, both enzyme activity and triglyceride hydrolysis are completely inhibited (348). Kompiang et al. (226) have shown that injecting antibody against lipoprotein lipase into roosters almost immediately increased plasma triglyceride concentration. Although the investigators did not measure lipoprotein lipase activity, they concluded that the instantaneous inhibition of triglyceride removal is a direct result of inhibition of the enzyme at sites within the plasma compartment readily accessible to immunoglobulins (33, 226). Indeed immunofluorescent techniques have recently shown binding of antibody to lipoprotein lipase at endothelial sites (235). Furthermore, as recently shown, the heparin-releasable hepatic lipase is located exclusively on the liver endothelial cells (400).

Chylomicrons attach to endothelial cells (41, 346, 356), become enmeshed in luminal projections of endothelial cells after intravenous injection, and are partially enveloped by these cells (Fig. 5). Present data suggest that chylomicrons and VLDL particles are too large to cross the capillary endothelium (41, 141, 261, 346, 355, 406, 410). Even in newborn animals, whose endothelial cells are not yet linked by tight junctions, the chylomicrons that pass through the gaps between cells are held back by the basement membrane and are thus prevented from entering the parenchyma (387). Hydrolysis of lipoprotein triglyceride would therefore have to occur at the luminal surface of endothelial cells. With histochemical techniques and light microscopy, early studies have localized lipoprotein lipase in the capillaries of adipose tissue (278). More detailed electron-microscope morphological studies in which lipoprotein lipase activity has been localized in adipose tissue by a modified Gomori dye technique show that reaction products are within vacuoles and vesicles of capillary endothelial cells and in the subendothelial space (41) and that no reaction product is in the capillary lumen or in or near fat cells. This study suggested that glycerides derived from chylomicrons are hydrolyzed in capillary endothelial cells and subendothelial spaces and that they cross the endothelium within a membrane-bounded system. Scow and co-workers (351) have suggested that in adipose tissue the products of lipolysis (fatty acids and monoglyceride) are transferred across the capillary wall by lateral movement in a continuous interface of various cell membranes to the endoplasmic reticulum of the fat cells, where they are reesterified. Monolayer studies of triglyceride hydrolysis with purified lipoprotein lipase show that free fatty acids and monoglyceride produced during lipolysis could move laterally in the interface and desorb from the surface when in contact with albumin (353).

ORIGIN OF ENDOTHELIAL LIPOPROTEIN LIPASE. The studies described above show that although heparin infusion releases the functional (endothelial) enzyme, considerable enzyme activity remains in the tissue (48, 129, 130, 177, 181, 337), suggesting that it is located at sites inaccessible to heparin. In fact lipoprotein lipase is present in isolated adipocytes (101, 336, 375, 376), heart mesenchymal cells (76, 77), myocytes (17, 81, 191), and mammary alveolar cells (83). However, whereas lipoprotein lipase activity is found in parenchymal cells maintained in tissue culture and might be the first expression of adipocytes in cultured fibroblasts (40, 101, 399), the enzyme is completely absent from cultured endothelial cells (199, 364, 404). Three primary cultures of endothelial cells isolated from bovine aorta (199), bovine pulmonary artery (364), and human umbilicus (404) contained no intrinsic lipoprotein lipase but could bind to purified lipoprotein lipase. Furthermore binding of enzyme to endothelial cells markedly stabilized its activity (364, 404) [purified lipoprotein lipase is very unstable in solution (122, 193, 205)]. These studies show that endothelial cells, although unable to synthesize lipoprotein lipase, can bind it (364), probably by means of heparan sulfate present on the surface of endothelial cells (64, 65, 407).

MECHANISM OF BINDING TO ENDOTHELIUM. A special role for a lipoprotein lipase–heparin interaction was evident from the earliest description of the enzyme, which was discovered in the circulation after heparin injection (169). The rapid release of the enzyme indicated that its location is close to the vascular lumen, suggesting that heparin interacts with the enzyme and releases it from the capillary endothelium (335). It was initially thought that heparin might be an integral part of the enzyme, necessary for catalytic activity (228); however, recent studies with purified preparations show that lipoprotein lipase contains less than 2% heparin and is fully active in its absence (204).

Studies during the last few years have clarified certain aspects of the heparin–lipoprotein lipase interaction. *1)* Purified lipoprotein lipase binds to heparin, heparan sulfate, or dermatan sulfate (31), suggesting that the iduronic acid present in these polysaccharides might play a role in the specific binding (300). The bond can be dissociated by high NaCl concentration, indicating an electrostatic interaction (26, 246). *2)* Heparan sulfate is the principal sulfated glycosaminoglycan of the glycocalyx of endothelial cells (64, 65, 407). *3)* Heparin binds specifically to the surface of various cell types (224, 246), including endothelial cells (150), and during this process displaces the endogenous glycosaminoglycan (234, 246). Based on these recent observations, Olivecrona et al. (300, 301) suggested the following scheme for the endothelial binding of lipoprotein lipase. Heparan sulfate occurs as a proteoglycan at the capillary endothelium. Its protein moiety is an integral part of the plasma membrane to which are anchored heparan sulfate chains 20–50 nm long. These polysaccharide chains in turn bind lipoprotein lipase. In this manner the enzyme may be able to interact with circulating lipoprotein particles at some distance from the plasma membrane (Fig. 4). Such a structural arrangement at the endothelium would explain the observation by Fielding and Higgins (130) that the kinetics of triglyceride hydrolysis by soluble lipoprotein lipase or endothelial enzyme are identical; furthermore the strong affinity between heparan sulfate and lipoprotein lipase would prevent detachment of the enzyme during its interaction with lipoprotein particles. Indeed little lipoprotein lipase is released into the circulation during assimilation of dietary fat (121). This model would also explain the short half-life of chylomicrons in the circulation, because several lipoprotein lipase molecules could simultaneously act on each lipoprotein particle (301). This theoretical scheme is strongly supported by studies of heparin–lipoprotein lipase interactions in cultured endothelial cells (364). These recent studies show that purified lipoprotein lipase attaches to endothelial cells through heparan sulfate on the cell surface and that adding heparin detaches lipoprotein lipase from the glycosaminoglycan and does not involve the release of a glycosaminoglycan–lipoprotein lipase complex.

Lipoprotein lipase–polysaccharide complexes are more resistant to inactivation than the free enzyme (204, 330). Binding purified lipoprotein lipase to endothelial cells stabilizes the enzyme, which is otherwise rapidly inactivated. Enzyme activity is equally enhanced when crude preparations of lipoprotein lipase are tested in the presence of heparin. The lipoprotein lipase–heparin complex is much more resistant to inactivation in vivo than when the enzyme is purified. Postheparin lipolytic activity has a half-life of 7–25 min in various species (417), whereas the purified enzyme is removed from the liver with a half-life in the circulation of ~1 min (402).

Heparan sulfate in the endothelial plasma membrane may be important in two additional aspects of lipoprotein lipase function. It may facilitate the last step in the transport of lipoprotein lipase from its site of synthesis to the luminal surface of the endothelium (301). Furthermore, because of electrostatic attraction between sulfated glycosaminoglycans and lipoproteins, it may enhance the interaction between lipoprotein lipase and circulating lipoprotein particles (203).

ROLE OF APOPROTEIN C-II. The requirement of serum proteins for optimal activity of lipoprotein lipase was established in the first studies of this enzyme (227, 230). This specific protein was identified as apoC-II, a polypeptide in the surface film of chylomicrons, VLDL, and HDL (127, 187, 239). The rate of triglyceride hydrolysis increases as a function of apoC-II concentration and is maximal at a 1:1 molar ratio of apoC-II to enzyme (82, 129). ApoC-II binds strongly to lipoprotein lipase (269), increasing the affinity of lipoprotein lipase for the lipid-water interface (29, 207, 349). Formation of the lipoprotein lipase–apoC-II complex is prevented by NaCl (126, 269), an inhibitor generally used to identify lipolytic activity as that of lipoprotein lipase. The apoC-II activation of lipolysis is inhibited by product (free fatty acid) accumulation at the site of lipolysis (299, 370). These in vitro studies suggest that apoC-II forms a complex with lipoprotein lipase at the surface of the endothelium, facilitating the hydrolysis of lipoprotein triglyceride (163, 370). Generally there is an excess of apoC-II on the surface of both chylomicrons and VLDL, suggesting that under normal conditions apoC-II is never rate limiting for extrahepatic lipolysis (256).

Recent studies with purified apoC-II have identified the specific functions of several of its regions (233). Table 9 summarizes these findings. ApoC-II is a peptide containing 78 amino acids; the first 50 NH$_2$-terminal amino acid residues are not involved in enzyme activation. The primary function of residues 43–50 appears to be lipid binding (208, 277) to phosphatidylcholine (70). Smith and Scow (370) proposed that this region retains apoC-II in the lipoprotein particle. Apparently a similar interaction with lipoprotein lipase exists because in the presence of high salt concentrations, which prevent activation of the enzyme by apoC-II, the enzyme nevertheless remains tightly bound to lipoproteins (126). The NH$_2$-terminal residues 58–78 are essential for lipoprotein lipase activation (70, 223, 282). Removing the COOH-terminal tripeptide Gly-Glu-Glu decreases the activation capacity by 95%. An electrostatic binding between the two COOH-terminal glutamic acid residues of apoC-II and positively charged regions of the enzyme that high concentrations of anions specifically disrupt has been suggested. Residues 55–67 probably interact specifically with the enzyme, changing the enzyme structure and thus stimulating enzyme activity (370).

ROLE OF APOPROTEIN E. ApoE (343) may play a role

402   HANDBOOK OF PHYSIOLOGY ~ THE RESPIRATORY SYSTEM I

FIG. 5. Attachment of circulating chylomicrons to capillary endothelium of various tissues. *A*: longitudinal section of capillary in lactating rat mammary gland taken 10 min after intravenous injection of chylomicrons (*Ch*). Many chylomicrons of various sizes are in capillary lumen (*Lu*). Cytoplasmic processes (*P*) extend from surface of endothelium (*E*) into capillary lumen. Chylomicrons in lumen are in contact with endothelial luminal surface (*large arrows*) and enmeshed by cytoplasmic processes (*small arrows*). *S*, secretory cell; *N*, nucleus; *B*, basement membrane; *ECS*, extracellular space; *L*, lipid droplet; *ER*, endoplasmic reticulum. × 10,000. (Micrograph courtesy of E. J. Blanchette-Mackie.) *B*: longitudinal section of capillary in interscapular brown adipose tissue of 8-day-old rat 3 min after intravenous injection of chylomicrons. Many chylomicrons are in capillary lumen in contact with the luminal surface of the endothelial cell and enmeshed by cytoplasmic processes of endothelium. Endothelial cell has basal processes (*BP*) that extend into extracellular space to adipocytes (*A*). *RBC*, erythrocytes; *M*, mitochondria. × 10,000. (Micrograph courtesy of E. J. Blanchette-Mackie.) *C*: cardiac muscle capillary. Section through profiles of two capillaries (*C*) containing chylomicrons from heart of a 24-h-fasted adult rat. Chylomicrons injected intravenously 2 min prior to fixation. Many cytoplasmic projections extend into capillary lumen making contact with chylomicron surfaces. Endothelial cell cytoplasm (*E*) contains numerous vesicles often open to either luminal or abluminal cell surface. *L*, myocyte lipid droplet; *My*, myocyte. × 17,000. (Micrograph courtesy of M. G. Wetzel.) *D*: endothelial cell from mainstem pulmonary artery of dog. Endothelial projections on luminal surface may be involved in entrapment of chylomicrons and lipid droplets. × 34,000. [From Smith and Ryan (371).] *E,F*: detail of chylomicron–capillary endothelium interaction. *E*: detail of capillary endothelium in interscapular brown adipose tissue of an 8-day-old rat taken 3 min after intravenous injection of chylomicrons. A chylomicron is in contact with endothelial cell surface at a point where cell is attenuated (*arrow*). Width of this small-diameter capillary is ~1 µm. × 90,000. (Micrograph courtesy of E. J. Blanchette-Mackie.) *F*: detail of capillary in lactating rat mammary gland 10 min after intravenous injection of chylomicrons. Endothelium shows vesicles (*v*) and a long cytoplasmic process that projects into capillary lumen enmeshing a chylomicron. *G*, glycogen; *Co*, collagen. × 80,000. (Micrograph courtesy of E. J. Blanchette-Mackie.)

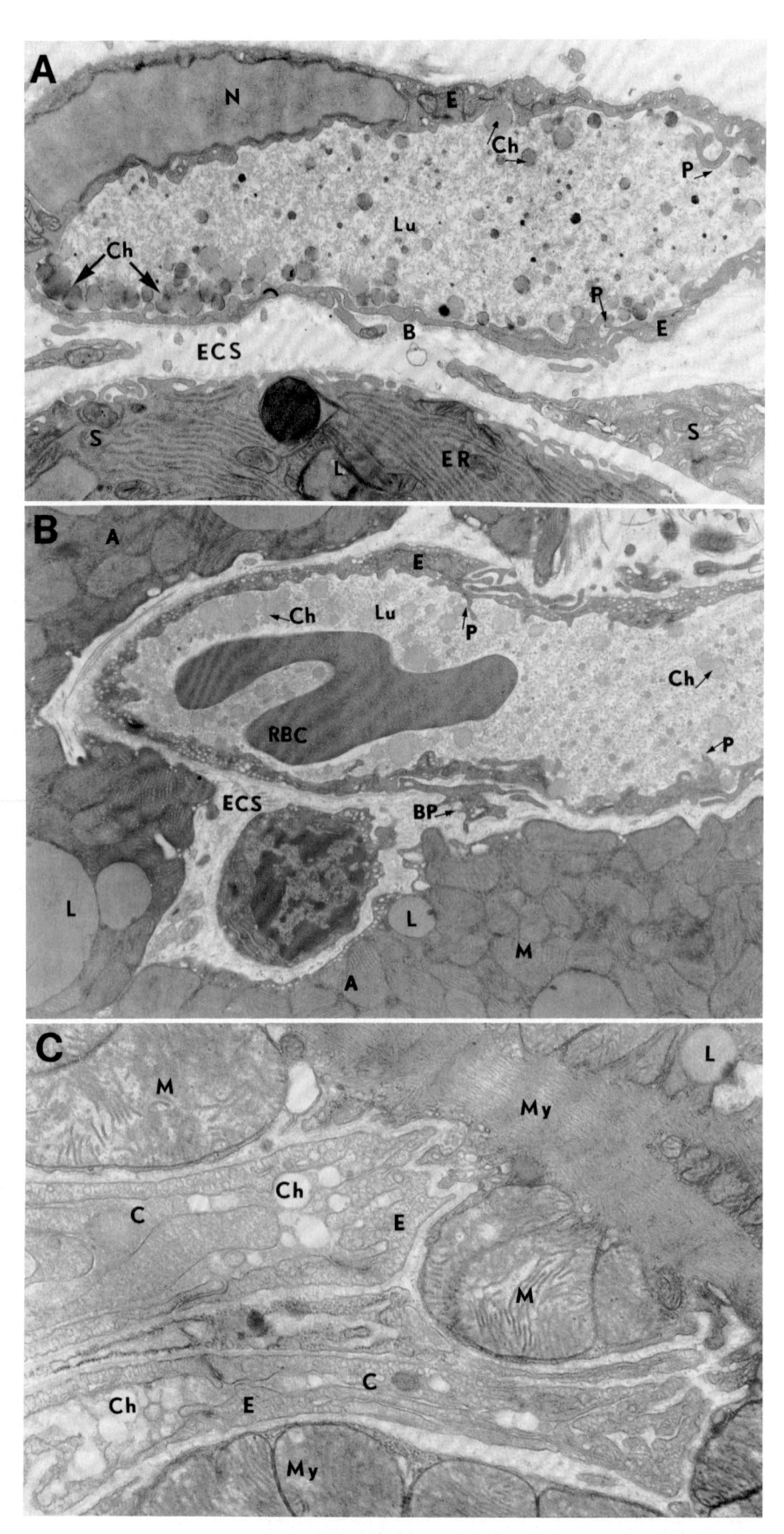

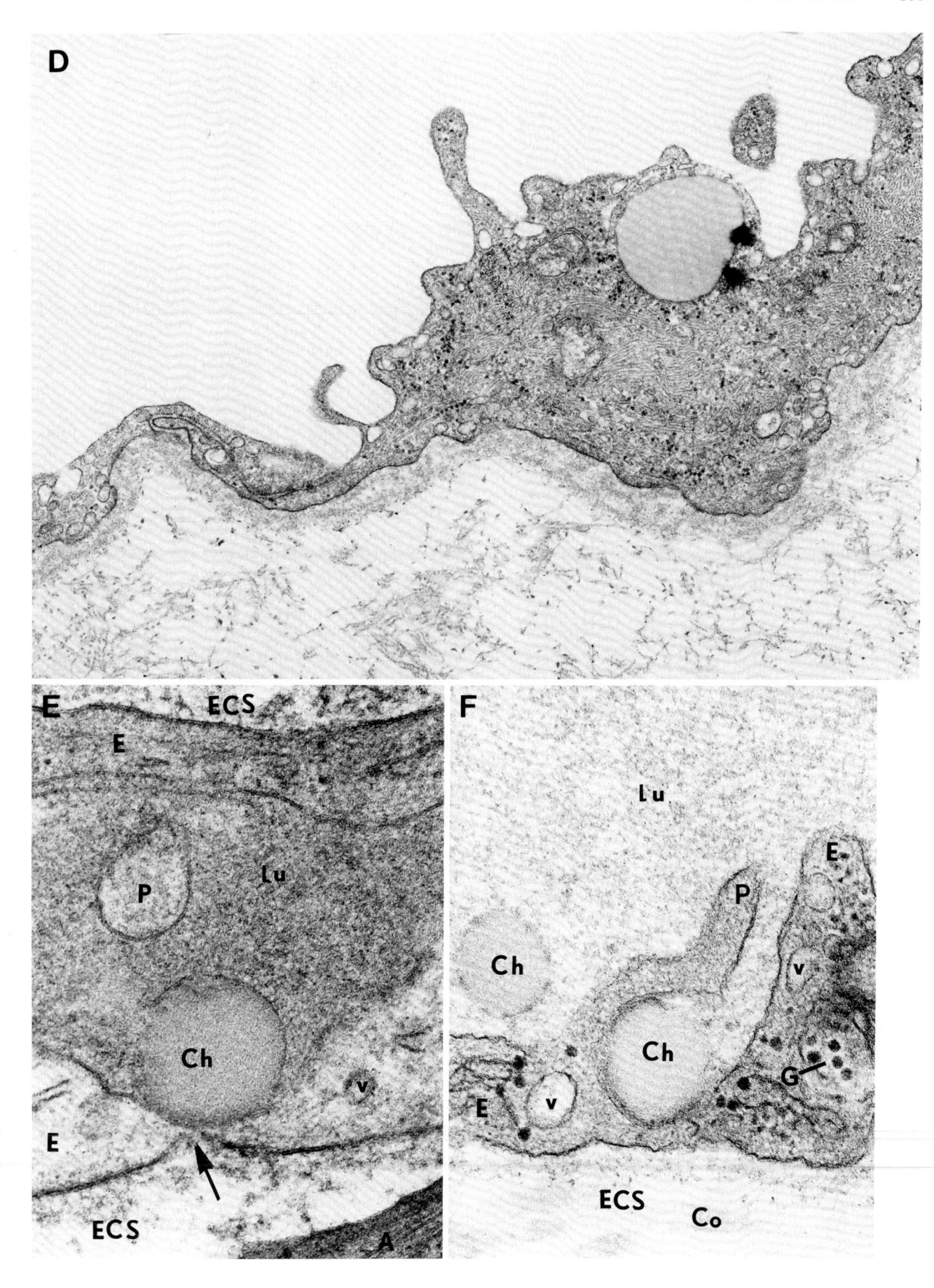

CHAPTER 12: LIPOPROTEINS AND LIPOPROTEIN LIPASE 403

TABLE 9. *Functions of Apoprotein C-II*

Peptide NH$_2$-Terminal Segment of Amino Acid	Function	Physiological Significance	Ref.
1–50	Phospholipid binding, especially 43–50	Interacts with lipoproteins and lipoprotein lipase	70, 208, 277
55–78	Change in lipoprotein lipase structure	Activates lipoprotein lipase	70, 223, 281
76–78	Ionic binding to lipoprotein lipase	Inhibited by anions	370

in the interaction between lipoprotein lipase and triglyceride-rich lipoproteins (86, 380). This recent suggestion is based on the following findings. Under physiological conditions apoE is the only apoprotein that binds to heparin (259, 358), and its binding to artificial substrates increases their hydrolysis by lipoprotein lipase (118). ApoE amounts to 15% of total VLDL apoprotein content (118); furthermore it is rapidly acquired by chylomicrons after they enter the circulation (202). Therefore, by attaching the lipoprotein particle to the capillary endothelium through a link between apoE and heparan sulfate, apoE may facilitate hydrolysis of lipoprotein triglyceride. Because lipoprotein lipase is present at the same site, this would affect the association between enzyme and circulating lipoprotein particles. In addition to its possible role in triglyceride removal, apoE is probably involved in the removal of cholesterol-rich lipoprotein remnants by the liver (184, 413).

Characteristics of Lipolytic Activity of Lipoprotein Lipase

Substrate specificity studies have shown a positional specificity for the primary ester bonds of triglycerides and diglycerides (275, 292). Fatty acid chain length and degree of unsaturation do not affect enzyme activity (276). In vitro the monoglycerides accumulate during hydrolysis of chylomicron triglyceride (128, 357); in vivo, however, the monoglycerides are hydrolyzed by monoglyceride hydrolase present in several tissues (164, 393, 403) and in platelets (63). Under certain conditions monoglycerides are hydrolyzed by lipoprotein lipase (27, 165).

Lipoprotein lipase has limited phospholipase activity, which enables it to hydrolyze the primary acyl bond of phosphatidylcholine and phosphatidylethanolamine (165, 354). Recent in vitro studies, however, show that purified lipoprotein lipase hydrolyzes ~40% of VLDL phospholipids, suggesting that the enzyme might contribute significantly to the catabolism of the surface coat of lipoproteins (108). Perhaps hydrolysis of phosphatidylcholine in the surface film of chylomicrons and VLDL exposes the neutral lipid core to the action of lipoprotein lipase; however, recent studies suggest that the surface film of lipoproteins contains significant amounts of triglyceride (368) that would thus be available to lipoprotein lipase even without prior hydrolysis of surface phospholipids.

Hydrolysis of phosphatidylcholine (165, 281, 383) and monoglyceride (27) is stimulated by apoC-II and inhibited by accumulation of free fatty acids. Recent studies on the mechanism of product inhibition (30) suggest that three factors cause inhibition. *1*) The products of lipolysis (free fatty acids and monoglycerides), being more surface active than the triglyceride substrate, concentrate at the lipid-water interface and displace the triglyceride (351). Also, because they are substrates of the enzyme, they competitively inhibit lipolysis. *2*) Accumulation of free fatty acids suppresses the activating effect of apoC-II. *3*) Free fatty acids bind to lipoprotein lipase (18, 29). Whether free fatty acids bind to the lipid binding region of the enzyme (28) is not known.

The strong product inhibition may regulate the level of lipoprotein hydrolysis at the capillary endothelium, ensuring that the production of free fatty acids does not exceed their uptake by the tissue (30). Suppression of the apoC-II effect is probably linked to weaker enzyme-particle binding, resulting in the detachment of the lipoprotein particle. Indeed individual lipoprotein particles may attach and detach several times to or from endothelium during hydrolysis of triglyceride (343).

LIPOPROTEIN LIPASE IN LUNG

The lungs have a unique location in the circulation; they receive the entire cardiac output and the lymphatic drainage of the gastrointestinal tract directly through the superior vena cava (136). The extensiveness of the pulmonary capillary bed (135), the small caliber of its vessels (135, 136), and the direct delivery to the lung of lymph rich in chylomicrons and VLDL suggest that the lung could be the site of the first step in the catabolism of triglyceride-rich lipoproteins. Furthermore triglyceride fatty acids might be important substrates for lung metabolism (120) and precursors of surfactant synthesis (283). Several groups (25, 52, 213, 286, 418, 419) have reported removal of circulating lipoprotein triglyceride by the lung. However, whereas some studies suggest that lipoprotein triglyceride is retained only temporarily and released later into the circulation (418, 419), others have shown that chylomicron triglyceride is hydrolyzed during uptake by the lung (213).

The endothelial cells of lung capillaries are joined by tight junctions (371) that prevent the uptake of lipoprotein particles; lipoprotein triglycerides (in chylomicrons and VLDL) therefore have to be hydrolyzed at the vascular endothelium before the uptake of triglyceride fatty acids into the lung. Lipoprotein lipase, the enzyme that controls the hydrolysis of triglyceride at the capillary wall, is therefore essential for the uptake of triglyceride fatty acids by the lung.

Although lipolytic activity was described in the lung as early as 1908 (341, 365), the nature of the lipolytic enzymes has not been well defined. Indeed most early reports have probably measured the activity of a second lipase active in the hydrolysis of intracellular lipid, i.e., leading to release of free fatty acids from the lung (188, 397) rather than uptake of triglyceride fatty acids from the circulation. The level of this second lipase amounts to ~20% of the total lipolytic activity of the lung (51, 183).

Early studies on the origin of the clearing factor (lipoprotein lipase) yielded conflicting results for the role of the lung. Anfinsen et al. (9) suggested that heart and lung have the greatest ability to initiate lipid clearing. Korn (227) on the other hand indicated that the lipolytic activity in the lung differs from lipoprotein lipase.

Tissue Distribution and Regulation of Activity

Evidence for the presence of lipoprotein lipase in the lung was first presented by Felts (120), who reported that VLDL triglyceride fatty acids are taken up by rabbit lung slices. Several reports have since confirmed the presence of lipoprotein lipase in the lung (1, 51, 88, 177, 308, 322). Recent studies (88) show that lipoprotein lipase activity is present in the lungs of many animal species (Table 10). There are, however, marked differences between species in the level of activity and the response to various stimuli (Table 10). For example, in mouse lung the enzyme is markedly affected by nutritional state (88), whereas in the rat the activity remains constant in fed and fasted animals (88, 177). Female mice have twice the activity level of males (88); however, in the rat the sex difference, although present, is less pronounced (181). Furthermore barbiturates inhibit lipoprotein lipase activity in mouse lung (367) but not in rat lung (99). Lipoprotein lipase in the lung has been studied most extensively in the rat (51, 99, 177, 181, 308, 322). Studies on the hormonal control of lipoprotein lipase

TABLE 10. *Lipoprotein Lipase Activity in Lung*

Species	Activity Level,* μmol FFA·g^{-1}·h^{-1}	Sex Differences	Nutrition	Ref.
Rat	10–30	Female ≥ Male	No effect	151, 177, 178
Mouse	15–40	Female > Male	Fasting	151
Rabbit	12		Fasting	151
Hamster	12	Male = Female	Fasting	151
Dog	14			388

* Activity level of fed males.   FFA, free fatty acid.   (Data from refs. 88, 177, 241.)

TABLE 11. *Regulation of Lipoprotein Lipase Activity in Rat Lung*

Condition or Treatment	Duration	Activity, % of Control	Ref.
Control*		100	308, 322
Glucocorticoids,* 200 μg·kg^{-1}·day^{-1}	8 days	170	
Thyroxine, 1 mg·kg^{-1}·day^{-1}	6 days	116	
Ovariectomy	3 wk	99	
Estradiol-17β, 250 μg·kg^{-1}·wk^{-1}	8 wk	100	181
Progesterone, 25 mg·kg^{-1}·wk^{-1}	8 wk	103	
Lactation	5–10 days	110	
Diabetes, streptozocin induced	7 days	120	
Alloxan diabetes	3 mo	185	308
Cold exposure, 4°C	1 day	186	322

Lipoprotein lipase activity quantitated in acetone ether powders or fresh homogenate of rat lung.   * Endothelial lipoprotein lipase activity released from perfused lung or lung slices by heparin was 15%–20% of total lung lipoprotein lipase (51, 177, 181).

activity in the lung show that activity increases after glucocorticoid administration (181) or exposure to low temperature (322), whereas thyroxine, sex hormones, and prolactin (lactation) do not affect enzyme activity [Table 11; (181)].

In the lung, as previously reported for other tissues, the enzyme is present at two sites: the parenchyma and endothelial surface (51, 84, 177, 181). Ten to twenty percent of the total lung enzyme is present in the endothelium at a site from which it is released within 2–5 min after heparin infusion. To assess the functional role of the endothelial enzyme in the lung, lipids were infused into an isolated, ventilated lung preparation of rats that received heparin 1 h before surgery (Fig. 6). The data show that loss of endothelial enzyme almost completely inhibits the hydrolysis of circulating triglycerides. Hydrolysis of diglycerides was reduced to 50% of its normal level, whereas the absence of endothelial lipoprotein lipase did not affect the hydrolysis of monoglycerides. These results confirm earlier reports of monoglyceride lipase in the lung (403) and suggest that in the lung, as in several other tissues (164, 393), the last step in the hydrolysis of circulating triglycerides (i.e., hydrolysis of monoglyceride) occurs deeper within the tissue (355) and is independent of endothelial lipoprotein lipase.

Lung Lipoprotein Lipase in Disease

The level of lipoprotein lipase in the lung has been measured in several clinical conditions.

DIABETES. Reports on lipid composition and the level of lipoprotein lipase activity in the lung in experimental diabetes conflict. The total lipid content of the lung in diabetic animals is not different from that in controls. However, whereas one study reports an in-

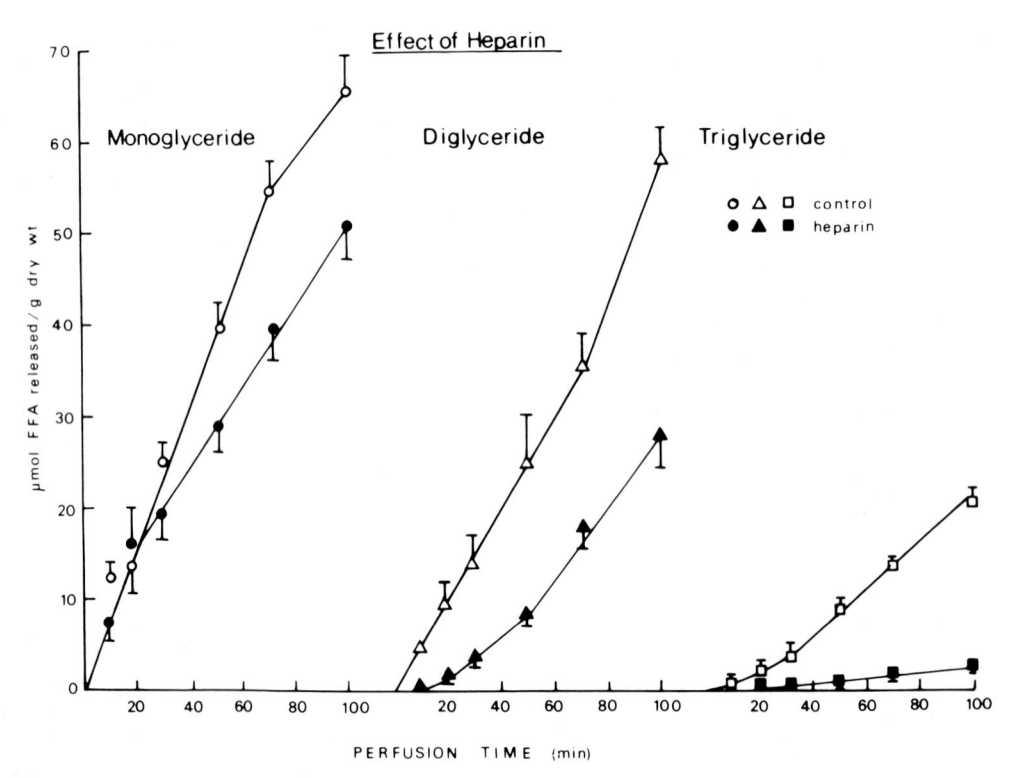

FIG. 6. Hydrolysis of glycerides by isolated perfused rat lung. Effect of loss of endothelial enzyme on rate of hydrolysis. Control, normal male Sprague-Dawley rats. Heparin, animals received 100 units/kg heparin 1 h before perfusion with tri-, di-, or monoglyceride. FFA, free fatty acid.

crease in lung phospholipids accompanied by a fall in triglyceride levels (384), several others report the opposite, i.e., a slight decrease in lung phospholipids and an increase in neutral fat (308, 329). These differences may be related to the species studied [rabbit (384) or rat (308, 329)]. A rise in lung neutral lipid in chronic alloxan diabetes has been ascribed to an increase in lipoprotein lipase activity (308). However, enzyme activity in acute streptozocin diabetes does not change [Table 11; (181)]. No conclusion can yet be reached about lipoprotein lipase activity in the diabetic lung, although lipid metabolism has been shown to depend on normal plasma insulin levels (282).

TRAUMA. Limited, nonhypotensive trauma (simple bone fracture) in the dog within 5 h markedly reduces heparin-releasable lipoprotein lipase in the lung. Concomitantly lung parenchymal enzyme increases (241). It is not known whether posttraumatic reduction in endothelial enzyme is common to other tissues or is limited to the lung. Catecholamine inhibition of enzyme release could increase parenchymal enzyme with concomitant reduction in enzyme release (14). The decrease in endothelial enzyme could also be the result of prolonged barbiturate anesthesia, which recently has been shown to markedly decrease heparin-releasable (endothelial) lipoprotein lipase in mouse lung (367). Such a decrease in functional enzyme could explain the pathogenesis of posttraumatic lipemia, which is mainly caused by high levels of VLDL (200).

Hillman and Le Quire (196) have suggested that adherence of VLDL to the pulmonary endothelium is a factor in the pathogenesis of fat embolism. It is conceivable that in the absence of lipoprotein lipase, VLDL are not released from a possible apoE-mediated link to the vascular endothelium (a step that usually follows lipolysis) and accumulate within capillaries. There is evidence that Intralipid particles (0.3–1.0 μm) and fat emulsion particles coalesce in situ in lipoprotein lipase–deficient lungs (99). Whether there is any relationship between low lipoprotein lipase activity, decreased availability of triglyceride fatty acids, and lower surfactant levels associated with certain types of trauma (99) cannot be answered at present.

SEVERE LIPEMIA. Loss of lipoprotein lipase from the lung has been reported in severe experimental hypertriglyceridemia (99). Release of the enzyme from the lung to the circulation was directly related to the circulating levels of VLDL and probably occurred as a result of the enzyme binding to lipoprotein particles at the endothelial surface. Such enzyme loss does not occur at normal plasma VLDL concentrations (333). Thus a decrease in lipoprotein lipase release from parenchyma to endothelium as a result of trauma (241) would lead to lipemia, and the rise in plasma VLDL levels would in turn deplete the endothelium of the already low levels of lipoprotein lipase, further impairing the clearing ability of the lung.

High levels of triglycerides in the lung vascular bed

have recently been implicated in pulmonary complications of newborn infants given parenteral nutrition containing Intralipid (10% soybean triglyceride emulsion) and in cases of acute pancreatitis in adults (219, 405). Because lipoprotein lipase is the key enzyme in the breakdown of circulating triglycerides (in lipoproteins and Intralipid particles), it is probably involved in these clinical conditions. In the first condition, triglycerides accumulate in the pulmonary circulation, eventually leading to pulmonary embolism and death (21, 93, 243) because of inefficient clearing due to low levels of lipoprotein lipase in preterm infants (8, 97, 361). In the second condition (acute pancreatitis), various degrees of respiratory failure are common (219, 405) but the pathogenesis of the pulmonary injury is unknown. Animal studies designed to mimic the clinical condition suggest that intravascular hydrolysis of triglycerides and release of free fatty acids in the lung vascular bed are the cause of the pulmonary injury that results in edema (221).

Accumulation of free fatty acids in the lung may markedly affect the turnover of elastin, influencing the structural integrity of the lung. A sudden rise in free fatty acid concentration in the lung vascular bed followed by diffusion of fatty acids into the interstitium could stimulate elastolysis and thus lead to pulmonary edema. Hydrolysis of elastin is markedly enhanced by hydrophobic anionic molecules, such as saturated and unsaturated fatty acids (214). Furthermore free fatty acids interfere with the synthesis of elastin by inhibiting the activity of lysyloxidase, an essential enzyme that controls cross-linking of elastin, the final step in elastin biosynthesis (215).

Origin

Recent studies on endothelial cell cultures derived from bovine pulmonary artery show that these cells do not synthesize the enzyme but have the capacity to bind it (364). Attachment of purified lipoprotein lipase to cultured endothelial cells markedly stabilizes the enzyme, which in free form is extremely unstable (364). In other tissues, such as heart and adipose tissue, the enzyme is synthesized by mesenchymal cells and then transported to the luminal surface of the capillary endothelium (76, 375). It is therefore tempting to suggest that mesenchymal cells like the recently described lipid interstitial cell (398) are the site of synthesis of lung lipoprotein lipase. This fibroblast appears in the lung after birth, is filled with lipid, and contains few other cytoplasmic organelles. The lipid composition of these cells is similar to that of serum lipids (262), suggesting that it is derived from lipoprotein triglyceride through the action of lipoprotein lipase. This fibroblast thus resembles the 3T3-Li fibroblast that differentiates into adipocytes (375). Indeed accumulation of fat in the 3T3 cell and its differentiation into adipocytes coincides with the appearance of lipoprotein lipase activity in the cell (375).

The main difference between the 3T3 cell and the lung lipid interstitial cell is that at weaning the former retains its fat and the latter loses its fat droplets. This could be related to the different functions of the cell in the two tissues—fat storage is the main function of adipose tissue; in the lung, triglyceride fatty acids are the energy source and precursors of phospholipids. Accumulation of fat in these cells between birth and weaning might be related to a higher influx of particulate lipoprotein triglyceride into the lung interstitium, because at this age the tight junctions are not yet fully developed in the endothelium and because the capillary basement membrane, the second barrier to particulate lipid (387), is incomplete (54). One may assume that, if indeed this cell synthesizes lipoprotein lipase in the developing lung, it can maintain this ability in the adult.

Functions

LIPID METABOLISM. As recently shown, the release of lipid components of lipoproteins other than triglycerides is related to the activity of lipoprotein lipase. Lipoprotein lipase activity in mammary tissue is related not only to the rate of chylomicron triglyceride uptake but also to the uptake of chylomicron cholesterol (423). Furthermore triglyceride depletion is associated with removal of phospholipid from circulating chylomicrons and VLDL (111). One may therefore assume that lipoprotein lipase facilitates the tissue uptake of the core components of lipoproteins (triglyceride fatty acids) and the surface film components (cholesterol and phosphatidylcholine). Whether this mechanism provides phospatidylcholine in addition to free fatty acids to the lung is unknown. It has recently been shown that 90% of surfactant cholesterol is derived from exogenous cholesterol supplied by serum lipoproteins (183a).

APOPROTEIN METABOLISM. ApoC, the major protein component of VLDL, has two important functions: 1) activation of lipoprotein lipase (239) and 2) inhibition of receptor-mediated hepatic uptake of cholesterol-rich lipoprotein remnants (413). Therefore it affects both the first step in lipoprotein catabolism (reduction of triglyceride core) and the final step (removal of lipoprotein remnants by liver). The main apoprotein components of LDL (apoB) and HDL (apoA-I and apoA-II) are catabolized with the lipoprotein particle. On the other hand the apoC group shuttles back and forth in the circulation between various lipoprotein classes and is not metabolized with a specific lipoprotein group; indeed little is known about its catabolism. Proteolysis of apoC in the isolated perfused lung has recently been reported (315, 373). There seems to be a link between lipoprotein lipase–mediated lipolysis (probably reduction of VLDL core) and concomitant production of apoprotein-containing free surface film. Thus a selective degradation of the protein portion of

VLDL occurred only when heparin was included in the perfusion medium. Because heparin rapidly releases endothelial lipoprotein lipase, the study indicates that the presence of lipoprotein lipase in the recycling perfusion medium is a prerequisite for the breakdown of apolipoproteins. Indeed the assumption that lipolysis precedes proteolysis of the apoprotein portion of the lipoproteins is based on the recent observation that breakdown of the purified, delipidated apoprotein by the isolated perfused lung occurs in the absence of heparin (373).

Lipoprotein lipase in the lung initiates the catabolism of circulating VLDL and chylomicrons by facilitating the removal of part of the lipid components; however, the concomitant breakdown of the C-II apoprotein moiety of the lipoprotein probably stops lipoprotein lipase activity by depriving the enzyme of its specific activator. Degradation of apoC-II in the lung could have important physiological functions. Proteolysis of apoC-II would prevent extensive lipolysis, preventing the production of free fatty acid levels that might exceed the capacity of the transport mechanism. Therefore under normal conditions free fatty acids would not diffuse into the interstitium where they could cause extensive structural damage.

The vascular system of the lung is much less susceptible to atherosclerosis than are the organs perfused by the systemic circulation (189); the difference in blood pressure can explain this phenomenon. It is not known whether the low incidence of atherosclerosis and the lung's high capacity for the catabolism of the protein moiety of VLDL are related. These observations suggest that lipoprotein lipase activity in the lung leads to the removal of only part of the lipid components of circulating lipoproteins before inactivation of the enzyme; this would lead to the formation of remnant particles that are relatively rich in triglycerides.

Zilversmit (420) has recently suggested that atherogenesis may result from the formation of cholesterol-rich remnants in proximity to the arterial endothelium where VLDL or chylomicrons are degraded by arterial lipoprotein lipase (98, 190). In support of this hypothesis are recent observations of chylomicron cholesterol uptake by endothelial (125, 134) and smooth muscle cells (137) and of a relationship between lipoprotein lipase activity and cholesterol deposition in arteries of cholesterol-fed rabbits (85). One may speculate that the triglyceride-rich remnants formed in the pulmonary circulation have a lower tendency to deposit in the arterial intima. Removal of apoC-II from the lipoprotein surface might also enhance hepatic receptor–mediated uptake and catabolism of triglyceride-rich lipoproteins.

The pulmonary microcirculation is the initial capillary bed traversed by newly formed VLDL. Therefore the lung may perform the first metabolic alterations of these molecules.

We thank Nancy Roberts, Deborah Washington, Cheryl Tillson, and Caricia Fisher for help in preparing the manuscript and Helen Bagdoian, MLS, and Ernest Lee, MLS, Georgetown University Medical Center Dahlgren Library for help with the literature search.

The authors' studies cited in this chapter are supported by National Institutes of Health Grant HL-19056.

REFERENCES

1. ABE, K., AND K. YOSHIMURA. Changes in lipoprotein lipase activity in tissues of rats exposed to cold of various durations. *J. Physiol. Soc. Jpn.* 34: 81–82, 1972.
2. AKANUMA, Y., AND J. A. GLOMSET. In vitro incorporation of cholesterol-^{14}C into very low density lipoprotein cholesteryl esters. *J. Lipid Res.* 9: 620–626, 1968.
3. ALAUPOVIC, P., G. KOSTNER, D. M. LEE, W. J. MCCONATHY, AND H. MAGNANI. Peptide composition of human plasma apolipoproteins A, B and C. *Expo. Annu. Biochim. Med.* 31: 145–160, 1972.
4. ALBERS, J. J., AND E. L. BIERMAN. The effect of hypoxia on uptake and degradation of low density lipoproteins by cultured human arterial smooth muscle cells. *Biochim. Biophys. Acta* 424: 422–429, 1976.
5. ALOUSI, A. A., AND S. MALLOV. Effects of hyperthyroidism, epinephrine, and diet on heart lipoprotein lipase activity. *Am. J. Physiol.* 206: 603–609, 1964.
6. ANDERSON, N. G., AND B. FAWCETT. An antichylomicronemic substance produced by heparin injection. *Proc. Soc. Exp. Biol. Med.* 74: 768–771, 1951.
7. ANDERSON, R. G. W., J. L. GOLDSTEIN, AND M. S. BROWN. Localization of low density lipoprotein receptors on plasma membrane of normal human fibroblasts and their absence in cells from a familial hypercholesterolemia homozygote. *Proc. Natl. Acad. Sci. USA* 73: 2434–2438, 1976.
8. ANDREW, G., G. CHAN, AND D. SCHIFF. Lipid metabolism in the neonate. I. The effects of Intralipid infusion on plasma triglyceride and free fatty acid concentrations in the neonate. *J. Pediatr.* 88: 273–278, 1976.
9. ANFINSEN, C. B., E. BOYLE, AND R. K. BROWN. The role of heparin in lipoprotein metabolism. *Science* 115: 583–586, 1952.
10. APPLEBAUM, D. M., A. P. GOLDBERG, O. J. PYKÄLISTÖ, J. D. BRUZELL, AND W. R. HAZZARD. Effect of estrogen on postheparin lipolytic activity: selective decline in hepatic triglyceride lipase. *J. Clin. Invest.* 59: 601–608, 1977.
11. ARGILES, J., AND E. HERRERA. Lipids and lipoproteins in maternal and fetus plasma in the rat. *Biol. Neonat.* 39: 37–44, 1981.
12. ARVIDSSON, E. O., AND P. BELFRAGE. Monoglyceride-protein interaction. The binding of monoolein to native human serum albumin. *Acta Chem. Scand.* 23: 232–236, 1969.
13. ASHBY, P., D. P. BENNETT, I. M. SPENCER, AND D. S. ROBINSON. Post-translational regulation of lipoprotein lipase activity in adipose tissue. *Biochem. J.* 176: 865–872, 1978.
14. ASHBY, P., AND D. S. ROBINSON. Effect of insulin, glucocorticoids and adrenaline on the activity of rat adipose-tissue lipoprotein lipase. *Biochem. J.* 188: 185–192, 1980.
15. AUGUSTIN, J., H. FREEZE, P. TEJADA, AND W. V. BROWN. A comparison of molecular properties of hepatic triglyceride lipase and lipoprotein lipase from human post-heparin plasma. *J. Biol. Chem.* 253: 2912–2920, 1978.
16. AUGUSTIN, J., AND H. GRETEN. Hepatic triglyceride lipase in tissue and plasma. *Prog. Biochem. Pharmacol.* 15: 5–40, 1979.
17. BAGBY, G. J., M. S. LIU, AND J. A. SPITZER. Lipoprotein lipase activity in rat heart myocytes. *Life Sci.* 21: 467–473, 1977.
18. BAGINSKY, M. L., AND W. V. BROWN. Differential characteristics of purified hepatic triglyceride lipase and lipoprotein lipase from human postheparin plasma. *J. Lipid Res.* 18: 423–

437, 1977.
19. BARR, D. P., E. M. RUSS, AND H. A. EDER. Protein-lipid relationships in human plasma. II. In atherosclerosis and related conditions. *Am. J. Med.* 11: 480–493, 1951.
20. BARRETT, M. D., AND R. A. BRADLEY. Lipid protein interactions. In: *Biochemistry of Disease. The Biochemistry of Atherosclerosis*, edited by A. M. Scanu, R. W. Wissler, and G. S. Getz. New York: Dekker, 1979, vol. 7, p. 96–106.
21. BARSON, A. J., M. L. CHISTWICK, AND C. M. DOIG. Fat embolism in infancy after intravenous fat infusions. *Arch. Dis. Child.* 53: 218–223, 1978.
22. BARTER, P. J., AND J. I. LALLY. In vitro exchanges of esterified cholesterol between serum lipoprotein fractions: studies of humans and rabbits. *Metabolism* 28: 230–236, 1979.
23. BASU, S. K., J. L. GOLDSTEIN, AND M. S. BROWN. Characterization of the low density lipoprotein receptor in membranes prepared from human fibroblasts. *J. Biol. Chem.* 253: 3852–3856, 1978.
24. BÉGIN-HEICK, N., AND H. M. C. HEICK. Increased lipoprotein lipase activity of skeletal muscle in cold-acclimated rats. *Can. J. Biochem.* 55: 1241–1243, 1977.
25. BELFRAGE, P., B. BORGSTRÖM, AND T. OLIVECRONA. The tissue distribution of radioactivity following the injection of varying levels of fatty acid labeled chylomicrons in the rat. *Acta Physiol. Scand.* 58: 111–123, 1963.
26. BENGTSSON, G., AND T. OLIVECRONA. Interaction of lipoprotein lipase with heparin-sepharose. Evaluation of conditions for affinity binding. *Biochem. J.* 167: 109–119, 1977.
27. BENGTSSON, G., AND T. OLIVECRONA. Apolipoprotein CII enhances hydrolysis of monoglycerides by lipoprotein lipase, but the effect is abolished by fatty acids. *FEBS Lett.* 106: 345–348, 1979.
28. BENGTSSON, G., AND T. OLIVECRONA. Binding of deoxycholate to lipoprotein lipase. *Biochim. Biophys. Acta* 575: 471–474, 1979.
29. BENGTSSON, G., AND T. OLIVECRONA. Lipoprotein lipase: some effects of activator proteins. *Eur. J. Biochem.* 106: 549–555, 1980.
30. BENGTSSON, G., AND T. OLIVECRONA. Lipoprotein lipase: mechanism of product inhibition. *Eur. J. Biochem.* 106: 557–562, 1980.
31. BENGTSSON, G., T. OLIVECRONA, M. HÖÖK, J. RIESENFELD, AND U. LINDAHL. Interaction of lipoprotein lipase with native and modified heparin-like polysaccharides. *Biochem. J.* 189: 625–633, 1980.
32. BENSADOUN, A., C. EHNHOLM, D. STEINBERG, AND W. V. BROWN. Purification and characterization of lipoprotein lipase from pig adipose tissue. *J. Biol. Chem.* 249: 2220–2227, 1974.
33. BENSADOUN, A., AND I. P. KOMPIANG. Role of lipoprotein lipase in plasma triglyceride removal. *Federation Proc.* 38: 2622–2626, 1979.
34. BENSON, J. D., A. BENSADOUN, AND D. COHEN. Lipoprotein lipase of ovarian follicles in the domestic chicken (*Gallus domesticus*). *Proc. Soc. Exp. Biol. Med.* 148: 347–350, 1975.
35. BERMAN, M., M. H. HALL III, R. I. LEVY, S. EISENBERG, D. W. BILHEIMER, R. D. PHAIR, AND R. H. GOEBEL. Metabolism of apoB and apoC lipoproteins in man: kinetic studies in normal and hyperlipoproteinemic subjects. *J. Lipid Res.* 19: 38–56, 1978.
36. BERNARD, C. Memorie sur le pancreas et sur le role du suc pancreatique dans les phenomens digestifs, particulierement dans la digestion des matiéres grasses neutres. *Compt. Rend. Suppl.* 43: 379–563, 1856.
37. BEZMAN, A., J. M. FELTS, AND R. J. HAVEL. Relation between incorporation of triglyceride-fatty acids and heparin released lipoprotein lipase from adipose tissue slices. *J. Lipid Res.* 3: 427–431, 1962.
38. BIERMAN, E. L., O. STEIN, AND Y. STEIN. Lipoprotein uptake and metabolism by rat aortic smooth muscle cells in tissue culture. *Circ. Res.* 35: 136–150, 1974.
39. BISHOP, C., T. DAVIES, R. F. GLASCOCK, AND W. A. WELCH. Studies on the origin of milk fat. A further study of bovine serum lipoproteins and an estimation of their contribution to milk fat. *Biochem. J.* 113: 629–633, 1969.
40. BJÖRNTORP, P., M. KARLSSON, H. PERTOFT, P. PETTERSSON, L. SJÖSTRÖM, AND U. SMITH. Isolation and characterization of cells from rat adipose tissue developing into adipocytes. *J. Lipid Res.* 19: 316–324, 1978.
41. BLANCHETTE-MACKIE, E. J., AND R. O. SCOW. Sites of lipoprotein lipase activity in adipose tissue perfused with chylomicrons. Electron microscope cytochemical study. *J. Cell Biol.* 51: 1–25, 1971.
42. BLANCHETTE-MACKIE, E. J., AND R. O. SCOW. Effects of lipoprotein lipase on the structure of chylomicrons. *J. Cell Biol.* 58: 689–708, 1973.
43. BLÁZQUEZ, E., L. A. LIPSHAW, M. BLÁZQUEZ, AND P. P. FOA. The synthesis and release of insulin in fetal, nursing and young adult rats: studies in vivo and in vitro. *Pediatr. Res.* 9: 17–25, 1975.
44. BLÁZQUEZ, E., T. SUGASE, M. BLÁZQUEZ, AND P. P. FOA. Neonatal changes in the concentration of rat liver cyclic AMP and of serum glucose, free fatty acids, insulin, pancreatic, and total glucagon in man and in the rat. *J. K. Med. Assoc.* 83: 957–967, 1974.
45. BORENSZTAJN, J. Lipoprotein lipase. In: *Biochemistry of Disease. Biochemistry of Atherosclerosis*, edited by A. M. Scanu, R. W. Wissler, and G. S. Getz. New York: Dekker, 1979, vol. 7, p. 231–245.
46. BORENSZTAJN, J., P. KEIG, AND A. H. RUBENSTEIN. The role of glucagon in the regulation of myocardial lipoprotein lipase activity. *Biochem. Biophys. Res. Commun.* 53: 603–608, 1973.
47. BORENSZTAJN, J., S. OTWAY, AND D. S. ROBINSON. Effect of fasting on the clearing factor lipase (lipoprotein lipase) activity of fresh and defatted preparations of rat heart muscle. *J. Lipid Res.* 11: 102–110, 1970.
48. BORENSZTAJN, J., AND D. S. ROBINSON. The effect of fasting on the utilization of chylomicron triglyceride fatty acids in relation to clearing factor (lipoprotein lipase) releasable by heparin in the perfused rat heart. *J. Lipid Res.* 11: 111–117, 1970.
49. BORENSZTAJN, J., M. S. RONE, S. P. BABIRAK, J. A. MCGARR, AND L. B. OSCAI. Effect of exercise on lipoprotein lipase activity in rat heart and skeletal muscle. *Am. J. Physiol.* 229: 394–397, 1975.
50. BORGSTRÖM, B. Digestion and absorption of lipids. In: *Gastrointestinal Physiology II*, edited by R. K. Crane. Baltimore, MD: University Park, 1976, vol. 12, p. 305–323. (Int. Rev. Physiol. Ser.)
51. BRADY, M., AND J. A. HIGGINS. The properties of the lipoprotein lipases of rat heart, lung and adipose tissue. *Biochim. Biophys. Acta* 137: 140–146, 1967.
52. BRAGDON, J. H., AND R. S. GORDON, JR. Tissue distribution of ^{14}C after intravenous injection of labeled chylomicrons and unesterified fatty acids in the rat. *J. Clin. Invest.* 37: 574–578, 1958.
53. BRECHER, P., AND H. T. KUAN. Lipoprotein lipase and acid lipase activity in rabbit brain microvessels. *J. Lipid Res.* 20: 464–471, 1979.
54. BRODY, J. S., AND C. VACCARO. Alterations in alveolar and capillary basement membrane during postnatal lung growth in the rat (Abstract). *Am. Rev. Respir. Dis.* 123: 231, 1981.
55. BROWN, M. S., S. E. DANA, AND J. L. GOLDSTEIN. Receptor-dependent hydrolysis of cholesteryl esters contained in plasma low density lipoprotein. *Proc. Natl. Acad. Sci. USA* 72: 2925–2929, 1975.
56. BROWN, M. S., J. R. FAUST, AND J. L. GOLDSTEIN. Role of the low density lipoprotein receptor in regulating the content of free and esterified cholesterol in human fibroblasts. *J. Clin. Invest.* 55: 783–793, 1975.
57. BROWN, M. S., AND J. L. GOLDSTEIN. Receptor-mediated control of cholesterol metabolism. *Science* 191: 150–154, 1976.
58. BROWN, M. S., P. T. KOVANEN, AND J. L. GOLDSTEIN. Re-

ceptor-mediated uptake of lipoprotein-cholesterol and its utilization for steroid synthesis in the adrenal cortex. *Recent Prog. Horm. Res.* 35: 215–257, 1979.
59. BROWN, M. S., P. T. KOVANEN, AND J. L. GOLDSTEIN. Evolution of the LDL receptor concept—from cultured cells to intact animals. *Ann. NY Acad. Sci.* 348: 48–68, 1980.
60. BROWN, M. S., P. T. KOVANEN, AND J. L. GOLDSTEIN. Regulation of plasma cholesterol by lipoprotein receptors. *Science* 212: 628–635, 1981.
61. BROWN, M. S., K. LUSKEY, H. A. BOHMFALK, J. HEGELSON, AND J. L. GOLDSTEIN. Role of the LDL receptor in the regulation of cholesterol and lipoprotein metabolism. In: *Lipoprotein Metabolism*, edited by H. Greten. Berlin: Springer-Verlag, 1976, p. 82–89.
62. BROWN, W. V., R. I. LEVY, AND D. S. FREDRICKSON. Further separation of the apoproteins of the human plasma very low density lipoproteins. *Biochim. Biophys. Acta* 200: 573–575, 1970.
63. BRY, K., T. KUUSI, L. C. ANDERSSON, AND P. K. J. KINNUNEN. Monoacylglycerol hydrolase in human platelets: effect of platelets on the hydrolysis of chylomicron acylglycerols by lipoprotein lipase in vitro. *FEBS Lett.* 106: 111–114, 1979.
64. BUONASSISI, V. Sulfated mucopolysaccharide synthesis and secretion in endothelial cell cultures. *Exp. Cell Res.* 76: 363–368, 1973.
65. BUONASSISI, V., AND M. ROOT. Enzymatic degradation of heparin-related mucopolysaccharides from the surface of endothelial cell cultures. *Biochim. Biophys. Acta* 385: 1–10, 1975.
66. CARDELL, R. R., JR., S. BADENHAUSEN, AND K. R. PORTER. Intestinal triglyceride absorption in the rat. An electron microscopical study. *J. Cell Biol.* 34: 123–155, 1967.
67. CAREW, T. E., S. B. HAYES, T. KOCHINSKY, AND D. STEINBERG. A mechanism by which high density lipoproteins may slow the atherogenic process. *Lancet* 1: 1315–1318, 1976.
68. CAREW, T. E., R. P. SAIK, K. H. JOHANSEN, C. A. DENNIS, AND D. STEINBERG. Low density and high density lipoprotein turnover following portacaval shunt in swine. *J. Lipid Res.* 17: 441–450, 1976.
69. CATAPANO, A. L., S. H. GIANTURCO, P. K. J. KINNUNEN, S. EISENBERG, A. M. GOTTO, JR., AND L. C. SMITH. Suppression of 3-hydroxy-3-methylglutaryl-CoA reductase by low density lipoproteins produced in vitro by lipoprotein lipase action on nonsuppressive very low density lipoproteins. *J. Biol. Chem.* 254: 1007–1009, 1979.
70. CATAPANO, A. L., P. K. J. KINNUNEN, W. C. BRECKENRIDGE, A. M. GOTTO, JR., R. L. JACKSON, J. A. LITTLE, L. C. SMITH, AND J. T. SPARROW. Lipolysis of ApoC-II deficient very low density lipoproteins. Enhancement of lipoprotein lipase action by synthetic fragments of ApoC-II. *Biochem. Biophys. Res. Commun.* 89: 951–957, 1979.
71. CHAJEK, T., AND S. EISENBERG. Very low density lipoproteins. Metabolism of phospholipids, cholesterol and apolipoprotein C in the isolated perfused rat heart. *J. Clin. Invest.* 61: 1654–1665, 1978.
72. CHAJEK, T., AND C. J. FIELDING. Isolation and characterization of a human serum cholesteryl ester transfer protein. *Proc. Natl. Acad. Sci. USA* 75: 3445–3449, 1978.
73. CHAJEK, T., O. STEIN, AND Y. STEIN. Interference with the transport of heparin-releasable lipoprotein lipase in the perfused rat heart by colchicine and vinblastine. *Biochim. Biophys. Acta* 388: 260–267, 1975.
74. CHAJEK, T., O. STEIN, AND Y. STEIN. Interaction of concanavalin A with membrane-bound and solubilized lipoprotein lipase of rat heart. *Biochim. Biophys. Acta* 431: 507–518, 1976.
75. CHAJEK, T., O. STEIN, AND Y. STEIN. Pre- and post-natal development of lipoprotein lipase and hepatic triglyceride hydrolase activity in rat tissues. *Atherosclerosis* 26: 549–561, 1977.
76. CHAJEK, T., O. STEIN, AND Y. STEIN. Lipoprotein lipase of cultured mesenchymal rat heart cells. I. Synthesis, secretion and releasability by heparin. *Biochim. Biophys. Acta* 528: 456–465, 1978.
77. CHAJEK, T., O. STEIN, AND Y. STEIN. Lipoprotein lipase of cultured mesenchymal rat heart cells. II. Hydrolysis of labeled very low density lipoprotein triacylglycerol by membrane-supported enzyme. *Biochim. Biophys. Acta* 528: 466–474, 1978.
78. CHAPMAN, M. J., G. L. MILLS, AND C. E. TAYLAUR. The effect of a lipid rich diet on the properties and composition of lipoprotein particles from the Golgi apparatus of guinea-pig liver. *Biochem. J.* 131: 177–185, 1973.
79. CHEUNG, A. H., A. BENSADOUN, AND C. F. CHENG. Direct solid phase radioimmunoassay for chicken lipoprotein lipase. *Anal. Biochem.* 94: 346–357, 1979.
80. CHILLIARD, Y., M. DORLEANS, AND P. MARAND-FEHR. Lipoprotein lipase activity in goat adipose tissue: comparison of three extraction methods. *Ann. Biol. Anim. Biochim. Biophys.* 17: 1021–1034, 1977.
81. CHOHAN, P., AND A. CRYER. The lipoprotein lipase (clearing-factor lipase) activity of cells isolated from rat cardiac muscle. *Biochem. J.* 174: 663–666, 1978.
82. CHUNG, J., AND A. M. SCANU. Isolation, molecular properties and kinetic characterization of lipoprotein lipase from rat heart. *J. Biol. Chem.* 252: 4202–4209, 1977.
83. CLEGG, R. A. Triacylglycerol hydrolysis by cells isolated from lactating rat mammary gland. *Biochim. Biophys. Acta* 663: 598–612, 1981.
84. COMPTON, S. K., M. HAMOSH, AND P. HAMOSH. Hydrolysis of triglyceride in the isolated, perfused rat lung. *Lipids* 17: 696–702, 1982.
85. COREY, J. E., AND D. B. ZILVERSMIT. Effect of cholesterol feeding on arterial lipolytic activity in the rabbit. *Atherosclerosis* 27: 201–212, 1977.
86. CRYER, A. Tissue lipoprotein lipase activity and its action in lipoprotein metabolism. *Int. J. Biochem.* 13: 525–541, 1981.
87. CRYER, A., AND H. M. JONES. Changes in the lipoprotein lipase (clearing-factor lipase) activity of white adipose tissue during development of the rat. *Biochem. J.* 172: 319–325, 1978.
88. CRYER, A., AND H. M. JONES. The distribution of lipoprotein lipase (clearing factor lipase) activity in the adiposal, muscular and lung tissues of 10 animal species. *Comp. Biochem. Physiol. B* 63: 501–505, 1979.
89. CRYER, A., A. MCDONALD, E. R. WILLIAMS, AND D. S. ROBINSON. Colchicine inhibition of the heparin-stimulated release of clearing-factor lipase from isolated fat-cells. *Biochem. J.* 152: 717–720, 1975.
90. CRYER, A., S. E. RILEY, E. R. WILLIAMS, AND D. S. ROBINSON. Effect of nutritional status on rat adipose tissue, muscle and post-heparin plasma clearing factor lipase activities: their relationship to triglyceride fatty acid uptake by fat-cells and to plasma insulin concentrations. *Clin. Sci. Mol. Med.* 50: 213–221, 1976.
91. CUNNINGHAM, V. J., AND D. S. ROBINSON. Clearing factor lipase in adipose tissue. Distinction of different states of the enzyme and the possible role of the fat cell in the maintenance of tissue activity. *Biochem. J.* 112: 203–209, 1969.
92. CUZNER, M. L., AND A. L. DAVISON. The lipid composition of rat brain myelin and subcellular fractions during development. *Biochem. J.* 106: 29–34, 1968.
93. DAHMS, B. B., AND T. C. HALPIN. Pulmonary arterial lipid deposit in newborn infants receiving intravenous lipid infusion. *J. Pediatr.* 97: 800–805, 1980.
94. DECKELBAUM, R. I., S. EISENBERG, M. FAINARU, Y. BARENHOLZ, AND T. OLIVECRONA. In vitro production of human plasma low density lipoprotein-like particles: a model for very low density lipoprotein catabolism. *J. Biol. Chem.* 524: 6079–6087, 1979.
95. DE GASQUET, P., AND E. PEQUIGNOT. Lipoprotein lipase activities in adipose tissues, heart and diaphragm of the genetically obese mouse (ob/ob). *Biochem. J.* 127: 445–447, 1972.
96. DE GASQUET, P., E. PEQUIGNOT-PLANCHE, N. T. TONNU, AND F. A. DIABY. Effect of glucocorticoids on lipoprotein lipase activity in rat heart and adipose tissue. *Horm. Metab. Res.* 7: 152–157, 1975.
97. DHANIREDDY, R., M. HAMOSH, K. N. SIVASUBRAMANIAN, P.

Chowdhry, J. Scanlon, and P. Hamosh. Postheparin lipolytic activity and Intralipid clearance in very low-birth-weight infants. *J. Pediatr.* 98: 617–622, 1981.
98. DiCorleto, P. E., and D. B. Zilversmit. Lipoprotein lipase activity in bovine aorta. *Proc. Soc. Exp. Biol. Med.* 148: 1101–1105, 1975.
99. Dimant, J., and E. Shafrir. Lipase activity in the lungs of rats subjected to experimental hypertriglyceridemia and fat embolism. *Isr. J. Med. Sci.* 10: 1551–1559, 1974.
100. Duksin, D., and P. Bornstein. Impaired conversion of procollagen to collagen by fibroblasts and bone treated with tunicamycin, an inhibitor of protein glycosylation. *J. Biol. Chem.* 252: 955–962, 1977.
101. Eckel, R. H., W. Y. Fujimoto, and J. D. Brunzell. Development of lipoprotein lipase in cultured 3T3-LI cells. *Biochem. Biophys. Res. Commun.* 78: 288–293, 1977.
102. Egelrud, T., and T. Olivecrona. The purification of a lipoprotein lipase from bovine skim milk. *J. Biol. Chem.* 247: 6212–6217, 1972.
103. Ehnholm, C., P. K. J. Kinnunen, J. K. Huttunen, E. A. Nikkila, and M. Ohta. Purification and characterization of lipoprotein lipase from pig myocardium. *Biochem. J.* 149: 649–655, 1975.
104. Ehnholm, C., W. Shaw, H. Greten, and W. V. Brown. Purification from human plasma of a heparin-released lipase with activity against triglyceride and phospholipids. *J. Biol. Chem.* 250: 6756–6761, 1975.
105. Eisenberg, S. Very-low density lipoprotein metabolism. *Prog. Biochem. Pharmacol.* 15: 139–165, 1979.
106. Eisenberg, S., D. W. Bilheimer, R. I. Levy, and F. T. Lindgren. On the metabolic conversion of human plasma very low density lipoprotein to low density lipoprotein. *Biochim. Biophys. Acta* 326: 361–377, 1973.
107. Eisenberg, S., and R. I. Levy. Lipoprotein metabolism. *Adv. Lipid Res.* 13: 1–89, 1975.
108. Eisenberg, S., and T. Olivecrona. Very low density lipoprotein. Fate of phospholipids, cholesterol and apolipoprotein C during lipolysis in vitro. *J. Lipid Res.* 20: 614–623, 1979.
109. Eisenberg, S., and D. Rachmilewitz. Metabolism of rat plasma very low density lipoprotein. I. Fate in circulation of the whole lipoprotein. *Biochim. Biophys. Acta* 326: 378–390, 1973.
110. Eisenberg, S., and D. Rachmilewitz. Metabolism of rat plasma very low density lipoprotein. II. Fate in circulation of apoprotein subunits. *Biochim. Biophys. Acta* 326: 391–405, 1973.
111. Eisenberg, S., and D. Rachmilewitz. The interaction of rat plasma very low density lipoproteins with lipoprotein lipase rich (post-heparin) plasma. *J. Lipid Res.* 16: 341–351, 1975.
112. Eisenberg, S., and D. Schurr. Phospholipid removal during degradation of rat very low density lipoprotein in vitro. *J. Lipid Res.* 17: 578–587, 1976.
113. Eisenberg, S., H. G. Windmueller, and R. I. Levy. Metabolic fate of rat and human lipoprotein apoproteins in the rat. *J. Lipid Res.* 14: 446–458, 1973.
114. Elphick, M. C., and D. Hull. Rabbit placental clearing-factor lipase and transfer to the foetus of fatty acids derived from triglycerides injected into the mother. *J. Physiol. London* 273: 475–487, 1977.
115. Enser, M. Clearing factor lipase in obese hyperglycemic mice (ob/ob). *Biochem. J.* 129: 447–453, 1972.
116. Evans, A. J. Lipoprotein lipase activity in adipose tissue of the domestic duck: the effect of age, sex and nutritional state. *Int. J. Biochem.* 3: 199–206, 1972.
117. Faergeman, O., and R. J. Havel. Metabolism of cholesteryl esters of rat very low density lipoproteins. *J. Clin. Invest.* 55: 1210–1218, 1975.
118. Fainaru, M., R. J. Havel, and K. Imaizumi. Apoprotein content of plasma lipoproteins of the rat separated by gel chromatography or ultracentrifugation. *Biochem. Med.* 17: 347–355, 1977.
119. Farrell, P. M., and M. Hamosh. The biochemistry of fetal lung development. *Clin. Perinatol.* 5: 197–229, 1978.
120. Felts, J. M. Biochemistry of the lung. *Health Phys.* 10: 973–979, 1964.
121. Felts, J. M., H. Itakura, and R. T. Crane. The mechanism of assimilation of constituents of chylomicrons, very low density lipoproteins and remnants—a new theory. *Biochem. Biophys. Res. Commun.* 66: 1467–1475, 1975.
122. Fielding, C. J. Inactivation of lipoprotein lipase in buffered saline solutions. *Biochim. Biophys. Acta* 159: 94–102, 1968.
123. Fielding, C. J. Purification of lipoprotein lipase from rat postheparin plasma. *Biochim. Biophys. Acta* 178: 499–507, 1969.
124. Fielding, C. J. Lipoprotein lipase: evidence for high- and low-affinity enzyme sites. *Biochemistry* 15: 879–884, 1976.
125. Fielding, C. J. Metabolism of cholesterol-rich chylomicrons. Mechanism of binding and uptake of cholesteryl esters by the vascular bed of the perfused rat heart. *J. Clin. Invest.* 62: 141–151, 1978.
126. Fielding, C. J., and P. E. Fielding. Mechanism of salt-mediated inhibition of lipoprotein lipase. *J. Lipid Res.* 17: 248–256, 1976.
127. Fielding, C. J., and P. E. Fielding. The activation of lipoprotein lipase by lipoprotein C (apo C II). In: *Cholesterol Metabolism and Lipolytic Enzymes*, edited by J. Polonovski. New York: Masson, 1977, p. 165–172.
128. Fielding, C. J., and P. E. Fielding. Characteristics of triacyglycerol and partial acylglycerol hydrolysis by human plasma lipoprotein lipase. *Biochim. Biophys. Acta* 620: 440–446, 1980.
129. Fielding, C. J., and R. J. Havel. Lipoprotein lipase. *Arch. Pathol. Lab. Med.* 101: 225–229, 1977.
130. Fielding, C. J., and J. M. Higgins. Lipoprotein lipase: comparative properties of the membrane-supported and solubilized enzyme species. *Biochemistry* 13: 4324–4330, 1979.
131. Fielding, C. J., I. Vlodavsky, P. E. Fielding, and D. Gospodarowicz. Characteristics of chylomicron binding and lipid uptake by endothelial cells in culture. *J. Biol. Chem.* 254: 8861–8868, 1979.
132. Fielding, P. E., and C. J. Fielding. A cholesteryl ester transfer complex in human plasma. *Proc. Natl. Acad. Sci. USA* 77: 3327–3330, 1980.
133. Fielding, P. E., V. G. Shore, and C. J. Fielding. Lipoprotein lipase: properties of the enzyme isolated from post-heparin plasma. *Biochemistry* 13: 4318–4323, 1974.
134. Fielding, P. E., V. G. Shore, and C. J. Fielding. Lipoprotein lipase: isolation and characterization of a second enzyme species from post heparin plasma. *Biochemistry* 16: 1896–1900, 1977.
135. Fishman, A. P. Dynamics of the pulmonary circulation. In: *Handbook of Physiology. Circulation*, edited by W. F. Hamilton. Washington, DC: Am. Physiol. Soc., 1963, sect. 2, vol. II, chapt. 48, p. 1667–1743.
136. Fishman, A. P., and G. G. Pietra. Handling of bioactive materials by the lung. *N. Engl. J. Med.* 291: 884–890, 1974.
137. Floren, C. H., J. J. Albers, and E. L. Bierman. Uptake of chylomicron remnants causes cholesterol accumulation in cultured human arterial smooth muscle cells. *Biochim. Biophys. Acta* 663: 336–349, 1981.
138. Forte, T., K. R. Norum, J. A. Glomset, and A. V. Nichols. Plasma lipoproteins in familial lecithin: cholesterol acyltransferase deficiency: structure of low and high density lipoprotein, as revealed by electron microscopy. *J. Clin. Invest.* 50: 1141–1148, 1971.
139. Fraser, R. Size and lipid composition of chylomicrons of different Svedberg units of flotation. *J. Lipid Res.* 11: 60–65, 1970.
140. Fredrickson, D. S., and R. S. Gordon, Jr. Transport of fatty acids. *Physiol. Rev.* 38: 585–630, 1958.
141. French, J. E. The behaviour of chylomicrons in the circulation: observations with the electron microscope. In: *Biochemical Problems of Lipids*, edited by A. C. Frazer. Amsterdam: Elsevier, 1963, p. 296–302. (Proc. Int. Conf. Biochem. Lipids, 7th.)

142. FRIEDMAN, G., O. STEIN, AND Y. STEIN. Lipoprotein lipase of cultured mesenchymal heart cells. III. Effect of glucocorticoids and insulin on enzyme formation. *Biochim. Biophys. Acta* 531: 222–232, 1978.
143. FRIEDMAN, H. I., AND R. R. CARDELL, JR. Effects of puromycin on the structure of rat intestinal epithelial cells during fat absorption. *J. Cell Biol.* 52: 15–40, 1972.
144. GAGE, S. H. The free granules (chylomicrons) of the blood as shown by the dark-field microscope. *Cornell Vet.* 10: 154–155, 1920.
145. GAGE, S. H., AND P. A. FISH. Fat digestion, absorption and assimilation in man and animals as determined by dark-field microscope and fat-soluble dye. *Am. J. Anat.* 34: 1–85, 1924.
146. GETZ, G. S., AND R. V. HAY. The formation and metabolism of plasma lipoproteins. In: *Biochemistry of Disease. The Biochemistry of Atherosclerosis*, edited by A. M. Scanu, R. W. Wissler, and G. S. Getz. New York: Dekker, 1979, vol. 7, p. 151–188.
147. GLANGEAUD, M. C., S. EISENBERG, AND T. OLIVECRONA. Very low density lipoprotein. Disassociation of apolipoprotein C during lipoprotein lipase induced lipolysis. *Biochim. Biophys. Acta* 486: 23–35, 1977.
148. GLASCOCK, R. F., V. A. WELCH, C. BISHOP, T. DAVIES, E. W. WRIGHT, AND R. C. NOBLE. An investigation of serum lipoproteins and their contribution to milk fat in the dairy cow. *Biochem. J.* 98: 149–156, 1966.
149. GLICKMAN, R. M., AND K. KIRSCH. The apoproteins of various size classes of human chylous fluid lipoproteins. *Biochim. Biophys. Acta* 371: 255–266, 1974.
150. GLIMELIUS, B., C. BUSCH, AND M. HOOK. Binding of heparin on the surface of cultured human endothelial cells. *Thromb. Res.* 12: 773–782, 1978.
151. GLOMSET, J. A. Lecithin:cholesterol acyltransferase. An exercise in comparative biology. *Prog. Biochem. Pharmacol.* 15: 41–66, 1979.
152. GOFMAN, J. W., F. T. LINDGREN, AND H. ELLIOTT. Ultracentrifugal studies of lipoproteins of human serum. *J. Biol. Chem.* 179: 973–979, 1949.
153. GOLDSTEIN, J. L., AND M. S. BROWN. Binding and degradation of low density lipoproteins by cultured human fibroblasts: comparison of cells from a normal subject and from a patient with homozygous familial hypercholesterolemia. *J. Biol. Chem.* 249: 5153–5162, 1974.
154. GOLDSTEIN, J. L., AND M. S. BROWN. Lipoprotein receptors, cholesterol metabolism, and atherosclerosis. *Arch. Pathol.* 99: 181–184, 1975.
155. GOLDSTEIN, J. L., AND M. S. BROWN. The low density lipoprotein pathway and its relation to atherosclerosis. *Annu. Rev. Biochem.* 46: 897–930, 1977.
156. GOLDSTEIN, J. L., S. E. DANA, J. R. FAUST, A. L. BEAUDET, AND M. S. BROWN. Role of lysosomal acid lipase in the metabolism of plasma low density lipoprotein. *J. Biol. Chem.* 250: 8487–8495, 1975.
157. GOTTO, A. M., R. I. LEVY, K. JOHN, AND D. G. FREDRICKSON. On the protein defect in abetalipoproteinemia *N. Engl. J. Med.* 284: 813–818, 1971.
158. GOTTO, A. M., JR., L. C. SMITH, AND B. ALLEN (editors). *Atherosclerosis*. New York: Springer-Verlag, 1980. (Proc. Int. Symp. Atherosclerosis, 5th, Houston, Texas.)
159. GREEN, H., AND M. MEUTH. An established pre-adipose cell line and its differentiation in culture. *Cell* 3: 127–133, 1974.
160. GREEN, P. H. R., R. M. GLICKMAN, C. D. SAUDEK, C. B. BLUM, AND A. R. TALL. Human intestinal lipoproteins. Studies in chyluric subjects. *J. Clin. Invest.* 64: 233–242, 1979.
161. GREEN, P. H. R., A. R. TALL, AND R. M. GLICKMAN. Rat intestine secretes discoid high density lipoprotein. *J. Clin. Invest.* 61: 528–534, 1978.
162. GREENFIELD, C. J., V. M. BARKETT, AND J. J. COALSON. The role of surfactant in the pulmonary response to trauma. *J. Trauma* 8: 735–741, 1968.
163. GRETEN, H., J. GROSSER, I. BECHT, O. SCHRECKER, K. PREISSNER, AND G. KLOSE. Enzymatic regulation of lipoprotein catabolism. In: *Atherosclerosis*, edited by A. M. Gotto, Jr., L. C. Smith, and B. Allen. New York: Springer-Verlag, 1980, p. 631–640. (Proc. Int. Symp. Atherosclerosis, 5th, Houston, Texas.)
164. GRETEN, H., B. WALTER, AND W. V. BROWN. Purification of a human post-heparin plasma triglyceride lipase. *FEBS Lett.* 27: 306–310, 1972.
165. GROOT, P. H. E., M. C. OERLEMANS, AND L. M. SCHEEK. Triglyceridase and phospholipase A1 activities of rat-heart lipoprotein lipase: influence of apolipoproteins C-II and C-III. *Biochim. Biophys. Acta* 530: 91–98, 1978.
166. GRUNDY, S. M., AND H. Y. I. MOK. Chylomicron clearance in normal and hyperlipidemic man. *Metabolism* 25: 1225–1239, 1976.
167. GUSTAFSON, A., I. KJELLMER, R. OLEGARD, AND L. VICTORIN. Nutrition in low-birth-weight infants. I. Intravenous injection of fat emulsion. *Acta Paediatr. Scand.* 61: 149–158, 1972.
169. HAHN, P. F. Abolishment of alimentary lipemia following injection of heparin. *Science* 98: 19–20, 1943.
170. HAHN, P. The postnatal development of hormone sensitive lipase in brown and white adipose tissue of the rat. *Experientia* 21: 634–635, 1965.
171. HALLBERG, D. Elimination of exogenous lipids from the blood stream. *Acta Physiol. Scand. Suppl.* 254: 1–23, 1965.
172. HAMILTON, R. L. Synthesis and secretion of plasma lipoproteins. *Adv. Exp. Med. Biol.* 26: 7–24, 1972.
173. HAMILTON, R. L., R. J. HAVEL, J. P. KANE, A. E. BLAUROCK, AND T. SATA. Cholestasis: lamellar structure of the abnormal human serum lipoprotein. *Science* 172: 475–478, 1971.
174. HAMILTON, R. L., M. C. WILLIAMS, C. J. FIELDING, AND R. J. HAVEL. Discoidal bilayer structure of nascent high density lipoproteins from perfused rat liver. *J. Clin. Invest.* 58: 667–680, 1976.
175. HAMOSH, M. Fat digestion in the newborn: role of lingual lipase and preduodenal digestion. *Pediatr. Res.* 13: 615–622, 1979.
176. HAMOSH, M., T. R. CLARY, S. S. CHERNICK, AND R. O. SCOW. Lipoprotein lipase activity of adipose and mammary tissue and plasma triglyceride in pregnant and lactating rats. *Biochim. Biophys. Acta* 210: 473–482, 1970.
177. HAMOSH, M., AND P. HAMOSH. Lipoprotein lipase in rat lung: the effect of fasting. *Biochim. Biophys. Acta* 380: 132–140, 1975.
178. HAMOSH, M., AND P. HAMOSH. The effect of estrogen on the lipoprotein lipase activity of rat adipose tissue. *J. Clin. Invest.* 55: 1132–1135, 1975.
179. HAMOSH, M., AND R. O. SCOW. Lipoprotein lipase activity in guinea pig and rat milk. *Biochim. Biophys. Acta* 231: 283–289, 1971.
180. HAMOSH, M., M. R. SIMON, H. CANTER, JR., AND P. HAMOSH. Lipoprotein lipase activity and blood triglyceride levels in fetal and newborn rats. *Pediatr. Res.* 12: 1132–1136, 1978.
181. HAMOSH, M., H. YEAGER, JR., Y. SHECHTER, AND P. HAMOSH. Lipoprotein lipase in rat lung. Effect of dexamethasone. *Biochim. Biophys. Acta* 431: 519–525, 1976.
182. HARLAN, W. R., JR., P. S. WINESETT, AND A. J. WASSERMAN. Tissue lipoprotein lipase in normal individuals and in individuals with exogenous hypertriglyceridemia and the relationship of this enzyme to assimilation of fat. *J. Clin. Invest.* 46: 239–247, 1967.
183. HARTIALA, J., J. VIIKARI, E. HIETANEN, H. TOIVONEN, AND P. UOTILA. Cigarette smoke affects lipolytic activity in isolated rat lungs. *Lipids* 15: 539–543, 1980.
183a.HASS, M. A., AND W. J. LONGMORE. Surfactant cholesterol metabolism of the perfused rat lung. *Biochim. Biophys. Acta* 573: 166–174, 1979.
184. HAVEL, R. J., Y. S. CHAO, E. E. WINDLER, L. KOTITE, AND L. S. GUO. Isoprotein specificity in the hepatic uptake of apolipoprotein E and the pathogenesis of familial dysbetalipoproteinemia. *Proc. Natl. Acad. Sci. USA* 77: 4349–4353, 1980.
185. HAVEL, R. J., J. L. GOLDSTEIN, AND M. S. BROWN. Lipopro-

teins and lipoprotein transport. In: *Metabolic Control of Disease*, edited by P. K. Bondy and L. E. Rosenberg. Philadelphia, PA: Saunders, 1980, p. 393–494.
186. HAVEL, R. J., J. P. KANE, AND M. L. KASHYAP. Interchange of apolipoproteins between chylomicrons and high density lipoproteins during alimentary lipemia in man. *J. Clin. Invest.* 52: 32–38, 1973.
187. HAVEL, R. J., V. G. SHORE, B. SHORE, AND D. M. BIER. Role of specific glycopeptides of human serum lipoproteins in the activation of lipoprotein lipase. *Circ. Res.* 27: 595–600, 1970.
188. HEINEMANN, H. O. Free fatty acid production by rabbit lung tissue in vitro. *Am. J. Physiol.* 201: 607–610, 1961.
189. HEINENMANN, H. O., AND A. P. FISHMAN. Nonrespiratory functions of mammalian lung. *Physiol. Rev.* 49: 1–47, 1969.
190. HENSON, L. C., AND M. C. SCHOTZ. Detection and partial characterization of lipoprotein lipase in bovine aorta. *Biochim. Biophys. Acta* 409: 360–366, 1975.
191. HENSON, L. C., M. C. SCHOTZ, AND I. HARARY. Lipoprotein lipase in cultured heart cells: characteristics and cellular location. *Biochim. Biophys. Acta* 487: 212–221, 1977.
192. HERNELL, O., T. EGELRUD, AND T. OLIVECRONA. Serum-stimulated lipases (lipoprotein lipases). Immunological cross reaction between the bovine and the human enzymes. *Biochim. Biophys. Acta* 381: 233–241, 1975.
193. HERNELL, O., AND T. OLIVECRONA. Human milk lipases. I. Serum-stimulated lipase. *J. Lipid Res.* 15: 367–374, 1974.
194. HIETANEN, E., AND M. R. C. GREENWOOD. A comparison of lipoprotein lipase activity and adipocyte differentiation in growing male rats. *J. Lipid Res.* 18: 480–490, 1977.
195. HIETANEN, E., AND J. HARTIALA. Developmental pattern of pulmonary lipoprotein lipase in growing rats. *Biol. Neonat.* 36: 85–91, 1979.
196. HILLMAN, J. W., AND V. S. LE QUIRE. Lipid metabolism and fat embolism after trauma: the contribution of serum lipoproteins to embolic fat. *Surg. Forum* 19: 465–467, 1968.
197. HO, Y. K., M. S. BROWN, H. J. KAYDEN, AND J. L. GOLDSTEIN. Binding, internalization, and hydrolysis of low density lipoprotein in long-term lymphoid cell lines from a normal subject and a patient with homozygous familial hypercholesterolemia. *J. Exp. Med.* 144: 444–455, 1976.
198. HOLLENBERG, C. H. The effect of incubation on the characteristics of the lipolytic activity of rat adipose tissue. *Can. J. Biochem. Physiol.* 40: 703–707, 1962.
199. HOWARD, B. V. Uptake of very low density lipoprotein triglyceride by bovine aortic endothelial cells in culture. *J. Lipid Res.* 18: 561–571, 1977.
200. HUTH, K. Fettstoffwechselstudien bei der experimentellen Fettembolie. *Neue Aspecte Transylol. Ther.* 5: 107–112, 1972.
201. IMAIZUMI, K., M. FAINARU, AND R. J. HAVEL. Composition of proteins of mesenteric lymph chylomicrons in the rat and alterations produced upon exposure of chylomicrons to blood serum and serum proteins. *J. Lipid Res.* 19: 712–722, 1978.
202. IMAIZUMI, K., R. J. HAVEL, M. FAINARU, AND J. L. VIGNE. Origin and transport of the A-I and arginine-rich apolipoproteins in mesenteric lymph of rats. *J. Lipid Res.* 19: 1038–1046, 1978.
203. IVERIUS, P. H. The interaction between human plasma lipoproteins and connective tissue glycosaminoglycans. *J. Biol. Chem.* 247: 2607–2613, 1972.
204. IVERIUS, P. H., U. LINDAHL, T. EGELRUD, AND T. OLIVECRONA. Effects of heparin on lipoprotein lipase from bovine milk. *J. Biol. Chem.* 247: 6610–6616, 1972.
205. IVERIUS, P. H., AND A. M. OSTLUND-LINDQVIST. Lipoprotein lipase from bovine milk, isolation procedure, chemical characterization and molecular weight analysis. *J. Biol. Chem.* 251: 7791–7795, 1976.
206. JACKSON, R. L., J. D. MORRISETT, AND A. M. GOTTO, JR. Lipoprotein structure and metabolism. *Physiol. Rev.* 56: 259–316, 1976.
207. JACKSON, R. L., F. PATTUS, AND G. DE HAAS. Mechanism of action of milk lipoprotein lipase at substrate interfaces: effects of apolipoproteins. *Biochemistry* 19: 373–378, 1980.
208. JACKSON, R. L., R. PATTUS, AND R. A. DEMEL. Interaction of plasma apolipoproteins with lipid monolayers. *Biochim. Biophys. Acta* 556: 369–387, 1979.
209. JANSEN, H., A. S. GARFINKEL, J. S. TWU, J. NIKAZY, AND M. C. SCHOTZ. Regulation of lipoprotein lipase immunological study of adipose tissue. *Biochim. Biophys. Acta* 531: 109–114, 1978.
210. JANSEN, H., H. STAM, C. KALKMAN, AND W. C. HULSMAN. On the dual location of lipoprotein lipase in rat heart: studies with a modified perfusion technique. *Biochem. Biophys. Res. Commun.* 92: 411–416, 1980.
211. JENSEN, G. L., D. L. BALY, P. M. BRANNON, AND A. BENSADOUN. Synthesis and secretion of lipolytic enzymes by cultured chicken hepatocytes. *J. Biol. Chem.* 255: 11141–11148, 1980.
212. JOHASSON, L., G. H. HANSSON, G. BONDJERS, G. BENGTSSON, AND T. OLIVECRONA. Immunochemical localization of lipoprotein lipase in human adipose tissue. *J. Lipid Res.* In press.
213. JONES, N. L., AND R. J. HAVEL. Metabolism of free fatty acids and chylomicron triglycerides during exercise in rats. *Am. J. Physiol.* 213: 824–828, 1967.
214. KAGAN, H. M., P. E. MILBURY, JR., AND D. M. KRAMSCH. A possible role for elastin ligands in the proteolytic degradation of arterial elastic lamellae in the rabbit. *Circ. Res.* 44: 95–103, 1979.
215. KAGAN, H. M., D. E. SIMPSON, AND L. TSENG. Substrate directed modulation of elastin oxidation by lysyl oxidase. *Connect. Tissue Res.* 8: 213–217, 1981.
216. KANE, J. P., D. A. HARDMAN, AND H. E. PAULUS. Heterogeneity of apolipoprotein B: isolation of a new species from human chylomicrons. *Proc. Natl. Acad. Sci. USA* 77: 2465–2469, 1980.
217. KEIG, P., AND J. BORENSZTAJN. Regulation of rat heart lipoprotein lipase activity during cold exposure. *Proc. Soc. Exp. Biol. Med.* 146: 890–893, 1974.
218. KEKKI, M. Lipoprotein lipase action determining plasma high density lipoprotein cholesterol level in adult normolipaemics. *Atherosclerosis* 37: 143–150, 1980.
219. KELLUM, J. M., JR., T. R. DE MEESTER, R. C. ELKINS, AND G. D. ZUIDEMA. Respiratory insufficiency secondary to acute pancreatitis. *Ann. Surg.* 175: 657–662, 1972.
220. KHOO, J. C., D. STEINBERG, B. THOMPSON, AND S. E. MAYER. Hormonal regulation of adipocyte enzymes. The effects of epinephrine and insulin on the control of lipase, phosphorylase kinase, phosphorylase and glycogen synthase. *J. Biol. Chem.* 248: 3823–3830, 1973.
221. KIMURA, T., J. K. TOUNG, S. MARGOLIS, W. R. BELL, AND J. L. CAMERON. Respiratory failure in acute pancreatitis: the role of free fatty acids. *Surgery* 87: 509–513, 1980.
222. KINNUNEN, P. K. J., J. K. HUTTUNEN, AND C. EHNHOLM. Properties of purified bovine milk lipoprotein lipase. *Biochim. Biophys. Acta* 450: 342–351, 1976.
223. KINNUNEN, P. K. J., R. L. JACKSON, L. C. SMITH, A. M. GOTTO, JR., AND J. T. SPARROW. Activation of lipoprotein lipase by native and synthetic fragments of human plasma apolipoprotein C-II. *Proc. Natl. Acad. Sci. USA* 74: 4848–4851, 1977.
224. KJELLEN, L., A. OLDEBERG, K. RUBIN, AND M. HOOK. Binding of heparin and heparan sulfate to rat liver cells. *Biochem. Biophys. Res. Commun.* 74: 126–133, 1977.
225. KNOX, A. M., R. G. STURTON, J. COOLING, AND D. N. BRINDLEY. Control of hepatic triacylglycerol synthesis. Diurnal variations in hepatic phosphatidate phosphohydrolase activity and in the concentrations of circulating insulin and corticosterone in rats. *Biochem. J.* 180: 441–443, 1979.
226. KOMPIANG, I. P., A. BENSADOUN, AND M. W. W. YANG. Effect of an anti-lipoprotein lipase serum on plasma triglyceride removal. *J. Lipid Res.* 17: 498–505, 1976.
227. KORN, E. D. Clearing factor, a heparin-activated lipoprotein lipase. *J. Biol. Chem.* 215: 1–14, 1955.
228. KORN, E. D. Inactivation of lipoprotein lipase by heparinase. *J. Biol. Chem.* 226: 827–832, 1957.

229. KORN, E. D. The assay of lipoprotein lipase in vivo and in vitro. *Methods Biochem. Anal.* 7: 145–192, 1959.
230. KORN, E. D., AND T. W. QUIGLEY, JR. Lipoprotein lipase of chicken adipose tissue. *J. Biol. Chem.* 226: 833–839, 1957.
231. KOSTNER, G., AND A. HOLASEK. Characterization and quantitation of the apolipoprotein from human chyle chylomicrons. *Biochemistry* 11: 1217–1223, 1972.
232. KOTLAR, T. J., AND J. BORENSZTAJN. Oscillatory changes in muscle lipoprotein lipase activity of fed and starved rats. *Am. J. Physiol.* 233 (*Endocrinol. Metab. Gastrointest. Physiol.* 2): E316–E319, 1977.
233. KOVANEN, P. T., S. K. BASU, J. L. GOLDSTEIN, AND M. S. BROWN. Low density lipoprotein receptors in bovine adrenal cortex. II. Low density lipoprotein binding to membranes prepared from fresh tissue. *Endocrinology* 104: 610–616, 1979.
234. KRAEMER, P. M. Heparin releases heparan sulfate from the cell surface. *Biochem. Biophys. Res. Commun.* 78: 1334–1340, 1977.
235. KRAUSS, R. M., H. G. WINDMUELLER, R. I. LEVY, AND D. S. FREDRICKSON. Selective measurement of two different triglyceride lipase activities in rat postheparin plasma. *J. Lipid Res.* 14: 286–295, 1973.
236. KRISHNAIAH, K. V., L. F. WALKER, J. BORENSZTAJN, G. SCHONFELD, AND G. S. GETZ. Apolipoprotein B variant derived from rat intestine. *Proc. Natl. Acad. Sci. USA* 77: 3806–3810, 1980.
237. KUUSI, T., P. K. KINNUNEN, C. EHNHOLM, AND E. A. NIKKILA. A simple purification procedure for rat hepatic lipase. *FEBS Lett.* 98: 314–318, 1979.
238. LANGER, T., W. STROBER, AND R. I. LEVY. The metabolism of low density lipoprotein in familial type II hyperlipoproteinemia. *J. Clin. Invest.* 51: 1528–1536, 1972.
239. LAROSA, J. C., R. I. LEVY, P. HERBERT, S. E. LUX, AND D. S. FREDRICKSON. A specific apoprotein activator for lipoprotein lipase. *Biochem. Biophys. Res. Commun.* 41: 57–62, 1970.
240. LAROSA, J. C., R. I. LEVY, H. G. WINDMUELLER, AND D. S. FREDRICKSON. Comparison of the triglyceride lipase of liver, adipose tissue and postheparin plasma. *J. Lipid Res.* 13: 356–363, 1972.
241. LEHR, L., H. NIEDERMULLER, AND G. HOFECKER. Changes in pulmonary lipoprotein lipase activity in dogs following experimental bone fracture: a new concept on the pathogenesis of post-traumatic impairment of lung surfactant synthesis and accumulation of fat in lung vessels? *Surgery* 81: 521–526, 1977.
242. LE MARCHAND, Y., A. SINGH, F. ASSIMACOPOULOS-JEANNET, L. ORCI, C. ROUILLER, AND B. JEANRENAUD. A role for the microtubular system in the release of very low density lipoprotein in perfused mouse livers. *J. Biol. Chem.* 248: 6862–6870, 1972.
243. LEVENE, M. I., J. S. WIGGLESWORTH, AND R. DESAI. Pulmonary fat accumulation after intralipid infusion in the preterm infant. *Lancet* 2: 815–818, 1980.
244. LEVY, R. I. The plasma lipoproteins: an overview. *Prog. Clin. Biol. Res.* 5: 25–42, 1976.
245. LEVY, R. I., D. W. BILHEIMER, AND S. EISENBERG. The structure and metabolism of chylomicrons and very low density lipoproteins (VLDL). In: *Plasma Lipoproteins*, edited by R. M. Smellie. London: Academic, 1971, p. 3–17. (Biochem. Soc. Symp. 33.)
246. LINDAHL, U., AND M. HOOK. Glycosaminoglycans and their binding to biological macromolecules. *Annu. Rev. Biochem.* 47: 385–417, 1978.
247. LINDER, C., S. S. CHERNICK, T. R. FLECK, AND R. O. SCOW. Lipoprotein lipase and uptake of chylomicron triglyceride by skeletal muscle of rats. *Am. J. Physiol.* 231: 860–864, 1976.
248. LINDGREN, F. T. The plasma lipoproteins: historical developments and nomenclature. *Ann. NY Acad. Sci.* 348: 1–15, 1980.
249. LINDGREN, F. T., AND A. V. NICHOLS. Structure and function of human lipoproteins. In: *Plasma Proteins. Biosynthesis, Metabolism, and Alterations in Disease*, edited by W. F. Putnam. New York: Academic, 1960, vol. 2, chapt. 1, p. 1–58.
250. LINDGREN, F. T., A. V. NICHOLS, AND F. M. KRAUSS. Structure, Function and Analysis. II. Clinical, Epidemiological and Metabolic Aspects. Champaign, IL: Am. Oil Chem. Soc., 1978. (Symp. High Density Lipoproteins.)
251. LIPPEL, K. (editor). *Report of the High-Density Lipoprotein Methodology Workshop.* Bethesda, MD: Natl. Inst. Health, 1979. (NIH Publ. 79-1661.)
252. LISCH, H. I., S. SEILER, L. REIDLER, AND H. BRAUNSTETNER. Assay and characterization of serum-stimulated lipolytic activity in homogenates of human adipose tissue. *Res. Exp. Med.* 170: 109–114, 1977.
253. LITHELL, H., AND J. BOBERG. Determination of lipoprotein lipase activity in human skeletal muscle tissue. *Biochim. Biophys. Acta* 528: 58–68, 1978.
254. LLOBERA, M., A. MONTES, AND E. HERRERA. Lipoprotein lipase activity in liver of the rat fetus. *Biochem. Biophys. Res. Commun.* 91: 272–277, 1979.
255. LUBCHENKO, L. O. Survival of the newborn infant. In: *Van Leeuwen's Newborn Medicine* (2nd ed.), edited by C. L. Paxson, Jr. Chicago, IL: Year Book, 1979, p. 1–20.
256. LUKENS, T. W., AND J. BORENSZTAJN. Action of lipoprotein lipase on apoprotein-depleted chylomicrons. *Biochem. J.* 175: 53–61, 1978.
257. MACHEBOEUF, M. Recherches sur les phosphoaminolipides et les stérides du sérum et du plasma sanguins: entraînement des phospholipides, des stérols et des stérides par les diverses fractions au cours du fractionnement des protéides du sérum. *Bull. Soc. Chim. Biol.* 11: 268–293, 1929.
258. MACHEBOEUF, M. Recherches sur les phosphoaminolipides et les stérides du sérum et du plasma sanguins: étude physicochimique de la fraction protéidique la plus riche en phospholipides et en stérides. *Bull. Soc. Chim. Biol.* 11: 485–503, 1929.
259. MACKINNON, N. O., AND A. CRYER. The interaction of very-low-density lipoproteins from pig and rat plasma with immobilized heparin. *Biochem. Soc. Trans.* 8: 373, 1980.
260. MAHLEY, R. W., AND K. H. WEISGRABER. An electrophoretic method for the quantitative isolation of human and swine plasma lipoproteins. *Biochemistry* 13: 1964–1969, 1974.
261. MAJNO, G. Ultrastructure of the vascular membrane. In: *Handbook of Physiology. Circulation*, edited by W. F. Hamilton. Washington, DC: Am. Physiol. Soc., 1965, sect. 2, vol. III, chapt. 64, p. 2293–2375.
262. MAKSVYTIS, H. J., C. VACCARO, AND J. S. BRODY. Isolation and characterization of the lipid-containing interstitial cell from the developing rat lung. *J. Clin. Lab. Invest.* 45: 248–259, 1981.
263. MALLOV, S., AND A. A. ALOUSI. Lipoprotein lipase activity of rat and human placenta. *Proc. Soc. Exp. Biol. Med.* 119: 301–306, 1965.
264. MARSH, J. B. Lipoproteins in a nonrecirculating perfusate of rat liver. *J. Lipid Res.* 15: 544–550, 1974.
265. MCBRIDE, O. W., AND E. D. KORN. The lipoprotein lipase of mammary gland and the correlation of its activity to lactation. *J. Lipid Res.* 4: 17–20, 1963.
266. MCCONATHY, W. J., AND P. ALAUPOVIC. Isolation and partial charcterization of apolipoprotein D: a new protein moiety of the human plasma lipoprotein system. *FEBS Lett.* 37: 178–182, 1973.
267. MCFARLANE, A. S. The behavior of pathological sera in the ultracentrifuge. *Biochem. J.* 29: 1175–1201, 1935.
268. MCGARRY, J. D., AND D. W. FOSTER. Regulation of ketogenesis and clinical aspects of the ketotic state. *Metabolism* 21: 471–489, 1972.
269. MILLER, A. L., AND L. C. SMITH. Activation of lipoprotein lipase by apolipoprotein glutamic acid. *J. Biol. Chem.* 248: 3359–3362, 1973.
270. MILLER, G. J., AND N. E. MILLER. Plasma high-density lipoprotein concentration and development of ischaemic heart-disease. *Lancet* 1: 16–19, 1975.
271. MILLER, N. E. The evidence for the antiatherogenicity of high density lipoprotein in man. *Lipids* 13: 914–919, 1978.
272. MILLER, N. E., D. B. WEINSTEIN, AND D. STEINBERG. Binding, internalization, and degradation of high density lipopro-

tein by cultured normal human fibroblasts. *J. Lipid Res.* 18: 438–450, 1977.
273. MINARI, O., AND D. B. ZILVERSMIT. Behavior of dog lymph chylomicron lipid constituents during incubation with serum. *J. Lipid Res.* 4: 424–436, 1963.
274. MJØS, O., O. FAERGEMAN, R. L. HAMILTON, AND R. J. HAVEL. Characterization of remnants produced during the metabolism of triglyceride-rich lipoproteins of blood plasma and intestinal lymph in the rat. *J. Clin. Invest.* 56: 603–615, 1975.
275. MORELY, N., AND A. KUKSIS. Positional specificity of lipoprotein lipase. *J. Biol. Chem.* 247: 6389–6393, 1972.
276. MORLEY, N., AND A. KUKSIS. Lack of fatty acid specificity in the lipolysis of oligo and polyunsaturated triacylglycerols by milk lipoprotein lipase. *Biochim. Biophys. Acta* 487: 332–342, 1977.
277. MORRISETT, J. D., R. L. JACKSON, AND A. M. GOTTO, JR. Lipid-protein interactions in the plasma lipoproteins. *Biochim. Biophys. Acta* 472: 93–133, 1977.
278. MOSKOWITZ, M. S., AND A. A. MOSKOWITZ. Lipase: localization in adipose tissue. *Science* 149: 72–73, 1965.
279. MOSTELLO, D. J., M. HAMOSH, AND P. HAMOSH. Effect of dexamethasone on lipoprotein lipase activity of fetal rat lung. *Biol. Neonat.* 40: 121–128, 1981.
280. MOXLEY, M. A., AND W. J. LONGMORE. Studies on the effects of alloxan and streptozotocyn induced diabetes on lipid metabolism in the isolated, perfused rat lung. *Life Sci.* 17: 921–925, 1975.
281. MUNTZ, H. G., N. MATSUOKA, AND R. L. JACKSON. Phospholipase activity of bovine milk lipoprotein lipase on phospholipid vesicles: influence of apolipoproteins C-II and C-III. *Biochem. Biophys. Res. Commun.* 90: 15–21, 1979.
282. MUSLINER, T. A., F. C. CHURCH, P. N. HERBERT, N. J. KINGSTON, AND R. S. SHULMAN. Lipoprotein lipase cofactor activity of a carboxyl terminal peptide of apolipoprotein CII. *Proc. Natl. Acad. Sci. USA* 74: 5358–5362, 1977.
283. NAIMARK, A. Cellular dynamics and lipid metabolism in the lung. *Federation Proc.* 32: 1967–1971, 1973.
284. NAKAI, T., P. S. OTTO, D. L. KENNEDY, AND T. F. WHAYNE, JR. Rat high density lipoprotein subfraction (HDL$_3$) uptake and catabolism by isolated rat liver parenchymal cells. *J. Biol. Chem.* 251: 4914–4921, 1976.
285. NELSON, G. J. (editor). *Blood Lipids and Lipoproteins: Quantitation, Composition, and Metabolism.* New York: Wiley, 1972.
286. NESTEL, P. J., R. J. HAVEL, AND A. BEZMAN. Sites of initial removal of chylomicron triglyceride fatty acids from the blood. *J. Clin. Invest.* 41: 1915–1921, 1962.
287. NIKKILA, E. A. Metabolic regulation of plasma high density lipoprotein concentrations. *Eur. J. Clin. Invest.* 8: 111–113, 1978.
288. NIKKILA, E. A., T. KUSSI, K. HARNO, M. TIKKANEN, AND M. R. TASKINEN. Lipoprotein lipase and hepatic endothelial lipase are key enzymes in the metabolism of plasma high density lipoproteins, particularly of HDL$_2$. In: *Atherosclerosis*, edited by A. M. Gotto, Jr., L. C. Smith, and B. Allen. New York: Springer-Verlag, 1980, p. 387–392. (Proc. Int. Symp. Atherosclerosis, 5th, Houston, Texas.)
289. NIKKILA, E. A., M. R. TASKINEN, AND M. KEKKI. Relation of plasma high-density lipoprotein cholesterol to lipoprotein lipase activity in adipose tissue and skeletal muscle of man. *Atherosclerosis* 29: 497–501, 1978.
290. NIKKILA, E. A., P. TORSTI, AND O. PENTTILA. The effect of exercise on lipoprotein lipase activity of rat heart, adipose tissue and skeletal muscle. *Metabolism* 12: 863–865, 1963.
291. NILSSON-EHLE, P. Human lipoprotein lipase activity: comparison of assay methods. *Clin. Chim. Acta* 54: 283–291, 1974.
292. NILSSON-EHLE, P., P. BELFRAGE, AND B. BORGSTRÖM. Purified human lipoprotein lipase: positional specificity. *Biochim. Biophys. Acta* 248: 114–120, 1971.
293. NILSSON-EHLE, P., A. S. GARFINKEL, AND M. C. SCHOTZ. Intra- and extracellular forms of lipoprotein lipase in adipose tissue. *Biochim. Biophys. Acta* 431: 147–156, 1976.
294. NILSSON-EHLE, P., A. S. GARFINKEL, AND M. C. SCHOTZ. Lipolytic enzymes and plasma lipoprotein metabolism. *Annu. Rev. Biochem.* 49: 667–693, 1980.
295. NOEL, S. P., AND D. RUBINSTEIN. Secretion of apolipoproteins in very low density and high density lipoproteins by perfused rat liver. *J. Lipid Res.* 15: 301–308, 1974.
296. NORUM, K. R., J. A. GLOMSET, A. V. NICHOLS, T. FORTE, J. J. ALBERS, W. C. KING, C. D. MITCHELL, K. R. APPLEGATE, E. L. GONG, V. CABANA, AND E. GJONE. Plasma lipoproteins in familial lecithin:cholesterol acyltransferase deficiency: effect of incubation with lecithin:cholesterol acyltransferase in vitro. *Scand. J. Clin. Lab. Invest. Suppl.* 142: 31–55, 1975.
297. OCKNER, R. K., F. B. HUGHES, AND K. J. ISSELBACHER. Very low density lipoproteins in intestinal lymph: role in triglyceride and cholesterol transport during fat absorption. *J. Clin. Invest.* 48: 2367–2373, 1969.
298. OLEGARD, R., A. GUSTAFSON, I. KJELLMER, AND L. VICTORIN. Nutrition in low birth weight infants. III. Lipolysis and free fatty acid elimination after intravenous administration of fat emulsion. *Acta Paediatr. Scand.* 64: 745–751, 1975.
299. OLIVECRONA, T., AND G. BENGTSSON. Molecular basis for the interaction of lipoprotein lipase with triglyceride-rich lipoproteins of the capillary endothelium. *INSERM Symp.* 87: 149–160, 1979.
300. OLIVECRONA, T., G. BENGTSSON, M. HOOK, AND U. LINDAHL. Physiologic implications of the interaction between lipoprotein lipase and some sulfated glycosaminoglycans. In: *Lipoprotein Metabolism*, edited by H. Greten. New York: Springer-Verlag, 1976, p. 13–19.
301. OLIVECRONA, T., G. BENGTSSON, S. E. MARKLUND, U. LINDAHL, AND M. HOOK. Heparin-lipoprotein lipase interactions. *Federation Proc.* 36: 60–65, 1977.
302. OLIVECRONA, T., T. EGELRUD, P. H. IVERIUS, AND U. LINDAHL. Evidence for an ionic binding of lipoprotein lipase to heparin. *Biochem. Biophys. Res. Commun.* 43: 524–529, 1971.
303. OLOFSSON, S., W. MCCONATHY, AND P. ALAUPOVIC. Isolation and partial characterization of an acidic lipoprotein from human high density lipoproteins. *Circulation* 56, Suppl. 3: 56, 1977.
304. OSTLUND-LINDQVIST, A. M. Properties of salt-resistant lipase and lipoprotein lipase purified from human post-heparin plasma. *Biochem. J.* 179: 555–559, 1979.
305. OTWAY, S., AND D. S. ROBINSON. The significance of changes in tissue clearing-factor lipase activity in relation to the lipaemia of pregnancy. *Biochem. J.* 106: 677–682, 1968.
306. PARKES, A. B., AND R. F. MAHLER. The nature of pig arterial lipase. *Atherosclerosis* 20: 281–286, 1974.
307. PARKIN, S. M., K. WALKER, P. ASHBY, AND D. S. ROBINSON. Effects of glucose and insulin on the activation of lipoprotein lipase and on protein synthesis in rat adipose tissue. *Biochem. J.* 188: 193–199, 1980.
308. PATHAK, R. M., V. S. SHEORAIN, G. K. KHULLER, AND D. SUBRAHMANYAM. Effect of alloxan-induced chronic diabetes on lipid composition and lipoprotein lipase activity of rat lung. *Biochem. Med.* 21: 215–219, 1979.
309. PATTEN, R. L. The reciprocal regulation of lipoprotein lipase activity and hormone-sensitive lipase activity in rat adipocytes. *J. Biol. Chem.* 245: 5577–5584, 1970.
310. PATTNAIK, N. M., AND D. B. ZILVERSMIT. Interaction of cholesteryl ester exchange protein with human plasma lipoproteins and phospholipid vesicles. *J. Biol. Chem.* 254: 2782–2786, 1979.
311. PEETERS, H. (editor). *The Lipoprotein Molecule.* New York: Plenum, 1978. (NATO Adv. Study Inst. Ser. A, Life Sci., vol. 15.)
312. PEQUIGNOT-PLANCHE, E., P. DE GASQUET, A. BOULANGE, AND N. T. TONNU. Lipoprotein lipase activity at onset of development of white adipose tissue in newborn rats. *Biochem. J.* 162: 461–463, 1977.
313. PERSSON, B. Lipoprotein lipase activity of human adipose tissue in health and in some diseases with hyperlipidemia as a common feature. *Acta Med. Scand.* 193: 457–462, 1973.
314. PERSSON, B., AND B. HOOD. Characterization of lipoprotein

lipase activity eluted from human adipose tissue. *Atherosclerosis* 12: 241–251, 1970.
315. PIETRA, G. G., L. G. SPAGNOLI, D. M. CAPUZZI, C. E. SPARKS, A. P. FISHMAN, AND J. B. MARSH. Metabolism of ^{125}I-labeled lipoproteins by the isolated rat lung. *J. Cell Biol.* 70: 33–46, 1976.
316. PLAAS, H. A. K., R. HARWOOD, AND A. CRYER. The lipoprotein lipase (clearing factor lipase) activity of bovine subcutaneous adipose tissue and isolated adipocytes. *Biochem. Soc. Trans.* 6: 596–598, 1978.
317. PLANCHE, E., A. BOULANGE, P. DE GASQUET, AND N. T. TONNU. Importance of muscle lipoprotein lipase in rats during suckling. *Am. J. Physiol.* 238 (*Endocrinol. Metab.* 1): E511–E517, 1980.
318. PYKÄLISTÖ, O. J., P. H. SMITH, AND J. D. BRUNZELL. Determinants of human adipose tissue lipoprotein lipase. *J. Clin. Invest.* 56: 1108–1117, 1975.
319. QUARFORDT, S. H., H. HILDERMAN, M. R. GREENFIELD, AND F. A. SHELBURNE. The effect of human arginine rich apoprotein on rat adipose lipoprotein lipase. *Biochem. Biophys. Res. Commun.* 78: 302–308, 1977.
320. RACHMILEWITZ, D., J. J. ALBERS, D. R. SAUNDERS, AND M. FAINARU. Apoprotein synthesis by human duodenojejunal mucosa. *Gastroenterology* 75: 677–682, 1978.
321. RACHMILEWITZ, D., AND M. FAINARU. Apolipoprotein A-I synthesis and secretion by cultured human intestinal mucosa. *Metabolism* 28: 739–743, 1979.
322. RADOMSKI, M. W., AND T. ORME. Response of lipoprotein lipase in various tissues to cold exposure. *Am. J. Physiol.* 220: 1852–1856, 1971.
323. REARDON, M. F., N. H. FIDGE, AND P. J. NESTEL. Catabolism of very low density lipoprotein B apoprotein in man. *J. Clin. Invest.* 61: 850–860, 1978.
324. REDGRAVE, T. G. Formation of cholesteryl ester-rich particulate lipid during metabolism of chylomicrons. *J. Clin. Invest.* 49: 465–471, 1970.
325. REDGRAVE, T. G. Association of Golgi membranes with lipid droplets (pre-chylomicrons) from within intestinal epithelial cells during absorption of fat. *Aust. J. Exp. Biol. Med. Sci.* 49: 209–224, 1971.
326. REDGRAVE, T. G. The role in chylomicron formation of phospholipase activity of intestinal Golgi membranes. *Aust. J. Exp. Biol. Med. Sci.* 51: 427–434, 1973.
327. REDGRAVE, T. G., AND D. M. SMALL. Transfer of surface components of chylomicrons to the high density lipoprotein fraction during chylomicron catabolism in the rat. *Circulation* 58, Suppl. 2: 11–14, 1978.
328. REICHL, D. Lipoprotein lipase activity in the adipose tissue of rats adapted to controlled feeding schedules. *Biochem. J.* 128: 79–87, 1972.
329. REINILA, A., V. A. KOIVISTO, AND H. K. AKERBLOM. Lipids in the pulmonary artery and the lungs of severely diabetic rats. *Diabetologia* 13: 305–310, 1977.
330. ROBINSON, D. S. Further studies on the lipolytic system induced in plasma by heparin injection. *Q. J. Exp. Physiol.* 41: 195–204, 1956.
331. ROBINSON, D. S. Changes in the lipolytic activity of the guinea pig mammary gland at parturition. *J. Lipid Res.* 4: 21–23, 1963.
332. ROBINSON, D. S. The clearing factor lipase and its action in the transport of fatty acids between the blood and the tissues. *Adv. Lipid Res.* 1: 133–182, 1963.
333. ROBINSON, D. S. The function of the plasma triglycerides in fatty acid transport. In: *Comprehensive Biochemistry. Lipid Metabolism*, edited by M. Florkin and E. H. Stotz. Amsterdam: Elsevier/North-Holland, 1970, sect. 4, vol. 18, p. 51–116.
334. ROBINSON, D. S., AND J. E. FRENCH. Heparin, the clearing factor lipase, and fat transport. *Pharmacol. Rev.* 12: 241–263, 1960.
335. ROBINSON, D. S., AND P. M. HARRIS. The production of lipolytic activity in the circulation of the hind limb in response to heparin. *Q. J. Exp. Physiol.* 44: 80–90, 1959.
336. RODBELL, M. Localization of lipoprotein lipase in fat cells of rat adipose tissue. *J. Biol. Chem.* 239: 753–755, 1964.
337. ROGERS, M. P., AND D. S. ROBINSON. Effects of cold exposure on heart clearing factor lipase and triglyceride utilization in the rat. *J. Lipid Res.* 15: 263–272, 1974.
338. ROHEIM, P. S., L. I. GIDEZ, AND H. A. EDER. Extrahepatic synthesis of lipoproteins of plasma and chyle: role of the intestine. *J. Clin. Invest.* 45: 297–300, 1966.
339. ROHEIM, P. S., D. E. HAFT, L. I. GIDEZ, A. WHITE, AND H. A. EDER. Plasma lipoprotein metabolism in perfused rat livers. II. Transfer of free and esterified cholesterol into the plasma. *J. Clin. Invest.* 42: 1277–1285, 1963.
340. SALAMAN, M. R., AND D. S. ROBINSON. Clearing factor lipase in adipose tissue. A medium in which the enzyme activity of tissue from starved rats increases in vitro. *Biochem. J.* 99: 640–647, 1966.
341. SAXL, P. Über Fett und Esterspaltung in den Geweben. *Biochem. Z.* 12: 343–360, 1908.
342. SCANU, A. M. Plasma lipoproteins: an introduction. In: *Biochemistry of Disease. The Biochemistry of Atherosclerosis*, edited by A. M. Scanu, R. W. Wiler, and G. S. Getz. New York: Dekker, 1979, vol. 7, p. 3–8.
343. SCHAEFER, E. J., S. EISENBERG, AND R. I. LEVY. Lipoprotein apoprotein metabolism. *J. Lipid Res.* 19: 667–687, 1978.
344. SCHAEFER, E. J., L. L. JENKINS, AND H. B. BREWER, JR. Human chylomicron apolipoprotein metabolism. *Biochem. Biophys. Res. Commun.* 80: 405–412, 1978.
345. SCHAEFER, E. J., AND R. I. LEVY. Composition and metabolism of high density lipoproteins. *Prog. Biochem. Pharmacol.* 15: 200–215, 1979.
346. SCHOEFL, G. I., AND J. E. FRENCH. Vascular permeability to particulate fat: morphological observations on vesicles of lactating mammary gland and of lung. *Proc. R. Soc. London Ser. B* 169: 153–165, 1968.
347. SCHONFELD, G., R. S. LEES, P. K. GEORGE, AND B. PFLEGER. Assay of total plasma apolipoprotein B concentration in human subjects. *J. Clin. Invest.* 53: 1458–1467, 1974.
348. SCHOTZ, M. C., J. S. TWU, M. E. PEDERSEN, C. H. CHEN, A. S. GARFINKEL, AND J. BORENSZTAJN. Antibodies to lipoprotein lipase: application to perfused heart. *Biochim. Biophys. Acta* 489: 214–224, 1977.
349. SCHRECKER, O., AND H. GRETEN. Activation and inhibition of lipoprotein lipase. Studies with artificial lipoproteins. *Biochim. Biophys. Acta* 572: 244–256, 1979.
350. SCHRIEBLER, T. H., AND H. H. WOLFF. Electronmicroskopische Untersuchungen am Herzmuskel der Ratte wahrend der Entwicklung, *Z. Zellforsch. Mikrosk. Anat.* 69: 22–40, 1966.
351. SCOW, R. O., E. J. BLANCHETTE-MACKIE, AND L. C. SMITH. Role of capillary endothelium in the clearance of chylomicrons. A model for lipid transport from blood by lateral diffusion in cell membranes. *Circ. Res.* 39: 149–162, 1977.
352. SCOW, R. O., AND S. S. CHERNICK. Mobilization, transport and utilization of free fatty acids. In: *Comprehensive Biochemistry. Lipid Metabolism*, edited by M. Florkin and E. H. Stotz. Amsterdam: Elsevier/North-Holland, 1970, sect. 4, p. 19–49.
353. SCOW, R. O., P. DESNUELLE, AND R. VERGER. Lipolysis and lipid movement in a membrane model: action of lipoprotein lipase. *J. Biol. Chem.* 254: 6456–6463, 1979.
354. SCOW, R. O., AND T. EGELRUD. Hydrolysis of chylomicron phosphatidyl choline in vitro by lipoprotein lipase, phospholipase A-2 and phopholipase C. *Biochim. Biophys. Acta* 431: 538–549, 1976.
355. SCOW, R. O., M. HAMOSH, E. J. BLANCHETTE-MACKIE, AND A. J. EVANS. Uptake of blood triglyceride by various tissues. *Lipids* 7: 497–505, 1972.
356. SCOW, R. O., C. R. MENDELSON, O. ZINDER, M. HAMOSH, AND E. J. BLANCHETTE-MACKIE. Role of lipoprotein lipase in the delivery of dietary fatty acids to lactating mammary tissue. In: *Dietary Lipids and Postnatal Development*, edited by C. Galli, G. Jacini, and A. Pecile. New York: Raven, 1973, p. 91–114.
357. SCOW, R. O., AND T. OLIVECRONA. Effects of albumin on products formed from chylomicron triacyglycerol by lipopro-

tein lipase in vitro. *Biochim. Biophys. Acta* 487: 472–486, 1977.
358. SHELBURNE, F. A., AND S. H. QUARFORDT. The interaction of heparin with an apoprotein of human very low density lipoprotein. *J. Clin. Invest.* 60: 944–950, 1977.
359. SHEMESH, M., A. BENSADOUN, AND W. HANSEL. Lipoprotein lipase activity in the bovine corpus luteum during the estrous cycle and early pregnancy. *Proc. Soc. Exp. Biol. Med.* 151: 667–669, 1976.
360. SHEN, B. W., A. M. SCANU, AND F. J. KEZDY. Structure of human serum lipoproteins inferred from compositional analysis. *Proc. Natl. Acad. Sci. USA* 74: 837–841, 1977.
361. SHENNAN, A. T., M. H. BRYAN, AND A. ANGEL. The effect of gestational age on Intralipid tolerance in newborn infants. *J. Pediatr.* 91: 134–137, 1977.
362. SHERRILL, B. C. Kinetic characteristics of the hepatic transport of chylomicron remnants. In: *Disturbances in Lipid and Lipoprotein Metabolism*, edited by J. M. Dietschy, A. M. Gotto, Jr., and J. A. Ontko. Bethesda, MD: Am. Physiol. Soc., 1978, chapt. 6, p. 99–109.
363. SHERRILL, B. C., T. L. INNERARITY, AND R. W. MAHLEY. Rapid hepatic clearance of the canine lipoproteins containing only the E apoprotein by a high affinity receptor. *J. Biol. Chem.* 255: 1804–1807, 1980.
364. SHIMADA, L., P. J. GILL, J. E. SILBERT, W. H. J. DOUGLAS, AND B. L. FANBURG. Involvement of cell surface heparan sulfate in the binding of lipoprotein lipase to cultured bovine endothelial cells. *J. Clin Invest.* 68: 995–1002, 1981.
365. SIEBER, N. Die Fettspaltung durch Lungengewebe. *Z. Physiol. Chem.* 55: 177–206, 1908.
366. SIGURDSSON, G., A. NICOLL, AND B. LEWIS. Conversion of very low density lipoprotein to low density lipoprotein: a metabolic study of apolipoprotein B kinetics in human subjects. *J. Clin. Invest.* 56: 1481–1490, 1975.
367. SKOWRONSKI, G. A., S. SHERR, AND S. B. GERTNER. Inhibition of lipoprotein lipase by barbiturates. *Federation Proc.* 40: 348, 1981.
368. SMALL, D. M. Membrane and plasma lipoproteins—bilayer to emulsion and emulsion to bilayer transition. In: *Proc. Int. Conf. on Biol. Membr.*, edited by K. Block, L. Bolio, and D. C. Tosten. Littleton, MA: PSG, 1981, chapt. 2, p. 11–34.
369. SMITH, L. C., H. J. POWNALL, AND A. M. GOTTO, JR. The plasma lipoproteins: structure and metabolism. *Annu. Rev. Biochem.* 47: 751–757, 1978.
370. SMITH, L. C., AND R. O. SCOW. Chylomicrons: mechanism of transfer of lipolytic products to cells. *Prog. Biochem. Pharmacol.* 15: 109–138, 1979.
371. SMITH, U., AND J. W. RYAN. Electron microscopy of endothelial and epithelial components of the lungs: correlations of structure and function. *Federation Proc.* 32: 1957–1966, 1973.
372. SNIDERMAN, A. D., T. E. CAREW, J. G. CHANDLER, AND D. STEINBERG. Paradoxical increase in rate of catabolism of low-density lipoproteins after hepatectomy. *Science* 183: 526–528, 1974.
373. SPARKS, C. E., J. L. DEHOFF, D. M. CAPUZZI, G. PIETRA, AND J. B. MARSH. Proteolysis of very low density lipoprotein in perfused lung. *Biochim. Biophys. Acta* 529: 123–130, 1978.
374. SPECTOR, A. A., K. JOHN, AND J. E. FLETCHER. Binding of long-chain fatty acids to bovine serum albumin. *J. Lipid Res.* 10: 56–67, 1968.
375. SPOONER, P. M., S. S. CHERNICK, M. M. GARRISON, AND R. O. SCOW. Development of lipoprotein lipase activity and accumulation of triacylglycerol in differentiating 3T3-Li adipocytes. Effects of prostaglandin $F_{2\alpha}$ 1-methyl-3-isobutylxanthine, prolactin, and insulin. *J. Biol. Chem.* 254: 1305–1311, 1979.
376. SPOONER, P. M., S. S. CHERNICK, M. M. GARRISON, AND R. O. SCOW. Insulin regulation of lipoprotein lipase activity and release in 3T3-Li adipocytes: separation and dependence of hormonal effects on hexose metabolism and synthesis of RNA and protein. *J. Biol. Chem.* 254: 10021–10029, 1979.
377. STEIN, O., AND Y. STEIN. Lipid synthesis, intracellular transport, storage and secretion. I. Electron microscopic radioautographic study of liver after injection of tritiated palmitate or glycerol in fasted and ethanol-treated rats. *J. Cell Biol.* 33: 319–339, 1967.
378. STEIN, O., AND Y. STEIN, High density lipoproteins reduce the uptake of low density lipoproteins by human endothelial cells in culture. *Biochim. Biophys. Acta* 431: 363–368, 1976.
379. STEIN, O., AND Y. STEIN. Catabolism of serum lipoproteins. *Prog. Biochem. Pharmacol.* 15: 216–237, 1979.
380. STEIN, Y., AND O. STEIN. Metabolism of plasma lipoproteins. In: *Atherosclerosis*, edited by A. M. Gotto, Jr., L. C. Smith, and B. Allen. New York: Springer-Verlag, 1980, p. 653–665. (Proc. Int. Symp. Atherosclerosis, 5th, Houston, Texas.)
381. STEINBERG, D. Origin, turnover and fate of plasma low density lipoprotein. *Prog. Biochem. Pharmacol.* 15: 166–199, 1979.
382. STEINGRIMSDOTTIR, L., J. A. BRASEL, AND M. R. C. GREENWOOD. Diet, pregnancy and lactation: effects on adipose tissue, lipoprotein lipase and fat cell size. *Metabolism* 29: 837–841, 1980.
383. STOCKS, J., AND D. J. GALTON. Activation of the phospholipase A1 activity of lipoprotein lipase by apoprotein C-II. *Lipids* 15: 186–190, 1980.
384. STRATTA-MONGA, P., G. GRASSINI, R. PIACENTINO, R. GARBAGNI, AND G. CARDELLINO. Changes in lung lipids induced by alloxan-diabetes and insulin hypoglycemia. *Minerva Med.* 64: 4411–4417, 1973.
385. STRAUSS, E. W. Morphological aspects of triglyceride absorption. In: *Handbook of Physiology. Alimentary Canal. Intestinal Absorption*, edited by C. F. Code. Washington, DC: Am. Physiol. Soc., 1968, sect. 6, vol. III, chapt. 71, p. 1377–1406.
386. SUDJIC, M. M., AND R. BOOTH. Activity of 3-hydroxy-3-methylglutaryl-coenzyme A reductase in brains of adult and 7-day-old rats. *Biochem. J.* 154: 559–560, 1976.
387. SUTER, E. R., AND G. MAJNO. Passage of lipid across vascular endothelium in newborn rats: an electron microscopic study. *J. Cell Biol.* 27: 163–177, 1965.
388. SVEDBERG, T., AND K. PEDERSON. The ultracentrifuge. In: *International Series of Monographs in Physics*, edited by R. H. Fowler and P. Kapitza. Oxford, UK: Clarendon, 1940.
389. SVEDBERG, T., AND H. RINDE. The ultracentrifuge, a new instrument for the determination of size and distribution of size of particles in amicroscopic colloids. *J. Am. Chem. Soc.* 46: 2677–2693, 1924.
390. SWAMINATHAN, N., AND F. ALADJEM. The monosaccharide composition and sequence of the carbohydrate moiety of human serum low density lipoproteins. *Biochemistry* 15: 1516–1522, 1976.
391. TALL, A. R., AND D. M. SMALL. Plasma high-density lipoproteins. *N. Engl. J. Med.* 299: 1232–1236, 1978.
392. TAN, M. H., T. SATA, AND R. J. HAVEL. The significance of lipoprotein lipase in rat skeletal muscles. *J. Lipid Res.* 18: 363–370, 1977.
393. TORNQVIST, H., P. NILSSON-EHLE, AND P. BELFRAGE. Enzymes catalyzing the hydrolysis of long-chain monoacylglycerides in rat adipose tissue. *Biochim. Biophys. Acta* 530: 474–486, 1978.
394. TORSTI, P. Thyroxine and the heart lipoprotein lipase. *Ann. Med. Exp. Biol. Fenn.* 43: 245–247, 1965.
395. TRIA, E., AND A. M. SCANU (editors). *Structural and Functional Aspects of Lipoproteins in Living Systems*. New York: Academic, 1969.
396. TWU, J. S., A. S. GARFINKEL, AND M. C. SCHOTZ. Rat heart lipoprotein lipase. *Atherosclerosis* 22: 463–472, 1975.
397. USPENSKII, V. I. Lipolytic activity of liver and lungs in experimental alloxan diabetes. *Federation Proc.* 24, Suppl. T43–T44, 1965.
398. VACCARO, C., AND J. S. BRODY. Ultrastructure of developing alveoli. I. The role of the interstitial fibroblast. *Anat. Rec.* 192: 467–480, 1978.
399. VAN, R. L. R., C. E. BAYLISS, AND D. A. K. RONCARI. Cytological and enzymological characterization of adult human adipocyte precursors in culture. *J. Clin. Invest.* 58: 699–704, 1976.

400. VAN BERKEL, T. J. C., J. F. KOSTER, AND W. C. HULSMANN. High density lipoprotein and low density lipoprotein catabolism by human liver and parenchymal and non-parenchymal cells from rat liver. *Biochim. Biophys. Acta* 486: 586–589, 1977.
401. VIRCHOW, R. Zur Entwickelungsgeschichte des Krebses nebst Bemerkungen über Fettbilung im Tierischen Korper und pathologische Resorbtion. *Virchows Arch. Pathol. Anat. Physiol.* 1: 94–203, 1847.
402. WALLINDER, L., G. BENGTSSON, AND T. OLIVECRONA. Rapid removal to the liver of intravenously injected lipoprotein lipase. *Biochim. Biophys. Acta* 575: 166–173, 1979.
403. WANG, M. C., AND H. C. MENG. Uptake and metabolism of alpha-monopalmitin by rat lung in vitro. *Lipids* 10: 721–725, 1975.
404. WANG-IVERSON, P., E. A. JAFFE, AND W. V. BROWN. Triglyceride hydrolysis by lipoprotein lipase bound to endothelilal cells in culture. In: *Atherosclerosis*, edited by A. M. Gotto, Jr. L. C. Smith, and B. Allen. New York: Springer-Verlag, p. 375–378. (Proc. Int. Symp. Atherosclerosis, 5th, Houston, Texas.)
405. WARSHAW, A. L., P. B. LESSER, M. RIE, AND D. J. CULLEN. The pathogenesis of pulmonary edema in acute pancreatitis. *Ann. Surg.* 182: 505–510, 1975.
406. WASSERMANN, F., AND T. F. MCDONALD. Electron microscopic study of adipose tissue (fat organs) with special reference to the transport of lipids between blood and fat cells. *Z. Zellforsch. Mikrosk. Anat.* 59: 326–357, 1963.
407. WASTESON, A., B. GLIMELIUS, C. BUSCH, H. WESTERMARK, H. HELDIN, AND B. NORLING. Effect of a platelet endoglycosidase on cell surface associated heparan sulphate of human cultured endothelial and glial cells. *Thromb. Res.* 11: 309–321, 1977.
408. WEIBEL, E. R. The ultrastructure of the alveolar capillary membrane or barrier. In: *The Pulmonary Circulation and Interstitial Space*, edited by A. P. Fishman and H. H. Hecht. Chicago, IL: Univ. of Chicago Press, 1969, p. 9–27.
409. WELD, C. B. Alimentary lipemia and heparin. *Can. Med. Assoc. J.* 51: 578, 1944.
410. WILLIAMSON, J. R. Adipose tissue: morphological changes associated with lipid mobilization. *J. Cell Biol.* 20: 57–74, 1964.
411. WILSON, D. E., C. M. FLOWERS, S. I. CARLILE, AND K. S. UDALL. Estrogen treatment and gonadal function in the regulation of lipoprotein lipase. *Atherosclerosis* 24: 491–499, 1976.
412. WILSON, D. E., P. H. SCHREIBMAN, A. C. BREWSTER, AND R. A. ARKY. The enhancement of alimentary lipemia by ethanol in man. *J. Lab. Clin. Med.* 75: 264–274, 1970.
413. WINDLER, E., Y. CHAO, AND R. J. HAVEL. Determinants of hepatic uptake of triglyceride-rich lipoproteins and their remnants in the rat. *J. Biol. Chem.* 255: 5475–5480, 1980.
414. WINDMUELLER, H. G., P. N. HERBERT, AND R. I. LEVY. Biosynthesis of lymph and plasma lipoprotein apoproteins by isolated perfused rat liver and intestine. *J. Lipid Res.* 14: 215–223, 1973.
415. WU, A. L., AND H. G. WINDMUELLER. Relative contributions by liver and intestine to individual plasma apolipoproteins in the rat. *J. Biol. Chem.* 254: 7316–7322, 1979.
416. WYNN, V., J. W. H. DOAR, G. L. MILLS, AND T. STOKES. Fasting serum triglyceride, cholesterol and lipoprotein levels during oral-contraceptive therapy. *Lancet* 2: 756–760, 1969.
417. YOSHITOSHI, Y., C. NAITO, H. OKANIWA, M. USUI, T. MOGAMI, AND T. TOMONO. Kinetic studies on metabolism of lipoprotein lipase. *J. Clin. Invest.* 42: 707–713, 1963.
418. ZAUNER, C. W., M. ARBORELIUS, JR., G. FEX, AND S. E. LINDELL. Pulmonary arterial-venous differences in lipids and lipid metabolites. *Federation Proc.* 40: 621, 1981.
419. ZAUNER, C. W., M. ARBORELIUS, JR., E. W. SWENSON, G. SUNDSTROM, S. E. LINDELL, AND M. FRIED. Arterial-venous differences across the lungs in plasma triglyceride concentration. *Respiration* 34: 2–8, 1977.
420. ZILVERSMIT, D. B. A proposal linking atherogenesis to the interaction of endothelial lipoprotein lipase with triglyceride-rich lipoproteins. *Circ. Res.* 33: 633–638, 1978.
421. ZILVERSMIT, D. B., L. B. HUGHES, AND J. BALMER. Stimulation of cholesterol ester exchange by lipoprotein-free rabbit plasma. *Biochim. Biophys. Acta* 409: 393–398, 1975.
422. ZINDER, O., M. HAMOSH, T. R. CLARY FLECK, AND R. O. SCOW. Effect of prolactin on lipoprotein lipase in mammary gland and adipose tissue of rats. *Am. J. Physiol.* 226: 744–748, 1974.
423. ZINDER, O., C. R MENDELSON, E. J. BLANCHETTE-MACKIE, AND R. O. SCOW. Lipoprotein lipase and uptake of chylomicron triacylglycerol and cholesterol by perfused rat mammary tissue. *Biochim. Biophys. Acta* 431: 526–537, 1976.
424. ZORRILLA, E., M. HULSE, A. HERNANDEZ, AND H. GERSHBERG. Severe endogenous hypertriglyceridemia during treatment with estrogen and oral contraceptives. *J. Clin. Endocrinol. Metab.* 28: 1793–1796, 1968.

CHAPTER 13

Regulation of airway secretions, ion transport, and water movement

JAY A. NADEL

JONATHAN H. WIDDICOMBE

ANTHONY C. PEATFIELD

Cardiovascular Research Institute and Departments of Medicine and Physiology, University of California, San Francisco, California

Department of Physiology, St. George's Hospital Medical School, London, England

CHAPTER CONTENTS

Airway Secretions
  Surface mucus
    Anatomy
    Physiology
  Submucosal glands
    Anatomy
    Physiology
  Effects of drugs and mediators
  Hypertrophy of mucus-secreting cells
    Human studies
    Animal studies
Ion Transport and Water Movement
  Introduction
  Mechanisms of ion transport
    Chloride secretion by dog tracheal epithelium
    Sodium absorption
    Other ion-transport processes
  Regulation of ion transport
  Relationship between ion transport and water movement

THE FLUID LINING THE AIRWAY is believed to consist of a superficial mucous gel phase and a lower, liquid sol phase. The cilia beat in the sol phase, and their tips make contact with and propel the viscous mucus up the airways, along with foreign materials trapped within the mucus. Ciliary activity and cough clear the secreted materials. [Ciliary activity is discussed in the chapter by Satir and Dirksen in this *Handbook*, and cough is discussed in the chapter by Leith, Sneddon, Butler, and Brain (120a) in the volume on the mechanics of breathing in this *Handbook* section on the respiratory system.] Where relevant their roles in the clearance of secretions are indicated. The symptomatology and pathology of various airway diseases, which suggest that abnormal secretion may play an important role in the evolution of these diseases, have been important motivators of research. The development of methods for obtaining and measuring the biochemical constituents of secreted materials has produced new insights into the regulation of airway secretions. Excellent reviews of the biochemistry of mucus are available (18, 38); consequently this is not covered in this chapter.

Secretory cells exist in the surface epithelium and in the submucosal glands, and secretory cell hypertrophy plays a conspicuous role in the pathology of chronic airway diseases. It is possible that bulk fluid production in the conducting airways occurs via gland secretion and that fine regulation of fluid occurs locally via active ion transport. The regulation of secretion and of ion transport has been reviewed elsewhere (220) and is discussed in detail in this chapter.

AIRWAY SECRETIONS

Surface Mucus

Respiratory tract mucus is synthesized and secreted by the cells of the surface epithelium and by the submucosal glands. Indeed in some species, such as the goose (155), rat (86), and rabbit (28), submucosal glands are scarce or absent; therefore the surface epithelial cells are presumably the primary source of mucus. In healthy adult humans the volume of the glands (down to 5th generation of bronchi) was calculated to be ~4 ml, with goblet cell volume ~1/40th of this value (161); potentially then, the submucosal glands probably make the greater contribution to the production of respiratory tract mucus.

ANATOMY. The lining of the mammalian trachea and bronchi is made up of a pseudostratified columnar epithelium containing a large variety of different cell types (32, 99). Of these cell types, three or four are believed to be secretory: goblet cells, serous cells, Clara cells, and possibly also ciliated cells.

Goblet cells. In 1867 Schulze (175) discovered goblet cells in the human bronchi and named them *Becherzellen*. The occurrence and distribution of goblet cells vary among species, but they rarely occur in the more distal airways except in chronic disease (195) or possibly after chronic irritation [in which case other cell types are believed to transform into goblet cells (100)]. Goblet cells are common in the human trachea and bronchi, with a density of ~6,800 cells/mm^2, and this can rise to ~10,000/mm^2 in patients with chronic bronchitis (59). They are rare or nonexistent in the bronchioles (160). The occurrence of tracheal goblet cells varies greatly among species. They are rare in the ferret (93), more numerous in the dog (185), and common in the cat (114) and rabbit (28). Ferrets have large numbers of goblet cells in the major bronchi (93). In the specific pathogen–free rat, goblet cells make up only 1% of the total number of epithelial cells at all levels of the trachea and bronchi (98), and they are also rare in the mouse (147). It appears then that the density of goblet cells in healthy individuals depends on the size of the airway: they are scarce or absent in small animals, and their numbers diminish from the caudal end of the trachea to the bronchioles in large animals. The ferret airway is an exception to this, but the paucity of goblet cells in the trachea is compensated for by the presence of a very large number of submucosal glands.

Goblet cells stain with Alcian blue (AB) and periodic acid–Schiff (PAS). The former stains mainly acidic glycoproteins and the latter mainly neutral glycoproteins. In the cat (114), dog (34, 186), and rabbit (150), acidic glycoproteins are the more common constituents of goblet cells, whereas in the rat, both neutral and acidic glycoprotein–staining goblet cells are readily observed. The staining characteristics of human goblet cells resemble those of the cat, showing a preponderance of cells containing mainly acidic glycoproteins (131). The submucosal glands in most species stain largely for neutral glycoproteins; consequently the histochemical properties of the two types of secretory cells suggest that they secrete different types of glycoprotein.

Rhodin and Dalhamn (168) and Jeffery and Reid (98) have described the ultrastructure of the cells of the rat airway in detail. Both groups describe the characteristic appearance of most goblet cell cytoplasm as occupied by large electron-lucent secretory granules, 0.5–1.5 µm in diameter. Goblet cells also contain smaller numbers of opaque granules, but these are more common in cat goblet cells (96).

The secretory process has not been studied in airway goblet cells, but it has been studied in goblet cells in the gut, where stimuli can be given to cause an observable release of granules. It was originally thought that the intestinal globlet cell secretions were apocrine (see ref. 72), but recent work suggests that the apical plasma membrane of the cells remains intact during both base-line secretion and secretion stimulated by acetylcholine (182). Autoradiographic studies with light and electron microscopes show that the secretory process is an extension of conventional exocytosis, in which one or more secretory granules fuse with the apical membrane at a single point and discharge their contents without interrupting the continuity of the plasma membrane. Mechanical irritation can damage the goblet cells so that they appear to be secreting by an apocrine mechanism (M. R. Neutra, unpublished observations), but whether an equivalent degree of mechanical stimulation occurs physiologically in vivo is not known. Goblet cells on the intestinal surface (as opposed to those in crypts) secrete in response to mustard oil (183) but not in response to pharmacological agents. In this respect they resemble mammalian airway goblet cells, which secrete in response to mustard oil (70) but do not respond to autonomic agonists (114). By analogy the airway goblet cell probably secretes by exocytosis of its granules, although there is no direct evidence for this. In birds such as the goose, where the only airway secretory cells are goblet cells, cholinergic agonists stimulate secretion (155). The goblet cells in these species may be innervated and act as the functional equivalent of the submucosal glands in mammals.

There have been no extensive autoradiographic studies on airway goblet cells. Lamb (114) reported that the cells took up radioactive sulfate given to the cat in vivo as the precursor sodium [^{35}S]sulfate, and this was confirmed by C. B. Basbaum (unpublished observations). However, in a later study using a similar technique, Jeffery (96) concluded that cat goblet cells did not take up [^{3}H]glucose or [^{35}S]sulfate to any marked degree, whereas goose goblet cells incorporated both of these radiolabeled precursors. In a limited study, rabbit tracheal goblet cells were shown to incorporate [^{35}S]sulfate (and probably also [^{3}H]glucose), but not very heavily (150). In a pilot experiment C. B. Basbaum (unpublished observations) found that the uptake of ^{35}S and its movement into the apical granules of cat goblet cells took between 6 and 24 h in vitro, compared with the maximum of 6 h allowed in the in vivo studies (114). Therefore the extent of radiolabel incorporation is unlikely to be sufficient for tagged mucins to be released from goblet cells during the in vivo experiments in the cat and rabbit. The evidence does support the fact that the acidic-staining glycoproteins of goblet cells are sulfated. Further autoradiographic studies are needed to elucidate the mechanism and time course of glycoprotein synthesis and turnover in epithelial goblet cells.

Epithelial serous cells. These cells were first described in the adult specific pathogen–free rat (98), in which they are the most common secretory cell in the extrapulmonary airways, comprising ~20% of the total cells. Serous cells decreased in frequency distally and were not observed at all in the bronchioles (100).

Epithelial serous cells are extremely rare in the mouse (147), but they have been observed in human fetal airways and in the cat (P. K. Jeffery, unpublished observations). In cats, however, the granules were more reminiscent of those found in goblet cells. Epithelial serous cells also occur in goose trachea, but they are rare (155).

Epithelial serous cells stain with both PAS and AB, suggesting the presence of both acidic and neutral glycoproteins. In their ultrastructural study of the rat, Jeffery and Reid (98) concluded that the serous cells were likely to be the same as the PAS-staining epithelial cells previously described by Jones and co-workers (105). The serous cells of the mouse stained with both AB and PAS (147), and no mention was made of the staining characteristics in the goose (155).

The epithelial serous cells resemble serous cells in the submucosal glands (98). The granules of epithelial serous cells are located mostly at the apical surface, are electron dense, and are ~600 nm in diameter (smaller than goblet cell granules). The cells have a filiform border, an irregularly shaped nucleus, and an electron-dense cytoplasm. There are no autoradiographic data available on epithelial serous cells, and it would be useful to have this data before physiological investigations of their secretory processes are carried out.

Epithelial serous cells have been found in quantity only in specific pathogen–free animals and the human fetus; consequently their function (if any) in the normal individual is unknown. Jeffery and Reid (98) postulated that they may be responsible for producing the low-viscosity periciliary liquid layer. Brandtzaeg (31) used immunohistochemical techniques to localize immunoglobulin A in specimens of the human nasal gland, the submandibular gland, and the intestinal wall (at biopsy) and suggested that epithelial serous cells are involved in the molecular completion and epithelial transfer of secretory immunoglobulin A. Clearly this role does not apply to human lower airways, because there is no evidence that such cells exist there. Jeffery and Reid (100) showed that on administering tobacco smoke to specific pathogen–free rats, the number of epithelial serous cells with electron-dense granules decreased and the number of goblet cells with electron-lucent granules increased. Cells containing both types of granules also became evident. They interpreted this finding as evidence that tobacco smoke caused a transformation of serous cells to goblet cells. So far as mucous secretion in the normal adult mammal is concerned, the most likely role for epithelial serous cells is as precursors to goblet cells. The lack of epithelial serous cells in normal human lower airways, however, means that such a transformation cannot explain the goblet cell hyperplasia found in people with chronic bronchitis (59, 70, 161, 203).

Clara cells. Kölliker (111) first described Clara cells in 1881. They are found only in airways ~1 mm in diameter, and so in large animals they do not extend into the bronchi (32). They extend proximally as far as the hilus in the rat (98) and to the trachea in the mouse (146).

Results from studies on whether Clara cells stain for mucous glycoproteins are contradictory. It is generally accepted that they do not stain with AB (146, 213), and whereas some workers claim that they stain with PAS (10), others have been unable to confirm this (113). In the mouse trachea, <2% of Clara cells contain electron-lucent granules like those found in goblet cells (147); therefore even if some of them do contain mucus they are unlikely to be a major source of airway mucus, particularly in the major airways of large mammals.

Clara cells, however, do contain two types of electron-dense granules (147) and also have other features of secretory cells; consequently their main function is almost certainly secretory (213). In the mouse trachea they constitute ~60% of the epithelial cells that project to the luminal surface (147); in the bronchioles of larger mammals most of the nonciliated cells are Clara cells (32), strongly suggesting that they are functionally important. It has been suggested that they may secrete a lipoprotein (10) that might act as a bronchiolar surfactant (58, 144). Clara cells have been observed to release their contents via merocrine (187) and apocrine (65) mechanisms. This and the fact that the cells contain more than one type of secretory granule suggest that the cells may well secrete at least two different products. Like epithelial serous cells, Clara cells may turn into goblet cells after the appropriate stimulation [e.g., with tobacco smoke (100)], or they may be precursors of ciliated and brush cells [as was proposed after exposing rats to nitrogen dioxide (66)]. In terms of mucous production, this transformation of Clara cells into goblet cells may be their most important role, but more evidence for this is required.

Ciliated cells. Ciliated cells are the most common epithelial cells in the airway; in the human there are nearly 5 times more ciliated cells than goblet cells. The cytoplasm of ciliated cells is lighter than that of the goblet cells because it contains fewer ribosomes. In addition, ciliated cells have no secretory granules (167). The structure of ciliated cells has been described in detail for many species (32) and is adapted to their function of activating and coordinating the cilia (171, 172); the mechanism for this is still poorly understood.

The ciliated cells do not stain with either AB or PAS, and so it is assumed that they neither contain nor secrete glycoprotein. Spicer and co-workers (186) demonstrated a layer of AB-staining material very close to the surface of the epithelial cells in dog and human trachea, a finding that has also been confirmed in the cat and goose (96). This layer of surface mucosubstance is thought to be stationary and may even be a glycocalyx, an integral component of the epithelial cells. The surface mucosubstance was also found with electron microscopy in the dog and rat (184). Its origin is obscure, and although it is sulfated it does not stain strongly with PAS and stains only weakly with AB, in sharp contrast with neighboring goblet cells, which take up both stains, and the submucosal glands, which are PAS positive. Spicer and co-workers (186) postulated (by exclusion) that the mucosubstance may be derived from the ciliated cells, even though ciliated cells do not stain, both because they are the most numerous cell type and because the mucosubstance is closely associated with them.

This surface mucosubstance has also been studied by autoradiography (96). In this study radiolabeled sulfate administered into the cat trachea in vivo was only slightly incorporated into the surface mucous layer and the epithelial cells in general but not specifically into the goblet cells. Tritiated glucose was incorporated into the surface mucosubstance and into the epithelial ciliated cells but only rarely into goblet cells. In the goose the surface mucosubstance did not label with [^{3}H]glucose and took up only small amounts of radiolabeled sulfate.

The anatomical evidence for the production of mucus by ciliated cells is circumspect: they neither contain secretory granules nor stain for mucins, but they do take up glycoprotein precursors. The surface mucosubstance must be formed somewhere, but its staining properties suggest that it is unlikely to be formed in either the goblet cells or the submucosal glands. Clearly, if the ciliated cells do synthesize and release glycoprotein, then they do so in a very different manner from the classic mucus-secreting cells of the large airways and gut. For example, they may simply incorporate preformed sulfated material onto the surface membrane.

Innervation. Since the studies of Florey and co-workers (70), it has been generally assumed that the mucus-secreting cells of the epithelium do not have any motor innervation. In most species, though not the mouse (146), epithelial nerves were observed in the tracheal epithelium, but most had the anatomical characteristics of sensory nerve endings (32, 167). Some species do have motor-type nerve endings. The rat, for example, has some axons containing dense-cored vesicles that are apparently adrenergic, as well as fewer axons containing agranular vesicles that are presumed to be cholinergic (97), although no synapses between nerve axons and epithelial cells have been observed. Motor nerve endings in the cat tracheal epithelium are nonexistent or extremely rare (46). Nerve axons that penetrate the epithelium have been reported in the goose, but they are infrequent (155). These axons contained neurosecretory vesicles (implying that they had motor functions), and they were seen close to ciliated, basal, and possible secretory cells. Small nerve fibers were seen in the tracheal epithelium of the domestic chicken, but they were presumed to be mainly afferent, although the possibility of a motor function was not excluded (201).

If any pattern is to be observed in the anatomy of airway innervation, it is that species with submucosal glands (e.g., human, dog, cat, and ferret) have a motor supply to the glands but not to surface (mucosal) epithelial secretory cells; in contrast, species without submucosal glands probably do have a motor supply to surface cells. In fact the mouse appears to have no nerve fibers in the large airways at all.

PHYSIOLOGY. The contribution of the epithelial secretory cells to the total amount of respiratory tract mucus is unknown, but the anatomical considerations cited in the previous section ensure that it varies considerably among species. Until more is known about the biochemistry and rheological properties of mucus derived from the epithelial cells and submucosal glands, any difference in function between mucus from the different sources remains obscure. The evidence shows that the mucins are chemically different and are subject to different control mechanisms. Physiological studies of epithelial mucus have concentrated on the possibility of its neurohumoral control and any role it might play in either the defense of the lungs in response to airway irritation or in the pathogenesis of disease.

Neurohumoral control. No study has conclusively shown that parasympathetic or sympathetic nerve stimulation or the administration of adrenergic or cholinergic drugs causes goblet cells to secrete [with depletion of their contents as the criterion for secretion (70, 77)]. Since the initial experiments of Florey et al. (70) on the cat, it has been assumed that goblet cells are not functionally innervated. The rabbit is an important species for the physiological investigation of goblet cell function because its large airways have goblet cells but almost no submucosal glands. Perry and Boyd (153) found that vagal stimulation more than doubled the output of respiratory tract fluid from the rabbit, and they postulated that this must have come from the goblet cells. It has been shown, however, that this stimulus elicits no increase in radiolabeled glycoprotein output from an enclosed rabbit tracheal segment (150). It is possible that Perry and Boyd's finding resulted from an increase in mucociliary transport rather than the appearance of newly secreted material. However, atropine inhibits the base-line rate of mucociliary transport in the rabbit trachea (112), so if this were the explanation, atropine might be expected to decrease the resting output of respiratory tract fluid from the rabbit. In fact atropine has no such effect (30). Boyd also tested the effect of acetylcholine injected subcutaneously (29) and found, even at near lethal doses, no consistent effect on respiratory tract fluid output; it is difficult to know how to interpret this. Administration of adrenergic and cholinergic agonists into the enclosed tracheal segment of the rabbit, or to tracheal explants, had no consistent effect on radiolabeled glycoprotein output (150).

In the goose, electrical stimulation of the ninth cranial nerve increased radiolabeled mucin output, and this was largely (but not completely) blocked by atropine (155). Although there was no evidence of the depletion of goblet cells, it was concluded from autoradiographic evidence and the fact that no other cells stained for mucins that this secretion was derived from goblet cells.

Physiological evidence for the neurohumoral control of goblet cell secretion in mammalian airways is still very equivocal. To date, light-microscopic studies have not demonstrated any gross anatomical or histochemical changes in goblet cell appearance that would reflect a level of secretion in progress comparable to that observed under the electron microscope in the gut. Detailed electron-microscopic studies of airway goblet cell secretion are needed. Until there is some specific method available to measure airway goblet cell secretion, their normal control mechanisms will be elusive. Sturgess and Reid (189) found that goblet cell hyperplasia occurred in the trachea and bronchial tissue of rats after daily injections of either isoproterenol or pilocarpine for 6 or 12 days. This is strong evidence that the cells are able to respond to autonomic factors, and it is likely that this anatomical change leads to an increase in the total goblet cell mucous output. Whether chronic adrenergic or cholinergic stimulation is responsible for goblet cell hyperplasia in humans is not known (see *Hypertrophy of Mucus-Secreting Cells*, p. 426).

Effects of irritants. A variety of irritants augment mucous secretion, as demonstrated by either volumetric measurement or glycoprotein output; among these irritants are mustard oil (70), ammonia vapor and cigarette smoke (169), serum (152), and carbon dust (151). In most of these cases the secretion could have come from the submucosal glands, the epithelial secretory cells, or both. The evidence for goblet cell involvement is scanty, again because there is no satisfactory method of demonstrating that an airway goblet cell is secreting. Florey and co-workers (70) claimed that mustard oil exhausted the submucosal glands in the cat and that some evidence indicated that the globlet cells were partly discharged, although complete exhaustion was never seen. Jeffery (96) found fewer goblet cells in a cat tracheal segment treated with ammonia than in a control segment, implying that some goblet cells were sufficiently depleted to prevent them from staining. Adler and co-workers (2) obtained a similar result after application of cholera toxin to explants of guinea pig trachea. Serum applied to rabbit tracheas in vitro caused a marked increase in radiolabeled glycoprotein output (150), suggesting that goblet cells are the source of the secretion and that the mechanism does not involve a reflex. Both serum- and ammonia-stimulated secretions (76, 78, 150) contain mucins with very high molecular weights ($M_r > 2 \times 10^6$) and take up AB, whereas pilocarpine-stimulated mucins (derived mainly from submucosal glands) have a more prominent, lower-molecular-weight component ($M_r \simeq 0.5 \times 10^6$) and stain with PAS. In summary, irritants almost certainly cause goblet cells to secrete, in addition to any other direct or reflex effects they may have on submucosal glands.

There is now some evidence that irritants, such as ammonia and serum, may also cause removal of the surface mucosubstance presumably derived from the ciliated cells. Gallagher and co-workers (76) found that after submucosal gland exhaustion by pilocarpine, ammonia released a heavily tritiated mucous component from the cat trachea. Autoradiography demonstrated that (in control tissue) little [^{3}H]glucose was incorporated into the submucosal glands or goblet cells but that most of it was taken up by the other ciliated epithelial cells. Similarly, serum also released a component that labeled strongly with tritium and that presumably originated from the same source (152).

The physiology of mucous secretion from epithelial cells is obscure, and several interesting questions may be asked. Why is there so much anatomical variation among species? In what way are submucosal glands important if the rabbit and rat can manage without them? How is mucous secretion controlled in those species where there appears to be no neural or pharmacological control mechanism for it? Why are there so few goblet cells in the ferret trachea? Such species differences are used to elucidate the mechanisms of airway mucous secretion, but they pose as many questions as they answer.

Submucosal Glands

ANATOMY. Many studies have focused on the neural control of the glands and the effects of mediators (especially mediators of inflammation). Although a few articles have covered the role of calcium and stimulus-secretion coupling in the regulation of airway gland secretion (39, 125), our understanding of exocrine gland regulations is better characterized in other secretory systems (see refs. 170a, 178, and 178a for a review of these concepts). The presence of submucosal glands varies among species: they are numerous in cats, pigs, ferrets, and healthy humans; rare in rabbits and guinea pigs; and nonexistent in geese (194). Thus sufficient differences in structure and function exist among species to make extrapolations of the results of these studies to humans unwarranted, and specific studies of human tissue are sorely needed. The distribution of mucus-secreting cells in a single species varies at different anatomical levels. Thus the ferret trachea contains many glands but only a few goblet cells. Almost the whole surface of the intrapulmonary bronchi and larger bronchioles is composed of goblet cells, but the bronchioles contain few glands (93). The gland system is made up of short funnel-shaped ducts leading to the airway surface; the duct is connected to collecting ducts, which in turn lead to mucous and serous tubules lined with mucous and serous cells, respectively (136). Contractions of myoepithelial cells (closely related to secretory cells) may aid secretion. Serous cells are characterized by electron-dense, discrete secretory granules; during stimulation, serous cells show loss of granules (a presumed index of protein secretion), diverticulation, and enlargement of their acinar lumina (15). The vacuolization of serous cells during stimulation is presumably caused by the secretion of ions and water (15). Protein and water secretion may be under separate control. Mucous cells are characterized by granules that are electron lucent and often confluent (135); during secretion the fused bilayers of adjacent membranes are believed to break down, causing membrane fusion (143).

PHYSIOLOGY. The development of new experimental methods has increased our understanding of the regulation of gland secretion. Radiolabeled precursors (e.g., ^{35}S) incorporated into mucins were used to identify the cellular sources of mucus; the secretion of these precursors, along with high-molecular-weight mucins, has aided in the study of gland secretion (188). The secretory rate of glands had long been a matter of conjecture, mainly because they were relatively inaccessible. A micropipette method has been developed for obtaining secretions from single gland ducts in cats (198). Anatomical and autoradiographical methods have also been used to study the location of specific receptors in gland cells (15).

Neural control. Autonomic nerves regulate the secretions from airway submucosal glands but not from surface goblet cells (see *Surface Mucus*, p. 419). Thus the glands are under parasympathetic, sympathetic, and nonadrenergic [vasoactive intestinal polypeptide (VIP)?] control.

Parasympathetic nerves. Parasympathetic nerve supply is via the vagus nerves, which end as varicosities containing small agranular vesicles near the gland tubules and ducts (138). Cholinergic and adrenergic varicosities were found near serous and mucous cells, with no selectivity of axons to either type of gland cell. Only 4% of the cholinergic varicosities occurred in close contact with gland cells; this suggests that any regulatory selectivity of specific cells likely depends on the distribution of receptors on the cells, rather than on the selectivity of innervation. In cats the resting secretory rate of individual glands is ~9 nl/min (198); the fact that atropine only slightly decreased the secretory rate suggests that tonic parasympathetic motor control of the glands plays a small role in resting secretion. Stimulation of the vagus nerves increased the rate of fluid secretion into pipettes (198) and ^{35}S-labeled mucins (48), effects that atropine abolished. These findings indicate that vagal muscarinic pathways stimulate fluid and mucin production from the glands. In vitro studies of the electrical transmural stimulation of ferret trachea nerves confirm the presence of parasympathetic nerves and muscarinic receptors (20). The vagal motor effects on gland secretion were potentiated by serotonin (156), possibly through an effect on airway mural ganglionic transmission. Muscarinic agonists appear to stimulate secretion from both serous and mucous cells (15); fluid flow from these cells increased markedly (198). However, the protein concentration (199) and the apparent viscoelastic properties of the secretions harvested in the micropipettes did not change (G. D. Leikauf, unpublished observations).

Various reflexes stimulate gland secretion. Among the most potent is irritation of the airway. Thus mechanical stimulation of the larynx increased the gland secretory rate via vagal pathways (83). In fact reflex gland secretion appears to be a part of the normal cough reflex and therefore assists in the removal of foreign irritants. Inflammation of the airway epithelium (e.g., in bronchitis) may reflexly stimulate excessive secretions from the glands. Epithelial inflammation might be the primary stimulus, causing the release of mediators that stimulate sensory nerve endings that reflexly produce excessive secretions. Stimulation of bronchial C fibers also increased gland secretion via a vagal reflex (50), and this is another pathway by which inflammation could cause excessive secretions. Hypoxia (47) and gastric stimulation (82) also increased the secretory flow from glands via vagal reflexes.

Sympathetic nerves. The sympathetic nerves also innervate glands. There are ~9 times more cholinergic (agranular) than adrenergic (dense-cored) varicosities near the glands (138). Because sympathetic nervous stimulation apparently produces as much secretion as vagal stimulation (20), it seems that the potency of neural control over effector cells depends mainly on the density of receptors and cells rather than on the numbers of nerve endings. Ninety-two percent of all axon bundles contained both adrenergic and cholinergic varicosities (138), a close contact that suggests that the nerves may interact. In fact Borson and Nadel (21) showed that stimulating the cholinergic nerves to glands inhibits adrenergic neurotransmission. Thus autonomic nervous stimulation may affect gland secretion directly or via an effect on other nerves.

Electrical stimulation of the thoracic sympathetic nerves increases both mucin (19) and fluid (20) production. A great deal of evidence shows that both α- and β-adrenergic agonists stimulate gland secretion with different, selective effects. The increased fluid flow from glands produced by sympathetic nerve stimulation is largely abolished by phentolamine, indicating that the effect is mainly due to α-adrenergic stimulation (20). This is confirmed by the fact that α-

adrenergic agonists are potent in causing fluid secretion from glands, whereas β-adrenergic agonists are not (20). On the other hand, both α- and β-adrenergic agonists stimulated ^{35}S-labeled mucin production (19). Other studies showed the α-adrenergic stimulation produced secretions with lower concentrations of protein (199) and sulfur (158) in fluid collected in micropipettes and markedly stimulated the release of lysozyme (196); β-adrenergic stimulation produced secretions with higher protein and sulfur concentrations in the secreted fluid but only small amounts of lysozyme. Anatomical studies suggest that α- and β-adrenergic stimulation produces selective effects on specific cell types. Thus Tom-Moy, Basbaum, and Nadel (196) used immunocytochemical methods to prove that lysozyme was localized selectively within the secretory granules of serous (but not mucous) cells, suggesting that α-adrenergic stimulation selectively depleted serous cells. Morphometric studies confirm that α-adrenergic agonists do in fact deplete serous cells, sparing the mucous cells (15). These morphological and biochemical differences in adrenergic responses are also reflected in changes in the viscoelastic behavior of mucus harvested in pipettes. Thus G. D. Leikauf (unpublished observations) found that β-adrenergic stimulation produced secretions of a higher apparent viscosity and lower elasticity than controls, α-adrenergic stimulation produced secretions of a lower apparent viscosity, and muscarinic stimulation produced no changes in viscoelastic behavior at all.

Nonadrenergic, noncholinergic nerves. Electron-microscopic studies indicate that varicosities containing large dense-cored vesicles are present in nerves located in the airway submucosa, and these are the suggested source of the nonadrenergic, noncholinergic nerves (14). Physiological evidence for this system's neural effects on gland secretion come from in vitro studies of transmural electrical stimulation of the nerves to the submucosal glands. Thus even after administering atropine, phentolamine, and propranolol, electrical stimulation still increased ^{35}S-labeled mucin secretion (19). The fact that tetrodotoxin abolished this effect implicates a neural role in the response. The mediator of this response is unknown, but VIP is a likely candidate because 1) immunocytochemical studies demonstrate the presence of nerves containing VIP in airway ganglia and in the submucosa of cats (197) and ferrets (14), 2) anatomical studies show vesicles containing VIP, and 3) VIP stimulated ^{35}S-labeled mucin production. This system's role in normal gland regulation is unknown.

Effects of Drugs and Mediators

Various drugs affect mucous secretion. In many cases the source of secretion (e.g., glands vs. surface cells) is not known and the mechanism of a drug's action is unclear. Various authors report differences that could be due to species differences or to the methods of study used, but these issues have not been widely explored.

The mediators most studied in airway regulation are those released in the airways by various "fixed" airway cells (e.g., mast cells) and circulating cells (e.g., neutrophils). These include preformed mediators stored within cells and released after the appropriate stimulation (e.g., histamine release from mast cells) and newly formed materials generated by the cells after stimulation (e.g., arachidonic acid metabolites). The sources of preformed mediators such as histamine are well known, but the metabolic pathways and interactions between cells of the arachidonic acid pathways are poorly understood. It is believed that in airways these mediators are mainly released from mast cells or from cells immobilized to the airways (e.g., neutrophils) due to the release of chemotactic factors from mast cells. However, the airway epithelial cells are the lining cells separating airway tissue from the environment, and we suggest that these cells act as sensors of toxic influences introduced into the airways. Thus on stimulation the epithelial cells are the logical cells to signal others and to mobilize airway defenses. They could release chemotactic mediators and bring neutrophils to the epithelium, then release other mediators and activate mast cells. Thus the airway epithelial cell is a good candidate to act as a "paracrine sensor," informing and mobilizing the airway cells and other cells (e.g., blood-borne cells).

Most studies involve administering agonists to secretory tissue in vitro and then measuring the secretory responses. Many inadequacies accompany such studies. *1*) Airway cells may convert the administered material to another, more or less potent material. *2*) In vitro studies eliminate other important interactions that might occur among cells. For example, leukotriene B_4 (LTB$_4$) is a potent chemotactic factor for leukocytes, and its release by airway cells stimulates chemotaxis and release of leukocyte isozymes. These isozymes could in turn have potent primary or secondary effects on secretory cells and other cells. *3*) Studies of administered mediators are often limited by the small amounts of mediators available (e.g., lipoxygenase products). This scarcity limits the scope of studies and therefore insights into mechanisms of action. *4*) Some mediators (e.g., those derived from lipoxygenase) lack specific antagonists; developing these antagonists would accelerate our understanding of the role of various mediators in these pathways. *5*) Most studies involve administering mediators in the tissue and are not physiological studies of mediator release from airway tissues. Because the structures of some of arachidonic acid's mediators have been described and specific radioimmunoassays have been developed, it is now possible to assess their biologic roles in both normal regulation and in disease.

Histamine (a preformed mediator) is released from mast cells after stimulation by specific antigens or other substances (e.g., 48/80), and its effects on secretion vary (139). Thus histamine had no effect on in vitro secretion in dogs or humans but did stimulate mucin production in cats and geese. One study reports that histamine stimulates the release of mucins from human airways by affecting receptors but that it is less potent than LTs or prostaglandins (PGs) (176).

In addition to primary effects on receptors in the gland cells themselves, mediators may also act on nervous pathways, secondarily affecting gland secretion. Thus bradykinin reflexly stimulated fluid production from airway submucosal glands in vivo (50) but had no significant effect on mucin release from explants (188). Bradykinin is released endogenously under various conditions and may play a role in the inflammatory process (159). The endogenous release of bradykinin could produce inflammatory changes and thereby modify autonomic responses. Recent evidence suggests that kinin receptors in the gut stimulate the production of PGE_2, which stimulates electrolyte secretion (68), and that kinins could operate in airways via similar indirect mechanisms. Basic polypeptides (e.g., kallidin and substance P) apparently stimulate mucous secretion in dogs, whereas hexadrimethrine (a kallidin antagonist) decreases it (13).

Two metabolic pathways of arachidonic acid metabolism have been described: the cyclooxygenase pathway (including PGs and their intermediates) and the lipoxygenase pathway (including LT derivatives, the major components of slow-reacting substance of anaphylaxis). Both of these pathways have been implicated in the regulation of airway secretions, but none of their effects are well characterized.

Most airway secretory studies of arachidonic acid metabolism have focused on the cyclooxygenase pathway, which produces various PGs and thromboxanes. Thus PGA_2, PGD_2, and $PGF_{2\alpha}$ increased mucin secretion in human airways, whereas PGE_2 reduced this secretion (128). One study found that indomethacin affected base-line mucin release, suggesting that lipoxygenase products generated by the airways regulate normal mucin production (176).

Products of the lipoxygenase pathway [mono- and dihydroxyeicosatetraenoic acid (HETE) and LTs] were shown to be potent mediators in allergic and inflammatory states, and these mediators also apparently affect secretion. Mono-HETE stimulates mucin secretion in human bronchi, and various synthetic HETEs (e.g., 5-, 8-, 11-, and 12-HETE) increase mucin release (176). Both LTC_4 and LTD_4 also increase mucin production even more potently than the HETEs. Of course, until the airway tissue's metabolism is better characterized, an understanding of the exact mode of action for these effects, as well as the interpretation of these findings, is limited.

Products of arachidonic acid metabolism have been studied principally as primary agonists. However, these materials might also operate by affecting the threshold of the target tissue (e.g., glands), thereby also affecting the tissue's responsiveness to other stimuli.

The role of preformed mediators and arachidonic acid metabolites in the changes in mucociliary clearance that accompany antigen-antibody responses induced by immunoglobulin E is unclear. The fact that nonselective antagonists of the lipoxygenase pathway prevent the mucociliary clearance changes seen experimentally in canine anaphylaxis suggests that these metabolites have important deleterious effects on either secretory or ciliary function (202).

Hypertrophy of Mucus-Secreting Cells

The association of sputum production with chronic lung disease [part of the definition of chronic bronchitis (133)] is well known (91a); Florey et al. (70), however, were the first to observe that this could be attributed to a hypertrophy of mucus-secreting cells as well as to an increase in their individual activity. Reid (160) carried out the first comprehensive study of necropsy specimens from patients with chronic bronchitis and showed that (among other pathological structural changes) both the number of epithelial goblet cells and the size of the submucosal glands in the bronchi increased. Florey et al. (70) also demonstrated (in animals) that chronic injections of formalin into the trachea resulted in goblet cell proliferation similar to that seen in chronic bronchitis, with the unstated hypothesis that the airway changes present in chronic bronchitis may also result from chronic irritation.

Because of the correlation between mucous cell hypertrophy and mucous hypersecretion, it has generally been assumed that hypertrophy necessarily leads to hypersecretion and that hypersecretion is caused by the increased activity of mucus-secreting cells. This need not be the case. The presence of mucous cell hypertrophy means that the rate of mucous synthesis over a given period has exceeded the rate of secretion, so that hypertrophy results when the rate of mucous synthesis increases faster than the rate of mucous secretion and also when a constant or increased rate of synthesis is accompanied by a downregulation of the secretory process. In this case overall hypersecretion may still be the final outcome, because the pool of available mucus is greater than normal.

Recent research has followed two lines: *1*) the epidemiology and quantification of mucous cell hypertrophy in humans with either chronic lung disease or who are exposed regularly to airway irritants and *2*) the time course and mechanisms of mucous cell hypertrophy in animals exposed to irritants and drugs.

HUMAN STUDIES. *Submucosal glands.* Methods of quantification of the degree of submucosal gland hypertrophy have been developed by Reid (161), Restrepo and Heard (166), de Haller and Reid (52), Dunnill et al. (56), and Alli (9). Comparisons of some of these methods (17, 190) indicate that the more time consuming and quantitative the method, the more accurate it is. The Dunnill point count (56) is recommended for the most accurate work, and the Reid index (52) is recommended for quantifying gross changes, because it takes much less time than other methods (190).

These methods were used to confirm the original observation of mucous gland hypertrophy in people with chronic bronchitis (52, 56, 84, 161, 166, 191). Hypertrophy has also been found in people with bronchiectasis (161), emphysema (87), asthma (190), carcinoma of the bronchus, pneumoconiosis and bronchopneumonia (69). Cystic fibrosis patients with chronic lung infections have a degree of submucosal gland hypertrophy similar to that present in adult chronic bronchitis (165).

The Reid index (161, 193) is the ratio of the height of a submucosal gland to the distance between the luminal edge of a cartilage ring and the surface epithelium (at the same place). In necropsy specimens from control human bronchi, the Reid index varied from 0.14 to 0.36, with a mean of 0.26. The values for bronchi from patients with chronic bronchitis (at least 5 yr) ranged from 0.41 to 0.79, with a mean of 0.59. There was no overlap between the two groups (161). On the other hand, other workers claim that there is a wide range of degree of hypertrophy in the general population and that such a clear distinction cannot be made (91, 192). Reid (161) also showed that the degree of hypertrophy (measured with Reid index) is associated with the amount of sputum produced daily. However, even in the submucosal glands of patients producing trace quantities of sputum, the gland-to-wall ratio might be significantly greater than in control tissue. This suggests that secretion increases considerably before sputum is produced. Presumably the mucociliary elevator removes the extra secretion, and only when it is overloaded is coughing elicited and sputum expectorated.

De Haller and Reid (52) compared the histochemistry of submucosal glands from the bronchi of patients with chronic bronchitis and from normal human bronchi. The proportion of mucous cells to serous cells is increased in the hypertrophied glands of patients with chronic bronchitis. Mucous cells contain an acid mucopolysaccharide that is resistant to neuraminidase, so that more mucus is secreted in chronic bronchitis than in normals and a greater proportion of it is resistant to neuraminidase. Thus the types of secretory cells appear to be normal, but they are present in different proportions, and this could alter the viscoelastic properties of the secreted mucus. These different cell types might represent different phases in the cycle of mucous elaboration, during which mucus may be discharged from the cell at any stage; consequently the different proportions of cell types need not necessarily reflect an abnormal cycle but could simply result from a quickening of the normal cycle (52).

Goblet cells. More detailed studies (36, 59, 60, 162) have been carried out since Florey et al. (70) and Reid (160) first observed goblet cell hypertrophy in chronic bronchitis. Chang (36) compared whole mounts of human bronchial epithelium (taken at autopsy) from smokers and nonsmokers and found a significantly greater number of distended goblet cells in the bronchi of the smokers. In some cases almost the whole surface was covered by goblet cells. Although few patients were studied, Chang (36) concluded that in bronchitis (but not in a variety of other lung diseases) there is a greater degree of goblet cell hyperplasia in smokers versus nonsmokers. Reid (162) looked at sections of human lung (various parts) taken from autopsies of 12 patients with chronic bronchitis. In each case the number of goblet cells in the peripheral airways increased, and in two cases there was a 1:1 ratio of goblet cells to other epithelial cells (vs. 1:20 or 1:30 in normal airways).

Ellefson and Tos (59, 60) conducted comprehensive studies and counted the number of goblet cells in whole mounts of human trachea and from human tracheal biopsies. They noted a slight tendency for goblet cell density to increase with increased cigarette consumption and an increased cell density in patients with a productive cough (59). In chronic tracheobronchitis, the mean goblet cell density was ~10,000/mm^2, compared with ~6,800/mm^2 in normal tracheas. The highest density found was ~13,750/mm^2 (60). Although this doubling of the number of goblet cells in the trachea would almost certainly result in differences in mucous production and a productive cough, if the normal proportion of goblet cells to ciliated cells is ~1:5 (167), then in the trachea of a patient with chronic bronchitis, the ratio would reach a maximum of 2:5. This is less than was reported in many less-quantitative studies. In two cases Florey et al. (70) reported finding only goblet cells; Chang (36) reported that goblet cells occupied the "whole surface" of the trachea; Reid (162) claimed a maximum ratio of goblet cells to other epithelial cells of ~1:1. There is no clear explanation for this variability, but it may reflect differences in patient selection; perhaps the differences indicate the need to carry out fully quantitative studies.

De Haller and Reid (52) briefly described the histochemistry of tracheal goblet cells in chronic bronchitis. Both control and diseased airway goblet cells contained AB-positive granules, whereas PAS-staining material was only observed at the base of goblet cells from the control subjects (not in chronic bronchitis). Whether this difference has any clinical significance is not known.

ANIMAL STUDIES. A variety of irritants and animals have been used to try to mimic the hypertrophy of mucus-secreting cells in chronic bronchitis. These include formalin in the cat (70); sulfur dioxide in the rat (115, 157, 163), dog (11, 35, 185), and lamb (130); and tobacco smoke in the mouse (121), rat (45, 88–90, 100, 102, 104, 105, 116), dog (149), and lamb (129, 130). Chlorine gas (61) and nitrogen dioxide (71) were also used as irritants in the rat. In all of these studies there was a demonstrable increase in goblet cell number, the size of the submucosal glands, or both. Protocols and doses varied among the studies, but 400 ppm of sulfur dioxide administered to rats for 3 h/day, 5 day/wk for 3 wk produced significant hypertrophy in goblet cells and submucosal glands (115). Similarly regimens for the administration of cigarette smoke also varied. Jones et al. (105) exposed rats to 25 cigarettes/day, 4 day/wk for 6 wk and found hypertrophy both in goblet cells and submucosal glands.

Hyperplasia in epithelial goblet cells is accompanied by a thickening of the airway epithelium, implying that the total number of cells increases (100, 104, 115, 116, 149). With chronic sulfur dioxide stimulation, however, not only are new cells formed but other epithelial cells (e.g., Clara cells) may be transformed into goblet cells (95); in addition, exposing rats to tobacco smoke provided evidence that epithelial serous cells may act as precursors to mucous cells (100).

A few investigators tried to follow the time course of any recovery by observing the structure of the airways at various intervals after removal of the irritant. With sulfur dioxide given to rats, there was no clear sign of any reversal of histological changes after 5 wk (115) or even after 3 mo (163). In a group of dogs exposed to tobacco smoke for 6 mo, there was evidence of recovery after 9 mo (149); Jones (102), however, noted the reversal of some histochemical changes in rats 9 days after cessation of exposure.

Although the observation that irritants cause mucous cell hypertrophy is well established, there are two fundamental questions, which have only partial answers: what is the mechanism of cell proliferation and how good a model of human chronic bronchitis is it?

Mechanism of hypertrophy. One possible mechanism for the histological changes observed after lung irritation is that irritation causes an excessive secretion that then acts as a nest for bacterial colonization and that secretory cell proliferation is secondary to this infection. The results of Reid (163) suggest that this is not the case, because she found no greater frequency of occurrence of organisms in the bronchi and lungs of animals exposed to sulfur dioxide than in control animals. On the other hand, Elmes and Bell (61) looked at the effect of chlorine gas on rats with a spontaneous pulmonary disease similar to human chronic bronchitis and found that chlorine only exacerbated changes that were already occurring, presumably due to the infection; they concluded that infection might be the primary cause of the changes and the irritation merely an adjuvant. However, this explanation begs the question. Might not the original spontaneous lung disease have resulted from another undetermined irritant that the rats were exposed to during their early development? Little of the more recent work in the field is specifically directed at the question of whether infection or hypertrophy comes first in chronic lung disease, but because hypertrophy can occur in disease-free animals exposed to irritants, it is now generally assumed that infection is a later stage in the etiology of chronic bronchitis.

Lane and Gordon (118) and Wells and Lamerton (204) suggest that cell proliferation might be the tissue's response to an initial killing and sloughing off of cells by the irritant. Lamb and Reid (115) noted an initial fall in goblet cell numbers that was followed by an increase in their numbers in the airways of rats exposed to sulfur dioxide. However, in their electron-microscopic study with specific pathogen–free rats, Jeffery and Reid (100) found no evidence of epithelial sloughing after exposure to tobacco smoke; cell hypertrophy, secretion, and proliferation were the earliest events noted.

Apart from an increase in the number of mucus-secreting cells, irritation also induces other histochemical changes in the lung. For example, there is an increase in the number of goblet cells containing acidic glycoproteins relative to the number containing neutral-staining glycoproteins (35, 89, 105, 115, 130, 185). In rats exposed to tobacco smoke, changes have been found within 20 h of the first exposure (102). In submucosal glands, there may also be a relative increase in acidic-staining (130) or neutral-staining (90) glycoproteins. Jones et al. (104) administered tobacco smoke to rats with and without the anti-inflammatory agent phenylmethyloxadiazole added to it and showed that the agent protected against goblet cell proliferation but not against the change in their staining characteristics. They used this as evidence that these two factors are affected by lung irritation but are under different control mechanisms.

Grieg et al. (88) investigated the effect of another anti-inflammatory agent, indomethacin (a PG-synthesis inhibitor), on goblet cell hyperplasia in rat airways. They showed that when injected intraperitoneally, indomethacin (like phenylmethyloxadiazole) inhibited the increase in numbers of epithelial mucous cells induced by chronic irritation with tobacco smoke but had no effect on intracellular mucin's change from acidic to neutral. The inhibition of hyperplasia was insignificant in the trachea but was significant in the lower airways, a fact that Grieg et al. (88) thought might be attributable to differences in the blood supply. Their explanation for these findings was that the indomethacin inhibited the rise in tissue levels of PGE that occurred during exposure to cigarette smoke. Prostaglandin E stimulates the adenylate cyclase receptor complex, causing a rise in intracellular cAMP that is associated with a cessation of cell division and a move toward cell differentiation (1). Thus the presence of indomethacin might be expected to inhibit mucous cell maturation. However, if this mechanism operates in the lung, exposure to tobacco smoke without indomethacin should cause a reduction in cell division, but the opposite is generally found to be true (100, 104, 204).

Another possible mechanism for mucus-secreting

cell hypertrophy is through the cells' constant stimulation during chronic irritation, in a manner similar to that of work hypertrophy in skeletal muscle. Acute irritation at various levels of the respiratory tract mainly causes reflex secretion of mucus from the trachea of the cat through parasympathetic pathways, but some sympathetic pathways may also be involved (154). Sturgess and Reid (189) injected rats with either isoproterenol or pilocarpine daily for 6–12 days, and the tracheobronchial tree was then examined histologically. Both agonists caused hypertrophy of the submucosal glands and epithelial goblet cells, but they resulted in different histological changes in the two groups of cells. This suggests that at least two different mechanisms were operating: isoproterenol caused an increase in the number of small acini in the submucosal glands and of goblet cells containing acidic glycoprotein, whereas pilocarpine induced an increase in the number of acini in large glands staining with PAS and in all types of goblet cells. The effect of these autonomic agonists on goblet cells was surprising, because they are not thought to be under neurohumoral regulation (see *Surface Mucus*, p. 419). Baskerville (16) carried out similar experiments, using only isoproterenol, in the pig (a species with an airway structure similar to that of humans). The increase in acidic glycoprotein relative to neutral glycoprotein in the mucous acini of the submucosal glands was comparable to that found in human chronic bronchitis (117). Similar changes were also reported in the glands of sheep exposed to sulfur dioxide (130). Chronic administration of methacholine chloride to dogs (for up to 3 mo) caused an increase in the activity of some glycosyltransferases in the tracheal tissue but not of fucosyltransferase (12). Assuming that these enzymes are involved in the synthesis of respiratory mucin, this study suggests that chronic cholinergic stimulation may influence the ability of respiratory tissue to alter the composition of mucins.

Kleinerman et al. (107) chronically administered methacholine to cats and noted an increase both in the size of bronchial submucosal glands and in the number of goblet cells (both relative to control animals). The staining characteristics of glycoproteins in the hypertrophied glands of the cat were normal, but the goblet cells contained a less acidic mucin than did control tissues. Confirming the suggestion of Baker et al. (12), these workers also demonstrated that glycoproteins collected in vitro from tissues chronically treated with methacholine had significantly greater amounts of sialic acid than was normal.

A neurally mediated mechanism for cell hypertrophy was implicated in the salivary glands of the rat. Increasing the work load of the parotid gland (via a bulk diet) increased mitosis and DNA content in the cells, an effect that could be prevented by removing the parasympathetic motor pathways to the gland prior to the diet change. The effects of sympathectomy were less pronounced (173). On the other hand, Muir et al. (137) stimulated the sympathetic and parasympathetic nerves to rat salivary glands for periods up to 1 h and demonstrated that the former caused an increase in the weights of the submaxillary and parotid glands and in their rates of cell division. Parasympathetic nerve stimulation had no such effects.

There is some evidence against the possibility of chronic stimulation causing hypertrophy via reflex activity. In one dog in which a tracheal pouch had been prepared, the long-term administration of sulfur dioxide caused hypertrophy of mucus-secreting cells in the remainder of the respiratory tract but not in the bypassed, innervated pouch (185). Lamb and Reid (115) believed that at least part of the action of sulfur dioxide is direct, because the number of goblet cells, as with other epithelial cells, decreases before increasing above normal levels.

In conclusion, it is not possible to say which of these mechanisms produces hypertrophy during chronic irritation of the airways. They are not mutually exclusive, so it is probable that mucous cell hypertrophy has a multifactorial etiology.

Experimental hypertrophy as a model for chronic bronchitis. The most noticeable histological features of human chronic bronchitis are submucosal gland hypertrophy and the proliferation of goblet cells, including their appearance in more peripheral airways (16). These changes are well established in the airways of animals exposed to chronic irritation (163, 164). In addition an increase in the proportion of intracellular material that is acidic rather than neutral occurs in both chronic bronchitis (52) and experimental hypertrophy (115). There is also an increase in mucins resistant to neuraminidase present in goblet cells in both conditions (115). Experiments with dogs compared the lung function of animals chronically exposed to sulfur dioxide with controls, and the observed changes reflect an obstruction of the airways similar to that noted in humans suffering from chronic obstructive airways disease (108). Although many studies, particularly by Reid and co-workers, use the rat, other authors contend that the pig (86, 103) and the dog (35, 212) provide better models of human airways (at least anatomically).

Not enough studies using autonomic agonists to induce airway secretory cell hyperplasia have been made to allow any firm conclusions concerning how representative these changes are of chronic bronchitis. However, Sturgess and Reid (189) and Baskerville (16) showed that the number of acidic-staining glycoproteins in the submucosal glands of rats and pigs, respectively, increased after chronic injections of isoproterenol, and they used this feature as further evidence for its similarity with chronic bronchitis. De Haller and Reid (52) noted that there was an increased proportion of mucous to serous cells in the submucosal glands in airways taken from patients with chronic bronchitis, although serous cells remained in the majority. M. Tom-Moy (unpublished observations) saw a similar change in the proportion of areas occupied by the two cell types in ferrets after chronic injections of isoproterenol.

Some workers studying chronic obstructive airways disease in animals compared the histological changes in it with those occurring in chronic bronchitis, and there are some notable similarities. Wheeldon and Pirie (212) studied dogs suffering from a condition they described as chronic bronchitis, although Chakrin and Saunders (35) claim that it is very rare in the dog. Jones et al. (103) studied the airways of pigs with enzootic pneumonia. Both groups of workers found submucosal gland hypertrophy, and histochemical analysis of the pig submucosal gland cells revealed changes comparable to those in human chronic bronchitis. However, the number of goblet cells in the pig decreased, and the authors postulated that the cells had probably discharged their contents and so were no longer visible.

In conclusion, the structural and histochemical changes occurring in the large airways during experimental hypertrophy generally compare well with those changes noted in human chronic bronchitis. However, as Reid (164) pointed out, an animal model of a human disease remains only a model, but the fact that chronic irritation of animal airways leads to changes similar to those in human chronic bronchitis is strong evidence that chronic exposure to irritants is an important component in the etiology of this disease in humans. There is still much to learn about the mechanisms of these changes, and animal models remain the best hope for furthering our understanding of chronic bronchitis.

ION TRANSPORT AND WATER MOVEMENT

Introduction

The water content of airway secretions is a critical factor in effective mucociliary clearance. First, the rheological properties of mucus depend on the degree of hydration. Second, the depth of the periciliary sol layer controls the cilia's ability to beat and contact the bottom of the mucous gel. Presumably, if the sol layer is too thin, the cilia cannot beat; if it is too deep, they beat, but they cannot move the mucous gel.

Thus the regulation of transepithelial water movement is important for proper airway function. In other epithelia, active ion transport underlies net transepithelial fluid movement (44, 92). The transfer of solute from one side of the epithelium to the other results in local osmotic gradients across the tissue, which then lead to transepithelial fluid movement (43, 54).

To determine if such active ion transport was present in airway epithelium, Olver and co-workers (145) mounted sheets of the posterior membranous portion of the dog's tracheal epithelium in Ussing chambers. They found that the tissue had a resistance (R) of 300–500 $\Omega \cdot cm^2$ and developed a spontaneous potential difference (PD) of ~30 mV (luminal side negative). The presence of this PD indicated that active transepithelial ion transport was present. To determine which ions were being actively transported, they applied Ussing's (200) short-circuit current (I_{sc}) technique. The principle of Ussing's method is that when current is passed across the epithelium so that the transepithelial PD = 0, no electrical driving force exists across the epithelium. If there are no hydrostatic or osmotic pressure differences across the tissue and the ion concentrations of the media bathing either side of the tissue are identical, then no forces exist to bring about the net movement of any ion by passive processes. If by using isotopes one detects the net movement of an ion across the epithelium, then this net movement must be due to active transport, i.e., the tissue metabolism provides the energy for net ion movement. Furthermore the sum of the current due to all active ion-transport processes is equal to the current needed to make PD = 0, i.e., the I_{sc}. Olver and co-workers (145) found an I_{sc} of ~100 $\mu A/cm^2$, which was entirely accounted for by a net movement of Cl toward the lumen and a smaller active transport of Na toward the serosa. There was thus no reason to postulate the existence of any other significant ion-transport processes. These results have been confirmed by other authors (4, 27, 218).

The results of Boucher et al. (22) indicate that the ion-transport processes found with Ussing chambers truly reflect those processes occurring in vivo; they found that the PD across the tracheal wall of anesthetized dogs was also ~30 mV (luminal side negative) and responded to drugs in the same way as tissues in vitro did.

Since the initial study of Olver et al. (145), the dog tracheal epithelium has become one of the better characterized Cl-secreting epithelia (75, 220). Ion transport across a number of other airway epithelia has also been described (26). Finally, the importance of active ion transport in the regulation of respiratory tract fluid production was established by studies where changes in ion transport produced predictable changes in transepithelial fluid flow (141, 210).

Mechanisms of Ion Transport

CHLORIDE SECRETION BY DOG TRACHEAL EPITHELIUM. The epithelia of the dog trachea and main stem bronchus and the fetal sheep trachea are the only airway epithelia known to show spontaneous Cl secretion (26, 27). Although amiloride induces Cl secretion in other airways (23, 24), normally their epithelia show only active Na absorption (26). The Cl secretion in dog tracheal epithelium is thus unusual. However, it has been studied in far greater detail than any other airway transport process.

On addition of 10^{-4} M ouabain to the serosal bath, the I_{sc}, active Na transport, and active Cl transport in dog tracheal epithelium all decline to zero within ~30 min (4, 218). Luminal ouabain is a far less potent inhibitor of ion transport (218). Potassium removal (another means of inhibiting Na^+-K^+-ATPase) has no effect in the luminal medium, but like ouabain it is a potent inhibitor of active ion transport when performed on the tissue's serosal face (211, 218). These results suggest that Na^+-K^+-ATPase in the basolateral membranes of the cells is essential for the active movement of both Na and Cl.

Sodium removal is another potent inhibitor of active Cl secretion. Replacing Na with choline nearly completely abolishes Cl transport (4, 218). This procedure is effective when done in both bathing media or in the serosal medium alone. Removing Na from the luminal solution has little effect on net Cl flux (J^{Cl}_{net}) (218). The primary action of Na removal on Cl fluxes is to reduce the flux of Cl from serosa to mucosa (J^{Cl}_{sm}) (127, 218). These results suggest that the entry of the actively transported Cl across the basolateral cell membranes is a Na-dependent process.

Thus active Cl secretion depends on functioning basolateral Na^+-K^+-ATPase and on the presence of Na in the serosal medium, features that are common to a large number of Cl-secreting tissues (73). A model for Cl secretion has been proposed that explains these findings (62, 179). A downhill electrochemical potential gradient for Na entry exists across the basolateral cell membranes. These membranes also possess carriers that mediate the linked entry of Na and Cl from the serosal medium. The energy in the transmembrane electrochemical Na gradient allows active Cl accumulation via the Na-linked influx process. An outwardly directed electrochemical gradient for Cl results, which leads to net Cl movement out of the cells across the apical membrane. The Na that entered with the Cl across the basolateral membrane returns to the serosa via Na pumps (Na^+-K^+-ATPase), which are only located on the basolateral membranes in dog tracheal epithelium (215) and most other epithelia (63). This scheme thus leads to electrogenic chloride secretion.

Most of the initial evidence for this model in dog tracheal epithelium was indirect and came from experiments using Ussing's I_{sc} technique. Attempts have been made to test this model with other methods. The model's important features that needed to be demonstrated were the presence of appropriate driving forces for Na entry and Cl exit across the basolateral and apical membranes, respectively, and the existence of linked entry of Na and Cl across the basolateral membrane. Approaches with intracellular microelectrodes and with isolated cells are now yielding important new information.

Isolated cells are important because they represent a preparation that, used with radioactive tracers, allows investigations of the exchange of ions across the basolateral membranes. In intact tissue sheets the basolateral membranes are separated from the bathing medium by a layer of collagenous connective tissue ~0.5–1 mm thick. This "dead space" precludes the investigation of ion exchange across the basolateral membranes. With isolated cells, however, the basolateral membranes are in direct contact with the bathing medium. We obtained a preparation of isolated cells from dog tracheal mucosa by exposing the tissue to Ca-free medium and collagenase (214). The three major cell types in intact epithelium (secretory, ciliated, and basal) are all present in approximately the same proportions as before dissociation. Other cell types are found in negligible amounts. The cells' viability is high, as judged by ciliary motion, the exclusion of vital dyes, high levels of oxygen consumption, and the incorporation of amino acids into protein. Furthermore the cells show no decline in viability for up to 6 h after isolation.

The intracellular levels of Na and K in these cells were $[Na]_i = 20$ and $[K]_i = 160$ mmol/liter cell H_2O. Ouabain (10^{-4} M) led to a virtually complete reversal of these levels. After 2 h of exposure, $[K]_i$ fell from 163 ± 4 to 43 ± 5 mmol/liter cell H_2O, whereas $[Na]_i$ rose from 22 ± 5 to 150 ± 8 mmol/liter cell H_2O (214). These results show that cells of the tracheal mucosa maintain the transmembrane Na gradient thought necessary for active Cl accumulation. The effect of ouabain on Na and K levels suggests (not surprisingly) that its inhibition of Cl transport in the intact tissue is due to an abolition of the basolateral Na gradient and the loss of the energy needed for the active accumulation of Cl.

The Cl content of our isolated cells was measured both by determining the equilibrium levels of ^{36}Cl uptake and by argentimetric titration. With ^{36}Cl uptake, $[Cl]_i = 50$ mmol/liter cell H_2O; with titration, $[Cl]_i = 60$ mmol/liter cell H_2O. Similar discrepancies between these two techniques have been reported for several other tissues (74, 80), and they are thought to be due to Cl binding. The lower estimate for $[Cl]_i$ (50 mmol/liter cell H_2O) predicts a membrane potential (E_m) of 23 mV if Cl is passively distributed according to the transmembrane electrical potential (activity coefficients of intracellular and extracellular Cl are assumed to be equal). Given the high viability of our cells, it seems probable that their E_m is closer to that of the short-circuited epithelium of ~60 mV (206). Thus it seems that the cells actively accumulate Cl.

Data from experiments with loop diuretics (217) suggest that this active accumulation of Cl involves NaCl cotransport. Loop diuretics inhibit the cotransport of Cl and cations (Na or Na + K) in a number of epithelial and nonepithelial tissues (148). Furosemide was shown to inhibit Cl secretion by dog tracheal epithelium from the serosal side but not from the luminal side (49, 127, 206). We confirmed this result and found that bumetanide and piretanide had similar effects (217). The diuretic MK-196 differs from other loop diuretics because it inhibits Cl secretion with equal potency from either side of the epithelium. It seems that loop diuretics did not affect Cl secretion via an action on Na^+-K^+-ATPase because *1*) they did not alter either the unidirectional or net Na fluxes; *2*) they did not affect amphotericin B's stimulation of Na transport; *3*) they did not cause significant changes in $[Na]_i$ or $[K]_i$; *4*) 10^{-3} M furosemide [as shown by Westenfelder et al. (211)] did not affect the activity of Na^+-K^+-ATPase isolated from dog tracheal epithelium; and *5*) ouabain, which inhibits Na^+-K^+-ATPase and causes increased intracellular Na levels (214), has a completely different action on the unidirectional Cl fluxes. Ouabain stops net Cl movement, predominantly by increasing the flux of Cl from mucosa to serosa (J_{ms}^{Cl}); it has little effect on J_{sm}^{Cl} (4, 218). In contrast all the loop diuretics caused significant reductions in both unidirectional Cl fluxes.

When added to isolated cells from dog tracheal epithelium, these diuretics decreased equilibrium ^{36}Cl levels from 47 to 28–35 meq/liter. The finding that these diuretics caused approximately equal decreases in the simultaneously determined influxes of Na and Cl indicated that this decline was due to the inhibition of linked Na and Cl entry (Fig. 1). In other epithelia and nonepithelial tissues, there is evidence that K is cotransported with Na and Cl in the ratio of 1:1:2 (Na:K:Cl). However, the removal of K from both the bathing media and the cells (by ouabain treatment) did not affect the influx of Na and Cl, which still could be inhibited by bumetanide (217). Thus in this tissue, Cl entry may involve a 1:1 cotransport of Na and Cl.

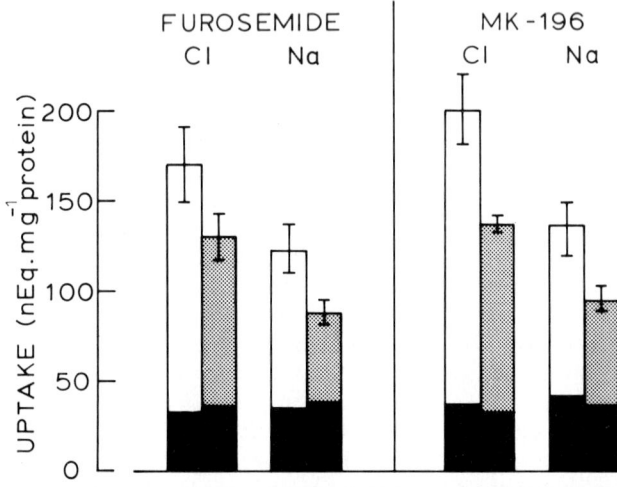

FIG. 1. Effects of furosemide and MK-196 on simultaneously determined influxes of ^{22}Na and ^{36}Cl by cells pretreated for 2 h with 10^{-4} M ouabain. *Open bars*, control uptake; *shaded bars*, uptake in presence of diuretics; *black bars*, extracellular uptakes expected in measured [^{14}C]sucrose spaces. Values are means ± SE; n = 5 (furosemide) and 4 (MK-196). Uptakes were for 2 min, during which time uptake is linear with time and reflects influx alone. Both diuretics caused statistically significant falls in Na and Cl influxes as determined by paired *t* test. [From Widdicombe et al. (217).]

Electrophysiological data also support the conclusion that loop diuretics inhibit an electrically neutral Cl entry process across the basolateral membranes of the cells. Thus Welsh (206) used equivalent circuit analysis to show that the inhibition of Cl secretion by furosemide has no effect on either the basolateral membrane resistance or electromotive force (emf). Assuming that the emf across the apical membrane (E_a) equals the Cl equilibrium potential (E_{Cl}), Welsh et al. (208) used tissues stimulated with epinephrine to estimate that furosemide caused a 50% decline in the aCl_i (intracellular activity of chloride), which agreed with the finding of decreased $[Cl]_i$ in isolated cells.

In other microelectrode studies on dog tracheal epithelium, Welsh et al. (208) used indomethacin-treated tissues to prevent the stimulation of Cl secretion by endogenously released PGs and found a transepithelial PD (ψ_t) of -10 mV and an apical membrane potential (ψ_a) of -42 mV. The basolateral membrane potential (ψ_b) was -52 mV (ψ_a is referred to the mucosal medium; ψ_b and ψ_t to the serosal medium). Stimulating Cl secretion with PGE_1 or epinephrine resulted in an increase in ψ_t, a depolarization of ψ_a, and no significant change in ψ_b. Detailed analysis of the time course of changes in ψ_a, ψ_b, and the fractional apical membrane resistance (F_R) [ratio of apical membrane resistance to transcellular resistance; $R_a/(R_a + R_b)$] revealed that after administering epinephrine, total resistance (R_T) and F_R declined rapidly over the first 20 s and ψ_b and ψ_a both depolarized (Fig. 2). These effects were thought to be due to increased Cl conductance (G_{Cl}) in the apical membrane, which caused F_R to fall and the potentials across both membranes to move toward the E_{Cl} for the cell, which was estimated to be about -24 mV. Although only the emf across the apical membrane was altered, one would expect changes in both ψ_a and ψ_b because the membranes are connected by a low-resistance paracellular shunt. Thus a change in emf at the apical membrane results in current flow within the epithelium that alters ψ_b. Studies with PGE_1 show that these effects did involve an increase in G_{Cl}. In Cl-containing medium, this drug mimics the effects of epinephrine. However, in Cl-free (SO_4^{2-} or gluconate) media, PGE_1 had no effect on ψ_t, ψ_a, or F_R. After this initial response, R_T continued to decline and F_R increased while both ψ_b and ψ_a hyperpolarized. Welsh et al. (208) suggested that these effects were due to increased basolateral membrane conductance. This would explain the continued decrease in R_T while F_R increased. Furthermore, if the conductance increase was to K, this would also explain the hyperpolarization of ψ_a and ψ_b, because these potentials would move toward the K equilibrium potential (E_K) of the cell (about -70 mV). Increased Cl secretion leads to increased Na pump activity because Na and Cl influxes are linked. Increased Na pump activity leads to increased K uptake, because the Na pump transports Na and K of epinephrine. The emf could then also be calculated, because the measured transmembrane potentials are the sum of the membrane emf and the voltage drop across the membrane resistance due to the flow of I_{sc} (e.g., $\psi_a = E_a - (I_{sc}R_a)$. Welsh et al. (209) found that tissues treated with indomethacin had an E_a of +11 mV and an R_a of 2,300 $\Omega \cdot cm^2$. The $E_b = -77$ mV and $R_b = 430$ $\Omega \cdot cm^2$. Epinephrine changed E_a to -30 mV without significantly affecting E_b. Both R_a and R_b decreased to 274 and 157 $\Omega \cdot cm^2$, respectively, and showed a significant inverse correlation with transport rate. The E_a correlated significantly with R_a. However, R_b and E_b were not correlated with one another. These results suggest that the apical membrane has both Cl and Na conductances and that the dominant factor regulating E_a under resting conditions is E_{Na}. After epinephrine stimulation G_{Cl} increases and E_a shifts toward E_{Cl}. The measured [Cl]$_i$ of 50 mM (214) predicts that $E_{Cl} = -23$ mV, which is close to the value E_a of -30 mV seen in the presence of epinephrine. If the decrease in R_b represents an increase in G_K, then the lack of correlation between E_b and R_b suggests that in the resting state $E_b \simeq E_K$ and that [K]$_i$ does not change much during stimulation. In fact measurements of aK$_i$ provide direct evidence for a close agreement between E_b and E_K, both before and after stimulation with epinephrine (180).

The findings that ψ_b is depolarized when [K] in the serosal medium is changed from 5.4 to 51 mM but that equivalent changes in serosal [Na] or [Cl] are without effect on ψ_b indicate that G_K is the predominant ion conductance in the basolateral membrane (205, 208).

On the other hand, the apical cell membrane appears to have a negligible G_K, in that changes in [K] in the luminal medium have no effect on ψ_a (205). The same conclusion can be reached less directly. If one assumes *1)* that the Na pump operates with a fixed stoichiometry of 3:2 (Na:K), *2)* that Na enters the cell only via the apical membrane Na conductance (G_{Na}) and the basolateral NaCl carrier, leaving only via the Na pump, and *3)* that Cl does not exit across the basolateral membranes, then the rate of pumped K entry should be two-thirds of the I_{sc}, or ~ 2 $\mu eq \cdot cm^{-2} \cdot h^{-1}$ (in a stimulated tissue). However, net K secretion is only 0.02–0.06 $\mu eq \cdot cm^{-2} \cdot h^{-1}$ (27, 205). In other words, most of the K pumped into the cells recycles across the cell's basolateral membranes, indicating that the G_K of the apical membranes is only $\sim 1\%$–3% of that of the basolateral membrane.

Ion-selective microelectrodes have been applied to the study of dog tracheal epithelium. Smith and Frizzell (180) found aK$_i$ to be 63 mM in the presence of indomethacin, falling to 52 mM after epinephrine stimulation. These levels are higher than predicted from the measured membrane potentials and demonstrate the active accumulation of K. The values of E_K calculated from aK$_i$ are -73 mV and -67 mV after indomethacin and epinephrine, respectively. These

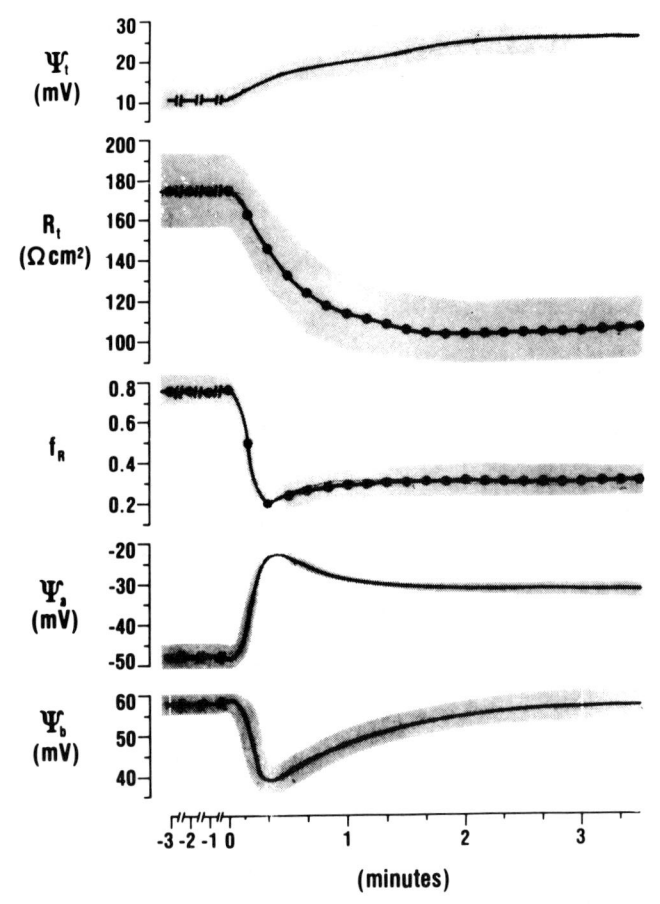

FIG. 2. Acute electrical response to stimulation with epinephrine. Time zero indicates onset of response to addition of epinephrine (10^{-6} M) to the submucosal solution. Total resistance (R_t) and fractional resistance (f_R) were measured at times indicated by *dots*. Transepithelial, apical, and basolateral membrane diffusive potentials (ψ_t, ψ_a, and ψ_b) were measured continuously. Values are means ± SE (*shaded area*). [From Welsh et al. (208).]

in a fixed 3:2 ratio (85). The suggested increase in basolateral K conductance (G_K) allows the increased amount of K pumped into the cells to leak back across the basolateral cell membranes without alteration in intracellular K content. The increase in G_K can thus be regarded as a volume regulatory response. Similar changes in G_K in response to Na pumping have been seen in Na-absorptive epithelia (174) and in nonepithelial tissues (33). Welsh et al. (208) also pointed out that an important feature of the increase in basolateral G_K is that the resulting hyperpolarization maintains the intracellular negativity that drives the downhill exit of Cl across the apical cell membrane. Shorofsky et al. (177) obtained results very similar to those of Welsh et al. (208).

Equivalent circuit analysis (209) has confirmed and extended these initial electrophysiological studies. Assuming that R_b and resistance of paracellular pathway (R_p) were unchanged during the first 10 s of the response to epinephrine, R_p was estimated from the values of R_T and F_R. Knowing R_p, it was possible to calculate R_a and R_b at different times after the addition values are close to values for E_b of −77 mV and −69 mV calculated by Welsh et al. (209), again suggesting that the basolateral membrane is selective for K. The value $[K]_i = 150$ mM calculated from chemical analysis converts to $aK_i = 112$ mM if one assumes that the intracellular activity coefficient is 0.75. This discrepancy between the aK_i determined by chemical analysis and by ion-selective microelectrodes has been described for a number of epithelia, and Civan (37) discusses its possible causes in detail. The true aK_i may lie between the values determined by these two techniques.

Intracellular Cl activity was measured (207) and equaled 37 mM, with an ψ_a of −60 mV. There was no change in aCl_i in tissues stimulated with epinephrine, but ψ_a declined to −46 mV. These values agree with the $aCl_i = 37$ mM predicted from the $[Cl]_i$ of isolated cells (217) and are 3.8 and 2.4 times the values expected for passive distribution according to the membrane potential. The aCl_i fell to 17 mM after removing Na from the bathing media, a level not statistically different from that expected from passive distribution. Bumetanide, a loop diuretic, also decreased aCl_i. These data again suggest the existence of NaCl cotransport in the basolateral membranes of dog tracheal epithelium. Similar Na-dependent accumulation of intracellular Cl has been described for the rat tracheal epithelium with Cl-sensitive microelectrodes (55).

To summarize these results, dog tracheal epithelium contains a Na^+-K^+-ATPase (211) that is located exclusively in the basolateral cell membranes (215). The resultant active uptake of K and the active extrusion of Na lead to an intracellular content of these ions that is above and below, respectively, the levels predicted by the intracellular potentials of −50 to −70 mV. The uptake of Cl across the basolateral membrane of the cells is linked to the movement of Na down its electrochemical potential gradient. This downhill movement of Na produces an active accumulation of Cl to levels greater than those predicted by ψ_a. Present evidence suggests that there is a 1:1 linkage between Na and Cl entry, rather than the 1:1:2 (Na:K:Cl) stoichometry described for some other tissues. Chloride now moves downhill across the apical cell membranes. Given the driving forces involved and the high permeability of this membrane to Cl, there is no reason to suggest that this movement occurs in any way other than passive diffusion (207). The two membranes differ markedly in their relative ionic permeabilities. The apical membrane is permeable to both Na and Cl but has a negligible G_K. The basolateral membrane, however, is K selective. This selectivity leads to a negative E_b value that then results in a hyperpolarization of the apical membrane, which provides the driving force for Cl exit from the cells. The stimulation of Cl secretion causes Na entry, stimulation of the Na pump, and increased uptake of K. The basolateral G_K, however, varies with the rate of Na pumping in such a way as to result in little change in $[K]_i$ with changes in active Cl secretion. This variation of G_K with the rate of Na pumping can thus be regarded as a volume-regulatory device.

SODIUM ABSORPTION. Dog tracheal epithelium shows active Na absorption proceeding at a rate about one-half to one-third that of active Cl secretion. Most other airway epithelia, however, show only Na absorption (26, 134). All the available evidence suggests that Na absorption by airway epithelia occurs according to the model of Koefoed-Johnsen and Ussing (110). This involves the passive entry of Na across the apical membrane down an electrochemical gradient, followed by its active extrusion across the basolateral cell membranes via Na^+-K^+-ATPase, which is located only in this membrane.

Work on epithelia in the dog trachea and bronchus suggests that the necessary driving forces for Na entry are present. Thus the interior of the cell is negative relative to the luminal medium (26, 64, 177, 208) and the intracellular Na concentration of isolated cells is low, ranging from 17 to 35 mM (26, 42, 214). As in other Na-absorbing epithelia, Na entry across the apical membranes appears to be sensitive to amiloride, because mucosal amiloride abolishes or reduces net Na absorption (23, 24, 109, 220). The presence of an amiloride-sensitive G_{Na} in the apical membrane is supported by electrophysiological data. Thus adding amiloride to canine bronchial epithelium results in a hyperpolarization of both membrane potentials and an increase in the R_a:R_b ratio (26). Similar results were reported for indomethacin-treated dog tracheal epithelium (209). The failure of Estep et al. (64) to record any marked changes after amiloride treatment might have been due to not pretreating their tissues with indomethacin; the apical membranes therefore may have had a high G_{Cl}, which might have obscured any changes caused by a reduction in the amiloride-sensitive G_{Na}. Support for an apical membrane G_{Na} is also provided by the findings that Na replacement in the mucosal medium increases F_R and causes hyperpolarization of ψ_a (26, 177, 205).

Amiloride seems to abolish Na absorption in most airway epithelia. This was shown in rabbit trachea (24), dog bronchus (25), and human bronchus (109). In all cases, the change in net Na movement exceeded the change in I_{sc}, and the difference was accounted for by the induction of net Cl secretion. Results from the dog bronchus are shown in Figure 3. It is uncertain how this increase in Cl secretion occurs. Boucher et al. (26) argue that Na-absorbing airway epithelia have lower $[Cl]_i$ and ψ_a than dog tracheal epithelium. These two factors mean that there is no driving force for net Cl movement across the apical membrane; aCl_i is at the level predicted for passive distribution according to ψ_a. The addition of amiloride reduces the total permeability to Na (P_{Na}) and leads to hyperpolarization of the apical membrane. This increase in negativity provides the driving force for net Cl movement

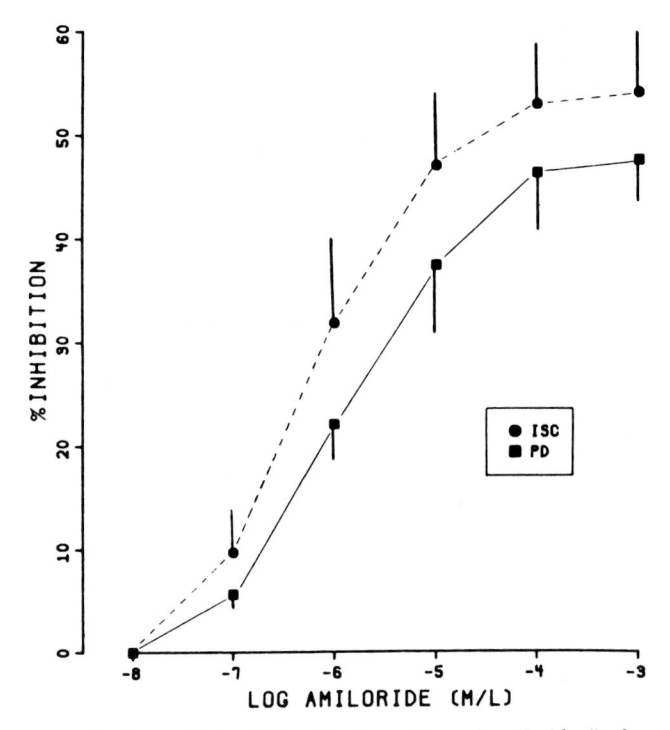

FIG. 3. Dose-effect relationship for action of amiloride (in luminal bathing solution) on bioelectric properties of excised canine bronchus. ISC, short-circuit current; PD, transepithelial electric potential difference. Values are means ± SE (vertical lines). Under resting conditions ISC is entirely accounted for by active Na absorption. Supramaximal doses of amiloride abolish active Na absorption, whereas ISC is only inhibited by 55%; this discrepancy is due to induction of Cl secretion. [From Boucher et al. (26). By permission of San Francisco Press, Box 6800, San Francisco, CA 94101.]

across the apical membrane and out of the cells.

Our initial report on the effects of amiloride on Na transport by dog tracheal epithelium (220) showed that 10^{-4} M amiloride reduced net Na absorption by one-half, due to a decline in J_{ms}^{Na}. The decline in J_{net}^{Na} was greater than the fall in I_{sc}, suggesting that Cl transport (which was not measured) may have increased. It was also found that J_{net}^{Na} after amiloride remained significantly greater than zero. Iodide and gluconate are not transported by dog tracheal epithelium (4, 219). After prolonged incubation (>1 h) in Cl-free media (in which either of these anions replaces Cl), I_{sc} declined to ~⅓ of its original value, and the I_{sc} response to isoproterenol [a stimulator of Cl secretion (5)] was negligible. Presumably under these circumstances, I_{sc} is entirely accounted for by net Na absorption. Amiloride inhibits this I_{sc} with a $K_d \simeq 10^{-6}$ M. However, only ~25%–50% of the I_{sc} is inhibited by supramaximal doses. This is true in either HCO_3^-- or Hepes-buffered media, thus ruling out the possibility that a stimulation of HCO_3^- secretion accompanies the inhibition of Na absorption. These data provide further evidence for the existence of amiloride-insensitive Na absorption in dog tracheal epithelium.

The exit of Na from the cells across the basolateral cell membranes is effected by Na^+-K^+-ATPase. Autoradiographic analysis of ouabain binding has localized the Na^+-K^+-ATPase in dog tracheal epithelium exclusively to the basolateral membranes (215). This is the side from which ouabain abolishes Na absorption in this tissue (218); it has little effect when added to the luminal solution. Submucosal ouabain inhibits active Na absorption across rabbit tracheal epithelium (24) and dog bronchial epithelium (27).

The limited data available suggest that airway Na absorption is unresponsive to either aldosterone or antidiuretic hormone, drugs that stimulate Na absorption in other epithelia (26). Amphotericin B causes large increases in active Na transport across dog tracheal epithelium (79) but does not affect I_{sc} across rabbit tracheal epithelium.

OTHER ION-TRANSPORT PROCESSES. Welsh (205) reported a small K secretion by dog tracheal epithelium of 0.04 μeq·cm^{-2}·h^{-1} that epinephrine barely affected. Boucher et al. (27) failed to detect any net K movement across epithelia from dog trachea or main stem bronchi but did detect a significant K secretion by bronchi of 0.035 μeq·cm^{-2}·h^{-1}. Increasing the permeability to K of the apical membrane of dog tracheal epithelium with amphotericin B (10^{-5} M) induces a K secretion of 0.86 μeq·cm^{-2}·h^{-1} (79).

Hydrogen ion secretion has not been measured in short-circuited airway epithelia. However, the replacement of HCO_3^- by Cl has no effect on I_{sc} across dog tracheal epithelium (4). The carbonic anhydrase inhibitor acetazolamide (10^{-4} M) is also without effect on I_{sc} (J. H. Widdicombe, unpublished observations). These results suggest that there is little active HCO_3^- or H transport by dog tracheal epithelium.

There is a small secretion of Ca across dog tracheal epithelium (1.51 neq·cm^{-2}·h^{-1}) that is approximately doubled by epinephrine (94).

Regulation of Ion Transport

A wide range of possible physiological and pathological mediators have been tested on the dog's tracheal epithelium. Fewer studies have been performed on other airway epithelia. In the dog tracheal epithelium, mediators can be divided into two classes: those stimulating Cl secretion with little effect on Na absorption and those causing an essentially electrically neutral movement of both Na and Cl toward the lumen.

Histamine (124) and acetylcholine (123) were the first putative mediators to be tested on dog tracheal epithelium. They caused essentially electrically neutral movement of Na and Cl. In short-circuited tissues, acetylcholine increased the unidirectional Cl flux toward the lumen in a dose-dependent manner. A dose of 5 × 10^{-5} M increased both net Na and net Cl movement toward the lumen by ~1.5 μeq·cm^{-2}·h^{-1}. These changes were due to increases in the fluxes of these ions toward the lumen; the unidirectional fluxes toward the submucosa were unchanged. Atropine ($\geq 10^{-8}$ M) abolished the changes in flux toward the lumen. Under open-circuit conditions, there were no detectable net movements of either Na or Cl; acetylcholine increased the movements of Na and Cl toward the lumen, resulting in a net secretion of these ions. The changes seen under open circuit were of similar magnitude to those under short circuit. In a second study Marin, Davis, and Nadel (124) obtained similar results with histamine. This drug (10^{-4} M) caused a relatively small change in I_{sc} (<0.5 μeq·cm^{-2}·h^{-1}), but without affecting the fluxes toward the serosa it caused an ~0.7 μeq·cm^{-2}·h^{-1} increase in net secretion of both Na and Cl in short-circuited tissues. Atropine (10^{-4} M) and burimamide (10^{-4} M) did not affect the response to histamine, but diphenhydramine (10^{-6} M) shifted the dose-response curve for I_{sc} to the right. Thus this response seemed to be mediated by H$_1$ receptors. Reducing the [Ca] in the bathing medium from 1.9 to 0 mM reduced the response in I_{sc} to histamine but not to acetylcholine (126). Histamine and acetylcholine do not change cAMP levels in the surface epithelium of the dog trachea (181).

Both histamine and acetylcholine stimulate gland secretion in the anterior portion of the dog trachea. Although the posterior membranous portion has fewer glands, it is not entirely gland free. The electrically silent movement of both Na and Cl toward the lumen under both open- and short-circuit conditions produced by these drugs may represent gland secretion.

Corrales, Nadel, and Widdicombe (40, 41) tested the mechanism by which glands may affect transepithelial J_{net}^{Na} and J_{net}^{Cl} fluxes in airways. We studied the cat because it contains more glands than the dog. Phenylephrine, a potent stimulator of gland secretion in cats (198), induced net secretory movements of both Na and Cl of ~10 μeq·cm^{-2}·h^{-1}. This was due to an increase in the unidirectional fluxes toward the lumen, and similar effects were seen under both open- and short-circuit conditions. One possible mechanism for the electrically silent movement of Na and Cl under short-circuit conditions is that the glandular epithelium secretes Cl, but due to geometrical considerations it is not fully short circuited during the passage of I_{sc}. Stimulation of Cl-secretion by phenylephrine (or by histamine or acetylcholine in the dog) could then increase PD across the gland epithelium and bring about net transepithelial movement of Na due to electrical forces. Chloride secretory processes have been described for a large number of epithelia (73) and generally involve a NaCl cotransport process in the basolateral membranes. Loop diuretics inhibit this cotransport process in a wide variety of epithelial and nonepithelial tissues (148). However, the phenylephrine-induced increases in Na and Cl secretion across cat tracheal epithelium were not blocked by either bumetanide (10^{-4} M) or furosemide (10^{-3} M) and neither was the output of fluid from the glands, as measured by our micropipette technique (198). Bromide can substitute for Cl in the Na-linked cotransport process in a wide range of epithelial and nonepithelial cells, but NO$_3$ and iodide cannot (67, 81, 132, 148, 217). Replacing Cl with any of these ions did not affect the increases in net Na secretion or gland fluid output produced by phenylephrine. We concluded that Na-linked secretion of Cl does not underlie the output of fluid from submucosal glands in the cat airway. It is possible that some undescribed ion transport process is responsible for the output of gland secretions. However, the contents of secretory granules could be hypertonic (142), and we never saw net NaCl secretion by cat tracheal epithelium without an increased output of nondialyzable, ^{35}SO$_4^{2-}$-labeled material (used as a marker of secretory granule discharge). We concluded that the release of osmotically active granule components into the gland lumen draws water by simple osmosis. This results in a NaCl gradient across the gland epithelium that leads to the net secretion of Na and Cl seen with phenylephrine in the cat and with histamine and acetylcholine in the dog.

The other secretagogues tested on dog tracheal epithelium are selective stimulators of Cl secretion. Sodium absorption is unchanged or declines slightly. The small decline in Na absorption might result from increased [Na]$_i$ secondary to raised Cl-linked Na entry.

Al-Bazzaz and Cheng (5) showed that adrenergic agents stimulated I_{sc} across dog tracheal epithelium with the following potency sequence: isoproterenol > epinephrine > norepinephrine > phenylephrine. The dissociation constant (K_d) for epinephrine was ~5 × 10^{-7} M. Flux data showed that the increase in I_{sc} of ~1.5 μeq·cm^{-2}·h^{-1} in response to epinephrine was due to stimulation of net Cl secretion; Na fluxes were unaffected. Propranolol abolished epinephrine's actions on I_{sc} and Cl fluxes. Epinephrine stimulated I_{sc} to the same extent in HCO$_3^-$-free media. Also replacement of Cl by SO$_4^{2-}$ greatly reduced the effects of epinephrine on I_{sc}. The effect of phenylephrine on I_{sc} was of small magnitude and short duration, and Al-Bazzaz and Cheng (5) did not detect any changes in net Cl secretion. The response in I_{sc} to phenylephrine was virtually abolished by propranolol. From these data they concluded that stimulation of β-adrenergic receptors led to increases in Cl secretion but that α-adrenergic receptors played no significant role in the regulation of ion transport by dog tracheal epithelium.

In other tissues, β-adrenergic agents act by raising intracellular levels of cAMP (170). The finding that addition of dibutyryl cAMP (10^{-3} M) to the submucosal bath stimulated net Cl secretion with little change in active Na absorption suggests that this might also be true for dog tracheal epithelium (3). The change in I_{sc} approximated the change in net Cl secretion. In the same study it was shown that in the presence of methylisobutylxanthine (MIX, 2 mM), a phosphodiesterase inhibitor, epinephrine increased the cAMP content of isolated cells from dog tracheal epithelium. Thus it seems that cAMP may act as a second messenger for β-adrenergic agents in the stimulation of Cl secretion across dog tracheal epithelium.

Al-Bazzaz and co-workers (8) provided an important advance in the understanding of how Cl secretion across dog tracheal epithelium may be regulated in vivo. They found that PGs stimulated Cl secretion and that indomethacin reduced the resting level of Cl secretion. Both PGE_1 and $PGF_{2\alpha}$ had the same effects when added to either the mucosal or serosal baths and caused dose-dependent increases in I_{sc}. The maximal response with both PGs was similar to that seen with epinephrine and was accounted for by an increase in Cl secretion. Both drugs also caused small falls in J_{net}^{Na} and J_{ms}^{Na}, although these changes in Na fluxes only reached statistical significance with PGE_1. Figure 4 shows that indomethacin (10^{-7}–10^{-6} M) caused a slow decline in I_{sc} to levels about one-half of base line after 1 h. Adding PGE_1 (in presence of indomethacin) increased I_{sc} and net Cl secretion to levels somewhat greater than achieved by PGE_1 alone. In a later study, Smith and co-workers (181) found that indomethacin reduced I_{sc} and intracellular cAMP content and also reduced spontaneous PGE_2 production to about one-fifth of its control level. Prolonged treatment with indomethacin reduced I_{sc} to levels expected with active Na absorption alone. Furthermore there was a significant correlation between the initial I_{sc} and the change in I_{sc} produced by indomethacin, with a slope not statistically different from one. This suggests that spontaneous variation in I_{sc} between tissues is due to variations in the level of PG-induced Cl secretion; Na absorption is probably relatively constant between tissues. Both PGE_1 and PGE_2 raised intracellular cAMP levels in isolated cells pretreated with MIX and in tissue sheets, whereas $PGF_{2\alpha}$ did not (8, 181). The possibility that $PGF_{2\alpha}$ might increase Cl secretion by elevating intracellular Ca levels was suggested by the fact that A 23187 (a Ca ionophore) stimulated Cl secretion to nearly the same extent as $PGF_{2\alpha}$ (6).

Other possible regulators of ion transport by dog tracheal epithelium have been described. The presence of material immunoreactive to VIP in nerves in the submucosa of dog airways (53) led us to investigate the effects of VIP on ion transport (140). This drug had little effect on I_{sc} unless the levels of Cl secretion were first reduced by indomethacin. Once Cl secretion was reduced we found that VIP stimulated Cl secretion with $K_d \simeq 10^{-8}$ M, and it was more effective from the serosal side than the luminal side. Maximal changes in Cl secretion and I_{sc} were ~1.5 $\mu eq \cdot cm^{-2} \cdot h^{-1}$; Na absorption was unaffected. Tetrodotoxin (10^{-6} M) did not affect VIP's actions, and neither did a combination of propranolol, phentolamine, and atropine; this suggests that VIP acts directly by interaction with receptors on the epithelial cells. J. H. Widdicombe (unpublished observations) found that VIP increased the cAMP levels of isolated cells from the tracheal epithelium, and immunocytochemical results support this finding (119). Under open-circuit conditions, VIP did not significantly affect either net Na or net Cl movements, suggesting that it probably plays only a minor role in the regulation of respiratory tract fluid levels.

We found that the peptides neurotensin, somatostatin, and bombesin did not affect ion transport (140). However, substance P produced a small transient stimulation of Cl secretion when added to the mucosal side of dog tracheal epithelium but had no effect when administered serosally (7). The smallness and "sidedness" of the response to substance P cast doubt on its having any physiological role in the regulation of airway ion transport.

Bradykinin is released by the lung parenchyma and airways (101), and we have investigated its actions on dog tracheal epithelium (120). Maximal changes in I_{sc} were the same no matter to which side of the tissue the drug was added (~30 $\mu A/cm^2$). However, the luminal response was transient and disappeared within ~5 min, whereas the serosal response was more prolonged. The K_d for luminal addition was $\simeq 10^{-9}$ M and the K_d for serosal addition was $\simeq 10^{-7}$ M. This difference might reflect a breakdown of the drug during passage through the submucosal collagen layers despite precautions taken against this by adding captopril, bacitracin, and an inhibitor of angiotensin-converting enzyme. Replacing Cl in the serosal bath with iodide or the addition of bumetanide (10^{-4} M) abolishes the response to bradykinin, suggesting that bradykinin acts by stimulating Cl secretion. Flux data

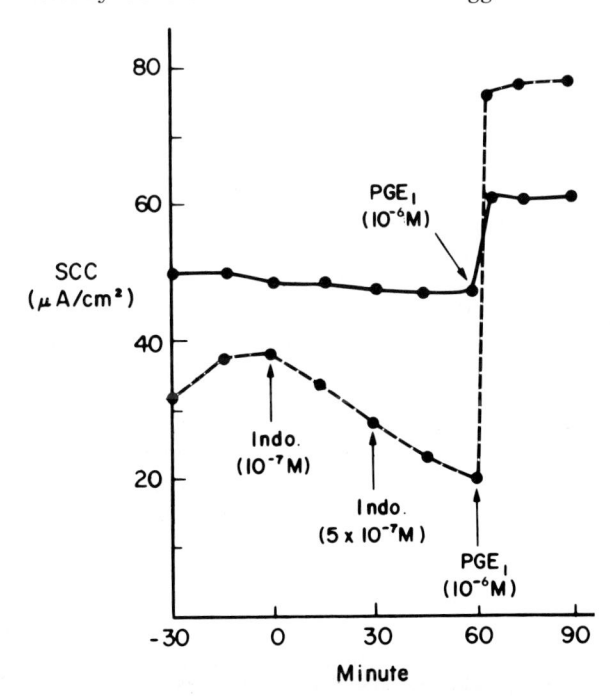

FIG. 4. Effect of indomethacin on short-circuit current (SCC) and subsequent response to prostaglandin E_1 (PGE_1; *broken line*). Both agents were added to mucosal reservoir. Control tissue (*solid line*) was treated with PGE_1 only. Note differences in SCC response to PGE_1. [From Al-Bazazz et al. (8).]

showed directly that increased Cl secretion accounted for the increase in I_{sc}. Bradykinin did not affect Na fluxes. Bradykinin's actions were not affected by tetrodotoxin or adrenergic and cholinergic blockers. Indomethacin (10^{-6} M) reduced the peak response in I_{sc} to serosal bradykinin from 1.1 ± 0.1 to 0.3 ± 0.1 μeq·cm^{-2}·h^{-1}, indicating that bradykinin may cause the release of PGs.

Smith et al. (181) investigated the relationship between cAMP levels and the stimulation of Cl secretion. Rather than use isolated cells pretreated with MIX (3), they measured cAMP levels in cells scraped from tissues mounted in Ussing chambers. They could therefore correlate changes in cAMP levels with changes in I_{sc}. They confirmed Al-Bazzaz's findings that epinephrine and PGE$_1$ increased I_{sc} and raised cellular cAMP levels. Theophylline also had these effects. Both PGF$_{2\alpha}$ and A 23187 increased I_{sc} but did not affect cAMP levels. Acetylcholine, histamine, and phenylephrine did not affect either variable. Smith et al. (181) found no correlation between I_{sc} and cAMP levels in either control or stimulated tissues. Also PGE$_1$ and epinephrine caused similar increases in I_{sc} but different increases in intracellular cAMP. Furthermore when they compared the increases in cAMP and I_{sc} to graded doses of epinephrine, they found that although both increased in a dose-dependent fashion, the dose-response curve for cAMP was displaced two log units to the right, so that increases in I_{sc} occurred without measurable changes in cAMP levels.

A large number of endogenous substances increase the secretion of Cl by dog tracheal epithelium. Some substances seem to raise intracellular cAMP levels, whereas others may act via other secondary messengers like [Ca]$_i$. In all cases the stimulation of Cl secretion is accompanied by decreased tissue resistance. In the cases where they were measured, mannitol fluxes (a marker of paracellular permeability) were unaffected or decreased (3, 8, 210). Thus the decrease in resistance presumably lies in the transcellular pathway. As with epinephrine (208), other secretagogues may act primarily by increasing the G_{Cl} of the apical membrane and the G_K of the basolateral membrane.

The evidence suggests that drugs that affect ion transport in vitro are also important in the regulation of ion transport in vivo. Boucher et al. (22) showed that the in vivo PD of dog tracheal epithelium was not significantly different from that seen in vitro (with Ussing chambers). Furthermore ouabain reduced this PD and amphotericin B increased it, again just as in vitro. They found that applying epinephrine and isoproterenol to the tracheal surface also increased the in vivo PD, but histamine and acetylcholine had no effect.

There are fewer studies on the regulation of ion transport by Na-absorbing epithelia. Boucher and Gatzy (25), using short-circuited segmental bronchi in the dog, found that cholinergic agents caused net movements of Cl, Na, and K to shift in a secretory direction. The movement of these ions from the mucosa to the serosa was unaffected. These results suggest that glandular secretion is superimposed on the base-line–active Na absorption, which is not itself affected by cholinergic agents. The effects of acetylcholine were blocked by atropine. The main effect of adrenergic agents (phenylephrine, epinephrine, and isoproterenol) on bronchial ion transport was an increase in conductance of up to 25% that was reflected in increases in both unidirectional Cl fluxes with no change in net Cl movement. Small decreases in Na absorption were seen with 10^{-5} M phenylephrine or isoproterenol but not with 10^{-3} M of either drug or with epinephrine (10^{-5} or 10^{-3} M). The use of phentolamine suggested that these drugs were not acting through α-receptors. These effects on bronchi contrasted with the effects on dog tracheal epithelium, where Boucher and Gatzy (25) confirmed the stimulation of Cl secretion reported earlier (5).

In the human bronchus, acetylcholine changes net movements of Cl and Na toward secretion by ~1.8 μeq·cm^{-2}·h^{-1}. Phenylephrine and isoproterenol (both 10^{-5} M) did not affect J_{net}^{Na} or J_{net}^{Cl} (109). Acetylcholine (10^{-4} M) did not affect ion transport in rabbit tracheal epithelium (51), possibly because rabbit tracheas lack glands.

The general picture that emerges from these studies is that neither cholinergic nor adrenergic agents greatly affect active Na absorption but that cholinergic agents induce an electrically neutral secretion of Na and Cl from submucosal mucous glands.

Relationship Between Ion Transport and Water Movement

Transepithelial fluid transport occurs in response to local osmotic gradients set up by active solute transport. Dog tracheal epithelium possesses both a secretory and an absorptive ion-transport process. Thus the net direction and volume of fluid flow across dog tracheal epithelium may be regulated by alterations in the relative magnitudes of Cl secretion and Na absorption.

To test this hypothesis, we (210) modified an apparatus described by Wiedner (221) that measures transepithelial water movement by an electrical method. A sheet of dog tracheal epithelium is mounted in this apparatus between two Lucite half-chambers. Warm, oxygenated Krebs-Henseleit solution is continuously circulated across the luminal face of the tissue. A tube attached to the luminal half-chamber is used to apply a hydrostatic pressure of 1 cmH$_2$O across the tissue, which holds it in place against a stainless steel screen and prevents flapping or bulging. The fluid on the closed serosal side of the tissue is introduced into a tube and layered with paraffin oil; then a capacitance probe is placed in the oil. The probe records the capacitance of the paraffin oil layer lying between the probe tip and the surface of the Krebs-Henseleit solution. As fluid moves across the tissue the Krebs-Henseleit solution moves up and down the tube and the thickness and capacitance of the oil layer changes. An indwelling Hamilton syringe in the closed chamber is used to calibrate the capacitance probe throughout an experiment by injecting or withdrawing 1–3 µl of the solution. Silver/silver Cl electrodes placed on either side of the tissue measure the transepithelial PD.

In our initial study with this apparatus we found that net fluid movement under resting conditions was not significantly different from zero. However, aminophylline (2×10^{-3} M), a drug that selectively stimulates active Cl secretion, always caused net fluid secretion. We also measured open-circuit Cl fluxes in paired tissues and found that there was no net movement of Cl under resting conditions but that there was a significant net movement of Cl toward the lumen after administering aminophylline. The relative sizes of the J_{net}^{Cl} and the fluid flow suggested that the secretion stimulated by aminophylline was approximately isosmotic with the bathing medium.

With a more sophisticated version of the original apparatus, we showed that under certain conditions active Na absorption can also cause transepithelial fluid movement (141). We used amphotericin B to stimulate Na absorption and measured ion fluxes or fluid flow across sheets of dog tracheal epithelium mounted in Ussing chambers or in our special apparatus, respectively. Under short-circuit conditions luminal amphotericin B (3×10^{-5} M) caused an inhibition of net Cl secretion and an increase in net Na absorption across paired tissues, thereby confirming an earlier study (79). In paired tissues under resting open-circuit conditions there was no significant transepithelial J_{net}^{Cl} or J_{net}^{Na}. Amphotericin B induced significant net fluxes of both Cl and Na toward the serosal side. In separate tissues from the same animals there was no significant transepithelial fluid movement under resting conditions. Amphotericin B caused a net absorption of fluid, and ouabain abolished the absorption of salt and fluid in amphotericin B–treated tissues. Figure 5 shows results from a typical experiment. We conclude that the stimulation of active Na transport by amphotericin B leads to fluid absorption.

These two studies on transepithelial water movement suggest that the movement of fluid across the dog tracheal epithelium in vivo may be dependent on a balance between active Cl secretion and active Na absorption.

We also investigated the fine structural changes produced during fluid absorption induced by amphotericin B (216). In five dogs we found that amphotericin B significantly increased the width of the lateral intercellular spaces in the center of the epithelium (halfway between basement and apical membranes)

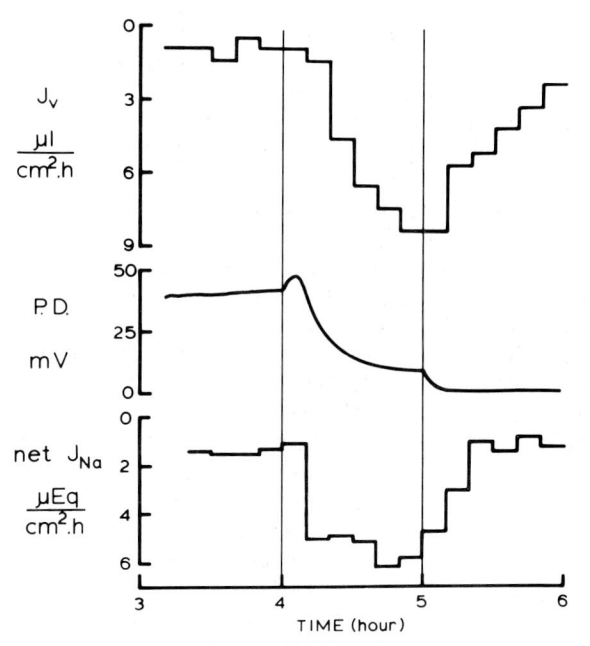

FIG. 5. Plots of changes in fluid volume flow (J_v) and net Na flux (J_{Na}) induced by adding amphotericin B (3×10^{-5} M) to luminal bath at 4 h and adding ouabain (10^{-2} M) to luminal bath at 5 h. Results are from single representative experiment. *Middle panel* shows record of transepithelial potential difference (PD) obtained from tissue mounted in volume-flow apparatus. [From Nathanson, Widdicombe, and Nadel (141).]

from 0.45 ± 0.24 to 1.94 ± 0.30 µm. There was also a corresponding reduction in cell width from 5.72 ± 1.32 to 4.31 ± 1.18 µm, which was not statistically significant. The increase in the fluid content of the lateral intercellular spaces led to a significant increase in cell height from 26.4 ± 3.8 to 37.0 ± 3.9 µm ($P < 0.05$, paired t test). When fluid absorption was inhibited by ouabain or by the replacement of luminal Na by choline, amphotericin B did not cause dilation of the lateral intercellular spaces. These data suggest that, as in other epithelia, a significant amount of transepithelial fluid flow passes down the lateral intercellular spaces and that these spaces may provide the local osmotic compartment that is responsible for linking transepithelial fluid movement to active ion transport.

Two other groups of workers directly measured fluid flow across airway epithelia. Durand et al. (57) mounted bovine tracheal epithelium in a modified Ussing chamber and connected the closed serosal chamber to a horizontal glass tube. They measured volume flow by using a photocell to record continuously the movement of the meniscus along the tube. They found $R \simeq 200 \, \Omega \cdot cm^2$ and PD $\simeq 30$ mV. No fluid flow was seen under base-line conditions or after histamine (10^{-4} M) was added. However, histamine doubled the hydraulic conductivity, as measured from fluid flows generated by adding sucrose to the bathing media. Loughlin et al. (122) introduced physiological saline into the lumen of a ferret trachea in vitro and then sandwiched the saline between layers of mineral oil. They measured fluid movement as the change in inulin concentration in the luminal fluid. Under resting conditions they found a significant net fluid absorption that carbamylcholine (10^{-6} M) converted to net secretion. Pretreatment with atropine prevented carbamylcholine's effect on this tissue.

An alternative to directly measuring volume flows is to measure net open-circuit ion fluxes across paired tissues mounted in Ussing chambers. Net movements of both Na and Cl in the same direction presumably reflect fluid movement. Assuming isotonicity of the transported fluid, an estimate of the volume flow can be made. Boucher et al. (26) report that epithelia from a number of airways show net absorption of both Na and Cl: adult sheep trachea and bronchi, monkey trachea, rabbit trachea, guinea pig trachea, human bronchi, and pig bronchi. In rabbit tracheal epithelium and dog bronchus, net Na and Cl absorption are equal at ~1.6 μeq·cm^{-2}·h^{-1} (24, 27). Assuming these flows represent an isotonic NaCl solution, then this corresponds to a volume flow of ~10 μl·cm^{-2}·h^{-1}. In the dog bronchus, ouabain reduces both net Na and net Cl movement to zero (27). The net Na absorption across human bronchi is ~1.5 μeq·cm^{-2}·h^{-1}, but net Cl movement is only 0.4 μeq·cm^{-2}·h^{-1} (109). There appears to be net Na absorption (~1.5 μeq·cm^{-2}·h^{-1}) in pig and rabbit nasal mucosa and human nasal polyps that is unaccompanied by Cl absorption (134). Boucher et al. (27) also found net Na absorption across dog tracheal epithelium unaccompanied by net Cl movement. Ouabain stopped this net Na movement but did not affect Cl movement, which was still not statistically different from zero. It should be pointed out that other workers have not detected net open-circuit Na absorption across dog tracheal epithelium (123, 141, 145, 220). What charges maintain electroneutrality in the face of the discrepancy between net open-circuit absorption of Na and Cl? It is not K secretion, which is <0.1 μeq·cm^{-2}·h^{-1} (27, 205). Bicarbonate absorption seems to be the only remaining candidate. Given the PD across dog tracheal epithelium and assuming that the permeability to HCO_3^- and Cl are equal, then a net HCO_3^- absorption of 0.4 μeq·cm^{-2}·h^{-1} is expected (27).

The picture emerging from studies of fluid movement is that airway epithelia under resting conditions show either negligible transepithelial fluid movement or are absorptive. The fluid absorbed may be solutions of NaCl, NaHCO$_3$, or both. The exact ratio of HCO_3^- and Cl absorbed presumably depends on whether active Cl secretion is present and on the relative permeability of the epithelium to HCO_3^- and Cl. The surface epithelium of dog trachea is unusual in that by increasing active Cl secretion it can cause fluid secretion. Net fluid movement toward the lumen of other species only occurs by the stimulation of gland secretion.

REFERENCES

1. ABELL, C. W., AND T. M. MONOHAN. The role of 3',5'-monophosphate in the regulation of mammalian cell division. *J. Cell Biol.* 59: 549–558, 1973.
2. ADLER, K. B., B. S. HARDWICK, AND J. E. CRAIGHEAD. Effect of cholera toxin on secretion of mucin by explants of guinea pig trachea. *Lab. Invest.* 45: 372–377, 1981.
3. AL-BAZZAZ, F. J. Role of cyclic AMP in regulation of chloride secretion by canine tracheal mucosa. *Am. Rev. Respir. Dis.* 123: 295–298, 1981.
4. AL-BAZZAZ, F. J., AND Q. AL-AWQATI. Interaction between sodium and chloride transport in canine tracheal mucosa. *J. Appl. Physiol.: Respirat. Environ. Exercise Physiol.* 46: 111–119, 1979.
5. AL-BAZZAZ, F. J., AND E. CHENG. Effect of catecholamines on ion transport in dog tracheal epithelium. *J. Appl. Physiol.: Respirat. Environ. Exercise Physiol.* 47: 397–403, 1979.
6. AL-BAZZAZ, F. J., AND T. JAYARAM. Ion transport by canine tracheal mucosa: effect of elevation of cellular calcium. *Exp. Lung Res.* 2: 121–130, 1981.
7. AL-BAZZAZ, F. J., AND J. KELSEY. Effect of substance P on ion transport by tracheal mucosa (Abstract). *Am. Rev. Respir. Dis.* 125: 243, 1982.
8. AL-BAZZAZ, F., V. P. YADAVA, AND C. WESTENFELDER. Modification of Na and Cl transport in canine tracheal mucosa by prostaglandins. *Am. J. Physiol.* 240 (*Renal Fluid Electrolyte Physiol.* 9): F101–F105, 1981.
9. ALLI, A. F. The radial intercepts method for measuring bronchial mucous gland volume. *Thorax* 30: 687–692, 1975.
10. AZZOPARDI, A., AND W. M. THURLBECK. The histochemistry of the nonciliated bronchiolar epithelial cell. *Am. Rev. Respir. Dis.* 99: 516–525, 1969.
11. BAKER, A. P., L. W. CHAKRIN, J. L. SAWYER, J. R. MUNRO, L. M. HILLEGASS, AND E. GIANNONE. Glycosyltransferases in canine respiratory tissue. Alterations in an experimentally induced hypersecretory state. *Biochem. Med.* 10: 387–399, 1974.
12. BAKER, A. P., L. W. CHAKRIN, AND J. R. WARDELL, JR. Chronic cholinergic stimulation of canine respiratory tissue. Its effect on the activities of glycosyltransferases and release of macromolecules. *Am. Rev. Repir. Dis.* 111: 423–431, 1975.
13. BAKER, A. P., L. M. HILLEGASS, D. A. HOLDEN, AND W. J. SMITH. Effect of kallidin, substance P, and other basic polypeptides on the production of respiratory macromolecules. *Am. Rev. Respir. Dis.* 115: 811–817, 1977.
14. BASBAUM, C. B., P. J. BARNES, M. A. GRILLO, J. H. WIDDICOMBE, AND J. A. NADEL. Adrenergic and cholinergic receptors in submucosal glands of the ferret trachea: autoradiographic localization. *Eur. J. Respir. Dis. Suppl.* 128: 433–435, 1983.
15. BASBAUM, C. B., I. UEKI, L. BREZINA, AND J. A. NADEL. Tracheal submucosal gland serous cells stimulated in vitro with adrenergic and cholinergic agonists: a morphometric study. *Cell Tissue Res.* 220: 481–498, 1981.
16. BASKERVILLE, A. The development and persistence of bronchial-gland hypertrophy and goblet-cell hyperplasia in the pig after injection of isoprenaline. *J. Pathol.* 119: 35–47, 1976.
17. BEDROSSIAN, W. M., A. E. ANDERSON, AND A. G. FORAKER. Comparison of methods for quantitating bronchial morphology. *Thorax* 26: 406–408, 1971.
18. BOAT, T. F., AND P. W. CHENG. Biochemistry of airway mucus secretions. *Federation Proc.* 39: 3067–3074, 1980.
19. BORSON, D. B., M. CHARLIN, B. D. GOLD, AND J. A. NADEL. Nonadrenergic noncholinergic nerves mediate secretion of macromolecules by tracheal glands of ferrets (Abstract). *Federation Proc.* 41: 1754, 1982.
20. BORSON, D. B., R. A. CHINN, B. DAVIS, AND J. A. NADEL.

Adrenergic and cholinergic nerves mediate fluid secretion from tracheal glands of ferrets. *J. Appl. Physiol.: Respirat. Environ Exercise Physiol.* 49: 1027–1031, 1980.
21. BORSON, D. B., AND J. A. NADEL. Cholinergic nerves inhibit adrenergic neurotransmission to tracheal submucosal glands of ferrets (Abstract). *Federation Proc.* 40: 254, 1981.
22. BOUCHER, R. C., JR., P. A. BROMBERG, AND J. T. GATZY. Airway transepithelial electric potential in vivo: species and regional differences. *J. Appl. Physiol.: Respirat. Environ. Exercise Physiol.* 48: 169–176, 1980.
23. BOUCHER, R. C., AND J. T. GATZY. Effect of amiloride (Am) and mucosal sodium removal on canine bronchial ion transport (Abstract). *Federation Proc.* 40: 447, 1981.
24. BOUCHER, R. C., AND J. T. GATZY. Characterization of Na^+ absorption across rabbit tracheal epithelium (Abstract). *Federation Proc.* 41: 1510, 1982.
25. BOUCHER, R. C., AND J. T. GATZY. Regional effects of autonomic agents on ion transport across excised canine airways. *J. Appl. Physiol.: Respirat. Environ. Exercise Physiol.* 52: 893–901, 1982.
26. BOUCHER, R. C., J. NARVARTE, C. COTTON, M. J. STUTTS, M. R. KNOWLES, A. L. FINN, AND J. T. GATZY. Sodium absorption in mammalian airways. In: *Fluid and Electrolyte Abnormalities in Exocrine Glands in Cystic Fibrosis*, edited by P. M. Quinton, J. R. Martinez, and U. Hopfer. San Francisco, CA: San Francisco Press, 1982, p. 271–287.
27. BOUCHER, R. C., M. J. STUTTS, AND J. T. GATZY. Regional differences in bioelectric properties and ion flow in excised canine airways. *J. Appl. Physiol.: Respirat. Environ. Exercise Physiol.* 51: 706–714, 1981.
28. BOYD, E. M. *Respiratory Tract Fluid*. Springfield, IL: Thomas, 1972.
29. BOYD, E. M., AND M. S. LAPP. On the expectorant action of parasympathomimetic drugs. *J. Pharmacol. Exp. Ther.* 87: 24–32, 1946.
30. BOYD, E. M., AND J. S. MUNRO. Ether anaesthesia and the output of fluids from the respiratory tract. *J. Pharmacol. Exp. Ther.* 79: 346–353, 1943.
31. BRANDTZAEG, P. Mucosal and glandular distribution of immunoglobulin components: differential localization of free and bound SC in secretory epithelial cells. *J. Immunol.* 112: 1553–1559, 1974.
32. BREEZE, R. G., AND E. B. WHEELDON. The cells of the pulmonary airways. *Am. Rev. Respir. Dis.* 116: 705–777, 1977.
33. CASTEELS, R., G. DROOGMANS, AND H. HENDRICKX. Electrogenic sodium pump in smooth muscle cells of the guinea-pig's taenia coli. *J. Physiol. London* 217: 297–313, 1971.
34. CHAKRIN, L. W., A. P. BAKER, S. S. SPICER, J. R. WARDELL, JR., N. DESANCTIS, AND C. DRIES. Synthesis and secretion of macromolecules by canine trachea. *Am. Rev. Respir. Dis.* 105: 368–381, 1972.
35. CHAKRIN, L. W., AND L. Z. SAUNDERS. Experimental chronic bronchitis. Pathology in the dog. *Lab. Invest.* 30: 145–154, 1974.
36. CHANG, S. C. Microscopic properties of whole mounts and sections of human bronchial epithelium of smokers and nonsmokers. *Cancer* 10: 1246–1262, 1957.
37. CIVAN, M. M. Intracellular activities of sodium and potassium. *Am. J. Physiol.* 234 (*Renal Fluid Electrolyte Physiol.* 3): F261–F269, 1978.
38. CLAMP, J. R., A. ALLEN, R. A. GIBBONS, AND G. P. ROBERTS. Chemical aspects of mucus. *Br. Med. Bull.* 34: 25–33, 1978.
39. COLES, S. J., J. JUDGE, AND L. REID. Differential effects of calcium ions on glycoconjugate secretion by canine tracheal explants. *Chest* 81, Suppl.: 34S–36S, 1982.
40. CORRALES, R. J., J. A. NADEL, AND J. H. WIDDICOMBE. Source of the fluid component of secretions from tracheal submucosal glands in cats. *J. Appl. Physiol.: Respirat. Environ. Exercise Physiol.* 56: 1076–1082, 1984.
41. CORRALES, R., J. H. WIDDICOMBE, AND J. A. NADEL. Relationship between mucus output and active Cl^- secretion in cat

tracheal epithelium. *Chest* 81, Suppl.: 7S–9S, 1982.
42. COTTON, C., AND J. GATZY. Electrolytes and sodium uptake in disaggregated canine tracheal epithelial cells (Abstract). *Federation Proc.* 41: 1260, 1982.
43. CURRAN, P. F., AND J. R. MACINTOSH. A model system for biological water transport. *Nature London* 193: 347–348, 1962.
44. CURRAN, P. F., AND A. K. SOLOMON. Ion and water fluxes in the ileum of rats. *J. Gen. Physiol.* 41: 143–168, 1957.
45. DALHAMN, T., AND U. PIRA. Isoelectric analysis of respiratory mucus from normal rats and rats exposed to tobacco smoke. *Am. Rev. Respir. Dis.* 119: 779–783, 1979.
46. DAS, R. M., P. K. JEFFERY, AND J. G. WIDDICOMBE. The epithelial innervation of the lower respiratory tract of the cat. *J. Anat.* 126: 123–131, 1978.
47. DAVIS, B., R. CHINN, J. GOLD, D. POPOVAC, J. G. WIDDICOMBE, AND J. A. NADEL. Hypoxemia reflexly increases secretion from tracheal submucosal glands in dogs. *J. Appl. Physiol.: Respirat. Environ. Exercise Physiol.* 52: 1416–1419, 1982.
48. DAVIS, B., M. MARIN, S. FISCHER, P. GRAF, J. WIDDICOMBE, AND J. A. NADEL. New method for study of canine mucous gland secretion in vivo: cholinergic regulation (Abstract). *Am. Rev. Respir. Dis.* 113: 257, 1976.
49. DAVIS, B., M. G. MARIN, I. UEKI, AND J. A. NADEL. Effect of furosemide on chloride ion transport and electrical properties of canine tracheal epithelium (Abstract). *Clin. Res.* 25: 132A, 1977.
50. DAVIS, B., A. M. ROBERTS, H. M. COLERIDGE, AND J. C. G. COLERIDGE. Reflex tracheal gland secretion evoked by stimulation of bronchial C-fibers in dogs. *J. Appl. Physiol.: Respirat. Environ. Exercise Physiol.* 53: 985–991, 1982.
51. DAVIS, J. D., R. C. BOUCHER, J. T. GATZY, AND P. A. BROMBERG. Pattern of salt transport in excised rabbit trachea (Abstract). *Physiologist* 23 (4): 100, 1980.
52. DE HALLER, R., AND L. REID. Adult chronic bronchitis: morphology, histochemistry and vascularization of the bronchial mucous glands. *Med. Thorac.* 22: 549–567, 1965.
53. DEY, R. D., W. A. SHANNON, JR., AND S. I. SAID. Localization of VIP-immunoreactive nerves in airways and pulmonary vessels of dogs, cats, and human subjects. *Cell Tissue Res.* 220: 231–238, 1981.
54. DIAMOND, J. M. Osmotic water flow in leaky epithelia. *J. Membr. Biol.* 51: 195–216, 1979.
55. DUFFEY, M. E., AND M. M. CLOUTIER. Intracellular chloride activities and active Cl secretion by rat trachea (Abstract). *Physiologist* 23(4): 62, 1980.
56. DUNNILL, M. S., G. R. MASSARELLA, AND J. A. ANDERSON. A comparison of the quantitative anatomy of the bronchi in normal subjects, in status asthmaticus, in chronic bronchitis, and in emphysema. *Thorax* 24: 176–179, 1969.
57. DURAND, J., W. DURAND-ARCZYNSKA, AND P. HAAB. Volume flow, hydraulic conductivity and electrical properties across bovine tracheal epithelium in vitro: effect of histamine. *Pfluegers Arch.* 392: 40–45, 1981.
58. EBERT, R. B., R. S. KRONENBERG, AND M. J. TERRACIO. Study of the surface secretion of the bronchiole using radioautography. *Am. Rev. Respir. Dis.* 114: 567–573, 1976.
59. ELLEFSEN, P., AND M. TOS. Goblet cells in the human trachea. Quantitative studies of normal tracheae. *Anat. Anz.* 130: 501–520, 1972.
60. ELLEFSEN, P., AND M. TOS. Goblet cells in human trachea: quantitative studies of a pathological biopsy material. *Arch. Otolaryngol.* 95: 547–555, 1972.
61. ELMES, P. C., AND D. BELL. The effects of chlorine gas on the lungs of rats with spontaneous pulmonary disease. *J. Pathol. Bacteriol.* 86: 317–329, 1963.
62. ERNST, S. A., AND J. W. MILLS. Basolateral plasma membrane localization of ouabain-sensitive sodium transport sites in the secretory epithelium of the avian salt gland. *J. Cell Biol.* 75: 74–94, 1977.
63. ERNST, S. A., AND J. W. MILLS. Autoradiographic localization of tritiated ouabain-sensitive sodium pump sites in ion trans-

porting epithelia. *J. Histochem. Cytochem.* 28: 72–77, 1980.
64. ESTEP, J. A., J. P. ZORN, AND M. G. MARIN. Effects of Cl⁻, Na⁺, and amiloride on the electrical properties of dog tracheal epithelium in vitro. *Am. Rev. Respir. Dis.* 126: 681–685, 1982.
65. ETHERTON, J. E., I. F. H. PURCHASE, AND B. CORRIN. Apocrine secretion in the terminal bronchiole of mouse lung. *J. Anat.* 129: 305–322, 1979.
66. EVANS, M. J., L. J. CABRAL-ANDERSON, AND G. FREEMAN. Role of the Clara cell in renewal of the bronchiolar epithelium. *Lab. Invest.* 38: 648–653, 1978.
67. EVELOFF, J., AND R. KINNE. Sodium-chloride transport in the medullary thick ascending limb of Henle's loop: evidence for a sodium-chloride cotransport system in plasma membrane vesicles. *J. Membr. Biol.* 72: 173–181, 1983.
68. FIELD, M., W. MUSCH, AND J. S. STOFF. Role of prostaglandins in the regulation of intestinal electrolyte transport. *Prostaglandins* 21, Suppl.: 73–79, 1981.
69. FIELD, W. E. H., E. N. DAVEY, L. REID, AND F. J. C. ROE. Bronchial mucous gland hypertrophy: its relation to symptoms and environment. *Br. J. Dis. Chest* 60: 66–80, 1966.
70. FLOREY, H., H. M. CARLETON, AND A. Q. WELLS. Mucus secretion in the trachea. *Br. J. Exp. Pathol.* 13: 269–284, 1932.
71. FREEMAN, G., AND G. B. HAYDON. Emphysema after low-level exposure to NO_2. *Arch. Environ. Health* 8: 125–128, 1964.
72. FREEMAN, J. A. Goblet cell fine structure. *Anat. Rec.* 154: 121–148, 1966.
73. FRIZZELL, R. A., M. FIELD, AND S. G. SCHULTZ. Sodium-coupled chloride transport by epithelial tissues. *Am. J. Physiol.* 236 (*Renal Fluid Electrolyte Physiol.* 5): F1–F8, 1979.
74. FRIZZELL, R. A., H. N. NELLANS, R. C. ROSE, L. MARKSCHEID-KASPI, AND S. G. SCHULTZ. Intracellular Cl concentrations and influxes across the brush border of rabbit ileum. *Am. J. Physiol.* 224: 328–337, 1973.
75. FRIZZELL, R. A., M. J. WELSH, AND P. L. SMITH. Hormonal control of chloride secretion by canine tracheal epithelium: an electrophysiological analysis. *Ann. NY Acad. Sci.* 372: 558–570, 1981.
76. GALLAGHER, J. T., R. L. HALL, P. K. JEFFERY, R. J. PHIPPS, AND P. S. RICHARDSON. The nature and origin of tracheal secretions released in response to pilocarpine and ammonia (Abstract). *J. Physiol. London* 275: 36P–37P, 1978.
77. GALLAGHER, J. T., P. W. KENT, M. PASSATORE, R. J. PHIPPS, AND P. S. RICHARDSON. The composition of tracheal mucus and the nervous control of its secretion in the cat. *Proc. R. Soc. London Ser. B* 192: 49–76, 1975.
78. GALLAGHER, J. T., P. W. KENT, R. J. PHIPPS, AND P. S. RICHARDSON. Influence of pilocarpine and ammonia vapour on the secretion and structure of cat tracheal mucins: differentiation of goblet and submucosal gland cell secretions. In: *Mucus in Health and Disease*, edited by M. Elstein and D. V. Parke. New York: Plenum, 1977, p. 91–102.
79. GATZY, J. T., AND R. C. BOUCHER. Amphotericin B and ion flow across canine trachea (Abstract). *Physiologist* 22 (4): 43, 1979.
80. GAYTON, D. C., AND J. A. M. HINKE. Evidence for the heterogeneous distribution of chloride in the barnacle muscle. *Can. J. Physiol. Pharmacol.* 49: 323–330, 1971.
81. GECK, P., C. PIETRZYK, B. C. BURCKHARDT, B. PFEIFFER, AND E. HEINZ. Electrically silent cotransport of Na⁺, K⁺ and Cl⁻ in Ehrlich cells. *Biochim. Biophys. Acta* 600: 432–447, 1980.
82. GERMAN, V. F., R. CORRALES, I. F. UEKI, AND J. A. NADEL. Reflex stimulation of tracheal mucus gland secretion by gastric irritation in cats. *J. Appl. Physiol.: Respirat. Environ. Exercise Physiol.* 52: 1153–1155, 1982.
83. GERMAN, V. F., I. F. UEKI, AND J. A. NADEL. Micropipette measurement of airway submucosal gland secretion: laryngeal reflex. *Am. Rev. Respir. Dis.* 122: 413–416, 1980.
84. GLYNN, A. A., AND L. MICHAELS. Bronchial biopsy in chronic bronchitis and asthma. *Thorax* 15: 142–152, 1960.
85. GLYNN, I. M., AND S. J. D. KARLISH. The sodium pump. *Annu. Rev. Physiol.* 37: 13–55, 1975.
86. GOCO, R. V., M. B. KRESS, AND O. C. BRANTIGAN. Comparison of mucus glands in the tracheobronchial tree of man and animals. *Ann. NY Acad. Sci.* 106: 555–571, 1963.
87. GREENBERG, S. D., S. F. BOUSHY, AND D. E. JENKINS. Chronic bronchitis and emphysema: correlation of pathologic findings. *Am. Rev. Respir. Dis.* 96: 918–928, 1967.
88. GRIEG, N., M. AYERS, AND P. K. JEFFERY. The effect of indomethacin on the response of bronchial epithelium to tobacco smoke. *J. Pathol.* 132: 1–9, 1980.
89. HAYASHI, M., G. C. SORNBERGER, AND G. L. HUBER. Differential response in the male and female tracheal epithelium following exposure to tobacco smoke. *Chest* 73: 515–518, 1978.
90. HAYASHI, M., G. C. SORNBERGER, AND G. L. HUBER. Morphometric analyses of tracheal gland secretion and hypertrophy in male and female rats after experimental exposure to tobacco smoke. *Am. Rev. Respir. Dis.* 119: 67–73, 1979.
91. HAYES, J. A. Distribution of bronchial gland measurements in a Jamaican population. *Thorax* 24: 619–622, 1969.
91a. HIPPOCRATES. *Regimen in Acute Diseases. XVII*, translated by W. H. S. Jones. London: Heinemann, 1923, p. 75–77.
92. HOUSE, C. R. *Water Transport in Cells and Tissues*. London: Arnold, 1974.
93. JACOB, S., AND S. PODDAR. Mucus cells of the tracheobronchial tree in the ferret (Abstract). *J. Anat.* 133: 691, 1981.
94. JAYARAM, T. H., AND F. J. AL-BAZZAZ. Calcium transport across canine tracheal mucosa: effect of epinephrine (Abstract). *Am. Rev. Respir. Dis.* 119: 319, 1979.
95. JEFFERY, P. K. Goblet Cell Increase in Rat Bronchial Epithelium Arising From Irritation or Drug Administration—an Experimental and Electron Microscopic Study. London: London Univ., 1973. Dissertation.
96. JEFFERY, P. K. Structure and function of mucus-secreting cells of cat and goose airway epithelium. In: *Respiratory Tract Mucus*, edited by R. Porter, J. Rivers, and M. O'Connor. Amsterdam: Elsevier, 1978, p. 5–20. (Ciba Found. Symp. 54.)
97. JEFFERY, P., AND L. REID. Intra-epithelial nerves in normal rat airways: a quantitative electron microscopic study. *J. Anat.* 114: 35–45, 1973.
98. JEFFERY, P. K., AND L. REID. New observations of rat airway epithelium: a quantitative and electron microscopic study. *J. Anat.* 120: 295–320, 1975.
99. JEFFERY, P. K., AND L. M. REID. Ultrastructure of airway epithelium and submucosal gland during development. In: *Lung Biology in Health and Disease. Development of the Lung*, edited by W. A. Hodson. New York: Dekker, 1977, vol. 6, chapt. 3, p. 87–134.
100. JEFFERY, P. K., AND L. REID. The effect of tobacco smoke, with or without phenylmethyloxadiazole (PMO), on rat bronchial epithelium: a light and electron microscopic study. *J. Pathol.* 133: 341–359, 1981.
101. JONASSON, O., AND E. L. BECKER. Release of kallikrein from guinea pig lung during anaphylaxis. *J. Exp. Med.* 123: 509–522, 1966.
102. JONES, R. The glycoproteins of secretory cells in airway epithelium. In: *Respiratory Tract Mucus*, edited by R. Porter, J. Rivers, M. O'Connor. Amsterdam: Elsevier, 1978, p. 175–188. (Ciba Found. Symp. 54.)
103. JONES, R., A. BASKERVILLE, AND L. REID. Histochemical identification of glycoproteins in pig bronchial epithelium: (a) normal and (b) hypertrophied from enzootic pneumonia. *J. Pathol.* 116: 1–11, 1975.
104. JONES, R., P. BOLDUC, AND L. REID. Protection of rat bronchial epithelium against tobacco smoke. *Br. Med. J.* 2: 142–144, 1972.
105. JONES, R., P. BOLDUC, AND L. REID. Goblet cell glycoprotein and tracheal gland hypertrophy in rat airways: the effect of tobacco smoke with or without the anti-inflammatory agent phenylmethyloxadiaxole. *Br. J. Exp. Pathol.* 54: 229–239, 1973.
107. KLEINERMAN, J., J. SORENSON, AND D. RYNBRANDT. Chronic bronchitis in the cat produced by chronic methacholine ad-

ministration (Abstract). *Am. J. Pathol.* 82: 45A, 1976.
108. KNIGHT, L., N. R. ANTHONISEN, W. ARKINSTALL, L. ENGEL, P. T. MACKLEM, R. R. MARTIN, L. W. CHAKRIN, AND J. R. WARDELL. The pathophysiology of an animal model for chronic bronchitis. *Am. Rev. Respir. Dis.* 107: 1081–1082, 1973.
109. KNOWLES, M. R., G. F. MURRAY, J. A. SHALLAL, J. T. GATZY, AND R. C. BOUCHER. Ion transport in excised human bronchi and its neurohumoral control. *Chest* 81, Suppl.: 11S–13S, 1982.
110. KOEFOED-JOHNSEN, V., AND H. H. USSING. The nature of the frog skin potential. *Acta Physiol. Scand.* 42: 298–308, 1958.
111. KÖLLIKER, A. Zur Kenntnis des Baves der Lunge des Menschen. *Verh. Physik. Med. Ges. Wurzburg* 16: 1–23, 1881.
112. KORDIK, P., E. BULBRING, AND J. H. BURN. Ciliary movement and acetylcholine. *Br. J. Pharmacol.* 7: 67–79, 1952.
113. KUHN, C., L. A. CALLAWAY, AND F. B. ASKIN. The formation of granules in the bronchiolar Clara cells of the rat. *J. Ultrastruct. Res.* 49: 387–400, 1974.
114. LAMB, D. The composition of tracheal mucus and the nervous control of its secretion in the cat (Appendix). *Proc. R. Soc. London Ser. B* 192: 72–76, 1975.
115. LAMB, D., AND L. REID. Mitotic rates, goblet cell increase and histochemical changes in mucus in rat bronchial epithelium during exposure to sulphur dioxide. *J. Pathol. Bacteriol.* 96: 97–111, 1968.
116. LAMB, D., AND L. REID. Goblet cell increase in rat bronchial epithelium after exposure to cigarette and cigar tobacco smoke. *Br. Med. J.* 1: 33–35, 1969.
117. LAMB, D., AND L. REID. Histochemical types of acidic glycoprotein produced by mucous cells of the tracheobronchial glands in man. *J. Pathol.* 98: 213–229, 1969.
118. LANE, B. P., AND R. E. GORDON. Regeneration of rat tracheal epithelium after mechanical injury. 1. The relationship between mitotic activity and cellular differentiation. *Proc. Soc. Exp. Biol. Med.* 145: 1139–1144, 1974.
119. LAZARUS, S. C., C. B. BASBAUM, P. J. BARNES, AND W. M. GOLD. Mapping of vasoactive intestinal peptide (VIP) receptors using cyclic AMP (cAMP) immunocytochemistry (Abstract). *Am. Rev. Respir. Dis.* 127, Suppl. 2: 274, 1983.
120. LEIKAUF, G. D., I. F. UEKI, J. A. NADEL, AND J. H. WIDDICOMBE. Bradykinin stimulation of active chloride transport in canine tracheal epithelium (Abstract). *Physiologist* 26(4): A-124, 1983.
120a. LEITH, D. E., S. L. SNEDDON, J. P. BUTLER, AND J. D. BRAIN. Cough. In: *Handbook of Physiology. Mechanics of Breathing*, edited by P. T. Macklem and J. Mead. Bethesda, MD: Am. Physiol. Soc., in press.
121. LEUCHTENBERGER, C., R. LEUCHTENBERGER, AND P. F. DOOLIN. A correlated histological, cytological, and cytochemical study of the tracheobronchial tree and lungs of mice exposed to cigarette smoke. *Cancer* 11: 490–506, 1958.
122. LOUGHLIN, G. M., G. A. GERENCSER, M. A. CROWDER, R. L. BOYD, AND J. A. MANGOS. Fluid fluxes in the ferret trachea. *Experientia* 38: 1451–1452, 1982.
123. MARIN, M. G., B. DAVIS, AND J. A. NADEL. Effect of acetylcholine on Cl⁻ and Na⁺ fluxes across dog tracheal epithelium in vitro. *Am. J. Physiol.* 231: 1546–1549, 1976.
124. MARIN, M. G., B. DAVIS, AND J. A. NADEL. Effect of histamine on electrical and ion transport properties of tracheal epithelium. *J. Appl. Physiol.: Respirat. Environ. Exercise Physiol.* 42: 735–738, 1977.
125. MARIN, M. G., J. A. ESTEP, AND J. P. ZORN. Effect of calcium on sulfated mucous glycoprotein secretion in dog trachea. *J. Appl. Physiol.: Respirat. Environ. Exercise Physiol.* 52: 198–205, 1982.
126. MARIN, M. G., AND M. M. ZAREMBA. Effect of calcium on ion transport and electrical properties of tracheal epithelium. *J. Appl. Physiol.: Respirat. Environ. Exercise Physiol.* 44: 900–904, 1978.
127. MARIN, M. G., AND M. M. ZAREMBA. Interdependence of Na⁺ and Cl⁻ transport in dog tracheal epithelium. *J. Appl. Physiol.: Respirat. Environ. Exercise Physiol.* 47: 598–603, 1979.

128. MAROM, Z., J. H. SHELHAMER, AND M. KALINER. Effects of arachidonic acid, monohydroxyeicosatetraenoic acid and prostaglandins on the release of mucous glycoproteins from human airways in vitro. *J. Clin. Invest.* 67: 1695–1702, 1981.
129. MAWDESLEY-THOMAS, L. E., AND P. HEALEY. Experimental bronchitis in lambs exposed to cigarette smoke. *Arch. Environ. Health* 27: 248–250, 1973.
130. MAWDESLEY-THOMAS, L. E., P. HEALEY, AND D. H. BARRY. Experimental bronchitis in animals due to sulphur dioxide and cigarette smoke. An automated quantitative study. In: *Inhaled Particles*, edited by W. H. Walton. Surrey, UK: Haessner Unwin, 1971, vol. III, p. 509–525.
131. MCCARTHY, C., AND L. REID. Intracellular mucopolysaccharides in the normal human bronchial tree. *Q. J. Exp. Physiol.* 49: 85–94, 1964.
132. MCROBERTS, J. A., S. ERLINGER, M. J. RINDLER, AND M. H. SAIER, JR. Furosemide-sensitive salt transport in the Madin-Darby canine kidney cell line. *J. Biol. Chem.* 257: 2260–2266, 1982.
133. Medical Research Council. Definition and classification of chronic bronchitis for clinical and epidemiological purposes. *Lancet* 1: 775–779, 1965.
134. MELON, J. Contributions à l'étude de l'activité secretoire de la muggneusse nasale. *Acta Oto-Rhino-Laryngol. Belg.* 22: 11–244, 1968.
135. MEYRICK, B., AND L. REID. Ultrastructure of cells in the human bronchial submucosal glands. *J. Anat.* 107: 281–299, 1970.
136. MEYRICK, B., J. M. STURGESS, AND L. REID. A reconstruction of the duct system and secretory tubules of the human bronchial submucosal gland. *Thorax* 24: 729–736, 1969.
137. MUIR, T. C., D. POLLOCK, AND C. J. TURNER. The effects of electrical stimulation of the autonomic nerves and of drugs on the size of salivary glands and their rate of cell division. *J. Pharmacol. Exp. Ther.* 195: 372–381, 1975.
138. MURLAS, C., J. A. NADEL, AND C. B. BASBAUM. A morphometric analysis of the autonomic innervation of cat tracheal glands. *J. Auton. Nerv. Syst.* 2: 23–37, 1980.
139. NADEL, J. A. Regulation of bronchial secretions. In: *Lung Biology in Health and Disease. Immunopharmacology of the Lung*, edited by H. H. Newball, New York: Dekker, 1983, vol. 19, p. 109–139.
140. NATHANSON, I., J. H. WIDDICOMBE, AND P. J. BARNES. Effect of vasoactive intestinal peptide on ion transport across the dog tracheal epithelium. *J. Appl. Physiol.: Respirat. Environ. Exercise Physiol.* 55: 1844–1848, 1983.
141. NATHANSON, I., J. H. WIDDICOMBE, AND J. A. NADEL. Effects of amphotericin B on ion and fluid movement across dog tracheal epithelium. *J. Appl. Physiol.: Respirat. Environ. Exercise Physiol.* 55: 1257–1261, 1983.
142. NEUTRA, M. R., AND J. L. MADARA. The structural basis of intestinal ion transport. In: *Fluid and Electrolyte Glands in Cystic Fibrosis*, edited by P. M. Quinton, J. R. Martinez, and U. Hopfer. San Francisco, CA: San Francisco Press, 1982, p. 194–226.
143. NEUTRA, M. R., AND S. F. SCHAEFFER. Membrane interactions between adjacent mucous secretion granules. *J. Cell Biol.* 74: 983–991, 1977.
144. NIDEN, A. H. Bronchiolar and large alveolar cell in pulmonary phospholipid metabolism. *Science* 158: 1323–1324, 1967.
145. OLVER, R. E., B. DAVIS, M. G. MARIN, AND J. A. NADEL. Active transport of Na⁺ and Cl⁻ across the canine tracheal epithelium in vitro. *Am. Rev. Respir. Dis.* 112: 811–815, 1975.
146. PACK, R. J., L. H. AL-UGAILY, AND G. MORRIS. The cells of the tracheobronchial epithelium of the mouse: a quantitative light and electron microscopy study. *J. Anat.* 132: 71–84, 1981.
147. PACK, R. J., L. H. AL-UGAILY, G. MORRIS, AND J. G. WIDDICOMBE. The distribution and structure of cells in the tracheal epithelium of the mouse. *Cell Tissue Res.* 208: 65–84, 1980.
148. PALFREY, H. C., AND P. GREENGARD. Hormone-sensitive ion transport systems in erythrocytes as models for epithelial ion

pathways. *Ann. NY Acad. Sci.* 372: 291–308, 1981.
149. PARK, S. S., Y. KIKKAWA, I. P. GOLDRING, M. M. DALY, M. ZELEFSKY, C. SHIM, M. SPIERER, AND T. MORITA. An animal model of cigarette smoking in beagle dogs. Correlative evaluation of effects on pulmonary function, defense, and morphology. *Am. Rev. Respir. Dis.* 115: 971–979, 1977.
150. PEATFIELD, A. C. The Control of Mucus Secretion Into the Lumen of the Trachea. London: London Univ., 1980. Dissertation.
151. PEATFIELD, A. C. Mucus secretion and its role in defence reflexes. In: *Advances in Physiologic Sciences. Respiration*, edited by I. Hutás and L. A. Debreczeni. Budapest: Pergamon, 1981, vol. 10, p. 519–528.
152. PEATFIELD, A. C., R. L. HALL, P. S. RICHARDSON, AND P. K. JEFFERY. The effect of serum on the secretion of radiolabeled mucous macromolecules into the lumen of the cat trachea. *Am. Rev. Respir. Dis.* 125: 210–215, 1982.
153. PERRY, W. F., AND E. M. BOYD. A method for studying expectorant action in animals by direct measurement of the output of respiratory tract fluids. *J. Pharmacol. Exp. Ther.* 73: 65–77, 1941.
154. PHIPPS, R. J., AND P. S. RICHARDSON. The effects of irritation at various levels of the airway upon tracheal mucus secretion in the cat. *J. Physiol. London* 261: 563–581, 1976.
155. PHIPPS, R. J., P. S. RICHARDSON, A. CORFIELD, J. T. GALLAGHER, P. K. JEFFERY, P. W. KENT, AND M. PASSATORE. A physiological, biochemical and histological study of goose tracheal mucin and its secretion. *Philos. Trans. R. Soc. London* 279: 513–540, 1977.
156. POPOVAC, D., R. CHINN, P. GRAF, J. NADEL, AND B. DAVIS. Serotonin potentiates nervous stimulation of mucus gland secretion in canine trachea in vivo (Abstract). *Physiologist* 22(4): 102, 1979.
157. QUEVAUVILLER, A., AND N. V. HUYEN. Hypersécrétion expérimentale du mucus bronchique chez le rat. I. Méthode d'appréciation anatomo-pathologique. *C. R. Soc. Biol. Paris* 160: 1845–1848, 1966.
158. QUINTON, P. M. Composition and control of secretions from tracheal bronchial submucosal glands. *Nature London* 279: 551–552, 1979.
159. REGOLI, D., AND J. BARABE. Pharmacology of bradykinin and related kinins. *Pharmacol. Rev.* 32: 1–46, 1980.
160. REID, L. Pathology of chronic bronchitis. *Lancet* 1: 275–278, 1954.
161. REID, L. Measurement of the bronchial mucous gland layer: a diagnostic yardstick in chronic bronchitis. *Thorax* 15: 132–141, 1960.
162. REID, L. Pathology of chronic bronchitis. In: *Bronchitis—An International Symposium*, edited by N. G. M. Orie and H. J. Shriter. Amsterdam: Van Gorcum, 1961, p. 137–147.
163. REID, L. An experimental study of hypersecretion of mucus in the bronchial tree. *Br. J. Exp. Pathol.* 44: 437–445, 1963.
164. REID, L. Evaluation of model systems for study of airway epithelium, cilia, and mucus. *Arch. Intern. Med.* 126: 428–434, 1970.
165. REID, L., AND R. DE HALLER. The bronchial mucous glands—their hypertrophy and change in intracellular mucus. *Mod. Probl. Paediatr.* 10: 195–199, 1967.
166. RESTREPO, G., AND B. E. HEARD. The size of bronchial glands in chronic bronchitis. *J. Pathol. Bacteriol.* 85: 305–310, 1963.
167. RHODIN, J. A. G. The ciliated cell. Ultrastructure and function of the human tracheal mucosa. *Am. Rev. Respir. Dis.* 93, Suppl.: 1–15, 1966.
168. RHODIN, J., AND T. DALHAMN. Electron microscopy of the tracheal ciliated mucosa in rat. *Z. Zellforsch. Mikrosk. Anat.* 44: 345–412, 1956.
169. RICHARDSON, P. S., R. J. PHIPPS, K. BALFRÉ, AND R. L. HALL. The roles of mediators, irritants and allergens in causing mucin secretion from the trachea. In: *Respiratory Tract Mucus*, edited by R. Porter, J. Rivers, and M. O'Connor. Amsterdam: Elsevier, 1978, p. 111–131. (Ciba Found. Symp. 54.)
170. ROBISON, G. A., R. W. BUTCHER, AND E. W. SUTHERLAND. *Cyclic AMP*. New York: Academic, 1971.
170a. RUBIN, R. P. Calcium-phospholipid interactions in secretory cells: a new perspective on stimulus-secretion coupling. *Federation Proc.* 41: 2181–2187, 1982.
171. SANDERSON, M. J., AND M. A. SLEIGH. Ciliary activity of cultured rabbit tracheal epithelium: beat pattern and metachrony. *J. Cell Sci.* 47: 331–347, 1981.
172. SATIR, P. How cilia move. *Sci. Am.* 231: 45–52, 1974.
173. SCHNEYER, C. A., AND H. D. HALL. Neurally mediated increase in mitosis and DNA of rat parotid with increase in bulk of diet. *Am. J. Physiol.* 230: 911–915, 1976.
174. SCHULTZ, S. G. Homocellular regulatory mechanisms in sodium-transporting epithelia: avoidance of extinction by "flush-through." *Am. J. Physiol.* 241 (*Renal Fluid Electrolyte Physiol.* 10): F579–F590, 1981.
175. SCHULZE, F. E. Epithel- und Drusenzellen. *Arch. Microsk. Anat. Entwicklungsmech.* 3: 137–197, 1867.
176. SHELHAMER, J. H., Z. MAROM, F. SUN, M. K. BACH, AND M. KALINER. The effects of arachinoids and leukotrienes on the release of mucus from human airways. *Chest* 81, Suppl.: 36S–37S, 1982.
177. SHOROFSKY, S. R., M. FIELD, AND H. FOZZARD. Electrophysiology of Cl secretion in canine trachea. *J. Membr. Biol.* 72: 105–116, 1983.
178. SILINSKY, E. M. Recent approaches to secretion and stimulus-secretion coupling. *Federation Proc.* 41: 2169–2171, 1982.
178a. SILINSKY, E. M. Properties of calcium receptors that initiate depolarization-secretion coupling. *Federation Proc.* 41: 2171–2180, 1982.
179. SILVA, P., J. STOFF, M. FIELD, L. FINE, J. N. FORREST, AND F. H. EPSTEIN. Mechanism of active chloride secretion by shark rectal gland: role of Na-K-ATPase in chloride transport. *Am. J. Physiol.* 233 (*Renal Fluid Electrolyte Physiol.* 2): F298–F306, 1977.
180. SMITH, P. L., AND R. A. FRIZZELL. Changes in intracellular K activities after stimulation of Cl secretion in canine tracheal epithelium (Abstract). *Chest* 81, Suppl.: 5S, 1982.
181. SMITH, P. L., M. J. WELSH, J. S. STOFF, AND R. A. FRIZZELL. Chloride secretion by canine tracheal epithelium: I. Role of intracellular cAMP levels. *J. Membr. Biol.* 70: 215–226, 1982.
182. SPECIAN, R. D., AND M. NEUTRA. Mechanism of rapid mucus secretion in goblet cells stimulated by acetylcholine. *J. Cell Biol.* 85: 626–640, 1980.
183. SPECIAN, R. D., AND M. R. NEUTRA. The surface topography of the colonic crypt in rabbit and monkey. *Am. J. Anat.* 160: 461–472, 1981.
184. SPICER, S. S., L. W. CHAKRIN, AND J. R. WARDELL, JR. Respiratory mucous secretion. In: *Sputum: Fundamentals and Clinical Pathology*, edited by M. J. Dulfano. Springfield, IL: Thomas, 1973, p. 22–68.
185. SPICER, S. S., L. W. CHAKRIN, AND J. R. WARDELL, JR. Effect of chronic sulfur dioxide inhalation on the carbohydrate histochemistry and histology of the canine respiratory tract. *Am. Rev. Respir. Dis.* 110: 13–24, 1974.
186. SPICER, S. S., L. W. CHAKRIN, J. R. WARDELL, JR., AND W. KENDRICK. Histochemistry of mucosubstances in the canine and human respiratory tract. *Lab. Invest.* 25: 483–490, 1971.
187. STINSON, S. F., AND C. G. LOOSLI. Ultrastructural evidence concerning the mode of secretion of electron-dense granules by Clara cells. *J. Anat.* 127: 291–298, 1978.
188. STURGESS, J., AND L. REID. An organ culture study of the effect of drugs on the secretory activity of the human bronchial submucosal gland. *Clin. Sci.* 43: 533–543, 1972.
189. STURGESS, J., AND L. REID. The effect of isoprenaline and pilocarpine on (a) bronchial mucus-secreting tissue and (b) pancreas, salivary glands, heart, thymus, liver and spleen. *Br. J. Exp. Pathol.* 54: 388–403, 1973.
190. TAKIZAWA, T., AND W. M. THURLBECK. Muscle and mucous gland size in the major bronchi of patients with chronic bronchitis, asthma, and asthmatic bronchitis. *Am. Rev. Respir. Dis.* 104: 331–336, 1971.

191. THURLBECK, W. M., AND G. E. ANGUS. The relationship between emphysema and chronic bronchitis as assessed morphologically. *Am. Rev. Respir. Dis.* 87: 815–819, 1963.
192. THURLBECK, W. M., AND G. E. ANGUS. A distribution curve for chronic bronchitis. *Thorax* 19: 436–442, 1964.
193. THURLBECK, W. M., G. E. ANGUS, AND J. A. P. PARÉ. Mucous gland hypertrophy in chronic bronchitis, and its occurrence in smokers. *Br. J. Dis. Chest* 57: 73–78, 1963.
194. THURLBECK, W. M., B. BENJAMIN, AND L. REID. Development and distribution of mucous glands in the foetal human trachea. *Br. J. Dis. Chest* 55: 54–64, 1961.
195. THURLBECK, W. M., D. MALAKA, AND K. MURPHY. Goblet cells in the peripheral airways in chronic bronchitis. *Am. Rev. Respir. Dis.* 112: 65–69, 1975.
196. TOM-MOY, M., C. B. BASBAUM, AND J. A. NADEL. Immunocytochemical localization of lysozyme in the ferret trachea (Abstract). *Physiologist* 23(4): 99, 1980.
197. UDDMAN, R., J. ALUMETS, O. DENSERT, R. HÅKANSON, AND F. SUNDLER. Occurrence and distribution of VIP nerves in the nasal mucosa and tracheobronchial wall. *Acta Oto-Laryngol.* 86: 443–448, 1978.
198. UEKI, I., V. F. GERMAN, AND J. NADEL. Micropipette measurement of airway submucosal gland secretion: autonomic effects. *Am. Rev. Respir. Dis.* 121: 351–357, 1980.
199. UEKI, I., AND J. A. NADEL. Differences in total protein concentration in submucosal gland fluid: α-adrenergic vs cholinergic (Abstract). *Federation Proc.* 40: 622, 1981.
200. USSING, H. H., AND K. ZERAHN. Active transport of sodium as the source of electric current in the short-circuited isolated frog skin. *Acta Physiol. Scand.* 23: 110–127, 1951.
201. WALSH, C., AND J. MCLELLAND. Intraepithelial axons in the avian trachea. *Z. Zellforsch. Mikrosk. Anat.* 147: 209–217, 1974.
202. WANNER, A., S. ZARZECKI, J. HIRSCH, AND S. EPSTEIN. Tracheal mucous transport in experimental canine asthma. *J. Appl. Physiol.* 39: 950–957, 1975.
203. WATSON, J. H. L., AND G. L. BRINKMAN. Electron microscopy of the epithelial cells of normal and bronchitic human bronchus. *Am. Rev. Respir. Dis.* 90: 851–866, 1964.
204. WELLS, A. B., AND L. F. LAMERTON. Regenerative response of the rat tracheal epithelium after acute exposure to tobacco smoke: a quantitative study. *J. Natl. Cancer Inst.* 55: 887–891, 1975.
205. WELSH, M. J. Evidence for basolateral membrane potassium conductance in canine tracheal epithelium. *Am. J. Physiol.* 244 (*Cell Physiol.* 13): C377–C384, 1983.
206. WELSH, M. J. Inhibition of chloride secretion by furosemide in canine tracheal epithelium. *J. Membr. Biol.* 71: 219–226, 1983.
207. WELSH, M. J. Intracellular chloride activities in canine tracheal epithelium. Direct evidence for sodium-coupled intracellular chloride accumulation in a chloride-secreting epithelium. *J. Clin. Invest.* 71: 1392–1401, 1983.
208. WELSH, M. J., P. L. SMITH, AND R. A. FRIZZELL. Chloride secretion by canine tracheal epithelium. II. The cellular electrical potential profile. *J. Membr. Biol.* 70: 227–238, 1982.
209. WELSH, M. J., P. L. SMITH, AND R. A. FRIZZELL. Chloride secretion by canine tracheal epithelium. III. Membrane resistances and electromotive forces. *J. Membr. Biol.* 71: 209–218, 1983.
210. WELSH, M. J., J. H. WIDDICOMBE, AND J. A. NADEL. Fluid transport across the canine tracheal epithelium. *J. Appl. Physiol.: Respirat. Environ. Exercise Physiol.* 49: 905–909, 1980.
211. WESTENFELDER, C., W. R. EARNEST, AND F. J. AL-BAZZAZ. Characterization of Na-K-ATPase in dog tracheal epithelium: enzymatic and ion transport measurements. *J. Appl. Physiol.: Respirat. Environ. Exercise Physiol.* 48: 1008–1019, 1980.
212. WHEELDON, E. B., AND H. M. PIRIE. Measurement of bronchial wall components in young dogs, adult normal dogs, and adult dogs with chronic bronchitis. *Am. Rev. Respir. Dis.* 110: 609–615, 1974.
213. WIDDICOMBE, J. G., AND R. J. PACK. The Clara cell. *Eur. J. Respir. Dis.* 63: 202–220, 1982.
214. WIDDICOMBE, J. H., C. B. BASBAUM, AND E. HIGHLAND. Ion contents and other properties of isolated cells from dog tracheal epithelium. *Am. J. Physiol.* 241 (*Cell Physiol.* 10): C184–C192, 1981.
215. WIDDICOMBE, J. H., C. B. BASBAUM, AND J. Y. YEE. Localization of Na pumps in the tracheal epithelium of the dog. *J. Cell Biol.* 82: 380–390, 1979.
216. WIDDICOMBE, J. H., A. A. GASHI, C. B. BASBAUM, AND I. T. NATHANSON. Structural changes associated with fluid absorption by dog tracheal epithelium. *Exp. Lung Res.* In press.
217. WIDDICOMBE, J. H., I. T. NATHANSON, AND E. HIGHLAND. Effects of "loop" diuretics on ion transport by dog tracheal epithelium. *Am. J. Physiol.* 245 (*Cell Physiol.* 14): C388–C396, 1983.
218. WIDDICOMBE, J. H., I. F. UEKI, I. BRUDERMAN, AND J. A. NADEL. The effects of sodium substitution and ouabain on ion transport by dog tracheal epithelium. *Am. Rev. Respir. Dis.* 120: 385–392, 1979.
219. WIDDICOMBE, J. H., AND M. J. WELSH. Anion selectivity of the chloride-transport process in dog tracheal epithelium. *Am. J. Physiol.* 239 (*Cell Physiol.* 8): C112–C117, 1980.
220. WIDDICOMBE, J. H., AND M. J. WELSH. Ion transport by the dog's tracheal epithelium. *Federation Proc.* 39: 3062–3066, 1980.
221. WIEDNER, G. Method to detect volume flows in the nanoliter range. *Rev. Sci. Instrum.* 47: 775–776, 1976.

CHAPTER 14

Macrophages in the respiratory tract

JOSEPH D. BRAIN | *Department of Environmental Science and Physiology, Harvard School of Public Health, Boston, Massachusetts*

CHAPTER CONTENTS

Classes of Pulmonary Macrophages
Origin of Pulmonary Macrophages
Fate of Pulmonary Macrophages
Harvesting Pulmonary Macrophages
Role of Pulmonary Macrophages
   Particle clearance
   Mucociliary transport
   Secretion and regulation
Measuring the Phagocytic Properties of Pulmonary Macrophages
   In situ
   In vitro
      Monolayer assays
      Suspension assays
Pathophysiology of Pulmonary Macrophages
   Emphysema
   Fibrosis
Conclusion

ALTHOUGH SIMILAR TO MACROPHAGES throughout the body—such as those present in the peritoneal cavity, bone marrow, and liver—pulmonary macrophages face unique challenges. Found on the inner surfaces of the respiratory tract, they come in contact with particles and pathogens contained in the inspired air. They are also exposed to higher oxygen pressures than their counterparts elsewhere in the body. Their mobility, phagocytic capacity, and bactericidal properties are essential to the maintenance of clean and sterile alveoli.

Because these cells are easily accessible by bronchopulmonary lavage, they have been studied extensively in vitro. Knowledge of the cell biology of phagocytic cells has been greatly extended by experiments with isolated pulmonary macrophages. Studies of these cells are of interest because their migratory patterns, phagocytic behavior, and secretory potential are pivotal events in the pathogenesis of pulmonary disease. Even though macrophages are an essential line of defense for airway and alveolar surfaces, they can also injure the host while exercising their defensive roles.

This chapter describes the major classes of pulmonary macrophages and discusses their origin, fate, recovery, and quantitation. Methods for quantifying their phagocytic function are also detailed. After discussing the role of pulmonary macrophages while emphasizing their protective posture, this chapter summarizes evidence that macrophages may also contribute to the pathogenesis of pulmonary diseases.

CLASSES OF PULMONARY MACROPHAGES

Pulmonary macrophages differ in their anatomical location as well as in their form and function. There are at least three types of pulmonary macrophages; the most prominent is the *alveolar macrophage*. Alveolar macrophages are large, mononuclear, phagocytic cells found on alveolar surfaces. They are not part of the continuous epithelial layer of type I and type II cells; rather, alveolar macrophages rest on this lining covered by surfactant. Figure 1 is a scanning electron micrograph of a human alveolar macrophage applied to type I cells above a capillary. Figure 2 reveals a dog alveolar macrophage moving along the air-blood barrier. Note the paucity of organelles in the trailing edge.

Another type of pulmonary macrophage is the *airway macrophage* (23). Airway macrophages can be found in both the large and small conducting airways. They may be present as passengers on the mucous escalator or may be found beneath the mucous lining adhering to the bronchial epithelium (140). These airway macrophages most likely are the result of alveolar-bronchiolar transport of alveolar macrophages, although it has been suggested that they are the product of direct migration of cells through the bronchial epithelium (28, 85). The number, appearance, and distribution of airway macrophages is markedly influenced by the method of fixation (23); intravascular perfusion is preferred.

Interstitial macrophages are the third type of pulmonary macrophage. They are found in the various connective tissue compartments of the lung, including alveolar walls, lymph nodes, and peribronchial and perivascular spaces. A typical interstitial macrophage in a human lung is shown in Figure 3. Connective tissue macrophages have been considered in detail by Sorokin and Brain (140). Wang (152) observed numerous macrophages subjacent to the mesothelial cell

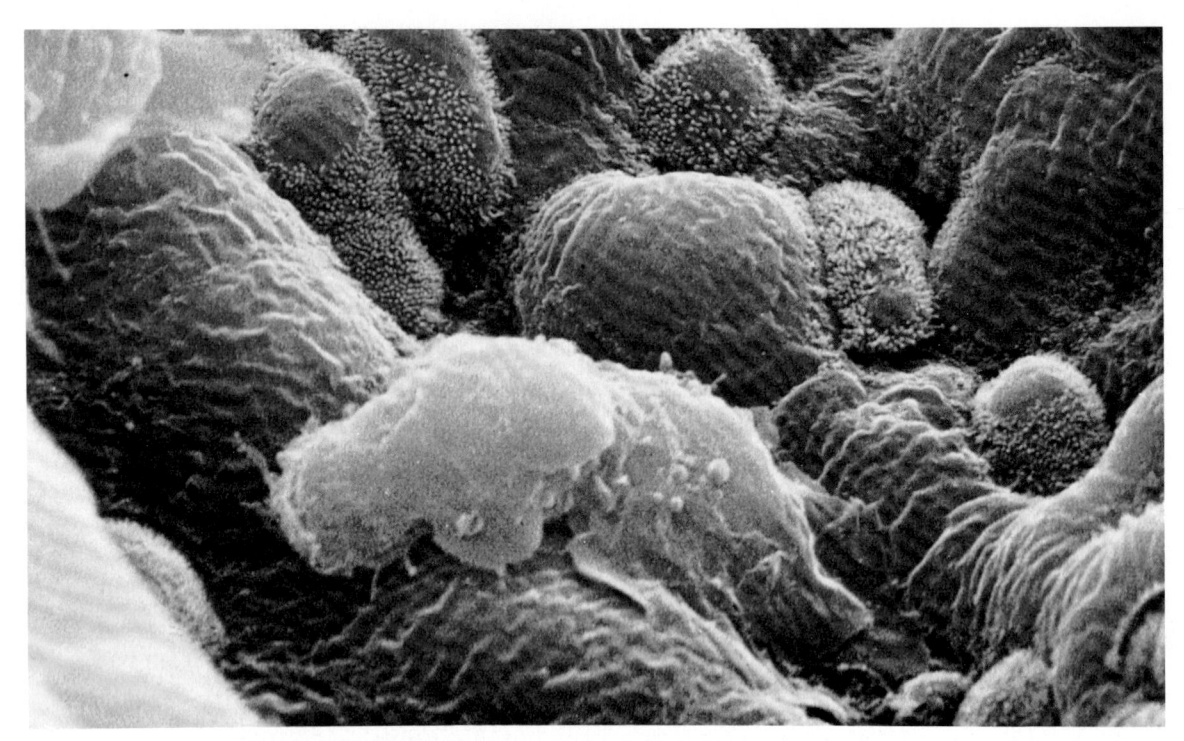

FIG. 1. Scanning electron micrograph showing human alveolar macrophage "climbing" over a capillary. Cell is clearly not part of the epithelial lining but is moving above it. The 5 cells in *upper part* of field with abundant microvilli are epithelial type II cells. × 3,700. (Micrograph courtesy of Dr. P. Gehr.)

layer of the pulmonary visceral pleura, particularly in the Kampmeier foci (small white patches found in the pleural folds of the lower mediastinum). These interstitial macrophages vary in appearance and, no doubt, in function as well. In lymph nodes, interstitial macrophages can frequently be found in close proximity to mast cells and lymphocytes.

In addition to these three primary types, other minor macrophage compartments exist. For example, macrophages are found in the pleural space where they not only serve a defensive role but may also act as miniature "roller bearings" that facilitate movements between the parietal and visceral pleura (3). There may also be a few intravascular macrophages similar to Kupffer cells in the hepatic sinusoids. In ruminants these macrophages are more prominent and may have an important functional role (153).

Macrophages from a single compartment need not be homogeneous. Heterogeneity is common in both structure and function. Many investigators have described considerable variability in macrophages recovered by bronchoalveolar lavage. Kavet and Brain (80) showed that the variabilty in the number of particles ingested per cell was greater than one would expect from the Poisson distribution. In other words some macrophages were more phagocytic than one would expect and others were less phagocytic. Parod and Brain (114) showed similar nonuniformity of phagocytic activity in lavaged macrophages using flow cytometry. Figure 4 illustrates the results of an experiment in which the theoretical and observed fraction of cells with x particles are shown. In this and all other similar experiments, the fractions of the cell population at the extremes of the distribution were higher than predicted. The Poisson distribution predicted that only ~1% of the cells would have no particles, but ~8% were empty. Similarly the number of cells that ingested 10 or more cells was much greater than expected.

Several investigators have used continuous-density centrifugation to separate macrophages into subpopulations. Holian et al. (75) and Dauber et al. (37) examined macrophages recovered by lavage from the lungs of normal guinea pigs. Using continuous-density gradients of colloidal silica, they divided the cells into six different fractions. They demonstrated that the cells in these fractions were different in both their morphological and cytochemical properties. The cells differed in their chemotactic responsiveness, the extent of pinocytosis, protein concentration, and the extent to which they released superoxide anions.

Monoclonal antibodies have also been used to characterize heterogeneity (99, 67). Godleski and Brain (56) described a specific antigen on the surface of hamster alveolar macrophages that is not present on macrophages from other organs. This antigen develops after macrophages emerge onto the alveolar surface. Monoclonal antibodies against this antigen have been produced. A flow cytometer/cell sorter was used to separate pulmonary macrophages into four subpopu-

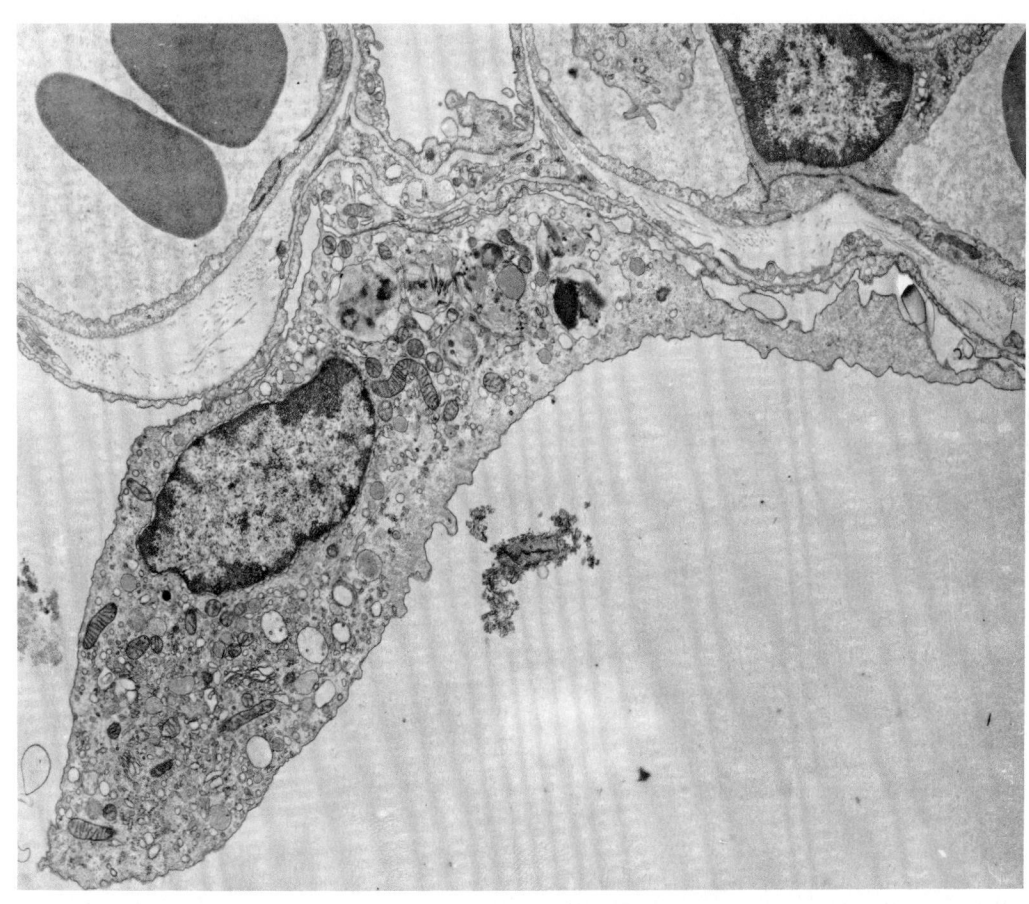

FIG. 2. Alveolar macrophage tightly applied to alveolar epithelium of a dog lung fixed by intratracheal instillation. Macrophage has a trailing pseudopodium and appears to be migrating toward the left. *Upper left* shows a capillary containing 2 erythrocytes. *Upper right* reveals a capillary with part of a white cell in the lumen and the nucleus of an endothelial cell directly to the right. × 7,000. (Micrograph courtesy of Dr. P. Gehr.)

lations that differed in both their length of time on the alveolar surface (as shown by [^{3}H]thymidine labeling) and the density of antigen on their plasma membrane (67).

ORIGIN OF PULMONARY MACROPHAGES

The origin and kinetics of pulmonary macrophages remain controversial. A primary question is whether they are normally derived directly from bone marrow via the blood monocytes or from an intrapulmonary population of macrophages and precursors capable of self-replication. Current evidence suggests that both pathways can occur, depending on the conditions. Alveolar macrophages are ultimately derived from cells in the bone marrow (55); however, this resident population can be maintained by proliferation of secondary-cell renewal systems within the lung. The notion that tissue macrophages always have monocytes as their immediate precursors is increasingly being challenged. Rather, the concept of a self-renewing resident macrophage population within the lungs seems likely. Data from parabiotic rats suggest that macrophage populations in unstimulated animals may be independent of circulating monocytes. Unilateral isotopic labeling in parabiotic rats showed the capability of cross-circulating labeled monocytes to emigrate from the blood in response to inflammation but failed to show their accumulation in normal resident macrophage populations. Intrapulmonary sources need not always be in the connective tissue. Even free alveolar macrophages may replicate. That alveolar macrophages are capable of cell division is demonstrated by Figure 5, which shows visible chromosomes in a macrophage recovered by lung lavage.

Bowden and Adamson (15a) presented data suggesting that cells in the pulmonary interstitial compartment are the primary site of proliferative activity leading to maintenance of and adaptive increases in the number of macrophages. After intratracheal administration of particulate loads, increased DNA synthesis and mitosis were seen in interstitial cells. These studies and other investigations in monocyte-free or-

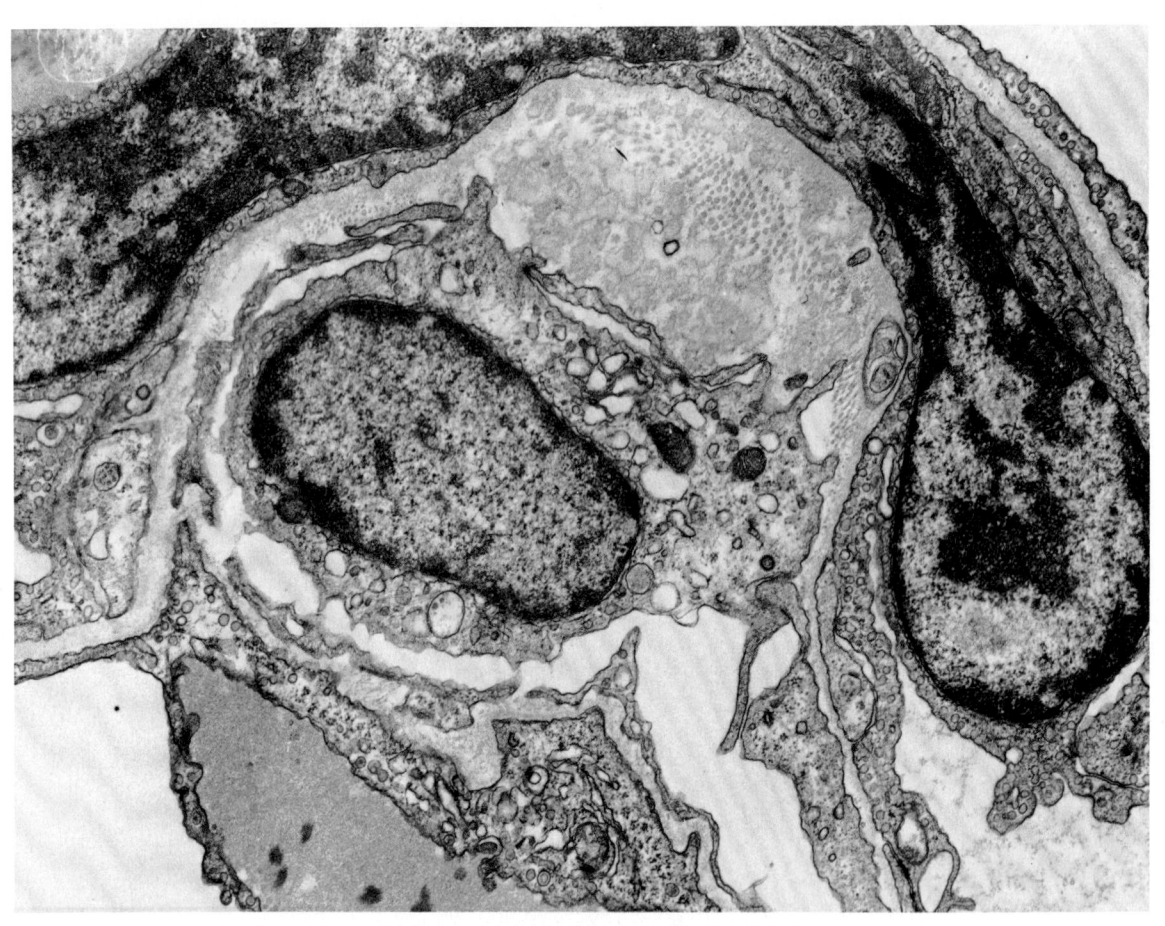

FIG. 3. Section of a human lung showing an interstitial macrophage in the *center*. To the *right* is the nucleus of an endothelial cell. *Above* and *right* of the macrophage is a bundle of collagen and elastin fibers. × 17,600. (Micrograph courtesy of Dr. P. Gehr.)

gan cultures suggest that with appropriate stimuli, macrophages in the interstitium reproduce and their progeny enter the air spaces.

Studies performed in animals with tuberculosis infection, however, showed that during chronic inflammatory processes, mononuclear cells were attracted to the area of the tubercle bacilli from the blood and became locally activated in the area surrounding the infection. There is growing recognition of the importance and strength of the response of monocytes to inflammatory stimuli. Influenced by lymphokines and ingested substances, these cells become rich in enzymes and microbicidal substances; they assume the properties of activated macrophages that can inhibit the growth of the tubercle bacilli. Thus although resident pulmonary macrophages defend the host against inhaled infectious and noninfectious particles, they play only a minor role in established chronic inflammation.

Observations in humans are consistent with these conclusions. Studies with incorporation of [^{3}H]thymidine have shown that human macrophages obtained by bronchopulmonary lavage are capable of limited proliferation. It has also been noted that patients with acute leukemia, who were under intensive chemotherapy and severely monocytopenic for several months, continued to have normal numbers of macrophages. Yet an ultimate bone marrow derivation of human

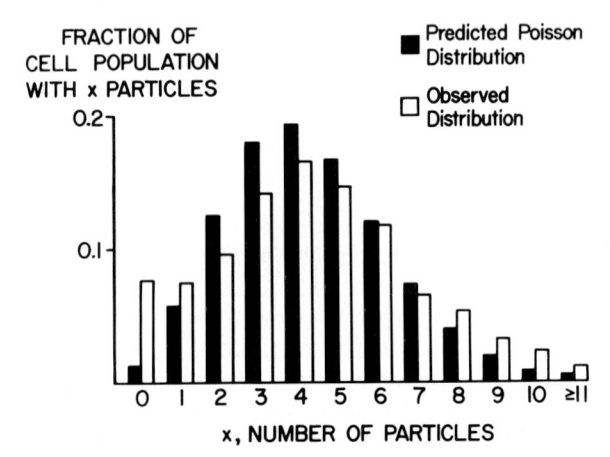

FIG. 4. Distribution of phagocytic ability in Syrian golden hamster macrophages. Cells were incubated in a balanced salt solution containing Ca^{2+} and Mg^{2+} (1 mM each) for 90 min; cells phagocytized an average of 4.3 particles per cell. *Solid bars*, theoretical fraction of cells with *x* particles as predicted by the Poisson formula. *Open bars*, fraction of cells with *x* particles actually observed. [From Parod and Brain (114).]

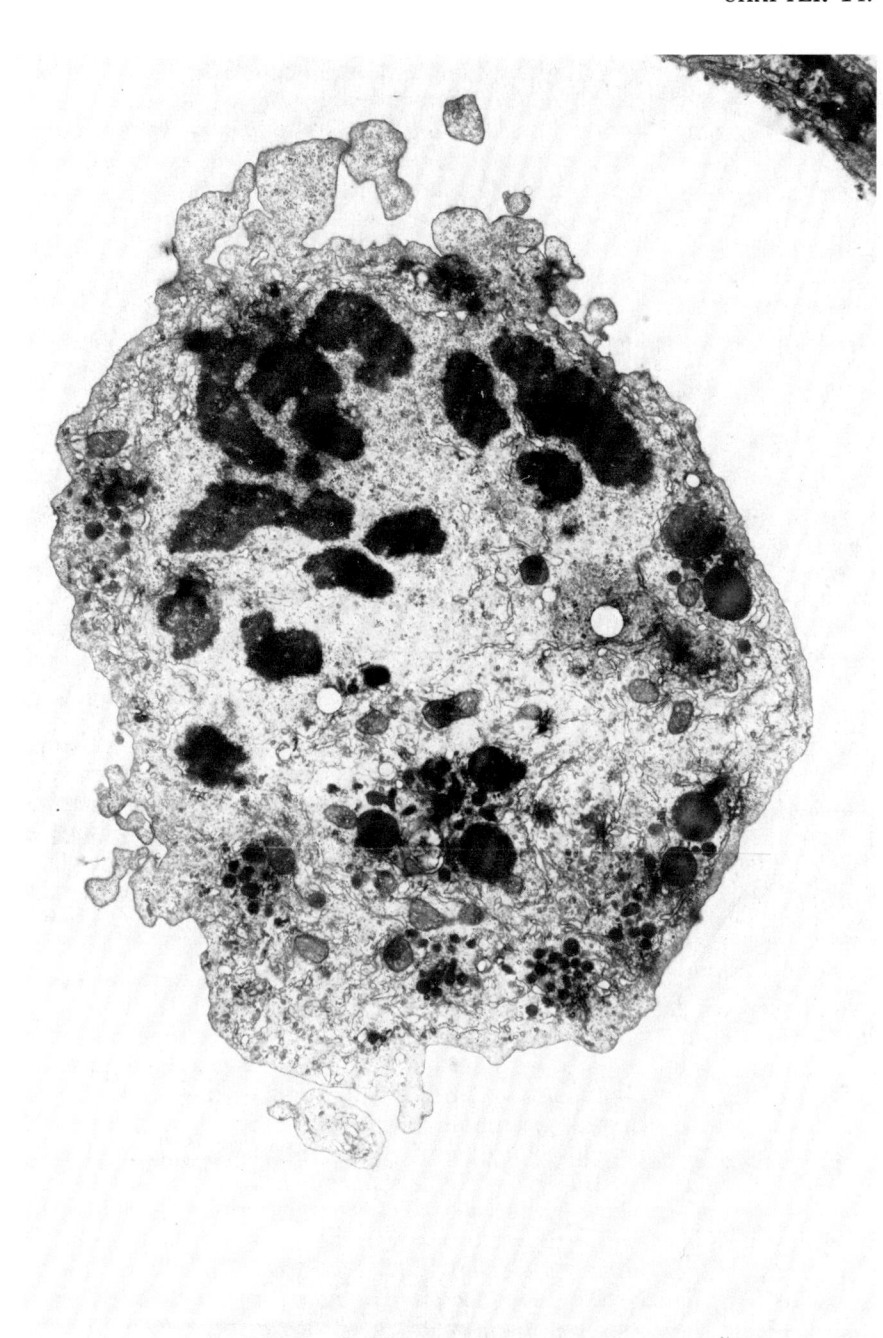

FIG. 5. Free alveolar macrophage in a mouse lung with chromosomes in its cytoplasm. Presence of such cells in mitosis shows that alveolar macrophages can divide and thus may help maintain the pool size of phagocytic cells. × 37,000. (Micrograph courtesy of Dr. M. Grant.)

macrophages is suggested by marrow transplant studies in which the donor and recipient were of different sexes. A fluorescent Y-chromosome marker was used to determine macrophage origin. One hundred days after transplantation in bone marrow, the macrophages in the transplant recipient were primarily of donor origin. Two mechanisms clearly exist for sustaining macrophage populations: 1) an influx of bone marrow–derived cells from the peripheral blood (14) and 2) self-replication in situ. What is not known is the relative importance of each mechanism under various physiological and pathological conditions.

Thus multiple strategies for maintaining the macrophage population in the lungs exist. In normal unchallenged animals, the immediate precursors are supplied by a cell renewal system in the pulmonary interstitium. Division of existing alveolar macrophages may also contribute to the maintenance of a pool of free cells. Demand for more macrophages as a result of infection or large numbers of inhaled particles may be met by 1) increased multiplication of free macrophages, 2) release of preexisting cells from reservoirs within the lungs, 3) increased production from macrophage precursors in the lung interstitium, and 4) an increased flux of monocytes from the blood to the lung.

FATE OF PULMONARY MACROPHAGES

Because differences exist among the classes of pulmonary macrophages, the fate of each must be considered separately. The possible destinations of alveolar macrophages have not been well described, but the possibilities are finite and easily enumerated. They may undergo alveolar-bronchiolar transport and be cleared from the lungs by mucociliary transport; they may enter the lymphatics or connective tissue; they may enter the circulation; or they may stay on the alveolar surface for extended periods, die there, disintegrate, and be ingested and digested by younger, more vigorous macrophages.

Some alveolar macrophages, once engorged with dust, find their way to the bronchioles and are then carried to the pharynx on the mucous blanket propelled by the cilia. Migration of macrophages through alveolar pores or through collateral pathways between adjacent bronchial paths also seems likely but is inadequately documented. In some fashion, however, macrophages move along the surfaces of alveoli and bronchioles to reach the mucous elevator.

The mechanisms responsible for the movement of macrophages to the bronchioles have not been identified. It is possible that macrophages exhibit directed locomotion because of a concentration gradient of a chemotactic factor. The phenomenon of chemotaxis has been extensively studied in vitro, particularly for neutrophils but less so for macrophages. No observations of alveolar macrophage movement in situ have been made and no evidence exists to suggest that other tropisms, such as geotropism, account for a purposeful migration of macrophages. There is little direct experimental evidence to suggest that the fluid lining of the alveolar regions moves mouthward, carrying macrophages with it, but some investigators have suggested this passive transport of cells as another mechanism.

A second possible route for the clearance of alveolar macrophages has been their direct entry into connective tissue and then into lymphatic pathways. The presence of particle-containing macrophages in these compartments has been suggested as evidence for this pathway. However, it is impossible to distinguish the entry of alveolar macrophages carrying particles from the passage of bare particles across airway and alveolar epithelium and their subsequent ingestion by connective tissue pulmonary macrophages already present there. During alveolar clearance some noningested particles may follow lymphatic channels from alveoli into the peribronchial, perivascular, or subpleural adventitias and thus penetrate into the connective tissue of the lung. They are then stored by resident macrophages. This route may be more pronounced when conditions favor increased permeability of the epithelium and the lymphatics (pulmonary edema). Then a greater number of particles might pass into these vessels through clefts between endothelial cells to be carried along lymphatic drainage paths until filtered out by macrophages located farther along in lymph nodes. Thus although inhaled particles can be found in connective tissue macrophages, little or no evidence exists that indicates movement of surface macrophages into connective tissue compartments. One cannot, however, totally exclude this possibility, although it must be an uncommon event. Yet it may be of consequence, because it could provide a pathway for pathogens and antigens in or on alveolar macrophages to meet reactive lymphocytes in the connective tissue.

HARVESTING PULMONARY MACROPHAGES

In vitro studies of pulmonary macrophages require the isolation of pure populations of macrophages from the lungs of animals and humans, but success in isolating pulmonary macrophages depends on the particular class involved. Alveolar macrophages, for example, represent a relatively accessible cell population. Unfortunately, airway and connective tissue macrophages in the lungs cannot be recovered with the same ease and purity.

No investigator has been able to prepare interstitial pulmonary macrophages with reasonable purity. Techniques for dissolving the lung and liberating individual cells have been developed (84), and intensive efforts have been made to separate certain lung cells, such as type II epithelial cells. However, interstitial macrophages are less numerous and little is known about the existence of unique physical or chemical properties that could be exploited in separating these cells. Conceivably their proclivity for attachment to glass or the identification of a specific surface receptor could be exploited. If a lung, well washed to eliminate many airway and alveolar macrophages, were dispersed, presumably those cells attaching to glass would be a population enriched in interstitial macrophages.

Airway macrophages may be isolated with somewhat greater ease. Isolated airway segments can be gently rinsed to recover the macrophages present on airway surfaces. This technique is adequate for recovering cells for morphological or histochemical analyses, but insufficient quantities are recovered for most biochemical or physiological studies. One can also attempt to lavage the airways and not the parenchyma. If the lungs are freed of gas and then carefully rinsed with small volumes of saline (1–3 times the volume of the dead space), it is mainly the airways that are rinsed. Appreciable interfacial tension between the injected saline and the airway surface, and the very modest inflating pressures associated with the small volumes injected, reduce the amount of saline reaching the parenchyma. It is also likely that the first few washes during lung lavage contain a higher percentage of airway macrophages than later washes, especially when a balanced salt solution including divalent cations is used.

Airway macrophages can also be recovered by collecting the free cells leaving the lungs via the trachea. Spritzer et al. (141) cannulated the esophagus and collected all swallowed material in a polyethylene bottle attached to a rat's flank. They recovered 1.245–2.47×10^6 macrophages per hour. Brain (16) developed a technique that permits the collection of diluted respiratory tract fluid from cats; 1.87–5.07×10^6 macrophages per hour were recovered from the lungs.

Regardless of the technique it is essential to recognize that the initial product is never pure. Desquamated airway epithelial cells (both ciliated and nonciliated), erythrocytes, neutrophils, and lymphocytes may be present in varying numbers. Differential counts should always be performed. For some applications macrophages should be purified by adhesion to glass, by density-gradient centrifugation, or by laser cell-sorter techniques.

Alveolar macrophages are traditionally recovered by bronchoalveolar lavage. After filling part or all of the lungs with saline via the airways, the fluid can be withdrawn. The recovered saline brings with it both cells and molecules contained in alveolar lining fluid, but not all free cells recovered by lung lavage meet the definition of alveolar macrophages discussed earlier. Some type I and type II pneumonocytes, airway epithelial cells, and contaminating red and white blood cells may also be harvested. Airway macrophages are always present; they are more prevalent in the initial washes and less so in the later washes. Lung lavages or washes to recover macrophages were first used by Gersing and Schumacher (54) and have been used extensively since the studies of LaBelle and Brieger (92, 93) and Myrvik et al. (110, 111). Brain and Frank (20–22) attempted to make the technique more sensitive and reproducible by utilizing multiple lung washes and by identifying and controlling the factors influencing macrophage yields.

Bronchoalveolar lavage is performed by cannulating the trachea (or by inserting a catheter through the trachea and wedging it in a bronchus), instilling wash solution, and then retrieving the lavage fluid by negative pressure. Excised lungs, whole lungs in situ, or parts of lungs in situ can be lavaged.

Excised lungs can be washed as follows. After dissecting the lungs free of other tissues, the trachea is cannulated with polyethylene tubing. Physiological saline flushes are used to harvest the free cells from the lungs. Repeated (6 or more) lavages with saline are recommended (20). During the washing procedure the excised lungs are suspended in physiological saline to eliminate hydrostatic gradients that might lead to uneven filling. When the washes are completed the lungs are fixed, sectioned, and stained for histological examination.

More frequently, lungs of small animals are washed in situ because the possibility of causing leaks in the lungs is reduced. After exsanguination the neck is opened and the trachea cannulated. The chest wall or diaphragm should be opened to allow the lungs to empty themselves of as much air as possible. Washes are then carried out as for excised lungs. In most mammalian species, yields are generally 3–15 million cells per gram lung for 12 washes.

Lungs of living animals may also be lavaged. This is convenient in large animals such as calves or dogs, although even small animals can be lavaged in vivo. After topical anesthesia of the upper airways, a cuffed endotracheal tube is introduced through the larynx and placed in the left or right bronchus or even in smaller airways. The cuff is then inflated to create a tight seal. The lung is freed of gas, if desired, by ventilation with pure oxygen for 15–20 min, producing a low lung volume by making the airway pressure negative (approx. -5 cmH$_2$O), and then occluding the airway. After a few minutes the remaining oxygen is absorbed. It is possible to lavage a lobe or lung without removing the gas; thus frequently this step is eliminated. The intubated lung or lobe may then be lavaged while the remaining lung meets the ventilatory demands of the animal. Animals tolerate the procedure better if the left lung or individual lobes are lavaged, because the right lung comprises ~60% of the total lung tissue. Smaller subdivisions of the lung may be lavaged by using smaller-caliber endotracheal tubes; tubes without inflatable cuffs may be simply wedged in an appropriately sized airway. Because only a small percentage of the total alveoli is washed, lavage of different lung segments can yield different results. This is especially likely if injury or disease is nonuniformly distributed in the lungs. Recoveries of injected saline may be less in animals possessing considerable collateral ventilation (e.g., the dog). Instilled saline not recovered is absorbed into the capillaries.

Similar procedures have been used to recover macrophages from humans and also to remove unwanted cells and secretions from small airways and parenchyma. With the advent of flexible fiberoptic bronchoscopy (128), access to the lower respiratory tract has become relatively easy and nontraumatic. Segmental lobes can be lavaged to obtain cytopathological material and bacteriological specimens. Typically a fiberoptic bronchoscope is introduced after premedication with atropine, meperidine, or diezepam, and topical anesthesia of the respiratory tract with a 2% lidocaine spray. Sterile saline can then be instilled and recovered through a bronchoscope placed in a pulmonary segment. The lavage procedure may be repeated several times. Lung lavage in humans generally uses volumes of 100–1,000 ml (30, 105). Depending on wash number, recovery of the instilled wash volume may be as low as 28% (39). Figure 6 shows an alveolar macrophage recovered from the lungs of a smoker. The cell is more activated and contains more lysosomes and phagocytized material than comparable cells from a nonsmoker.

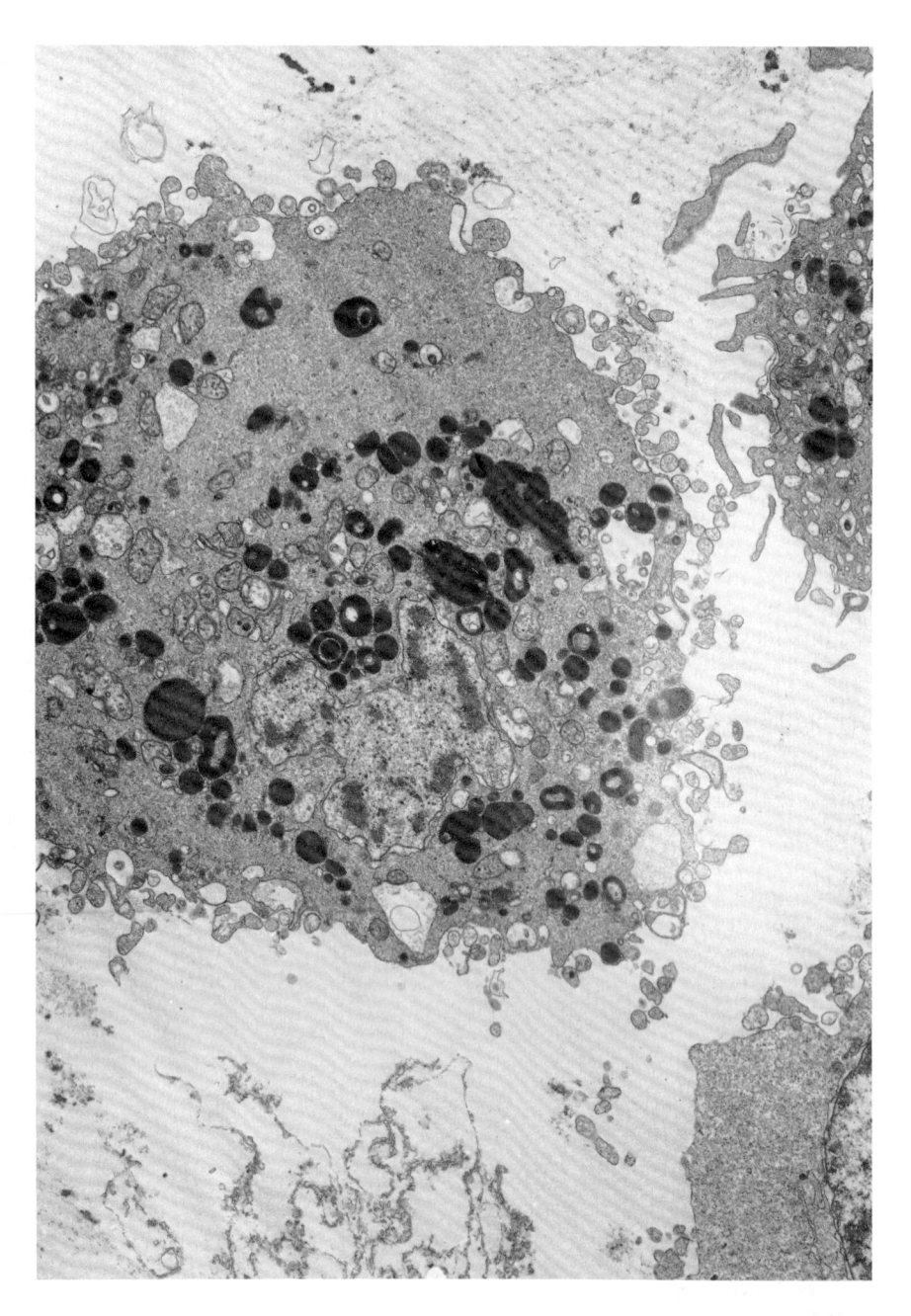

FIG. 6. Human alveolar macrophage obtained by bronchoalveolar lavage of a smoker's lung. Compared to that of a non-smoker, lysosomal compartment is greatly expanded and consists mainly of hetero-lysosomes, some possessing clear lipid-rich centers. × 11,000. (Micrograph courtesy of Dr. M. Grant.)

To obtain quantitatively consistent recoveries of macrophages it is necessary to control all aspects of the harvesting procedure. Brain and Frank (20) examined the effects of freeing gas in the lungs, length of postmortem delay time, wash volume, leakage, pathological changes, and number of washes. Another paper reported the effects of age, sex, lung weight, and body weight on the number of free cells recovered (21). Additional observations dealt with the effects of wash osmolarity and temperature and the washing cycle duration (22). Mechanical factors are also involved in the recovery of free cells from the alveolar surface and airways. Massaging the excised lungs or the chest wall when lungs are washed in situ increases macrophage recovery.

Examining the impact of procedural variables has provided some clues to physiological questions. For example, experiments with varied washing fluid compositions have given insight into the surface forces existing between the alveolar macrophages and the alveolar wall (22). Those experiments show that Ca^{2+} and Mg^{2+} are responsible for the differences in cell yields between a balanced salt solution and physiological saline; Ca^{2+} and Mg^{2+} critically influence the adhesive forces that exist between alveolar macrophages and the alveolar wall. This effect of divalent cations is particularly prominent in small rodents such as rats, hamsters, and mice but is also seen in cats and rabbits. Figure 7 shows two washout curves for hamsters. The average number of macrophages recovered per wash is plotted against the wash number. In lungs washed six times with a balanced salt solution containing Ca^{2+} and Mg^{2+} very few cells are recovered. Only when the lungs are washed six more times with 0.85% NaCl (lacking divalent cations) are adhesive forces between macrophages and the alveolar epithelium interrupted, and only then are large numbers of macrophages harvested.

Lung lavage is often used to quantify changes in macrophage pool size after aerosol challenge, lung infection, or lung injury. Lung lavage is more reliable and sensitive with repeated washes. The mean cumulative yield increases at a faster rate than the standard error (17). Although individual washes vary, differences tend to cancel each other so that the cumulative total yield becomes less variable. Lungs should be washed at least six times to achieve maximum sensitivity.

It is not surprising that a cell system so intimately involved with the disposal of inhaled materials responds to the quantity of particles presented to it. More than 60 years ago, Permar (117) stated that foreign particulate material introduced into the lungs increased the rate of production of phagocytes. Since then many other investigators have reported changes in macrophage pool size in response to particle challenge. Yevich (166) reported an increase in the number of rat alveolar spaces that contained macrophages after exposure to aerosols of oil or diatomaceous earth. Bingham et al. (13) reported that exposure to lead sesquioxide resulted in decreased numbers of alveolar macrophages. Gross et al. (66) reported significant increases in pulmonary macrophages after massive intratracheal instillations of silicon dioxide and antimony trioxide. Brain (16, 17) exposed hamsters and rats to a wide variety of particulates, including carbon, coal dust, barium sulfate, triphenyl phosphate, chrysotile, iron oxide, and cigarette smoke and observed increased macrophage numbers. Beck, Brain, and Bohannon (11) described changes in macrophage populations after exposing hamsters to iron oxide, aluminum oxide, volcanic ash, and α-quartz (silica). Macrophages in humans also respond to chronic exposure to inhaled tobacco smoke (118). Brain (17) observed that smaller particles tend to be more effective stimuli than larger particles. The number of macrophages released may be related more to particle number or particle surface area than to particle mass. In experiments with coal-dust suspensions instilled into hamsters, identical masses of particles smaller than 0.053 mm produced twice the response of particles larger than 0.25 mm.

When attempting to interpret changes in the number of macrophages present in the lungs, one must be aware of the assumptions implicit in the technique of lung washing and hence realize its limitations. The ratio of the cells harvested to those actually present is usually assumed to be the same in controls and in experimental exposure groups, but it is always possible that the experimental treatment has influenced the efficiency of recovery. If the experimental procedure provokes an inflammatory response, bronchoconstriction, or atelectasis, the efficiency of cell harvest may be altered.

The pool size of macrophages, like any other biological pool, is dynamically determined. The equilibrium number of cells present at any time is a function of the input and output history of the pool. For example, if pool size decreases, it may be due to decreased production, recruitment of free cells, or accelerated clearance of free cells from the lungs. If both input and output of free cells increase, pool size can remain constant despite increased release of alveolar macrophages onto the lung surface. Accelerated or depressed lysis of macrophages also influences the equilibrium number of free cells.

ROLE OF PULMONARY MACROPHAGES

Particle Clearance

Macrophages are usually credited with keeping the surfaces of the lungs clean and sterile. They ingest inhaled pathogens and particles as well as endogenous effete cells and even "worn-out" surfactant (43). Several reviews are available (15, 16, 24, 73, 74).

Although large numbers of infectious particles are continuously deposited in the lungs, the alveolar surface is usually sterile (97). The phagocytic and lytic

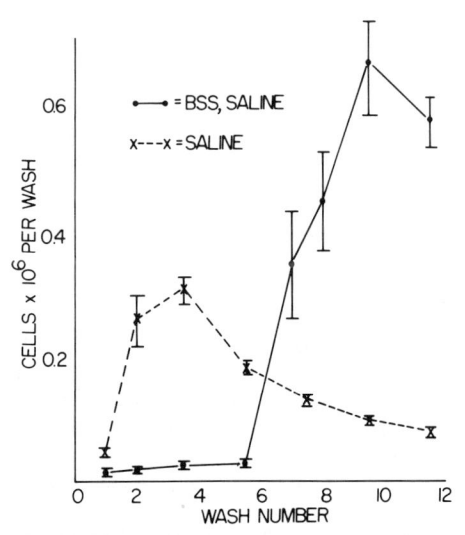

FIG. 7. Yield of cells per wash recovered from hamster lungs washed with either saline (0.85% NaCl) or BSS (balanced salt solution containing Ca^{2+} and Mg^{2+}). *Dashed line*, 12 saline washes; *solid line*, 6 BSS washes followed by 6 saline washes. Means ± SE. [From Brain et al. (24).]

potentials of pulmonary macrophages provide most of the bactericidal properties of the lungs. Macrophages are also responsible for ingesting and killing viruses (125, 126). During acute infection or injury they are also supplemented by other leukocytes. Increased inert or infectious particles stimulate the recruitment of additional macrophages. Like other phagocytes, alveolar macrophages are rich in lysosomes, subcellular organelles 0.5 µm or less in diameter. Exposure to inhaled particles also increases the amount of lysosomes in alveolar macrophages. Sorokin (138, 139) used electron microscopy and histochemistry to describe the activation of macrophages and the dynamics of lysosomal elements after exposure to iron oxide aerosols. The lysosomes attach themselves to the phagosomal membrane surrounding the ingested pathogen. Then the lysosomal and phagosomal membranes become continuous and the lytic enzymes kill and digest the bacteria. Macrophages are responsible for the intracellular killing of parasites such as African trypanosomes and malarial parasites (132); lung macrophages are also involved in the response to viral infections (123, 125, 126). Among the enzymes known to be present in lysosomes are proteases (120), acid ribonuclease (35), β-glucuronidase (98), acid phosphatase (35, 98), lysozyme (137), β-galactosidase (164), and phospholipases (49).

More important to the microbicidal activity of macrophages than lytic enzymes are the oxygen-dependent cytotoxic systems. Although best described in neutrophils (9, 88), these mechanisms are also present in pulmonary macrophages. Phagocytosis triggers increased oxygen consumption and the generation of oxygen radicals such as superoxide (O_2^-), hydroxyl radicals, singlet oxygen, and hydrogen peroxide. These highly reactive oxygen derivatives modify macromolecules of pathogens. Lipids, proteins, and nucleic acids may be modified by myeloperoxidase and halide-mediated oxygen-dependent reactions (88). Damaging oxidizing agents can also include several halogen derivatives such as chlorine and hypochlorous acid. Macrophages also contain ingredients that can protect them against the damaging effects of these oxidizing agents. Protective substances include vitamin E, ascorbic acid, the glutathione redox system, and catalase and superoxide dismutase.

A recent review by Elsbach and Weiss (44) also emphasized the oxygen-independent microbicidal systems in phagocytes. Certain bactericidal proteins have been identified that act specifically against certain gram-negative bacteria. Elsbach and Weiss (44) describe a granule-associated protein in neutrophils that causes susceptible bacteria to lose their ability to multiply. This change is associated with an increase in the permeability of the cell wall and activation of degradative enzymes in the bacterial envelope that act on phospholipids and peptidoglycan. Patterson-Delafield et al. (116) described cytotoxic arginine-rich proteins recovered from rabbit alveolar macrophages similar to those seen in rabbit neutrophils. In purified form, two of these are potently microbicidal for *Candida albicans*.

Pulmonary macrophages not only ingest and kill pathogens but also deal with nonliving insoluble dust and debris. Figure 8 shows how iron oxide previously instilled into the lungs can be seen in membrane-bound vesicles in the macrophage cytoplasm. This function is essential, because rapid endocytosis of insoluble particles presents particle penetration through the alveolar epithelia and facilitates alveolar-bronchiolar transport. Schiller (130) and Sorokin and Brain (140) found little evidence that macrophages laden with dust can reenter the alveolar wall; only free particles appear to penetrate. Thus phagocytosis plays an important role in the prevention of particle entry into the fixed tissues of the lung. Once particles leave the alveolar surface and penetrate below the epithelial barriers (type I and II cells), their removal is slowed. In humans, those remaining on the surface are cleared with biological half times estimated to be from days to months, whereas particles that have penetrated into interstitial and lymphatic tissues are cleared more slowly with half times ranging to as much as thousands of days. Therefore the extent to which macrophages influence the probability of particle penetration into fixed tissues is critical in determining the clearance times of particles from the nonciliated regions of the lungs.

Many test materials have been used to describe the pathways of particle clearance in the respiratory tract. Iron oxide is convenient because it can be readily generated in various forms by combustion of iron pentacarbonyl (26, 148). It is easily seen in the light microscope when stained by the Prussian blue reaction and in the electron microscope because of its electron density. Sorokin and Brain (140) used both of these microscopic techniques to study particle clearance in the lungs of mice after they were exposed to an aerosol of submicrometric hematite (Fe_2O_3) (mass median aerodynamic diam = 0.31 µm, geometric SD = 1.25). The animals were serially killed up to 14 mo after inhalation exposure. Initially particles that deposit on airways were swept toward the pharynx by mucociliary movements. Examination of the lung sections clearly showed three phases of clearance. Particles depositing on alveolar surfaces were rapidly ingested by alveolar macrophages. This phase was virtually complete in 24 h. The second phase was characterized by the gradual migration of particle-laden alveolar macrophages toward ciliated bronchiolar surfaces. These cells were also swept toward the pharynx by ciliary action but appeared to move much more slowly than uningested particles. Clearance by this pathway continued for several months. The third (or chronic) phase began when particles appeared within macrophages in the connective tissue of the lungs; these particles persisted

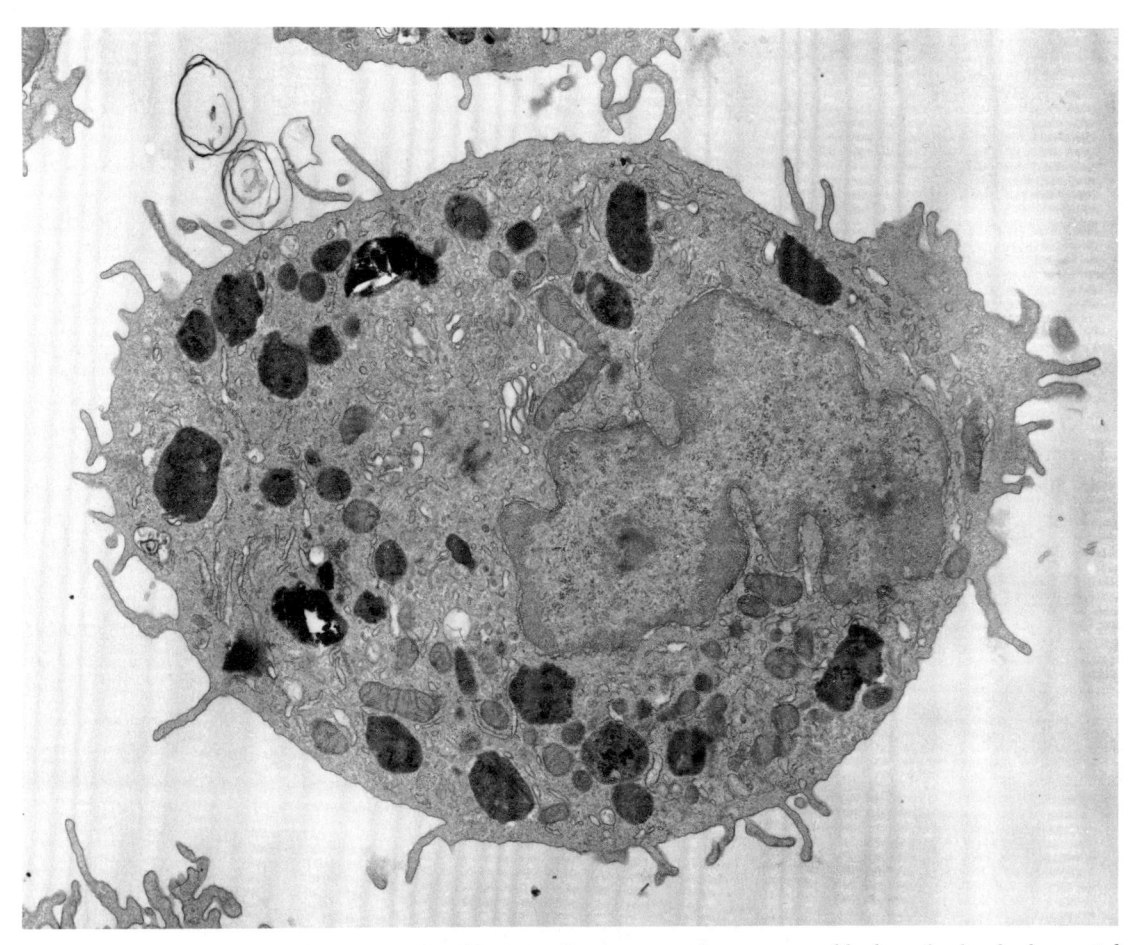

FIG. 8. Hamster alveolar macrophage recovered by bronchoalveolar lavage 1 day after the animal received an intratracheal instillation of magnetite (Fe_3O_4). These particles of iron oxide can be seen in phagosomes on *left side* of the cell; because they absorb electrons efficiently they appear black. Small pseudopods extend from the plasma membrane. × 12,400. (Micrograph courtesy of Dr. P. Gehr.)

for long periods but were slowly dissolved. The rate of solubilization depends critically on the particle size; smaller particles with correspondingly greater surface area dissolve faster. Light microscopy was the most useful in delineating these phases, whereas electron microscopy permitted the description of the ultrastructure of phagosomes and lysosomes. Sorokin (138, 139) recently further characterized dynamics of lysosomal formation and fusion after exposure to inhaled iron oxide aerosol.

Macrophages ingest almost any foreign material reaching the alveoli, such as aspirated cod liver or mineral oil. They also engulf endogenous materials such as red cells that may be present after pulmonary hemorrhage caused by increased pulmonary capillary pressure subsequent to left heart failure. In fact, an early synonym for alveolar macrophages was "heart failure cells." Finally, macrophages may ingest endogenous cells and materials even without pathological provocation. Effete epithelial cells and excess or inactive pulmonary surfactant are also probably ingested and degraded by macrophages. It is likely that alveolar macrophages even ingest other dead or damaged macrophages. To exercise these responsibilities, macrophages must move about on the alveolar surface. As shown in Figure 9, the macrophages also extend pseudopods over the epithelium in search of particles and pathogens.

Mucociliary Transport

Although macrophages have a key role in removing deposited particles from the lungs, they do not function in isolation. Other mechanisms also facilitate the clearance of particles from the respiratory tract. Highly soluble particles dissolve rapidly and are absorbed into the blood from the respiratory tract. Their metabolism and excretion resemble those of an intravenously injected dose of the same material. Cough should be mentioned because it is important when normal clearance mechanisms are depressed or absent and when excess secretions are present. Irritation of the nose induces powerful physiological reflexes, including sneezing, an effective means of removing un-

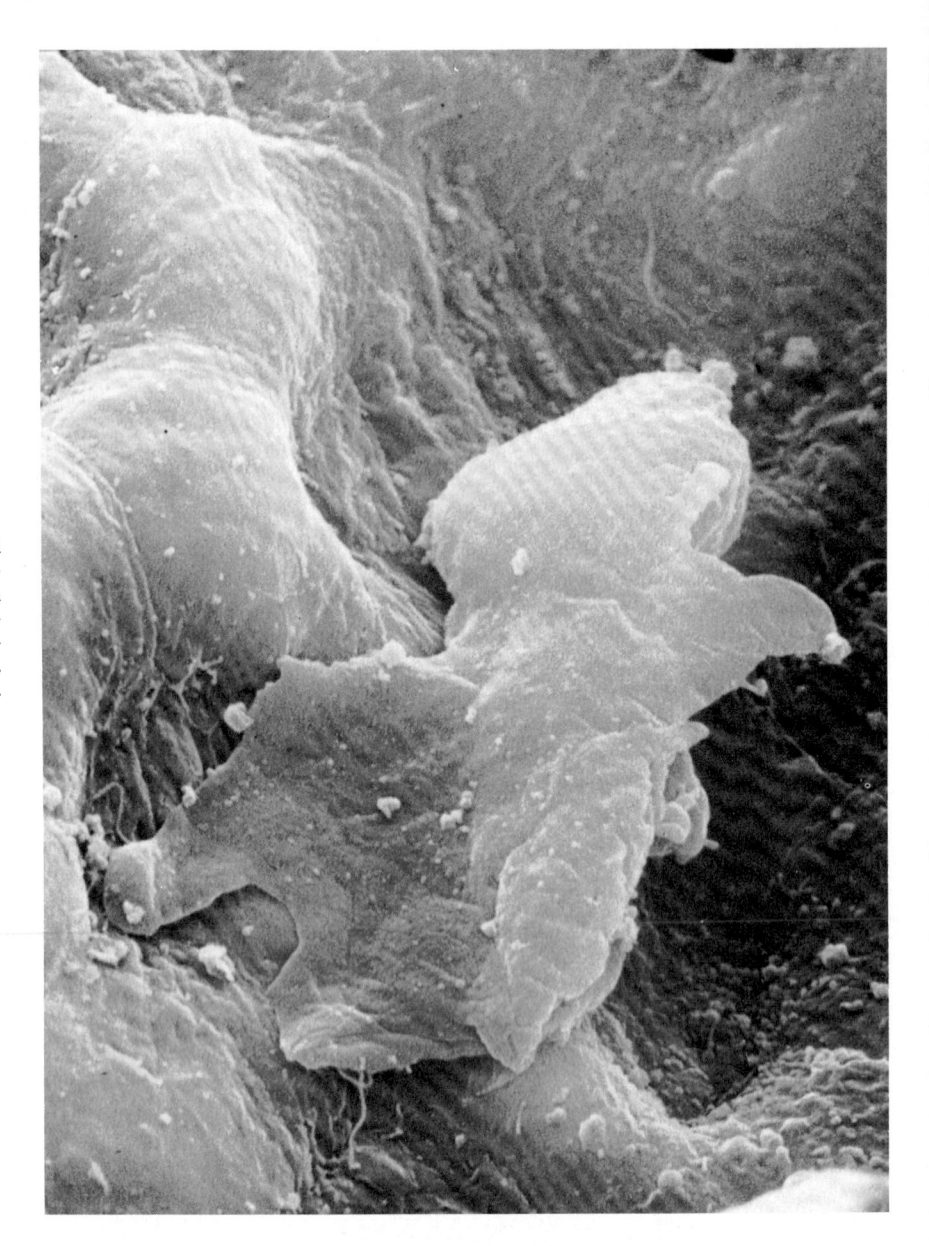

FIG. 9. Scanning electron micrograph of horse lung revealing a macrophage moving on surface of the alveolar epithelium that overlies the capillaries. Note prominent ridge in the *upper left*. Two pseudopods that are being extended can be seen. × 5,200. (Micrograph courtesy of Dr. P. Gehr.)

wanted particles from the nose. Similarly the laryngeal epithelium and the airways contain cough and irritant receptors. Coughing creates airway narrowing as well as maximal expiratory flows. Then the very high linear velocities that are created are able to move mucus and debris along the airways (101). However, in normal humans the major way of cleaning the airways is by mucociliary transport.

Much of the surface of the respiratory tract from the nose to the terminal bronchioles is covered with a mucous membrane composed of pseudostratified ciliated columnar epithelium. The term *pseudostratified* is used because there appear to be several layers of epithelial cells, as indicated by the nuclei found at different levels. Serial secretions, however, show that each cell touches the basement membrane. The primary cell type is the ciliated columnar cell, which has numerous cilia extending from its free surface into the tracheal lumen. Krahl (89) estimates that there are ~270 cilia on each ciliated columnar cell or 1,800 million cilia per centimeter of mucosal surface. Also present in the airways are characteristic mucus-secreting cells called goblet cells. Chronic irritation of the tracheal or bronchial mucosa can lead to an increasing number of goblet cells.

Even more important in terms of the mass of secretions present are the submucosal glands that in contrast to goblet cells are more influenced by the parasympathetic nervous sytem. The combined secretions of the goblet cells, submucosal glands, and other cells form a fluid layer located around and above the cilia that is moved mouthward by the cilia. The fluid also contains cells, debris, alveolar lining fluid, and secretions of airway cells and glands.

Particles that deposit on the mucous blanket covering pulmonary airways and the nasal passages are moved toward the pharynx by the cilia, which beat ~1,000 times per minute. Cells and particles that have been transported from the nonciliated alveoli to the ciliated airways are also carried with the moving carpet of mucus. At the pharynx, mucus, cells, and debris coming from the nasal cavities and the lungs meet, mix with salivary secretions, and enter the gastrointestinal tract after being swallowed. The particles are removed with half times from minutes to hours. There is little time for solubilization of slowly dissolving materials. In contrast, particles deposited in the nonciliated compartments have much longer residence times; there, small differences in in vivo solubility can have great significance.

A number of factors can affect the speed of mucous flow by either influencing the cilia or by altering the properties of the mucus. These aspects of ciliary action may be affected: number of strokes per minute, amplitude of each stroke, time course and form of each stroke, length of the cilia, ratio of ciliated to nonciliated area, and susceptibility of the cilia to intrinsic and extrinsic agents that modify their rate and quality of motion. The characteristics of the mucus are frequently of critical importance. The thickness of the mucous layer and its rheological properties may vary widely. Several investigators, beginning with the classic work of Lucas and Douglas (106), have shown that the mucous carpet is divided into two distinct layers. There is an outer, viscous mucous layer that comes in contact with the cilia only during their active stroke. Underneath the viscous layer is a more fluid layer (the periciliary fluid) that surrounds the cilia and provides a relatively frictionless medium in which the cilia move. The thickness and quality of these two layers could have profound effects on the effective action of the cilia. For example, slight drying could increase the viscosity of the mucous layer without affecting the underlying cilia, and yet ciliary action might be less effective in moving the upper mucous layer. Or the fluid layer may become too thick; it could then elevate the viscous mucous sheet so that the cilia would fail to make contact with it and thus be unable to propel it. Several investigators have demonstrated circumstances in which the functional changes observed in mucociliary transport were primarily attributable to alterations in the character of the mucosal secretions and not to a direct injury to the ciliary mechanism.

Many studies do not characterize ciliary motility and the quantity and rheological properties of the mucus separately. In most cases the interaction of the two processes, mucous transport, is the measured variable. Most evidence suggests that mucous secretion is a more sensitive process than ciliary activity. In many instances the quantity and rheological characteristics of the polymeric gel that constitutes mucus may be affected independently of any change in the cilia.

Secretion and Regulation

Abundant evidence indicates that macrophages have many functions in addition to phagocytosis. Macrophages secrete a variety of substances that interact with multienzyme cascades and with other cells such as lymphocytes, fibroblasts, and other macrophages. Thus the macrophage both responds to and regulates its external environment. Werb (158) reviewed materials secreted by macrophages (Table 1). Interactions between alveolar macrophages and lymphocytes may be involved in the suppression or induction of immunological pulmonary disease. Shellito et al. (133) recently demonstrated that murine alveolar macrophages differ significantly from peritoneal macrophages in both lymphocyte binding and their ability to stimulate lymphocyte proliferation. Unanue (145) reviewed other aspects of the immunoregulatory function of the macrophage and described factors that regulate the expression of I-region–associated antigens by macrophages. Macrophages are involved in the presentation of antigens and interact with the helper-inducer set of T lymphocytes. Finally, interactions between macrophages and lymphocytes are modified by exposure to inhaled particles such as tobacco smoke (41).

As discussed in *Emphysema*, p. 465, and *Fibrosis*, p. 466, some of these secretions are involved in connective tissue turnover, for example, collagenase, elastase, and lysosomal enzymes. Other secretions affect lymphoid cells by helping to regulate mitogenesis and differentiation. Macrophages release additional products such as interferon, fibronectin, lysozyme, certain components of complement, and antiproteases that are involved in defense processes.

Other biologically active materials secreted by macrophages include an angiogenesis factor, plasminogen activator, prostaglandins, nucleosides, cyclic nucleotides, pyrogens, granulopoietins, and factors influencing fibroblast proliferation and tumor growth. Still other agents may interact with humoral enzyme systems such as the clotting, complement, fibrinolytic, and kinin-generating systems. Macrophages are known to secrete plasminogen activator, a variety of oxygenation products of arachidonic acid such as prostaglandins F_2 and E_2 and thromboxane B_2 (38). Finally, macrophages secrete a number of components of complement, interleukin 1, and a variety of modulators of cellular behavior such as mitogens for T and B cells, thymic maturation factor, and stimulants of collagen synthesis and angiogenesis (38).

Pulmonary macrophages are also involved in the induction and expression of several forms of cell-mediated and humoral immunity; they are essential for delayed hypersensitivity reactions and may be involved in allograft rejection and the pathogenesis of autoimmune diseases. The response of macrophages in the lung to antigens in the respiratory tract may

TABLE 1. *Secreted Products of Macrophages*

A. Proteins and Peptides		
Enzymes	Plasma proteins	Factors regulating cellular functions

Neutral proteinases
  Plasminogen activator
  Metal-dependent elastase
  Collagenase (types I–, II–, III–specific)
  Collagenase (type V–specific)
  Cytolytic proteinase
Lysozyme
Lipoprotein lipase
Arginase
Phosphatases
Acid hydrolases
	α_2-Macroglobulin
	Fibronectin
	Transcobalamin II
	Apolipoprotein E
	Coagulation proteins
	  Tissue thromboplastin
	  Factor V
	  Factor VII
	  Factor IX
	  Factor X
	Complement components
	  C1
	  C2
	  C3
	  C4
	  C5
	  Properidin
	  Factor B
	  Factor D
	  C3b inactivator
	  β_1H (C3b inactivator accelerator)
		Interleukin 1 (endogenous pyrogen)
		Angiogenesis factor
		Factors promoting proliferation of:
		  Fibroblasts
		  Endothelial cells
		Interferon
		Factors inhibiting proliferation of:
		  Tumor cells
		  Listeria monocytogenes

B. Low-Molecular-Weight Substances		
Reactive metabolites of oxygen	Bioactive lipids	Nucleotide metabolites
Superoxide anion Hydrogen peroxide	Prostaglandin E_2 6-Ketoprostaglandin $F_{1\alpha}$ Thromboxane B_2 Leukotriene C (slow-reacting substance of anaphylaxis) 12-Hydroxyeicosatetraenoic acid Others	cAMP Thymidine Uracil Uric Acid

From Werb (158).

vary. They may prevent excessive antigen stimulation by ingesting and catabolizing inhaled foreign proteins and antigens derived from bacteria, viruses, fungi, and other microbes. Alternatively they may preserve and present antigens to lymphocytes and act cooperatively with components of the immune system (145).

There is considerable evidence that macrophages may also be involved in the detection and destruction of neoplastic cells (102). More than two decades ago, Gorer (60) noted that macrophages are prominent during the rejection of tumor cells. Since then other investigators have shown that macrophages can selectively damage tumor cells (45, 61). The stimulation of macrophages by infection can further enhance the ability of macrophages to prevent tumor growth (71, 83). Unfortunately there is little evidence that macrophage-mediated destruction of large tumor burdens may be an effective way of treating cancer. In most tumors the number of macrophages is too low to result in the destruction of all tumor cells, even when the macrophages are activated to an optimal tumoricidal state (48). Lung cancer remains a very untreatable disease.

MEASURING THE PHAGOCYTIC PROPERTIES OF PULMONARY MACROPHAGES

In Situ

The capacity of the lung to ingest and kill pathogens via its macrophages has been widely studied. The progress of intrapulmonary bacterial killing can be assayed by counting bacterial colony-forming units (CFU) in pour-plate cultures containing samples of lung homogenates from animals killed at various times after a bacterial aerosol exposure. The results are then compared to the number of CFU seen immediately after the bacterial challenge. This technique was first developed by Laurenzi et al. (95). The extent of bacterial survival at any time can be expressed as the CFU divided by the CFU at 0 h. To simultaneously study killing and physical clearance from the lungs, Green and Kass (65) incorporated ^{32}P into *Staphylococcus aureus* and *Proteus mirabilis* aerosols and found that for both species 80%–85% of the initial radioactivity remained in the lungs at 4 h. However, at that time, only 8.7% of the *Staphylococcus aureus* and 23.4% of the *Proteus mirabilis* organisms present at 0 h were still able to form colonies. Thus the disappearance of CFU could be largely accounted for by intrapulmonary killing rather than physical removal.

Green and Goldstein (63) refined the assay by normalizing the CFU counted from a lung sample to the ^{32}P activity remaining in the same set of lungs. The great advantage of this approach is that it permits a correction for interanimal variability in aerosol deposition, a major cause of variation. Because of differences in animal activity, size, chamber temperature, and other factors, different animals may have widely varying amounts of bacteria deposited in their lungs. Histological evidence by Green and Kass (65) and later by Goldstein et al. (59) pointed undeniably to the macrophage as the premier effector of intrapulmonary bactericidal activity. By carefully counting intracellular and extracellular staphylococci in fixed sections of the right lung and counting CFU from homogenates of the left lung of mice, Goldstein et al. (59) showed that bacterial ingestion by macrophages always preceded their killing.

The colony-counting technique has been used extensively to study the effects of toxic agents, clinical syndromes, and environmental factors on intrapulmonary killing. For example, Green and Kass (64) demonstrated the depressant effects of ethanol and hypoxia. Other depressants include NO_2 (58), cigarette smoke (96, 142), cold stress (65a), and radiation (86). Goldstein et al. (59) showed that the toxic effects of ozone on killing were more a consequence of defects in intracellular bactericidal activity than impaired bacterial ingestion. These distinctions should be made whenever possible.

Quantitating the rate of particle ingestion per se in intact lungs is elusive because of the difficulty of making direct observations of macrophages and particles in the respiratory tract. It is possible to utilize morphometric approaches and serial killing to estimate the rate at which free particles are transferred to intracellular sites. Brain and Corkery (19) devised a technique for estimating the extent of in situ phagocytosis of radioactive particles administered to rodents by intratracheal instillation or inhalation. Their approach is based on analysis of how particles and macrophages wash out of the lung during repeated lung lavage. They established that pulmonary lavage removes macrophages in a pattern distinctly different from that of free particles (those not associated with macrophages or fixed tissues).

Within hours after intratracheal instillation of ^{198}Au colloid, Brain and Corkery (19) observed that the curve describing the washout of radioactivity began to lose the shape characteristic of free particles and started to mimic the washout of the macrophages; this suggests a transfer of particles from the free state to a cell-associated state. A mathematical curve fitting gave rise to an index (λ) that is the fraction of particles phagocytosed. Although there is considerable animal-to-animal variability, λ is usually ~50%–75% by 2 h, greater than 95% by 10 h, and nearly 100% at 24 h.

This assay has proven useful to examine the impact of particles on the function of pulmonary macrophages in vivo. Brain and Corkery (19) examined the effects of preexposure to iron oxide, colloidal carbon, and coal dust on the endocytosis of colloidal gold. For all three materials endocytosis measured 2 h after exposure was significantly depressed. However, when the hamsters were given the test gold particles 24 h after exposure, only the coal-dust group exhibited depressed endocytosis. They concluded that all dusts can competitively inhibit endocytosis, but only some exhibit a sustained toxic effect on macrophage function. Beck, Brain, and Bohannon (11) incorporated the λ-assay into a comprehensive in vivo hamster bioassay designed to assess the toxicity of particulates for the lungs. As shown in Figure 10 the λ-assay discriminates between relatively nontoxic dusts such as iron oxide and aluminum oxide and the highly fibrogenic dust α-quartz. Its cytotoxicity for macrophages is reflected by the depression in λ. At the highest dose, <30% of the gold was ingested in 90 min, compared to >60% in the controls.

A novel approach to studying macrophage function in situ was recently described. Brain et al. (18) and Gehr et al. (53) reported how both phagocytosis of iron oxide particles and macrophage motility can be monitored noninvasively by magnetometric methods.

When magnetic forms of iron oxide are instilled or inhaled into the lungs, the retained particles can be used as an in vivo tracer for phagocytosis, cytoplasmic motility, and particle clearance. These particles can be magnetized and aligned by an external magnetic field; the remanent magnetism coming from them can then be measured at the surface of a human's or animal's chest. Immediately after magnetization the field from the lungs begins to decay (relaxation). Interestingly the characteristics of this decay change after exposure. In order to observe relaxation at any specific time, the chest is merely remagnetized and the remanent field monitored. Relaxation is caused by the random reorientation of particles away from their initially aligned state. In vivo experiments suggest that the rotational forces applied to the particles come largely from intracellular movements of phagosomes and lysosomes that contain the particles (18, 52, 53). It is believed that these movements arise from contractions of the cytoskeleton, which orchestrate cell motion required for functions such as phagocytosis, secretion, and ameboid movement. The hypothesis that organelle motion is a dominant mechanism for relaxation has now been confirmed in studies of hamster pulmonary macrophages observed in vitro [(51, 146, 147); I. Nemoto, H. Toyotama, and J. D. Brain, unpublished observations]. Cultured macrophages that had previously ingested magnetic particles ex-

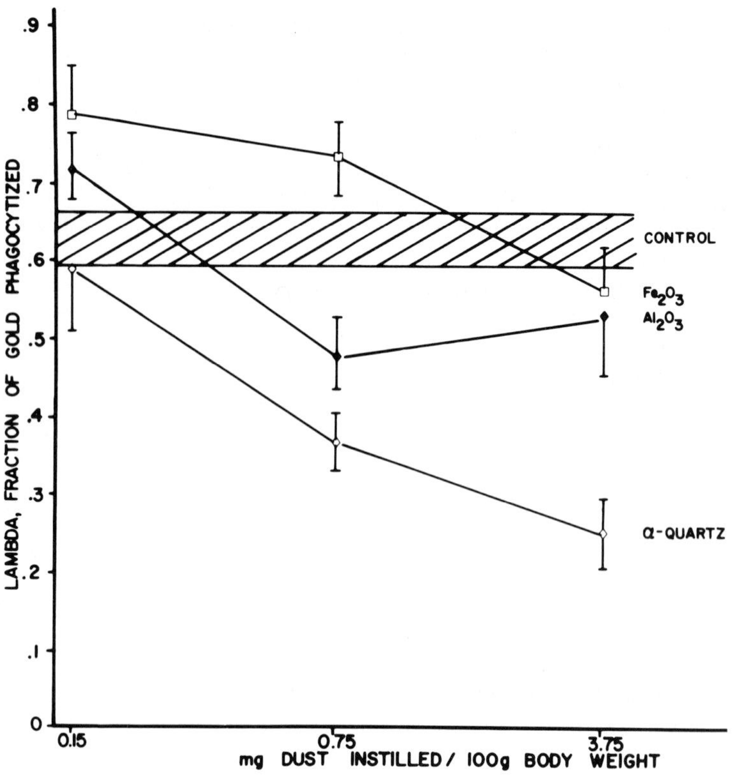

FIG. 10. Dose-response curve for λ-assay 1 day after exposure to iron oxide, aluminum oxide, or α-quartz. Fraction of gold ingested was measured 90 min after its instillation. Wilcoxon rank-sum test used to compare experimental groups and saline-only controls. Means ± SE. $P < 0.01$ for 0.75 and 3.75 mg α-quartz, $P < 0.01$ for 0.75 mg aluminum oxide, $P < 0.05$ for 0.15 mg iron oxide; all other data points not significantly different from control value ($P < 0.05$). [From Beck, Brain, and Bohannon (11).]

hibited relaxation quantitatively similar to that seen in vivo, demonstrating that cardiac and respiratory movements are not essential for particle misalignment. Cytochalasin B (51) or D (146, 147) slowed relaxation as did cold, formalin fixation, or nocodazole (146). Each of these interventions compromises the contractile capabilities of the cytoskeleton. Nemoto, Toyotama, and Brain (unpublished observations) reported similar results and demonstrated temperature dependence of relaxation over a wide range.

In rabbits exposed to magnetic iron oxide (γ-Fe$_2$O$_3$) and then measured periodically, the exponential decay constant of the first 2 min of relaxation changed rapidly during the first 24 h and thereafter remained fairly constant (18). Similar changes in the time course of relaxation were found in hamsters (53). These results correlate well with morphological findings that phagocytosis proceeds rapidly toward completion during the first 24 h after aerosol deposition. In addition to the morphological evidence for this, the progress of phagocytosis was quantified by using the λ-technique. One hour after instillation of colloidal gold into rabbits 27% of it had been phagocytized; after 16 h 91% had been ingested (18). Relaxation parameters, such as the half time for the decay, continued to change for weeks after initial deposition of the particles. This may indicate changes in the proportions of the total particle burden located in various pulmonary compartments (e.g., macrophages and connective tissue) (18, 53).

The remanent field immediately after magnetization, before relaxation occurs, is proportional to the amount of magnetic material remaining in the lungs. This measurement, repeated over weeks or months, describes a clearance curve. It requires several seconds to move an animal or subject from the magnetizing field to the probe of the measuring device, and of course some relaxation has ensued. To estimate the initial field, the data from the first one or two minutes of relaxation are fit to the equation $B = B_0 e^{-\lambda_0 t}$, in which B is the field strength at time t after magnetization, λ_0 is the decay constant, and B_0 is the field strength at the time the magnet was removed. Clearance has been described in rabbits and hamsters (18, 53) and in humans (34). The studies in humans compared the clearance kinetics of magnetic dust in smokers and nonsmokers; the former were shown to clear their burden of magnetic dust significantly more slowly over one year. In long-term studies such as these, magnetic iron oxide is less harmful than radioactively tagged particles.

In Vitro

A wide variety of methods is available to assess in vitro endocytosis in macrophages. A review describing the merits and limitations of different approaches has been published by Kavet and Brain (81). Once harvested, phagocytic cells are usually studied in one of two ways: as adherent monolayers or as cells in suspension. Certain principles apply to endocytic assays regardless of which type of culture system is employed.

First, one should characterize the cell population

introduced into the incubation medium. It is important to quantify *1)* the number (or concentration) of cells present, *2)* their identity, and *3)* the fraction of phagocytes that is viable. Particle uptake per cell (or per cell mass) will be improperly estimated if nonmacrophages or nonviable macrophages are included. The recovered cells should be purified or appropriate corrections should be made when the endocytic rates are calculated.

Second, in both suspension and monolayers it is necessary to be able to *1)* arrest phagocytosis and *2)* separate the cells from unphagocytized particles. With monolayers these two aims are simultaneously achieved with a thorough rinse of the coverslip or culture dish. In a suspension system, arrest and separation usually require a two-step process. Phagocytic arrest can be accomplished by rapidly chilling the culture, by adding inhibitors such as iodoacetate, sodium fluoride, or *N*-ethylmaleimide, or by diluting suspensions to the point at which the probability of cell-particle contact approaches zero. When the cells and particles in suspension assays have different densities and/or sedimentation rates, separation of arrested cells from remaining free particles can be accomplished by centrifugation. Filtration can also be used to separate cells and free particles, provided that all cells are trapped by the filter and all free particles pass through.

MONOLAYER ASSAYS. Mononuclear phagocytes characteristically settle and attach to glass or plastic surfaces. After attachment the cells spread on the surface and send out cytoplasmic projections that help anchor the cells. Once established, macrophage monolayers can be sustained for days or weeks, but it is important to recognize and experimentally control for the effects of different culture conditions. A period of 30–60 min is usually more than enough to allow all of the deposited cells to establish contact with the coverslip or the surface of the Petri dish. Inevitably a variable fraction of macrophages does not attach at all or strongly enough to withstand a subsequent rinse. After rinsing the monolayer free of unattached phagocytic cells as well as erythrocytes and lymphocytes, a particle challenge is introduced. At the termination of the exposure period the monolayer is rinsed free of substrate and the amount of ingestion measured.

Phagocytic assays often exploit the ease with which monolayers can be prepared for light microscopy. After fixation and staining procedures one can count the number of particles ingested by each cell or the percentage of macrophages containing substrate. Another common approach is to incubate with radioactive particles and count the activity remaining in the monolayer after it has been thoroughly rinsed. Unfortunately such assay procedures do not always include a technique to adequately discriminate between particles internalized and those merely adsorbed to the plasma membrane.

Monolayers can also be used to examine bacterial killing. The killing is usually followed by counting bacterial CFU recovered from the monolayers. After the desired challenge period the monolayer is rinsed and transferred to a medium containing a drug (e.g., bacteria-specific antibiotic) that inactivates extracellular organisms but does not penetrate phagocyte membranes to affect those phagocytosed. Before they are assayed on agar pour plates, intracellular microbes are first released from macrophages by sonication, freezing-thawing, or hypotonic disruption. Bacteria are thus freed of the intracellular environment in which multiplication might be restricted and allowed to grow colonies under optimal conditions. Also, organisms that may have existed intracellularly in clumps are dispersed so that each may form its own colony. Time-dependent killing curves are then generated. An alternative method relies on the ability of dividing microorganisms to incorporate radiolabeled nucleotides when synthesizing nucleic acids. By radioautography one can count the number of microbes per macrophage that have engaged in DNA synthesis. This method has two disadvantages: *1)* procedures are lengthy (weeks), and *2)* it cannot distinguish between stasis and killing (i.e., an intracellular microorganism might survive for a while without synthesizing nucleic acids).

SUSPENSION ASSAYS. A major advantage of studying phagocytosis in suspension is that it can include the phagocytes that might rinse away in a monolayer system either by failure to attach or by detaching at a later stage. Shaking suspension systems provide a further advantage; when phagocytes are cultured on glass or plastic substrates they spread and in some instances crawl along the substrate surface. The extent of cellular motility in these systems depends on culture conditions and also on inherent cellular characteristics. Thus contact between particles and cells (and therefore ingestion) can be influenced by the cells' motile characteristics. In suspension systems, cell-particle contact is determined primarily by collision probabilities (150) and is likely independent of motility. However, one of the limitations of incubating in suspension is that long-term cultures (days or weeks) are impractical because phagocytic cells start to plate out even when constantly agitated in siliconized vessels. Therefore most assays are usually based on culture durations of no longer than 2–3 h. Although their significance is unclear, several methodical and physiological differences have been observed between suspended and adherent macrophages (119).

Once cells are separated from the particles, several methods are available to quantify the amount of ingested material in the purified cell fractions. One approach is to use radiolabeled particles; if the specific activity (i.e., activity per unit particle mass) and cell number or protein mass are known, the average amount of substrate phagocytosed per cell or per milligram cell protein is easily computed (150). Quite often only relative indices of phagocytosis are needed and uptake is expressed as radioactive counts per minute per cell rather than as mass ingested per cell. Other widely used methods rely on the use of a particle that can be extracted in a solubilized form from the cells and spectrophotometrically analyzed.

A new assay for pulmonary macrophage endocytosis that uses flow cytometry was recently developed (114). Macrophages recovered by lung lavage are incubated with fluorescent latex particles. Then a cytofluorograph is used to characterize the uptake of particles by small samples of pulmonary macrophages. A linear relationship exists between the number of fluorescent latex particles and the fluorescent intensity associated with each cell up to 47 particles per cell. Particle uptake is significantly inhibited by removing divalent cations with ethylenediaminetetraacetic acid and lowering the incubation temperature.

As shown in Figure 11, this assay has been used to examine the effect of temperature and divalent cations on the uptake of latex beads (114). Particle uptake was examined at three different incubation temperatures both with and without Ca^{2+} and Mg^{2+}. Under all conditions the uptake of particles began immediately with no suggestion of an initial lag phase. In the presence of Ca^{2+} and Mg^{2+} the mean number of particles per cell after 90 min of incubation was significantly reduced when incubation temperature was lowered to 24°C and 3°C. This effect was particularly apparent at 3°C. At all three temperatures the uptake of particles increased significantly from 5 to 90 min of incubation. The uptake of particles by macrophages incubated in a balanced salt solution without Ca^{2+} and Mg^{2+} was significantly less than the uptake of particles with these cations.

PATHOPHYSIOLOGY OF PULMONARY MACROPHAGES

In addition to a variety of protective postures that help the host, macrophages may also participate in the pathogenesis of lung disease. Inhaled toxic, radioactive, or carcinogenic particles become concentrated in pulmonary macrophages because macrophages are actively phagocytic. What begins as a diffuse and even exposure becomes highly localized and nonuniform. "Hot spots" of high dosage are formed that may exceed the thresholds for certain effects and cause damage. Macrophages may also metabolize chemicals and change them to a more toxic form.

When macrophages adhere to the airway epithelium they may increase epithelial exposure to inhaled toxic materials. More importantly, this close association with the bronchial epithelium can lead to transbronchial transport of inhaled particles and subsequent reingestion by connective tissue macrophages (154). These cells, like their relatives in the alveolar and airway compartments, also segregate, retain, and perhaps metabolize carcinogenic and other toxic particles.

Hot spots may be associated with damage to the epithelial barriers and thus with enhanced epithelial

FIG. 11. Effect of temperature and divalent cations on uptake of fluorescent latex particles as measured with a dual-laser flow cytometer. Experiments performed by adding a 0.01 ml aliquot of cells (at 0 min) to 3 ml of balanced salt solution (BSS) containing particles. At indicated times, 1 aliquot of the cell-particle suspension was analyzed. *Closed symbols* represent data from cells incubated in BSS containing Ca^{2+} and Mg^{2+} (1 mM each); *open symbols* represent data from cells incubated in BSS without added Ca^{2+} and Mg^{2+} and 0.1 mM ethylenediaminetetraacetic acid. Incubation temperatures: 37°C (*circles*), 24°C (*triangles*), and 3°C (*squares*). Each data point is mean of 4 experiments; SE averaged 10% of means. [From Parod and Brain (114).]

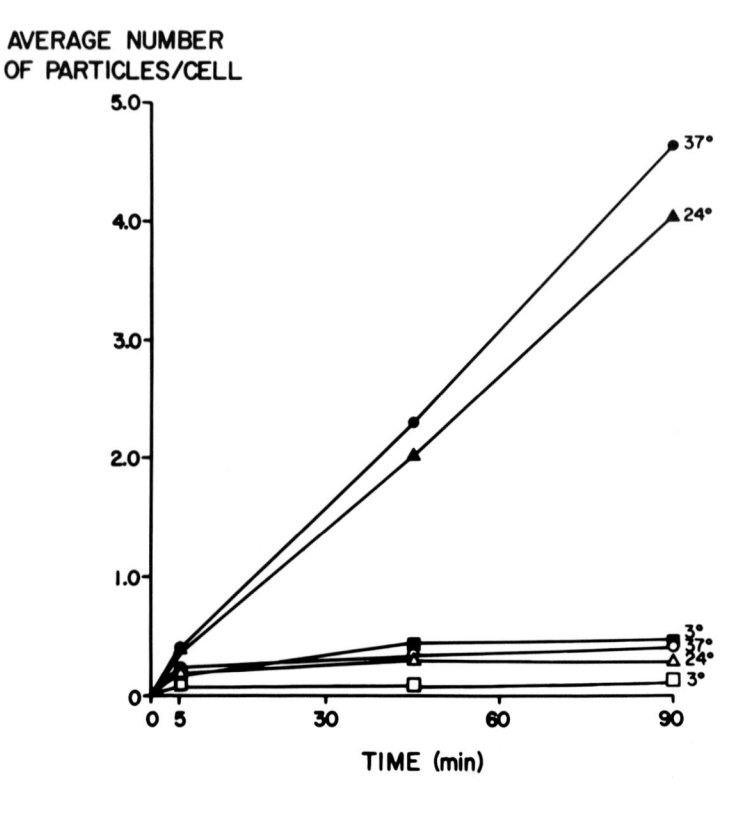

transport. These in turn could lead to increased access of toxic particles to the connective tissue compartment. Epithelial defenses may also be breached at the alveolar level; because of lymphatic pathways, particles may end up in similar sites. Particles gaining access to the lymphatics are cleared slowly, thus increasing their contribution to the pathogenesis of many lung diseases. Years after exposure to particles these connective tissue burdens may constitute the major reservoir of retained particles. Connective tissue macrophages may contribute to progressive damage by concentrating and storing potent toxic particles for long periods.

Another way in which macrophages may be involved is through diminution or failure of their defensive role. Several investigators, using in vivo and in vitro bactericidal and phagocytic assays, have shown that macrophage function can be compromised by environmental insults and pathological changes. Such diverse agents as silica, immunosuppressives, ethanol intoxication, cigarette smoke, air pollution, and oxygen toxicity can depress the ability of pulmonary macrophages to protect their host. Sometimes the agent or factor acts directly on the macrophage, producing a damaged or even a dead cell. For example, the ingestion of lead oxide particles is followed by swelling of the mitochondria, nuclear membrane, and endoplasmic reticulum as well as the appearance of precipitation complexes within the nuclear chromatin and cytoplasm (42). In other cases (e.g., high concentrations of inhaled particles) the mechanism can be competitive inhibition in which the phagocytic machinery becomes saturated even in the absence of cytotoxicity. In other instances, particularly those situations involving pulmonary edema or altered acid-base balance, the macrophages may be undamaged but their activity may be depressed because of an indirect effect on their milieu, the airway or alveolar microenvironment. Nonetheless it is important to realize that macrophage failure or damage is not always a cause of the disease in question; in many instances, alterations in macrophage function may simply reflect the onset and progression of the disease. For example, changes in macrophage activity during pulmonary edema associated with oxygen toxicity fall into this class. It may not be the macrophage's failure to ingest particles or bacteria that causes the edema, but rather the reverse.

There are situations in which pulmonary macrophages not only fail but contribute directly to the pathogenesis of pulmonary diseases. Two important examples involve pulmonary connective tissue (68, 144). Connective tissue proteins have an essential role in lung structure and function. Collagen and elastin help maintain alveolar, airway, and vascular stability, limit lung expansion, and contribute to lung recoil at all lung volumes. Two groups of lung disease are associated with aberrations of normal collagen and elastin balance: emphysematous and fibrotic disorders.

Emphysema

Because of growing understanding of the pathogenesis of emphysema, attention has been focused on the balance between elastase and antielastase in the respiratory tract (135). Elastase is one of many enzymes involved in the intracellular killing and digestion of pathogens. It is also involved in wound healing, for example, disposal of damaged cells and debris. Although these enzymes constitute an important aspect of the lung's defensive posture, when kept in a chronically activated state their digestive capacity may damage pulmonary tissues. Release of lysosomal enzymes, particularly proteases, from activated macrophages and leukocytes promotes the development of emphysema. Release is a consequence of cell death, cell injury, exocytosis, or regurgitation while feeding. Increased deposition of particles acts to recruit additional macrophages and thus may reinforce the effect.

Interest in proteolytic injury was stimulated because of knowledge about pulmonary emphysema associated with inborn α-antitrypsin–inhibitor deficiency in humans (94). Imbalances between proteolytic activity and its inhibition have important implications as a general mechanism of lung injury. Macrophages secrete enzymes capable of connective tissue degradation. Both collagenase and elastase activity can be detected in fluids from macrophage cultures (151, 159, 160, 163). The release of both enzymes is stimulated by cell activation and phagocytosis. Enzyme secretion is stimulated by cytochalasin B, colchicine, and vinblastine. There is evidence that exposure to smoke causes increased synthesis and release of elastolytic enzymes from these cells (90, 124). Importantly, culture media from alveolar macrophages of smokers demonstrated greater elastase activity than those obtained from nonsmokers. These findings tend to confirm the suspected role of macrophages in the pathogenesis of pulmonary emphysema in smokers. Generally macrophages contribute less elastase to lavage fluid than do neutrophils. However, connective tissue macrophages that can release elastase in close contact with elastin may be very important. Smoke and other pollutant particles characteristic of work and urban environments also act to recruit more cells, activate them, and release proteolytic enzymes. Smokers have higher levels of elastase activity in bronchoalveolar lavage fluid than nonsmokers (77). For all of these outcomes the extent of damage depends on the number of additional macrophages recruited, the extent of their activation, and the degree to which elastase and other toxic materials are secreted or released from macrophages. Pathogenesis of emphysema may also be facilitated by damage to epithelial barriers, which provides greater access of elastase to elastin.

Several animal models have been produced that support the proteolytic theory of emphysema. A lesion very similar to emphysema can be produced by intratracheal instillation or aerosolization of nonspecific proteolytic enzymes such as papain or by elastase (78, 79, 136). Homogenates of neutrophils or pulmonary macrophages have a similar effect (108, 156), as does elastase present in purulent sputum (103, 104). In all of these models the lesion is usually characterized by an initial phase of enzymatic degradation of elastin in the lungs, a subsequent resynthesis to control levels, and then a more gradual architectural derangement leading to expanded air spaces and/or destruction of alveoli.

The role of antiprotease should be noted. Porcine pancreatic elastase instilled into hamsters with no serum or serum from α_1-antitrypsin–deficient people results in a lesion resembling emphysema. However, identical amounts of pancreatic elastase added with serum from normal individuals results in no change. Thus the maintenance of a normal balance between elastase and elastase inhibitors is critical. The body's defenses against excessive elastase levels include inhibitors present in alveolar and airway lining fluid, and the ingestion and degradation of elastase by macrophages. Macrophages bind neutrophil elastase although some of the enzyme may remain active.

Therapies should focus on the reduction of unopposed proteases and attempt either to 1) regulate the production and release of neutrophil and macrophage proteases or 2) augment inhibitor activity by stimulating endogenous production through the use of synthetic antielastase agents or through replacement therapy utilizing elastase recovered from blood or other biological fluids.

This chapter has described how reactive metabolites of oxygen such as superoxide anions, hydroxyl radicals, and hydrogen peroxide are used by macrophages and neutrophils to kill microorganisms. However, these agents may also cause damage. For example, they may damage cell membranes or essential metabolic enzymes; they may reduce the activity of endogenous protease inhibitors and thus allow the activity of extracellular proteases to go unchecked. Oxygen radicals may also have an indirect effect by damaging other phagocytic cells and causing release of toxic and proteolytic enzymes. Weitberg et al. (157) recently demonstrated that human phagocytes that produce oxygen radicals may also produce cytogenic damage in cultured mammalian cells. Conceivably, chronic inflammatory states characterized by persistent increases in macrophages may contribute to cancer by this mechanism.

Fibrosis

Fibrogenesis also involves macrophage damage. Dead or dying macrophages may release a substance or substances that can attract fibroblasts and elicit fibrogenic responses. Dust particles of appropriate size, shape, chemical composition, and durability may deposit on alveolar surfaces and stimulate production of excess collagen in the alveolar wall. In such fibrotic diseases as asbestosis and silicosis, progressive fibrogenesis may continue long after inhalation of dust particles has stopped. Excessive collagen or alterations in types of collagen may make the lungs stiffer than normal, severely decreasing the vital capacity and increasing the muscular forces required for breathing.

Asbestos, glass, and other fibrous dusts have been shown to stimulate collagen synthesis (40, 122). Fibers longer than 5 μm are sometimes incompletely ingested by macrophages (5) and may lead to macrophage death or release of mediators. Growth of fibroblasts in vitro has been shown to require a solid supporting particle of critical minimum dimensions (107).

There is some evidence that fibrogenesis may involve macrophages and occur as a two-step process (8, 70). This especially applies to highly fibrogenic particles such as silica, which have very symmetrical shapes. Silica has not been shown to exert a direct stimulatory effect on fibroblasts. Rather the interaction of a particle with a macrophage is thought to release factors that stimulate local production of collagen by fibroblasts. It is unlikely that macrophages differentiate into collagen-synthesizing fibroblasts (6, 127), and the addition of silica to cultured fibroblasts does not stimulate collagen biosynthesis or release (122).

Several investigators have produced evidence showing that macrophages can produce a factor or factors that in turn influence the proliferation (100) and biosynthetic activity (4) of fibroblasts. After adding silica particles to mouse macrophages, Heppleston and Styles (70) reported the presence of a factor that stimulated chick fibroblasts to produce collagen. Burrell and Anderson (31) showed the same response with rabbit pulmonary macrophages and WI-38 fibroblasts. Allison (7) summarized other experiments in his laboratory supporting the two-stage theory of fibrogenesis by utilizing an in vivo preparation. Aalto and Kulonen (1) reported that macrophages damaged by quartz in vitro release factors that stimulate collagen synthesis by fibroblasts in culture. By using a diffusion chamber implanted into mouse peritoneal cavities, Bateman et al. (10) observed that when mouse peritoneal macrophages were incubated with either chrysotile asbestos or silica, factors that diffused through a Nucleopore membrane produced fibrosis. It is possible that generation of similar fibrogenesis-stimulating factors by quartz-damaged pulmonary macrophages in vivo may play a role in the development of fibrosis in the lungs, but such factors have not yet been isolated from the developing silicotic lung (121).

Diffusion chambers bounded by Millipore filters were placed in the peritoneal cavities of mice for a month or more. If the chambers contained only peritoneal macrophages or silica particles, no fibrogenesis occurred, but if both silica and peritoneal macrophages were placed in the chamber, the result was a marked thickening of the parietal and visceral pleura with significant collagen deposition beneath the mesothelial cells. Allison (7) concluded that "a factor released from surviving macrophages stimulated by silica passes out of the diffusion chamber and stimulates collagen synthesis by fibroblasts."

Silica and asbestos present the added hazard of being cytotoxic to alveolar macrophages. Within a few minutes they can lyse cells by direct interaction with the plasma membrane or, if successfully ingested, within several hours cause rupture of secondary lysosomes, releasing lysosomal hydrolases into the cytoplasm (8). Yeager et al. (165) demonstrated that short-fiber chrysotile asbestos is cytotoxic for human alveolar macrophages studied in vitro. When similar effects occur in vivo, the resulting dead macrophages can become focal points for further fibrogenesis. In addition the particles are released anew on the alveolar surface to cause more irritation. Not all published experiments, however, support the two-stage theory. Harington et al. (69) added culture medium from hamster macrophages incubated with silica and observed decreased collagen biosynthesis. Additional research is needed to explore these possible species differences.

The responses of the lung to inhaled antigens and allergens and the area of environmental allergic respiratory disease are also emerging as important areas that may involve macrophages. Considerable evidence is available showing that inhaled organic chemicals, dusts, molds, and animal proteins can cause a variety of lung responses such as allergic asthma, extrinsic allergic alveolitis, immune complex disease, and other phenomena. Excellent discussions of these diseases are available that suggest that macrophages may sometimes be involved (87). Little is known about the degradation of proteins deposited on the respiratory tract surfaces. No doubt in many instances macrophages and pulmonary clearance defend the body against excessive antigenic stimulation. However, there may also be circumstances in which clearance pathways cooperate with the immune system and preserve and present immunogenic molecules to the immune system. Thus the issue of how and when pulmonary macrophages suppress or enhance the immunogenicity of antigens must be confronted.

Other pulmonary diseases may also involve macrophages. Pulmonary-alveolar proteinosis, a disease characterized by the presence of lipoproteinaceous material in the alveoli, may alter macrophage function (73, 74). Golde et al. (57) suggested that phagocytosis of excessive quantities of the characteristic lipoproteinaceous material may damage macrophages and contribute to the frequent infectious complications of this disease. Similar alterations in macrophage function can be produced by drug-induced phospholipidoses. For example, Ferin (47) described alterations in macrophage function caused by chlorphentermine. The resulting phospholipidosis suppressed alveolar clearance of a test particle. Gee et al. (50) speculated on possible relationships between sarcoidosis and macrophages. They noted that the disease is often associated with elevations of serum levels of lysozyme and/or angiotensin-converting enzyme. Gee et al. (50) believe that the elevated lysozyme levels are caused by increased secretion of the enzyme by monocytes and lung macrophages. In addition human pulmonary macrophages recovered from patients with sarcoid have more angiotensin-converted enzyme than those recovered from normals. They believe there is evidence for macrophage activation in sarcoidosis.

CONCLUSION

Macrophages serve as a key element in the defense of alveolar and airway surfaces. They are also capable of injuring the host while exercising their defensive role. Investigations should continue into the ultrastructural and biochemical features of normal pulmonary macrophages as well as their alterations after exposure to physical, chemical, and infectious agents.

REFERENCES

1. AALTO, M., AND E. KULONEN. Fractionation of connective-tissue-activating factors from the culture medium of silica-treated macrophages. *Acta Pathol. Microbiol. Scand. Sect. C* 87: 241–250, 1979.
2. ADAMS, D. O. Macrophage activation and secretion. Summary. *Federation Proc.* 41: 2193–2197, 1982.
3. AGOSTONI, E. Mechanics of the pleural space. *Physiol. Rev.* 52: 57–128, 1972.
4. AHO, S., AND E. KULONEN. Effect of silica-liberated macrophage factors on protein synthesis in cell-free systems. *Exp. Cell Res.* 104: 31–38, 1977.
5. ALLISON, A. C. Experimental methods—cell and tissue culture: effects of asbestos particles on macrophages, mesothelial cells and fibroblasts. In: *Biological Effects of Asbestos*, edited by P. Bogovski, J. C. Gilson, V. Timbrell, and J. C. Wagner. Lyons, France: IARC, 1973, p. 89–93.
6. ALLISON, A. C. Pathogenic effects of inhaled particles and antigens. *Ann. NY Acad. Sci.* 221: 299–308, 1974.
7. ALLISON, A. C. Mechanisms of macrophage damage in relation to the pathogenesis of some lung diseases. In: *Lung Biology in Health and Disease. Respiratory Defense Mechanisms*, edited by J. D. Brain, D. F. Proctor, and L. M. Reid. New York: Dekker, 1977, vol. 5, pt. 2, chapt. 26, p. 1075–1102.
8. ALLISON, A. C., J. S. HARINGTON, AND M. BIRBECK. An examination of the cytotoxic effects of silica on macrophages. *J. Exp. Med.* 124: 141–154, 1966.
9. BABIOR, B. M. The role of oxygen radicals in microbial killing by phagocytes. In: *The Reticuloendothelial System: A Comprehensive Treatise. Biochemistry and Metabolism*, edited by A. J. Sbarra and R. R. Strauss. New York: Plenum, 1980, vol. 2, p. 339–354.
10. BATEMAN, E. D., R. J. EMERSON, AND P. J. COLE. A study of macrophage-mediated initiation of fibrosis by asbestos and silica using a diffusion chamber technique. *Br. J. Exp. Pathol.* 63: 414–425, 1982.
11. BECK, B. D., J. D. BRAIN, AND D. BOHANNON. An in vivo

hamster bioassay to assess the toxicity of particulates for the lungs. *Toxicol. Appl. Pharmcol.* 66: 9-29, 1982.
12. BESTERMAN, J. M., AND R. B. LOW. Endocytosis: a review of mechanisms and plasma membrane dynamics. *Biochem. J.* 210: 1-13, 1983.
13. BINGHAM, E., E. A. PFITZER, W. BARKLEY, AND E. P. RADFORD. Alveolar macrophages: reduced number in rat after prolonged inhalation of lead sesquioxide. *Science* 162: 1297-1299, 1968.
14. BLUSSÉ, A., AND R. VAN FURTH. Origin, kinetics, and characteristics of pulmonary macrophages in the normal steady state. *J. Exp. Med.* 149: 1504-1518, 1979.
15. BOWDEN, D. H. The alveolar macrophage. *Curr. Top. Pathol.* 55: 1-36, 1973.
15a. BOWDEN, D. H., AND I. Y. R. ADAMSON. Adaptive responses of the pulmonary macrophagic system to carbon. I. Kinetic studies. *Lab. Invest.* 38: 422-431, 1978.
16. BRAIN, J. D. Free cells in the lungs: some aspects of their role, quantitation, and regulation. *Arch. Intern. Med.* 126: 477-487, 1970.
17. BRAIN, J. D. The effects of increased particles on the number of alveolar macrophages. In: *Inhaled Particles III*, edited by W. H. Walton. London: Unwin, 1971, p. 209-225.
18. BRAIN, J. D., S. B. BLOOM, P. A. VALBERG, AND P. GEHR. Behavior of magnetic dusts in the lungs of rabbits correlates with phagocytosis. *Exp. Lung Res.* 6: 115-131, 1984.
19. BRAIN, J. D., AND G. C. CORKERY. The effect of increased particles on the endocytosis of radiocolloids by pulmonary macrophages in vivo: competitive and toxic effects. In: *Inhaled Particles IV*, edited by W. H. Walton. Oxford, UK: Pergamon, 1977, p. 551-564.
20. BRAIN, J. D., AND N. R. FRANK. Recovery of free cells from rat lungs by repeated washings. *J. Appl. Physiol.* 25: 63-69, 1968.
21. BRAIN, J. D., AND N. R. FRANK. The relation of age to the number of lung free cells, lung weight, and body weight in rats. *J. Gerontol.* 23: 58-62, 1968.
22. BRAIN, J. D., AND R. FRANK. Alveolar macrophage adhesion: wash electrolyte composition and free cell yield. *J. Appl. Physiol.* 34: 75-80, 1973.
23. BRAIN, J. D., P. GEHR, AND R. I. KAVET. Airway macrophages: the importance of the fixation method. *Am. Rev. Respir. Dis.* 129: 823-826, 1984.
24. BRAIN, J. D., J. J. GODLESKI, AND S. P. SOROKIN. Structure, origin and fate of the macrophage. In: *Lung Biology in Health and Disease. Respiratory Defense Mechanisms*, edited by J. D. Brain, D. F. Proctor, and L. M. Reid. New York: Dekker, 1977, vol. 5, pt. 2, chapt. 20, p. 849-852.
25. BRAIN, J. D., D. W. GOLDE, G. M. GREEN, D. J. MASSARO, P. A. VALBERG, P. A. WARD, AND Z. WERB. Biologic potential of pulmonary macrophages. *Am. Rev. Respir. Dis.* 118: 435-443, 1978.
26. BRAIN, J. D., P. A. VALBERG, S. P. SOROKIN, AND W. C. HINDS. An iron oxide aerosol suitable for animal exposures. *Environ. Res.* 7: 13-26, 1974.
27. BRODY, A. P., AND G. S. DAVIS. Alveolar macrophage toxicology. In: *Mechanisms in Respiratory Toxicology*, edited by H. Witschi and P. Nettesheim. Boca Raton, FL: CRC, 1982, vol. 2, p. 3-28.
28. BRUNDELET, J. P. Experimental study of the dust clearance mechanism of the lung. I. Histological study in rats of the intrapulmonary bronchial route of elimination. *Acta Pathol. Microbiol. Scand. Suppl.* 175: 1-141, 1965. Dissertation.
29. BURNS, C. A., AND A. ZARKOWER. Increased alveolar macrophage effector cell function after intratracheal instillation of particulates. *J. Clin. Lab. Immunol.* 10: 107-112, 1983.
30. BURNS, D. M., D. SHURE, R. FRANCOZ, M. KALAFER, J. HARREL, K. WITZTUM, AND K. M. MOSER. The physiologic consequences of saline lobar lavage in healthy human adults. *Am. Rev. Respir. Dis.* 127: 695-701, 1983.
31. BURRELL, R., AND M. ANDERSON. The induction of fibrosis by silica-treated alveolar macrophages. *Environ. Res.* 6: 389-394, 1973.
32. CAMPBELL, E. J. Human leukocyte elastase, cathepsin G, and lactoferrin: family of neutrophil granule glycoproteins that bind to an alveolar macrophage receptor. *Proc. Natl. Acad. Sci. USA* 79: 6941-6945, 1982.
33. CAMPBELL, E. J., R. R. WHITE, R. M. SENIOR, AND R. J. RODRIQUEZ. Receptor-mediated binding and internalization of leukocyte elastase by alveolar macrophages in vitro. *J. Clin. Invest.* 64: 824-833, 1979.
34. COHEN, D., S. ARAI, AND J. D. BRAIN. Smoking impairs long-term dust clearance from the lungs. *Science* 204: 514-517, 1979.
35. COHN, Z. A., AND E. WIENER. The particulate hydrolases of macrophages. I. Comparative enzymology, isolation, and properties. *J. Exp. Med.* 18: 991-1008, 1963.
36. CORSTVET, R. E., J. A. RUMMAGE, AND J. T. HOMER. Recovery of pulmonary alveolar macrophages from nonanesthetized calves. *Am. J. Vet. Res.* 43: 2253-2254, 1982.
37. DAUBER, J. H., A. HOLIAN, M. E. ROSEMILLER, AND R. P. DANIELE. Separation of bronchoalveolar cells from the guinea pig on continuous density gradients of Percoll: morphology and cytochemical properties of fractionated lung macrophages. *J. Reticuloendothel. Soc.* 33: 119-126, 1983.
38. DAVIES, P. Secretory functions of mononuclear phagocytes: overview and methods for preparing conditioned supernatants. In: *Method for Studying Mononuclear Phagocytes*, edited by D. O. Adams, P. J. Edelson, and H. Koren. New York: Academic, 1981, p. 549-560.
39. DAVIS, G. S., M. S. GIANCOLA, M. C. COSTANZA, AND R. B. LOW. Analyses of sequential bronchoalveolar lavage samples from healthy human volunteers. *Am. Rev. Respir. Dis.* 126: 611-616, 1982.
40. DAVIS, J. K. G. Are ferruginous bodies an indication of atmospheric pollution by asbestos? In: *Biological Effects of Asbestos*, edited by P. Bogovski, J. C. Gilson, V. Timbrell, and J. C. Wagner. Lyons, France: IARC, 1973, chapt. 11, p. 238-242.
41. DESHAZO, R. D., D. E. BANKS, J. E. DIEM, J. A. NORDBERG, Y. BASER, D. BEVIER, AND J. E. SALVAGGIO. Bronchoalveolar lavage cell—lymphocyte interactions in normal nonsmokers and smokers. Analysis with a novel system. *Am. Rev. Respir. Dis.* 127: 545-548, 1983.
42. DEVRIES, C. R., P. INGRAM, S. R. WALKER, R. W. LINTON, W. F. GUTKNECHT, AND J. D. SHELBURNE. Acute toxicity of lead particulates on pulmonary alveolar macrophages. Ultrastructural and microanalytical studies. *Lab. Invest.* 48: 35-44, 1983.
43. ECKERT, H., M. LUX, AND B. LACHMANN. The role of alveolar macrophages in surfactant turnover. *Lung* 161: 213-218, 1983.
44. ELSBACH, P., AND J. WEISS. A reevaluation of the roles of the O_2-dependent and O_2-independent microbicidal systems of phagocytes. *Rev. Infect. Dis.* 5: 843-853, 1983.
45. EVANS, R., AND P. ALEXANDER. Cooperation of immune lymphoid cells with macrophages in tumor immunity. *Nature London* 228: 620-622, 1972.
46. FELS, A. O., N. A. PAWLOWSKI, E. B. CRAMER, T. K. C. KING, Z. A. COHN, AND W. A. SCOTT. Human alveolar macrophages produce leukotriene B$_4$. *Proc. Natl. Acad. Sci. USA* 79: 7866-7870, 1982.
47. FERIN, J. Alveolar macrophage mediated pulmonary clearance suppressed by drug-induced phospholipidosis. *Exp. Lung Res.* 4: 1-10, 1982.
48. FIDLER, I. J., AND G. POSTE. Macrophages and cancer metastasis. In: *Macrophages and Natural Killer Cells*, edited by S. J. Normann and E. Sorkin. New York: Plenum, 1982, p. 65-75.
49. FRANSON, R. C., AND M. WAITE. Lysosomal phospholipases A$_1$ and A$_2$ of normal and bacillus Calmette Guerin-induced alveolar macrophages. *J. Cell Biol.* 56: 621-627, 1973.
50. GEE, J. B. L., P. T. BODEL, S. K. ZORN, L. M. HINMAN, C. A. STEVENS, AND R. A. MATTHAY. Sarcoidosis and mononuclear phagocytes. *Lung* 155: 243-253, 1978.

51. GEHR, P., J. D. BRAIN, AND S. B. BLOOM. Magnetometry: a tool to study intracellular movement (Abstract). *J. Cell Biol.* 97: 194a, 1983.
52. GEHR, P., J. D. BRAIN, S. B. BLOOM, AND P. A. VALBERG. Magnetic particles in the liver: a probe for cell function. *Nature London* 302: 336–338, 1983.
53. GEHR, P., J. D. BRAIN, I. NEMOTO, AND S. B. BLOOM. Behavior of magnetic particles in hamster lungs: estimates of clearance and cytoplasmic motility. *J. Appl. Physiol.: Respirat. Environ. Exercise Physiol.* 55: 1196–1202, 1983.
54. GERSING, R., AND H. SCHUMACHER. Experimentelle Untersuchungen über die Staubphagozytose. *Beitr. Silikose-Forsch.* 25: 31–34, 1955.
55. GODLESKI, J. J., AND J. D. BRAIN. The origin of alveolar macrophages in mouse radiation chimeras. *J. Exp. Med.* 136: 630–643, 1972.
56. GODLESKI, J. J., AND J. D. BRAIN. Natural and induced antisera specific for pulmonary macrophages. *Lung.* In press.
57. GOLDE, D. W., M. TERRITO, T. N. FINLEY, AND M. C. CLINE. Defective lung macrophages in pulmonary alveolar proteinosis. *Ann. Intern. Med.* 85: 304–309, 1976.
58. GOLDSTEIN, E., M. C. EAGLE, AND P. D. HOEPRICH. Effect of nitrogen dioxide on pulmonary bacterial defense mechanisms. *Arch. Environ. Health* 26: 202–204, 1973.
59. GOLDSTEIN, E., W. LIPPERT, AND D. WARSHAUER. Pulmonary alveolar macrophage. Defender against bacterial infection of the lung. *J. Clin. Invest.* 54: 519–528, 1974.
60. GORER, P. A. Some recent work on tumour immunity. *Adv. Cancer Res.* 4: 149–169, 1956.
61. GRANGER, G. A., AND R. S. WEISER. Homograft target cells: contact destruction in vitro by immune macrophages. *Science* 151: 97–99, 1966.
62. GRANT, M. M., S. P. SOROKIN, AND J. D. BRAIN. Lysosomal enzyme activities in pulmonary macrophages from rabbits breathing iron oxide. *Am. Rev. Respir. Dis.* 120: 1003–1012, 1979.
63. GREEN, G. M., AND E. GOLDSTEIN. A method for quantitating intrapulmonary bacterial inactivation in individual animals. *J. Lab. Clin. Med.* 68: 669–677, 1966.
64. GREEN, G. M., AND E. H. KASS. Factors influencing the clearance of bacteria by the lung. *J. Clin. Invest.* 43: 769–776, 1964.
65. GREEN, G. M., AND E. H. KASS. The role of the alveolar macrophage in the clearance of bacteria from the lung. *J. Exp. Med.* 119: 167–176, 1964.
65a.GREEN, G. M., AND E. H. KASS. The influence of bacterial species on pulmonary resistance to infection in mice subjected to hypoxia, cold stress and ethanolic intoxication. *Br. J. Exp. Pathol.* 46: 360–366, 1965.
66. GROSS, P., R. T. P. DETREVILLE, E. B. TOLKER, M. KASCHAK, AND M. A. BABYAK. The pulmonary macrophage response to irritants. An attempt at quantitation. *Arch. Environ. Health* 18: 174–185, 1969.
67. HARBISON, M. L., J. J. GODLESKI, M. MORTARA, AND J. D. BRAIN. Correlation of age and surface antigen in hamster alveolar macrophages. *Lab. Invest.* 50: 653–658, 1984.
68. HARINGTON, J. S., AND A. C. ALLISON. Tissue and cellular reactions to particles, fibers, and aerosols retained after inhalation. In: *Handbook of Physiology. Reactions to Environmental agents,* edited by D. H. K. Lee, H. L. Falk, and S. D. Murphy. Bethesda, MD: Am. Physiol. Soc., 1977, sect. 9, chapt. 17, p. 263–283.
69. HARINGTON, J. S., M. RITCHIE, P. C. KING, AND K. MILLER. The in vitro effects of silica-treated hamster macrophages on collagen production by hamster fibroblasts. *J. Pathol.* 109: 21–37, 1973.
70. HEPPLESTON, A. G., AND J. A. STYLES. Activity of a macrophage factor in collagen formation by silica. *Nature London* 214: 521–524, 1967.
71. HIBBS, J. B., JR., L. H. LAMBERT, JR., H. LEWIS, AND J. S. REMINGTON. Possible role of macrophage mediated nonspecific cytotoxicity in tumour resistance. *Nature London New Biol.* 235: 48–50, 1972.
72. HINMAN, L. J., C. A. STEVENS, R. A. MATTHAY, AND B. L. GEE. Elastase and lysozyme activities in human alveolar macrophages. *Am. Rev. Respir. Dis.* 121: 263–271, 1980.
73. HOCKING, W. G., AND D. W. GOLDE. The pulmonary-alveolar macrophage (first of two parts). *N. Engl. J. Med.* 301: 580–587, 1979.
74. HOCKING, W. G., AND D. W. GOLDE. The pulmonary-alveolar macrophage (second of two parts). *N. Engl. J. Med.* 301: 639–645, 1979.
75. HOLIAN, A., J. H. DAUBER, M. S. DIAMOND, AND R. P. DANIELE. Separation of bronchoalveolar cells from the guinea pig on continuous gradients of Percoll: functional properties of fractionated lung macrophages. *J. Reticuloendothel. Soc.* 33: 157–164, 1983.
76. HUNNINGHAKE, G. W., J. E. GADEK, S. V. SZAPIEL, I. J. STRUMPF, O. KAWANAMI, V. J. FERRANS, B. A. KEOGH, AND R. G. CRYSTAL. The human alveolar macrophage. In: *Methods in Cell Biology,* edited by C. C. Harris, B. F. Trump, and G. D. Stoner. New York: Academic, 1980, vol. 21, p. 95–112.
77. JANOFF, A., L. RAJU, AND R. DEARING. Levels of elastase activity in bronchoalveolar lavage fluids of healthy smokers and nonsmokers. *Am. Rev. Respir. Dis.* 127: 540–544, 1983.
78. JOHANSON, W. G., JR., AND A. K. PIERCE. Effects of elastase, collagenase, and papain on structure and function of rat lungs in vitro. *J. Clin. Invest.* 51: 288–293, 1972.
79. KAPLAN, P. D., C. KUHN, AND J. A. PIERCE. The induction of emphysema with elastase. I. The evolution of the lesion and the influence of serum. *J. Lab. Clin. Med.* 82: 349–356, 1973.
80. KAVET, R. I., AND J. D. BRAIN. Phagocytosis: quantification of rates and intercellular heterogeneity. *J. Appl. Physiol.: Respirat. Environ. Exercise Physiol.* 42: 432–437, 1977.
81. KAVET, R. I., AND J. D. BRAIN. Methods to quantify endocytosis: a review. *J. Reticuloendothel. Soc.* 27: 201–221, 1980.
82. KAVET, R. I., J. D. BRAIN, AND D. J. LEVENS. Characteristics of pulmonary macrophages lavaged from hamsters exposed to iron oxide aerosols. *Lab. Invest.* 38: 312–319, 1978.
83. KELLER, R. Mechanisms by which activated macrophages destroy syngeneic rat tumor cells in vitro. Cytokinetics, noninvolvement of T-lymphocytes and effects of metabolic inhibitors. *Immunology* 27: 285–291, 1974.
84. KIKKAWA, Y., AND K. KONEDA. The type II epithelial cell of the lung. I. Method of isolation. *Lab. Invest.* 30: 76–84, 1974.
85. KILBURN, K. H. Functional morphology of the distal lung. *Int. Rev. Cytol.* 37: 153–270, 1974.
86. KIM, M., E. GOLDSTEIN, J. P. LEWIS, W. LIPPERT, AND D. WARSHAUER. Murine pulmonary alveolar macrophages: rates of bacterial ingestion, inactivation and destruction. *J. Infect. Dis.* 133: 310–320, 1976.
87. KIRKPATRICK, C. H., AND H. Y. REYNOLDS (editors). *Lung Biology in Health and Disease. Immunologic and Infectious Reactions in the Lung.* New York: Dekker, 1976, vol. 1.
88. KLEBANOFF, S. J. Myeloperoxidase-mediated cytotoxic systems. In: *The Reticuloendothelial System: A Comprehensive Treatise. Biochemistry and Metabolism,* edited by A. J. Sbarra and R. R. Strauss. New York: Plenum, 1980, p. 279–308.
89. KRAHL, V. E. Microstructure of the lung. *Arch. Environ. Health* 6: 43–51, 1963.
90. KUHN, C., III, AND R. M. SENIOR. The role of elastase in the development of emphysema. *Lung* 155: 188–197, 1978.
91. KUHN, C., III, R. M. SENIOR, AND J. A. PIERCE. The pathogenesis of emphysema. In: *Mechanisms in Respiratory Toxicology,* edited by H. Witschi and P. Nettesheim. Boca Raton, FL: CRC, 1982, vol. 2, p. 155–211.
92. LABELLE, C. W., AND H. BRIEGER. Synergistic effects or aerosols. II. Effects on rate of clearance from the lung. *Arch. Indust. Health* 20: 100–105, 1959.
93. LABELLE, C. W., AND H. BRIEGER. The fate of inhaled particles in the early post-exposure period. *Arch. Environ. Health* 1: 432–437, 1960.

94. LAURELL, C. B., AND S. ERIKSSON. The electrophoretic α_1-globulin pattern of serum in α_1-antitrypsin deficiency. *Scand. J. Clin. Lab. Invest.* 15: 132–140, 1963.
95. LAURENZI, G. A., L. BERMAN, M. FIRST, AND E. H. KASS. A quantitative study of the deposition and clearance of bacteria in the murine lung. *J. Clin. Invest.* 43: 759–768, 1964.
96. LAURENZI, G. A., J. J. GUARNERI, R. B. ENDRIGA, AND J. P. CAREY. Clearance of bacteria by the lower respiratory tract. *Science* 142: 1572–1573, 1963.
97. LAURENZI, G. A., R. T. POTTER, AND E. H. KASS. Bacteriological flora of the lower respiratory tract. *N. Engl. J. Med.* 265: 173–178, 1961.
98. LEAKE, E. S., D. GONZALES-OJEDA, AND Q. N. MYRVIK. Enzymatic differences between normal alveolar macrophages and oil-induced peritoneal macrophages obtained from rabbits. *Exp. Cell Res.* 35: 553–561, 1964.
99. LEBLANC, P. A., S. W. RUSSELL, AND S.-M. T. CHANG. Mouse mononuclear phagocyte antigenic heterogeneity detected by monoclonal antibodies. *J. Reticuloendothel. Soc.* 32: 219–231, 1982.
100. LEIBOVICH, S. J., AND R. ROSS. A macrophage-dependent factor that stimulates the proliferation of fibroblasts in vitro. *Am. J. Pathol.* 84: 501–514, 1976.
101. LEITH, D. E. Cough. In: *Lung Biology in Health and Disease. Respiratory Defense Mechanisms*, edited by J. D. Brain, D. F. Proctor, and L. M. Reid. New York: Dekker, 1977, vol. 5, pt. 2, chapt. 15, p. 545–592.
102. LEVY, M. H., AND E. F. WHEELOCK. The role of macrophages in defense against neoplastic disease. *Adv. Cancer Res.* 20: 131–163, 1974.
103. LIEBERMAN, J. Involvement of leukocytic proteases in emphysema and antitrypsin deficiency. *Arch. Environ. Health* 27: 196–200, 1973.
104. LIEBERMAN, J., AND M. A. GAWAD. Inhibitors and activators of leukocytic proteases in purulent sputum: digestion of human lung and inhibition by alpha$_1$-antitrypsin. *J. Lab. Clin. Med.* 77: 713–727, 1971.
105. LOW, R. B., G. S. DAVIS, AND M. S. GIANCOLA. Biochemical analyses of bronchoalveolar lavage fluids of normal healthy volunteers. *Am. Rev. Respir. Dis.* 118: 863–876, 1978.
106. LUCAS, A. M., AND L. C. DOUGLAS. Principles underlying ciliary activity in the respiratory tract. II. A comparison of nasal clearance in man, monkey, and other mammals. *Arch. Otolaryngol.* 20: 518–541, 1934.
107. MAROUDAS, N. G. Chemical and mechanical requirements for fibroblast adhesion. *Nature London* 244: 353–354, 1973.
108. MASS, B., I. IKEDA, D. R. MERANZE, G. WEINBAUM, AND P. KIMBEL. Induction of experimental emphysema: cellular and species specificity. *Am. Rev. Respir. Dis.* 106: 384–391, 1974.
109. MCGOWAN, S. E., P. J. STONE, J. D. CALORE, G. L. SNIDER, AND C. FRANZBLAU. The fate of neutrophil elastase incorporated by human alveolar macrophages. *Am. Rev. Respir. Dis.* 127: 449–455, 1983.
110. MYRVIK, Q. N., E. S. LEAKE, AND B. FARISS. Studies on pulmonary alveolar macrophages from the normal rabbit: a technique to procure them in a high state of purity. *J. Immunol.* 86: 128–132, 1961.
111. MYRVIK, Q. N., E. S. LEAKE, AND B. FARISS. Lysozyme content of alveolar and peritoneal macrophages from the rabbit. *J. Immunol.* 86: 133–136, 1961.
112. NAKANE, P. K., AND G. B. PIERCE. Enzyme-labeled antibodies: preparation and application for the localization of antigens. *J. Histochem. Cytochem.* 14: 929–931, 1966.
114. PAROD, R. J., AND J. D. BRAIN. Uptake of latex particles by macrophages: characterization using flow cytometry. *Am. J. Physiol.* 245 (*Cell Physiol.* 14): C220–C226, 1983.
115. PAROD, R. J., AND J. D. BRAIN. Uptake of latex particles by pulmonary macrophages: role of calcium. *Am. J. Physiol.* 245 (*Cell Physiol.* 14): C227–C234, 1983.
116. PATTERSON-DELAFIELD, J., D. SZLAREK, R. J. MARTINEZ, AND R. I. LEHRER. Microbicidal cationic proteins of rabbit alveolar macrophages: amino acid composition and functional attributes. *Infect. Immun.* 31: 723–731, 1981.
117. PERMAR, H. H. The development of the mononuclear phagocyte of the lung. *J. Med. Res.* 42: 147–162, 1920.
118. PLOWMAN, P. N. The pulmonary macrophage population of human smokers. *Ann. Occup. Hyg.* 25: 393–405, 1982.
119. POFIT, J. F., AND P. R. STRAUSS. Membrane transport by macrophages in suspension and adherent to glass. *J. Cell Physiol.* 92: 249–255, 1977.
120. PRATT, S. A., M. H. SMITH, A. J. LADMAN, AND T. N. FINLEY. The ultrastructure of alveolar macrophages from human cigarette smokers and nonsmokers. *Lab. Invest.* 24: 331–338, 1971.
121. REISER, K. M., AND J. A. LAST. Silicosis and fibrogenesis: fact and artifact. *Toxicology* 13: 51–72, 1979.
122. RICHARDS, R. J., AND T. G. MORRIS. Collagen and mucopolysaccharide production in growing lung fibroblasts exposed to chrysotile asbestos. *Life Sci.* 12: 441–451, 1973.
123. RODGERS, B. C., AND C. A. MIMS. Role of macrophage activation and interferon in the resistance of alveolar macrophages from infected mice to influenza virus. *Infect. Immun.* 36: 1154–1159, 1982.
124. RODRIGUEZ, R. J., R. R. WHITE, R. M. SENIOR, AND E. A. LEVINE. Elastase release from human alveolar macrophages: comparison between smokers and non-smokers. *Science* 198: 313–314, 1977.
125. ROSE, R. M., C. CRUMPACKER, J. L. WANER, AND J. D. BRAIN. Murine cytomegalovirus pneumonia: description of a model and investigation of pathogenesis. *Am. Rev. Respir. Dis.* 125: 568–573, 1982.
126. ROSE, R. M., C. CRUMPACKER, J. L. WANER, AND J. D. BRAIN. Treatment of murine cytomegalovirus pneumonia with acyclovir and interferon. *Am. Rev. Respir. Dis.* 127: 198–203, 1983.
127. ROSS, R., N. B. EVERETT, AND R. TYLER. Wound healing and collagen formation. VI. The origin of the wound fibroblast studied in parabiosis. *J. Cell Biol.* 44: 645–654, 1970.
128. SACKNER, M. A. Bronchofiberscopy. *Am. Rev. Respir. Dis.* 111: 62–88, 1975.
129. SCHAFFNER, T., H. U. KELLER, M. W. HESS, AND H. COTTIER. Macrophage functions in antimicrobial defense. *Klin. Wochenschr.* 60: 720–726, 1982.
130. SCHILLER, E. Inhalation, retention, and elimination of dusts from dogs' and rats' lungs with special reference to the alveolar phagocytes and bronchial epithelium. In: *Inhaled Particles and Vapours*, edited by C. N. Davies. London: Pergamon, 1961, p. 342–344.
131. SENIOR, R. M., E. J. CAMPBELL, AND B. VILLIGER. Obtaining and culturing human and animal alveolar macrophages. In: *Methods for Studying Mononuclear Phagocytes*, edited by E. O. Adams, P. J. Edelson, and H. Koren. New York: Academic, 1982, p. 69–84.
132. SETHI, K. K. Intracellular killing of parasites by macrophages. *Clin. Immunol. Allergy* 2: 541–565, 1982.
133. SHELLITO, J., J. L. CALDWELL, AND H. B. KALTREIDER. Immune functions of murine alveolar macrophages: binding of lymphocytes and support of lymphocyte proliferation. *Exp. Lung Res.* 4: 93–107, 1983.
134. SLAUSON, D. O. The mediation of pulmonary inflammatory injury. In: *Advances in Veterinary Science and Comparative Medicine*, edited by C. E. Cornelius, C. F. Simpson, and D. L. Dungworth. New York: Academic, 1982, vol. 26, p. 99–153.
135. SNIDER, G. L. Emphysema. *Clin. Chest. Med.* 4: 327–499. Philadelphia, PA: Saunders, 1983.
136. SNIDER, G. L., J. A. HAYES, C. FRANZBLAU, H. M. KAGAN, P. S. STONE, AND A. L. KORTHY. Relationship between elastolytic activity and experimental emphysema-inducing properties of papain preparations. *Am. Rev. Respir. Dis.* 110: 254–262, 1974.
137. SORBER, W. A., E. S. LEAKE, AND Q. N. MYRVIK. Isolation and characterization of hydrolase-containing granules from rabbit lung macrophages. *J. Reticuloendothel. Soc.* 16: 184–

192, 1974.
138. SOROKIN, S. P. Dynamics of lysosomal elements in pulmonary alveolar macrophages. I. The postactivation lysosomal cycle. *Anat. Rec.* 206: 117–143, 1983.
139. SOROKIN, S. P. Dynamics of lysosomal elements in pulmonary alveolar macrophages. II. Transitory intracytoplasmic events in activated cells. *Anat. Rec.* 206: 145–170, 1983.
140. SOROKIN, S. P., AND J. D. BRAIN. Pathways of clearance in mouse lungs exposed to iron oxide aerosols. *Anat. Rec.* 181: 581–626, 1975.
141. SPRITZER, A. A., J. A. WATSON, J. A. AULD, AND M. A. GUETTHOFF. Pulmonary macrophage clearance. The hourly rates of transfer of pulmonary macrophages to the oropharynx of the rat. *Arch. Environ. Health* 17: 726–730, 1968.
142. SPURGASH, A., R. EHRLICH, AND R. PETZOLD. Effect of cigarette smoke on resistance to respiratory infection. *Arch. Environ. Health* 16: 385–390, 1968.
143. STEINMAN, R. M., I. S. MELLMAN, W. A. MULLER, AND Z. A. COHN. Endocytosis and the recycling of plasma membrane. *J. Cell Biol.* 96: 1–27, 1983.
144. TURINO, G. M., J. R. RODRIGUEZ, L. M. GREENBAUM, AND I. MANDL. Mechanisms of pulmonary injury. *Am. J. Med.* 57: 493–505, 1974.
145. UNANUE, E. R. Symbiotic relationships between macrophages and lymphocytes. In: *Macrophages and Natural Killer Cells*, edited by S. J. Normann and E. Sorkin. New York: Plenum, 1982, p. 49–63.
146. VALBERG, P. A. Endosome motion and rheology in lung macrophages after maghemite phagocytosis (Abstract). *J. Cell Biol.* 97: 426a, 1983.
147. VALBERG, P. A. Magnetometry of ingested particles in pulmonary macrophages. *Science.* 224: 513–516, 1984.
148. VALBERG, P. A., AND J. D. BRAIN. Generation and use of three types of iron-oxide aerosol. *Am. Rev. Respir. Dis.* 120: 1013–1024, 1979.
149. VALBERG, P. A., J. D. BRAIN, AND D. KANE. Effects of colchicine or cytochalasin B on pulmonary macrophage endocytosis in vivo. *J. Appl. Physiol.: Respirat. Environ. Exercise Physiol.* 50: 621–629, 1981.
150. VALBERG, P. A., B.-H. CHEN, AND J. D. BRAIN. Endocytosis of colloidal gold by pulmonary macrophages. *Exp. Cell Res.* 141: 1–14, 1982.
151. WAHL, L. M., S. M. WAHL, S. E. MERGENHAGEN, AND G. R. MARTIN. Collagenase production by lymphokine-activated macrophages. *Science* 187: 261–263, 1975.
152. WANG, N. The regional differences of pleural mesothelial cells in rabbits. *Am. Rev. Respir. Dis.* 110: 623–633, 1974.
153. WARNER, A. P., AND J. D. BRAIN. Intravascular pulmonary macrophages in ruminants actively participate in reticuloendothelial clearance of particles (Abstract). *Federation Proc.* 43: 1001, 1984.
154. WATSON, A. Y., AND J. D. BRAIN. Uptake of iron oxide aerosols by mouse airway epithelium. *Lab. Invest.* 40: 450–459, 1979.
155. WATSON, A. Y., AND J. D. BRAIN. The effect of SO_2 on the uptake of particles by mouse bronchial epithelium. *Exp. Lung Res.* 1: 67–87, 1980.
156. WEINBAUM, G., V. MARCO, T. IKEDA, B. MASS, D. R. MERANZE, AND P. KIMBEL. Enzymatic production of experimental emphysema in the dog. Route of exposure. *Am. Rev. Respir. Dis.* 109: 351–357, 1974.
157. WEITBERG, A. B., S. A. WEITZMAN, M. DESTREMPES, S. A. LATT, AND T. P. STOSSEL. Stimulated human phagocytes produce cytogenetic changes in cultured mammalian cells. *N. Engl. J. Med.* 308: 25–29, 1983.
158. WERB, Z. How the macrophage regulates its extracellular environment. *Am. J. Anat.* 166: 237–256, 1983.
159. WERB, Z., AND S. GORDON. Elastase secretion by stimulated macrophages. Characterization and regulation. *J. Exp. Med.* 142: 361–377, 1975.
160. WHARTON, W. Human macrophage-like cell line U937-1 elaborates mitogenic activity for fibroblasts. *J. Reticuloendothel. Soc.* 33: 151–156, 1983.
161. WHITE, R., A. JANOFF, R. GORDON, AND E. CAMPBELL. Evidence for in vivo internalization of human leukocyte elastase by alveolar macrophages. *Am. Rev. Respir. Dis.* 125: 779–781, 1982.
162. WHITE, R., D. LEE, G. S. HABICHT, AND A. JANOFF. Secretion of alpha-1-protease inhibitor by cultured rat alveolar macrophages. *Am. Rev. Respir. Dis.* 123: 447–449, 1981.
163. WHITE, R., H. S. LIN, AND C. KUHN III. Elastase secretion by peritoneal exudative and alveolar macrophages. *J. Exp. Med.* 146: 802–808, 1977.
164. YARBOROUGH, D. J., O. T. MEYER, A. M. DANNENBERG, JR., AND B. PEARSON. Histochemistry of macrophage hydrolases. III. Studies of β-galactosidase, β-glucuronidase and aminopeptidase with indolyl and naphthyl substrates. *J. Reticuloendothel. Soc.* 4: 390–408, 1967.
165. YEAGER, H., JR., D. A. RUSSO, M. YAÑEZ, D. GERARDI, R. P. NOLAN, E. KAGAN, AND A. M. LANGER. Cytotoxicity of a short-fiber chrysotile asbestos for human alveolar macrophages: preliminary observations. *Environ. Res.* 30: 224–232, 1983.
166. YEVICH, P. P. Lung structure—relation to response to particulate. *Arch. Environ. Health* 10: 37–43, 1965.

CHAPTER 15

Function-structure correlations in cilia from mammalian respiratory tract

PETER SATIR | Department of Anatomy, Albert Einstein College of Medicine, Bronx, New York

ELLEN ROTER DIRKSEN | Department of Anatomy, University of California School of Medicine, Los Angeles, California

---

CHAPTER CONTENTS

Distribution and General Organization of Cilia
Ciliogenesis
Axoneme
Ciliary Membrane
    Ciliary crown
    Freeze-fracture studies and membrane organization
    Ciliary necklace
Sliding-Microtubule Mechanism
    Geometry of sliding
    Direct examination of sliding
    Structure and function of the dynein arm
    Human dynein
Control of Sliding
    Mutant studies
    Sliding and switching mechanisms
    Calcium ions and ciliary arrest
    Membrane control of calcium ion concentration
    Calmodulin
Ciliary Beat
Mucociliary Transport
    Periciliary fluid
    Mucous layer
Function of Metachronism
Factors Influencing Mucociliary Clearance
    Effects of sympathomimetic and parasympathomimetic drugs
    Effect of local anesthetics
    Relationship of drug effects to axonemal controls
Ciliary Dysfunction in Humans
    Genetic and structural implications
Summary

SINCE CILIA WERE FIRST DESCRIBED in protozoa by van Leeuwenhoek approximately 300 years ago, sporadic attempts have been made to understand their function. The role of cilia in human respiratory physiology has been investigated since the early nineteenth century, when Purkinje and Valentin described moving respiratory cilia and Sharpey advanced the concept of mucociliary transport (33). Nevertheless the details of the relationships between structure and function in cilia from the mammalian respiratory tract have been hard to obtain, partly because of the lack of accessibility of these cilia and the difficulty of maintaining normal physiological conditions during experimental procedures and partly because their relatively short length and small diameter make microscopic observation difficult. Since the advent of modern techniques for studying cell biology, especially electron microscopy, subcellular fractionation, and new methods of biochemical analysis, our knowledge of ciliary structure and function has expanded. Much of the new understanding has been derived from studies on the cilia of invertebrates, with the assumption that mammalian cilia behave more or less similarly. One basis for this assumption is the common ultrastructure of all somatic cilia so far examined (25). Only within the last few years has it been possible to demonstrate that the basic mechanisms are similar for all cilia and to study the detailed organization and action of cilia from the mammalian respiratory tract. With this new understanding, human ciliary mutants have been discovered, which has given us new means of analyzing human ciliary function.

DISTRIBUTION AND GENERAL ORGANIZATION OF CILIA

The distribution of cilia in the human respiratory tract, as in most mammals, is quite extensive. Cilia line the epithelium of the respiratory mucosa from the nasal passages to the respiratory bronchioles, where they are involved in the movement of the mucous blanket, which catches airborne particles. Figure 1 from a recent review (56) diagrams the general organization of the respiratory tree and indicates mucus-transport velocities and ciliary-beat frequencies based on experiments on rat lung (36). The principal feature of the mucociliary escalator is that mucus is propelled with increasing velocity from all parts of the respiratory tract to the oropharynx.

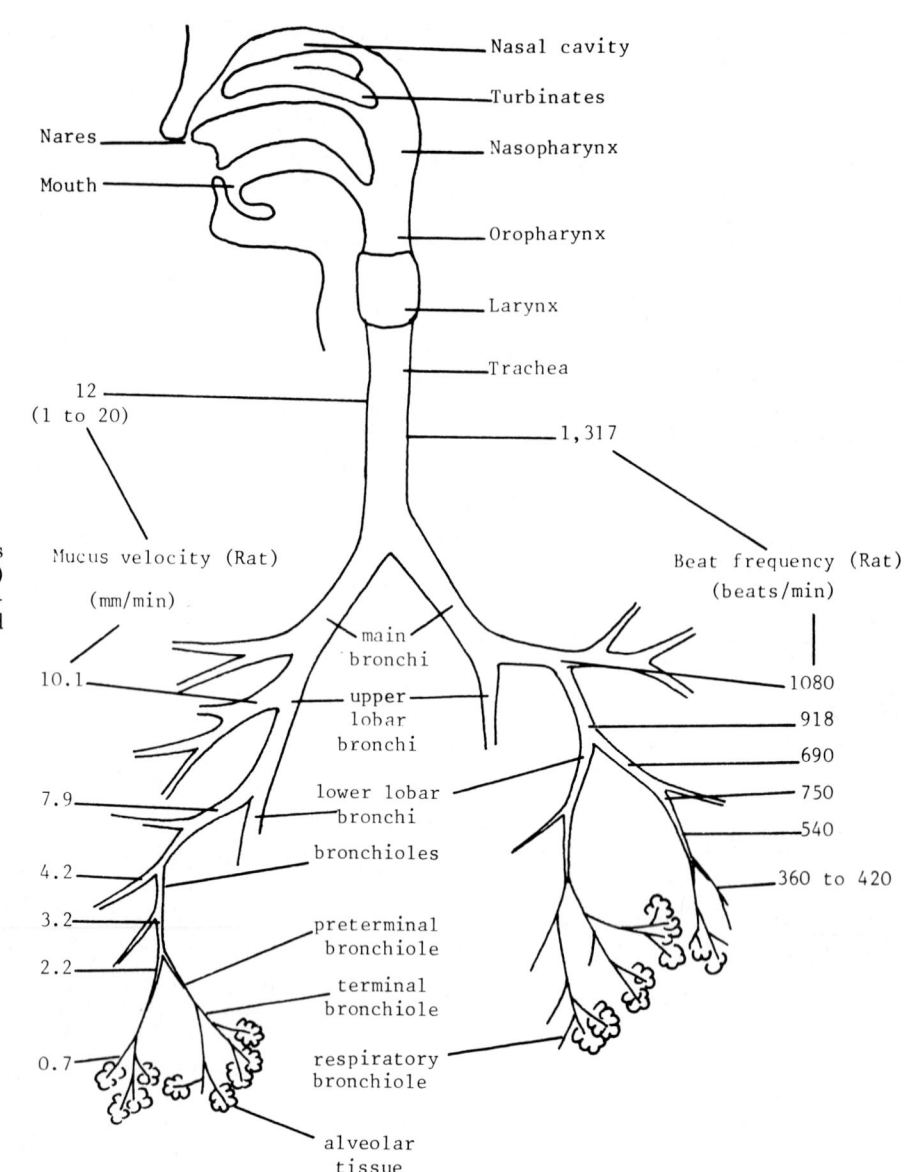

FIG. 1. Mucus-transport velocities (*left*) and ciliary beat frequencies (*right*) at different levels of mammalian respiratory tract. [From Sanderson and Sleigh (56).]

The individual components of the mucociliary system have been studied in some detail (55, 56). A typical ciliated epithelial cell of the mammalian respiratory system bears 250–300 cilia at its apical border (Figs. 2 and 3). Depending on the animal and the level of the respiratory tree, the percentage of ciliated cells varies. In humans the cilia of the upper respiratory passages are so thick they appear to carpet the entire surface, even though numerous other nonciliated cell types are present; in the larger airways the cilia extend ~10 μm from the cell surface. In other mammals (e.g., the rabbit) the cilia are shorter.

The cilia are spaced uniformly along the cell surface in a relaxed hexagonal lattice. Interspersed between adjacent cilia are slender microvilli, which in rabbits are about one-third as long as the cilia (Fig. 3). Each cilium is ~0.25 μm in diameter and is composed of two major elements, a microtubule-containing axoneme ~0.2 μm in diameter ensheathed by a specialized extension of the cell membrane, the ciliary membrane. The ciliary membrane ends at the surface proper, whereas the axonemal microtubules continue downward into the cell cortex to become the basal body. The basal body consists of a cylinder whose walls are nine interconnected triplet microtubules. Connected to one side of the basal body is the basal foot (Fig. 3). The basal foot of normal respiratory tract cilia points toward the oropharynx, i.e., in the direction in which the cilia move the mucous sheet.

CILIOGENESIS

During cell differentiation the basal bodies attach to the cell surface and give rise to the ciliary axoneme, which grows outward in coordination with the mem-

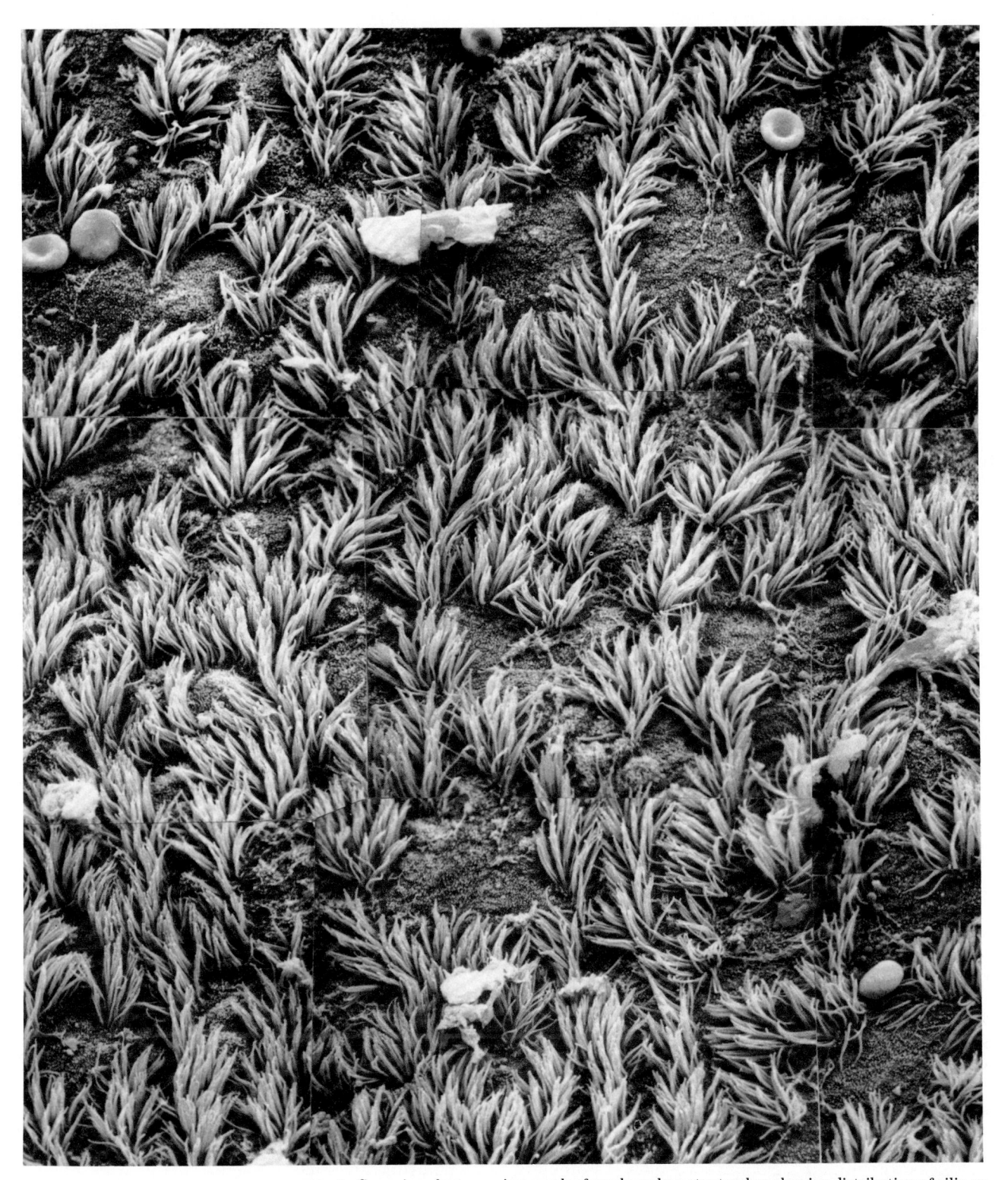

CHAPTER 15: FUNCTION-STRUCTURE CORRELATIONS IN CILIA 475

FIG. 2. Scanning electron micrograph of newborn hamster trachea showing distribution of cilia on the epithelium. × 1,900.

brane. The basal bodies are assembled (through a complex sequence of events) from precursor structures associated with centrioles (18, 20, 21). The sequence of basal body morphogenesis and subsequent ciliary outgrowth is similar whether it occurs during embryogenesis or cell renewal as a consequence of normal sloughing of the epithelium or of pathological response (22). Not all the cilia of a cell emerge at the same

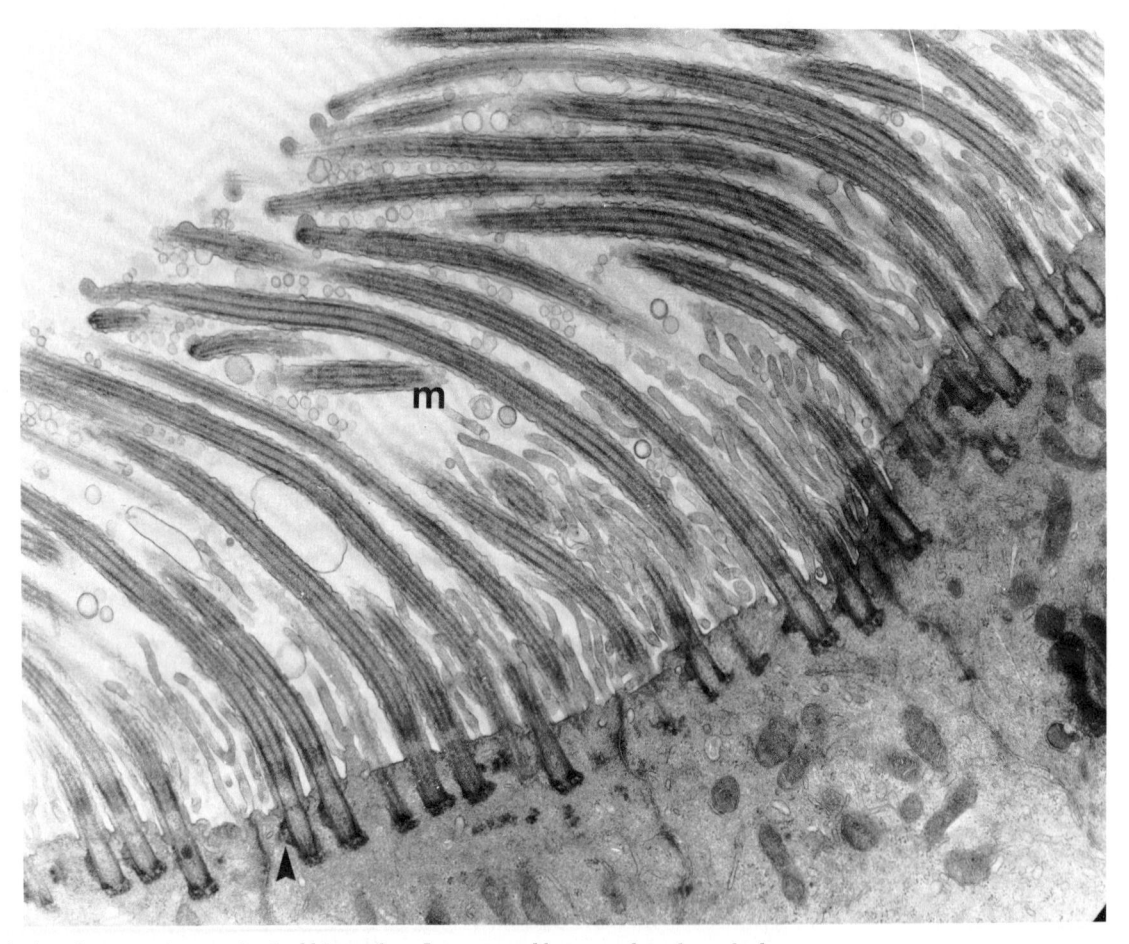

FIG. 3. Transmission electron micrograph of rabbit trachea. Interspersed between densely packed cilia are many thin microvilli (*m*). Basal feet (*arrowhead*) on cilia point to the left and indicate effective stroke direction. Majority of cilia lie in a gentle curve representing a position near beginning of the recovery stroke. × 16,000.

time; cilia probably first grow out at the periphery of the cell and later in the center (19).

AXONEME

The general ultrastructure of respiratory tract cilia is well known (52) and corresponds to what is understood about all motile somatic cilia. The axoneme consists of the established 9 + 2 pattern, 9 microtubular doublets located in a circle around a central pair of single microtubules (Fig. 4*A*). A single complete microtubule (~24 nm diam) consists of a cylinder whose wall is composed of 13 protofilaments (Fig. 4*B*); each protofilament consists of chains of ~5-nm subunits of tubulin, a ubiquitous self-assembling ~50,000-dalton protein that occurs in several slightly differing forms (53). Each doublet consists of two subfibers: subfiber A (a complete microtubule with 13 protofilaments) and subfiber B (a partial microtubule with 10 or 11 protofilaments). The doublets are linked by several series of permanent and transient bridges, including circumferential interdoublet links, radial spokes from the doublets to the central sheath surrounding the central microtubules, and dynein arms. Although a direct analysis of the biochemistry of mammalian respiratory tract cilia has not been done, in other species the biochemistry of the axoneme is quite complex; at least 150 proteins, of which tubulin is the most abundant, have been identified in two-dimensional gels of isolated axonemes (50). Each axoneme substructure is composed of many polypeptides whose order of attachment is important for proper assembly and function of the substructure (e.g., ~17 different polypeptides comprise a single radial spoke). This complexity provides very powerful genetic and biochemical regulation of the axoneme.

The axoneme alone is responsible for ciliary motility. Treatment of cilia with nonionic detergents destroys the integrity of the ciliary membrane but causes little, if any, substantial change in the axoneme proper. These membraneless axonemes beat normally when placed in appropriate solutions containing approximately millimolar concentrations of Mg^{2+} and

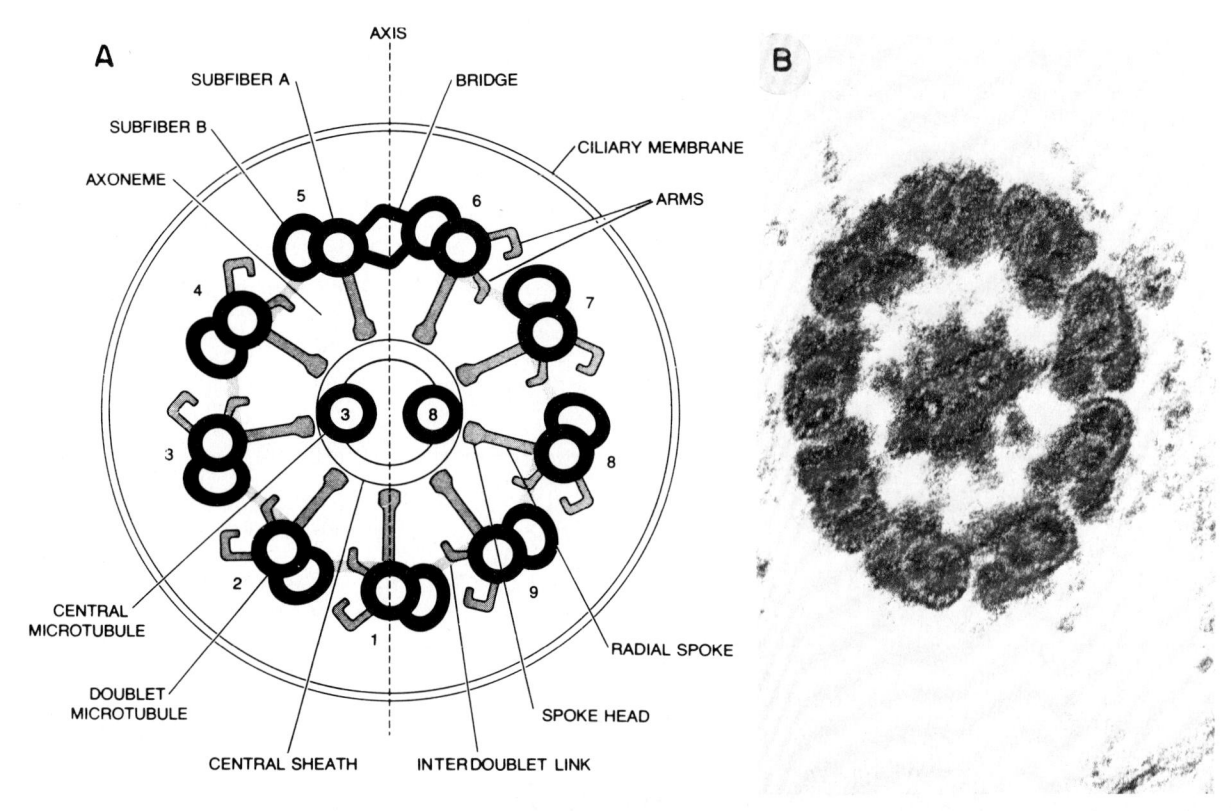

FIG. 4. *A*: axoneme as viewed from base to tip. *B*: isolated axoneme prepared by removing ciliary membrane and staining with tannic acid to demonstrate the number of protofilaments in microtubules and other details of axonemal organization. × 300,000. [*A* from Satir (60a).]

ATP as essential components. For instance, when Triton X-100 is used to remove the membranes from cilia isolated from ciliated cells of the respiratory tract of rabbits, the axonemes reactivate in a solution containing 2.5 mM Mg^{2+}, 2 mM ATP, 75 mM KCl (to adjust the ionic strength), and 0.1% 2-mercaptoethanol (to maintain the SH groups of enzymes such as dynein in a reduced state) in Tris-HCl buffer at pH 8.0 (24). In the absence of ATP there is no reactivation.

CILIARY MEMBRANE

The ciliary axoneme is completely enclosed by what first appears to be a simple extension of the cell membrane (Fig. 5). As just noted this membrane can be removed with detergents. In addition, X-ray diffraction of cilia indicates that the membrane shares certain characteristics with nerve myelin (69). This demonstrates that the composition of the ciliary membrane is similar to that of other membranes in being composed of a lipid bilayer into which proteins or glycoproteins can be intercalated. In the intact cell the ciliary membrane maintains and regulates the ionic environment, the concentrations of ATP and divalent cations, and the conditions for normal enzymatic activity of the axoneme. The membrane provides a means for the control of ciliary activity by the cell and organism.

Under unusual and some pathological conditions, ciliary resorption is seen. When chemical carcinogens cause resorption in tracheal epithelium, the ciliary membrane appears to be digested in autophagic vacuoles (22). In resorptive processes of simpler cilia, e.g., *Naegleria* or *Chlamydomonas*, the membrane is probably able to rejoin the undifferentiated cell membrane and be reutilized without breakdown.

Ciliary Crown

The cilium tapers at the tip. In mammalian cilia the taper is blunt, ~0.5 μm, often ending in a specialized structure, the ciliary crown [Fig. 5*A*; (23)]. The ciliary crown inserts into the membrane and is attached to a dense plaque between the axoneme and membrane. This crown appears to be tightly bound to the ends of the microtubules; when the ciliary membrane is removed by nonionic detergent the crown remains attached to the axoneme (17, 39). Similar extracellular coats are usually glycoproteins. Because the tip of the cilium is the portion in direct contact with the overlying mucous blanket, specific interactions between the mucus and ciliary crown have been postulated.

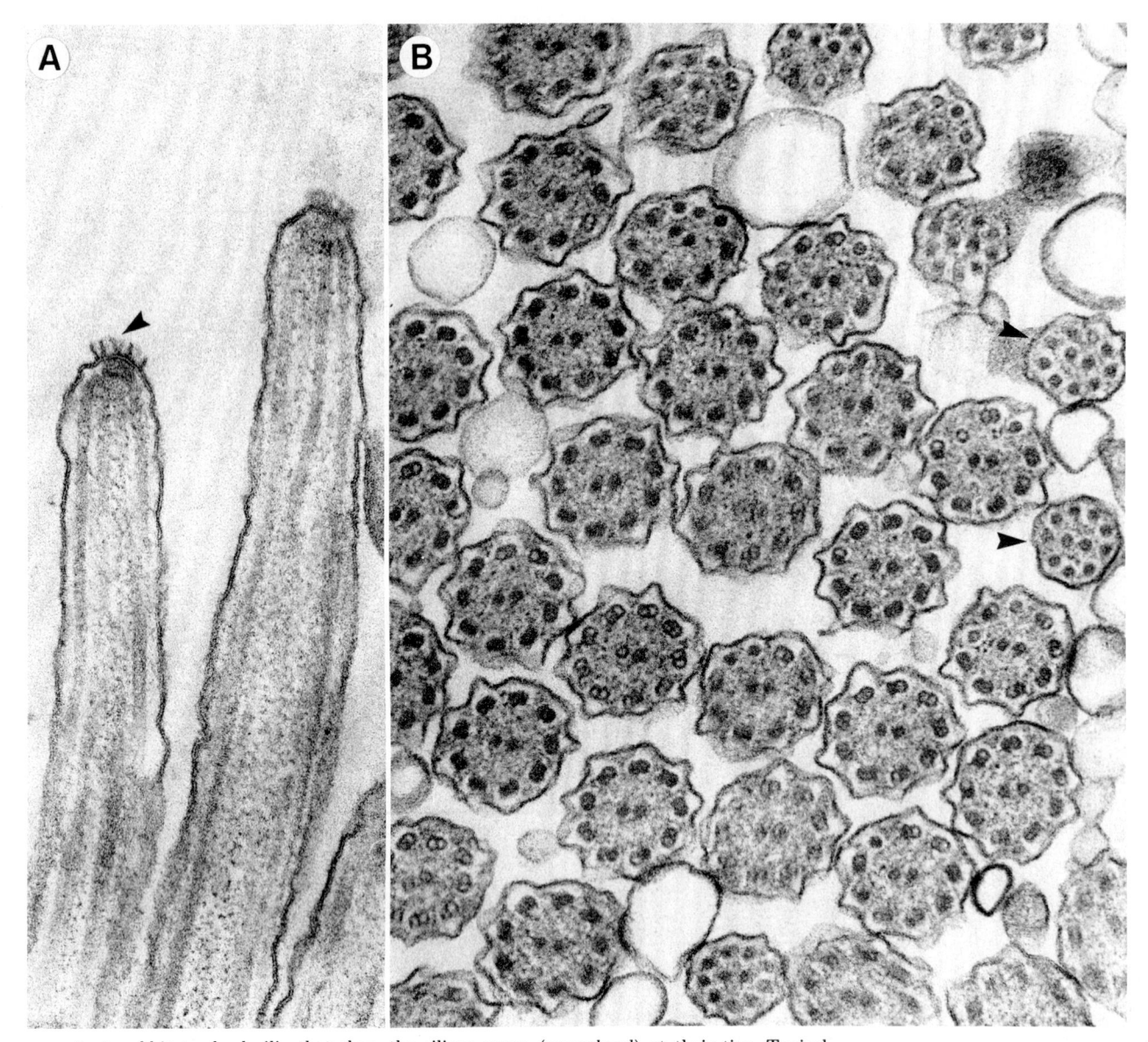

FIG. 5. *A*: rabbit tracheal cilia that show the ciliary crown (*arrowhead*) at their tips. Typical trilaminar unit membrane encloses each cilium. × 93,000. *B*: rabbit tracheal cilia in cross-section, demonstrating a few reduced tips with 9 single microtubules (*arrowheads*). × 81,000.

Freeze-Fracture Studies and Membrane Organization

Freeze-fracture studies have revealed that the ciliary membrane is nearly devoid of intramembrane particles for much of its length, especially when compared with the rich particle array displayed in other cell surface specializations, such as the microvilli (62). Researchers interpret the lack of particles along the ciliary membrane to mean that the membrane interior is largely unbroken lipid bilayer and that the membrane has severely restricted permeability and transport properties. However, recent studies on protozoan ciliary membranes have shown that the protein composition of the membrane is rather complex. In such cilia the membrane contains a variety of ion channels, enzymes, and antigenic determinants (1, 47); therefore the freeze-fracture appearance may be somewhat deceptive. The possibility that there are many classes of specific receptor molecules in the otherwise structurally homogenous ciliary membrane may be particularly important. These receptors must couple the environmental stimuli to the ciliary axonemal machinery. A 10-μm cilium has a membrane surface area of ~8 μm^2, a large area that may facilitate interaction and exchange with the environment.

Ciliary Necklace

On some invertebrate cilia, particles appear in patches or rows corresponding to the microtubules. Such specializations are rare for the few mammalian

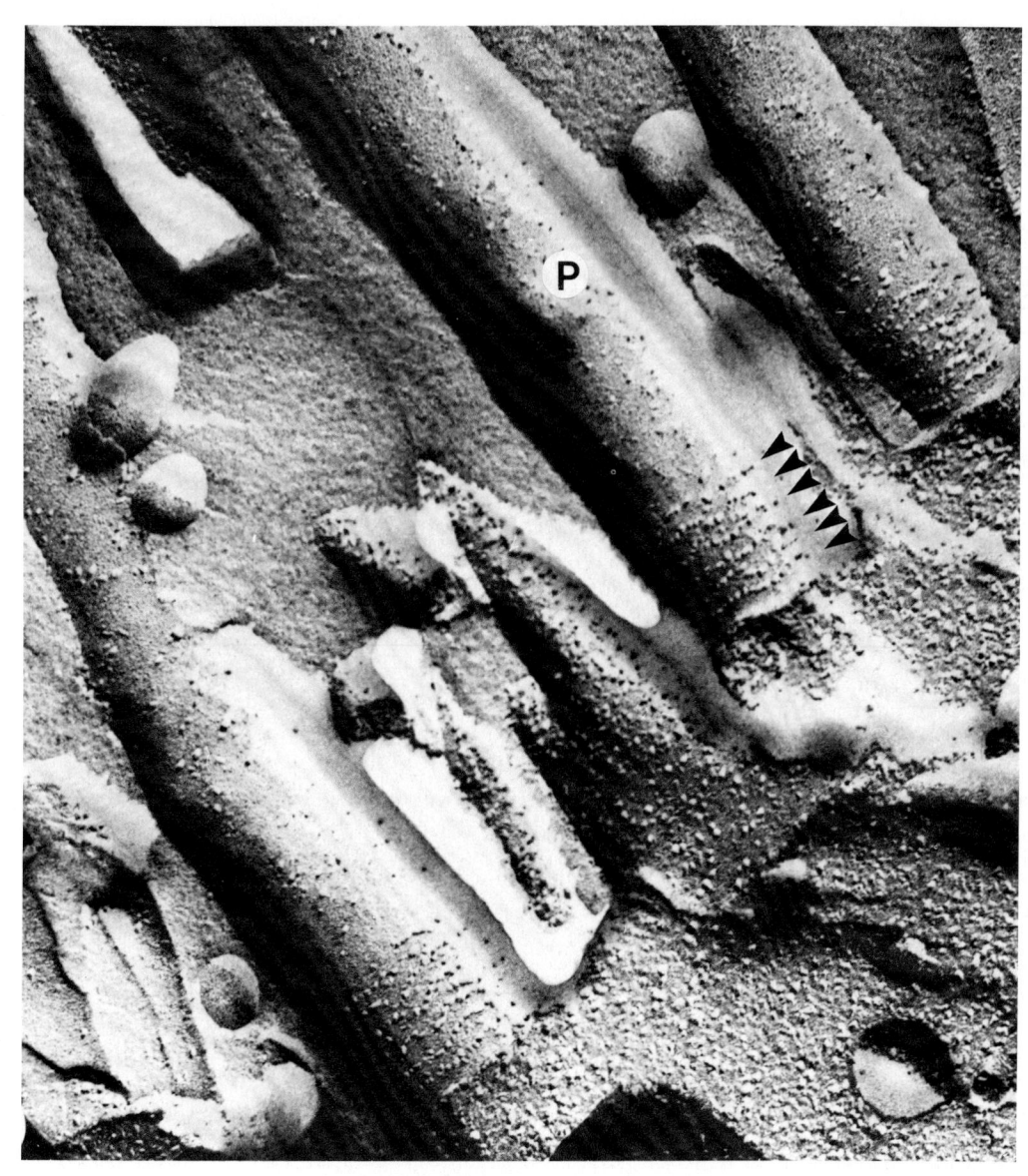

FIG. 6. Freeze-fracture image of rat tracheal cilia. At the base of each cilium there is a ciliary necklace. Six necklace strands are labeled (*arrowheads*) on the protoplasmic fracture face (*P*). × 80,000. [From Gilula and Satir (31).]

somatic ciliary membranes thus far examined by freeze fracture. However, a unique membrane specialization, the ciliary necklace, is revealed on all somatic cilia at the cilium base where the centriole attaches to the cell membrane (31). The number of strands on a mature cilium shows phylogenetic specificity; the largest number of strands thus far seen, up to 11, is found in rat tracheal or mouse oviduct cilia (Fig. 6). The ciliary necklace is part of a microtubule-membrane complex that extends from the midwall of each doublet and ends in the membrane. This complex gives a characteristic cross-sectional appearance to thin sections of cilia containing the necklace.

Although the function of the ciliary necklace is unknown, the surface properties of the necklace region clearly differ from the remainder of the ciliary membrane. For example, cationized ferritin binds preferentially to this region (5). Because pretreatment with neuraminidase or protease blocks this binding, the binding sites for polycationic ferritin appear to be negatively charged glycoproteins or mucopolysaccharides. These substances can also be detected at the necklace surface by lectins (57). The necklace particles bind concanavalin A and wheat germ agglutinin but not certain other lectins, suggesting that the intramembrane particles associated with the necklace are highly specified with respect to their sugar moieties. The ciliary crown also exhibits this specific binding.

The ciliary necklace appears to be an important attachment region for the developing cilium. As a basal body matures and takes its position at the apex of the cell, the formation of the ciliary necklace precedes the emergence of the axonemal doublets (46). As the cilium matures, more strands are added to the necklace. Deciliation occurs just above the necklace; thus the necklace remains with the cell body (58) and may play a role in the positioning of the basal body and in subsequent ciliogenetic events.

A recurrent suggestion is that the ciliary necklace may be involved in sensory transducing mechanisms during normal ciliary beat. One reason for this suggestion is that the necklace is part of the ciliary structure in nonmotile cilia, such as those of the retinal rods, that have become specialized sensory organelles. In cochlear hair cells the axoneme is lost in some mammals, including humans, but the ciliary necklace remains.

Mycoplasma infection of mammalian respiratory epithelium causes ciliostasis and damage to the epithelium (13). To be fully pathogenic the organism must specifically attach to the host cell surface by means of a special organelle; this attachment occurs between cilia. Inspection of freeze-etched replicas from experimentally infected epithelia show that the ciliary necklace undergoes severe deterioration within 24 h, whereas control tissues show no change. Therefore the disruption of the ciliary necklace appears to be associated with the onset of ciliary immotility.

SLIDING-MICROTUBULE MECHANISM

Ciliary motion is based on the sliding of the doublet axonemal microtubules with respect to each other. The action of the dynein arms, which are the axonemal ATPase, produces the sliding. Although the biochemistry of dynein in different species is still to be resolved, the overall mechanism of microtubule sliding and the activity cycle of the dynein arms that produces this sliding remain essentially constant for all 9 + 2 axonemes.

The sliding-microtubule model of ciliary activity is based on two lines of experimental evidence. The first concerns the behavior of the doublets as the cilium bends. Satir (59, 60) examined the tips of certain invertebrate cilia to show that the pattern of doublet termination is geometrically consistent with the conclusion that microtubules remain at constant length throughout the beat cycle. A general sliding equation has been derived from such geometrical considerations, where the displacement (Δl) of a doublet is related to bend angle ($\Sigma \alpha$)

$$\Delta l = d_n \Sigma \alpha \qquad (1)$$

and d_n is a constant indicating the effective axonemal diameter for the particular doublet. The second line of evidence, that of Summers and Gibbons (73, 74), demonstrates that ATP produces disintegration of the axoneme when the ciliary membrane is removed by detergent and trypsin is used to digest the interdoublet links and radial spokes. Without these constraining structures, ATP causes the axonemal doublets to telescope apart because the dynein arms on one doublet (N) push the adjacent doublet (N + 1) in a consistent direction.

Geometry of Sliding

In the mussel gill cilia, which were used as a model for constructing the geometry of sliding, all doublets contain B subfibers that are equal in length but shorter than A subfibers, which vary greatly in length. Because of this architecture, tips with fewer than 9 A subfibers are seen, regardless of bend position. In active mammalian cilia, A subfibers seem more equal in length, and tips with fewer than 9 A subfibers are not often seen; however, a number of 8 + 2 and 6 + 2 ciliary tip images are seen in mouse oviduct (23), and corresponding images are seen in tracheal cilia (63). Therefore the principles in Equation 1 probably hold for mammalian and invertebrate cilia. One reason for the paucity of reduced tips in mammalian cilia may be the intermittent nature of the activity of these cilia. However, a second possibility is that because the ciliary microtubules of the mammalian respiratory tract usually terminate in a specialized crown-plaque complex they may be fixed at both ends. For a sliding mechanism to generate a single bend, sliding fixed axonemal microtubules would have to twist during beating, absorbing the potential tip displacement (17, 34), so that only minimal displacements would usually be seen. This possibility requires further study.

When reactivated by ATP, single rabbit tracheal axonemes that have attached themselves at both ends generate sinusoidal waves consistent with balanced sliding, where without twist a bend in one direction must be balanced by a bend in the opposite direction. This conforms to the necessary constraints imposed by the geometry of sliding and to similar tests in invertebrates (67). These geometrical considerations come closest to predicting the sliding displacements that must occur in cilia of a living cell during beating.

Additional geometric tests of sliding, with radial-spoke periodicity as an intrinsic marker of distance for each doublet microtubule, have been made in invertebrate cilia (82). The radial spokes, which originate at subfiber A and extend toward the central axis of the axoneme, occur unevenly spaced in groups of three; the greater spacing (~36 nm) between successive spokes of the same group is closer to the cilium base and the smaller spacing (~24 nm) is closer to the ciliary tip. The distance between successive spoke triplets is ~48 nm. This intricate periodicity is maintained for all doublets studied along both straight and bent regions of a cilium, which makes even minimal contraction of the axoneme improbable. Furthermore displacements of the axonemal doublets predicted by Equation 1 occur locally, and as predicted Δl remains constant along straight regions of the axoneme. Preliminary data for respiratory tract cilia demonstrate that similar triplet spoke-group spacing occurs.

Direct Examination of Sliding

Summers and Gibbons (73, 74) first demonstrated that sliding and bending of doublet microtubules, which normally occur together in a beating cilium, may be uncoupled by treatment of the axoneme with proteolytic enzymes such as trypsin. After this treatment the axoneme no longer beats when ATP is added, but the interaction between the dynein arms and microtubules is preserved and can be studied further.

When ATP is added the trypsin-treated axonemes disintegrate by sliding, elongating to as much as 8–9 times the original axonemal length as doublets are extended (Fig. 7).

Dirksen and Zeira (24) likewise recently directly demonstrated sliding of cilia in the respiratory tract of mammals. Experimentally this preparation is more difficult to handle. Disintegration by sliding occurs if quiescent trypsin-digested axonemes are treated with ATP or if trypsin is added to ATP-reactivated axonemes (Fig. 7B).

For both invertebrate and mammalian cilia such preparations have been subjected to ultrastructural analysis. In trypsin-treated axonemes of *Tetrahy-*

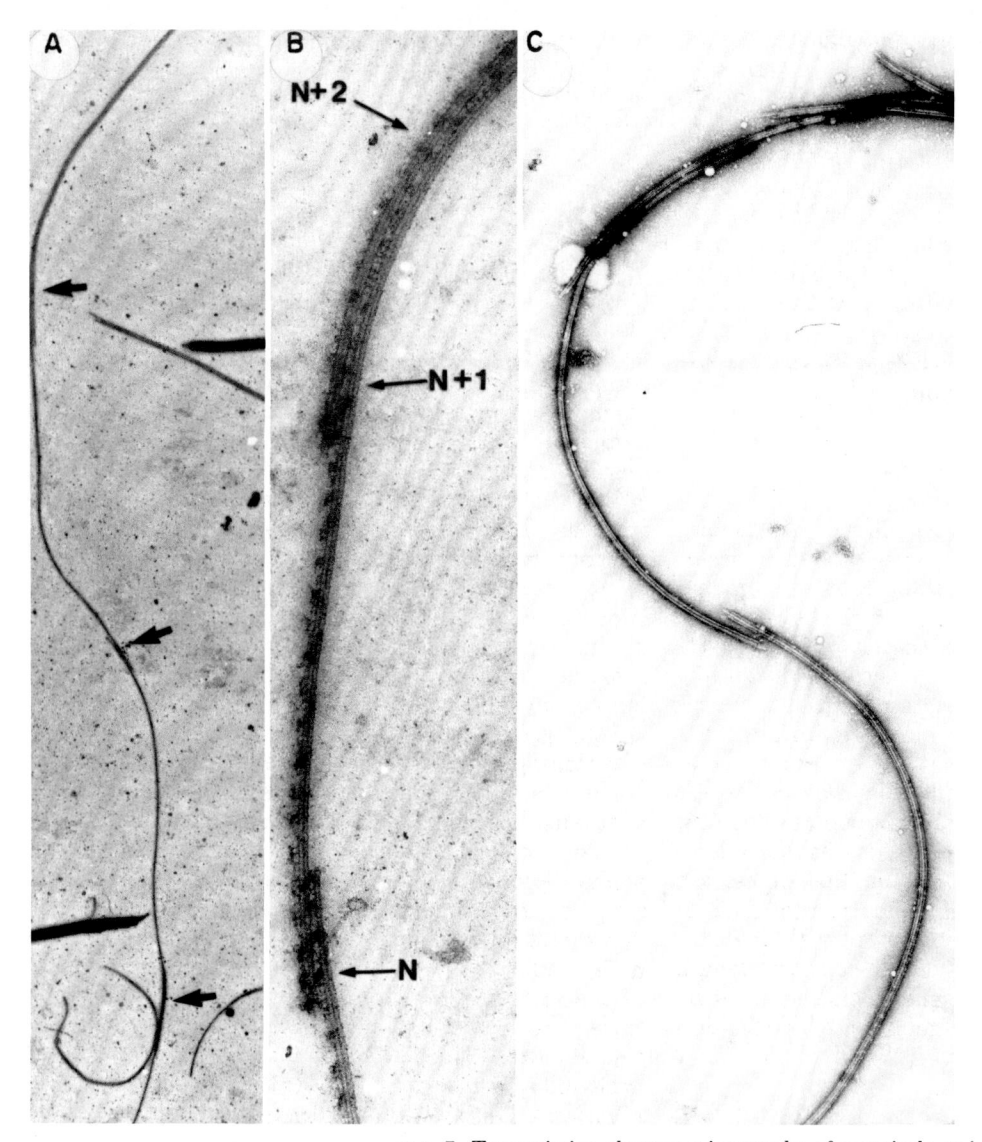

FIG. 7. Transmission electron micrographs of negatively stained preparations of ciliary doublet microtubules, showing sliding after addition of ATP. A: low magnification of a *Tetrahymena* preparation including regions of overlap of individual doublets (*arrows*) in a telescoping axoneme. × 9,500. B: *Tetrahymena* cilia doublets at a higher magnification to demonstrate direction of sliding and doublets numbered N, N + 1, N + 2. The A subfibers of each doublet are marked by the spoke group repeat. × 50,000. C: rabbit tracheal ciliary doublets with overlap as in B. × 26,000. (Micrographs A and B courtesy of W. Sale.)

mena, sliding is circumferentially isotropic, i.e., at least seven and possibly all nine doublet microtubules are capable of unidirectional sliding. The dynein arms can be visualized in preparations such as that in Figure 7; thus doublets N and N + 1 may be determined (54).

Structure and Function of the Dynein Arm

The mechanochemical cycle of a typical dynein arm is shown in Figure 8 (66), which indicates two successive binding sites on subfiber B of doublet N + 1. In the absence of ATP a 21-nm-long arm is bound to the distal site. When ATP is added the arm is released and then shortens to create an interdoublet gap of ~10 nm. The arm then reextends. In its fully extended position it is 26 nm long and tilted toward the base at a 40° angle. The dynein arm reattaches to subfiber B at the more proximal site; reextension and reattachment require ATP hydrolysis. The arm then returns to the rigor position by relative sliding of doublets N and N + 1 by ~16 nm. Although during a sliding disintegration doublets could be ejected from either the tip or the base of the axoneme, doublet N always pushes doublet N + 1 toward the axoneme tip because of the polarity of the dynein-arm cycle.

With minor modification and despite some differences in position and in biochemistry, probably all arms of a single axoneme perform this cycle during ciliary beat. For example, when the outer arms of an axoneme are extracted, if the axoneme is subsequently reactivated by ATP it will beat with half the normal frequency. As outer arms are successively re-added, beat frequency returns proportionally, implying that the amount of dynein and beat are correlated even if only the inner row of arms is present (28). Thus the rate of microtubule sliding is probably proportional to the number of dynein arms. Yano and Miki-Noumura (83) have recently confirmed this.

Each dynein arm is composed of several subunits. There are probably three large globular domains in a single arm (37). Based on rapid-freeze replica techniques (32), negative stain, and unstained images of isolated dynein, several different models for the three-dimensional organization of these globular domains in relation to arm structure have been proposed. Isolated dynein is also complex chemically. For example, in sea urchin sperm tails, dynein, which has a molecular weight of ~1 million, probably consists of two ATPase heavy chains (Aα, Aβ), each greater in molecular weight than 250,000, together with several intermediate- and light-chain components (8). In some species the numbers and sizes of the ATPase heavy chains as well as the associated components of lower molecular weight differ between the inner and outer rows of arms. The enzymatic characteristics of the dynein ATPases have been studied in some detail (29, 81). One important feature of the ATPase is its extreme sensitivity to vanadate, an analogue of phos-

FIG. 8. Mechanochemical cycle of dynein arm. Two successive binding sites on subfiber B of doublet N + 1 are indicated. *A*: 21-nm-long arm is bound to distal site in the absence of ATP (rigor). *B*: addition of ATP causes release and maximal shortening of arm to open an ~10-nm interdoublet gap. Release is independent of hydrolysis of ATP. *C*: arm reextends. In its fully extended position, arm is ~26-nm long and tilts basally at an ~40° angle. *D*: arm reattaches to subfiber B at the more proximal site. Reextension and reattachment require hydrolysis of ATP, but point at which product release occurs is speculative. *E*: arm returns to the rigor equilibrium position by relative sliding of doublets N and N + 1 by 16 nm. [From Satir et al. (66).]

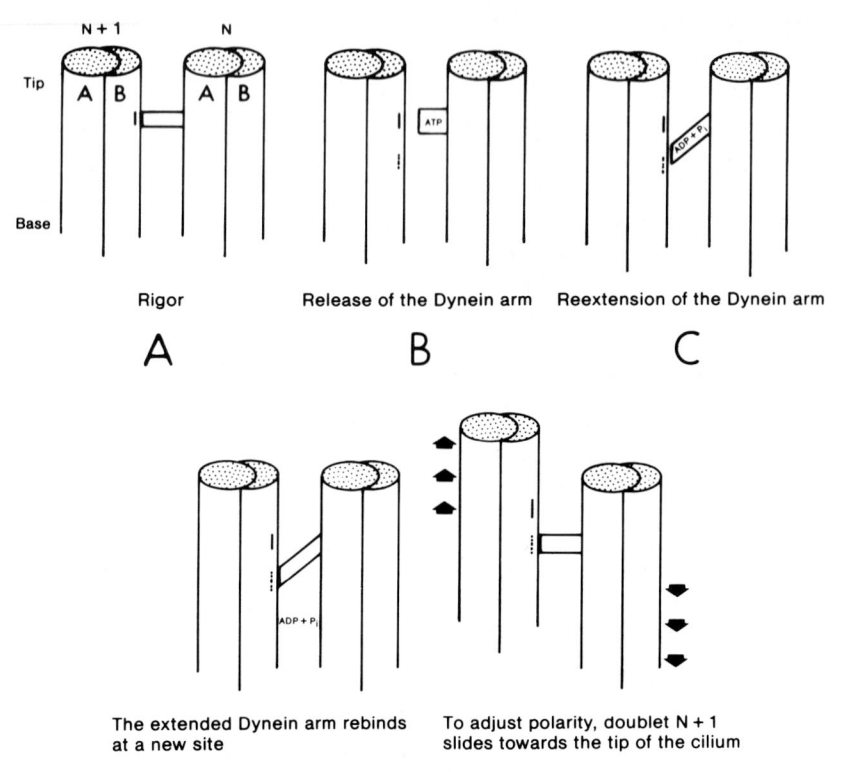

phate (26, 30). As a corollary, micromolar concentrations of vanadate inhibit ATP reactivation of axonemes by interrupting the arm cycle.

Both ends of a single dynein arm may interact with the tubulin lattice of the axonemal microtubules. It is not clear why the attachment to subfiber A is relatively permanent, whereas the attachment to subfiber B is cyclic. When isolated dynein arms are reattached to axonemal microtubules previously stripped of their dynein, the arms rebind to both subfiber A and B. The binding to subfiber B is probably more sensitive to ATP addition than is the binding to subfiber A because in certain experiments the arms are released preferentially from subfiber B (75).

Human Dynein

Despite the extensive biochemical and structural studies of the dynein arm in invertebrate cilia, little comparable information exists about the dyneins of human cilia. Dynein arms, however, appear structurally normal on motile human sperm. Electron-microscopic histochemistry indicates that ATPase activity is associated with the arms. The flagella of normal human sperm possess a complement of polypeptides of high molecular weight that migrate electrophoretically, as do the dyneins of invertebrate and other mammalian sperm (7). At least four bands appear in the dynein region of the electrophoretic gels. Mutant sperm lacking dynein arms (see CILIARY DYSFUNCTION IN HUMANS, p. 490) lack several of these bands in gel electrophoresis. It seems reasonable to anticipate that the mechanochemical cycle of dynein in invertebrate cilia applies to human and other mammalian cilia.

CONTROL OF SLIDING

An understanding of the sliding mechanism is necessary but not sufficient for understanding how mammalian cilia beat. Sliding in the intact cilium is converted into bending; a series of sequential waves of bending propagates along the axoneme. Because sliding is preserved in protease-treated axonemes, whereas the control system that converts sliding into bending is destroyed, it is easier to obtain information on sliding than on the control system. The radial spokes and circumferential interdoublet links, which are lost with protease digestion, probably form important parts of the regulatory system that produces the propagating bending waves.

Part of the function of the control system must be to limit sliding. Another part must be to restore displaced doublets to their original positions. These properties are lost after protease digestion. One way to sort out the different functions of the control system is to follow the course of axoneme digestion by different proteases. The changes as digestion proceeds are measured as effects on ciliary-beat form and frequency. For example, elastase digestion produces axonemes whose sliding velocity is nearly constant but whose bending amplitude gradually increases. This suggests that elastase probably does not appreciably affect sliding but does affect the form of beat (10). The interdoublet links also seem to be particularly sensitive to digestion by elastase. On the other hand trypsin digestion is much less specific and affects the degree of sliding and bending differently. This suggests that the interdoublet links are the elastic girdle of the axoneme and are important in the regulation of the amplitude of bends during beat.

The radial spokes are in a position to provide precise local regulation of sliding. For example, radial spokes in bent regions of beating cilia seem to be attached not only to subfiber A of the axonemal microtubules but also to the central sheath (82). This attachment is transitory, and in straight regions of the axoneme the radial spokes are free at their distal end. Sliding occurs parallel to the longitudinal axis of the axoneme, whereas bending occurs perpendicular to that axis. The latter is the direction in which the radial spokes project (see Fig. 4), suggesting that the radial spokes are elements in transducing sliding into local bending, i.e., in bend generation and propagation.

Mutant Studies

Some of the most impressive evidence regarding the function of the radial spokes and central sheaths comes from studies of mutants of the green alga *Chlamydomonas*, which lack either radial spokes or central-sheath projections. These mutants are immotile, although only single polypeptides (among the many that comprise the spokes and sheaths) differ from the wild type (50). After treatment with detergent, axonemes from these cells fail to beat on addition of ATP. After digestion of the axonemes with trypsin, however, addition of ATP is followed as usual by sliding disintegration; i.e., the sliding system is operational. That part of the control system that restrains unlimited sliding, presumably the circumferential interdoublet links, must also be operational because the undigested axonemes do not slide apart. However, the part of the control system that is involved with bend generation and propagation is missing, as expected from the lack of radial-spoke–central-sheath interaction. A complication in this simplified scheme of radial-spoke function for these *Chlamydomonas* mutants is that suppressors have been found where motility returns, whereas the proteins and structures associated with the mutation remain missing (42). The significance of this finding is unclear, but one possibility is that the control system is redundant and correlated with more than one specific set of structures. As we indicate in CILIARY DYSFUNCTION IN HUMANS, p. 490, a parallel series of mutants occurs in human cilia.

Sliding and Switching Mechanisms

Another function of the control system must be to permit the axonemal doublets to slide asynchronously. The trypsin-treated axonemes always show a single polarity of active sliding. In an intact cilium this must mean that all the doublets do not work at the same time, because synchronous activity of the nine doublets around the circumference of the axoneme would cancel out effective movement. Ultrastructural analysis indicates that the important doublet asynchrony takes place between doublets 1–4 and 6–9 (65), implying that not all doublets moving tipward in each portion of the beat cycle are active. As the effective stroke progresses, doublets 1–4 are active, but doublets 4–7 actually move tipward. As the recovery stroke progresses, doublets 6–9 are active but doublets 9, 1, and 2 move tipward.

The central sheath consists of a series of projections 16 nm apart. Each sheath projection is related only to a subset of microtubule doublets so that the radial-spoke heads arising from doublets 1–5 and 6–9 abut against different projections. This arrangement would be expected if the central-sheath–radial-spoke complex provided a switching mechanism for turning on and off active sliding in these microtubule-doublet subsets. This model of sequential activity during ciliary beat has been called the switch-point hypothesis (64). Whether the switching mechanism is activated by biochemical modifications of the axonemal proteins, by mechanical or elastic feedback loops, or by a combination of biochemical and mechanical properties of the axonemal proteins is not clear.

Calcium Ions and Ciliary Arrest

It has been known for some time that Ca^{2+} affects ciliary activity. For example, axonemes of the lateral cilia of the mussel gill reactivate and beat normally when the Ca^{2+} concentration surrounding the axoneme is $<10^{-7}$ M but are arrested when the concentration is increased to $\sim 10^{-6}$ M (79). All the lateral cilia then stop in one position, near the beginning of their effective stroke. One interpretation of this observation is that one of the switching mechanisms of the axoneme is Ca^{2+} sensitive and that this switch may be blocked by increasing the axonemal Ca^{2+} concentration so that either doublets 6–9 remain active or doublets 1–4 fail to become active. As a result the cilia move to the arrest position from every beat position and are caught there.

The ATP-induced sliding of axonemes after trypsin treatment is not affected by increases in Ca^{2+} concentration far greater than those necessary to inhibit beating. This suggests that the Ca^{2+} does not operate on the dynein system directly but probably on those components of the control system that are digested by trypsin.

In the lateral cilia the switching mechanism is also sensitive to high concentrations of external vanadate and to azide (78). In the presence of these agents the cilia arrest in a different position, near the beginning of their recovery stroke. This arrest is postulated to occur because either doublets 1–4 remain active or doublets 6–9 fail to become active. Although vanadate and azide are nonphysiological agents, they act as probes for studying this alternate non-Ca^{2+}-sensitive switch position.

The Ca^{2+} threshold for arrest of mammalian cilia seems to be several orders of magnitude higher than the threshold of the lateral cilia of the mussel (27). The biochemical basis for this difference is not clear, and the physiological effects of internal Ca^{2+} concentration on mammalian cilia remain controversial.

Membrane Control of Calcium Ion Concentration

With high concentrations of Ca^{2+} in the surrounding medium, the axonemal Ca^{2+} concentration is maintained at a low level by the ciliary and surrounding cell membranes, which pump Ca^{2+} from the axoneme. With electrical or mechanical stimulation the membrane depolarizes, the pumps are effectively overcome, and the concentration of free Ca^{2+} around the axoneme rises. Stimulation can occur by a variety of modes directly at the ciliary membrane or at the basal pole of the cell (see FACTORS INFLUENCING MUCOCILIARY CLEARANCE, p. 487). When the membrane repolarizes, the concentration of Ca^{2+} falls and the normal ciliary state is restored.

To produce this sequence of events the membrane contains voltage-sensitive Ca^{2+} channels, which respond to membrane depolarization, and Ca^{2+} pumps, which are presumably Ca^{2+}-ATPase. In *Paramecium* the voltage-sensitive Ca^{2+} channels and several Ca^{2+}-ATPases have been found in isolated ciliary membranes prepared by deciliation (1, 47). The Ca^{2+} channels must be primarily in the ciliary membrane, because they are greatly reduced in the cell body membrane after deciliation. The Ca^{2+} pumps occur both in ciliary and cell body membranes. Histochemical localization of Ca^{2+} has shown deposits along the cytoplasmic surface of the ciliary membrane, particularly at the ciliary necklace (61). Because the ciliary necklace remains with the cell body, this localization suggests that the necklace might be a Ca^{2+} pump; however, the enzymatic composition of the necklace remains unknown.

Calmodulin

The Ca^{2+} sensor of the ciliary axoneme is probably calmodulin, a Ca^{2+}-binding protein of 17,000 daltons analogous to muscle troponin C. Calmodulin occurs ubiquitously in mammalian tissues where it provides Ca^{2+} regulation of many enzymatic processes, including activation of brain phosphodiesterase (see refs. 14 and 45 for reviews). Calmodulin is localized in protozoan cilia (43) and binds Ca^{2+} in a range of concentrations appropriate to the action of the Ca^{2+} switch.

CILIARY BEAT

Mammalian cilia, like other cilia, beat with a propulsive effective stroke and a recovery stroke (Fig. 9). In rabbit tracheal cilia the beat cycle begins with the recovery stroke (55, 56). In this stroke a bend at the base of the cilium enlarges and propagates toward the ciliary tip. The cilium is inclined at an angle of 30°–40° to the cell surface so the ciliary tip sweeps through a clockwise arc as seen from above. The recovery stroke merges into the effective stroke without pause. During the effective stroke the cilium moves back to the starting position in a plane perpendicular to the cell surface. The recovery stroke lasts nearly twice as long as the effective stroke. A rest phase of variable duration occurs at the end of the effective stroke. This form of beat is essentially the same in human respiratory tract cilia (44).

Two bent regions form during the beat cycle; these are in opposite directions and generally of somewhat different magnitudes. They are analogous to the principal and reverse bends that occur during motion of the spermatozoan flagella. This asymmetric-bend formation is thought to correspond to different amounts of sliding on the two sides of the ciliary axoneme (i.e., doublets 1–4 vs. 6–9). Because of asymmetry the effective stroke is predominantly vertical and the cilium is extended from the cell surface by almost its full length. In contrast the recovery stroke is more horizontal and the cilium lies much closer to the cell surface. This distinction provides the hydrodynamic basis for ciliary propulsion because the effective stroke carries along with it a larger volume of material than does the recovery stroke (9). Viscous forces are much more important than inertial forces in ciliary motion. This has at least two implications: *1*) the material moved by the cilia is "clawed" forward; i.e., the cilium operates in a medium in a fashion that corresponds to a human body swimming in molasses, and *2*) when the cilia stop moving, the material stops almost simultaneously.

MUCOCILIARY TRANSPORT

In 1934 Lucas and Douglas (40) first proposed the conventional model for mucociliary transport. In this model, the fluid covering the epithelium consists of two layers (Fig. 10). The lower layer, which bathes the cilia and in which they beat freely, is a less viscous or periciliary layer; the upper layer is a highly viscous mucous layer (51).

Mucociliary transport depends not only on the beat characteristics of the cilia but also on the composition and thickness of the periciliary and of the mucous layer. Under optimal conditions in the respiratory tract, mucus is propelled at velocities of 10 mm/min by cilia beating at ~20 Hz.

Periciliary Fluid

The periciliary fluid resembles interstitial fluid. It consists of a watery solution of materials secreted by the submucosal glands and surface goblet cells of the respiratory epithelium. It is free of glycoproteins, is similar in viscosity to serum, and provides a substrate on which the mucous layer floats. Materials from the external environment may penetrate through the mucus into the periciliary layer to interact with the ciliary membrane.

The height of the periciliary layer is probably significant because it determines the position of intersection between the mucous blanket and the ciliary stroke. In their recovery stroke, cilia lie entirely within the layer (Fig. 10). Variability in the ionic and molecular composition of the periciliary fluid or in the quantity of secretion affects the activity of the cilia or

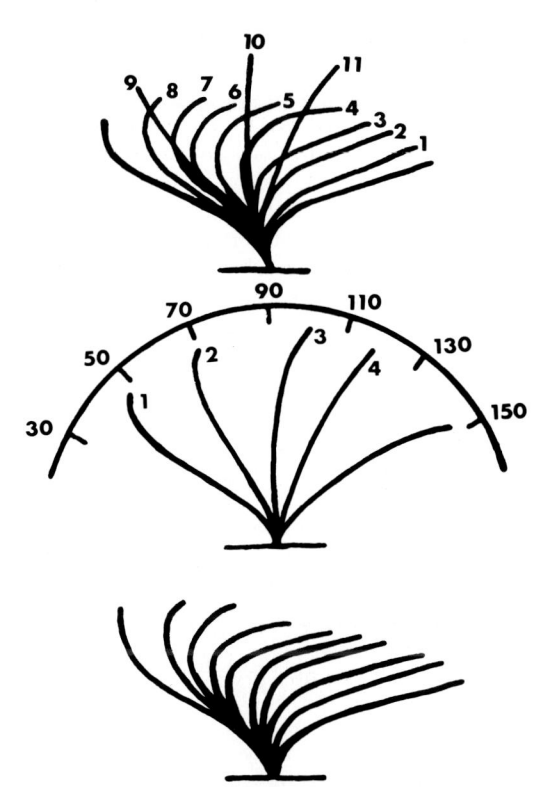

FIG. 9. *Top*, series of profiles of rabbit tracheal cilia traced from high-speed cinematographic film (250 frames/s) shows the change in shape of each cilium at intervals of 4 ms during recovery and effective strokes of the beat cycle. *Middle*, angular position (in degrees) of cilium at different stages of effective stroke. These profiles are a composite of several beat cycles of different cilia because it was not possible to trace successive stages of movement of a single cilium through an entire beat. *Bottom*, profiles of recovery stroke taken from scanning electron micrographs. [From Sanderson and Sleigh (55).]

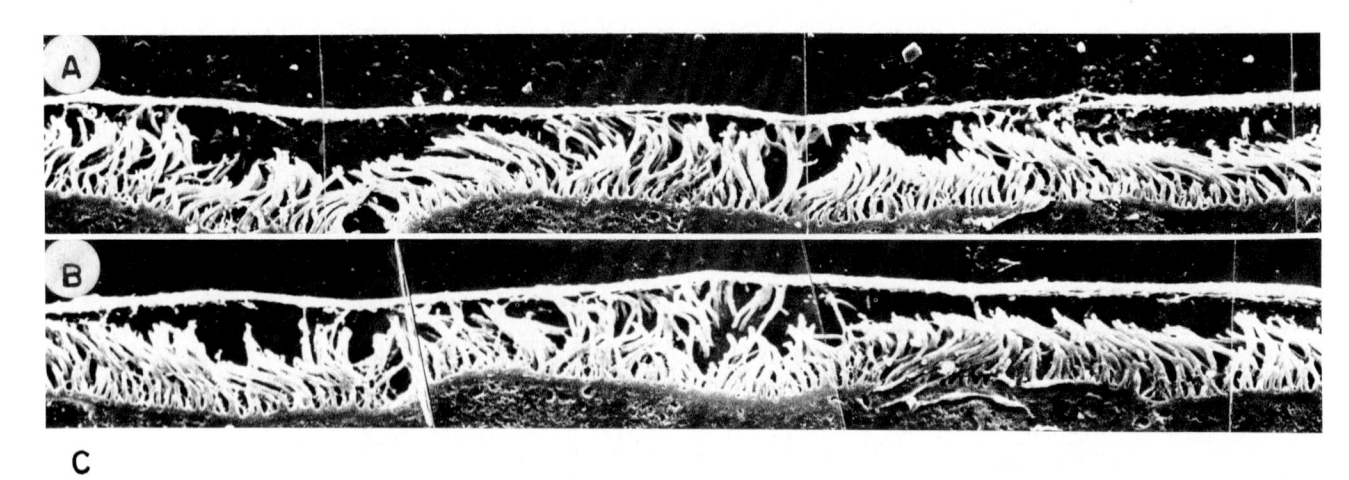

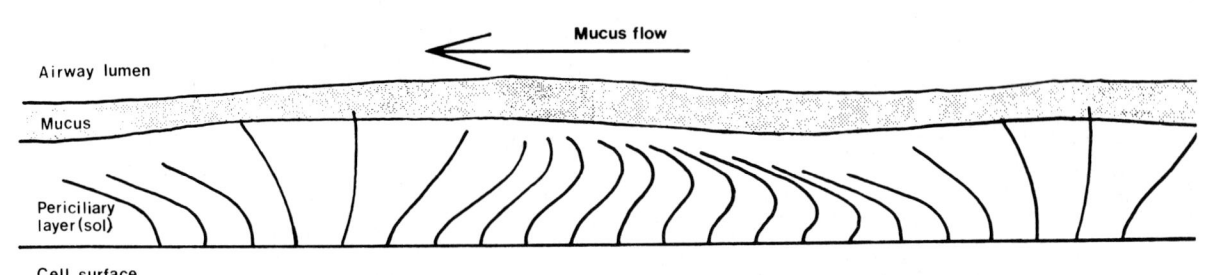

FIG. 10. Demonstration of relationship between propulsive cilia and overlying mucus during the 2 phases of the beat cycle. *A, B*: scanning electron micrographs of 2 consecutive sections (1 μm thick). Overlying mucus is preserved as a thin continuous sheet. Cilia are seen in profile in various beat positions underneath sheet. *C*: diagrammatic reconstruction of the relationship. Recovery strokes of cilia occur within the periciliary layer, whereas the effective stroke penetrates, lifts, and propels the mucus. [From Sanderson and Sleigh (56).]

the overall efficiency of transport. The periciliary fluid is continuously stirred by ciliary action; however, this stirring by itself does not produce directed mucociliary transport.

Mucous Layer

The mucous layer is moved by the cilia. The extent to which the mucus is a continuous blanket over the periciliary surface is unclear; some have found the mucous layer to be distributed in patches over the epithelium (35), whereas others have found a more continuous mucous blanket [Fig. 11; (41, 70)].

Mucus is a viscoelastic non-Newtonian gel, and its rheological properties depend on the elongated glycosylated macromolecules comprising it. A major constituent is a ~500,000-dalton glycoprotein.

The cilia must make direct contact with the mucus to transfer enough momentum to the layer to move the mucus. This contact is accomplished during the effective stroke of the cilia; as the cilia become more vertically oriented their tips reach through the periciliary fluid to penetrate the mucus (Fig. 10). At the end of the effective stroke the cilia withdraw from the mucus. Ciliary penetration into the mucous layer and consequent mucous transport are inhibited if the mucus is too highly cross-linked; also the transfer of momentum is ineffectual and movement ceases if the mucus is too weakly cross-linked (68).

FUNCTION OF METACHRONISM

For cilia to effectively move the mucous blanket they must move in a manner that minimizes their mutual interference. A beating cilium influences its neighbor through the medium, in this case the periciliary fluid. This cilium in turn acts on its neighboring cilium and so on, so that a field of cilia becomes coordinated by hydrodynamic coupling. Because each cilium is forced to beat somewhat out of phase with many of its nearest neighbors, moving waves of ciliary activity are produced. The waves of activity moving over the field are metachronal waves. This activity has been studied mainly in water-propelling cilia where the metachronal waves are very prominent (4) but where the organization is somewhat different from that of the mammalian respiratory tract (55).

Metachronal-wave characteristics are related to a number of parameters of tissue organization; the most important are the length and spacing of the cilia, the pattern of the beat, and the viscosity of the medium that bathes the cilia. In tracheal epithelium isolated

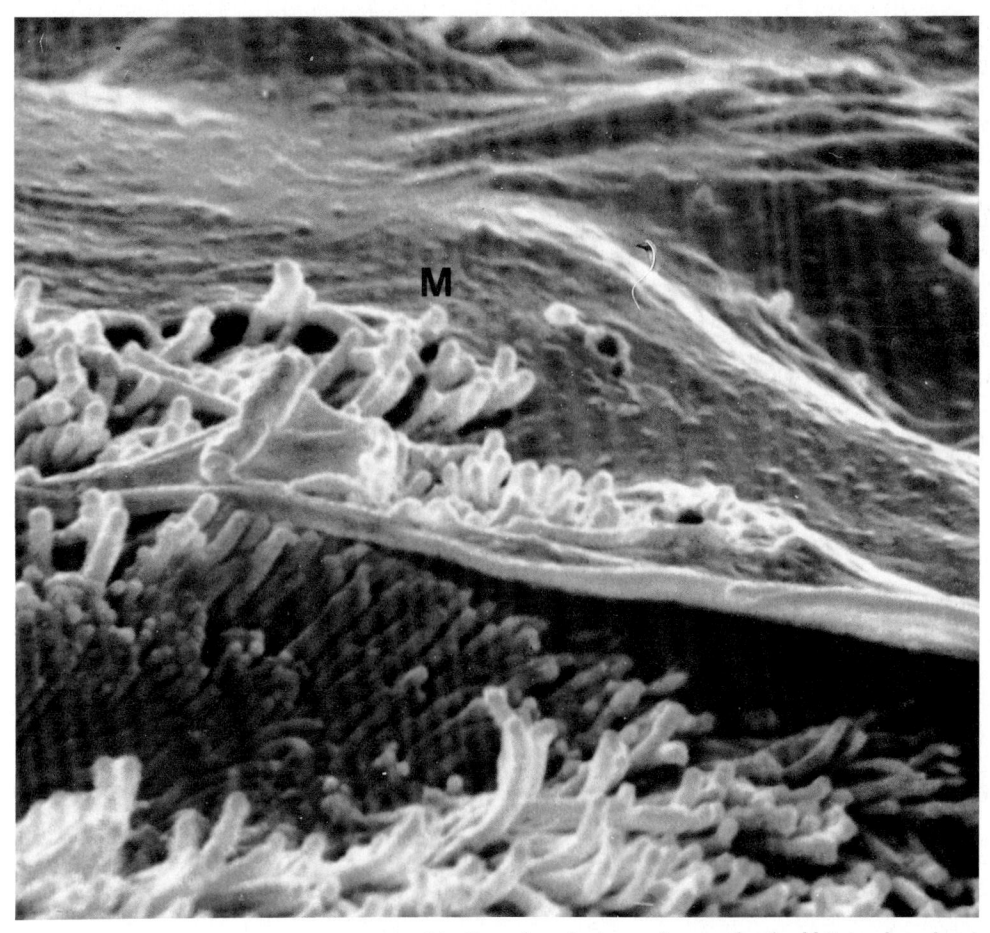

FIG. 11. Scanning electron micrograph of rabbit trachea showing details of the mucous blanket over the ciliated epithelium. Mucus (M) is situated at tips of the cilia. × 13,500. [From Sturgess (70).]

from the rabbit and maintained in culture for a number of days, cinematographic records show that at any given time only a small number of cilia are actively beating and that these cilia are clustered in discrete areas of activity. The active cilia are surrounded by large numbers of cilia arrested near the beginning of the recovery stroke so that their tips point in the direction of mucous transport (56). The films show metachronal waves, small recurrent ripples of activity, passing over clusters of three or four cells. As these ripples sweep along, all cilia on the cell cluster become active in succession.

Scanning electron microscopy (Fig. 12) reveals the highly characteristic appearance of each metachronal wave of the rabbit respiratory epithelium (55). Areas of activity are seen as hollow spaces with central areas surrounded by cilia whose tips point in different directions; the recovery phase of each beating cilium begins at some distance from the center of the hollow. A bend progressing from the ciliary base to its tip draws the cilium backward and sideways; the tip describes a clockwise arc as viewed from above. In the effective stroke the cilia rise above the other cilia and can be more readily observed.

These well-defined active areas display antilaeoplectic metachronism; i.e., if one faces in the direction in which the wave is traveling, the effective stroke occurs backward and to the left. Unlike water-propelling cilia, which normally are continuously active and whose hydrodynamic coupling involves both the effective and recovery strokes, tracheal cilia are hydrodynamically coupled only through their recovery strokes in the periciliary layer. For a cilium to contribute to mucous transport it must first become active, then complete a recovery stroke (which activates the neighboring cilia to generate the metachronal wave), and then begin the effective stroke (which serves to propel the mucous blanket). This sequence seems advantageous because with the recovery stroke initiating the cycle many cilia begin beating before the mucus imposes restraints. In addition the downstream orientation of the ciliary tips produces a nonslip surface to prevent the counterflow of mucus.

FACTORS INFLUENCING MUCOCILIARY CLEARANCE

About 50% of the particulate matter introduced into the respiratory tract of healthy individuals is cleared

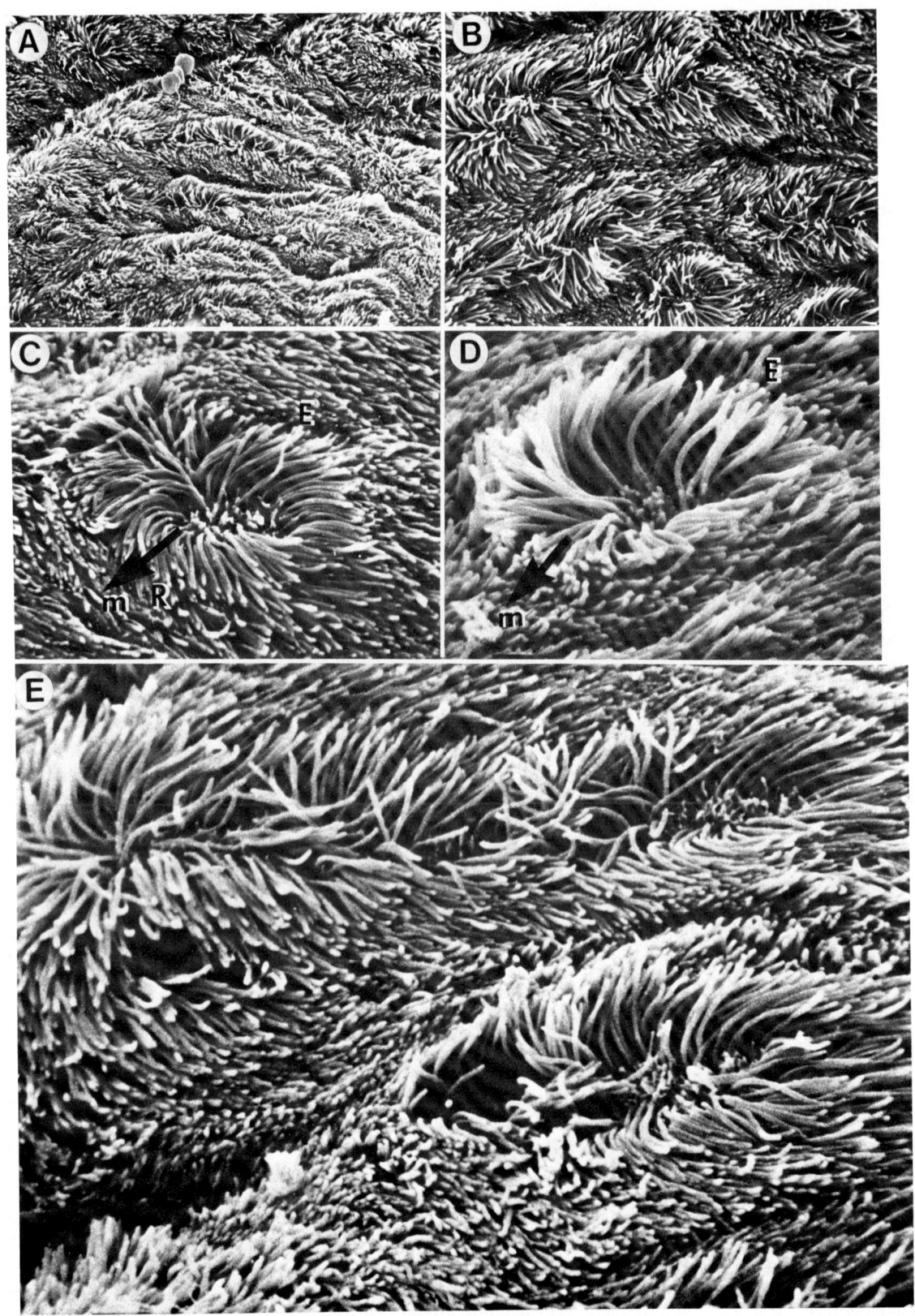

FIG. 12. Scanning electron micrographs of rabbit tracheal ciliated epithelia showing different areas of activity. *A, B*: numerous independent patches of activity that are restricted to areas at the crest of irregular surface undulations. *A*: × 600. *B*: × 1,200. *C, D*: higher magnification of individual areas of activity show resting cilia lying in position reached at end of previous effective stroke. In each patch of beating cilia various stages of the beat cycle surround a central hollow. Cilia at lower and left edges of formation are performing a recovery stroke (*R*) when viewed from above. Metachronal wave (*m*) that results moves toward the *bottom left* of the micrographs. Curved effective stroke (*E*) moves across the hollow from left to right. *C*: × 3,000. *D*: × 4,800. *E*: large areas of activity are seen in this figure. × 3,900. [From Sanderson and Sleigh (55).]

in 30 min by ciliary action. However, there are large individual variations in clearance rate, and a number of physiological factors, including sleep, age, and exercise, influence mucociliary transport. Environmental agents, such as tobacco smoke, carbon dust, and sulfur dioxide, and many pharmacological agents also affect mucociliary clearance (11). As indicated previously, normal mucociliary clearance depends on a number of interrelated factors, including an intact epithelium with coordinated functioning cilia, the composition and height of the periciliary layer, the optimal rheological properties of the mucus, and the right amount of mucus. Clearance is not a direct measure of ciliary activity. It involves complex physiological events, including autonomic nervous system control and mediation of muscle contraction, vascular permeability, and mucous and fluid secretion in the respiratory tract. Nerve endings penetrate into the respiratory epithelium and may influence all these processes. Many drugs also affect more than one process. Because of the heterogeneous nature of the respiratory epithelium and the variety of locations beneath the epithelium on which the nervous system can act, it has been very difficult to sort out unequivocally the effects of pharmacological agents, neurotransmitters, and other substances on the various components involved in clearance.

Another important influence on ciliary activity that is related to secretion and clearance is the active transport of ions across the respiratory epithelium. The net transport of ions, particularly Cl^-, is toward the periciliary layer (48). As a consequence of local osmotic gradients created by this transport, water crosses the epithelium and becomes part of the solution surrounding the cilia. Many drugs, including acetylcholine, epinephrine, histamine, prostaglandin, and aminophylline, increase net ion and water transport toward the airway lumen. Some of these substances also affect ciliary activity directly (80).

Effects of Sympathomimetic and Parasympathomimetic Drugs

In animal experiments, adrenergic agents such as epinephrine, isoproterenol, or β-adrenergic agonists that have predominantly β_2-activity stimulate overall mucociliary transport rates. They seem to be important in determining the composition of the periciliary layer by causing serous cells to secrete large volumes of fluid low in protein concentration and containing lysozyme. The β-adrenergic stimulation selectively depletes mucous cells so that only small amounts of fluid with a high protein concentration are produced. One effect of the β-adrenergic agonist isoproterenol is directly on the cilia. In monolayer cultures of respiratory epithelium, 10^{-7} M isoproterenol increases the frequency of ciliary beating; this effect is β-adrenergic specific because 10^{-7} M propranolol blocks the increase in frequency (77). A difficulty with laser-scattering spectroscopy used in this study and other methods used to measure changes in ciliary activity after drug application in explanted materials is that only one parameter, the frequency, is generally being measured. It would also be desirable to know the number of cilia that are beating and the nature of ciliary coordination.

Cholinergic agents stimulate ciliary activity directly (15). Stimulation by these agents depletes both mucous and serous cells, presumably affecting the composition of both mucus and the periciliary layer. Cholinergic antagonists such as atropine impair mucous transport. A direct action by these antagonists on ciliary activity has not been established.

Effect of Local Anesthetics

The local anesthetics have been shown to be cilioinhibitory, possibly due to a generalized ciliotoxic effect. In explants from punch biopsies of human tracheal or bronchial epithelium in tissue culture medium, a large number of local anesthetics with various concentrations (0.05% for dibucaine hydrochloride, 5% for lidocaine, 10% for cocaine) depressed ciliary activity (16). How local anesthetics exert this effect is speculative.

Relationship of Drug Effects to Axonemal Controls

Some effects of drugs on the ciliary beat—particularly the methylxanthines, serotonin, the prostaglandins, and the β-adrenergic agonists—are apt to be mediated via the adenyl cyclase–cAMP system. The hypothesis to account for this mediation stipulates that cyclase activity at the cell membrane is stimulated by the action of the drugs, resulting in an increase in the concentration of intracellular cAMP and stimulation of cAMP-dependent protein kinases; these kinases then phosphorylate specific proteins (76). An attractive feature of this hypothesis is that with the cilium a drug could interact with receptors both at the base of the ciliated cell and on the ciliary membrane itself. For example, the lateral cilia of the mussel gill are innervated at their bases and respond to the neurotransmitters serotonin or dopamine, applied either by nervous stimulation or exogenously in the bathing fluid (49). Axonemal proteins appear to be phosphorylated under certain conditions in some cilia, but the effect of phosphorylation of particular proteins on ciliary beat is still unsettled. Perhaps these proteins are the proteins of the switching mechanisms discussed previously (see *Sliding and Switching Mechanisms*, p. 484). It is also possible that Ca^{2+} and cAMP exert opposite effects on phosphorylation, because Ca^{2+}-calmodulin activates phosphodiesterase, which breaks down cAMP.

CILIARY DYSFUNCTION IN HUMANS

Based on the description of human ciliary mutants (2) the role of immotile cilia in causing human disease has become apparent. It has also become clear that ciliary dysfunction is not per se a fatal disease. The first mutants to be described had axonemes lacking dynein arms [see Fig. 14B; (3)]. Male patients with this structural abnormality were infertile because their sperm were immotile. It was natural to ask whether cilia other than sperm tails were affected. This proved to be true. Because of the absence of motile cilia, these individuals had had chronic infections of the upper and lower airways since childhood. Moreover ~50% of the first patients examined had situs inversus. The combination of situs inversus, bronchiectasis, and chronic sinusitis has been known for some time as Kartagener's syndrome (38). This syndrome is caused by a generalized ciliary structural defect rather than by immunological, secretory, or other causes. In addition it is evident why males with Kartagener's syndrome are also infertile.

Kartagener's triad is only one expression of the immotile cilia syndrome. Table 1 presents clinical data on 14 people (age 25–40) with the immotile cilia syndrome (2). The sine qua non of this syndrome is chronic bronchitis, rhinitis, and sinusitis, which develop early in life. There is no correlation between the occurrence of the syndrome and smoking or the inhalation of other environmental pollutants or respiratory irritants. All the males are sterile, whereas the females are not. The ability to bear children suggests that the motility of the oviduct cilia is not crucial for female fertility or for keeping the oviducts free from infection. However, because of the small number of women examined it is not known whether the syndrome is associated with reduced fertility. Otitis sometimes occurs as part of this syndrome, presumably because cilia line the eustachian tube. Situs inversus occurs in ~50% of these patients, regardless of sex.

Respiratory clearance is virtually absent in patients with immotile ciliary disease (Fig. 13). During 2 h, only ~8% of inhaled test particles are cleared from the tracheobronchial tract of these patients compared with an average 62% clearance for healthy subjects. In other disease states, such as environmentally induced chronic bronchitis, asthma, or cystic fibrosis, mucociliary clearance is impaired and coughing is the mechanism that removes material from the respiratory tract. In the immotile cilia syndrome, respiratory clearance is also accomplished by coughing. Coughing is a potent substitute for ciliary action because, as shown in Figure 13, 30% clearance is effected within a few minutes (12).

TABLE 1. *Clinical Data on 14 Persons With Immotile-Cilia Syndrome*

	Age	Bronchitis, Rhinitis, Sinusitis	Otitis	Situs Inversus	Sterility	Smoking
Male	37	+	+	+	+	−
	33	+	−	−	+	−
	32	+	−	+	+	+
	32	+	−	−	+	−
	41	+	+	−	+	Ex-smoker
	40	+	+	+	+	+
	25	+	−	+	+	+
	25	+	+	−	+	−
	31	+	−	−	+	−
	34	+	+	+	+	−
Female	28	+	+	+	[a]	−
	39	+	−	+	2 children	+
	32	+[b]	+	+	1 child	Ex-smoker
	27	+	+	+	[c]	+

[a] Patient has tried to become pregnant for 3.5 yr without success. [b] No clear evidence of sinusitis. [c] Has not tried to become pregnant. [Adapted from Afzelius (2).]

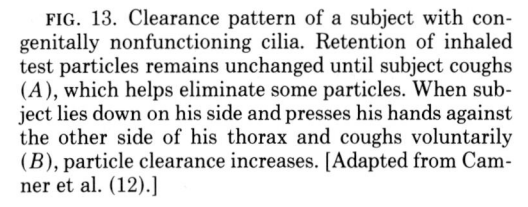

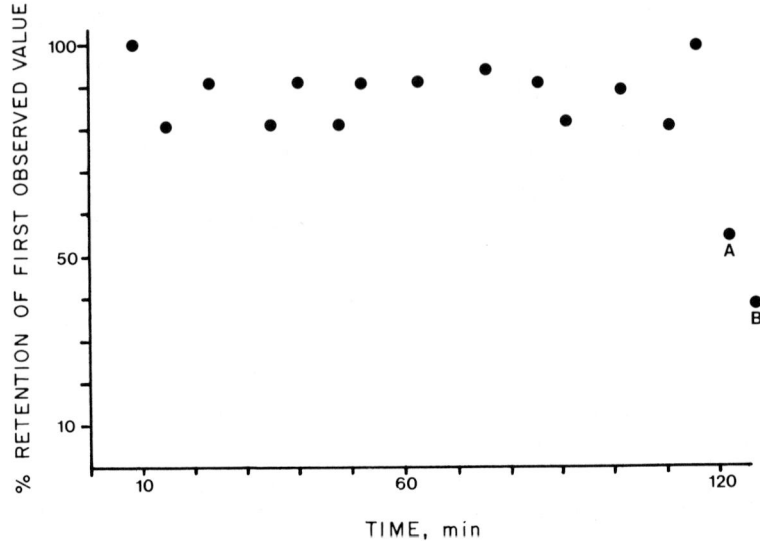

FIG. 13. Clearance pattern of a subject with congenitally nonfunctioning cilia. Retention of inhaled test particles remains unchanged until subject coughs (*A*), which helps eliminate some particles. When subject lies down on his side and presses his hands against the other side of his thorax and coughs voluntarily (*B*), particle clearance increases. [Adapted from Camner et al. (12).]

Genetic and Structural Implications

The immotile cilia syndrome has a familial basis; thus siblings are sometimes affected. The underlying defect in this syndrome appears to be one of a series of autosomal recessive mutations, because parents of children with the syndrome do not have a higher incidence of ciliary-based diseases than does the general population. Because there are so many structures comprising the axoneme and because they require multiple gene products for their correct assembly and function, it is not surprising that immotile cilia arise from a variety of mutations and therefore are genetically heterogeneous. As more families with the syndrome are diagnosed many different structural defects are being identified. In some affected individuals the cilia show transposition of a peripheral doublet to the center and a missing or defective central pair [Fig. 14D; (71)]. Individuals whose cilia lack radial spokes have also been described [Fig. 14C; (6, 72)]. As a result of these defects the cilia are immotile even though their dynein arms are apparently present. On other patients with immotile cilia, no structural abnormalities of the ciliary axoneme have been found. Sometimes the organization of the basal bodies seems abnormal and the basal feet point in many directions. However, because genetic effects are not necessarily structural, it is reasonable to expect that in some individuals with immotile cilia the structure of the cilia will be entirely normal.

The parallel between the immotile cilia syndrome in humans and ciliary mutants in the green alga *Chlamydomonas* is particularly striking. We have described above (see *Mutant Studies*, p. 483) the radial-spoke–central-sheath defect in *Chlamydomonas*. Other mutants that give rise to the paralyzed phenotype include dynein-arm mutants, central pair mutants, and developmentally abnormal mutants. Moreover it has proved relatively easy to relate the *Chlamydomonas* abnormalities to the molecular defects that interrupt the ciliary beat. Therefore the mechanisms responsible for the immotile cilia syndrome in humans probably are analogous to those that have been identified for this protistan cell. In *Chlamydomonas* several of the mutations that have been carefully analyzed involve a single or very few polypeptides. Alterations in a polypeptide can affect an entire pathway of assembly of an axonemal structure such as a radial spoke or dynein arm. Single-gene mutations appear to be sufficient to produce immotile cilia in humans.

This reasoning also strongly supports the idea that the details of the motility mechanism in human cilia are identical to those described for invertebrate and protistan cilia. Without dynein arms, immotility would presumably result because the interaction between dynein arms and the sliding of microtubules powers the human ciliary beat. The radial-spoke deficiency would cause immotility because of impairment of the radial-spoke–central-sheath interaction so that sliding would not be properly converted into bending.

We have noted (see MUCOCILIARY TRANSPORT, p. 485) there is an interplay of many factors in tracheobronchial clearance mechanisms. In some diseases, such as cystic fibrosis, ciliary beat may not per se be impaired. Certain environmental agents may produce chronic respiratory disease by acting on the ciliated cells over a period of time, changing beat characteristics, metachronal coordination, or the number of cilia that are beating. With the knowledge of the molecular mechanisms of ciliary activity obtained mainly from the extensive work on invertebrate and protistan cilia, it is now beginning to be possible to uncover the precise physiological role of cilia in respiration as well as in other bodily processes. The immotile cilia syndrome has allowed us to dissect the role that genetic and structural defects of cilia, rather than secretory malfunctions or environmental challenges, play in the development of respiratory disease (47a, 47b).

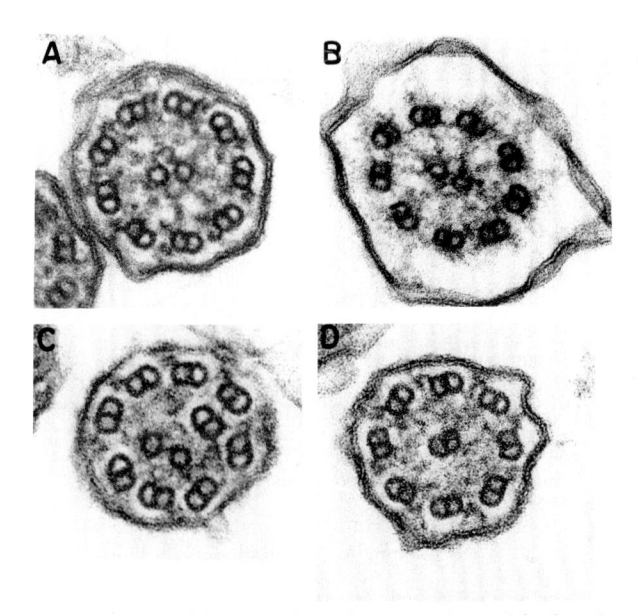

FIG. 14. *A*: normal human cilium from a patient with chronic bronchitis. × 122,000. *B*: human cilium from a patient whose cilia lack dynein arms. × 122,000. *C*: human cilium with radial spokes missing; central pair of single microtubules is eccentric and one of the outer doublets is displaced toward axoneme center. × 122,000. *D*: cross-section of a human cilium, transposition mutant. In the region of transposition, one of the outer doublets moves to the center. Central pair of microtubules is missing. × 130,000. (Courtesy of J. Sturgess.)

SUMMARY

The ultrastructure and mechanism of ciliary motility in humans and other organisms, such as simple protists and invertebrates, are quite similar wherever they have been studied. The mechanism of ciliary motility is based on doublet sliding, which is converted into propagated repetitive bending. Normal ciliary function depends on complex assembly processes to produce the axonemal structures responsible for sliding and bending. Dynein is a key element of the mechanochemical transducing system that generates the energy for axonemal function. The ciliary membrane is also an important component in the control of ciliary function by the cell and the organism, as it is the intermediary between the axoneme and the environment. Cations such as Ca^{2+} and metabolites such as cAMP are mediators of this control.

Mammalian cilia, like other cilia, beat with a metachronism that allows effective movement of the mucous blanket of the respiratory tract. In healthy individuals, ciliary activity accomplishes respiratory clearance. In the genetic diseases characterized by immotile cilia, clearance is impaired or is totally absent and coughing may substitute for ciliary action. Immotile human cilia are the result of a variety of mutations that often affect the correct assembly of axonemal structures such as the dynein arms or radial spokes. Therefore dissection of the genetic and environmental components of the mucociliary system is now possible. In the final analysis mucociliary clearance depends on factors such as the rheology and amount of mucus, the ionic composition of the periciliary layer, the integrity of the epithelium, the control by the autonomic nervous system, and ciliary action.

We thank our many colleagues (credited individually in the figure legends) for providing illustrations of their work. Drs. Michael Sanderson and Jennifer Sturgess also provided important counsel and discussion, particularly on the sections relating to their original findings and interpretations. We thank Stephen Lebduska and Michael Zeira for their considerable technical support and Christine Hubertus for help with the preparation of the manuscript.

This study was supported by National Institutes of Health Grants HL-22560 and HL-23428.

REFERENCES

1. ADOUTTE, A., R. RAMANATHAN, R. M. LEWIS, R. R. DUTE, K.-Y. LING, C. KUNG, AND D. L. NELSON. Biochemical studies of the excitable membrane of *Paramecium tetraurelia*. III. Proteins of cilia and ciliary membranes. *J. Cell Biol.* 84: 717–738, 1980.
2. AFZELIUS, B. A. The immotile-cilia syndrome and other ciliary diseases. *Int. Rev. Exp. Pathol.* 19: 1–43, 1979.
3. AFZELIUS, B. A., R. ELIASSON, O. JOHNSEN, AND C. LINDHOLMER. Lack of dynein arms in immotile human spermatozoa. *J. Cell Biol.* 66: 225–232, 1975.
4. AIELLO, E., AND M. A. SLEIGH. The metachronal wave of lateral cilia of *Mytilus edulis*. *J. Cell Biol.* 54: 493–506, 1972.
5. ANDERSON, R. G. W., AND C. HEIN. Distribution of anionic sites on the oviduct ciliary membrane. *J. Cell Biol.* 72: 482–492, 1977.
6. ANTONELLI, M., A. MODESTI, M. DE ANGELIS, P. MARCOLINI, N. LUCARELLI, AND S. CRIFO. Immotile cilia syndrome: radial spokes deficiency in a patient with Kartagener's triad. *Acta Paediatr. Scand.* 70: 571–573, 1981.
7. BACCETTI, B., A. G. BURRINI, V. PALLINI, AND T. RENIERI. Human dynein and sperm pathology. *J. Cell Biol.* 88: 102–107, 1981.
8. BELL, C. W., E. FRONK, AND I. R. GIBBONS. Polypeptide subunits of dynein 1 from sea urchin sperm flagella. *J. Supramol. Struct.* 11: 311–317, 1979.
9. BLAKE, J. R., AND M. A. SLEIGH. Hydromechanical aspects of ciliary propulsion. In: *Swimming and Flying in Nature*, edited by T. Y. Wu, C. J. Brokaw, and C. Brennen. New York: Plenum, 1975, p. 185–210.
10. BROKAW, C. J. Elastase digestion of demembranated sperm flagella. *Science* 207: 1365–1367, 1980.
11. CAMNER, P. Clearance of particles from the human tracheobronchial tree. *Clin. Sci.* 59: 79–84, 1980.
12. CAMNER, P., B. MOSSBERG, AND B. A. AFZELIUS. Evidence of congenitally nonfunctioning cilia in the tracheobronchial tract in two subjects. *Am. Rev. Respir. Dis.* 112: 807–809, 1975.
13. CARSON, J. L., A. M. COLLIER, AND W. A. CLYDE, JR. Ciliary membrane alterations occurring in experimental *Mycoplasma pneumoniae* infection. *Science* 206: 349–351, 1979.
14. CHEUNG, W. Y. Calmodulin plays a pivotal role in cellular recognition. *Science* 207: 19–27, 1980.
15. CORSSEN, G., AND C. R. ALLEN. Acetylcholine: its significance in controlling ciliary activity of human respiratory epithelium in vitro. *J. Appl. Physiol.* 14: 901–904, 1959.
16. CORSSEN, G., AND C. R. ALLEN. Cultured human respiratory epithelium: its use in the comparison of the cytotoxic properties of local anesthetics. *Anesthesiology* 21: 237–243, 1960.
17. DENTLER, W. L. Microtubule-membrane interactions in cilia and flagella. *Int. Rev. Cytol.* 72: 1–47, 1981.
18. DIRKSEN, E. R. Centriole morphogenesis in developing ciliated epithelium of the mouse oviduct. *J. Cell Biol.* 51: 286–302, 1971.
19. DIRKSEN, E. R. Ciliogenesis in the mouse oviduct: a scanning electron microscope study. *J. Cell Biol.* 62: 899–904, 1974.
20. DIRKSEN, E. R. Assembly of the microtubular organelles, centrioles and cilia. In: *Cell Reproduction*, edited by E. R. Dirksen, D. Prescott, and C. F. Fox. New York: Academic, 1978, p. 315–336.
21. DIRKSEN, E. R., AND T. T. CROCKER. Centriole replication in differentiating ciliated cells of mammalian respiratory epithelium: an electron microscopic study. *J. Microsc.* 5: 629–656, 1965.
22. DIRKSEN, E. R., AND T. T. CROCKER. Ultrastructural alterations produced by polycyclic aromatic hydrocarbons on rat tracheal epithelium in organ culture. *Cancer Res.* 28: 906–923, 1968.
23. DIRKSEN, E. R., AND P. SATIR. Ciliary activity in the mouse oviduct as studied by transmission and scanning electron microscopy. *Tissue Cell* 4: 389–404, 1972.
24. DIRKSEN, E. R., AND M. ZEIRA. Microtubule sliding in cilia of the rabbit trachea and oviduct. *Cell Motil.* 1: 247–260, 1981.
25. FAWCETT, D. W., AND K. R. PORTER. A study of the fine structure of ciliated epithelia. *J. Morphol.* 94: 221–281, 1954.
26. FLAVIN, M., T. MARTENSEN, J. NATH, AND T. KOBAYASHI. Inhibition of dynein ATPase by vanadate, and its possible use as a probe for the role of dynein in cytoplasmic motility. *Biochem. Biophys. Res. Commun.* 81: 1313–1318, 1978.
27. FREEDMAN, R. I., M. ZEIRA, AND E. ROTER DIRKSEN. Some aspects of the regulation of ciliary activity in mammalian somatic cells. *J. Submicrosc. Cytol.* 15: 97–100, 1983.
28. GIBBONS, B. H., AND I. R. GIBBONS. The effect of partial extraction of dynein arms on the movement of reactivated sea-urchin sperm. *J. Cell Sci.* 13: 337–357, 1973.
29. GIBBONS, I. R. Studies on the adenosine triphosphatase activity of 14S and 30S dynein from cilia of *Tetrahymena*. *J. Biol. Chem.* 241: 5590–5596, 1966.
30. GIBBONS, I. R., M. P. COSSON, J. A. EVANS, B. H. GIBBONS, B. HOUCK, K. H. MARTINSON, W. S. SALE, AND W.-J. Y. TANG. Potent inhibition of dynein adenosinetriphosphatase and of the motility of cilia and sperm flagella by vanadate. *Proc. Natl. Acad. Sci. USA* 75: 2220–2224, 1978.

31. GILULA, N. B., AND P. SATIR. The ciliary necklace. A ciliary membrane specialization. *J. Cell Biol.* 53: 494–509, 1972.
32. GOODENOUGH, U. W., AND J. E. HEUSER. Substructure of the outer dynein arm. *J. Cell Biol.* 95: 798–815, 1982.
33. GRAY, J. *Ciliary Movement.* London: Cambridge Univ. Press, 1928.
34. HOLWILL, M. E. J., H. J. COHEN, AND P. SATIR. A sliding microtubule model incorporating axonemal twist and compatible with three-dimensional ciliary bending. *J. Exp. Biol.* 78: 265–280, 1979.
35. IRAVANI, J., AND G. N. MELVILLE. Mucociliary function in the respiratory tract as influenced by physicochemical factors. *Pharmacol. Ther.* 2: 471–492, 1976.
36. IRAVANI, J., AND A. VAN AS. Mucus transport in the tracheobronchial tree of normal and bronchitic rats. *J. Pathol.* 106: 81–93, 1972.
37. JOHNSON, K. A., AND J. S. WALL. Structural and mass analysis of dynein by scanning transmission electron microscopy. *J. Submicrosc. Cytol.* 15: 181–186, 1983.
38. KARTAGENER, M. Zur Pathogenese der Bronchiektasien: Bronchiektasien bei Situs viscerum inversus. *Beitr. Klin. Tuberk. Spezifischen Tuberk. Forsch.* 83: 489–501, 1933.
39. KUHN, C., AND W. ENGLEMAN. The structure of the tips of mammalian respiratory cilia. *Cell Tissue Res.* 186: 491–498, 1978.
40. LUCAS, A. M., AND L. C. DOUGLAS. Principles underlying ciliary activity in the respiratory tract. II. A comparison of nasal clearance in man, monkey and other mammals. *Arch. Otolaryngol.* 20: 518–541, 1934.
41. LUCHTEL, D. Extracellular lining layer of pulmonary airways. In: *Mechanism and Control of Ciliary Movement*, edited by C. Brokaw and P. Verdugo. New York: Liss, 1982, p. 77–81.
42. LUCK, D. J. L., B. HUANG, AND C. J. BROKAW. A regulatory mechanism for flagellar function is revealed by suppressor analysis in *Chlamydomonas*. In: *Mechanism and Control of Ciliary Movement*, edited by C. Brokaw and P. Verdugo. New York: Liss, 1982, p. 159–164.
43. MAIHLE, N. J., J. R. DEDMAN, A. R. MEANS, J. G. CHAFOULAS, AND B. H. SATIR. Presence and indirect immunofluorescent localization of calmodulin in *Paramecium tetraurelia*. *J. Cell Biol.* 89: 695–699, 1981.
44. MARINO, M. M., AND E. AIELLO. Cinemicrographic analysis of beat dynamics of human respiratory cilia. In: *Mechanism and Control of Ciliary Movement*, edited by C. Brokaw and P. Verdugo. New York: Liss, 1982, p. 35–40.
45. MEANS, A. R., AND J. DEDMAN. Calmodulin—an intracellular calcium receptor. *Nature London* 285: 73–77, 1980.
46. MENCO, B. P. M. Qualitative and quantitative freeze-fracture studies on olfactory and respiratory epithelial surfaces of frog, ox, rat, and dog. IV. Ciliogenesis and ciliary necklaces (including high-voltage observations). *Cell Tissue Res.* 212: 1–16, 1980.
47. MERKEL, S. J., E. S. KANESHIRO, AND E. I. GRUENSTEIN. Characterization of the cilia and ciliary membrane proteins of wild-type *Paramecium tetraurelia* and a pawn mutant. *J. Cell Biol.* 89: 206–215, 1981.
47a. MYGIND, N., M. H. NIELSEN, AND M. PEDERSEN (editors). Kartagener's syndrome and abnormal cilia. *Eur. J. Respir. Dis. Suppl.* 127: 1–167, 1983.
47b. MYGIND, N., F. V. RASMUSSEN, AND F. MOLGAARD (editors). Cellular and neurogenic mechanisms in nose and bronchi. *Eur. J. Respir. Dis. Suppl.* 128, pts. 1 and 2: 1–557, 1983.
48. NADEL, J. A., B. DAVIS, AND R. J. PHIPPS. Control of mucous secretion and ion transport in airways. *Annu. Rev. Physiol.* 41: 369–381, 1979.
49. PAPARO, A., M. D. HAMBURG, AND E. H. COLE. Catecholamine influence on unit activity of the visceral ganglion of the mussel *Mytilus edulis*, and the control of ciliary movement—I. *Comp. Biochem. Physiol. C* 51: 35–40, 1975.
50. PIPERNO, G., B. HUANG, AND D. L. LUCK. Two dimensional analysis of flagellar proteins from wild type and paralyzed mutants of *Chlamydomonas reinhardtii*. *Proc. Natl. Acad. Sci. USA* 74: 2045–2050, 1977.

51. PROCTOR, D. F. Historical background. In: *Lung Biology in Health and Disease. Respiratory Defense Mechanisms*, edited by J. D. Brain, D. F. Proctor, and L. M. Reid. New York: Dekker, 1977, vol. 5, pt. I, chapt. 1, p. 3–24.
52. RHODIN, J. A. G. Ultrastructure and function of the human tracheal mucosa. *Am. Rev. Respir. Dis.* 93: 1–15, 1966.
53. ROBERTS, K., AND J. S. HYAMS (editors). *Microtubules.* New York: Academic, 1981, 595 p.
54. SALE, W. S., AND P. SATIR. Direction of active sliding of microtubules in *Tetrahymena* cilia. *Proc. Natl. Acad. Sci. USA* 74: 2045–2049, 1977.
55. SANDERSON, M. J., AND M. A. SLEIGH. Ciliary activity of cultured rabbit tracheal epithelium: beat pattern and metachrony. *J. Cell Sci.* 47: 331–347, 1981.
56. SANDERSON, M. J., AND M. A. SLEIGH. The function of respiratory tract cilia. In: *The Lung and Its Environment*, edited by G. Bonsignore and G. Cumming. New York: Plenum, 1982, p. 81–120.
57. SANDOZ, D., E. BOISVIEUX-ULRICH, AND B. CHAILLY. Relationships between intramembrane particles and glycoconjugates in the ciliary membrane of the quail oviduct. *Biol. Cell.* 36: 267–280, 1979.
58. SATIR, B., W. S. SALE, AND P. SATIR. Membrane renewal after dibucaine deciliation of *Tetrahymena*. Freeze-fracture technique, cilia, membrane structure. *Exp. Cell Res.* 97: 83–91, 1976.
59. SATIR, P. Studies on cilia. II. Examination of the distal region of the ciliary shaft and the role of the filaments in motility. *J. Cell Biol.* 26: 805–834, 1965.
60. SATIR, P. Studies on cilia. III. Further studies on the cilium tip and a "sliding filament" model of ciliary motility. *J. Cell Biol.* 39: 77–94, 1968.
60a. SATIR, P. How cilia move. *Sci. Am.* 231: 44–52, 1974.
61. SATIR, P. Production and arrest of ciliary motility. In: *Contractile Systems in Non-Muscle Tissues: Proceedings*, edited by S. V. Perry, A. Margreth, and R. S. Adelstein. Amsterdam: Elsevier/North-Holland, 1976, p. 263–273.
62. SATIR, P. Microvilli and cilia: surface specializations of mammalian cells. In: *Mammalian Cell Membranes. The Diversity of Membranes*, edited by G. A. Jamieson and D. M. Robinson. London: Butterworths, 1977, vol. 2, p. 323–357.
63. SATIR, P. Structural basis of ciliary movement. *Environ. Health Perspect.* 35: 77–82, 1980.
64. SATIR, P. Mechanisms and controls of ciliary motility. In: *Prokaryotic and Eukaryotic Flagella*, edited by W. B. Amos and J. G. Duckett. Cambridge, UK: Cambridge Univ. Press, 1982, p. 179–201.
65. SATIR, P., AND W. S. SALE. Tails of *Tetrahymena*. *J. Protozool.* 24: 498–501, 1977.
66. SATIR, P., J. WAIS-STEIDER, S. LEBDUSKA, A. NASR, AND J. AVOLIO. The mechanochemical cycle of the dynein arm. *Cell Motil.* 1: 303–327, 1981.
67. SHINGYOJI, C., A. MURAKAMI, AND K. TAKAHASHI. Local reactivation of Triton-extracted flagella by iontophoretic application of ATP. *Nature London* 265: 269–270, 1977.
68. SILBERBERG, A. Rheology of mucus, mucociliary interaction and ciliary activity. In: *Mechanism and Control of Ciliary Movement*, edited by C. Brokaw and P. Verdugo. New York: Liss, 1982, p. 25–28.
69. SILVESTER, N. R. The cilia of *Tetrahymena pyriformis*: X-ray diffraction by the ciliary membrane. *J. Mol. Biol.* 8: 11–19, 1964.
70. STURGESS, J. M. The mucous lining of major bronchi in the rabbit lung. *Am. Rev. Respir. Dis.* 115: 819–827, 1977.
71. STURGESS, J. M., J. CHAO, AND J. A. P. TURNER. Transposition of ciliary microtubules. *N. Engl. J. Med.* 303: 318–322, 1980.
72. STURGESS, J. M., J. CHAO, J. WONG, N. ASPIN, AND J. A. P. TURNER. Cilia with defective radial spokes: a cause of human respiratory disease. *N. Engl. J. Med.* 300: 53–56, 1979.
73. SUMMERS, K. E., AND I. R. GIBBONS. Adenosine triphosphate-induced sliding of tubules in trypsin-treated flagella of sea-urchin sperm. *Proc. Natl. Acad. Sci. USA* 68: 3092–3096, 1971.
74. SUMMERS, K. E., AND I. R. GIBBONS. Effects of trypsin digestion on flagellar structures and their relationship to motility. *J.*

Cell Biol. 58: 618–629, 1973.
75. TAKAHASHI, M., AND Y. TONOMURA. Binding of 30S dynein with the B-tubule of the outer doublet of axonemes from *Tetrahymena pyriformis* and the adenosine triphosphate-induced dissociation of the complex. *J. Biochem. Tokyo* 84: 1339–1355, 1978.
76. TASH, J. S., AND A. R. MEANS. Regulation of protein phosphorylation and motility of sperm flagella by cAMP and calcium (Abstract). *J. Cell Biol.* 91: 335a, 1981.
77. VERDUGO, P., N. T. JOHNSON, AND P. Y. TAM. β-Adrenergic stimulation of respiratory ciliary activity. *J. Appl. Physiol.: Respirat. Environ. Exercise Physiol.* 48: 868–871, 1980.
78. WAIS-STEIDER, J., AND P. SATIR. Effect of vanadate on gill cilia: switching mechanism in ciliary beat. *J. Supramol. Struct.* 11: 339–347, 1979.
79. WALTER, M. F., AND P. SATIR. Calcium control of ciliary arrest in mussel gill cells. *J. Cell Biol.* 79: 110–120, 1978.
80. WANNER, A. State of the art. Clinical aspects of mucociliary transport. *Am. Rev. Respir. Dis.* 116: 73–125, 1977.
81. WARNER, F. D., AND D. R. MITCHELL. Dynein: the mechanochemical coupling adenosine triphosphatase of microtubule-based sliding filament mechanisms. *Int. Rev. Cytol.* 66: 1–43, 1980.
82. WARNER, F. D., AND P. SATIR. The structural basis of ciliary bend formation. *J. Cell Biol.* 63: 35–63, 1974.
83. YANO, Y., AND T. MIKI-NOUMURA. Recovery of sliding ability in arm-depleted flagellar axonemes after recombination with extracted dynein 1. *J. Cell Sci.* 48: 223–235, 1981.

CHAPTER 16

Blood coagulation and fibrinolysis

ROBERT W. COLMAN
ANDREI Z. BUDZYNSKI

Thrombosis Research Center, Temple University School of Medicine, Philadelphia, Pennsylvania

CHAPTER CONTENTS

Congenital Deficiencies in Initiation of Blood Coagulation
    Factor XII
    Plasma prekallikrein
    Plasma kininogens
    Interaction of contact-system proteins
    Factor XI
    Factor IX
    Factor VIII
Relationship of Intrinsic and Extrinsic Blood Coagulation
    Factor X
    Factor VII
    Thromboplastin
Regulation of Prothrombin Activation
    Prothrombin
    Factor V
    Coagulant phospholipid surfaces
    Calcium ions
    Thrombin formation
    Thrombin specificity
    Regulation of thrombin activity
    Heparin and antithrombin III
    Interaction of thrombin with fibrin
    Nonmammalian inhibitors of thrombin
    Thrombinlike enzymes in snake venoms
Electron Microscopy of Fibrinogen
Fibrinogen Structure
    Model of fibrinogen molecule
    Conversion of fibrinogen to fibrin clot
    Polymerization sites
    Cross-linking of fibrin
Interaction of Fibrinogen with Plasma Proteins
Interaction of Fibrinogen with Cells
Degradation by Proteases Other than Plasmin
Degradation of Fibrinogen and Fibrin by Plasmin
    Role of fibrin in clot formation and lysis
Plasminogen and Plasmin
    Plasminogen activators
    Inhibitors of plasminogen and plasmin
    Physiological fibrinolysis

BLOOD NORMALLY CIRCULATES through endothelium-lined vessels without coagulation, platelet activation, or appreciable hemorrhage. Injury to the vessels triggers the hemostatic process. Platelets adhere to damaged endothelium or exposed subendothelium and change shape preparatory to aggregation and secretion of intracellular contents. At the same time plasma proteins react with the subendothelium, resulting in activation of the contact phase of coagulation. Investigators have studied blood coagulation reactions in vitro because it is difficult to reduce this complex reaction to its component parts in vivo. A formidable body of knowledge has accumulated; this chapter presents the highlights. The chapter by Ross and Schwartz in this *Handbook* deals with platelets and vessels and is complementary.

A major paradox that has baffled investigators and clinicians is that the events that appear to initiate coagulation in vitro may not be the same as those involved in in vivo hemostasis. Researchers have recently made important advances in the study of proteins involved in the early response to foreign surfaces (56, 250, 369, 594). It is now known that three proteins are involved in the initiating steps of the intrinsic pathway: Hageman factor, prekallikrein, and high-molecular-weight (HMW) kininogen. Lack of any one of these three proteins results in slow generation of thrombin and a prolonged in vitro clotting time or partial thromboplastin time. Nevertheless a deficiency of any of these three proteins does not lead to a defect in hemostasis. In contrast a disorder in other factors that lie further along the intrinsic pathway of blood coagulation (e.g., factors XI, VIII, IX) is associated with a similar prolongation of the clotting time or partial thromboplastin time, resulting in a bleeding diathesis (537). Although they are not well defined, alternative pathways to the activation of factor XI must exist.

CONGENITAL DEFICIENCIES IN INITIATION OF BLOOD COAGULATION

The in vitro system has been investigated by experiments with plasma from individuals deficient in specific clotting factors and with purified coagulation proteins. Ratnoff and Colopy (538) identified a patient (whose surname, Hageman, is the eponym for factor XII) who had a markedly prolonged partial thromboplastin time and lacked a plasma factor that bound to surfaces and was active at the initiating step of the coagulation cascade (540). Plasma deficient in Hageman factor was subsequently shown to possess a profound abnormality of surface-dependent fibrinolysis (255) and did not generate bradykinin on incubation with glass beads or kaolin (370–372, 374). In 1965 Hathaway et al. (223) described a coagulation defect characterized by a prolonged activated partial thromboplastin time in a family named Fletcher. Increasing the incubation time with the activating surface corrected the defect (223, 224), suggesting that the defect resulted in an abnormal rate of contact activation. Wuepper (693) subsequently identified the protein missing in Fletcher plasma as prekallikrein. Fletcher plasma displays abnormal surface-activated kinin formation and fibrinolysis, which purified human prekallikrein corrects (672, 695). Thus prekallikrein is an important determinant of the rate of Hageman factor activation but an absolute requirement for kinin generation (568), because kallikrein is the plasma enzyme that digests kininogen to generate bradykinin (107, 667).

Extensive studies on the interaction of Hageman factor and prekallikrein in the initiation of plasma proteolysis appeared to have reached a consensus by 1974 (107). However, evidence soon suggested that an additional plasma cofactor is required for both Hageman factor activation and expression of activity (581, 669). Later studies confirmed that HMW kininogen corrected the deficient activation of prekallikrein (669) and the defective activation of factor XI (582) in purified systems. Asymptomatic individuals were discovered [e.g., Williams (108), Fitzgerald (571), and Flaujeac (305)] who had prolonged activated partial thromboplastin time, decreased surface-activated fibrinolysis, grossly defective prekallikrein activation, and absent kinin formation (108, 130, 305, 571). Purified HMW kininogen corrected all the defects in Williams and Flaujeac plasma. Williams plasma was completely devoid of functional or antigenic kininogen (108). Fitzgerald plasma (657) had 50% of the normal concentration of low-molecular-weight (LMW) kininogen but no detectable HMW kininogen; Flaujeac plasma had 8% of the normal plasma kininogen (130, 305). Abnormal coagulation tests, fibrinolysis, and kinin generation were the hallmark of each deficient plasma.

Factor XII

Hageman factor (factor XII) is a single-chain polypeptide of β-globulin mobility (Fig. 1). Its molecular weight is 85,000 and the isoelectric point for human Hageman factor is between 6.1 and 6.5; however, considerable charge heterogeneity was observed with a pH range of 5.9–7.0 (98). In plasma the concentration of factor XII by quantitative radial immunodiffusion has been estimated to be 29 μg/ml (15–47 μl/ml) (550). This level has been confirmed by radioimmunoassay (570). Traditionally factor XII can be assayed on a functional basis by a modification of the partial thromboplastin time (527) with Hageman factor–de-

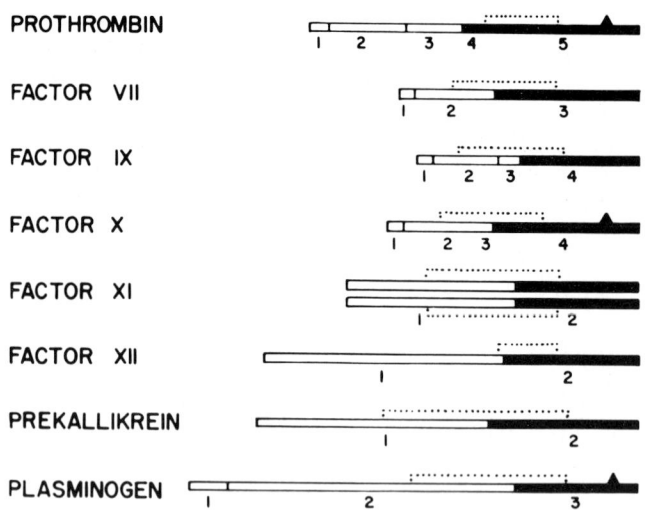

FIG. 1. Stick models of zymogens involved in coagulation, kinin formation, and fibrinolysis. *Dark bars*, polypeptide chain containing the active-site serine. *Dotted lines*, 1 or more disulfide bridges. Numbers, zymogen domains, in most cases defined by sites of proteolytic cleavage. Bar size is roughly proportional to molecular weight. *Dark triangles*, location of active serine residue. Domain 1 of prothrombin, factor VII, IX, and X contains the Gla residues responsible for Ca^{2+} binding and thus phospholipid attachment. Domain 1 in factor XI, XII, and prekallikrein represents the heavy chain, probably the site of attachment to negatively charged surfaces. Domain 1 in plasminogen represents the peptide cleaved by plasmin to convert Glu-plasminogen to Lys-plasminogen. Domain 3 of prothrombin is the factor V–binding site and is cleaved from domain 2 by thrombin. In factors IX and X, bonds between domain 2 and 3 are cleaved during zymogen activation. In prothrombin, cleavage between dark and light halves of the molecule by factor Xa is not sufficient to form thrombin but does remove prothrombin from its phospholipid attachment. Cleavage between domain 4 and 5 to form 2-chain thrombin forms the active enzyme. In all other cases zymogen conversion to enzyme occurs by cleavage between dark and light portions to form 2 polypeptide chains connected by disulfide bridges. Only factor XI exists as a dimer; thus factor XIa has 2 identical active sites. [From Jackson and Nemerson (262a). Reproduced with permission from the *Annual Review of Biochemistry*, vol. 49, © 1980 by Annual Reviews Inc.]

ficient plasma as the substrate. Ratnoff and Saito (541) used chromogenic substrates of a synthetic peptide to assay activated Hageman factor. Hageman factor protein can be assayed immunologically with monospecific antisera (550, 570). However, immunologic assays do not yield information on the activation state of Hageman factor.

Contact with negatively charged surfaces or addition of a protease that produces enzymatic cleavage can activate factor XII. These two mechanisms have been referred to as surface and fluid-phase activation (541). Nonphysiological substances with negative surface charge that activate factor XII include glass, kaolin, celite, dextran sulfate, and ellagic acid (535); biological components include articular cartilage, crude collagen preparations (536), skin (462), fatty acids (125, 371), calcium pyrophosphate and urate (282), and L-homocysteine (536). The physiological activator may be present in the subendothelial vascular basement membrane (218); however, the exact component of connective tissue responsible for factor XII activation is unknown. Early studies showed that Hageman factor was activated by merely binding to the negatively charged surface. The binding or consequences thereof allowed some conformational change in the molecule, which exposed an active site (541). The finding of increased hydrophobicity (159) and a change in the circular dichroism spectrum (400) supports the occurrence of conformational changes in surface-bound Hageman factor. Autoactivation or the presence of trace quantities of proteolytic enzymes could also explain the evidence that binding of Hageman factor to a negatively charged surface alone without proteolytic cleavage is sufficient to fully activate the molecule. Optimal activation may also require limited proteolytic cleavage. Initial cleavage leads to a two-chain form of activated factor XII (factor XIIa) still linked by disulfide bridges, which remains bound to the surface and exhibits potent coagulant activity. Additional proteolysis leads to a second form of activated Hageman factor (factor XIIf), which has a molecular weight of 28,000 and has lost its coagulant activity because of the cleavage of the 52,000-M_r polypeptide that had attached it to the surface. The enzyme factor XIIf in the fluid phase is a potent activator of prekallikrein.

One of the major inhibitors of activated Hageman factor (167) and Hageman factor fragments (585) is the inhibitor of the activated first component of complement (C$\overline{1}$-INH). Molecular weights and plasma concentration of clotting-factor inhibitors are shown in Table 1. Antithrombin III also binds and inactivates Hageman factor fragments, although the inactivation observed appeared much slower than that obtained with comparable concentrations of C$\overline{1}$-INH (615). Heparin appeared to accelerate the binding and inactivation of Hageman factor by antithrombin III in purified systems, but suprapharmacological concentrations are required and the effect is not significant in plasma.

Impaired synthesis in liver disease decreases factor XII. Hageman factor is also mildly diminished in states in which activation of the intrinsic system occurs, such as hypotensive septicemia, hyperacute renal allograft rejection, and nephrotic syndrome. In these situations the cause of the decrease in factor XII levels is not known but may be due to clearance in vivo or combination with protease inhibitors after conversion to an activated enzyme.

Plasma Prekallikrein

Plasma prekallikrein circulates in the blood as a single-chain precursor (Fig. 1) with a molecular weight of 88,000 (355, 589). However, only 25% exists as free prekallikrein (587) because approximately 75% circulates bound to HMW kininogen (354). Prekallikrein has an isoelectric point of 8.5–9.0 and the mobility of

TABLE 1. *Plasma Concentration of Coagulation and Fibrinolytic Inhibitors*

Inhibitor	M_r	mg/100 ml	µM
Antithrombin III	65,000	29 ± 2.9	4.5
α_2-Macroglobulin	725,000	260 ± 70	3.6
C1-esterase inactivator	104,000	23 ± 3.0	2.3
α_1-Protease inhibitor	54,000	290 ± 45	54.0
Inter-α-antitrypsin	169,000	50 ± 2.5	3.0
α_1-Antichymotrypsin	69,000	49 ± 6.5	7.0
α_2-Antiplasmin	70,000	7 ± 1.5	1.0
Histidine-rich glycoprotein	60,000	9 ± 4.5	1.5

a fast γ-globulin. The conversion of prekallikrein to kallikrein can be catalyzed by factor XIIa or XIIf with the cleavage of a single peptide bond, which forms a 55,000-M_r heavy chain (355) that is still attached by disulfide bonds to a 32,000-M_r chain in the case of factor XIIa. The light chain contains the active-site serine. Kallikrein can then cleave at least four substrates in plasma: factor XII (20, 97), plasminogen (103), HMW kininogen (265, 266), and prorenin (477, 590). When purified kallikrein is added to plasma it is rapidly inactivated to an equal extent by two plasma protease inhibitors: α_2-macroglobulin inhibits the kinin-forming activity of kallikrein but only partially inhibits its esterolytic activity (220) and its amidolytic activity (578) by forming a covalent complex with kallikrein (220); C$\overline{1}$-INH (192) forms a 1:1 stoichiometric complex with kallikrein (577) such that both its proteolytic and amidolytic activity are inhibited. Antithrombin III also inhibits kallikrein but is slow even in the presence of heparin (306). The α_2-antiplasmin (567) and α_1-protease inhibitors (176, 578) are also inefficient inhibitors.

When prekallikrein is activated because of pathophysiological changes in human disease, the conversion of prekallikrein to kallikrein decreases the concentration of prekallikrein as measured by enzymatic or coagulant assays. The kallikrein formed combines rapidly with its plasma inhibitors, leading to the inactivation of kallikrein and a reduction in plasma inhibitory activity. The resulting complexes may circulate (109) and are detectable antigenically with antibodies directly against either C$\overline{1}$-INH or kallikrein. Thus, although the functional level may decrease, the antigenic levels are unchanged. Colman et al. (109) documented such a sequence of events in typhoid fever: the decrease in prekallikrein or kallikrein inhibitory activity and appearance of enzyme-inhibitor complexes parallel the fever and positive blood cultures that appear in the acute phase of the disease. Activation of prekallikrein and decrease of plasma kallikrein inhibitory activity have also been described in hypotensive septicemia, hyperacute renal allograft rejection, nephrotic syndrome, and myocardial ischemia. In addition an isolated decrease of prekallikrein presumably due to decreased hepatic synthesis with normal levels of kallikrein inhibitory activity occurs in cirrhosis and dengue fever. Colman (107a) recently reviewed the prekallikrein changes in congenital and acquired diseases.

Plasma Kininogens

The kininogens are substrates in plasma from which vasoactive peptides such as bradykinin, lysylbradykinin, and other kinins are released. The kininogenases are kinin-forming enzymes that are derived from plasma (kallikrein, plasmin) or glandular tissue (salivary glands, pancreas, kidney). Jacobsen and Kriz (265, 266) described two different forms of purified human kininogens (I and II) and showed that there is an HMW kininogen that is rapidly cleaved by plasma kallikrein and an LMW kininogen that is more readily cleaved by a tissue kallikrein. The discovery of plasma deficient in all kininogen (108) or HMW kininogen (571, 657) demonstrated that two forms of kininogen do exist in native plasma.

Purified HMW kininogen migrates as an α-globulin with an isoelectric point of 4.3 and occurs as a single polypeptide chain with a molecular weight of 120,000 (212). In plasma the concentration is 80 μg/ml or 20% of the total kininogen. In human plasma, LMW kininogen (240 μg/ml) is a single polypeptide chain with a molecular weight of 52,000 on sodium dodecyl sulfate (SDS)–polyacrylamide gel electrophoresis (212). Its isoelectric point is 4.7 and it migrates as a β_1-globulin. Both kininogens are glycoproteins. Human plasma kallikrein has been shown to cleave HMW kininogen to release bradykinin (512), forming a two-chain, disulfide-linked molecule containing a heavy chain with an apparent molecular weight of 65,000 and a light chain with an apparent molecular weight of 44,000 (284). In human and bovine kininogens the light chain possesses the major antigenic determinants that distinguish HMW from LMW kininogen (283, 292, 385) and the coagulant activity site (642). The light chain of HMW kininogen is also responsible for the complex formed with kallikrein (111, 576, 578).

Interaction of Contact-System Proteins

Although the binding of Hageman factor to a negatively charged surface may allow activation of Hageman factor by conformational changes or by autoactivation, the enzyme in plasma primarily responsible for cleavage and activation of human Hageman factor is plasma kallikrein. Thus in prekallikrein-deficient plasma the binding of Hageman factor to the surface occurred normally, but the cleavage and presumably activation was retarded compared to normal plasma (549). Because Hageman factor and prekallikrein render each other active by specific limited proteolytic cleavage, Cochrane et al. (97) proposed a theory of reciprocal activation in which Hageman factor and prekallikrein interact and become active. This concept appears to apply to both the fluid and solid (surface-bound) phase (97, 206, 549). The initial event(s) that triggers cleavage or activation of either Hageman factor or prekallikrein is not known. The presence of HMW kininogen is critical for the rate of factor XII activation. For a fixed quantity of surface-bound Hageman factor, the subsequent activation of prekallikrein appeared proportional to the quantity of HMW kininogen added (206, 207, 339, 401, 681). However, there appears to be an optimal concentration of HMW kininogen, and excess HMW kininogen is inhibitory (207, 339, 401).

The fact that prekallikrein circulates in a complex with HMW kininogen (354, 587) helps us understand the role of HMW kininogen in prekallikrein activation (Fig. 2). The main effect of HMW kininogen in prekallikrein activation is to place this Hageman factor substrate on the surface in an optimal position for its subsequent interaction with Hageman factor (548). In the absence of HMW kininogen, much less prekallikrein is bound to the surface (680) and neither activation of Hageman factor nor activation of prekallikrein proceeds at a normal rate. The augmentation of the rate of activation and cleavage of prekallikrein by activated Hageman factor in the presence of HMW kininogen may therefore reflect an effect on the binding of prekallikrein. However, HMW kininogen does not adsorb to activating surfaces in the absence of factor XII. For HMW kininogen to adsorb to kaolin with its complexed prekallikrein and factor XI, the procofactor HMW kininogen must first be cleaved by kallikrein to its heavy ($M_r = 65,000$) and light ($M_r = 56,000$) chains (589c). These interactions allow coordination of adsorption of the four contact-system proteins.

Several studies (339, 401, 402) have also indicated that HMW kininogen enhances the function of activated Hageman factor in converting prekallikrein to kallikrein in both purified systems and in plasma. In a purified system, recent studies have shown (588) that HMW kininogen at relatively low concentrations can prevent the loss of factor XIIf and kallikrein on polypropylene surfaces, apparently potentiating kallikrein formation. Other proteins can also prevent surface adsorption but at higher concentrations. The apparent potentiation of factor XIIf of the activation of prekallikrein in plasma by HMW kininogen is largely due to protection against protease inhibitors. The prekallikrein–HMW kininogen complex facilitates surface-bound Hageman factor activation. The kallikrein–HMW kininogen complex decreases the rate of kallikrein inactivation by $\overline{C1}$-INH (576). The light-chain domains of kallikrein interact with the light chain of HMW kininogen to form a complex with a dissociation constant (K_d) of 0.75 μM. This complex also protects kallikrein against inhibition by α_2-macroglobulin (578).

Recent data show that the amount of functional prekallikrein available is directly related to the

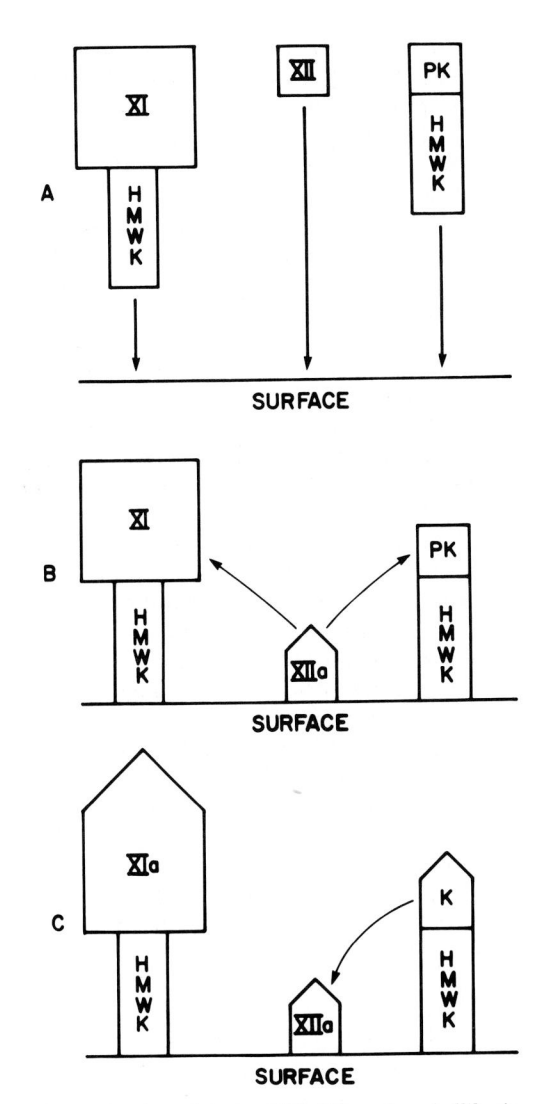

FIG. 2. Contact activation of factor XII, XI, and prekallikrein (PK). *A*: factor XII from the blood fluid phase binds directly to a foreign negatively charged surface. Factor XI–high-molecular-weight kininogen (HMWK) complex and prekallikrein-HMWK complex each bind to the surface via HMWK. *B*: factor XII is converted to active enzyme factor XIIa by autoactivation and/or a conformational change. Factor XIIa then enzymatically catalyzes conversion of its substrates factor XI and prekallikrein to active enzymes. *C*: active enzymes XIa and kallikrein (K) remain attached to HMWK and to surface. About half of the kallikrein molecules dissociate and may attack factor XIIa to yield factor XII fragments, which dissociate from the surface. Kallikrein may also attack factor XII zymogen to cleave it to an active enzyme during a positive feedback reaction.

amount of HMW kininogen and inversely proportional to the amount of inhibitor present (576). Surface activation of prekallikrein is suboptimal in normal plasma. Removal of $\overline{C1}$-INH or addition of purified HMW kininogen enhances the activation (587). Moreover, activation of prekallikrein by a surface proceeds at a similar rate with or without HMW kininogen in inhibitor-depleted normal plasma. In kininogen-deficient plasma both functional and immunochemical assays show low prekallikrein activity. However, the addition of HMW kininogen corrects the decrease in prekallikrein activity, indicating that the usual assay requires the prekallikrein–HMW kininogen complex to yield a normal value. The reactions in the functional assays of prekallikrein involve the activation of factor XII by conformational change after exposure to a surface and/or cleavage by kallikrein, which involves the cofactor HMW kininogen. This protein is necessary for the activation and the activity of factor XII. Prekallikrein conversion to kallikrein acts as a feedback, hastening the conversion of factor XII to activated factor XII. The prekallikrein–HMW kininogen complex also appears to demonstrate enhanced immunoreactivity compared to free prekallikrein.

Factor XI

Rosenthal et al. (564) first reported a new congenital hemorrhagic disease that was distinct from factor VIII and IX deficiencies. The syndrome was thought to be due to deficiency of plasma thromboplastin antecedent (now known as factor XI). Nossel (461) soon presented evidence that factor XI was activated by another enzyme. Ratnoff et al. (539) identified the enzyme as activated factor XII. Thus factor XI is a substrate and the product is activated factor XI (factor XIa). The molecular weight of human factor XI has been estimated at 175,000 by gel filtration (228, 431) and 150,000 by SDS–polyacrylamide gel electrophoresis (57, 278, 302, 694). Amino acid and carbohydrate composition data (302) suggest that the true molecular weight is 120,000–125,000, including 5% carbohydrate. The isoelectric point of factor XI is estimated as 8.9–9.1 (228).

When factor XI is treated with reducing agents (694), its molecular weight is reduced to 80,000 (57, 278). Native factor XI thus exists as a dimer, with two subunits linked by disulfide bonds (see Fig. 1). Purified factor XI is converted to a proteolytic enzyme on exposure to activated factor XII (57, 278, 302, 694). Factor XIa promotes clot formation in factor XI–deficient plasma in the absence of kaolin and possesses esterolytic activity (278, 302). Neither Ca^{2+} nor phospholipid is required for the conversion of factor XI to factor XIa. Without reduction the activation of factor XI to XIa does not change its molecular weight. After reduction, factor XIa appears as two (57, 694) components with molecular weights of approximately 50,000 and 35,000 in place of the single component with a molecular weight of approximately 80,000 that is seen in reduced factor XI (57, 278, 302, 694). The appearance of these two chains parallels the generation of clotting activity (57). Cleavage of each of the 80,000-M_r subunits present in the native dimeric molecule into disulfide-linked heavy and light chains therefore results in the conversion of factor XI to XIa, which takes up tritiated diisopropylfluorophosphate

(DFP) to form a single diisopropylphosphoserine residue per light chain or two serines per mole of enzyme. The amino acid sequence in the light chain shows strong homology to the corresponding sequences of factors XIIa, XIa, Xa, and thrombin (302).

Thompson et al. (641) discovered that factor XI exists in normal plasma as a bimolecular complex with HMW kininogen. This indicates that the true substrate of activated factor XII in plasma is the factor XI–HMW kininogen complex. Most of the factor XI in plasma is bound to the surface through HMW kininogen (680). After cleavage to factor XIa the complex remains surface bound. In order to activate a factor XI–kininogen complex, therefore, activated factor XII must come in contact with another complex. In addition kallikrein that has either dissociated from the surface or been activated in the fluid phase may be able to cleave surface-bound factor XII molecules that are in proximity to the factor XI–HMW kininogen complex. Factor XIa behaves as a serine protease and has esterolytic activity toward esters of lysine and arginine (93). It also has strong amidolytic activity toward pyroglutamylprolylarginyl-p-nitroanilide (589d), which has allowed development of an amidolytic assay. Factor XIa is inhibited by a number of plasma inhibitors; α_1-protease inhibitor is the most important of these (90), but $\overline{\text{C1}}$-INH (6), antithrombin III (120, 302), and α_2-antiplasmin (567) also inhibit factor XIa. Recently quantitative data indicate that α_1-protease accounts for 68% of the inhibitory activity of plasma, antithrombin III accounts for 16%, and $\overline{\text{C1}}$-INH and α_2-antiplasmin account for the remainder (589b). Furthermore the light chain of HMW kininogen protects against all those inhibitors (589b).

Factor IX

The next steps in the hemostatic system involve reactions leading to the formation of factor IXa. There are thought to be two pathways. The intrinsic pathway begins in the contact phase; its product, factor XIa, converts factor IX to IXa in the presence of Ca^{2+} (Fig. 3). This serine protease hydrolyzes factor X to Xa in the presence of the protein cofactor (coagulant factor VIII), phospholipid, and Ca^{2+}. These proteins of the intrinsic pathway were associated with three diseases generically called hemophilias, i.e., deficiencies of factor VIII, factor IX, and factor XI. Both factor VIII and IX deficiencies are classic genetic disorders involving the absence or abnormality of these specific proteins inherited by a sex-linked (X-linked) recessive mechanism.

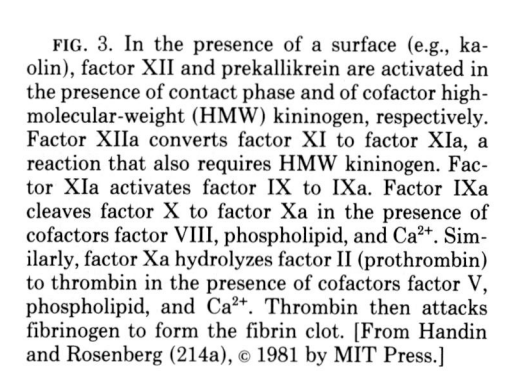

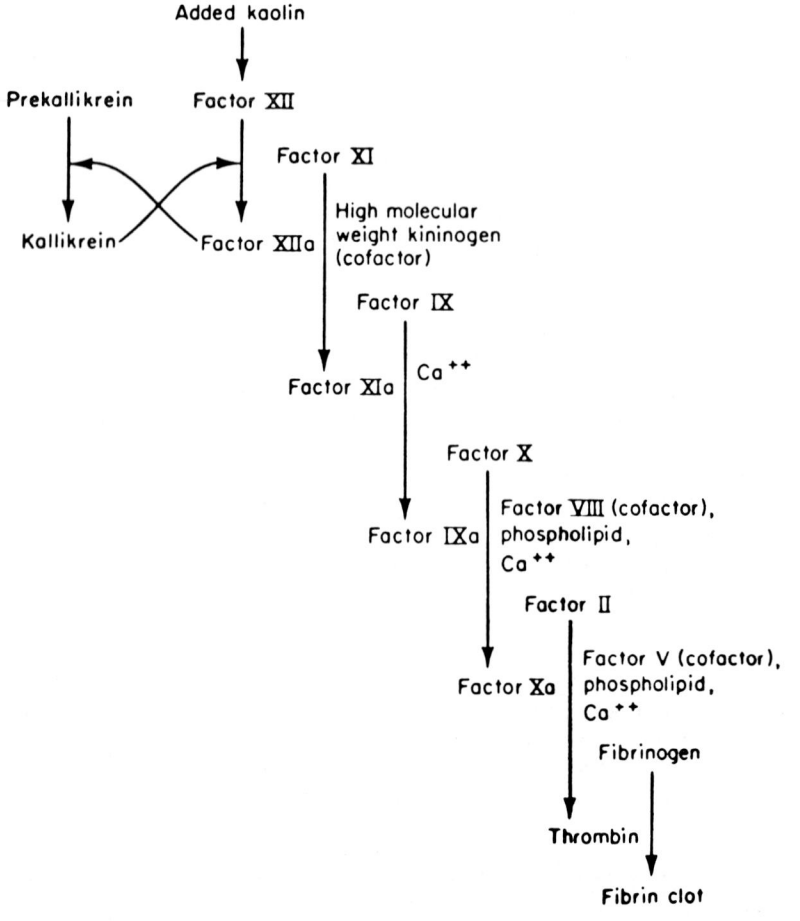

FIG. 3. In the presence of a surface (e.g., kaolin), factor XII and prekallikrein are activated in the presence of contact phase and of cofactor high-molecular-weight (HMW) kininogen, respectively. Factor XIIa converts factor XI to factor XIa, a reaction that also requires HMW kininogen. Factor XIa activates factor IX to IXa. Factor IXa cleaves factor X to factor Xa in the presence of cofactors factor VIII, phospholipid, and Ca^{2+}. Similarly, factor Xa hydrolyzes factor II (prothrombin) to thrombin in the presence of cofactors factor V, phospholipid, and Ca^{2+}. Thrombin then attacks fibrinogen to form the fibrin clot. [From Handin and Rosenberg (214a), © 1981 by MIT Press.]

The description of hemophilia as a clinical entity first appeared in the Talmud. In 1803 J.C. Otto (482), a Philadelphia physician, published a description of hemophilia. A century later it was realized that there are two forms of hemophilia and each is caused by the lack of a different protein in the blood. The two most common coagulation disorders are hemophilia A and hemophilia B (501). Although the clinical symptoms of hemophilia A and B may be similar, blood from one type can correct the coagulation time of blood from an individual with the other type (3, 37). Factor IX deficiency was called Christmas disease by Biggs and her colleagues (36), after the first of their patients with the disease. The factor was designated factor IX by an international nomenclature committee (692).

Human factor IX is a single-chain glycoprotein (see Fig. 1) containing approximately 20% carbohydrate (including hexose, N-acetylhexosamine, and N-acetylneuraminic acid) and present in plasma at 4 µg/ml. Human factor IX has a molecular weight of 55,000. Factor IX contains 12 γ-carboxyglutamic acid residues per mole (62, 126, 177, 478). The γ-carboxyglutamic acid residues are critical in the binding of Ca^{2+} to factor IX and are required for the interaction of factor IX with phospholipid vesicles. Human factor IX shows sequence homology with the other vitamin K–dependent proteins, particularly in the NH_2-terminal domain of the heavy chain containing the active-site region. Accordingly it has been suggested that a common ancestor zymogen of the vitamin K–dependent proteins gave rise to these remaining similar proteins (178, 281).

Factor IX functions in the intrinsic pathway of blood coagulation where it is activated by factor XIa to factor IXa ($M_r = 45,000$) and an activation glycopeptide ($M_r = 10,000$). This reaction has an absolute requirement for divalent metal ions such as Ca^{2+} and phospholipids. The result of the activation is the conversion of factor IX to a serine protease. Two internal peptide bonds are hydrolyzed in human factor IX during this reaction. The heavy and light chains of factor IXa are held together by a disulfide bond(s). The light chain ($M_r = 17,000$) originates from the NH_2-terminal portion of the zymogen molecule; the heavy chain ($M_r = 28,000$) originates from the COOH-terminal region. The first cleavage between an Arg-Val bond is the critical event in the activation reaction leading to the formation of an ion pair between the newly generated valine residue and the aspartic acid residue adjacent to the active-site serine. This intramolecular rearrangement is analogous to the activation mechanism that has been established for the pancreatic serine proteases (605, 625). Factor IX also contains the three amino acids histidine, aspartic acid, and serine that comprise the charge-relay network system (54, 387, 602, 605).

Factor IX is also activated by tissue factor and factor VIIa (480), providing a second mechanism for the activation of factor IX and bypassing the contact-activation system involving factor XIa. Although the rate of activation of factor IX by tissue factor and factor VIIa is 7 times slower than that of the activation of factor X by the intrinsic pathway (268), the relative importance of these two pathways is unknown under physiological conditions. Factor IXa in the presence of activated factor VIII, Ca^{2+}, and phospholipid converts factor X to factor Xa (Fig. 3). The cleavage between Arg-51 and Ile-52 forms factor Xa. Activated factor VIII forms a complex with factor IXa in the presence of Ca^{2+} and phospholipid. Factor IXa is readily inhibited by antithrombin III, a reaction accelerated several hundredfold by the presence of heparin (303). A one-to-one molar complex of enzyme and inhibitor is formed that is stable to boiling in the presence of SDS.

Factor IX is depressed in the plasma of some patients with hepatocellular disease, suggesting that the liver is the site of synthesis. Because factor IX is a vitamin K–dependent protein, synthesis of the biologically active protein is decreased by the administration of warfarin. Plasma from five patients receiving this drug contained antigenically detectable factor IX antigen, which has a more rapid electrophoretic mobility than that of normal factor IX; this increase in electrophoretic mobility probably represents a decrease in carboxylation (475). In warfarin overdose a decreased level of biologically active factor IX is found in plasma. In contrast the acquired factor IX deficiency associated with nephrotic syndrome may result from urinary loss (439). Factor IX concentrates may be necessary in addition to vitamin K to treat these conditions.

Factor VIII

Factor VIII (antihemophilic factor) is critical in blood coagulation, as is apparent from the severe bleeding disorder in patients with severe classic hemophilia (hemophilia A) who lack this protein. A component of normal plasma, designated antihemophilic globulin (500), shortens the clotting time of hemophilic blood (2). This protein, defined as factor VIII by the International Committee on Thrombosis and Haemostasis (692), has recently been designated VIII:C (458). This molecule should be distinguished from the protein with which it circulates in a complex, the large glycoprotein necessary for normal primary hemostasis that is referred to as factor VIII–related protein (VIIIR) or von Willebrand's factor. The observation that hemophilic plasmas have normal or increased levels of a factor VIII–like protein (detected by immunoassays with rabbit antibodies to purified human factor VIII) suggested the distinction between the two proteins (698). Although the observations were interpreted initially as evidence for synthesis of an abnormal factor VIII in hemophilia, the evidence now overwhelmingly favors the existence of two distinct proteins circulating as a complex in plasma. Chromatography or centrifugation in high-ionic-strength buffers (such as 1 M NaCl or 0.24 M CaCl$_2$) can separate the two proteins (551, 674, 675, 698).

Immunologic separation of VIII:C from VIIIR has been achieved (697). Less immunoadsorption of VIII:C than VIIIR antigenic determinants (VIIIR:Ag) was observed when solid-phase rabbit antibody to factor VIII was used. At physiological ionic strength a complex of VIII:C and VIIIR is formed (503). At least three different methods have been used to separate VIII:C from other plasma proteins. Purification of intact factor VIII complex is followed by its dissociation in high salt buffers so that VIII:C is separated from VIIIR (113, 542, 551, 631, 698). The second approach used agarose-bound antibody to VIIIR (240, 296, 503, 650) or agarose-bound VIIIR (243). A third purification method employed polyelectrolyte (270a, 297) and standard ion-exchange (499) resins that have different adsorption properties for VIII:C and VIIIR. None of these methods is fully satisfactory. The lability of VIII:C most likely results from proteolytic degradation (650). There is general agreement that plasmin inactivates VIII:C and that the rate of loss depends on the enzyme concentration (16, 398, 499). Activated protein C may be more effective. The effect of thrombin on VIII:C is the best studied instance of enzyme modification of this coagulation factor; these data are considered later in this section.

Reducing agents have a marked effect on VIIIR structure. The function of VIIIR, measured as the protein's ability to aggregate platelets in the presence of ristocetin (VIIIR:RC), is also decreased by reduction. The activity of VIII:C is quite stable under these conditions. Reduction inactivates 95% of VIIIR:RC in purified human factor VIII complex and modifies the structure of the VIIIR protein toward smaller multimers and toward the 240,000-M_r subunit and its dimer (115). The VIII:C levels were unchanged after a 2-h incubation in these experiments. Although VIII:C is partially inactivated only when plasma is treated with very high concentrations of 1,4-dithiothreitol (4 mM), it is less affected by reducing agents than other coagulation factors (52). Intact thiol groups appear to have an important role in VIII:C function because a variety of thiol inhibitors inactivate VIII:C (17). The stability of VIII:C also depends on pH and Ca^{2+} concentrations; VIII:C is most stable at neutral pH and there is marked loss below pH 6 and above pH 8 (673, 677, 689). Calcium concentration is important as well, because ethylenediaminetetraacetate (EDTA)-anticoagulated plasma and ion-exchange resin-treated plasma lose VIII:C when compared to citrate-anticoagulated plasma (673).

The VIII:C has a molecular weight of 293,000 ± 23,000 on Sephadex G-200 gel filtration, is relatively stable, is inhibited by human antibodies to factor VIII (551), and is activated by thrombin (552, 650, 677). The lability of highly purified VIII:C has prevented accurate measurement of its specific activity. The plasma concentration of VIII:C is less than 100 ng/ml. The VIII:C (separated from VIIIR) is bound by concanavalin A–agarose and is eluted with the sugar α-D-glucopyranoside (650). This strongly suggests that VIII:C is a glycoprotein and has carbohydrate groups that bind to concanavalin A. Not surprisingly some bacterial glycosidases and oxidases inactivate VIII:C (18, 180).

Human antibodies to VIII:C do not form immunoprecipitates when tested with plasma or with factor VIII concentrates. The human antibodies form stable immune complexes with VIII:C (323, 324), and the antibodies are typically bivalent immunoglobulin G. However, the reactants are present in extremely low concentrations and may have been below the threshold for immunochemical detection. Human antibody to VIII:C has a greater affinity for VIII:C than VIII:C has for VIIIR, allowing separation of the soluble immune complex (antibody-VIII:C) from VIIIR. Immunization with intact factor VIII complex elicits antibodies that form immunoprecipitates with VIIIR:Ag (40, 247, 656). Rabbits may form both precipitating antibodies to VIIIR and neutralizing antibodies to VIII:C (285). Insolubilized rabbit antisera bind the factor VIII complex, removing both VIII:C and VIIIR from plasma (240, 296, 503, 650, 697). Antibody neutralization assays have been carried out with some success. Plasma from approximately 10% of hemophiliacs with mild (10%) or moderate (2%) disease neutralizes naturally occurring antibodies against VIII:C. These plasmas have been designated cross-reacting material-positive (CRM$^+$) or hemophilia A$^+$. Plasma from the other 90% of the hemophilic patients failed to neutralize the human antibodies and has been characterized as CRM$^-$ or hemophilia A$^-$. The insensitivity and poor precision of antibody neutralization assays have been overcome, allowing the development of quantitative immunoradiometric assays (239, 325, 504, 547) for VIII:C antigenic determinants (VIII:CAg). There is excellent correlation of VIII:CAg content with VIII:C coagulant activity in both normal plasma and in the plasma from patients with severe von Willebrand's disease, suggesting that patients with severe von Willebrand's disease may synthesize VIII:C but that because it is inactivated, plasma levels are low.

The primary site of VIII:C synthesis is not known. However, recent liver perfusion studies suggest that this organ releases VIII:C under appropriate conditions. A potent human antibody to VIII:C completely inactivated the VIII:C, and a protein synthesis inhibitor blocked the VIII:C rise (488). The liver seemed able to release VIII:C, but it apparently does not do so unless VIIIR is present.

The participation of VIII:C in a complex with factor IXa, phospholipid, and Ca^{2+} is important in the conversion of factor X to Xa by the enzyme factor IXa (231, 244, 479, 583). Both antibody to factor IX and antibody to VIII:C can individually inhibit the factor X activator (479). Measurement of the release of tritium-labeled activation peptide demonstrated that factor IXa can activate factor X slowly in the presence of phospholipid and Ca^{2+}, even though factor VIII is absent, but that factor VIII markedly enhances this reaction (252). This complex is analogous to that composed of factor Xa, factor Va, phospholipid, and Ca^{2+}, i.e., prothrombinase (154).

The activity of VIII:C is enhanced when plasma or factor VIII concentrates are incubated with small amounts of thrombin (481, 534), which suggests that thrombin activation is essential for VIII:C to accelerate factor X proteolysis. The rate of factor Xa formation was proportional to the amount of thrombin-activated factor VIII. Thrombin activation of VIII:C was also demonstrated when factor Xa generation was assayed by an amidolytic procedure that used a synthetic tripeptide chromogenic substrate (467). Highly purified VIII:C has a molecular weight of 290,000 on Sephadex G-200 gel filtration in 1 M NaCl. After incubation with diluted thrombin the active fractions have increased VIII:C and an apparent molecular weight of 150,000, indicating that VIII:C fragmentation accompanies activation. When concentrated thrombin is used, rapid activation of VIII:C is followed by inactivation; most of the nonfunctional protein has a molecular weight of 100,000–130,000. The inactivation is probably due to activated protein C. In similar studies with highly purified bovine VIII:C, Vehar and Davie (652) noted that incubation with thrombin was followed by an increase in VIII:C activity and a decrease in the molecular weight of the protein on SDS-polyacrylamide gel electrophoresis.

RELATIONSHIP OF INTRINSIC AND EXTRINSIC BLOOD COAGULATION

Activation of the extrinsic coagulation system can circumvent the need for the first six proteins of the intrinsic pathway (Fig. 4). This system involves exposure of blood to tissue factor, a lipoprotein that (in addition to Ca^{2+} and factor VII) is required for the conversion of factor X to Xa. These intrinsic and extrinsic systems provide alternative mechanisms of activating factor X to Xa, the active enzyme that participates in blood coagulation. However, their separation may not be as complete as first believed; fragments of factor XII (Hageman factor) formed by kallikrein cleavage of the protein in the presence of HMW kininogen can increase the activity of factor VII 40-fold and therefore enormously amplify extrinsic activation. Furthermore there are many backward reactions operating in factor X activation (e.g., the conversion of factor IX to IXa and factor VII to VIIa by factor Xa) that occur in purified systems. The role of these positive feedbacks in vivo is still unclear.

Factor X

Human factor X is a zymogen of a 62,000-M_r serine protease (see Fig. 1). Factor Xa is composed of two

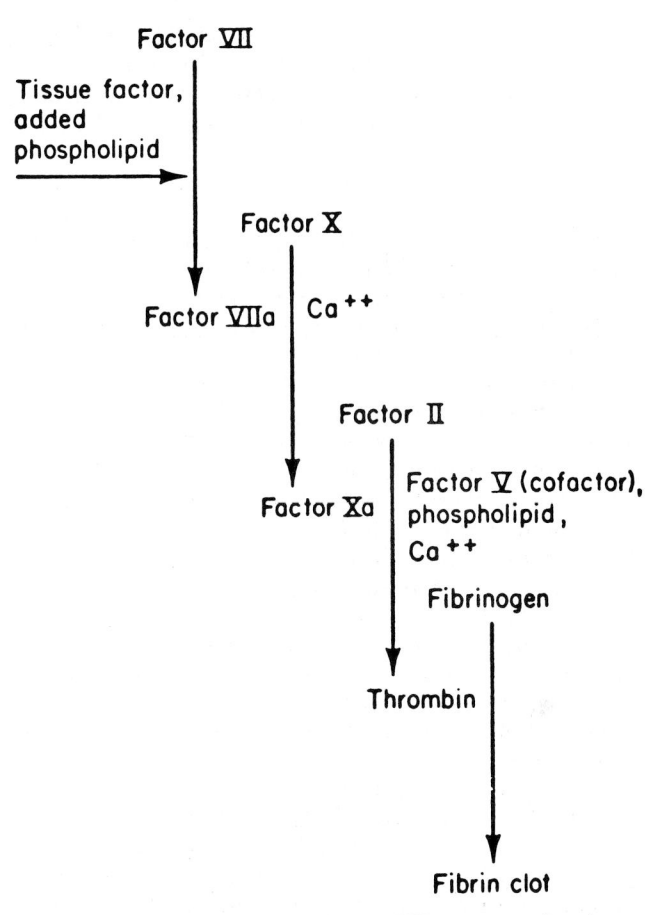

FIG. 4. Extrinsic coagulation. Factor VII is converted to factor VIIa by autoactivation, factor XIIa, or in a feedback reaction by factor Xa. Factor VIIa in presence of tissue factor and Ca^{2+} can convert factor X to factor Xa. Once factor Xa is formed, pathway is identical to intrinsic coagulation (see Fig. 3). [From Rosenberg (560a), © 1981 by MIT Press.]

polypeptide chains, a 56,000-M_r heavy chain and 16,000-M_r light chain, joined by a disulfide bond (179, 260). The amino acid sequence of both chains of bovine factor X has been determined (146, 645). The heavy chain contains hexose, hexosamine, and neuraminic acid residues with a total carbohydrate content of 15%. Factor X possesses considerable sequence homology with factors II, VII, and IX, which has led some workers to postulate a common genetic ancestor.

The ability of factor X to bind Ca^{2+} is due to the presence of γ-carboxyglutamic acid, whose two free carboxy groups act as negative ligands for Ca^{2+}. Eleven of the first 38 amino acids in the NH$_2$-terminal region of the light chain of bovine factor X are γ-carboxyglutamic acids (62). Reduced vitamin K is required for the carboxylation of glutamic acid, which is a postribosomal modification of glutamic acid. Treatment of patients or cows (616, 618) with dicumarol results in the synthesis of abnormal forms of factor X antigen, which do not bind Ca^{2+} and display increased anodal electrophoretic mobility.

Factor Xa is a trypsinlike enzyme that hydrolyzes

peptide bonds containing arginine, which contributes the carboxyl group. The active center of factor Xa includes a nucleophilic serine (Ser-233) and a charge-relay system of amino acids Asp-138 and His-93 (645).

Factor VII

The single plasma protein that functions exclusively in the extrinsic system is factor VII. In the presence of tissue factor this protein bypasses the first six proteins in the intrinsic system and can activate factor X to Xa. Factor VII is a 47,000-M_r glycoprotein, as determined by SDS–polyacrylamide gel electrophoresis. A single-chain form may be isolated in the presence of inhibitors of trypsinlike serine proteases (cf. Fig. 1); however, in the absence of inhibitors a two-chain form that is joined by disulfide bonds is found. The single-chain zymogen factor VII is converted to two-chain α-VIIa; the molecular weights of the two chains are 29,500 and 23,500, with the carbohydrate and the nucleophilic serine on the heavy chain. The single chain form appears to possess coagulant activity, but its activity increases up to 120-fold when it is converted to the two-chain form (531). Much evidence suggests that the zymogen itself possesses enzymatic activity. Factor VII and α-VIIa both incorporate DFP, but the rate constant for the enzyme is only 4–5 times that of the zymogen. Both esterase and coagulant activity increase as factor VII is converted to the two-chain form (701). The heavy chain of α-VIIa can undergo further cleavage by factor Xa at an Arg-Gly bond, yielding a 17,000-M_r chain and a 12,500-M_r chain (532). The 12,500-M_r chain contains the nucleophilic serine, but the three-chain form (known as β-VIIa) has no coagulant activity and undergoes no further cleavage.

Thromboplastin

The activation of factor X by α-VIIa requires thromboplastin, a membrane lipoprotein present in brain, lung, and placenta. Extraction with detergents or organic solvents dissociates the thromboplastin into its apoprotein (tissue factor) and phospholipid components, neither of which alone possesses coagulant activity (254, 444, 626). Nemerson and Pitlick (445) found that the apoprotein, tissue factor, of bovine lung consists of two HMW species. Recombination of apoprotein and phospholipid in the presence of sodium deoxycholate restored coagulant activity. Phosphatidylethanolamine and phosphatidylcholine were both effective, although reduced phosphatidylcholine and lysophosphatidylcholine had no activity. A ratio of 7.5 to 10 mg phospholipid per milligram of protein was optimal. Bjorklid et al. (43) purified tissue factor from human brain and found a molecular weight of 52,000 on SDS–polyacrylamide gel electrophoresis. Both phosphatidylethanolamine and phosphatidylcholine form complexes with tissue factor that are stable. Lysophosphatidylcholine does not form complexes, and reduced phosphatidylcholine forms complexes only at very high lipid-to-protein ratios (517). Binding of phospholipid to tissue factor is thus necessary for tissue factor coagulant activity. In the absence of phospholipids, no interaction occurs between human tissue factor and either human factor Xa or a factor VII (42). The activation of factor X occurs concomitantly with hydrolysis of a specific Arg-Ile bond, resulting in the loss of a peptide with a molecular weight of approximately 11,000, termed the *activation peptide*. At high concentrations of factor VIIa and tissue factor most of the factor X is rapidly converted to α-Xa (M_r = 34,300) and then undergoes autocatalytic conversion to β-Xa (M_r = 29,600). At low concentrations of factor VIIIa and tissue factor the conversion of factor X to α-Xa occurs more slowly. The amount of α-Xa thus formed feeds back on the remaining factor X, converting it to an intermediate. The α-Xa then acts on the intermediate and on itself to form β-Xa.

REGULATION OF PROTHROMBIN ACTIVATION

Rapid prothrombin activation to form thrombin in plasma involves five components. Only the proteolytic enzyme factor Xa is necessary for thrombin generation, but the extremely slow rate of prothrombin activation by factor Xa alone emphasizes the role of the other three activator components: factor Va, phospholipids, and Ca^{2+} (Fig. 3). Factor V, after activation by thrombin (factor Va), functions in a manner analogous to a receptor on the platelet membrane and binds factor Xa and prothrombin (151, 409). Phospholipids, which exist in aqueous solution as molecular bilayers, provide a model membrane to which the protein molecules bind (263, 702). Calcium ions are required for both factor Xa and prothrombin binding to the phospholipid membrane surface (28, 156, 157, 496). This Ca^{2+}-mediated binding requires the presence of γ-carboxyglutamic acid in the protein (617).

The modification (carboxylation) of specific glutamic acid residues in these proteins (352, 442, 617) requires reduced vitamin K during their biosynthesis in the liver (155, 264). The functional consequence of oral anticoagulant action is elimination of the Ca^{2+}-mediated association of the vitamin K–dependent clotting factors with the phospholipids of the cell membrane (156). The interactions among the components of the complex prothrombin activation system enhance the rate of thrombin formation (154, 409), providing a mechanism by which rapid thrombin formation can occur as part of the hemostatic response. Such explosive thrombin formation occurs where negatively charged phospholipids are available (566, 703).

Prothrombin

The prothrombin molecule is a single polypeptide chain that can be divided into two approximately equal parts, the "pro" portion and the thrombin portion

(Fig. 5). The pro portion, which is derived from the NH$_2$-terminal end of prothrombin, has a molecular weight of 35,000 (154). The pro half of prothrombin may be further divided into the fragment 1 region (residues 1–156), which contains two carbohydrate side chains, and the fragment 2 region (residues 157–274). Both fragment 1 and fragment 2 regions contain very similar triple disulfide loops; thus their tertiary structures may be very similar, although their primary structures are different. The NH$_2$-terminal end of fragment 1 contains all ten of the γ-carboxyglutamic acid residues. The net distribution of charged amino

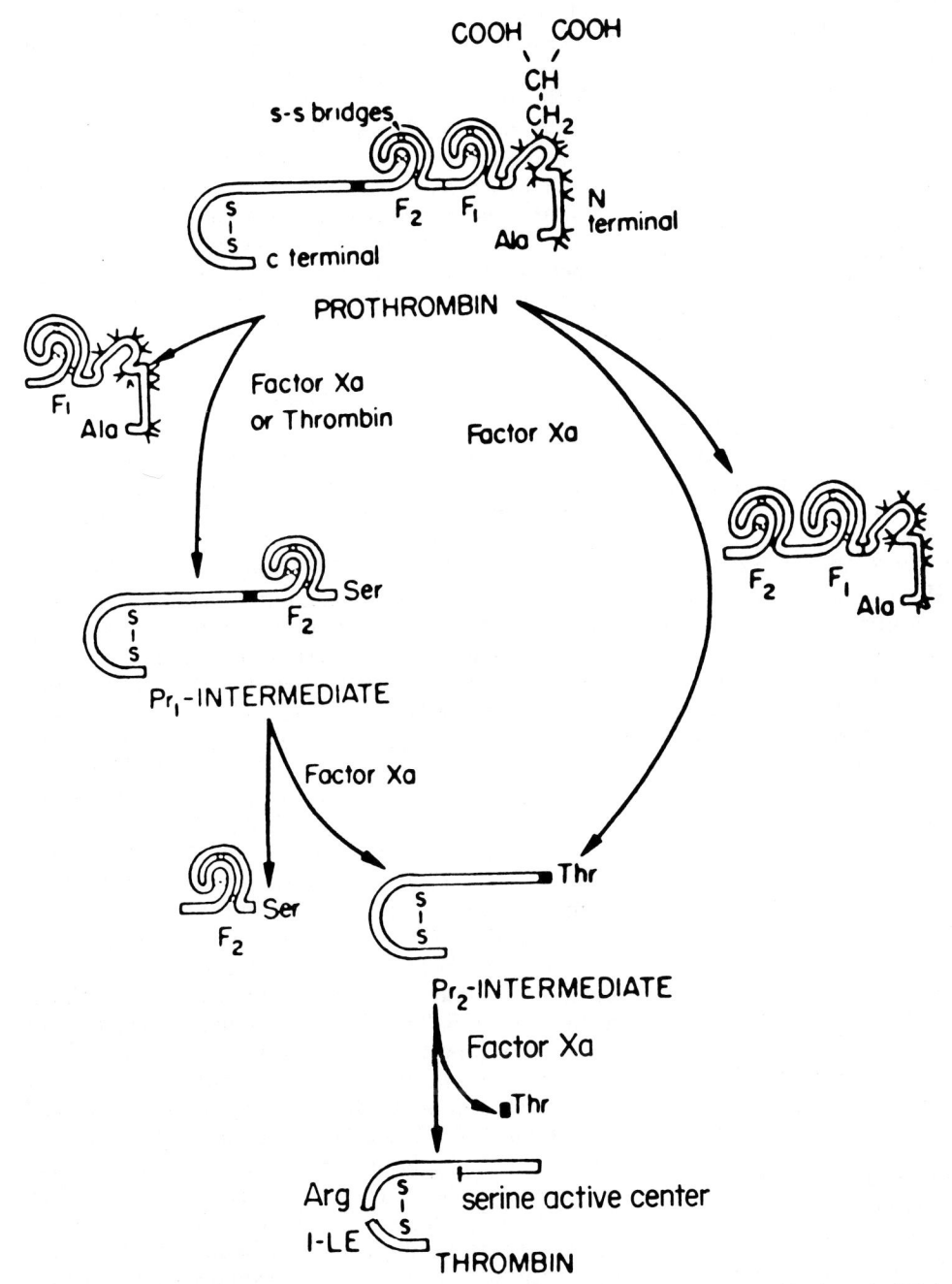

FIG. 5. Prothrombin activation. Prothrombin is activated to thrombin initially by right-hand pathway. The NH$_2$-terminal (N-terminal) "pro" piece containing fragment 1 (F$_1$) and fragment 2 (F$_2$) is cleaved by factor Xa. Prothrombin 2 (Pr$_2$ intermediate) results, which in turn is cleaved by factor Xa at an Ile-Arg bond to yield a serine active center on the larger polypeptide chain (β-chain) and a small α-chain still attached by a disulfide bridge. Left-hand pathway may operate in the test tube once thrombin is formed with cleavage between fragment 1 and fragment 2 preceding final cleavage between fragment 2 and Pr$_2$ intermediate, but only the right-hand pathway occurs at in vivo Ca^{2+} concentration.

acids in prothrombin results in the pro half having a net negative charge (i.e., relatively acidic) and the thrombin half having a slight net positive charge.

Factor V

Bovine factor V has been isolated as a single-chain glycoprotein (M_r = 300,000–330,000) (110, 148, 211, 448, 573, 608) with a carbohydrate content of approximately 15%–20%. Incubation of factor V with thrombin or an activation from Russell's viper venom generates activated factor V and also results in a series of proteolytic cleavages in the factor V molecule (128, 148, 251, 574). Transient products can be observed by SDS–polyacrylamide gel electrophoresis that have molecular weights of approximately 200,000 and 150,000 (148, 446, 543, 574). Two final major products with molecular weights of 70,000 and 100,000 (148) make up factor Va. Another product that has an approximate molecular weight of 150,000 is an activation polypeptide that is rich in carbohydrate. Several other components with molecular weights less than 70,000 also occur. The activated form of protein C degrades factor Va (286). Factor V is particularly susceptible to inactivation by many proteases (104, 105).

Incubation of factor V with thrombin or an enzyme from Russell's viper venom results in a marked increase in the factor V activity in bioassays with factor V–deficient plasma (574). Functionally this activation process results in conversion to factor Va, a form that binds both prothrombin (151) and factor Xa (174). Miletich et al. (408, 409) demonstrated that activation of factor V is necessary for it to function as a factor Xa receptor on platelets, suggesting that factor V is simply a procofactor (Fig. 6). Bovine factor V activity depends on the presence of a single Ca^{2+} ion, which can be removed only with strong chelators such as EDTA in the presence of denaturing agents such as urea (205). Addition of Ca^{2+} restores activity. Interestingly, removal of sialic acid residues from factor V appears to enhance its activity (211), although oxidation or removal of galactose inactivates the molecule (573). Two-chain factor Va can be dissociated into its constituent polypeptide chains by removing divalent cations (148). The dissociated product is without biologic activity, but incubation with Mn^{2+} and/or Ca^{2+} can regenerate the biologic activity (148, 205). The carbohydrate moiety has been implicated in factor V binding to zwitterionic lipids (276, 277, 573). The molecular mechanism(s) by which factor Va increases the rate of prothrombin activation has not been clearly demonstrated, although effects on both the formation of the enzyme-substrate complex (prothrombin–factor Xa) and the efficiency of proteolysis by factor Xa have been reported (106, 653).

Coagulant Phospholipid Surfaces

Phospholipids exist in aqueous solutions as lamellar aggregates or bilayers (263) due to the exclusion of hydrophobic residues (such as the fatty acyl chains of lipids) from the aqueous environment. The polar head groups of the phospholipids are in contact with the aqueous solution. Such bilayer structures constitute a major structural component of cellular membranes and subcellular organelles. Phospholipid activity in blood coagulation has two structural requirements: *1*) some of the molecules of the bilayer must have a net negative charge (27, 497), and *2*) the fatty acyl chains must be in a liquid crystalline (melted) state. Studies on the lipids of cell membranes indicate that specific phospholipids are asymmetrically distributed between the two halves of the bilayer, with the negatively charged lipids predominantly on the inside face (566). Experiments with right-side-out and inside-out erythrocyte membranes have demonstrated that the right-side-out membranes are inactive in shortening the recalcification time of plasma, whereas inside-out membranes have a marked effect (703).

Calcium Ions

Calcium ions participate in virtually every reaction in the coagulation system, including direct effects on proteolytic enzymes, on proteins binding to phospholipid, on association and dissociation of subunits of oligomeric proteins, and on platelet aggregation and release reactions. In prothrombin activation, Ca^{2+} alters the rate of prothrombin cleavage by both factor Xa and thrombin; it affects factors V and Va, most probably by affecting factor Va–subunit interactions (148, 574); it mediates the binding of prothrombin and

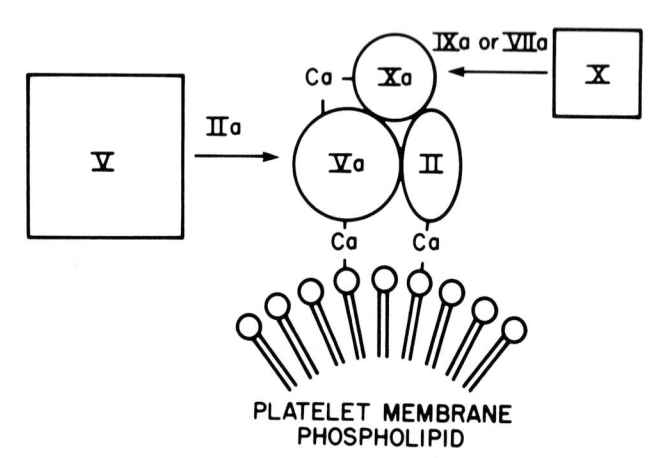

FIG. 6. Formation of receptor on platelets and phospholipids by attachment of factor Va required to bind factor Xa. Factor V is converted by thrombin (factor IIa) to factor Va. Factor Va in the presence of Ca^{2+} binds to phospholipid micelle or platelet membrane. Prothrombin (factor II) binds to phospholipid through Ca^{2+} attached to the fragment 1 domain containing Gla residues. Factor Xa is formed from factor X via either the intrinsic pathway (factor IXa) or the extrinsic pathway (factor VIIa). Factor Xa then binds to factor Va and phospholipid markedly accelerates its ability to cleave factor II to IIa.

factor Xa to the membrane surface of the phospholipid bilayer. All current evidence suggests that Ca^{2+} (23, 127, 156, 157, 263, 440, 442) serves as a bridge between the γ-carboxyglutamic acid domain and either carboxylate or phosphate moieties from the phospholipid head groups. Calcium ions may induce conformational changes in the γ-carboxyglutamic acid domains prior to Ca^{2+}-mediated binding to phospholipids (441). Interestingly, at 1.3 mM Ca^{2+} (the physiological concentration), exposed phospholipid surfaces are almost exactly one-half saturated with prothrombin (237, 238, 240), thus making this process spontaneous when the appropriate phospholipid membrane surfaces are exposed to blood.

Thrombin Formation

Factor Xa hydrolyzes two peptide bonds in prothrombin (9, 10, 138, 152, 261, 262, 490, 619). The first peptide bond cleaved is the Arg-Thr bond (Arg51-Thr52) between the pro (prothrombin fragment 1–2) half and the thrombin-forming (prethrombin fragment 2) half of the molecule (see Fig. 5). The second bond cleaved is the Arg-Ile peptide bond (Arg49-Ile50) between the A and B chains of thrombin. This order of bond cleavage in prothrombin by factor Xa is unaffected by factor Va phospholipids and Ca^{2+} (149, 150, 153, 261, 262, 409), indicating that the function of these components is not to change the order of bond cleavage. Aronson et al. (12) observed identical products of prothrombin cleavage by factor Xa both in vivo in systems containing chemically homogeneous proteins and ex vivo in whole blood that clots in a test tube. Thrombin can also cleave an Arg-Ser bond in prothrombin, giving rise to prothrombin fragment 1 and prethrombin fragment 1. However, this cleavage, although experimentally useful, is physiologically insignificant because it does not occur in whole plasma or blood (12) and because it is suppressed by Ca^{2+}. Prothrombin fragment 1 contains the γ-carboxyglutamic acid domain and is responsible for binding to Ca^{2+} and thus to phospholipid ions. Prothrombin fragment 2 is required for interaction with factor Va. The acceleration caused by phospholipids may in vivo be provided by the platelet membrane (Fig. 6).

Once thrombin is generated from its precursor, prothrombin, it plays a variety of roles in the hemostatic mechanism and potentially plays a number of roles in other physiological processes. Thrombin is a serine protease and cleaves peptide bonds involving discrete arginine residues (72, 143, 350, 351, 640). Thrombin possesses extensive selectivity; this limited specificity allows thrombin to regulate the hemostatic process. Gladner and Laki (194) and Miller and Van Vunakis (410) identified thrombin as a member of the serine protease class of proteases and demonstrated that a DFP-sensitive peptide containing an active-site serine equivalent to Ser-195 of chymotrypsin is present in the thrombin catalytic site. Glover and Shaw (195) later demonstrated that the equivalent to His-57 in chymotrypsin was also present in a selected peptide region of the thrombin sequence. During coagulation thrombin converts fibrinogen into fibrin and is associated with the activation of protein C and factors V, VIII, and XIII. In addition the enzyme binds to platelet membranes and is partly responsible for platelet activation and aggregation.

The primary structure of bovine thrombin has been elucidated (256, 351) and studies of the primary structure have been reported for the human enzyme. The complete primary structure of human prethrombin 2, which is the immediate precursor of human thrombin, has also been elucidated. Human prethrombin 2 bears considerable homology with its bovine counterpart. The B (heavy) chain contains a highly reactive serine residue in the amino acid sequence -Asp-Ser-Gly- (residues 204–206) that forms a catalytic site with the so-called charge-relay system (143, 350). Once the active site is generated, however, human thrombin recognizes as a substrate its own A chain and cleaves the A chain at position Arg13-Thr14; the stable form of human α-thrombin consists of an A chain of only 36 residues (138). Considerable homology exists between thrombin and chymotrypsin with conservation of approximately 30% of the residues. It is likely, however, that the primary binding site for substrates in the thrombin molecule is similar to that of trypsin and chymotrypsin; however, unlike these two pancreatic enzymes, thrombin must possess secondary binding sites that confer the unique specificity observed for the enzyme.

Thrombin Specificity

Thrombin has a preferential proteolytic specificity for the cleavage of arginine peptide bonds (144). However, many arginine-containing bonds are not susceptible to hydrolysis by thrombin; this implies a more limited specificity of the enzyme. Human blood proteins in which the site of thrombin cleavage of the polypeptide chains has been identified include fibrinogen, Aα-Arg16-Gly17 and Bβ-Arg14-Gly15 (47); factor XIII, Arg36-Gly37 (633); prothrombin, Arg51-Thr52 (11) and Arg155-Ser156 (662); thrombin, Aα-Arg13-Thr14 (72); antithrombin III, Arg385-Ser386 (273); C3a component of complement, Arg69-Ala70; pituitary growth hormone, Arg134-Thr135 (201); and apolipoprotein C3, Arg40-Gly41 (613). Porcine secretion contains a phenylalanine residue nine amino acids to the left of the cleaved peptide bond Arg14-Asp15 (438); a similar spacing between phenylalanine and arginine residues is present in human fibrinopeptide A, but an aromatic amino acid in such an arrangement is not a prerequisite in many other susceptible proteins. The data on amino acid sequences on either side of the thrombin-susceptible peptide bond revealed no unique requirements for contiguous residues. Frequently occurring nonpolar amino acids immediately to the left of the susceptible arginine and polar residues to the right are not always found rigorously in the sequence of all cleaved bonds. The unique requirements of the amino acid sequence of the contiguous residues that define the thrombin-susceptible bonds in proteins are not known.

It has been found through trial and error that substituted esters of arginine [e.g., α-N-tosylarginine methyl ester (600) or α-N-benzoylarginine esters] are good substrates for thrombin. The derivatives have been used for the quantitative assay for many years. After recognition that arginine is an essential amino acid in the cleaved bond (47) and subsequent studies on the relationship between the sequence of fibrinopeptide A analogues and the kinetics of hydrolysis by thrombin (333–335, 579), many peptides were synthesized in an effort to formulate a specific substrate for thrombin. Tripeptides containing the COOH-terminal group of arginine in an amide bond with a chromophore or fluorescent derivative [chromogenic (632) and fluorogenic (419) substrates, respectively] have been developed and are used for quantitative determination of amidolytic activity of thrombin. These peptides usually have nonpolar amino acid residues to the left of arginine, e.g., D-phenylalanylpipecolylarginyl-p-nitroaniline and N-benzylphenylalanylvalylarginyl-p-nitroaniline (26, 49, 92). The chromogenic substrates are very useful for the laboratory assessment of thrombin activity. The yellow p-nitroaniline cleaved from a virtually colorless substrate provides a quick and sensitive assay.

The specificity of thrombin for fibrinogen [Michaelis constant (K_m) for clotting = 10^{-6} M] appears to depend on the primary structure of the cleaved Aα- and Bβ-polypeptide chains rather than on their conformation (47). The observation that thrombin can cleave fibrinopeptides from denatured fibrinogen or from the reduced and isolated Aα- and Bβ-chains supports this hypothesis. Out of 136 arginyl peptide bonds, only four are cleaved in fibrinogen. The part of the fibrinogen molecule participating in the attachment of thrombin through binding sites may be the Aα- and Bβ-chains. Comparing the amino acid sequences of fibrinopeptide A from many animal species showed the presence of phenylalanine in position 9 to the left of the cleaved arginine (45). Such homology is absent in fibrinopeptides B and a few other proteins cleaved by thrombin. Other investigators suggest a noncovalent binding of thrombin to the substrate through a glutamic or aspartic acid residue or their respective amines in positions 6, 7, or 8 to the right of the susceptible bond (664). No direct experimental evidence supports this view. Studies on the kinetics of the thrombin-catalyzed cleavage of fibrinopeptide A from synthetic peptides indicated that Aα-Phe8-Arg23 is a much better substrate than Aα-Ala10-Arg23 (579). Similar work with fragments of the fibrinogen Aα-chain suggest that thrombin binds within the sequence Aα-Ala1-Arg23 with a possible localization in Aα-Phe8-Arg16. The binding was strengthened by Aα-Pro34-Lys44 and Aα-Cys45-Met51. The primary binding site appears to reside in the Aα-chain in residues 1–23 and is associated with the cleavage of fibrinopeptides; the secondary binding site has also been postulated in the first 51 amino acid residues of the Aα-chain (238). After the cleavage of fibrinopeptides A and B, thrombin remains attached to the binding sites; this interaction would explain the phenomenon recognized long ago that fibrin decreased thrombin concentration in the clot supernate (140, 246, 591, 683). Gorman (198) proposed that the interaction of fibrinogen with thrombin may involve multiple secondary binding sites. Direct tests of the thrombin-concentration dependence of binding indicate two classes of binding sites: *1*) a high-affinity site with an acidic dissociation constant (K_a) of 4.8×10^5 M^{-1} and a 0.35 maximum molar binding ratio of thrombin to fibrin, and *2*) a low-affinity site with K_a of 6.8×10^4 M^{-1} and a 1.6 maximum molar binding ratio (338). Whether the two classes of binding sites are related to the cleavages of fibrinopeptides A or B is not known.

Regulation of Thrombin Activity

Thrombin is an important regulatory enzyme in hemostasis. Its action affects both cells and blood proteins. The regulatory function results from the limited specificity of thrombin for few macromolecular substrates. Thrombin binds to platelets (190, 646, 678, 691), stimulating aggregation and secretion. Thrombin also enhances proliferation of human endothelial cells in the presence of fibroblast growth factor (61, 75, 76, 84, 200, 382); initiates fibrinogen clotting; activates factor V (148, 446, 449, 574), factor VIII (16), factor XIII (633), and protein C (286); and inactivates factor VIIIa (16). There is some disagreement in the literature whether factor Va is inactivated (148, 574) or unaffected (446) by incubation with thrombin. Proteolytic cleavage by thrombin after the activation of factor V is not responsible for the decrease in activity that has been observed in some studies, because hirudin does not block the loss of activity. The protein C in some thrombin preparations may play a role. Under physiological conditions a reversible binding to fibrin regulates the activity of thrombin (338) and the formation of a covalent product with antithrombin III regulates an irreversible inhibition (461). Thrombin generated in the whole blood is also consumed in the process of binding to platelets, endothelial cells, and various other cells. The relatively limited capacity of the cellular binding does not seem to play a primary role in the regulation of thrombin activity in vivo. The major regulator of thrombin is the plasma protease inhibitor antithrombin III. The formation of thrombin–antithrombin III complex is greatly accelerated in the presence of heparin, which catalytically increases the inactivating function of antithrombin III (41, 332, 461, 592). Although heparin interacts in purified systems with thrombin (460, 461), the main anticoagulant function of heparin in the blood is expressed through the enhancement of antithrombin III reactivity. Two other plasma inhibitors, α_2-macroglobulin (311) and α_1-protease inhibitor (384), inhibit thrombin in purified systems; however, their significance in the regulation of thrombin activity in vivo is questionable (137).

Heparin and Antithrombin III

Heparin is a highly sulfated mucopolysaccharide with widely varying molecular weights. Heparin can be extracted from a variety of organs, including the liver, lungs, and intestine (147). Attachment of a carbohydrate linkage region to serine residues of a specific extended sequence of alternating residues of serine and glycine residues initiates the biosynthesis of heparin. The synthesis depends on the action of four specific enzymes (glycosyltransferases), which use uridine 5′-diphosphate (UDP) sugars as their substrates (559). The polymer chain of the mucopolysaccharide is completed by the alternate attachment of N-acetylglucosamine and glucuronic acid and is controlled by two specific glycosyltransferases that utilize UDP-N-acetylglucosamine and UDP–glucuronic acid. Thus each postsynthetic modification is controlled by a specific enzyme and is only initiated when the preceding reaction has been completed. Glucosamine residues are partially N-deacetylated, and the exposed amino groups are then sulfated. Glucuronic acid residues then may be epimerized to iduronic acid residues. An N-sulfated glucosamine residue on uronic acid stimulates this conversion. The iduronic acid residues are partially esterified with sulfate at the C-2 position. Finally the glucosamine moieties are sulfated at the C-6 position.

The final product, macromolecular heparin (696), consists of individual chains with molecular weights of 60,000–100,000 that are composed of many combinations of uronic acid and glucosamine residues. Once formed the proteoglycan can be hydrolyzed by lysosomal proteolytic enzymes, endoglycosidases that can cleave the mucopolysaccharide chain between glucuronic acid and glucosamine residues (242, 468) and exoglycosidases that cleave monosaccharides from the nonreducing ends of the complex carbohydrate (450).

Heparin has been isolated from a variety of species, including invertebrates, aquatic mammals, and humans (121, 141, 267, 622). In most instances the lung or intestinal mucosa has been utilized (141). Extraction of heparin involves homogenization, proteolytic digestion, differential precipitation with quaternary ammonium salts, and chromatography of the substances on anion-exchange resins (141). The purified heparins contain single polysaccharide chains with molecular weights up to 35,000. The average molecular weight of these preparations is approximately 12,000 (622). Approximately 25% of the polysaccharide chains bear the protein linkage regions. The remainder have free uronic acid or glucosamine at the end of the chain. Cleavage of the large polysaccharide chains of the native macromolecular heparin at multiple sites forms these heparin species.

As expected, heparin derived from all known sources is composed of alternating uronic acid and glucosamine moieties. The uronic acid and glucosamine moieties are linked via alternating β-D and α-D 1-4 bonds (267). The former may exist as iduronic acid-2-sulfate, glucuronic acid, or nonsulfated iduronic acid. Heparin derived from porcine or bovine intestine contains more sulfated iduronic acid than glucuronic acid. The glucosamine residues may be N-sulfated, N-acetylated, or have free amino groups. Furthermore these moieties may have a free hydroxyl group at position C-6 or be sulfated at this position. Mucopolysaccharide obtained from porcine or beef intestine possesses 4 times the N-sulfated glucosamine as N-acetylated glucosamine moieties; that from bovine lung has 10 times as much N-sulfated glucosamine as N-acetylated glucosamine. Heparin derived from porcine or bovine intestine or bovine lung has a slight preponderance of sulfated glucosamine over nonester sulfated glucosamine groups (90, 507, 639). The disaccharide unit iduronsyl-2-sulfate glucosamine-2,6 disulfate represents the major structural element of all heparin preparations (280). However, a variety of other disaccharides are present within mucopolysaccharide preparations (601). Heparin is present within aqueous solutions as a loose helical coil with the sulfate and COOH-terminal groups directed into the aqueous environment. The precise structure of a given turn of the helical coil depends on the monosaccharide sequence in that region.

Mucopolysaccharides exhibit heterogeneity in molecular weight, ratios of glucuronic acid to iduronic acid, ratios of ester and N-sulfation, and amounts of N-acetylation (91, 245, 321). The anticoagulant potency is not tightly correlated with any of these properties. However, when Lam et al. (310) fractionated heparin by binding it to excess antithrombin, they found two distinct populations of heparin that differed greatly in their ability to bind to antithrombin. Two-thirds of the unfractionated heparin was unable to complex with antithrombin and was responsible for less than 15% of the anticoagulant activity. One-third of the unfractionated heparin bound tightly to antithrombin. The fraction possessed more than 85% of the total anticoagulant activity (310). Heparin isolated from many organs (including the human lung) behaves similarly (403).

Active heparin species, after fractionation on antithrombin, are still heterogeneous in molecular weight, varying from 7,000 to 20,000 (561). Those with molecular weights of 7,000 vary in specific activity from 35 to 400 units/mg, whereas those with molecular weights of 20,000 are more homogeneous and possess specific activities of 700–750 units/mg. Both of these forms of heparin interact similarly with antithrombin (561, 563).

To appreciate the functional properties of heparin with regard to the coagulation pathway, the biochemistry and physiology of its cofactor, plasma antithrombin, must be considered. Early reports (112, 418) indicated that thrombin lost activity when added to serum. It was then recognized (59) that heparin had anticoagulant activity only in the presence of a plasma protein, heparin cofactor. Kinetic studies (416, 666) demonstrated that antithrombin and heparin cofactor activity are closely related and that heparin accelerates the inactivation of thrombin by antithrombin. Abildgaard (1) isolated a human plasma, α_2-globulin, that exhibited both activities. Rosenberg and Damus (562) purified large amounts of human antithrombin and presented evidence that the plasma heparin cofactor activity was present in the same molecule.

Antithrombin III, or heparin cofactor, is considered the most important inhibitor of the later stages of the blood coagulation mechanism (222, 560). The single-chain protein ($M_r = 65,000$) ranges from 18 to 30 mg/dl plasma (3–5 μM) (222), which is more than enough to inhibit all the thrombin that can be formed from prothrombin (1.5 μM) (160). Antithrombin inhibits many serine proteases to varying degrees in addition to thrombin, e.g., the coagulation factors IXa and Xa (560, 615). Antithrombin III also inhibits plasma kallikrein (306), factor VIIa (196), factor XIa (120, 589a),

and plasmin in vitro (222, 306), but the inactivation is slow and incomplete even in the presence of heparin.

Heparin alters the reaction rate but not the affinity. The reaction between antithrombin and thrombin, or factor Xa, is enhanced at least a thousandfold by heparin. The data indicate that each antithrombin molecule binds one enzyme molecule. This stoichiometry is unchanged by heparin; however, the complex formation with heparin is so rapid that the rate is difficult to measure (562). The active site of thrombin is required for formation of the antithrombin-enzyme complex, because the addition of DFP, which alkylates the active-site serine, totally inhibits the reaction (Fig. 7). Rosenberg and Damus (562) further demonstrated that the active-site serine of thrombin interacts with a critical arginyl residue in antithrombin to form a covalent bond. The complex resists denaturing agents but is cleaved by hydroxylamine, suggesting an ester linkage in the inhibitor–acyl enzyme complex (83, 489). Chemical modification of the lysyl residues of antithrombin (positively charged sites that bind the negatively charged heparin molecule) prevents binding of heparin to antithrombin; heparin's ability to enhance thrombin inactivation was decreased when it was added to the modified antithrombin. However, other studies indicate that heparin also interacts with thrombin (208); the exact mechanism of the inhibition of thrombin by antithrombin is still unclear.

The association between familial antithrombin deficiency and recurrent venous thromboembolism indicates the importance of antithrombin in the regulation of the coagulation system (358). In this autosomal dominant trait, antithrombin concentration ranged from 25% to 50% of normal. Some estimates

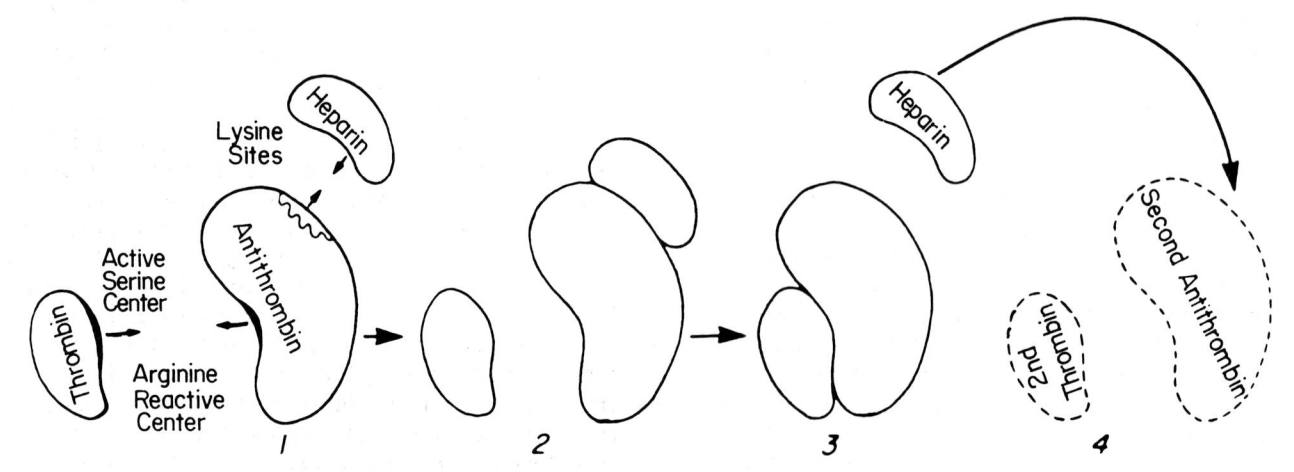

FIG. 7. Mechanism of thrombin inhibition by heparin–antithrombin III. Antithrombin III (antithrombin on figure), the major inhibitor of thrombin in plasma, serves as substrate for thrombin. 1) Active site of thrombin containing reactive serine attacks a peptide bond adjacent to an arginine residue in antithrombin III. Covalent ester bond forms to stabilize the complex. 2) Heparin can markedly accelerate this reaction by combining with antithrombin III at lysine-binding sites and inducing a conformational change on the inhibitor. 3) Heparin dissociates after combination of thrombin with antithrombin III. 4) Heparin can then accelerate the combination of a 2nd molecule of antithrombin III with thrombin, thus acting in a catalytic fashion. [From Rosenberg (560a), © 1981 by MIT Press.]

place the prevalence of heterozygous antithrombin deficiency at approximately 1/5,000 of the population (598); however, this is not the general experience. Clinical characteristics, shared by affected individuals with inherited antithrombin deficiency, include the onset of thrombosis (usually venous) between the ages of 10 and 30 yr. The affected individual presents with thrombophlebitis of the deep veins of the legs and with frequent pulmonary embolism. Predisposing events include surgery, pregnancy, trauma, and infection. Because of their depressed antithrombin levels, patients may appear to be heparin resistant and may require large amounts of heparin for adequate anticoagulation. The concentration of the inhibitor in some individuals with familial antithrombin deficiency increases after therapy with warfarin (358). In the majority of the families studied the immunologic and functional levels of antithrombin are depressed simultaneously (508). Variants have been reported with normal levels of the antithrombin antigen but low levels of functional inhibitory activity (386).

Why does a 50% concentration of antithrombin III predispose to thrombosis? With an animal model there is an inverse relationship between factor Xa inhibitory activity and the extent of thrombi formation (193). Paradoxically, heparin administration is associated with a progressive reduction in the functional and immunologic concentration of antithrombin (359). Whether this change predisposes to the thrombosis that may rarely occur during heparin therapy is not known.

Interaction of Thrombin With Fibrin

The recognition that thrombin is removed from clotting blood or plasma and adsorbed on fibrin clot led to the description of fibrin as an antithrombin (140). The association with fibrin occurs most likely via the secondary binding sites of thrombin but not through the catalytic site, because covalent modification of the active center with DFP does not affect the binding to fibrin (338). Bound thrombin, with full clotting activity, can be recovered after fibrin clot lysis by plasma. The binding of thrombin to fibrin in vivo may play an important regulatory role in the availability of the biologically active enzyme. On generation of thrombin in the blood the enzyme is bound initially to fibrinogen, which is then converted to fibrin. Thrombin remains reversibly attached to these proteins during the conversion and at the same time is protected from inactivation by antithrombin III. Thrombin bound to the platelet membrane receptor is similarly protected from inactivation by antithrombin III (604, 646). Bound thrombin is slowly released from the clot into the liquid phase to either activate more fibrinogen and platelets or to be inactivated by antithrombin III. Defective thrombin binding to fibrin clots occurs in some patients with fibrinolytic states or in some congenital dysfibrinogenemias. Under these conditions the balance between the free and bound enzyme is altered and thrombotic episodes may occur even without activation of other blood clotting factors.

Nonmammalian Inhibitors of Thrombin

A selective and potent inhibitor of thrombin, hirudin, is found in the saliva of the leech *Hirudo medicinalis*. Hirudin specifically inhibits thrombin (380, 381) and is the main anticoagulant of the leech, preventing the ingested blood from clotting. Hirudin is a polypeptide with a molecular weight of approximately 10,000. Bagdy et al. (22) have partially determined its amino acid sequence. The binding affinity of hirudin [inhibition constant (K_i) = 63 pM] is the highest known for thrombin (160). Parker and Mant (498) found a polypeptide similar to hirudin in the salivary gland of the tsetse fly *Glossina morsitans morsitans*. Interestingly the saliva of the giant South American leech *Haementeria ghilianii* does not contain any hirudinlike thrombin inhibitor; instead a fibrinogenolytic mechanism accomplishes the anticoagulation of blood (67).

Thrombinlike Enzymes in Snake Venoms

Snake venoms are a rich source of proteolytic enzymes. Some venoms induce the clotting of blood, plasma, and purified fibrinogen. This effect prompted the name *thrombinlike enzymes* for the active agents, and this misnomer is widely spread in the literature. The primary structure of fibrinogen-clotting enzymes from snake venoms is being actively investigated; the data will permit conclusions about amino acid sequence homology with that of human thrombin. Except for clotting of fibrinogen most of these enzymes are functionally different from thrombin: they are not inhibited by antithrombin III in the absence or presence of heparin, they do not activate clotting factors, and they do not aggregate blood platelets (593). Clotting of fibrinogen or plasma occurs with snake venoms from most of the *Crotalidae* group. Most of the *Elapidae* and *Viperidae* group venoms do not contain coagulant activity, with the exception of three *Elapidae* venoms and two *Viperidae* venoms (258, 476), which have marginal and perhaps indirect clotting activity.

The interest in thrombinlike enzymes developed because the blood of patients bitten by poisonous snakes was often unclottable for many days (546). Subsequent work in vitro with purified snake venom enzymes demonstrated specific cleavages in fibrinogen. Fibrinogen-clotting enzymes isolated from various snake venoms are valuable tools in studies on the structure and function of many proteins including fibrinogen. Some purified venom enzymes have prevented increased blood clottability in patients with thrombotic disorders by degrading fibrinogen in the circulation and activating fibrinolysis (30, 316, 623). Ancrod, an enzyme from the *Agkistrodon rhodostoma* venom, initiates fibrin polymerization by the cleavage of fibrinopeptide A only (158) but also causes significant degradation of the α-chain of fibrin (391, 584). Reptilase from *Bothrops jararaca* and batroxobin from *Bothrops atrox* also cleave fibrinopeptide A (39, 48, 182, 322) and form fine-structured clots that appear to contain fibrin monomers in an end-to-end arrangement (322). Fibrinogen-clotting activity was demonstrated in the venom of *Crotalus adamanteus*, the eastern diamondback rattlesnake. At least two enzyme species were found (378, 509) with specific clotting activity comparable to that of reptilase and batroxobin. The loss of fibrinopeptide B prior to the loss of fibrinopeptide A by the action of venom enzyme of the snake *Agkistrodon contortrix contortrix* does not induce fibrin polymerization above 25°C, but below this temperature clotting occurs (595), indicating that the loss of fibrinopeptide B reveals a binding site. Although fibrinogen-clotting activity was found in most of the *Crotalidae* venoms, these venom enzymes have not been as well characterized as those from the *Bothrops* or *Agkistrodon* genera.

ELECTRON MICROSCOPY OF FIBRINOGEN

Fibrinogen is a plasma glycoprotein consisting of three pairs of polypeptide chains. The concentration of fibrinogen in plasma varies from 175 to 350 mg/dl, with the mean value 260 mg/dl or 7 μM. The shape of the fibrinogen molecule has been debated for years. The trinodular structure seen originally by Hall and Slayter (214) in shadow-casting electron microscopy was not readily accepted (425). Negative-staining techniques were used to detect the presence of large globular structures with diameters of 23 nm (294, 526). The use of high concentrations of proteins and inorganic reagents may have formed the protein artifacts in these studies. The globular structure of fibrinogen is not compatible with hydrodynamic data and with properties of derivatives cleaved by some proteolytic enzymes. Recent electron-microscope patterns of fibrinogen obtained with either shadow casting or negative-staining techniques (168, 298, 682) support the trinodular shape of fibrinogen as shown in Figure 8. The molecule has an overall length of 45 nm and is composed of three nodules, two lateral (6.5 mm diam) and one central (5 nm diam). A thin filament approximately 15 nm long and 1–3 nm thick connects the nodules. The electron-microscope techniques examined the dehydrated fibrinogen molecule; thus the trinodular structure may not apply to the explanation of some properties of fibrinogen in aqueous solutions.

Electron-microscope patterns of crystallized clottable fragments derived by limited proteolysis provide further evidence of a nodular fibrinogen molecule (99, 648, 671). The trinodular model of the fibrinogen molecule is generally accepted. The model is useful because it is a simple explanation of the fibrin polymerization process and consistent with chemical data showing three domains (nodules) corresponding to the terminal plasmin-degradation products, fragments D and E (131, 181, 365, 518)

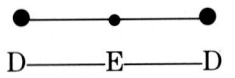

●———●———●
D———E———D

In this model the large end nodules correspond to the D domains and the central nodule to the E domain.

A refreshing approach to the shape of the fibrinogen molecule used freeze-etching electron microscopy to study the replicas of the molecule in the hydrated state in a water solution. The patterns had a banana-like shape without accentuation of any nodules or domains (19). These patterns of fibrin oligomers have not been published. Data from hydrodynamic measurements of model particles (326), from small-angle X-ray scattering (327), and from neutron small-angle scattering (377) support the flexible bananalike shape of fibrinogen in solution. These studies also indicate that the unusually high viscosity of fibrinogen solutions does not result from an extraordinary asymmetry, as formerly presumed, but from a very high degree of hydration. One gram of fibrinogen can bind as much as 4 g of water (19), compared to the frequently reported value of approximately 0.3 g of water per gram for many proteins. The structural characteristics associated with the unusual hydration of fibrinogen remain unexplained.

FIBRINOGEN STRUCTURE

Physical properties of fibrinogen are well established. The sedimentation constant $s_{20,w}$ is in the range of 7.6 to 8.6 (81, 271). The partial specific volume $\bar{v}$ is 0.725 g/ml^3 (8, 81, 290), and the diffusion coefficient is 1.98×10^{-7} cm^2/s (81, 603). The limiting viscosity number η is 0.24 (603, 627), a very high figure indicating either great asymmetry of the molecule (axial ratio 1:30) or an unusually high degree of hydration. The molecular weight for fibrinogen of 340,000 has been accepted on the basis of diffusion and sedimentation (81, 271, 603) and supported by sedimentation equilibrium data (145) and the sum of the molecular weights of the polypeptide chains, as determined by SDS–polyacrylamide gel electrophoresis (396, 399). Spectropolarimetric measurements revealed the presence of approximately 35% of an α-helical form (253, 404), which is irreversibly denatured in 5 M guanidine hydrochloride or in 5–10 M urea. Most of the α-helical structure of fibrinogen is recovered in fragment D (64).

Unraveling the amino acid sequence of human fibrinogen took 35 years, starting with paper chromatography of amino acid mixtures recovered from acid hydrolysate (23) and ending in 1979 with modern techniques of amino acid sequencing (136, 347). Only

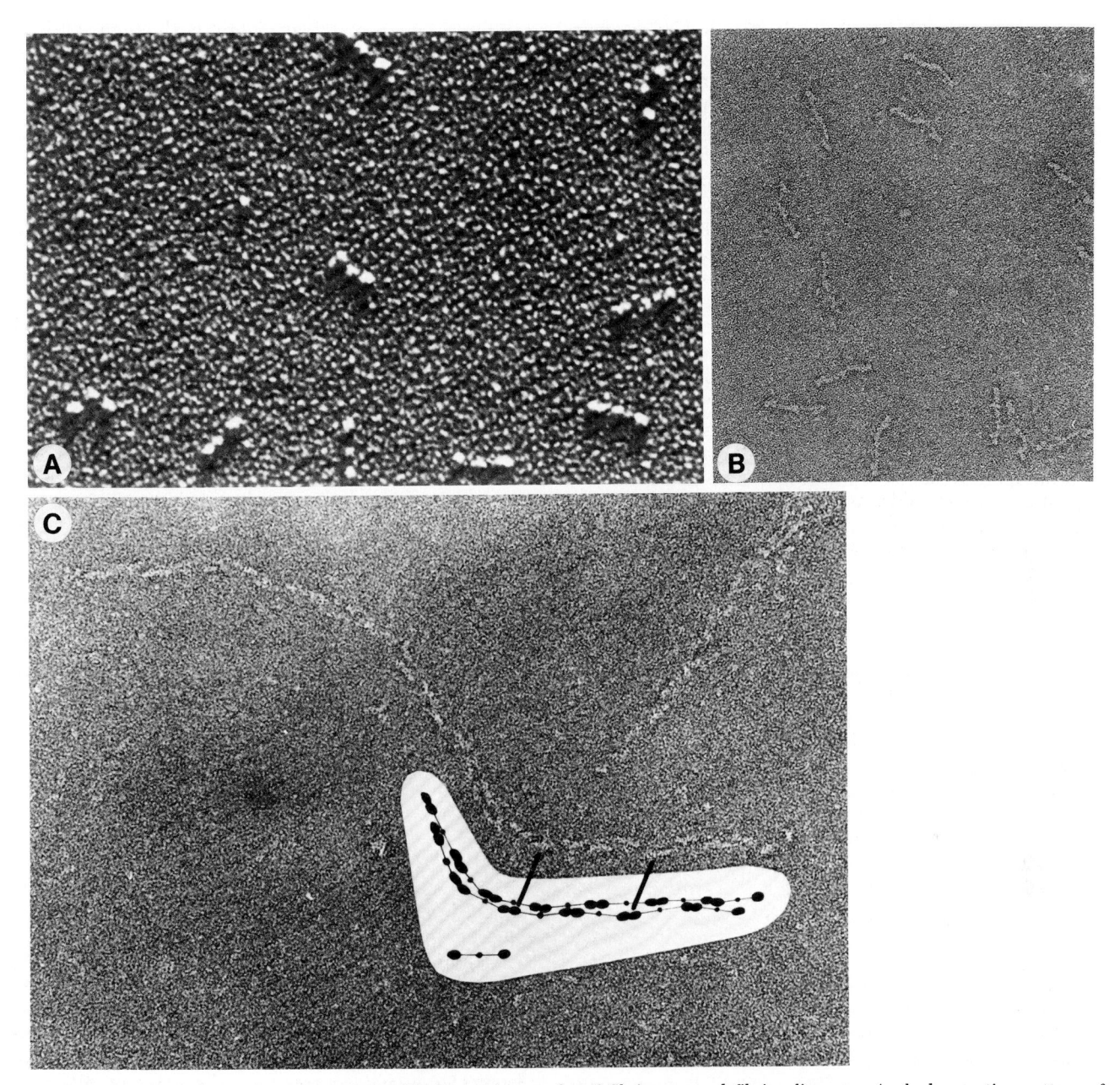

FIG. 8. Electron micrographs of fibrinogen and fibrin oligomers. A: shadow-casting pattern of fibrinogen demonstrating appearance of trinodular molecules. Technique did not permit visualization of connections between central and outer nodules. × 215,000. B: specimen stained negatively with uranyl acetate confirms elongated trinodular shape of fibrinogen molecules. Flexibility of molecules and thickness of connector that links nodules are apparent. × 194,000. C: fibrin oligomer, a protofibril, stained negatively. Interpretive drawing indicates half-staggered overlap of fibrin monomers, which form 2 parallel strands. Staggered association is basis of a 22.5-nm periodicity of fibrin fibers. Arrows, end-to-end junctions of outer nodules in adjacent fibrin monomers. × 194,000. [A from Hall and Slayter (214); B from Williams (682); C from Hantgan et al. (215).]

minor discrepancies remain in the sequence of the Aα- and Bβ-chains. Nucleotide sequencing of cDNAs corresponding to the individual fibrinogen chains will probably resolve these discrepancies. Chung et al. (88) have sequenced cDNA for bovine Bβ-chain and Crabtree and Kant (116) have cloned cDNAs for the Aα-, Bβ-, and γ-chains of rat fibrinogen.

There are three pairs of polypeptide chains in the fibrinogen molecule: the human Aα-chain (610 amino acids; M_r = 68,000), the Bβ-chain (461 amino acids; M_r = 58,000), and the γ-chain (411 amino acids; M_r = 47,000). Variants of the γ-chain have been reported differing in charge (414, 426) or molecular weight (172, 690); the γ-chain apparently has an extension with a molecular weight of approximately 3,000 at the COOH terminal. Extensive homology was found between the Bβ- and γ-chains (233) and some homology with the Aα-chains (665), which supports the popular concept that vertebrate fibrinogen evolved from a common single polypeptide chain ancestor. Carbohydrate moieties ($M_r \sim 2,500$) are attached at Bβ-Asn364 (234) and at γ-Asn52 (257, 414). The presence of a carbohydrate side chain attached to the Aα-chain has not been demonstrated. The addition of carbohydrate is a posttranslational modification catalyzed by several enzymes that complete the structure of this glycoprotein containing 3.5% carbohydrate. In liver disease (383, 491) and in hepatoma (202) an increased amount of sialic acid and galactose was reported in fibrinogen, resulting in a prolonged thrombin clotting time. Removal of sialic acid by neuraminidase shortened the clotting time in proportion to the number of sialic acid residues removed. Fetal fibrinogen also has elevated sialic acid content and delayed clotting, which partial removal of sialic acid corrected (188). Recently Gati and Straub (191) described a subpopulation of the normal fibrinogen polypeptide chains with a different sialic acid content in the Bβ- and γ-chains. In each of these chains two major species were found with approximately one or two residues of sialic acid per chain. This observation, implying the presence of branched oligosaccharides, has been confirmed by the demonstration (459) that the Bβ- and γ-chains contain biantennary oligosaccharide of the same sequence after removal of the terminal sialic acid

ical reactions of the protein. The model reflects a dimeric trinodular elongated form in which a thin long connector links the two larger COOH-terminal domains with the smaller NH₂-terminal domain (Fig. 9); it was suggested that the chains in the connector are folded into supercoiled α-helices (135). The molecule probably has a twofold axis of symmetry, by analogy with the conformation of immunoglobulins determined by X-ray diffraction (606). Thrombin cleaves fibrinopeptides A and B from the NH₂ terminals of the Aα- and Bβ-chains, respectively. This reaction exposes polymerization sites *A* and *B* in the central domain (473); a complementary binding site *a* is present in fibrinogen on the γ-chain without any thrombin action (474). The model also indicates the four rings, each involving six cysteine residues, that may tighten the entry sites of the connector to the domains and the three disulfide bridges that link the two halves of the molecule through the α—α and γ=γ covalent bonds. Four carbohydrate moieties are attached to the Bβ- and γ-chains. Cross-link sites reside in the COOH terminals of the Aα- and γ-chains and include donor (lysine) and acceptor (glutamine). The large portion of the COOH terminal of the Aα-chain may loosely fill the space and entrap large amounts of water in all directions outward from the three nodular domains and connectors.

Conversion of Fibrinogen to Fibrin Clot

It has long been postulated that fibrinogen transition to fibrin occurs in two steps catalyzed by throm-

$$\text{Gal}\beta \to \text{GlcNAc}\beta \to \text{Man}\alpha 1 \searrow$$
$$\substack{6 \\ 3}\text{Man}\beta 1 \to 4\text{GlcNAc}\beta 1 \to 4\text{GlcNAc}\beta \to \text{Asn}$$
$$\text{Gal}\beta \to \text{GlcNAc}\beta \to \text{Man}\alpha 1 \nearrow$$

The number of free sulfhydryl groups in the fibrinogen molecule is less than one (77, 232, 342); thus cysteine residues are involved in the formation of disulfide bonds. There are 29 disulfide bonds per fibrinogen molecule with known locations (233); only three (Aα-Cys28, γ-Cys8, and γ-Cys9) link the two halves of the dimeric molecule (51). These three disulfide bonds are stable and do not undergo disulfide exchange (44, 69). Two disulfide rings in each half of the fibrinogen molecule, 111 amino acid residues apart in the Aα- and γ-chains and 112 residues apart in the Bβ-chain, are unique structural features (135). The three polypeptide chains are bound together at junctions involving six cysteine residues. Disulfide bonds do not appear to directly affect the phenomenon of clottability: reduction under nondenaturing conditions of 10 disulfide bonds does not abolish thrombin clottability of the reduced fibrinogen (69).

Model of Fibrinogen Molecule

Doolittle (131) proposed a model of the fibrinogen molecule on the basis of physical properties and chem-

bin (309). Studies have demonstrated that the first step involves a limited proteolytic cleavage of the fibrinogen molecule; the second step involves a spontaneous specific association of the resulting species.

Thrombin releases two molecules of fibrinopeptide A from the Aα-chain and two molecules of fibrinopeptide B from the Bβ-polypeptide chain (53); this converts fibrinogen to fibrin monomer (Fig. 10). Thrombin releases fibrinopeptide A much faster than fibrinopeptide B (34). Fibrin monomers polymerize spontaneously to form a three-dimensional fibrin network. Years of investigation have not explained why fibrinogen remains in an aqueous solution and fibrin monomer polymerizes. Fibrinopeptide cleavage is needed for the clotting phenomenon, the formation of highly organized fibrin fibers. Electron microscopy reveals a 24-nm periodicity (corresponding to half the length of the fibrinogen molecule) and a few other repetitive cross-striation patterns (215). Fibrinogen precipitation with protamine sulfate or basic proteins shows the same periodicity in the precipitate (620, 621), indicating binding sites in fibrinogen that help

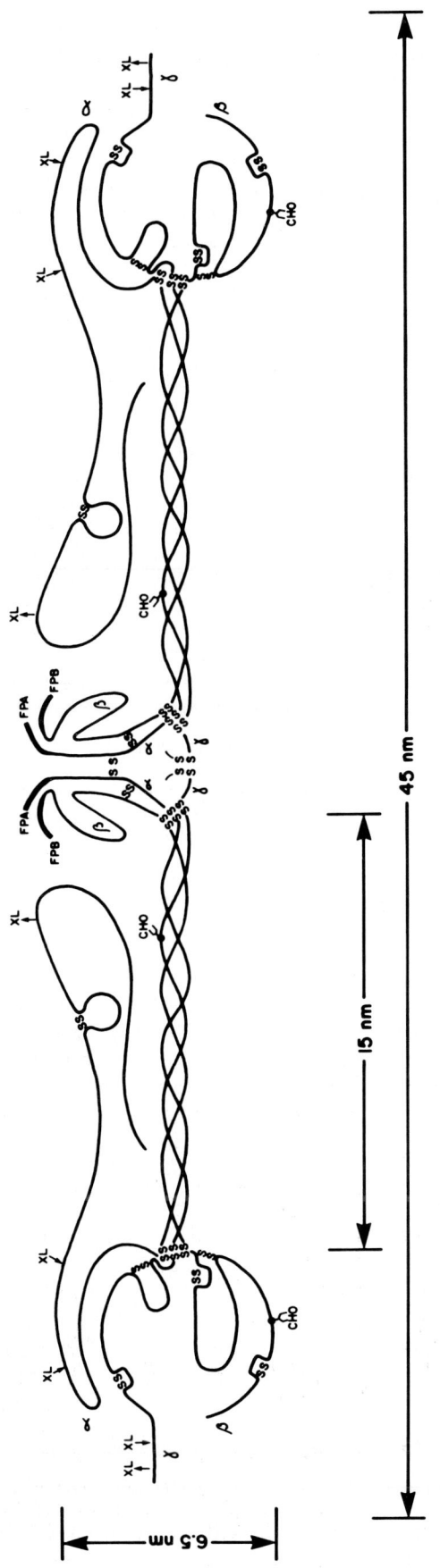

FIG. 9. Model of fibrinogen molecule. Dimeric structure of molecule with probable rotational symmetry. Overall length, ~45 nm; connector length, 15 nm; diameter of outer nodules, 6.5 nm; $M_r = 340,000$. Two pairs of 3 polypeptide chains; thrombin cleaves fibrinopeptides A and B (FPA and FPB, thickened segments) from NH$_2$ terminals of Aα- and Bβ-chains, respectively; γ-chain is not affected by thrombin. Four oligosaccharides (CHO), each $M_r \sim 2,500$, are attached to the Bβ- and γ-chains, endowing fibrinogen as a glycoprotein. There are 29 disulfide bonds (SS), 3 of which link 2 halves of the fibrinogen molecule: 1 bond is between Aα-chains and 2 bonds between γ-chains. Sites available for factor XIIIa–catalyzed cross-linking between lysine donors (XL, *arrow pointing upward*) and glutamine acceptors (XL, *arrow pointing downward*) are located in COOH terminals of Aα- and γ-chains. COOH terminals of Bβ- and γ-chains and adjacent part of connector are cleaved by plasmin as fragment D; corresponding portion of fibrinogen molecule is depicted by electron microscopy as outer nodule and defined as the structural D domain. NH$_2$ terminals of all 3 chains and adjacent part of connector are removed by plasmin as fragment E; this region is demonstrated on electron micrographs of fibrinogen as the central nodule and is called E domain. COOH terminals of Aα-chains (polar appendages) are loosely structured and possibly fill the space around connector.

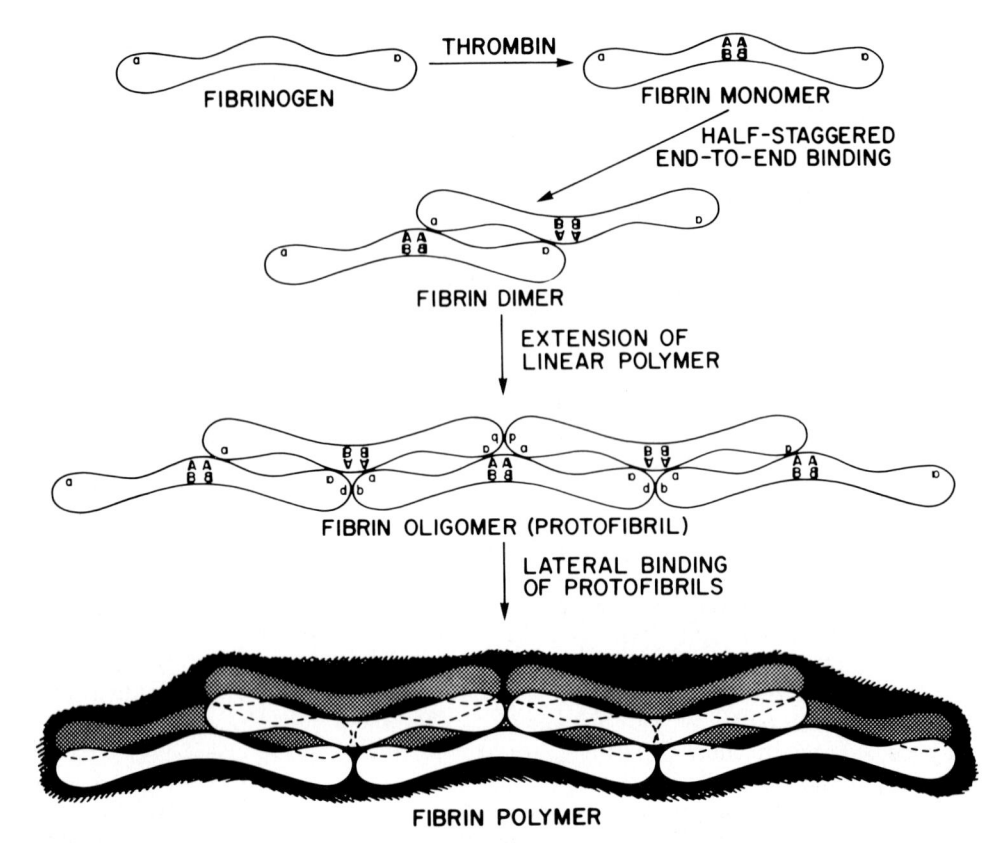

FIG. 10. Formation of fibrin. Driving force for assembly of fibrin network originates from specific association of complementary binding sites. One polymerization site (*a*) is present on fibrinogen molecule D domain. Complementary sites (*A*) are activated by thrombin in fibrin E domain. Due to a probable rotational symmetry, right half of fibrin molecule is a mirror reflection of left half. Binding between *a* and *A* sites on 2 fibrin monomer molecules forms 2 links that hold molecules in a half-staggered orientation. Extension of this process leads to end-to-end polymerization and generation of protofibrils. A new polymerization site (*bb*) appears on fibrin oligomer, probably because of alignment of 2 D domains; this site is apparently absent in fibrin monomer or dimer. A complementary site (*B*) is present in E domain of fibrin. Binding of *a* and *A* sites may propagate formation of linear fibrin protofibrils, whereas binding of *bb* with 2 *B* sites may be responsible for side-to-side coalescence of protofibrils.

to organize the molecules even without the cleavage of fibrinopeptides. Electron-microscope patterns of short oligomers of fibrin (215, 298) support the hypothesis that fibrin monomers assemble into fibers by a half-staggered overlap of the polymerizing units (161). The organization of fibrin monomers into a fibrin network may take place in two steps: an end-to-end alignment of monomers followed by a lateral aggregation of the fibrin strands (161). A speculative hypothesis suggests that the loss of fibrinopeptide A may initiate the end-to-end associations, whereas the cleavage of fibrinopeptide B may enable the side-to-side interactions (322). Both steps were observed by electron microscopy. A half-staggered association forms the first fibrin dimer (Fig. 10); successive addition of monomers to each end of the growing polymer results in the elongation of the fibrin strand, forming a protofibril of two half-staggered linear polymers (216). The arrangement of monomers in protofibrils implies that the polymerization could have occurred by a direct end-to-end linkage; however, this is not possible. In the second step of clot formation the individual protofibrils aggregate by side-to-side interactions, regardless of whether both fibrinopeptides are cleaved or fibrinopeptide A only (216). However, the formation of transparent or opaque clots after differential cleavage of fibrinopeptides A and B by proteases from certain snake venoms indicates an important role of fibrinopeptide B in the molding of fibrin structure (50, 472, 595). Fibrin I (which lacks only fibrinopeptide A) is more susceptible to proteolytic degradation than fibrin II (which lacks both fibrinopeptides A and B); this is evidence of the significant role of fibrinopeptide B cleavage in fibrin structure (304, 472, 519).

Polymerization Sites

Two sets of polymerization sites are thought to be involved in fibrin formation (50, 473). One set (*A, a* in Fig. 10) operates after the cleavage of fibrinopeptide A by thrombin. The association of the complementary sites A (in the NH$_2$-terminal domain) and a (in the COOH-terminal domain) results in half-staggered end-to-end polymerization and protofibril formation (215). In the linear polymer a new bivalent site bb occurs that is not functional in fibrin monomers (470, 473). Whether the formation of the bb site depends on the cleavage of fibrinopeptide B is not known. The release of fibrinopeptide B, however, activates site B (in the NH$_2$-terminal domain) complementary to bb. The binding of the bb site on protofibril with two B sites on another fibrin polymer represents the mechanism of side-to-side aggregation of protofibrils, resulting in thickening of fibrin strands and visible gelation.

Recently investigators have focused on localizing the regions of the fibrinogen or fibrin monomer molecule that participate in polymerization. Chemical modification of carboxylic acid groups (312), the amide groups of glutamine (132), histidine (161, 627), tyrosine (511, 607, 627), and lysine (80, 510) residues resulted in polymerization inhibition. These amino acids may either participate in the binding regions or may be located in their proximity, interfering with normal polymerization processes.

As an alternative, degradation products of fibrinogen and fibrin were used to localize binding regions. Early observations noted that fragment D inhibited fibrin monomer polymerization (314, 315), implying the presence of a binding region on this degradation product. Using insolubilized fibrin monomer, Matthias et al. (389, 390) suggested that the COOH terminal of the γ-chain remnant of fragment D may contain a polymerization site (301). Olexa and Budzynski (474) recently demonstrated that the site a resides in the 38 COOH-terminal residues of the γ-chain.

The location of the binding site in the NH$_2$-terminal domain of fibrin monomer is being actively pursued. Kudryk et al. (300) used insolubilized fibrinogen to imply that either the NH$_2$-terminal of the Bβ-chain or the COOH terminal of the γ-chain of the NH$_2$-terminal disulfide knot is necessary for polymerization. Abnormal fibrinogen Detroit (353) has a functional binding site in the fragment D domain but a defective site in the NH$_2$-terminal domain (299). This fibrinogen variant contains a single amino acid substitution, Aα-Arg19→Ser, suggesting that the binding site is at or near residue 19 on the Aα-chain (299). Recently, Laudano and Doolittle (318) provided evidence that the tripeptide Gly-Pro-Arg, which is contiguous with fibrinopeptide A, binds to fibrinogen and inhibits fibrin monomer polymerization. The tetrapeptide Gly-His-Arg-Pro, contiguous with fibrinopeptide B, binds also to fibrinogen (319), and Ca^{2+} increases the binding (320). Thus the cleavage of fibrinopeptides A and B by thrombin exposes polymerization sites in the α- and β-chains of fibrin. An important feature of the activation is the formation of a free α-amino group on glycine, because chemical modification of this group abolished the binding function (249, 319).

Cross-Linking of Fibrin

The final step in blood coagulation is the stabilization of the fibrin clot (308, 341, 343, 586). The enzyme involved, factor XIII, is activated by thrombin, which converts the inactive zymogen in the blood and platelets (586) into a Ca^{2+}-dependent transglutaminase (119, 166). The enzyme is unique in the coagulation system because it is not a serine protease but contains a free sulfhydryl group of cysteine in the catalytic site (89). The mechanism of factor XIIIa action involves the formation of a covalent amide bond between the γ-carbonyl group of glutamine and the ϵ-amino group of lysine. In the reaction glutamine is considered the amide acceptor and lysine the donor. The new bond, ϵ-(γ-glutamyl)lysine, has a cross-linking function because these residues are located in different polypeptide chains (515). The reaction is very specific: few glutamine or lysine residues are susceptible to cross-linking. However, comparing amino acid sequences around the cross-linking sites in the α- and γ-chains did not reveal any unique structures.

Fibrinogen can be slowly cross-linked by factor XIIIa (169, 275); thus cross-linking sites are exposed even without the removal of fibrinopeptides. Fowler et al. (169) found trinodular molecules cross-linked through the outer nodules in an end-to-end nonoverlapping fashion in an elegant electron-microscope study. This reaction, however, is not the main route under physiological conditions, because thrombin required for the activation of factor XIII also converts fibrinogen to fibrin. The substrate important for hemostasis is fibrin. The initial fast reaction links two γ-chains from two different fibrin monomer molecules aligned in an antiparallel arrangement. Each chain contributes γ-Gln398 and γ-Lys406 (located 14 and 6 residues from the COOH terminal, respectively), forming a γ-chain dimer (85, 134, 399). After completion of γ-chain dimerization a much slower process of α-chain polymerization occurs (397, 399). Two physiologically important glutamine residues, γ-Gln328 and Aα-Gln366, have been identified as amide acceptors (136); another glutamine residue, Aα-Gln237, may be involved in the cross-linking of the α-chain to other proteins (133, 175). Lysine residue Aα-Lys508 is a predominant cross-linking donor site; Aα-Lys556 and Aα-Lys562 probably also contribute to the formation of α-chain polymers (82). The greatly different rates of γ-chain dimerization and α-chain polymerization imply that in the fibrin protofibrils the COOH terminals of the γ-chains are already aligned. However, the long COOH terminals of the α-chains seem to be loosely spaced around protofibrils. Perhaps the coalescence into thicker fibers is required to bring the donor and acceptor residues in close proximity to be cross-linked. Four to six ε-(γ-glutamyl)lysine bonds were found per molecule of fibrin monomer in cross-linked blood clots and thrombi (516). Gaffney et al. (186) found all γ- and α-chains in cross-linked forms in fibrin from patients with venous and arterial thromboembolism.

INTERACTION OF FIBRINOGEN WITH PLASMA PROTEINS

The purification of fibrinogen from human and animal plasma with a variety of procedures established that certain proteins are difficult to remove, although the solubility, molecular weight, and overall charge of these proteins differed greatly from those of fibrinogen. The development of sensitive function-specific techniques and immunologic assays demonstrated contamination of fibrinogen preparations with plasma fibronectin (452), plasminogen (391), von Willebrand's factor (451), and factor XIII (341, 451). These observations imply that some contaminants may not be just trapped nonspecifically during the purification procedures but may persistently accompany fibrinogen due to a specific affinity. Fibrinogen interaction with some plasma proteins may be a prelude to either formation or dissolution of clots. The association with fibrinogen is not easily broken during fractionation with ammonium sulfate, sodium sulfate, glycine, or low concentrations of ethanol; however, ion-exchange and affinity chromatography does disrupt the interaction. The fibrinogen affinity for plasma proteins reflects properties that have not been clearly recognized in the past.

The binding of fibrinogen with fibrin monomer is the major associative function of fibrinogen (597). Soluble complexes of various molecular weights were formed between fibrinogen and fibrin monomers, which lack either fibrinopeptide A or both fibrinopeptides A and B. The fibrin monomer formed a clot on dissociation; thus it was postulated that the soluble complexes play a regulatory role in clot deposition. Fibrin kept soluble was ready for deposition at a site where the dissociation could occur (337, 597). Attempts to detect and measure intravascular coagulation produced a voluminous literature on the presence of soluble fibrin in a variety of diseases. The results indicate that the presence of soluble fibrin complexes in the circulation accompanies thromboembolic phenomena. The diagnostic value of the complexes in disseminated intravascular coagulation or hypercoagulable states is disputed, however (31, 348, 433). Gel-filtration chromatography is one of the most common methods for analysis (164, 313, 437), although it can detect only stable and cross-linked complexes. The latter may be formed in the liquid phase under the combined action of thrombin, factor XIIIa, and plasmin on fibrinogen without previous deposition of a clot (213). The molecular composition of fibrinogen-fibrin monomer complexes is not fully clarified, despite many studies (164, 597, 609), because of the many possible interactions between different fibrin monomers. A controversy concerning which fibrin-degradation products participate in soluble complexes further complicates the situation (317, 609). Although experiments support the existence of fibrinogen-fibrin monomer complexes, their structure and properties are not fully understood.

Plasma fibronectin is a 440,000-M_r glycoprotein composed of two polypeptide chains held together by disulfide bonds at the COOH terminals and having the NH$_2$-terminal sequence Pyr-Ala-Glu (259, 423). This protein (cold-insoluble globulin) is the major nonclottable component of Cohn fraction I; in the cold it coprecipitates with fibrinogen (421). Polymeric forms of this protein were found in tissues and adherent cells of vertebrates; therefore the universal name *fibronectin* was proposed, denoting that it binds to fibrous proteins, in particular collagen and fibrin (651). The binding is mediated partly by the formation of factor XIIIa–catalyzed cross-linking bonds (429, 430). Cryoprecipitates in plasma are more abundant in the presence of heparin, which potentiates the coprecipitation of fibrinogen and fibronectin. The COOH terminal of the fibrinogen Aα-chain may account for the precipitation with fibronectin (614). Fibronectin has been demonstrated in human platelets (522), but it does not seem to significantly affect fibrinogen binding to platelet membrane receptors (452, 700). The association of fibronectin with fibrinogen has been reported in some diseases (424). Plasma fibrinogen is heterogeneous and even after purification has two major species ($M_r \sim 340,000$ and $M_r \sim 320,000$) (451). After separation in SDS–polyacrylamide gel electrophoresis, a heparin-precipitable fraction at 2°C from normal human plasma contained only the HMW fibrinogen species (614). The LMW species lacked the Aα-chain COOH-terminal peptide ($M_r \sim 13,200$) (427), implying that a fibronectin-binding site may be localized in this missing polypeptide chain segment. Fibrin binding to fibronectin occurs via cross-linking bonds catalyzed by factor XIIIa. An NH$_2$-terminal 27,000-M_r fragment of fibronectin cleaved by either trypsin (430) or plasmin (270) contains the glutaminyl residues of the participating acceptor. The same structural region is involved in cross-linking with collagen and binding of bacteria. Cross-linked heteropolymers of fibrin and fibronectin enhance in tissue culture the attachment and spreading of cells (209). This observation may be relevant for adhesion and migration of cells proliferating during wound healing.

Fibrinogen interaction with von Willebrand's factor has not been studied. However, this factor has some structural and functional similarities with fibronectin: both proteins have polypeptide chain subunits of similar size, and the binding of von Willebrand's factor to collagen has been demonstrated (328, 466). The latter phenomenon may reflect the mechanism of platelet adhesion to subendothelial tissue.

The binding of plasminogen with fibrinogen and fibrin is well documented. This specific association occurs through lysine-binding sites on the plasminogen molecule (533, 612, 643). The interaction with plasminogen is important for the initiation of fibrinolysis on the clot surface. Deutsch and Mertz (124) used affinity chromatography on lysine-Sepharose to easily separate plasminogen from fibrinogen.

Because both fibrinogen and fibrin are substrates for factor XIIIa, a binding with this enzyme is anticipated. Factor XIII may also interact with fibrinogen through its binding site(s); however, direct evidence of this is lacking.

INTERACTION OF FIBRINOGEN WITH CELLS

Because of its asymmetric shape and high degree of hydration, fibrinogen increases the viscosity of the blood. Fibrinogen in the blood interacts with erythrocytes and affects their aggregation, often by forming rouleaux. This effect depends on the fibrinogen concentration and probably results from its absorption on the surface of erythrocytes. The erythrocyte aggregates in the large blood vessels are broken apart as the shear rate increases; the extent of aggregation is inversely proportional to the velocity of blood flow. The association between fibrinogen and erythrocytes does not appear to be strong. Extensive washing of whole blood clots removes almost all erythrocytes from the fibrin network. In contrast, platelet remnants in blood clots usually adhere to the fibrin network, indicating a strong interaction between these thrombi elements.

Evidence shows that unactivated platelets do not react with fibrinogen in blood or purified systems. However, ADP-activated platelets require fibrinogen for aggregation (118, 611). The promotion of platelet aggregation is a hemostatic function of fibrinogen that is not dependent on its conversion to fibrin by thrombin. In the plasma of patients with congenital afibrinogenemia, ADP-activated platelets aggregate poorly (676). Suspensions of washed or gel-filtered human platelets aggregate slightly, if at all, in high concentrations of aggregating agents. The addition of fibrinogen to such suspensions restores platelet aggregability to the level found in normal platelet-rich plasma (436, 454, 636). Monovalent Fab antifibrinogen antibody fragment, which inhibits fibrin polymerization but not the release of fibrinopeptides, prevents platelet aggregation by thrombin (647). These observations suggest a direct role for fibrinogen in platelet aggregation and utilization of fibrinogen either from the extracellular pool or after secretion from α-granules (60). The intact polypeptide chains of fibrinogen are required for platelet aggregation, because fragment X is significantly less potent (451). Platelets stimulated by ADP (33, 376, 435, 505) or epinephrine (33, 524) expose specific Ca^{2+}-dependent fibrinogen receptor. There is a correlation between the amount of bound fibrinogen and the extent of platelet aggregation (506). Because intact platelets do not interact with fibrinogen, the binding sites on the surface may be covered by membrane proteins. On activation a shape change occurs, followed by metabolic and secretory changes. These events may expose the binding sites to the surrounding milieu. Attempts to solve this problem used proteolytic digestion with chymotrypsin (204, 452) or pronase (452) to remove the membrane proteins. Such platelets agglutinate in the presence of fibrinogen by a direct mechanism that is independent of platelet metabolic energy and ADP but requires Ca^{2+}. Kornecki et al. (295) demonstrated two classes of fibrinogen receptors of high (K_d = 21 nM; n = 960–1,860) and low (K_d = 8.4 μM; n = 88,000–400,000) affinity. Most studies showed a direct correlation between the amount of bound fibrinogen and the rate of platelet aggregation, supporting the dependence of aggregation on the occupancy of the specific receptors by fibrinogen. Furthermore as a bivalent molecule fibrinogen may link the adjacent platelets in the presence of Ca^{2+}, inducing the phenomenon of aggregation.

Platelet membrane glycoproteins II_b and III_a may act as a fibrinogen-binding site because on membrane activation by thrombin the two glycoproteins form clusters, as demonstrated by immunoelectron microscopy (525). Glycoproteins II_b or III_a are missing in platelets from patients with Glanzmann's thrombasthenia. Such platelets do not aggregate with ADP and lack fibrinogen receptor (295, 453).

The bivalent structure of the fibrinogen molecule seems to play an essential role in the link between two cells, perhaps through its binding to membrane glycoproteins. A second suggestion is that fibrinogen interaction with cell surface fibronectin may mediate cell-to-surface and cell-to-cell attachments (651). A third possibility is the binding of fibrinogen to cell actomyosin and contractile proteins, as in clot retraction, which occurs in the presence of platelets, fibroblasts (454), and leukocytes but not erythrocytes (456).

The agglutinating function of fibrinogen is also expressed in its interaction with certain strains of staphylococci that clump in the presence of this protein. The reaction occurs at fibrinogen concentrations as low as 0.1 μg/ml. Hawiger et al. (227) developed a staphylococcal clumping test to quantify fibrinogen. The molecular basis of staphylococcal clumping is attributable primarily to the bivalent, dimeric structure of fibrinogen. Reduced and carboxymethylated human fibrinogen binds to staphylococci but does not induce clumping (226). The clumping activity of fragment X isolated from advanced digests of fibrinogen has decreased more than the clumping activity of its less-degraded counterpart; the binding of their chains is significantly decreased compared with that of fibrinogen.

DEGRADATION BY PROTEASES OTHER THAN PLASMIN

The COOH terminal of the Aα-chain is attacked first by many proteases. The rapid degradation of this chain agrees with its probable exposure on the surface of the fibrinogen and fibrin molecules. Fibrinogen-degradation products cleaved by other proteases and the sequence of their appearance are different from those observed in plasmic digests; the only exception is trypsin. Most studies concentrated on the phenomenology of degradation and the fate of biologic functions but did not isolate and characterize the products. Trypsin rapidly cleaves fibrinopeptides A and B and will clot fibrinogen at low temperatures (4); the subsequent degradation resembles that of plasmin even in the demonstration of similar X, Y, D, and E groups of derivatives (363, 407). Mihalyi and Godfrey (405) isolated a late trypsin-degradation product with physicochemical properties similar to those of plasmic fragment D. Chymotrypsin degradation is kinetically different (406), apparently because of its specificity for cleaving peptide bonds of nonpolar amino acids. Chymotrypsin degrades the fragment D domain to peptides that do not precipitate with antifibrinogen antiserum, but the fragment E domain is resistant (363). Recently interest was directed to the proteolytic enzymes derived from cells, particularly from leukocytes, because in vivo a number of cells invade clots and may contribute to fibrin dissolution. The investigations did not determine the relative lytic effect of cellular enzymes as compared with the effect of the activation of the plasminogen in the clot. The studies showed, however, that the qualitative degradation pathway of fibrinogen is different from the degradation pathway catalyzed by plasmin. Human peripheral blood leukocytes degrade fibrinogen in an entirely different pattern compared with the degradation of plasmin (523). The Aα-, Bβ-, and γ-chains are cleaved; the initial products are larger than fragment X, not clottable by thrombin, and have potent anticoagulant activity. Bilezikian and Nossel (38) confirmed and extended these observations, showing that both fibrinopeptides A and B were removed with attached segments of the α- and β-chains, respectively. The specificity of the leukocyte proteases for fibrinogen is unique. Fibrinogen digestion with elastaselike neutral protease isolated from human granulocytes produced comparable results (203). Purified human neutrophil neutral protease also attacks initially the Aα-chain; however, the degradation products do not have anticoagulant properties (670).

The salivary glands of the giant South American leech *Haementeria ghilianii* contain in the cytosol fraction a fibrinolytic anticoagulant, hementin (68). Hementin is a proteolytic enzyme that degrades fibrinogen and fibrin, even in the presence of the protease inhibitors occurring in human plasma (67). The enzyme has the same affinity for human fibrinogen and fibrin. It cleaves fibrinogen initially in the Aα-chain and then the γ-chain, yielding characteristic HMW fragments that are different from the fragments caused by plasmin digestion of fibrinogen.

Some snake venoms contain proteases that degrade fibrinogen and fibrin. In some instances these venoms do not have agents that clot fibrinogen. These proteases usually degrade significantly only the Aα-chain; however, enzymes from two snake venoms cleave the Bβ-chain faster than the Aα-chain (Table 2). The venom of the western diamondback rattlesnake, from which four different venom proteases were isolated, is an exception; proteases II and III degrade fibrinogen in plasma in the presence of protease inhibitors, rendering it unclottable by a cleavage of the Bβ-chain without degradation of the Aα- and γ-chains (494).

TABLE 2. *Fibrinogenolytic Enzymes in Snake Venoms*

Species	Common Name	Enzyme	M_r	Chain Cleaved	Ref.
Agkistrodon contortrix mokasen	Northern copperhead	Fibrinogenase	22,900	Aα	417
Agkistrodon acutus	Sharp-nosed pit viper	Fibrinolytic	24,100	Aα	483, 484
Trimeresurus mucrosquamatus	Chinese habu	α-Fibrinogenase	22,400	Aα	486, 487
		β-Fibrinogenase	26,000	Bβ, then Aα	
Trimeresurus gramineus	Green tree viper	α-Fibrinogenase	23,500	Aα	485
		β-Fibrinogenase	25,000	Bβ, then Aα	
Crotalus atrox	Western diamondback rattlesnake	Fibrinolytic	21,500 60,000		24, 25
Crotalus atrox	Western diamondback rattlesnake	Fibrinogenolytic proteases			494
		I	19,500	Aα	
		II	24,000	Bβ	
		III	28,500	Bβ	
		IV	45,000	Aα	

This unique action indicates the importance of the Bβ-chain in fibrin polymerization and clot formation.

DEGRADATION OF FIBRINOGEN AND FIBRIN BY PLASMIN

The interest in proteolytic degradation of fibrinogen developed from observations that plasmin digestion of fibrinogen formed products with anticoagulant activity (455, 649). Thus degradation of fibrinogen by plasmin (the enzyme formed during activation of the fibrinolytic system) could counteract and balance the clot-forming effect of thrombin generated in the activated coagulation system. To characterize the degradation products and explain their anticoagulant activities, plasmic digests of human fibrinogen were separated by ion-exchange chromatography. Five fractions were isolated: fragments A, B, C, D, and E (464, 465). Fragments D and E are the major end products; fragments A, B, and C are LMW remnants of the Aα- and Bβ-chains. Intermediate products, fragments X and Y, were recognized and characterized later (70, 366-368). The sequential degradation of fibrinogen by plasmin was observed; the proposed asymmetric scheme of digestion (360, 367) is illustrated in Figure 11. The initial cleavages in the fibrinogen molecule occur at the COOH terminal of the Aα-chain (187, 412) and at the NH$_2$ terminal of the Bβ-chain (307, 596), which are the most susceptible regions for enzymatic hydrolysis. As a result the 250,000-M_r fragment X (368) is formed. This derivative is heterogeneous (163, 422, 599) but remains clottable with thrombin. Next an asymmetric cleavage of fragment X occurs, which splits peptide bonds in the Aα-, Bβ-, and γ-chains approximately in the middle of the supercoiled connector (Fig. 11), resulting in the formation of 155,000-M_r fragment Y (368) and 103,000-M_r fragment D (364, 520, 521), neither of which is clottable by thrombin. Furthermore proteolysis by plasmin results in the second asymmetric split, which degrades fragment Y into 45,000-M_r fragment E (364, 518) and another fragment D molecule. The asymmetric scheme of fibrinogen degradation by plasmin required that two fragment D molecules form from one fibrinogen molecule. Experiments have verified the suggestion that fibrinogen has two fragment D domains and one fragment E domain. Subsequently the close structural relationship between fragment E and the NH$_2$-terminal disulfide knot was established (46): these two degradation products have similar NH$_2$-terminal amino acids; similar contents of cysteine, tyrosine, and tryptophan; similar molecular weights; and form immunoprecipitation lines of identity with antiserum against fibrinogen (361, 365). The most important conclusion concerning fragment E and the NH$_2$-terminal disulfide knot was the realization of their common origin from the NH$_2$-terminal domain of the fibrinogen molecule. This was a landmark in the understanding of fibrinogen structure, which consists of six polypeptide chains linked at their NH$_2$ terminals. A study showing 2 mol of fibrinopeptide A in fragments X and Y (66) and a demonstration of fragment Y asymmetry by electron microscopy (170) support this fibrinogen model.

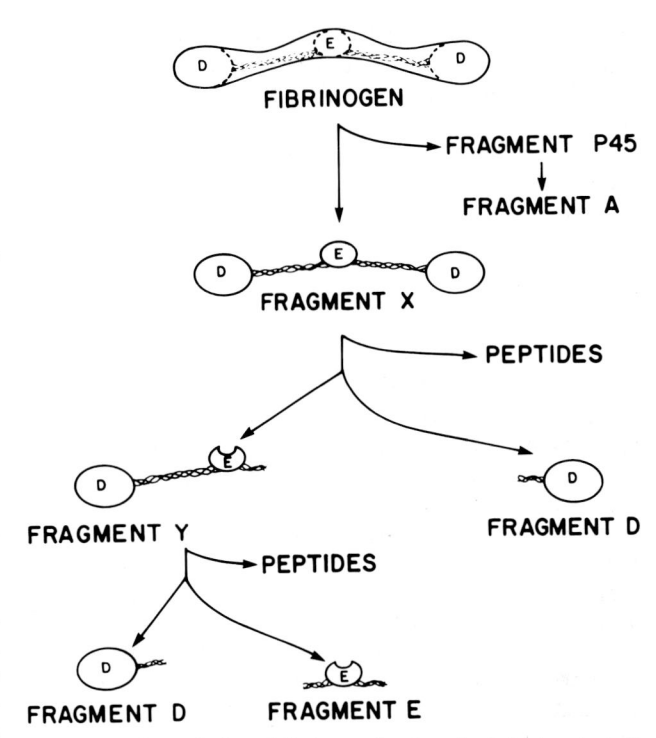

FIG. 11. Degradation of fibrinogen by plasmin. Initial proteolytic attack removes the COOH terminal of Aα-chain as fragment P45 and its degradation product fragment A. Fragment X is a group of derivatives, the less degraded of which are coagulable by thrombin. Fragments X and Y are cleaved asymmetrically to form terminal degradation products, fragments D and E. From 1 fibrinogen molecule 2 molecules of fragment D and 1 of fragment E are formed.

Fragments D and E account for approximately 75% of the fibrinogen molecule. Another 25% is recovered in heterogeneous derivatives of a large, COOH-terminal segment of the Aα-chain, the so-called polar appendage (131). One of these derivatives is fragment P45 (175), a large 45,000-M_r segment of a single polypeptide chain. This fragment is expected from the reaction: fibrinogen → fragment X + 2 fragments P45. This degradation product was seen in early plasmic digests of fibrinogen on SDS-polyacrylamide gel electrophoresis (175, 413), and a partial purification of this fragment was reported (65, 235, 659). A terminal degradation product of fragment P45 is 21,000-M_r fragment A (217, 235, 634, 635).

Several approaches were used to localize fragment D in the COOH-terminal domain of the fibrinogen molecule. The origin of fragment D was postulated and accepted before the amino acid sequence of this part of fibrinogen was known. Evidence is also provided from calculations of molecular weights of fragments D (M_r = 103,000) and E (M_r = 45,000) derived from the cleavage of fragment Y ($M_r = 155,000$) (360). This is supported by the observation with SDS–polyacrylamide gel electrophoresis that one γ-chain in fragment Y is the same as in fibrinogen (66, 181, 411, 518) and by the presence of the COOH-terminal sequence of the Bβ-chain in this fragment. The determination of the amino acid sequence of the COOH terminal of human and bovine fibrinogen γ-chain showed that lysine residues in position 6 from the terminal and glutamine residues in position 14 are involved in the formation of factor XIIIa–catalyzed ε-(γ-glutamyl)lysine cross-link bonds (85). The demonstration that fragment D can be cross-linked by factor XIIIa and form fragment DD is proof of the origin of the fragment from the COOH terminal of the fibrinogen molecule (521). Although the Bβ-chain COOH terminal does not have any measurable function, its presence in fragment D was initially deduced from the distribution of molecular weight between fragments D and E (66, 181, 187, 411, 518). The final proof came from the amino acid sequences of the Bβ-chain terminals in fragment D and fibrinogen, which were identical.

It is evident from the polypeptide chain composition of fragments X, Y, D, E, and A, and of cyanogen bromide derivatives (which have been cleaved at methionine residues) that almost the entire fibrinogen molecule can be recovered in HMW degradation products. Proteolytic degradation of fibrinogen does not seem to induce significant changes of conformation; the degradation products retain several functions of the parent fibrinogen molecule.

Fibrin is the main target for plasmin in the blood clot. Plasmic degradation products of non-cross-linked fibrin are very similar to those of fibrinogen (including fragments X, Y, D, and E) except for the absence of the fibrinopeptides (63, 139, 520). Apparently the conversion of fibrinogen to fibrin produces no significant change of conformation. However, plasmic products derived from cross-linked fibrin are different because of the presence of the γ-chain dimers and α-chain polymers in the fibrin network. The α-chain polymers are quite susceptible to plasmic digestion and are degraded to a heterogeneous group of LMW fragments (175, 217, 635). From the remaining partially digested fibrin, intermediate HMW products are cleaved (5, 544) and characterized by the presence of unruptured connectors between the domains of fragments D and E, e.g., the complex DY/YD (171, 173). Plasmin degrades these species to a (DD)E complex, a primary soluble degradation product of cross-linked fibrin (183, 187, 199, 251, 471). The γ-chain dimers bound covalently by ε-(γ-glutamyl)lysine cross-link bonds between different fibrin molecules (85, 399) are the structural basis of the plasmin-resistant fragment DD species (183, 251, 293, 364, 520, 521), which are noncovalently bound to fragment E in the (DD)E complex. Plasmic degradation of cross-linked fibrin also differs from that of non-cross-linked fibrin or fibrinogen in that unique species of fragment E are formed, i.e., fragments E_1 ($M_r \sim 60,000$), E_2 ($M_r \sim 55,000$), and E_3 ($M_r \sim 50,000$) (471). Fragments E_1 and E_2 can bind to fragment DD, forming a (DD)E complex; fragment E_3 cannot (470). It appears that fragments E_1 and E_2 either are not formed or are readily degraded during plasmic digestion of fibrinogen or non-cross-linked fibrin. Thus plasmic digestion of cross-linked fibrin proceeds according to the scheme shown in Figure 12.

The scheme outlines the proteolysis of preformed fibrin by plasmin. However, in physiological or pathological situations in vivo there is a dynamic state between fibrin formation and lysis. The initial attack of thrombin on fibrinogen removes fibrinopeptide A, and fibrin I polymer is formed. Further action of thrombin occurs at a solid-liquid interphase, resulting in removal of fibrinopeptide B and formation of fibrin II. However, plasmin competes with thrombin for the NH_2 terminal of the Bβ-chain, although for different peptide bonds. If plasmin acts on fibrin I before thrombin it cleaves a segment Bβ-Pyr1-Arg42, containing fibrinopeptide B; this prevents further consolidation of the clot. Plasmin cleavage of fibrin I may regulate the formation of fibrin II and the relative rates of proteolysis of the Bβ-chain by thrombin, and plasmin may determine the occurrence of thrombotic disease (463).

Role of Fibrin in Clot Formation and Lysis

Experiments indicate that fibrin structure directly participates in the last stage of blood coagulation and in the activation of the fibrinolytic system. Fibrin is not a mere physical plug formed at the site of the injured blood vessel to arrest hemorrhage. Highly organized fibrin fibers in the clot possess exposed specific binding sites that interact with enzymes and cofactors.

The binding of thrombin with fibrin (338) fulfills a dual role, removing free enzyme from the site of thrombus formation and protecting bound active thrombin from irreversible inactivation by antithrombin III. An analogous interaction probably occurs with factor XIIIa; however, supportive data are not available. Three Ca^{2+}-binding sites demonstrated on fibrinogen (375, 528) are most likely to be present in fibrin as well. Thus fibrin could play a Ca^{2+}-mediated regulatory role in hemostasis, as exemplified by the regulation of factor XIII activation by Ca^{2+} bound to fibrinogen (117). The binding of fibrinogen to the activated platelets followed by its conversion to fibrin may result in the incorporation of all or part of the platelet membranes into the clot, probably endowing it with immobilized platelet receptors. All these phenomena render the fibrin clot surface thrombogenic.

At the same time a counteracting process takes place in fibrin. The clot has specific binding functions toward several components of the fibrinolytic system.

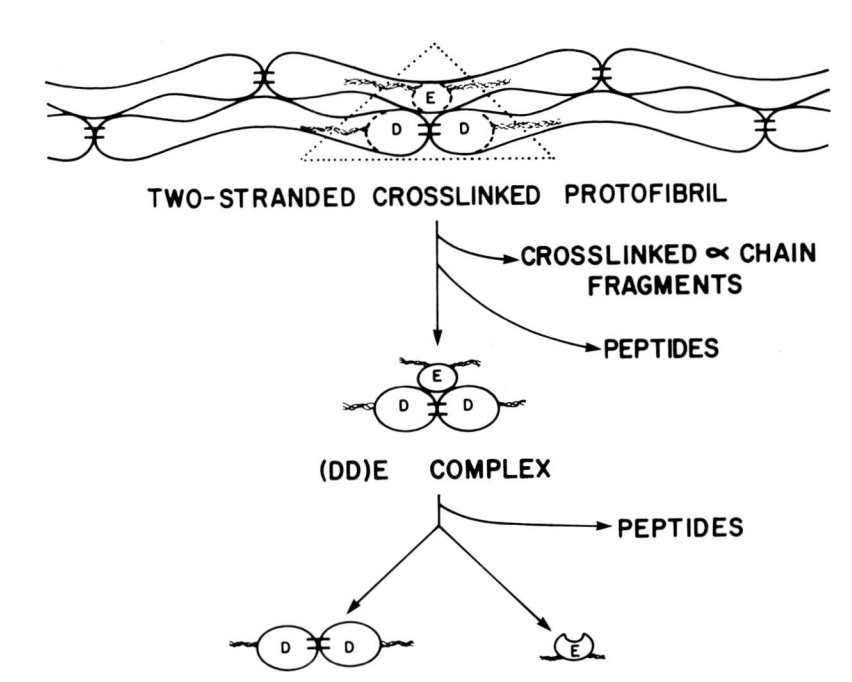

FIG. 12. Degradation of cross-linked fibrin by plasmin. Initial enzyme action cleaves cross-linked α-chain COOH-terminal fragments as a mixture of derivatives. Next exposed connectors are disrupted and a (DD)E complex liberated. Components of the complex are derived from 3 different fibrin monomer molecules and 2 fragments D are kept together by covalent cross-link bonds. Fragment E in the complex still has A and B polymerization sites; however, after long proteolysis with plasmin the sites are damaged and the complex falls apart.

Again, the role of fibrin appears to be twofold: it serves as a cofactor in the activation process and protects bound active fibrinolytic enzymes from inactivation by plasma inhibitors of proteases. The network of fibrin fibers is significant in the regulation of the coagulation and fibrinolytic systems.

PLASMINOGEN AND PLASMIN

Human plasminogen is a circulating single-chain glycoprotein with a molecular weight of approximately 92,000 [Figs. 1 and 13; (93, 556, 644, 661, 686)]. Its concentration in plasma is 20 mg/dl or 2.2 µM (529, 699). The site of plasminogen biosynthesis was controversial for decades until a recent report demonstrated its synthesis by primary cultures of rat hepatocytes (55). Plasminogen exists in two major forms, which differ in molecular weight and NH$_2$-terminal residues: the native protein has glutamic acid (Glu-plasminogen); however, a degraded form (M_r = 84,000) contains lysine (Lys-plasminogen) (93, 556, 644, 686). Magnusson et al. (351) elucidated the complete amino acid sequence of Glu-plasminogen; it is characterized by five homologous disulfide loop structures called "krinkles." As shown in Figure 13, plasmin can convert Glu-plasminogen to Lys-plasminogen by the cleavage at the Lys78-Lys79 bond with the release of the preactivation peptide (93, 556, 660, 661, 686). The Lys-plasminogen is further cleaved at Arg560-Val561 to form the active enzyme plasmin (393, 628, 661, 686). The release of the preactivation peptide is not mandatory, because a single cleavage at Arg560-Val561 can convert Glu-plasminogen to Glu-plasmin (628, 629). The activation of Lys-plasminogen by urokinase (87) or streptokinase (688) occurs much faster than that of Glu-plasminogen. The final product of activation, plasmin, is a serine protease composed of two polypeptide chains, a heavy A chain and a light B chain, linked by two disulfide bonds; the B chain contains the enzyme's catalytic site (210, 557, 630). The action of the enzyme is confined to hydrolysis of lysine and arginine peptide bonds. Although the most susceptible physiological substrate for plasmin is fibrin, the enzyme (a protease of broad specificity) digests many proteins. With an increased generation of plasmin in the circulation several proteins are cleaved, including fibrinogen (455); factors V (129), VIII (16, 499), and XII (279); components of the complement system (514); and some hormones such as ACTH, glucagon, and somatotropin (415).

Plasminogen has affinity for fibrin via structures called lysine-binding sites (533, 612, 643); Lys-plasminogen has a higher affinity than the intact Glu-plasminogen. The lysine-binding sites are in the A chain of plasmin (553); one site has high affinity (K_d = 9 µM) and four sites low affinity (K_d = 5 mM) for ε-aminocaproic acid (86). The latter compound inhibits plasminogen binding to fibrin.

Plasminogen Activators

Three different pathways may accomplish activation of plasminogen (101). *1*) Intrinsic activation involves components present in precursor forms in the blood. *2*) Extrinsic activation utilizes activators from cells and tissues, including the vessel wall. *3*) Exogenous activation occurs in therapeutic situations in

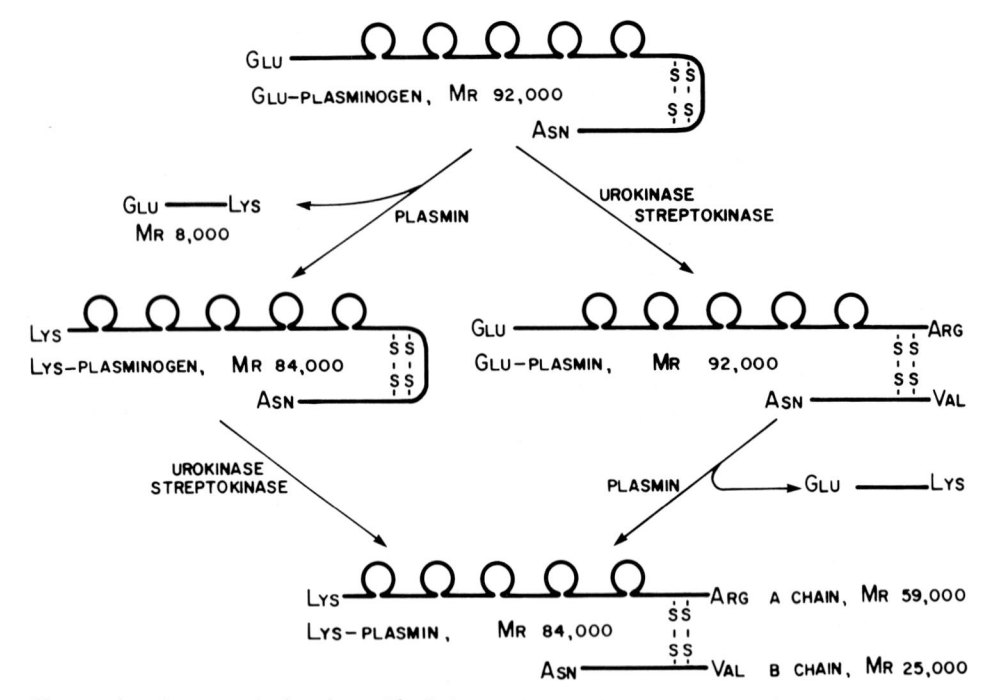

FIG. 13. Plasminogen activation. Human plasminogen, a single polypeptide chain protein, contains 790 amino acid residues, NH$_2$-terminal glutamic acid, 5 homologous loop structures ("krinkles"), and 24 disulfide bonds. On action of plasmin on Glu-plasminogen a cleavage at Lys76-Lys77 occurs, releasing NH$_2$-terminal peptide and yielding Lys-plasminogen. Cleavage of the Arg560-Val561 bond by activators results in formation of Lys-plasmin, composed of 2 chains (A and B) linked by 2 disulfide bonds. Lys-plasminogen activation seems approximately 10 times faster than that of Glu-plasminogen. In presence of plasmin inhibitors the cleavage of NH$_2$-terminal peptide is significantly decreased and Glu-plasmin (potentially convertible into Lys-plasmin) is formed.

which urokinase or streptokinase are infused. All studied activators generate plasmin by the cleavage of the Arg560-Val561 peptide bond in plasminogen.

Intrinsic activators of plasminogen originate from contact-phase activation of blood coagulation. In purified systems kallikrein (103), factor XIa (356), and factor XIIa (197) can each activate plasminogen to plasmin. Kallikrein is more potent in purified systems than factor XIa (356); when the concentration of prekallikrein (which is 10 times higher than the concentration of factor XI in plasma) is considered, kallikrein accounts for 90% of Hageman factor–dependent fibrinolysis. Plasminogen activation by factor XIIa requires too high a concentration of this enzyme to be physiologically significant. Because factor XII, HMW kininogen, and prekallikrein are required for the formation of kallikrein in plasma, defects of contact-phase–activated fibrinolysis are not surprising in plasma lacking prekallikrein [Fletcher factor; (569, 672)], HMW kininogen [Williams factor; (108, 130, 305, 571)], and factor XII (255). The quantitative contribution of contact-phase–mediated plasminogen activation to physiological fibrinolysis is unknown. In addition, intrinsic activators that do not depend on contact activation of blood coagulation and may be related to circulatory urokinase exist in plasma.

Extrinsic activators in the tissue of most organs in various amounts (14) are usually tissue bound and require harsh conditions for extraction. The amount of the activator seems to correlate with the degree of vascularization of the organ tissue. The activators from human lung (554), human seminal plasma (13), human cervical cells (35), and pig heart (100) seem to be serine proteases ($M_r \sim 60,000$) composed of two polypeptide chains linked by disulfide bonds. Extrinsic plasminogen activators are found in the blood after exercise or during stasis due to venipuncture. These activators differ from urokinase and may be the released vascular activator, perhaps the activator synthesized in the endothelial cells (345, 493). Blood and tissue plasminogen activators have affinity for fibrin, which potentiates the activation process (74, 658). The regulation mechanism of the vascular activator is poorly understood but is being intensely investigated; it may be the key to the regulation of the fibrinolytic response in vivo.

Exogenous activators are usually urokinase and streptokinase. Urokinase, a plasminogen activator first isolated from urine and more recently purified from tissue culture renal cells (610), is a trypsinlike enzyme. Urokinase is a far more potent activator of plasminogen than kallikrein and factor XIa when tested by lysis of radioactive fibrin (356). Urokinase has been purified as two species, a heavy 54,000-M_r form and a light 31,600-M_r form (71, 329, 331, 660). The light form is believed to be an enzymatically active degradation product of the heavy form (330, 331). Both species consist of a single polypeptide chain with common amino acid sequences (330, 679). Urokinase appears to have an affinity for fibrinogen and fibrin (237, 288) and thus may be able to activate plasminogen in or near the thrombus (86). The purified enzyme has been successfully used in thrombolytic therapy; its use for the treatment of other forms of thrombotic disease is under evaluation (274, 362, 495, 654).

Streptokinase is a 47,000-M_r glycoprotein (123, 637) isolated from cultures of Lancefield group C strain of β-hemolytic streptococci. Streptokinase is not an enzyme; it forms a 1:1 stoichiometric complex with plasminogen, in which the catalytic-site serine residue of the plasminogen moiety becomes available (580). The complex is primarily responsible for the activation of plasminogen (392, 580). Complex formation is followed by a series of proteolytic cleavages of both components: plasminogen is converted to plasmin, and streptokinase is cleaved to a 37,000-M_r polypeptide chain (393). Streptokinase is the most widely used thrombolytic agent because it is far less expensive and much easier to obtain than urokinase. The drug is, however, antigenic in humans and may produce pyrogenic and other toxic side effects.

Inhibitors of Plasminogen and Plasmin

The characterization of inhibitors of plasminogen activation is still incomplete. Differentiation between the inhibitors of activation and inhibitors of plasmin, which is the product of the first reaction, is difficult. A direct measurement of the Arg-Val bond cleavage in plasminogen and an assessment of the generated plasmin activity are helpful.

Inhibitors of intrinsic activators of plasminogen have been recognized in human plasma: C1-esterase inhibitor (289), an inhibitor of factor XIIa–induced fibrinolysis (229), antithrombin III–heparin complex (236), and α_2-macroglobulin (394). However, the role and contribution of intrinsic activators and inhibitors to physiological fibrinolysis is not known.

Inhibitors of vascular and tissue activators of plasminogen have been identified, but the lack of established knowledge about the structure and function of vascular and tissue activators hampers further studies. Agents with antifibrinolytic activity have been characterized whose mechanism of action depends on an interaction with plasminogen lysine-binding sites (612), which decreases the affinity of activators for plasminogen. Aminocarboxylic acids that bind specifically with these sites include lysine, ϵ-aminocaproic acid (often called 6-aminohexanoic acid), and trans-4-(aminomethyl)cyclohexanecarboxylic acid (tranexamic acid) (379, 643). The antifibrinolytic effect of the last two compounds after administration to humans and animals is well recognized; these compounds have been used therapeutically to control increased activation of the fibrinolytic system. A histidine-rich glycoprotein from human plasma (225, 230) was found to bind to human plasminogen; the protein has high affinity for plasminogen and plasmin lysine-binding sites with K_d values of 1.1 μM and 0.9 μM, respectively (336). This protein acts like ϵ-aminocaproic acid and may be a physiological modulator of plasminogen activation.

Streptokinase is inhibited in human plasma by antibodies that are probably induced by previous infections with β-hemolytic streptococci. The concentration of streptokinase antibodies greatly varies between normal persons and even more in patients. For example, the amount of streptokinase required to neutralize the circulating antibodies in normal healthy persons varied between 25,000 and 3,000,000 units (655); however, administration of 350,000 units of streptokinase neutralized the circulating antibodies in 95% of normal persons. The use of streptokinase as a thrombolytic agent in patients suffering from thromboembolic disease requires neutralization of the circulating antibodies prior to the effective activation of plasminogen.

The inhibition of urokinase in the circulation is not well understood. Plasma protease inhibitors [α_2-antiplasmin (420), α_2-macroglobulin (469), α_1-protease inhibitor (96), and antithrombin III (95)] inhibit urokinase slowly but probably none of the inhibitors has significant effect in vivo. Because the biologic half-life of urokinase in humans is short, ($\sim$15 min) the clearance mechanism may be important in the regulation of urokinase activity in vivo (165). Demonstration of urokinase inactivation by cytosol from endothelial cells implies the contribution of the blood vessel wall in the regulation of the local fibrinolytic activity (346).

Plasmin is affected by several protease inhibitors occurring in human plasma. The inhibition of the enzyme in a purified system was demonstrated with α_2-antiplasmin, α_2-macroglobulin, α_1-protease inhibitor, antithrombin III, inter-α-trypsin inhibitor, and C1-esterase inhibitor. Under physiological conditions in the normal blood only the first two inhibitors are significant in the inactivation of plasmin (see Table 1). A fast-acting inactivator of plasmin is α_2-antiplasmin (101, 420, 434), a single-chain 70,000-M_r glycoprotein immunochemically different from other plasma protease inhibitors. It forms a covalently bound 1:1 stoichiometric complex with plasmin (420, 684). The concentration of α_2-antiplasmin in normal plasma ($\sim$1 μM) indicates that this inhibitor neutralizes approximately 50% of the plasmin that can be generated from the circulating plasminogen (2.2 μM). After exhaustion of α_2-antiplasmin the remaining plasmin is inhibited by a slow reaction with α_2-macroglobulin (101, 219, 434). This inhibitor, a two-chain dimeric 725,000-M_r glycoprotein (272, 558), forms a noncovalent complex with plasmin that contains more than one enzyme molecule per molecule of α_2-macroglobulin and has some esterase and proteolytic activity (221). Plasma concentration of α_2-macroglobulin is 3 μM; thus it is sufficiently high to neutralize the remaining plasmin after saturation of α_2-antiplasmin inhibitory capacity.

Physiological Fibrinolysis

Fibrinolysis is a defense mechanism that controls in the organism the deposition of fibrin in the circulation and in tissues. Fibrinolysis is also involved in other biologic systems, e.g., wound healing and tissue repair (15), malignant cell transformation (545), macrophage function (545), and ovulation and embryo implantation (624). The complex mechanisms that trigger activation of fibrinolysis are not well understood. Activation of blood coagulation is paralleled by fibrinolysis activation. Direct activation of plasminogen by kallikrein and factor XIa would bypass the vascular activator pathway (278). Activation of clotting factors and generation of fibrin may play a role in stimulation of vascular activator secretion from the endothelial cells. Trace amounts of thrombin, however, suppress the fibrinolytic potential of cultured endothelial cells by a rapid decrease of intracellular plasminogen activator activity (344). In addition, activation of fibrinolysis may be under neurohormonal control by the secretion of a plasminogen activator releasing hormone that would act on the endothelial cells (79).

Some clinical observations are compatible with a conclusion that thrombotic disease and atherosclerosis may accompany decreased fibrinolytic activity and defects or abnormalities of plasminogen or its activators (7, 58, 78, 82, 94, 458, 492, 502, 513, 565, 688). However, a congenital deficiency of α_2-antiplasmin is manifested by a bleeding tendency (291).

The activation of the fibrinolytic system in vivo is compatible with the increased level of plasminogen activators in the circulation and preparedness for lysis rather than with degradation of plasma proteins (Fig. 14). Plasminogen is poorly activated in the liquid phase by its activators because of low affinity and low concentration of the zymogen, which may be partially complexed with histidine-rich glycoprotein. The sur-

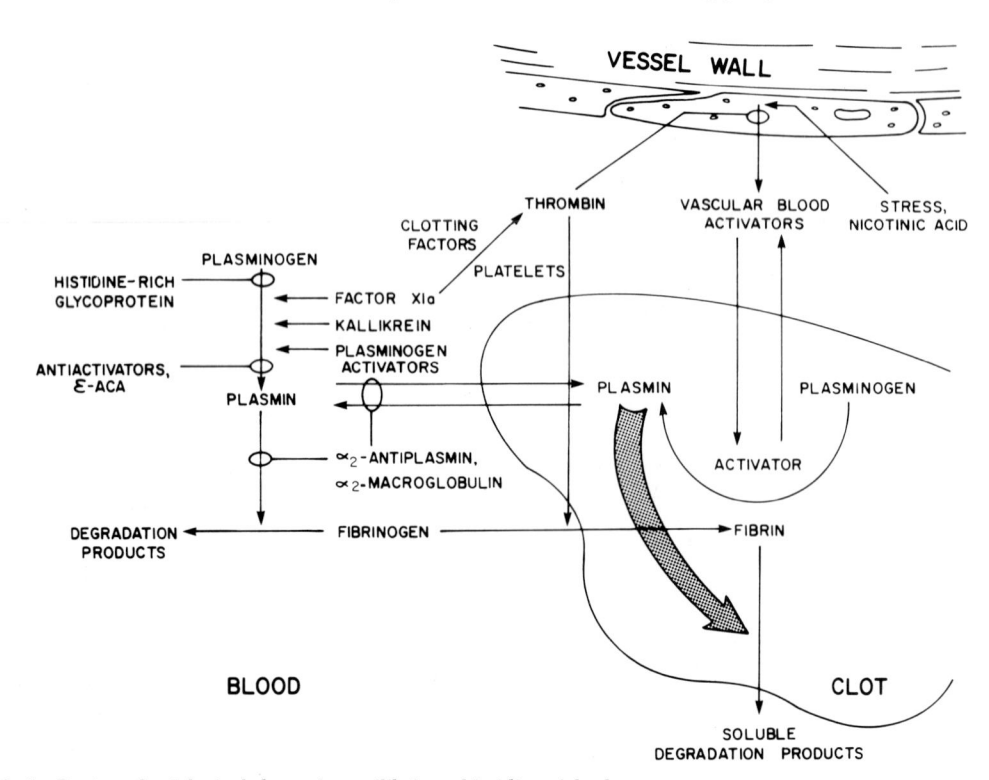

FIG. 14. Physiological fibrinolysis. During physiological dynamic equilibrium, histidine-rich glycoprotein and other antiactivators regulate interaction of plasminogen in blood with plasminogen activators. Even if minute amounts of plasmin are generated (e.g., after release of vascular plasminogen activator following stress) the enzyme is promptly inactivated by α_2-antiplasmin. On activation of the blood coagulation system, fibrin clot is formed, which not only strongly binds vascular plasminogen activator and plasminogen from blood but also significantly accelerates the activation rate. Resulting plasmin is protected from inhibitors while attached to fibrin. Enzyme is inactivated by α_2-antiplasmin and α_2-macroglobulin after proteolytic dissolution of fibrin and liberation into the liquid phase of blood. Thus the fibrin network catalyzes initiation and regulation of fibrinolysis. Kallikrein and factor XIa can activate plasminogen in the liquid phase, but their role appears less significant and not specifically associated with fibrin clot.

face and specific binding sites of fibrin are central to the entire mechanism of fibrinolysis (114, 685). Plasminogen and its activator attached to the lysine-binding sites on fibrin would accomplish at least three objectives: *1)* a specific spatial orientation placing the molecules optimally for the proteolytic cleavage of plasminogen by activator and the formation of plasmin; *2)* a high concentration of the reactants on the fibrin fiber to increase the rate of both the plasminogen activation and proteolytic degradation of the very support—fibrin; and *3)* protection of the active plasmin from destruction by α_2-antiplasmin. Plasmin that is released from the dissolved fibrin is rapidly inactivated by α_2-antiplasmin in the circulation. The inhibitor, which diffuses from the blood into clot, not only has an impaired access to the fibrin-bound plasmin, but is also inactivated in a process of cross-linking with fibrin by factor XIIIa (572). Approximately 50% of the circulating plasminogen is expected to be complexed with the specific plasma inhibitor because of the plasminogen concentration in plasma (~2 μM) and the interaction between its high-affinity lysine-binding site and histidine-rich glycoprotein ($K_d \sim 1$ μM) (336). This regulatory interaction would decrease the available free-plasminogen concentration and result in an antifibrinolytic effect.

Clearly other components contribute to the dissolution of blood clots in vivo. Platelets are incorporated into clots and provide their activators (340, 638) and inhibitors (122, 142, 189, 395, 432, 584) to the process of fibrinolysis. The physiological significance of these agents is uncertain, and there are differences of opinion as to whether platelets accelerate or inhibit clot lysis. Factor XIIIa cross-links fibrin, rendering it less susceptible to lysis; in addition, platelet factor XIII has an antiplasmin activity (395). Cellular fibrinolysis may offer an alternative fibrinolytic pathway because leukocyte proteases can degrade fibrinogen. The role of phagocytosis for the dissolution of fibrin needs to be adequately addressed.

Research was supported in part by Grants HL-14217 and HL-24365 from the National Heart, Lung, and Blood Institute and by Grant 1420 from the Council for Tobacco Research.

REFERENCES

1. ABILDGAARD, U. Highly purified antithrombin 3 with heparin cofactor activity prepared by disc electrophoresis. *Scand. J. Clin. Lab. Invest.* 21: 89–91, 1968.
2. ADDIS, T. The pathogenesis of hereditary haemophilia. *J. Pathol. Bacteriol.* 15: 427–452, 1911.
3. AGGELER, P. M., S. G. WHITE, M. B. GLENDENING, E. W. PAGE, T. B. LEAKE, AND G. BATES. Plasma thromboplastin component (PTC) deficiency: a new disease resembling hemophilia. *Proc. Soc. Exp. Biol. Med.* 79: 692–694, 1952.
4. ALEXANDER, B., A. RIMON, AND E. KATCHALSKI. Action of water-insoluble trypsin derivatives on fibrinogen clottability. *Thromb. Diath. Haemorrh.* 16: 507–525, 1966.
5. ALKJAERSIG, N., A. DAVIES, AND A. FLETCHER. Fibrin and fibrinogen proteolysis products: comparison between gel filtration and SDS polyacrylamide electrophoresis analysis. *Thromb. Haemost.* 38: 524–535, 1977.
6. AMIR, J., J. PENSKY, AND O. D. RATNOFF. Plasma inhibition of activated plasma thromboplastin antecedent (factor XIa) in pregnancy. *J. Lab. Clin. Med.* 79: 106–112, 1972.
7. AOKI, N., M. MOROI, Y. SAKATA, N. YOSHIDA, AND M. MATSUDA. Abnormal plasminogen. A hereditary molecular abnormality found in a patient with recurrent thrombosis. *J. Clin. Invest.* 61: 1186–1195, 1978.
8. ARMSTRONG, S. H., M. J. E. BUDKA, K. C. MORRISON, AND M. HASSON. Preparation and properties of serum and plasma proteins. XII. The refractive properties of human plasma and certain purified fractions. *J. Am. Chem. Soc.* 69: 1747–1753, 1947.
9. ARONSON, D. L. N-terminal amino acid changes during the conversion of human prothrombin to thrombin. *Proc. Congr. Int. Soc. Hematol.* 2: 309–314, 1962.
10. ARONSON, D. L. N-terminal amino acid formed during the activation of prothrombin. *Nature London* 194: 475–478, 1962.
11. ARONSON, D. L., A. P. BALL, R. B. FRANZA, T. E. HUGLI, AND J. W. FENTON II. Human prothrombin fragments F1 ($\alpha\beta$) and F2: preparation and characterization of structural and biological properties. *Thromb. Res.* 20: 239–253, 1980.
12. ARONSON, D. L., L. STEVON, A. P. BALL, B. R. FRANZA, JR., AND J. S. FINLAYSON. Generation of the combined prothrombin activation peptide (F1-2) during the clotting of blood and plasma. *J. Clin. Invest.* 60: 1410–1418, 1977.
13. ASTEDT, B., B. BLADH, L. HOLMBERG, AND P. LIEDHOLM. Purification of plasminogen activator(s) from human seminal plasma. *Experientia* 32: 148–149, 1976.
14. ASTRUP, T. Tissue activators of plasminogen. *Federation Proc.* 25: 42–51, 1966.
15. ASTRUP, T. Fibrinolysis—an overview. In: *Progress in Chemical Fibrinolysis and Thrombolysis*, edited by J. F. Davidson, R. M. Rowan, M. M. Samama, and P. C. Desnoyers. New York: Raven, 1978, vol. 3, p. 1–57.
16. ATICHARTAKARN, V., V. J. MARDER, E. P. KIRBY, AND A. Z. BUDZYNSKI. Effects of enzymatic degradation on the subunit composition and biologic properties of human factor VIII. *Blood* 51: 281–297, 1978.
17. AUSTEN, D. E. G. Thiol groups in the blood clotting action of factor VIII. *Br. J. Haematol.* 19: 477–484, 1970.
18. AUSTEN, D. E. G., AND E. BIDWELL. Carbohydrate structure in factor VIII. *Thromb. Diath. Haemorrh.* 28: 464–472, 1972.
19. BACHMANN, L., W. W. SCHMITT-FUMIAN, R. HAMMEL, AND K. LEDERER. Size and shape of fibrinogen. I. Electron microscopy of the hydrated molecule. *Makromol. Chem.* 176: 2603–2618, 1975.
20. BAGDASARIAN, A., B. LAHIRI, AND R. W. COLMAN. Origin of the high molecular weight activator of prekallikrein. *J. Biol. Chem.* 248: 7742–7747, 1973.
21. BAGDASARIAN, A., B. LAHIRI, R. C. TALAMO, P. Y. WONG, AND R. C. COLMAN. Immunochemical studies of plasma kallikrein. *J. Clin. Invest.* 54: 1444–1454, 1974.
22. BAGDY, D., E. BARABAS, L. GRÁF, T. E. PETERSEN, AND S. MAGNUSSON. Hirudin. *Methods Enzymol.* 45: 669–678, 1976.
23. BAILEY, K. The proteins of skeletal muscle. *Adv. Protein Chem.* 1: 289–317, 1944.
24. BAILLIE, A. J., AND A. K. SIM. Activation of the fibrinolytic enzyme system in laboratory animals and in man. A comparative study. *Thromb. Diath. Haemorrh.* 25: 499–506, 1971.
25. BANG, N. U. A molecular structural model of fibrin based on electron microscopy of fibrin polymerization. *Thromb. Diath. Haemorrh. Suppl.* 13: 73–80, 1964.
26. BANG, N. U., AND L. E. MATTLER. Thrombin sensitivity and specificity of three chromogenic peptide substrates. In: *The Chemistry and Biology of Thrombin*, edited by R. L. Lundblad,

J. W. Fenton II, and K. G. Mann. Ann Arbor, MI: Ann Arbor Science, 1977, p. 305–310.
27. BANGHAM, A. D. A correlation between surface charge and coagulant action of phospholipid. *Nature London* 192: 1197–1198, 1961.
28. BARTON, P. G., AND D. J. HANAHAN. Some lipid-protein interactions involved in prothrombin activation. *Biochim. Biophys. Acta* 187: 319–327, 1969.
29. BELITSER, V. A., T. V. VARETSKA, AND V. P. MANJAKOV. On the model for the fibrinogen molecule. Consecutive stages of fibrin polymerization. *Thromb. Res.* 2: 567–578, 1973.
30. BELL, W. R., W. R. PITNEY, AND J. F. GOODWIN. Therapeutic defibrination in the treatment of thrombotic disease. *Lancet* 1: 490–493, 1968.
31. BENABID, Y., E. CONCORD, AND M. SUSCILLON. Soluble fibrin complexes: separation as a function of pH and characterization. *Thromb. Haemost.* 37: 144–153, 1977.
32. BENNETT, B., AND O. D. RATNOFF. Studies on the response of patients with classic hemophilia to transfusion with concentrates of antihemophilic factor. A difference in the half-life of an antihemophilic factor as measured by procoagulant and immunologic techniques. *J. Clin. Invest.* 51: 2593–2596, 1972.
33. BENNETT, J. S., AND G. J. VILAIRE. Exposure of platelet fibrinogen receptors by ADP and epinephrine. *J. Clin. Invest.* 64: 1393–1401, 1979.
34. BETTELHEIM, F. R. The clotting of fibrinogen. II. Fractionation of peptide material liberated. *Biochim. Biophys. Acta* 19: 121–130, 1956.
35. BIGBEE, W. L., AND R. H. JENSEN. Characterization of plasminogen activator in human cervical cells. *Biochim. Biophys. Acta* 540: 285–294, 1978.
36. BIGGS, R., A. S. DOUGLAS, R. G. MACFARLANE, J. V. DACIE, W. R. PITNEY, C. MERSKEY, AND J. R. O'BRIEN. Christmas disease: a condition previously mistaken for haemophilia. *Br. Med. J.* 2: 1378–1381, 1952.
37. BIGGS, R., AND R. G. MACFARLANE. The reaction of haemophilic plasma to thromboplastin. *J. Clin. Pathol.* 4: 455–459, 1951.
38. BILEZIKIAN, S. B., AND H. L. NOSSEL. Unique pattern of fibrinogen cleavage by human leukocyte proteases. *Blood* 50: 21–28, 1977.
39. BILEZIKIAN, S. B., H. L. NOSSEL, V. P. BUTLER, JR., AND R. E. CANFIELD. Radioimmunoassay of human fibrinopeptide B and kinetics of fibrinopeptide cleavage by different enzymes. *J. Clin. Invest.* 56: 438–445, 1975.
40. BIRD, P., AND C. R. RIZZA. A method for detecting factor VIII clotting activity associated with factor VIII-related antigen in agarose gels. *Br. J. Haematol.* 31: 5–12, 1975.
41. BJÖRK, I., AND B. NORDENMAN. Acceleration of the reaction between thrombin and antithrombin III by non-stoichiometric amounts of heparin. *Eur. J. Biochem.* 68: 507–511, 1976.
42. BJORKLID, E., E. STORM, B. ØSTERUD, AND H. PRYDZ. The interaction of the protein and phospholipid components of tissue thromboplastin (factor III) with the factors VII and X. *Scand. J. Haematol.* 14: 65–70, 1975.
43. BJORKLID, E., E. STORM, AND H. PRYDZ. The protein component of human brain thromboplastin. *Biochem. Biophys. Res. Commun.* 55: 969–976, 1973.
44. BLOMBÄCK, B., M. BLOMBÄCK, W. FINKBEINER, A. HOLMGREN, B. KOWALSKA-LOTH, AND G. OLOVSON. Enzymatic reduction of disulfide bonds in fibrinogen by the thioredoxin system. I. Identification of reduced bonds and studies on reoxidation process. *Thromb. Res.* 4: 55–75, 1974.
45. BLOMBÄCK, B., M. BLOMBÄCK, AND N. J. GRONDAHL. Studies on fibrinopeptides from mammals. *Acta Chem. Scand.* 19: 1789–1791, 1965.
46. BLOMBÄCK, B., M. BLOMBÄCK, A. HENSCHEN, B. HESSEL, S. IWANAGA, AND K. R. WOODS. N-terminal disulfide knot of human fibrinogen. *Nature London* 218: 130–134, 1968.
47. BLOMBÄCK, B., M. BLOMBÄCK, B. HESSEL, AND S. IWANAGA. Structure of N-terminal fragments of fibrinogen and specificity of thrombin. *Nature London* 215: 1445–1448, 1967.

48. BLOMBÄCK, B., M. BLOMBÄCK, AND I. M. NILSSON. Coagulation studies on "Reptilase" an extract of the venom from *Bothrops jararaca*. *Thromb. Diath. Haemorrh.* 1: 76–86, 1957.
49. BLOMBÄCK, B., B. HESSEL, D. HOGG, AND G. CLAESON. Substrate specificity of thrombin on proteins and synthetic substrates. In: *The Chemistry and Biology of Thrombin*, edited by R. L. Lundblad, J. W. Fenton II, and K. G. Mann. Ann Arbor, MI: Ann Arbor Science, 1977, p. 275–290.
50. BLOMBÄCK, B., B. HESSEL, D. HOGG, AND L. THERKILDSEN. A two-step fibrinogen-fibrin transition in blood coagulation. *Nature London* 275: 501–505, 1978.
51. BLOMBÄCK, B., B. HESSEL, S. IWANAGA, J. REUTERBY, AND M. BLOMBÄCK. Primary structure of human fibrinogen and fibrin. I. Cleavage of fibrinogen with cyanogen bromide. Isolation and characterization of NH_2-terminal fragments of the alpha (A) chain. *J. Biol. Chem.* 247: 1496–1512, 1972.
52. BLOMBÄCK, B., B. HESSEL, G. SAVIDGE, L. WIKSTRÖM, AND M. BLOMBÄCK. The effect of reducing agents on factor VIII and other coagulation factors. *Thromb. Res.* 12: 1177–1194, 1978.
53. BLOMBÄCK, B., AND I. YAMASHINA. On the N-terminal amino acids in fibrinogen and fibrin. *Ark. Kemi* 12: 299–319, 1958.
54. BLOW, D. M., J. J. BIRKTOFT, AND B. S. HARTLEY. Role of a buried acid group in the mechanism of action of chymotrypsin. *Nature London* 221: 337–341, 1969.
55. BOHMFALK, J. F., AND G. M. FULLER. Plasminogen is synthesized by primary cultures of rat hepatocytes. *Science* 209: 408–410, 1980.
56. BORDET, J., AND O. GENOU. Recherches sur la coagulation du sang et les serums anticoagulant. *Ann. Inst. Pasteur Paris* 15: 129–144, 1901.
57. BOUMA, B. N., AND J. H. GRIFFIN. Human blood coagulation factor XI: purification properties and mechanism of activation by activated XII. *J. Biol. Chem.* 252: 6432–6437, 1977.
58. BRAKMAN, P., O. K. ALBRECHTSEN, AND T. ASTRUP. A comparative study of coagulation and fibrinolysis in blood from normal men and women. *Br. J. Haematol.* 12: 74–85, 1966.
59. BRINKHOUS, K. M., H. P. SMITH, E. D. WARNER, AND W. H. SEEGERS. The inhibition of blood clotting: an unidentified substance which acts in conjunction with heparin to prevent the conversion of prothrombin into thrombin. *Am. J. Physiol.* 125: 683–687, 1939.
60. BROEKMAN, M. J., R. I. HANDIN, AND P. COHEN. Distribution of fibrinogen, and platelet factors 4 and XIII in subcellular fractions of human platelets. *Br. J. Haematol.* 31: 51–55, 1975.
61. BUCHANAN, J. M., L. B. CHEN, AND B. R. ZETTER. Reaction of thrombin with fibroblasts and mouse splenocytes. In: *The Chemistry and Biology of Thrombin*, edited by R. L. Lundblad, J. W. Fenton II, and K. G. Mann. Ann Arbor, MI: Ann Arbor Science, 1977, p. 519–530.
62. BUCHER, D., E. NEBELIN, J. THOMSEN, AND J. STENFLO. Identification of γ-carboxyglutamic acid residues in bovine factors IX and X, and in a new vitamin K-dependent protein. *FEBS Lett.* 68: 293–297, 1976.
63. BUDZYNSKI, A. Z. Structure of fibrinogen in relation to its proteolytic degradation products. *Postepy Hig. Med. Dosw.* 23: 293–369, 1969.
64. BUDZYNSKI, A. Z. Difference in conformation of fibrinogen degradation products as revealed by hydrogen exchange and spectropolarimetry. *Biochim. Biophys. Acta* 229: 663–671, 1971.
65. BUDZYNSKI, A. Z., R. T. JOSEPH, S. A. OLEXA, AND S. NIEWIAROWSKI. Binding functions of the fibrinogen molecule (Abstract). *Federation Proc.* 38: 996, 1979.
66. BUDZYNSKI, A. Z., V. J. MARDER, AND J. R. SHAINOFF. Structure of plasmic degradation products of human fibrinogen. Fibrinopeptide and polypeptide chain analysis. *J. Biol. Chem.* 249: 2294–2302, 1974.
67. BUDZYNSKI, A. Z., S. A. OLEXA, B. S. BRIZUELA, R. T. SAWYER, AND G. S. STENT. Anticoagulant and fibrinolytic properties of salivary proteins from the leech *Haementeria ghilianii*. *Proc. Soc. Exp. Biol. Med.* 168: 266–275, 1981.

68. BUDZYNSKI, A. Z., S. A. OLEXA, AND R. T. SAWYER. Composition of salivary gland extracts from the leech *Haementeria ghilianii*. *Proc. Soc. Exp. Biol. Med.* 168: 259–265, 1981.
69. BUDZYNSKI, A. Z., AND M. STAHL. Partial reduction of bovine fibrinogen by some sulfhydryl compounds. *Biochim. Biophys. Acta* 175: 282–289, 1969.
70. BUDZYNSKI, A. Z., M. STAHL, M. KOPEC, Z. S. LATALLO, Z. WEGRZYNOWICZ, AND E. KOWALSKI. High molecular weight products of the late stage of fibrinogen proteolysis by plasmin and their structural relation to the fibrinogen molecule. *Biochim. Biophys. Acta* 147: 313–323, 1967.
71. BURGES, R. A., K. W. BRAMMER, AND J. D. COOMBES. Molecular weight of urokinase. *Nature London* 208: 894–896, 1965.
72. BUTKOWSKI, R. J., J. ELION, M. R. DOWNING, AND K. G. MANN. The primary structure of human prothrombin 2 and α-thrombin. *J. Biol. Chem.* 252: 4942–4957, 1977.
73. BUTKOWSKI, R. J., J. ELION, M. R. DOWNING, AND K. G. MANN. Primary structure of human thrombin (Abstract). *Federation Proc.* 35: 1765, 1976.
74. CAMIOLO, S. M., S. THORSEN, AND T. ASTRUP. Fibrinogenolysis and fibrinolysis with tissue plasminogen activator, urokinase, streptokinase-activated human globulin, and plasmin. *Proc. Soc. Exp. Biol. Med.* 138: 277–280, 1971.
75. CARNEY, D. H., AND D. D. CUNNINGHAM. Cell surface action of thrombin is sufficient to initiate division of chick cells. *Cell* 14: 811–823, 1978.
76. CARNEY, D. H., K. C. GLENN, AND D. D. CUNNINGHAM. Conditions which affect initiation of animal cell division by trypsin and thrombin. *J. Cell. Physiol.* 95: 13–22, 1978.
77. CARTER, J. R., AND E. D. WARNER. Evaluation of disulfide bonds and sulfhydryl groups in the blood clotting mechanism. *Am. J. Physiol.* 179: 549–556, 1954.
78. CASH, J. D. A new approach to studies of the fibrinolytic enzyme system in man. *Am. Heart J.* 75: 424–428, 1968.
79. CASH, J. D. Control mechanism of activator release. In: *Progress in Chemical Fibrinolysis and Thrombolysis*, edited by J. F. Davidson, R. M. Rowan, M. M. Samama, and P. D. Desnoyers. New York: Raven, 1978, vol. 3, p. 65–75.
80. CASPARY, E. A. Studies on the acetylation of human fibrinogen. *Biochem. J.* 62: 507–512, 1956.
81. CASPARY, E. A., AND R. A. KEKWICK. Some physicochemical properties of human fibrinogen. *Biochem. J.* 67: 41–48, 1957.
82. CHAKRABARTI, R., G. R. FEARNLEY, E. D. HOCKING, A. DELITHEOS, AND G. M. CLARKE. Fibrinolytic activity related to age in survivors of myocardial infarction. *Lancet* 1: 573–574, 1966.
83. CHANG, T.-L., R. D. FEINMAN, B. H. LANDIS, AND J. W. FENTON II. Antithrombin reactions with α- and γ-thrombins. *Biochemistry* 18: 113–119, 1979.
84. CHEN, L. B., AND J. B. BUCHANAN. Mitogenic activity of blood components. I. Thrombin and prothrombin. *Proc. Natl. Acad. Sci. USA* 72: 131–135, 1975.
85. CHEN, R., AND R. F. DOOLITTLE. γ-γ cross-linking sites in human and bovine fibrin. *Biochemistry* 10: 4487–4491, 1971.
86. CHESTERMAN, C. N., M. J. ALLINGTON, AND A. A. SHARP. Relation of plasminogen activator to fibrin. *Nature London* 238: 15–16, 1972.
87. CHRISTENSEN, U. Kinetic studies of the urokinase-catalysed conversion of NH_2-terminal glutamic acid plasminogen to plasmin. *Biochim. Biophys. Acta* 481: 638–647, 1977.
88. CHUNG, D. W., M. W. RIXON, R. T. A. MACGILLIVRAY, AND E. W. DAVIE. Characterization of a cDNA clone coding for the β-chain of bovine fibrinogen. *Proc. Natl. Acad. Sci. USA* 78: 1466–1470, 1981.
89. CHUNG, S. I., M. C. LEWIS, AND J. E. FOLK. Relationships of the catalytic properties of human plasma and platelet transglutaminases (activated blood coagulation factor XIII) to their subunit structures. *J. Biol. Chem.* 249: 940–950, 1974.
90. CIFONELLI, J. A. Heparin: structure, function and clinical implications. Relation of chemical structure of heparin to its anticoagulant activity. In: *The Chemistry of Heparin*, edited by R. A. Bradshaw and S. Wessler. New York: Plenum, 1975, p. 95–103.
91. CIFONELLI, J. A., AND J. KING. Structural studies on heparins with unusually high N-acetylglucosamine contents. *Biochim. Biophys. Acta* 320: 331–340, 1973.
92. CLAESON, G., L. AURELL, G. KARLSON, AND P. FRIBERGER. Substrate structure and activity relationship. In: *New Methods for the Analysis of Coagulation Using Chromogenic Substrates*, edited by I. Witt. Berlin: de Gruyter, 1977, p. 39–54.
93. CLAEYS, G., AND J. VERMYLEN. Physico-chemical and proenzyme properties of NH_2-terminal glutamic acid and NH_2-terminal lysine plasminogen. Influence of 6-aminohexanoic acid. *Biochim. Biophys. Acta* 342: 351–359, 1974.
94. CLAYTON, J. K., J. A. ANDERSON, AND G. P. MCNICOL. Preoperative prediction of postoperative deep vein thrombosis. *Br. Med. J.* 2: 910–912, 1976.
95. CLEMMENSEN, I. Inhibition of urokinase by complex formation with human antithrombin III in absence and presence of heparin. *Thromb. Haemost.* 39: 616–623, 1978.
96. CLEMMENSEN, I., AND F. CHRISTENSEN. Inhibition of urokinase by complex formation with human alpha 1-antitrypsin. *Biochim. Biophys. Acta* 249: 591–599, 1976.
97. COCHRANE, C. G., S. D. REVAK, AND K. D. WUEPPER. Activation of Hageman factor in solid and fluid phases. *J. Exp. Med.* 138: 1564–1569, 1973.
98. COCHRANE, C. G., K. D. WUEPPER, B. S. AIKEN, S. D. REVAK, AND H. L. SPIEGELBERG. The interaction of Hageman factor and immune complexes. *J. Clin. Invest.* 51: 2736–2745, 1972.
99. COHEN, C., AND N. M. TOONEY. Crystallization of modified fibrinogen. *Nature London* 251: 659–660, 1974.
100. COLE, E. R., AND F. W. BACHMAN. Purification and properties of a plasminogen activator from pig heart. *J. Biol. Chem.* 252: 3729–3737, 1977.
101. COLLEN, D. Identification and some properties of a new fast-reacting plasmin inhibitor in human plasma. *Eur. J. Biochem.* 69: 209–216, 1976.
102. COLLEN, D. On the regulation and control of fibrinolysis. *Thromb. Haemost.* 43: 77–89, 1980.
103. COLMAN, R. W. Activation of plasminogen by human plasma kallikrein. *Biochem. Biophys. Res. Commun.* 35: 273–279, 1969.
104. COLMAN, R. W. The effect of proteolytic enzymes on bovine factor V. I. Kinetics of activation and inactivation by bovine thrombin. *Biochemistry* 8: 1438–1444, 1969.
105. COLMAN, R. W. The effect of proteolytic enzymes on factor V. II. Kinetics of activation and inactivation by papain, plasmin, and other proteolytic enzymes. *Biochemistry* 8: 1445–1450, 1969.
106. COLMAN, R. W. Factor V: an activator of factor Xa in the absence of prothrombin. *Br. J. Haematol.* 19: 675–684, 1970.
107. COLMAN, R. W. Formation of human plasma kinin. *N. Engl. J. Med.* 291: 509–515, 1974.
107a. COLMAN, R. W. Deficiencies of factor XII, prekallikrein and high molecular weight kininogen. In: *Hemostasis and Thrombosis: Basic Concepts and Clinical Practice*, edited by R. W. Colman, J. Hirsch, V. Marder, and E. Salvman. Philadelphia, PA: Lippincott, 1982, p. 1–17.
108. COLMAN, R. W., A. BAGDASARIAN, R. C. TALAMA, C. F. SCOTT, M. SEAVEY, J. A. GUIMARAES, J. V. PIERCE, AND A. P. KAPLAN. Williams trait. Human kininogen deficiency with diminished levels of plasminogen proactivator and prekallikrein associated with abnormalities of the Hageman factor-dependent pathways. *J. Clin. Invest.* 56: 1650–1662, 1975.
109. COLMAN, R. W., R. EDELMAN, C. F. SCOTT, AND R. H. GILMAN. Plasma kallikrein activation and inhibition during typhoid fever. *J. Clin. Invest.* 61: 287–296, 1978.
110. COLMAN, R. W., J. MORAN, AND G. PHILIP. Kinetic properties and molecular size of thrombin-activated factor V. *J. Biol. Chem.* 245: 5941–5946, 1970.
111. COLMAN, R. W., M. SCHAPIRA, AND C. F. SCOTT. Regulation of the formation and inhibition of human plasma kallikrein. *Ann. NY Acad. Sci.* 370: 261–270, 1981.
112. CONTEJEAN, C. Recherches sur les injections intraveineuses

de peptone et leur influence sur la coagulabilité du sang chez le chien. *Arch. Physiol. Norm. Pathol.* 7: 45–48, 1895.
113. COOPER, H. A., AND R. H. WAGNER. The defect in hemophilic and von Willebrand's disease plasmas studied by a recombination technique. *J. Clin. Invest.* 54: 1098–1099, 1974.
114. CORCORAN, D. H., E. W. FERGUSON, L. J. FRETTO, AND P. A. MCKEE. Localization of a cross-link donor site in the alpha-chain of human fibrin. *Thromb. Res.* 19: 883–888, 1980.
115. COUNTS, R. B., S. L. PASKELL, AND S. K. ELGEE. Disulfide bonds and the quaternary structure of factor VIII/von Willebrand factor. *J. Clin. Invest.* 62: 702–708, 1978.
116. CRABTREE, G. R., AND J. A. KANT. Molecular cloning of cDNA for the α, β and γ chains of rat fibrinogen. *J. Biol. Chem.* 256: 9718–9723, 1981.
117. CREDO, R. B., C. G. CURTIS, AND L. LORAND. Ca^{2+}-related regulatory function of fibrinogen. *Proc. Natl. Acad. Sci. USA* 75: 4234–4237, 1978.
118. CROSS, M. J. Effect of fibrinogen on the aggregation of platelets by adenosine diphosphate. *Thromb. Diath. Haemorrh.* 12: 524–527, 1964.
119. CURTIS, C. G., K. L. BROWN, R. B. CREDO, R. A. DOMANIK, A. GRAY, P. STENBERG, AND L. LORAND. Calcium dependent unmasking of active center cysteine during activation of fibrin stabilizing factor. *Biochemistry* 13: 3774–3780, 1974.
120. DAMUS, P. S., M. HICKS, AND R. D. ROSENBERG. Anticoagulant activity of heparin. *Nature London* 246: 355–359, 1973.
121. DANISHEFSKY, I., H. STEINER, A. BELLA, AND A. FRIEDLANDER. Investigations on the chemistry of heparin. *J. Biol. Chem.* 244: 1741–1745, 1969.
122. DEN OTTOLANDER, G. J. H., B. LEIJNSE, AND M. M. J. CREMER-ELFRINK. Plasmatic and platelet anti-plasmins and anti-activators. *Thromb. Diath. Haemorrh.* 18: 404–415, 1967.
123. DERENZO, E. C., P. K. SIITERI, B. L. HUTCHING, AND P. H. BELL. Preparation and certain properties of highly purified streptokinase. *J. Biol. Chem.* 242: 533–542, 1967.
124. DEUTSCH, D. G., AND E. MERTZ. Plasminogen: purification from human plasma by affinity chromatography. *Science* 170: 1095–1096, 1970.
125. DIDISHEIM, P., AND R. S. MIBASHA. Activation of Hageman factor (factor XII) by long chain saturated fatty acids. *Thromb. Diath. Haemorrh.* 9: 346–353, 1963.
126. DISCIPIO, R. G., AND E. W. DAVIE. Characterization of protein S, a γ-carboxyglutamic acid containing protein from bovine and human plasma. *Biochemistry* 18: 899–904, 1979.
127. DOMBROSE, F. A., S. N. GITEL, K. ZAWALICH, AND C. M. JACKSON. The association of bovine prothrombin fragment 1 with phospholipid: quantitative characterization of the Ca^{2+} ion-mediated binding of prothrombin fragment 1 to phospholipid vesicles and a molecular model for its association with phospholipid. *J. Biol. Chem.* 254: 5027–5040, 1979.
128. DOMBROSE, F. A., T. YASUI, Z. ROUBAL, AND W. H. SEEGERS. Ac-globulin (factor V): preparation of a practical product. *Prep. Biochem.* 2: 381–396, 1972.
129. DONALDSON, V. H. Effect of plasmin in vitro on clotting factors in plasma. *J. Lab. Clin. Med.* 56: 644–651, 1960.
130. DONALDSON, V. H., H. I. GLUECK, M. A. MILLER, H. Z. MOVAT, AND F. HABEL. Kininogen deficiency in Fitzgerald trait: role of high molecular weight kininogen in clotting and fibrinolysis. *J. Lab. Clin. Med.* 89: 327–337, 1976.
131. DOOLITTLE, R. F. Structural aspects of the fibrinogen to fibrin conversion. *Adv. Protein Chem.* 27: 1–109, 1973.
132. DOOLITTLE, R. F., K. G. CASSMAN, R. CHEN, J. J. SHARP, AND G. L. WOODING. Correlation of the mode of fibrin polymerization with the pattern of cross-linking. *Ann. NY Acad. Sci.* 202: 114–126, 1972.
133. DOOLITTLE, R. F., K. G. CASSMAN, B. A. COTTRELL, AND S. J. FRIEZNER. Amino acid sequence studies on the α chain of human fibrinogen. Isolation and characterization of two linked α-chain cyanogen bromide fragments from fully cross-linked fibrin. *Biochemistry* 16: 1715–1719, 1977.
134. DOOLITTLE, R. F., R. CHEN, AND F. LAU. Hybrid fibrin proof of the intermolecular nature of crosslinking units. *Biochem. Biophys. Res. Commun.* 44: 94–100, 1971.
135. DOOLITTLE, R. F., D. M. GOLDBAUM, AND L. R. DOOLITTLE. Designation of sequences involved in the "coiled-coil" interdomainal connections in fibrinogen: construction of an atomic scale model. *J. Mol. Biol.* 120: 311–325, 1978.
136. DOOLITTLE, R. F., K. W. K. WATT, B. A. COTTRELL, D. D. STRONG, AND M. RILEY. The amino acid sequence of the α-chain of human fibrinogen. *Nature London* 280: 464–468, 1979.
137. DOWNING, M. R., J. W. BLOOM, AND K. G. MANN. Comparison of the inhibition of thrombin by three plasma protease inhibitors. *Biochemistry* 17: 2649–2653, 1978.
138. DOWNING, M. R., R. J. BUTKOWSKI, M. M. CLARK, AND K. G. MANN. Human prothrombin activation. *J. Biol. Chem.* 250: 8897–8906, 1975.
139. DUDEK, G. A., M. KLOCZEWIAK, A. Z. BUDZYNSKI, Z. S. LATALLO, AND M. KOPEC. Characterization and comparison of macromolecular end products of fibrinogen and fibrin proteolysis by plasmin. *Biochim. Biophys. Acta* 214: 44–51, 1970.
140. EAGLE, H. Studies on blood coagulation. II. The formation of fibrin from thrombin and fibrinogen. *J. Gen. Physiol.* 18: 547–555, 1935.
141. EHRLICH, J., AND S. S. STIVALA. Chemistry and pharmacology of heparin. *J. Pharm. Sci.* 62: 517–521, 1969.
142. EKERT, H., I. FRIEDLANDER, AND R. M. HARDISTY. The role of platelets in fibrinolysis. Studies on the plasminogen activator and antiplasmin activity of platelets. *Br. J. Haematol.* 18: 575–584, 1970.
143. ELION, J., M. R. DOWNING, R. J. BUTKOWSKI, AND K. G. MANN. Structure of human thrombins: comparison with other serine preteases. In: *The Chemistry and Biology of Thrombin*, edited by R. L. Lundblad, J. W. Fenton II, and K. G. Mann. Ann Arbor, MI: Ann Arbor Science, 1977, p. 97–111.
144. ELMORE, D. T. The enzymic properties of thrombin and factor Xa. *Biochem. Soc. Trans.* 1: 1191–1194, 1973.
145. ENDRES, G. F., AND H. A. SCHERAGA. Molecular weight of bovine fibrinogen by sedimentation equilibrium. *Arch. Biochem. Biophys.* 144: 519–528, 1971.
146. ENFIELD, D. L., K. H. ERICSSON, K. A. WALSH, H. NEURATH, AND K. TITANI. Bovine factor X_1 (Stuart factor). Primary structure of the light chain. *Proc. Natl. Acad. Sci. USA* 72: 16–19, 1975.
147. ENGELBERG, H. *Heparin: Metabolism, Physiology and Clinical Application.* Springfield, IL: Thomas, 1963.
148. ESMON, C. T. The subunit structure of thrombin-activated factor V. Isolation of activated factor V, separation of subunits and reconstitution of biological activity. *J. Biol. Chem.* 254: 964–973, 1979.
149. ESMON, C. T., AND C. M. JACKSON. The conversion of prothrombin to thrombin. III. The factor Xa-catalyzed activation of prothrombin. *J. Biol. Chem.* 249: 7782–7790, 1974.
150. ESMON, C. T., AND C. M. JACKSON. The conversion of prothrombin to thrombin. IV. The function of the fragment 2 region during activation in the presence of factor V. *J. Biol. Chem.* 249: 7791–7797, 1974.
151. ESMON, C. T., W. G. OWEN, D. L. DUIGUID, AND C. M. JACKSON. The action of thrombin on blood clotting factor V: conversion of factor V to a prothrombin-binding protein. *Biochim. Biophys. Acta* 310: 289–294, 1973.
152. ESMON, C. T., W. G. OWEN, AND C. M. JACKSON. The conversion of prothrombin to thrombin. II. Differentiation between thrombin- and factor Xa-catalyzed proteolyses. *J. Biol. Chem.* 249: 606–611, 1974.
153. ESMON, C. T., W. G. OWEN, AND C. M. JACKSON. The conversion of prothrombin to thrombin. V. The activation of prothrombin by factor Xa in the presence of phospholipid. *J. Biol. Chem.* 249: 7798–7807, 1974.
154. ESMON, C. T., W. G. OWEN, AND C. M. JACKSON. A plausible mechanism for prothrombin activation by factor Xa, factor Va, phospholipid, and calcium ions. *J. Biol. Chem.* 249: 8045–8047, 1974.

155. ESMON, C. T., J. A. SADOWSKI, AND J. W. SUTTIE. A new carboxylation reaction. The vitamin K-dependent incorporation of $H^{14}CO_3$ into prothrombin. *J. Biol. Chem.* 250: 4744–4748, 1975.

156. ESMON, C. T., J. W. SUTTIE, AND C. M. JACKSON. The functional significance of vitamin K action, difference in phospholipid binding between normal and abnormal prothrombin. *J. Biol. Chem.* 250: 4095–4099, 1975.

157. ESNOUF, M. P., AND F. JOBIN. Lipids in prothrombin conversion. *Thromb. Diath. Haemmorrh. Suppl.* 17: 103–110, 1965.

158. EWART, M. R., M. W. C. HATTON, J. M. BASFORD, AND K. S. DODGSON. The proteolytic action of arvin on human fibrinogen. *Biochem. J.* 118: 603–609, 1970.

159. FAIR, B. D., H. SAITO, O. D. RATNOFF, AND W. B. RIPPON. Detection by fluorescence of structural changes accompanying the activation of Hageman factor (factor XII). *Proc. Soc. Exp. Biol. Med.* 155: 199–202, 1977.

160. FENTON, J. W., II, B. H. LANDIS, D. A. WALZ, D. H. BING, R. D. FEINMAN, M. P. ZABINSKI, S. A. SONDER, L. J. BERLINER, AND J. S. FINLAYSON. Human thrombin: preparative evaluation, structural properties and enzymic specificity. In: *The Chemistry and Physiology of the Human Plasma Proteins*, edited by D. H. Bing. New York: Pergamon, 1979, p. 151–183.

161. FERRY, J. D. The mechanism of polymerization of fibrinogen. *Proc. Natl. Acad. Sci. USA* 38: 566–569, 1952.

162. FILIP, D. J., J. D. ECKSTEIN, AND J. J. VELTKAMP. Hereditary antithrombin III deficiency and thromboembolic disease. *Am. J. Hematol.* 1: 343–349, 1976.

163. FLETCHER, A. P., N. ALKJAERSIG, S. FISHER, AND S. SHERRY. The proteolysis of fibrinogen by plasmin: the identification of thrombin-clottable fibrinogen derivatives which polymerize abnormally. *J. Lab. Clin. Med.* 68: 780–802, 1966.

164. FLETCHER, A. P., N. ALKJAERSIG, J. O'BRIEN, AND V. G. TULEVSKI. Blood hypercoagulability and thrombosis. *Trans. Assoc. Am. Physicians* 83: 159–167, 1970.

165. FLETCHER, A. P., N. ALKJAERSIG, S. SHERRY, E. GENTON, J. HIRSH, AND F. BACHMANN. The development of urokinase as a thrombolytic agent. Maintenance of a sustained thrombolytic state in man by its intravenous infusion. *J. Lab. Clin. Med.* 65: 713–731, 1965.

166. FOLK, J. E., AND S. I. CHUNG. Molecular and catalytic properties of transglutaminases. *Adv. Enzymol. Relat. Areas Mol. Biol.* 38: 109–191, 1973.

167. FORBES, C. D., J. PENSKY, AND O. D. RATNOFF. Inhibition of activated Hageman factor and activated plasma thromboplastin antecedent by purified serum C1 inactivator. *J. Lab. Clin. Med.* 76: 809–815, 1970.

168. FOWLER, W. E., AND H. P. ERICKSON. Trinodular structure of fibrinogen. Confirmation by both shadowing and negative stain electron microscopy. *J. Mol. Biol.* 134: 241–249, 1979.

169. FOWLER, W. E., H. P. ERICKSON, R. R. HANTGAN, J. MCDONAGH, AND J. HERMANS. Cross-linked fibrinogen dimers demonstrate a feature of the molecular packing in fibrin fibers. *Science* 211: 287–289, 1981.

170. FOWLER, W. E., L. J. FRETTO, H. P. ERICKSON, AND P. A. MCKEE. Electron microscopy of plasmic fragments of human fibrinogen as related to trinodular structure of the intact molecule. *J. Clin. Invest.* 66: 50–56, 1980.

171. FRANCIS, C. W., V. J. MARDER, AND G. H. BARLOW. Plasmic degradation of crosslinked fibrin. Characterization of new macromolecular soluble complexes and a model for their structure. *J. Clin. Invest.* 66: 1033–1043, 1980.

172. FRANCIS, C. W., V. J. MARDER, AND S. E. MARTIN. Demonstration of a large molecular weight variant of the γ chain of normal human plasma fibrinogen. *J. Biol. Chem.* 255: 5599–5604, 1980.

173. FRANCIS, C. W., V. J. MARDER, AND S. E. MARTIN. Plasmic degradation of crosslinked fibrin. I. Structural analysis of the particulate clot and identification of new macromolecular soluble complexes. *Blood* 56: 456–464, 1980.

174. FREEMAN, J. P., M. C. GUILLIN, A. BEZEAUD, AND C. M. JACKSON. Activation of bovine blood coagulation factor V. A prerequisite for it to bind both prothrombin and factor Xa (Abstract). *Federation Proc.* 36: 675, 1977.

175. FRETTO, L. J., E. W. FERGUSON, H. M. STEINMAN, AND P. A. MCKEE. Localization of the α-chain cross-link acceptor sites of human fibrin. *J. Biol. Chem.* 253: 2184–2195, 1978.

176. FRITZ, H., G. WUNDERER, K. KUMMER, N. HEIMBURGER, AND E. WERLE. α1-Antitrypsin und C 1-Inaktivator: Progressiv-Inhibitoren für Serumkallikreine von Mensch und Schwein. *Hoppe-Seyler's Z. Physiol. Chem* 353: 906–910, 1972.

177. FRYKLUND, L., H. BORG, AND L.-O. ANDERSSON. Amino-terminal sequence of human factor IX: presence of γ-carboxyl glutamic acid residues. *FEBS Lett.* 65: 187–189, 1976.

178. FUJIKAWA, K., M. H. COAN, D. L. ENFIELD, I. K. TITAN, L. H. ERICSSON, AND E. W. DAVIE. A comparison of bovine prothrombin, factor IX (Christmas factor), and factor X (Stuart factor). *Proc. Natl. Acad. Sci. USA* 71: 427–430, 1974.

179. FUJIKAWA, K., M. E. LEGAZ, AND E. W. DAVIE. Bovine factors X_1 and X_2 (Stuart factor): isolation and characterization. *Biochemistry* 11: 4882–4891, 1972.

180. FUKUI, H., S. MIKAMI, T. OKUDA, N. MURASHIMA, T. TAKASE, AND A. YOSHIOKA. Studies of von Willebrand factor: effects of different kinds of carbohydrate oxidases, SH-inhibitors and some other chemical reagents. *Br. J. Haematol.* 36: 259–270, 1977.

181. FURLAN, M., AND E. A. BECK. Plasmic degradation of human fibrinogen. I. Structural characterization of degradation products. *Biochim. Biophys. Acta* 263: 631–644, 1972.

182. FURLAN, M., T. SEELICH, AND E. A. BECK. Clottability and cross-linking reactivity of fibrin(ogen) following differential release of fibrinopeptides A and B. *Thromb. Haemost.* 36: 582–592, 1976.

183. GAFFNEY, P. J., AND M. BRASHER. Subunit structure of the plasmin-induced degradation products of crosslinked fibrin. *Biochim. Biophys. Acta* 295: 308–313, 1973.

184. GAFFNEY, P. J., AND M. BRASHER. Mode of action of ancrod as a defibrinating agent. *Nature London* 251: 53–54, 1974.

185. GAFFNEY, P. J., M. BRASHER, AND F. JOE. Further physicochemical and immunological data concerning the D-dimer complex. *Thromb. Haemost.* 38: 226–227, 1977.

186. GAFFNEY, P. J., M. BRASHER, K. LORD, C. J. L. STRACHAN, A. R. WILKINSON, V. V. KAKKAR, AND M. F. SCULLY. Fibrin subunits in venous and arterial thromboembolism. *Cardiovasc. Res.* 10: 421–426, 1976.

187. GAFFNEY, P. J., AND P. DOBOS. A structural aspect of human fibrinogen suggested by its plasmin degradation. *FEBS Lett.* 15: 13–16, 1971.

188. GALANAKIS, D. K., AND M. W. MOSESSON. Correction of the delayed fibrin aggregation of fetal fibrinogen by partial removal of sialic acid (Abstract). *Thromb. Haemost.* 42: 79, 1979.

189. GANGULY, P. A low molecular weight antiplasmin of human blood platelets. *Clin. Chim. Acta* 39: 466–468, 1972.

190. GANGULY, P., AND W. J. SONNICHSEN. Binding of thrombin to human platelets and its possible significance. *Br. J. Haematol.* 34: 291–301, 1976.

191. GATI, W. P., AND P. W. STRAUB. Separation of both the Bβ- and the γ-polypeptide chains of human fibrinogen into two main types which differ in sialic acid content. *J. Biol. Chem.* 253: 1315–1321, 1978.

192. GIGLI, I., J. W. MASON, R. W. COLMAN, AND K. F. AUSTEN. Interaction of plasma kallikrein with CT inactivator. *J. Immunol.* 104: 574–581, 1970.

193. GITEL, S. N., R. C. STEPHENSON, AND S. WESSLER. In vitro and in vivo correlation of clotting protease activity. Effect of heparin. *Proc. Natl. Acad. Sci. USA* 74: 3028–3032, 1977.

194. GLADNER, J. A., AND K. LAKI. The inhibition of thrombin by diisopropylphosphofluoridate. *Arch. Biochem. Biophys.* 62: 501–506, 1956.

195. GLOVER, G., AND E. SHAW. The purification of thrombin and isolation of a peptide containing the active-center histidine. *J. Biol. Chem.* 246: 4594–4601, 1971.

196. GODAL, H. C., M. RYGH, AND K. LAAKE. Progressive inactivation of purified factor VII by heparin and antithrombin III. *Thromb. Res.* 5: 773–775, 1974.
197. GOLDSMITH, G. H., H. SAITO, AND O. D. RATNOFF. The activation of plasminogen by Hageman factor (factor XII) and Hageman factor fragments. *J. Clin. Invest.* 62: 54–60, 1978.
198. GORMAN, J. J. Inhibition of human thrombin assessed with different substrates and inhibitors. Characterization of fibrinopeptide binding interaction. *Biochim. Biophys. Acta* 412: 273–282, 1975.
199. GORMSEN, J., AND C. FEDDERSEN. Demonstration of different D and E antigenic intermediates during plasmin degradation of non-stabilized and stabilized fibrin clots. *Scand. J. Haematol.* 10: 337–348, 1973.
200. GOSPODAROWICZ, D., K. D. BROWN, C. R. BIRDWELL, AND B. R. ZETTER. Control of proliferation of human vascular endothelial cells. Characterization of the response of human umbilical vein endothelial cells to fibroblast growth factor, epidermal growth factor, and thrombin. *J. Cell Biol.* 77: 774–788, 1978.
201. GRAF, L., E. BARAT, J. BORVENDEG, I. HERMANN, AND A. PATTLEY. Action of thrombin on ovine, bovine and human pituitary growth hormones. *Eur. J. Biochem.* 64: 333–340, 1976.
202. GRALNICK, H. R., H. GIVELBER, AND E. ABRAMS. Dysfibrinogenemia associated with hepatoma. *N. Engl. J. Med.* 299: 221–226, 1978.
203. GRAMSE, M., C. BINGENHEIMER, W. SCHMIDT, R. EGBRING, AND K. HAVEMANN. Degradation products of fibrinogen by elastase-like neutral protease from human granulocytes. *J. Clin. Invest.* 61: 1027–1033, 1978.
204. GREENBERG, J. P., M. A. PACKHAM, M. A. GUCCIONE, J. HARFENIST, J. L. ORR, R. L. KINLOUGH-RATHBONE, D. W. PERRY, AND J. F. MUSTARD. The effect of pretreatment of human and rabbit platelets with chymotrypsin on their responses to human fibrinogen and aggregating agents. *Blood* 54: 754–765, 1979.
205. GREENQUIST, A. C., AND R. W. COLMAN. Factor V, a calcium containing protein. *Blood* 46: 769–782, 1975.
206. GRIFFIN, J. H. The role of surface in the surface-dependent activation of Hageman factor (blood coagulation factor XII). *Proc. Natl. Acad. Sci. USA* 75: 1998–2002, 1978.
207. GRIFFIN, J. H., AND C. G. COCHRANE. Mechanisms for the involvement of high molecular weight kininogen in surface dependent reactions of Hageman factor. *Proc. Natl. Acad. Sci. USA* 73: 2554–2558, 1976.
208. GRIFFITH, J. J. Kinetic analysis of the heparin-enhanced antithrombin III/thrombin reaction. Reaction rate enhanced by heparin-thrombin association. *J. Biol. Chem.* 254: 12044–12049, 1979.
209. GRINNELL, F., M. FELD, AND D. MINTER. Fibroblast adhesion to fibrinogen and fibrin substrata: requirement for cold-insoluble globulin (plasma fibronectin). *Cell* 19: 517–525, 1980.
210. GROSKOPF, W. R., B. HSIEH, L. SUMMARIA, AND K. C. ROBBINS. Studies on the active center of human plasmin. The serine and histidine residues. *J. Biol. Chem.* 244: 359–365, 1969.
211. GUMPRECHT, J. G., AND R. W. COLMAN. Role of sialic acid in the function of bovine factor V. *Arch. Biochem. Biophys.* 169: 278–286, 1975.
212. HABAL, F. M., B. J. UNDERDOWN, AND H. Z. MOVAT. Further characterization of human plasma kininogens. *Biochem. Pharmacol.* 24: 1241–1243, 1975.
213. HAFTER, R., R. VON HUGO, AND H. GRAEF. Origin of soluble crosslinked fibrin oligomers: an in vitro study. *Thromb. Haemost.* 42: 275–276, 1979.
214. HALL, C. E., AND H. S. SLAYTER. The fibrinogen molecule: its size, shape and mode of polymerization. *J. Biophys. Biochem. Cytol* 5: 11–15, 1959.
214a. HANDIN, R. I., AND R. D. ROSENBERG. Hemorrhagic disorders. III. Disorders of primary and secondary hemostasis. In: *Hematology*, edited by W. S. Beck. Cambridge, MA: MIT Press, 1981, chapt. 28, p. 425–439.
215. HANTGAN, R. R., W. FOWLER, H. ERICKSON, AND J. HERMANNS. Fibrin assembly: a comparison of electron microscopic and light-scattering results. *Thromb. Haemost.* 44: 119–124, 1980.
216. HANTGAN, R. R., AND J. HERMANS. Assembly of fibrin. A light scattering study. *J. Biol. Chem.* 254: 11272–11281, 1979.
217. HARFENIST, E. J., AND R. E. CANFIELD. Degradation of fibrinogen by plasmin. Isolation of an early cleavage product. *Biochemistry* 14: 4110–4117, 1975.
218. HARPEL, P. C. Studies on the interaction between collagen and a plasma kallikrein-like activity. Evidence for a surface-active enzyme system. *J. Clin. Invest.* 51: 1813–1822, 1972.
219. HARPEL, P. C. Human α_2-macroglobulin. *Methods Enzymol.* 45: 639–652, 1976.
220. HARPEL, P. C. Circulating inhibitors of human plasma, kallikrein. In: *Chemistry and Biology of the Kallikrein-Kinin System in Health and Disease*, edited by J. J. Pisano and K. F. Austen. Washington, DC: US Govt. Printing Office, 1977, p. 169–177. (Fogarty Int. Ctr. Proc. 27.)
221. HARPEL, P. C., AND M. W. MOSESSON. Degradation of human fibrinogen by plasmin α_2-macroglobulin-enzyme complexes. *J. Clin. Invest.* 52: 2175–2184, 1973.
222. HARPEL, P. C., AND R. D. ROSENBERG. α_2-Macroglobulin and antithrombin-heparin cofactor: modulators of hemostatic and inflammatory reactions. *Prog. Hemostasis Thromb.* 3: 145–189, 1976.
223. HATHAWAY, W. E., L. P. BELHANSEN, AND H. S. HATHAWAY. Evidence for a new plasma thromboplastin factor. I. Case report, coagulation studies and physicochemical properties. *Blood* 26: 521–532, 1965.
224. HATTERSLEY, P. G., AND D. HAYSE. Fletcher factor deficiency. A report of three unrelated cases. *Br. J. Haematol.* 18: 411–416, 1970.
225. HAUPT, H., AND N. HEIMBURGER. Humanserumproteine mit hoher Affinität zu Carboxymethylcellulose. I. Isolierung von Lysozym, C1q und zwei bisher unbekannten α-Globulinen. *Hoppe-Seyler's Z. Physiol. Chem.* 353: 1125–1132, 1972.
226. HAWIGER, J., D. K. HAMMOND, S. TIMMONS, AND A. Z. BUDZYNSKI. Interaction of human fibrinogen with staphylococci: presence of a binding region on normal and abnormal fibrinogen variants and fibrinogen derivatives. *Blood* 51: 799–812, 1978.
227. HAWIGER, J., S. NIEWIAROWSKI, V. GUREWICH, AND D. P. THOMAS. Measurement of fibrinogen and fibrin degradation products in serum by staphylococcal clumping test. *J. Lab. Clin. Med.* 75: 93–108, 1970.
228. HECK, L. W., AND A. P. KAPLAN. Substrates of Hageman factor. I. Isolation and characterization of human factor XI (PTA) and inhibition of the activated enzyme by alpha 1-antitrypsin. *J. Exp. Med.* 140: 1615–1621, 1974.
229. HEDNER, U., AND G. MARTINSSON. Inhibition of activated Hageman factor (factor XIIa) by an inhibitor of plasminogen activation (PA-inhibitor). *Thromb. Res.* 12: 1015–1023, 1978.
230. HEIMBURGER, N., H. HAUPT, T. KRANZ, AND S. BAUDNER. Humanserumproteine mit hoher Affinität zu Carboxymethylcellulose II. Physikalisch-chemische und immunologische Charakterisierung eines histidinreichen 3,8S-α_2-Glykoproteins (CM-Protein I). *Hoppe-Seyler's Z. Physiol. Chem.* 353: 1133–1140, 1972.
231. HEMKER, H. C., M. J. P. KAHN, AND P. P. DEVILEE. The adsorption of coagulation factors onto phospholipid. Its role in the reaction mechanism of blood coagulation. *Thromb. Diath. Haemorrh.* 24: 214–223, 1970.
232. HENSCHEN, A. Number and reactivity of disulfide bonds in fibrinogen and fibrin. *Ark. Kemi* 22: 355–374, 1964.
233. HENSCHEN, A. Disulfide bridges and molecular symmetry in fibrinogen (Abstract). *Thromb. Haemost.* 42: 14, 1979.
234. HENSCHEN, A., AND F. LOTTSPEICH. Sequence homology be-

tween γ-chain and β-chain in human fibrin. *Thromb. Res.* 11: 869–880, 1977.
235. HESSEL, B. On the structure of the COOH-terminal part of the Aα chain of human fibrinogen. *Thromb. Res.* 7: 75–87, 1975.
236. HIGHSMITH, R. F., AND R. D. ROSENBERG. The inhibition of human plasmin by human antithrombin-heparin cofactor. *J. Biol. Chem.* 249: 4335–4338, 1974.
237. HISANO, S. Immunofluorescence study on thrombolysis with special reference to the patterns of distribution and the contents of fibrin, plasminogen, α_2-macroglobulin and urokinase in artificial thrombi. *Thromb. Haemost.* 39: 53–60, 1978.
238. HOGG, D. H., AND B. BLOMBÄCK. The mechanism of the fibrinogen-thrombin reaction. *Thromb. Res.* 12: 953–964, 1978.
239. HOLMBERG, L., L. BORGE, R. LJUNG, AND I. M. NILSSON. Measurement of antihaemophilic factor A antigen (VIII:CAg) with a solid phase immunoradiometric method base on homologous non-haemophilic antibodies. *Scand. J. Haematol.* 23: 17–24, 1979.
240. HOLMBERG, L., AND R. LJUNG. Purification of factor VIII:C by antigen-antibody chromatography. *Thromb. Res.* 12: 667–675, 1978.
241. HOLMBERG, L., AND I. M. NILSSON. AHF-related protein in clinical praxis. *Scand. J. Haematol.* 12: 221–231, 1974.
242. HORNER, A. A. Enzymic depolymerization of macromolecular heparin as a factor in control of lipoprotein lipase activity. *Proc. Natl. Acad. Sci. USA* 69: 3469–3473, 1972.
243. HOROWITZ, B., A. LIPPIN, AND K. R. WOODS. Purification of low molecular weight factor VIII by affinity chromatography using factor VIII-sepharose. *Thromb. Res.* 14: 463–475, 1979.
244. HOUGIE, C., K. W. E. DENSON, AND R. BIGGS. A study of the reaction product of factor VIII and factor IX by gel filtration. *Thromb. Diath. Haemorrh.* 18: 211–222, 1967.
245. HOVINGH, P., AND A. LINKER. Enzymatic degradation of heparin and heparitin sulfate. *J. Biol. Chem.* 245: 6170–6175, 1980.
246. HOWELL, W. H. The preparation and properties of thrombin, together with observations on antithrombin and prothrombin. *Am. J. Physiol.* 26: 453–473, 1910.
247. HOYER, L. W. Specificity of precipitating antibodies in immunologic identification of antihaemophilic factor. *Nature London New Biol.* 245: 49–51, 1973.
248. HOYER, L. W. Von Willebrand's disease. In: *Progress in Hemostasis and Thrombosis*, edited by T. H. Spaet. New York: Grune & Stratton, 1976, vol. III, p. 231–287.
249. HSIEH, K., M. S. MUDD, AND G. D. WILNER. Fibrin polymerization. I. Alkylating peptide inhibitors of fibrin polymerization. *J. Med. Chem.* 24: 322–327, 1981.
250. HUBBARD, D., AND G. L. LUCAS. Ionic charges of glass surfaces and other materials, and their possible role in the coagulation of blood. *J. Appl. Physiol.* 15: 265–270, 1960.
251. HUDRY-CLERGEON, G., L. PATUREL, AND M. SUSCILLION. Identification d'un compléxe (D-D) ... E dans les produits de dégradation de la fibrine bovine stabilisée par la facteur XIII. *Pathol. Biol.* 22: 47–52, 1974.
252. HULTIN, M. B., AND Y. NEMERSON. Activation of factor X by factors IXa and VIII; a specific assay for factor IXa in the presence of thrombin-activated factor VIII. *Blood* 52: 928–940, 1978.
253. HUSEBY, R. M., AND M. MURRAY. Molecular structure of fibrinogen. I. Helical content and the role of the tyrosine moiety in the fibrinogen molecule. *Biochim. Biophys. Acta* 133: 243–250, 1967.
254. HVATUM, M., AND H. PRYDZ. Studies on tissue thromboplastin—its splitting into two separable parts. *Thromb. Diath. Haemorrh.* 21: 217–222, 1969.
255. IATRIDIS, S. G., AND J. H. FERGUSON. Active Hageman factor. A plasma lysokinase of the human fibrinolytic system. *J. Clin. Invest.* 41: 1277–1287, 1962.
256. ITTYERAH, R., R. RAWALA, AND R. W. COLMAN. Immunochemical studies of factor V of bovine platelets. *Eur. J. Biochem.* 120: 235–241, 1981.
257. IWANAGA, S., B. BLOMBÄCK, N. GRONDAHL, B. HESSEL, AND P. WALLEN. Amino acid sequence of the N-terminal part of the γ-chain in human fibrinogen. *Biochim. Biophys. Acta* 160: 280–283, 1968.
258. IWANAGA, S., G. OSHIMA, AND T. SUZUKI. Proteinases from the venom of *Agkistrodon halys blomhoffi*. *Methods Enzymol.* 45: 459–468, 1976.
259. IWANAGA, S., K. SUZUKI, AND S. HASHIMOTO. Bovine plasma cold-insoluble globulin: gross structure and function. *Ann. NY Acad. Sci.* 312: 56–72, 1978.
260. JACKSON, C. M. Characterization of two glycoprotein variants of bovine factor X and demonstration that the factor X zymogen contains two polypeptide chains. *Biochemistry* 11: 4873–4882, 1972.
261. JACKSON, C. M., C. T. ESMON, S. N. GITEL, W. G. OWEN, AND R. A. HENRIKSEN. The conversion of prothrombin to thrombin: the function of the propiece of prothrombin in prothrombin and related coagulation factors. *Boerhaave Ser.* 10: 59–88, 1975.
262. JACKSON, C. M., C. T. ESMON, AND W. G. OWEN. The activation of bovine prothrombin. In: *Proteases and Biological Control*, edited by E. Reich, D. B. Rifkin, and E. Shaw. New York: Cold Spring Harbor, 1975, vol. 2, p. 95–109. (Cold Spring Harbor Conf. Cell Proliferation.)
262a. JACKSON, C. M., AND Y. NEMERSON. Blood coagulation. *Annu. Rev. Biochem.* 49: 765–811, 1980.
263. JACKSON, C. M., W. G. OWEN, S. N. GITEL, AND C. T. ESMON. The chemical role of lipids in prothrombin activation. *Thromb. Diath. Haemorrh. Suppl.* 57: 273–293, 1974.
264. JACKSON, C. M., AND J. W. SUTTIE. Recent developments in understanding the mechanism of vitamin K antagonist drug action and the consequences of vitamin K action in blood coagulation. In: *Progress in Hematology*, edited by E. B. Brown. New York: Grune & Stratton, 1977, vol. X, p. 233–259.
265. JACOBSEN, S. Substrates from plasma kinin-forming enzymes in human, dog, and rabbit plasmas. *Br. J. Pharmacol.* 26: 403–411, 1966.
266. JACOBSEN, S., AND M. KRIZ. Some data on two purified kininogens from human plasma. *Br. J. Pharmacol.* 29: 25–36, 1967.
267. JEANLOZ, R. W. Heparin: structure, function and clinical implications. In: *The Chemistry of Heparin*, edited by R. A. Bradshaw and S. Wessler. New York: Plenum, 1975, p. 3–17.
268. JESTY, J., AND S. A. SILVERBERG. Kinetics of the tissue factor-dependent activation of coagulation factors IX and X in a bovine plasma system. *J. Biol. Chem.* 254: 12337–12345, 1979.
269. JESTY, J., A. K. SPENCER, AND Y. NEMERSON. The mechanism of action of factor X. Kinetic control of alternative pathways leading to the formation of activated factor X. *J. Biol. Chem.* 249: 5614–5622, 1974.
270. JILEK, F., AND H. HORMANN. Cold-insoluble globulin: cyanogen bromide and plasminolysis fragments containing a label introduced by transamidation. *Hoppe-Seyler's Z. Physiol. Chem.* 358: 1165–1168, 1977.
270a. JOHNSON, A. J., V. E. MACDONALD, M. SEMAR, J. E. FIELD, J. SHUCK, C. LEWIS, AND J. BRIND. Preparation of the major plasma fractions by solid-phase polyelectrolytes. *J. Lab. Clin. Med.* 92: 194–210, 1978.
271. JOHNSON, P., AND E. MIHALYI. Physicochemical studies of bovine fibrinogen. I. Molecular weight and hydrodynamic properties of fibrinogen and fibrinogen cleaved by sulfite in 5M guanidine HCl solution. *Biochim. Biophys. Acta* 102: 467–475, 1965.
272. JONES, J. M., J. M. CREETH, AND R. A. KEKWICK. Thiol reduction of human α_2-macroglobulin. The subunit structure. *Biochem. J.* 127: 187–197, 1972.
273. JÖRNVAL, H., W. W. FISH, AND I. BJÖRK. The thrombin cleavage site in bovine antithrombin. *FEBS Lett.* 106: 358–362, 1979.
274. KAKKAR, V. V., AND M. F. SCULLY. Thrombolytic therapy.

Br. Med. Bull. 34: 191–199, 1978.
275. KANAIDE, H., AND J. R. SHAINOFF. Cross-linking of fibrinogen and fibrin by fibrin-stabilizing factor (factor XIIIa). *J. Lab. Clin. Med.* 85: 574–597, 1975.
276. KANDALL, C. L., S. B. SHOHET, T. K. AKINBAMI, AND R. W. COLMAN. Determinants of the formation and activity of factor V-phospholipid complexes. I. Influence of phospholipid structure. *Thromb. Diath. Haemorrh.* 34: 256–270, 1975.
277. KANDALL, C. L., S. B. SHOHET, T. K. AKINBAMI, AND R. W. COLMAN. Determinants of the formation and activity of factor V-phospholipid complexes. II. Molecular properties of the complexes. *Thromb. Diath. Haemorrh.* 34: 271–284, 1975.
278. KAPLAN, A. P. Initiation of the intrinsic coagulation and fibrinolytic pathways of man: the role of surfaces, Hageman factor, prekallikrein, high molecular weight kininogen, and factor XI. In: *Progress in Hemostasis and Thrombosis*, edited by T. H. Spaet. New York: Grune & Stratton, 1978, vol. IV, p. 127–175.
279. KAPLAN, A. P., AND K. F. AUSTEN. The fibrinolytic pathway of human plasma. Isolation and characterization of the plasminogen proactivator. *J. Exp. Med.* 136: 1378–1393, 1972.
280. KARAPALLY, J. C., AND C. P. DIETRICH. A uronic acid isomerase in *Flavobacterium* heparinum. *Can. J. Biochem.* 48: 164–177, 1970.
281. KATAYAMA, K., L. H. ERICSSON, D. L. ENFIELD, K. A. WALSH, H. NEURATH, E. W. DAVIE, AND K. TITANI. Comparison of amino acid sequence of bovine coagulation factor IX (Christmas factor) with that of other vitamin K-dependent plasma proteins. *Proc. Natl. Acad. Sci. USA* 76: 4990–4993, 1979.
282. KELLERMEYER, R. W., AND R. T. BRECKENRIDGE. The inflammatory process in acute gouty arthritis. I. Activation of Hageman factor by sodium urate crystals. *J. Lab. Clin. Med.* 65: 307–315, 1965.
283. KERBIRIOU, D. M., B. N. BOUMA, AND J. H. GRIFFIN. Immunochemical studies of human high molecular weight kininogen and of its complexes with plasma prekallikrein or kallikrein. *J. Biol. Chem.* 255: 3952–3958, 1980.
284. KERBIRIOU, D. M., AND J. H. GRIFFIN. Human high molecular weight kininogen. Studies on structure-function relationships and of proteolysis of the molecule occurring during contact activation of plasma. *J. Biol. Chem.* 254: 12020–12027, 1979.
285. KERNOFF, P. B. A., AND C. R. RIZZA. The specificity of antibodies to factor VIII produced in the rabbit after immunization with human cryoprecipitate. *Thromb. Diath. Haemorrh.* 29: 652–660, 1973.
286. KISIEL, W., W. M. CANFIELD, L. H. ERICSSON, AND E. W. DAVIE. Anticoagulant properties of bovine plasma protein C following activation by thrombin. *Biochemistry* 16: 5824–5831, 1977.
287. KISIEL, W., K. FUJIKAWA, AND E. W. DAVIE. Activation of bovine factor VII (Proconvertin) by factor XII (activated Hageman Factor). *Biochemistry* 16: 4189–4194, 1977.
288. KJELDGAARD, N. O., AND J. PLOUG. Urokinase an activator of plasminogen activation. *Biochim. Biophys. Acta* 24: 283–289, 1957.
289. KLUFT, C. Elimination of inhibition in euglobulin fibrinolysis by use of flufenamate: involvement of C1-inactivator. *Haemostasis* 6: 351–369, 1977.
290. KOENIG, V. L. Partial specific volume for some porcine and bovine plasma protein fractions. *Arch. Biochem. Biophys.* 25: 241–245, 1950.
291. KOIE, K., T. KAMIYA, K. OGATA, AND J. TAKAMATSU. α_2-Plasmin-inhibitor deficiency (Miyasato disease). *Lancet* 2: 1334–1336, 1978.
292. KOMIYA, M., H. KATO, AND T. SUZUKI. Homology between bovine high molecular weight and low molecular weight kininogen. *Biochem. Biophys. Res. Commun.* 49: 1438–1443, 1972.
293. KOPEĆ, M., E. TEISSEYRE, G. DUDEK-WOJCIECHOWSKA, M. KLOCZEWIAK, A. PANKIEWICZ, AND Z. S. LATALLO. Studies on the "Double D" fragment from stabilizing bovine fibrin. *Thromb. Res.* 2: 283–291, 1973.

294. KÖPPEL, G. Electron microscopic investigation of the shape of fibrinogen nodules: a model for certain proteins. *Nature London* 212: 1608–1609, 1966.
295. KORNECKI, E., S. NIEWIAROWSKI, T. A. MORINELLI, AND M. KLOCZEWIAK. Effects of chymotrypsin and adenosine diphosphate on the exposure of fibrinogen receptors on normal human and Glanzmann's thrombasthenia. *J. Biol. Chem.* 256: 5695–5701, 1981.
296. KOUTTS, J., N. GUDE, AND B. G. FIRKIN. The dynamic interrelationship between factor VIII and von Willebrand factor. *Thromb. Res.* 8: 533–541, 1976.
297. KOUTTS, J., J. M. LAVERGNE, AND D. MEYER. Immunological evidence that human factor VIII is composed of two linked moieties. *Br. J. Haematol.* 37: 415–428, 1977.
298. KRAKOW, W., G. F. ENDRES, B. M. SIEGEL, AND H. A. SCHERAGA. An electron microscopic investigation of the polymerization of bovine fibrin monomer. *J. Mol. Biol.* 71: 95–103, 1972.
299. KUDRYK, B., B. BLOMBÄCK, AND M. BLOMBÄCK. Fibrinogen Detroit: an abnormal fibrinogen with non-functional NH$_2$-terminal polymerization domain. *Thromb. Res.* 9: 25–36, 1976.
300. KUDRYK, B. J., D. COLLEN, K. R. WOODS, AND B. BLOMBÄCK. Evidence for localization of polymerization sites in fibrinogen. *J. Biol. Chem.* 249: 3322–3325, 1974.
301. KUDRYK, B., J. REUTERBY, AND B. BLOMBÄCK. Adsorption of plasmic Fragment D to thrombin modified fibrinogen-sepharose. *Thromb. Res.* 2: 297–304, 1973.
302. KURACHI, K., AND E. W. DAVIE. Activation of human factor XI (plasma thromboplastin antecedent) by factor XIIa (activated Hageman factor). *Biochemistry* 16: 5831–5837, 1977.
303. KURACHI, K., K. FUJIKAWA, G. SCHMER, AND E. W. DAVIE. Inhibition of bovine factor IXa and factor Xaβ by antithrombin III. *Biochemistry* 15: 373–377, 1976.
304. KWAAN, H. C., G. H. BARLOW, AND N. SUWANWELA. Fibrinogen and its derivatives in relationship to ancrod and reptilase. *Thromb. Res.* 2: 123–136, 1973.
305. LACOMBE, N. J. Deficit constitutional en un nouveau facteur de la coagulation intervenant au niveau de contact: le facteur "Flaujeac." *C. R. Acad. Sci. Ser. D* 280: 1039–1041, 1975.
306. LAHIRI, B., A. B. BAGDASARIAN, B. MITCHELL, R. C. TALAMO, R. W. COLMAN, AND R. D. ROSENBERG. Antithrombin-heparin cofactor: an inhibitor of plasma kallikrein. *Arch. Biochem. Biophys.* 175: 737–747, 1976.
307. LAHIRI, B., AND J. R. SHAINOFF. Fate of fibrinopeptides in the reaction between human plasmin and fibrinogen. *Biochim. Biophys. Acta* 303: 161–170, 1972.
308. LAKI, K., AND L. LORAND. On the solubility of fibrin clots. *Science* 108: 280, 1948.
309. LAKI, K., AND W. F. H. M. MOMMAERTS. Transition of fibrinogen to fibrin as a two-step reaction. *Nature London* 156: 664, 1945.
310. LAM, L. H., J. E. SILBERT, AND R. D. ROSENBERG. The separation of active and inactive forms of heparin. *Biochem. Biophys. Res. Commun.* 69: 570–577, 1976.
311. LANCHANTIN, G. F., M. L. PLESSET, J. A. FRIEDMANN, AND D. W. HART. Dissociation of esterolytic and clotting activities of thrombin by trypsin-binding macroglobulin. *Proc. Soc. Exp. Biol. Med.* 121: 444–449, 1966.
312. LASKOWSKI, M., S. EHRENPREIS, T. H. DONNELLY, AND H. A. SCHERAGA. Equilibria in the fibrinogen-fibrin conversion. V. Reversibility and thermodynamics of the proteolytic action of thrombin on fibrinogen. *J. Am. Chem. Soc.* 82: 1340–1348, 1960.
313. LATALLO, Z. S. Formation and detection of fibrinogen derived complexes. *Thromb. Diath. Haemorrh.* 34: 677–685, 1975.
314. LATALLO, Z. S., A. Z. BUDZYNSKI, B. LIPINSKI, AND E. KOWALSKI. Inhibition of thrombin and of fibrin polymerization, two activities derived from plasmin-digested fibrinogen. *Nature London* 203: 1184–1185, 1964.
315. LATALLO, Z. S., A. P. FLETCHER, N. ALKJAERSIG, AND S. SHERRY. Influence of pH, ionic strength, neutral ions, and

thrombin on fibrin polymerization. *Am. J. Physiol.* 202: 675–680, 1962.

316. LATALLO, Z. S., AND S. LOPACIUK. New approach to thrombolytic therapy. The use of defibrase in connection with streptokinase. *Thromb. Diath. Haemorrh. Suppl.* 56: 253–255, 1973.

317. LATALLO, Z. S., L. E. MATTLER, N. U. BANG, M. S. HANSEN, AND M. L. CHANG. Analysis of soluble fibrin complexes by agarose gel chromatography and protamine sulfate gelation. *Biochim. Biophys. Acta* 420: 69–80, 1976.

318. LAUDANO, A. P., AND R. F. DOOLITTLE. Synthetic peptide derivatives that bind to fibrinogen and prevent the polymerization of fibrin monomers. *Proc. Natl. Acad. Sci. USA* 75: 3085–3089, 1978.

319. LAUDANO, A. P., AND R. F. DOOLITTLE. Studies on synthetic peptides that bind to fibrinogen and prevent fibrin polymerization. Structural requirements, number of binding sites and species differences. *Biochemistry* 19: 1013–1019, 1980.

320. LAUDANO, A. P., AND R. F. DOOLITTLE. Influence of calcium ion on the binding of fibrin amino terminal peptides to fibrinogen. *Science* 212: 457–459, 1981.

321. LAURENT, T. C. Studies on fractioned heparin. *Arch. Biochem. Biophys.* 92: 224–231, 1961.

322. LAURENT, T. C., AND B. BLOMBÄCK. On the significance of the release of two different peptides from fibrinogen during clotting. *Acta Chem. Scand.* 12: 1875–1877, 1958.

323. LAVERGNE, J. M., D. MEYER, AND H. REISNER. Characterization of human anti-factor VIII antibodies purified by immune complex formation. *Blood* 48: 931–939, 1976.

324. LAZARCHICK, J., AND L. W. HOYER. The properties of immune complexes formed by human antibodies to factor VIII. *J. Clin. Invest.* 60: 1070–1079, 1977.

325. LAZARCHICK, J., AND L. W. HOYER. Immunoradiometric measurement of the factor VIII procoagulant antigen. *J. Clin. Invest.* 62: 1048–1052, 1978.

326. LEDERER, K. Grösse und Gestalt des Fibrinogenmoleküls. 3. Hydrodynamische Studien. *Makromol. Chem.* 176: 2641–2653, 1975.

327. LEDERER, K., AND R. HAMMEL. Grösse und Gestalt des Fibrinogenmoleküls. 2. Röntgenkleinwinkelstreuung an verdünnten Losungen. *Makromol. Chem.* 176: 2619–2639, 1975.

328. LEGRAND, Y. J., A. RODRIGUEZ-ZEBALLOS, G. KARTALIS, F. FAUVEL, AND J. P. CAEN. Adsorption of factor VIII antigen-activity complex by collagen. *Thromb. Res.* 13: 909–911, 1978.

329. LESUK, A., L. TERMINIELLO, AND J. H. TRAVER. Crystalline human urokinase: some properties. *Science* 147: 880–881, 1965.

330. LESUK, A., L. TERMINIELLO, J. H. TRAVER, AND J. L. GROFF. Biochemical and biophysical studies of human urokinase. *Thromb. Diath. Haemorrh.* 18: 293–294, 1967.

331. LESUK, A., L. TERMINIELLO, J. H. TRAVER, AND J. L. GROFF. Proteolytic degradation of human urokinase to active fragments (Abstract). *Federation Proc.* 26: 647, 1967.

332. LI, E. H. H., J. W. FENTON II, AND R. D. FEINMAN. The role of heparin in the thrombin-antithrombin III reaction. *Arch. Biochem. Biophys.* 175: 153–159, 1976.

333. LIEM, R. K. H., R. H. ANDREATTA, AND H. A. SCHERAGA. Mechanism of action of thrombin on fibrinogen. II. Kinetics of hydrolysis of fibrinogen-like peptides by thrombin and trypsin. *Arch. Biochem. Biophys.* 147: 201–213, 1971.

334. LIEM, R. K. H., AND H. A. SCHERAGA. Mechanism of action of thrombin on fibrinogen. III. Partial mapping of the active sites of thrombin and trypsin. *Arch. Biochem. Biophys.* 158: 387–395, 1973.

335. LIEM, R. K. H., AND H. A. SCHERAGA. Mechanism of action of thrombin on fibrinogen. IV. Further mapping of the active sites of thrombin and trypsin. *Arch. Biochem. Biophys.* 160: 333–339, 1974.

336. LIJNEN, H. R., M. HOYLAERTS, AND D. COLLEN. Isolation and characterization of a human plasma protein with affinity for the lysine binding sites in plasminogen. *J. Biol. Chem.* 255: 10214–10222, 1980.

337. LIPINSKI, B., A. WEGRZYNOWICZ, A. Z. BUDZYNSKI, M. KO-PEĆ, Z. S. LATALLO, AND E. KOWALSKI. Soluble unclottable complexes formed in the presence of fibrinogen degradation products (FDP) during the fibrinogen-fibrin conversion and their potential significance in pathology. *Thromb. Diath. Haemorrh.* 17: 65–77, 1967.

338. LIU, C. Y., H. L. NOSSEL, AND K. L. KAPLAN. The binding of thrombin by fibrin. *J. Biol. Chem.* 254: 10421–10425, 1979.

339. LIU, C. Y., C. F. SCOTT, A. BAGDASARIAN, J. V. PIERCE, A. P. KAPLAN, AND R. W. COLMAN. Potentiation of the function of Hageman factor fragments by high molecular weight kininogen. *J. Clin. Invest.* 60: 7–17, 1977.

340. LOCKHART, M. S., P. C. COMP, AND F. B. TAYLOR, JR. Role of platelets in lysis of dilute plasma clots: requirement for metabolically active platelets. *J. Lab. Clin. Med.* 94: 285–294, 1979.

341. LOEWY, A. G., K. DUNATHAN, R. KRIEL, AND H. L. WOLFINGER, JR. Fibrinase. I. Purification of substrate and enzyme. *J. Biol. Chem.* 236: 2625–2633, 1961.

342. LOEWY, A. G., J. A. GALLANT, AND K. DUNATHAN. Fibrinase. IV. Effect on fibrin solubility. *J. Biol. Chem.* 236: 2648–2655, 1961.

343. LORAND, L., AND K. KONISHI. Activation of the fibrin-stabilizing factor of plasma by thrombin. *Arch. Biochem.* 105: 58–67, 1964.

344. LOSKUTOFF, D. J. Effect of thrombin on the fibrinolytic activity of cultured bovine endothelial cells. *J. Clin. Invest.* 61: 329–332, 1979.

345. LOSKUTOFF, D. J., AND T. S. EDGINGTON. Synthesis of a fibrinolytic activator and inhibitor by endothelial cells. *Proc. Natl. Acad. Sci. USA* 74: 3903–3907, 1977.

346. LOSKUTOFF, D. J., AND T. S. EDGINGTON. An inhibitor of plasminogen activator in rabbit endothelial cells. *J. Biol. Chem.* 256: 4142–4145, 1981.

347. LOTTSPEICH, F., AND A. HENSCHEN. Completion of amino acid sequences in fibrinogen (Abstract). *Thromb. Haemost.* 42: 13, 1979.

348. LUND, P. K., F. BROSSTAD, AND P. KIERULF. Detection of soluble fibrin in plasma using fibrinogen Sepharose columns. *Thromb. Res.* 11: 907–912, 1977.

350. MAGNUSSON, S., T. E. PETERSEN, L. SOTTRUP-JENSEN, AND H. CLAEYS. Complete primary structure of prothrombin: isolation, structure and reactivity of ten carboxylated glutamic acid residues and regulation of prothrombin activation by thrombin. In: *Proteases and Biological Control*, edited by E. Reich, D. B. Rifkin, and E. Shaw. New York: Cold Spring Harbor, 1975, p. 123–149. (Cold Spring Harbor Conf. Cell Proliferation.)

351. MAGNUSSON, S., L. SOTTRUP-JENSEN, T. E. PETERSEN, G. DUDEK-WOJCIECHOWSKA, AND H. CLAEYS. Homologous "krinkle" structures common to plasminogen and prothrombin. Substrate specificity of enzymes activating prothrombin and plasminogen. In: *Proteolysis and Physiological Regulation*, edited by D. W. Ribbons and K. Brew. New York: Academic, 1976, vol. 11, p. 203–238.

352. MAGNUSSON, S., L. SOTTRUP-JENSEN, T. E. PETERSEN, H. R. MORRIS, AND A. DELL. Primary structure of the vitamin K-dependent part of prothrombin. *FEBS Lett.* 44: 189–193, 1974.

353. MAMMEN, E. F., A. S. PRASAD, M. I. BARNHART, AND C. C. AU. Congenital dysfibrinogenemia: fibrinogen Detroit. *J. Clin. Invest.* 48: 235–249, 1969.

354. MANDLE, R. J., JR., R. W. COLMAN, AND A. P. KAPLAN. Identification of prekallikrein and high molecular weight kininogen as a complex in human plasma. *Proc. Natl. Acad. Sci. USA* 73: 4179–4183, 1976.

355. MANDLE, R. J., JR., AND A. P. KAPLAN. Hageman factor substrates. Human plasma prekallikrein: mechanism of activation by Hageman factor and participation in Hageman factor-dependent fibrinolysis. *J. Biol. Chem.* 252: 6097–7001, 1977.

356. MANDLE, R. J., JR., AND A. P. KAPLAN. Hageman-factor-

dependent fibrinolysis: generation of fibrinolytic activity by the interaction of human activated factor XI and plasminogen. *Blood* 54: 850–862, 1979.

357. MANN, K. G., AND C. W. BATT. The molecular weights of bovine thrombin and its primary autolysis products. *J. Biol. Chem.* 244: 6555–6557, 1969.

358. MARCINIAK, E., C. H. FARLEY, AND P. A. DeSIMONE. Familial thrombosis due to antithrombin III deficiency. *Blood* 43: 219–231, 1974.

359. MARCINIAK, E., AND J. P. GOCKERMAN. Heparin-induced decrease in circulating antithrombin III. *Lancet* 2: 581–584, 1977.

360. MARDER, V. J. Immunologic structure of fibrinogen and its plasmin degradation products. Theoretical and clinical considerations. In: *Fibrinogen*, edited by K. Laki. New York: Dekker, 1968, p. 339–358.

361. MARDER, V. J. Identification and purification of fibrinogen degradation products produced by plasmin. Considerations on the structure of fibrinogen. *Scand. J. Haematol. Suppl.* 13: 21–36, 1971.

362. MARDER, V. J. The use of fibrinolytic agents: choice of patient, drug administration, laboratory monitoring. *Ann. Intern. Med.* 90: 802–808, 1979.

363. MARDER, V. J., AND A. Z. BUDZYNSKI. The structure of the fibrinogen degradation products. In: *Progress in Hemostasis and Thrombosis*, edited by T. H. Spaet. New York: Grune & Stratton, 1974, vol. 2, p. 141–174.

364. MARDER, V. J., A. Z. BUDZYNSKI, AND G. H. BARLOW. Comparison of the physicochemical properties of fragment D derivatives of fibrinogen and fragment D-D of cross-linked fibrin. *Biochim. Biophys. Acta* 427: 1–14, 1976.

365. MARDER, V. J., A. Z. BUDZYNSKI, AND H. L. JAMES. High molecular weight derivatives of human fibrinogen produced by plasmin. III. Their NH$_2$-terminal amino acids and comparison with the "NH$_2$-terminal disulfide knot." *J. Biol. Chem.* 247: 4775–4781, 1972.

366. MARDER, V. J., AND N. R. SHULMAN. High molecular weight derivatives of human fibrinogen produced by plasmin. II. Mechanism of their anticoagulant activity. *J. Biol. Chem.* 244: 2120–2124, 1969.

367. MARDER, V. J., N. R. SHULMAN, AND W. R. CARROLL. The importance of intermediate degradation products of fibrinogen in fibrinolytic hemorrhage. *Trans. Assoc. Am. Physicians* 53: 156–167, 1967.

368. MARDER, V. J., N. R. SHULMAN, AND W. R. CARROLL. High molecular weight derivatives of human fibrinogen produced by plasmin. I. Physicochemical and immunological characterization. *J. Biol. Chem.* 244: 2111–2119, 1969.

369. MARGOLIS, J. Glass surface and blood coagulation. *Nature London* 178: 805–806, 1956.

370. MARGOLIS, J. Plasma pain-producing substance and blood clotting. *Nature London.* 180: 1464–1465, 1957.

371. MARGOLIS, J. Activation of permeability factor in plasma by contact with glass. *Nature London* 180: 635–636, 1958.

372. MARGOLIS, J. Activation of plasma by contact with glass. Evidence for a common reaction which releases plasma kinin and initiates coagulation. *J. Physiol. London* 144: 1–22, 1958.

373. MARGOLIS, J. Activation of Hageman factor by saturated fatty acids. *Aust. J. Exp. Biol. Med. Sci.* 40: 505–513, 1962.

374. MARGOLIS, J. The interrelationship of coagulation of plasma and release of peptides. *Ann. NY Acad. Sci.* 104: 133–145, 1963.

375. MARGUERIE, G., G. CHAGNIEL, AND M. SUSCILLON. The binding of calcium to bovine fibrinogen. *Biochim. Biophys. Acta* 490: 94–103, 1977.

376. MARGUERIE, G. A., E. F. PLOW, AND T. S. EDGINGTON. Human platelets possess an inducible and saturable receptor specific for fibrinogen. *J. Biol. Chem.* 254: 5357–5363, 1979.

377. MARGUERIE, G., AND H. B. STUHRMANN. A neutron small-angle scattering study of bovine fibrinogen. *J. Mol. Biol.* 102: 143–156, 1976.

378. MARKLAND, F. S., AND P. S. DAMUS. Purification and properties of a thrombin-like enzyme from the venom of *Crotalus adamanteus* (Eastern diamondback rattlesnake). *J. Biol. Chem.* 246: 6460–6473, 1971.

379. MARKUS, G., J. L. DePASQUALE, AND F. C. WISSLER. Quantitative determination of the binding of epsilon-aminocaproic acid to native plasminogen. *J. Biol. Chem.* 253: 727–732, 1978.

380. MARKWARDT, F. Hirudin as an inhibitor of thrombin. *Methods Enzymol.* 19: 924–932, 1970.

381. MARKWARDT, F., AND P. WALSMANN. Die Reaktion zwischen Hirudin and Thrombin. *Z. Physiol. Chem.* 312: 85–98, 1958.

382. MARTIN, B. M., AND J. P. QUIGLEY. Binding and uptake of thrombin: possible role in the thrombin-induced mitogenesis of chick embryo fibroblasts. In: *The Chemistry and Biology of Thrombin*, edited by R. L. Lundblad, J. W. Fenton II, and K. G. Mann. Ann Arbor, MI: Ann Arbor Science, 1977, p. 531–544.

383. MARTINEZ, J., J. E. PALASCAK, AND D. KWASNIAK. Abnormal sialic acid content of the dysfibrinogenemia associated with liver disease. *J. Clin. Invest.* 61: 535–538, 1978.

384. MATHESON, N. R., AND J. TRAVIS. Inactivation of human thrombin in the presence of human α_1-proteinase inhibitor. *Biochem. J.* 159: 495–502, 1976.

385. MATHESON, R. T., D. R. MILLER, M. J. LACOMBE, Y. HAN, S. IWANGA, H. KATO, AND K. WUEPPER. Flaujeac factor deficiency reconstruction with highly purified bovine high molecular weight kininogen and delineation of a new permeability enhancing peptide released by plasma kallikrein from bovine high molecular weight kininogen. *J. Clin. Invest.* 58: 1395–1406, 1976.

386. MATSUO, T., Y. OHKI, S. KONDO, AND O. MATUSO. Familial antithrombin III deficiency in a Japanese family. *Thromb. Res.* 16: 815–823, 1979.

387. MATTHEWS, B. W., P. G. SIGLER, R. HENDERSON, AND D. M. BLOW. Three-dimensional structure of tosyl-α-chymotrypsin. *Nature London* 214: 652–654, 1967.

388. MATTHIAS, F. R., AND D. L. HEENE. Comparative adsorption studies between fibrinogen and its degradation products and fibrinmonomer produced by reptilase and thrombin. *Thromb. Res.* 3: 745–749, 1973.

389. MATTHIAS, F. R., D. L. HEENE, AND E. KONRADI. Behavior of fibrinogen and fibrinogen degradation products (FDP) towards insolubilized fibrinogen and fibrinmonomer. *Thromb. Res.* 3: 657–664, 1973.

390. MATTHIAS, F. R., D. L. HEENE, AND Z. WEGRZYNOWICZ. Reduction of insolubilized fibrinogen. *Thromb. Res.* 4: 803–808, 1974.

391. MATTOCK, P., AND M. P. ESNOUF. Differences in the subunit structure of human fibrin formed by the action of arvin, reptilase and thrombin. *Nature London New Biol.* 233: 277–279, 1971.

392. McCLINTOCK, D. K., AND P. H. BELL. The mechanism of activation of human plasminogen by streptokinase. *Biochem. Biophys. Res. Commun.* 43: 694–702, 1971.

393. McCLINTOCK, D. K., M. E. ENGLERT, C. DZIOBKOWSKI, E. H. SNEDEKER, AND P. H. BELL. Two distinct pathways of the streptokinase-mediated activation of highly purified human plasminogen. *Biochemistry* 13: 5334–5344, 1974.

394. McCONNELL, D. J. Inhibitors of kallikrein in human plasma. *J. Clin. Invest.* 51: 1611–1623, 1972.

395. McDONAGH, J., T. H. KIESSELBACH, AND R. H. WAGNER. Factor XIII and antiplasmin activity in human platelets. *Am. J. Physiol.* 216: 508–513, 1969.

396. McDONAGH, J., H. MESSEL, R. P. McDONAGH, JR., G. MURANO, AND B. BLOMBÄCK. Molecular weight analysis of fibrinogen and fibrin chains by an improved sodium dodecyl sulfate gel electrophoresis method. *Biochim. Biophys. Acta* 257: 135–142, 1972.

397. McDONAGH, R. P., JR., J. McDONAGH, M. BLOMBÄCK, AND B. BLOMBÄCK. Crosslinking of human fibrin: evidence for intermolecular crosslinking involving α-chains. *FEBS Lett.* 14: 33–36, 1971.

398. McKee, P. A., J. C. Andersen, and M. E. Switzer. Molecular structural studies of human factor VIII. *Ann. NY Acad. Sci.* 240: 8–33, 1975.
399. McKee, P. A., P. Mattock, and R. L. Hill. Subunit structure of human fibrinogen, soluble fibrin, and cross-linked insoluble fibrin. *Proc. Natl. Acad. Sci. USA* 66: 738–744, 1970.
400. McMillan, C. R., H. Saito, O. D. Ratnoff, and A. G. Waltan. The secondary structure of human Hageman factor (factor XII) and its alteration by activating agents. *J. Clin. Invest.* 54: 1326–1335, 1974.
401. Meier, H. L., J. V. Pierce, R. W. Colman, and A. P. Kaplan. Activation and function of human Hageman factor. The role of high molecular weight kininogen and prekallikrein. *J. Clin. Invest.* 60: 18–31, 1977.
402. Meier, H. L., C. F. Scott, R. Mandel, Jr., M. E. Webster, J. V. Pierce, R. W. Colman, and A. P. Kaplan. Requirements for contact activation of human Hageman factor. *Ann. NY Acad. Sci.* 283: 93–103, 1977.
403. Metcalf, D. D., R. A. Lewis, J. F. Silbert, R. D. Rosenberg, S. I. Wasserman, and K. R. Austen. Isolation and characterization of heparin from the human lung. *J. Clin. Invest.* 64: 1537–1543, 1979.
404. Mihalyi, E. Physicochemical studies of bovine fibrinogen. III. Optical rotation of the native and denatured molecule. *Biochim. Biophys. Acta* 102: 487–499, 1965.
405. Mihalyi, E., and J. E. Godfrey. Digestion of fibrinogen by trypsin. II. Characterization of the large fragment obtained. *Biochim. Biophys. Acta* 67: 90–103, 1963.
406. Mihalyi, E., and J. E. Godfrey. Kinetic studies of the digestion of fibrinogen by α-chymotrypsin. *Biochim. Biophys. Acta* 132: 94–103, 1967.
407. Mihalyi, E., R. M. Weinberg, D. W. Towne, and M. E. Friedman. Proteolytic fragmentation of fibrinogen. I. Comparison of the fragmentation of human and bovine fibrinogen by trypsin or plasmin. *Biochemistry* 15: 5372–5381, 1976.
408. Miletich, J. P., C. M. Jackson, and P. W. Majerus. Interaction of coagulation factor Xa with human platelets. *Proc. Natl. Acad. Sci. USA* 74: 4033–4036, 1977.
409. Miletich, J. P., C. M. Jackson, and P. W. Majerus. Properties of the factor X binding site on human platelets. *J. Biol. Chem.* 253: 6908–6916, 1978.
410. Miller, K. D., and H. Van Vunakis. The effects of diisopropylfluorophosphate on the proteinase and esterase activities of thrombin and on prothrombin and its activators. *J. Biol. Chem.* 223: 227–237, 1956.
411. Mills, D. A. Molecular model for the proteolysis of human fibrinogen by plasmin. *Biochim. Biophys. Acta* 263: 619–630, 1972.
412. Mills, D. A., and S. Karpatkin. Heterogeneity of human fibrinogen: possible relation to proteolysis by thrombin and plasmin as studied by SDS-polyacrylamide gel electrophoresis. *Biochem. Biophys. Res. Commun.* 40: 206–211, 1970.
413. Mills, D. A., and S. Karpatkin. The initial macromolecular derivatives of human fibrinogen produced by plasmin. *Biochim. Biophys. Acta* 271: 163–173, 1972.
414. Mills, D. A., and I. E. Liener. Partial chemical characterization of the isolated γ-chain of human fibrinogen. *Arch. Biochem. Biophys.* 130: 629–635, 1969.
415. Mirsky, I. A., G. Perisutti, and N. C. Davis. Destruction of glucagon, adrenocorticotropin and somatotropin by human blood plasma. *J. Clin. Invest.* 38: 14–20, 1959.
416. Monkhouse, F. C., E. S. France, and W. H. Seegers. Studies on the antithrombin and heparin cofactor activities of a fraction adsorbed from plasma by aluminum hydroxide. *Circ. Res.* 3: 337–341, 1955.
417. Moran, J. B., and C. R. Geren. Characterization of a fibrinogenase from northern copperhead (*Agkistrodon contortrix mokasen*) venom. *Biochim. Biophys. Acta* 659: 161–168, 1981.
418. Morawitz, P. *The Chemistry of Blood Coagulation*. Springfield, IL: Thomas, 1968.
419. Morita, T., H. Kato, S. Iwanaga, K. Takada, T. Kimura, and S. Sakakibara. New fluorogenic substrates for α-thrombin, factor Xa, kallikreins and urokinase. *J. Biochem. Tokyo* 82: 1495–1498, 1977.
420. Moroi, M., and N. Aoki. Isolation and characterization of alpha2-plasmin inhibitor from human plasma. A novel proteinase inhibitor which inhibits activator-induced clot lysis. *J. Biol. Chem.* 251: 5956–5965, 1976.
421. Morrison, P. R., J. T. Edsall, and S. G. Miller. Cold-insoluble globulin. *J. Am. Chem. Soc.* 70: 3103–3108, 1948.
422. Mosesson, M. W., N. Alkjaersig, B. Sweet, and S. Sherry. Human fibrinogen of relatively high solubility. Comparative biophysical, biochemical and biological studies with fibrinogen of lower solubility. *Biochemistry* 6: 3279–3287, 1967.
423. Mosesson, M. W., A. B. Chen, and R. M. Huseby. The cold-insoluble globulin of human plasma: studies of its essential structural features. *Biochim. Biophys. Acta* 386: 509–524, 1975.
424. Mosesson, M. W., R. W. Colman, and S. Sherry. Chronic intravascular coagulation syndrome. *N. Engl. J. Med.* 278: 815–821, 1968.
425. Mosesson, M. W., J. Escaig, and G. Feldmann. Electron microscopy of metal-shadowed fibrinogen molecules deposited at different concentrations. *Br. J. Haematol.* 43: 469–477, 1979.
426. Mosesson, M. W., J. S. Finlayson, and R. A. Umfleet. Human fibrinogen heterogeneities. III. Identification of γ-chain variants. *J. Biol. Chem.* 247: 5223–5227, 1972.
427. Mosesson, M. W., D. K. Galanakis, and J. S. Finlayson. Comparison of human plasma fibrinogen subfractions and early plasmic fibrinogen derivatives. *J. Biol. Chem.* 249: 4656–4664, 1974.
428. Mosher, D. F. Cross-linking of cold-insoluble globulin by fibrin-stabilizing factor. *J. Biol. Chem.* 250: 6614–6621, 1975.
429. Mosher, D. F. Action of fibrin-stabilizing factor on cold-insoluble globulin and α_2-macroglobulin in clotting plasma. *J. Biol. Chem.* 251: 1639–1645, 1976.
430. Mosher, D. F., P. E. Schad, and J. M. Vann. Cross-linking of collagen and fibronectin by factor XIIIa. Localization of participating glutaminyl residues to a tryptic fragment of fibronectin. *J. Biol. Chem.* 255: 1181–1188, 1980.
431. Movat, H. Z., and A. H. Ozge-Anwar. The contact phase of blood coagulation: clotting factors XI and XII, their isolation and interaction. *J. Lab. Clin. Med.* 84: 861–867, 1974.
432. Mui, P. T. K., H. L. James, and P. Ganguly. Isolation and properties of a low molecular weight antiplasmin of human blood platelets and serum. *Br. J. Haematol.* 29: 627–637, 1975.
433. Muller-Berghaus, G., I. Mahn, and W. Krell. Formation and dissociation of soluble fibrin complexes in plasma at 20°C and at 37°C. *Thromb. Res.* 14: 561–572, 1979.
434. Müllertz, S., and I. Clemmensen. The primary inhibitor of plasmin in human plasma. *Biochem. J.* 159: 545–553, 1976.
435. Mustard, J. F., M. A. Packham, R. L. Kinlough-Rathbone, D. W. Perry, and E. Regoeczi. Fibrinogen and ADP induced platelet aggregation. *Blood* 52: 452–466, 1978.
436. Mustard, J. F., D. W. Perry, N. G. Ardlie, and M. A. Packham. Preparations of suspensions of washed platelets from humans. *Br. J. Haematol.* 22: 193–204, 1972.
437. Musumeci, V., D. Culasso, and P. Boni. A rapid chromatographic method for quantitation of high molecular weight fibrinogen derivatives in plasma. *Thromb. Haemost.* 39: 555–563, 1978.
438. Mutt, V., S. Magnusson, J. E. Jorpes, and E. Dahl. Structure of porcine secretin. I. Degradation with trypsin and thrombin. Sequence of the tryptic peptides. The C-terminal residue. *Biochemistry* 4: 2358–2362, 1965.
439. Natelson, E. A., E. C. Lynch, R. A. Hettig, and C. P. Alfrey. Acquired factor IX deficiency in the nephrotic syndrome. *Ann. Intern. Med.* 73: 373–379, 1970.
440. Nelsestuen, G. L., and M. Broderius. Interaction of prothrombin and blood-clotting factor X with membranes of varying composition. *Biochemistry* 16: 4172–4177, 1977.
441. Nelsestuen, G. L., M. Broderius, and G. Martin. Role of

γ-carboxyglutamic acid. An unusual protein transition required for the calcium-dependent binding of prothrombin to phospholipid. *J. Biol. Chem.* 251: 5648–5656, 1976.
442. NELSESTUEN, G. L., AND T. K. LIM. Equilibria involved in prothrombin- and blood-clotting factor X-membrane binding. *Biochemistry* 16: 4164–4171, 1977.
443. NELSESTUEN, G. L., T. H. ZYTKOVICZ, AND J. B. HOWARD. The mode of action of vitamin K. Identification of γ-carboxyglutamic acid as a component of prothrombin. *J. Biol. Chem.* 249: 6347–6350, 1974.
444. NEMERSON, Y. Characteristics and lipid requirements of coagulant proteins extracted from brain and lung: the specificity of the protein component of tissue factor. *J. Clin. Invest.* 48: 322–331, 1969.
445. NEMERSON, Y., AND F. A. PITLICK. Purification and characterization of the protein component of tissue factor. *Biochemistry* 9: 5100–5105, 1970.
446. NESHEIM, M. E., AND K. G. MANN. Thrombin-catalyzed activation of single chain bovine factor V. *J. Biol. Chem.* 254: 1326–1334, 1979.
448. NESHEIM, M. E., K. H. MYMEL, L. HIBBARD, AND K. G. MANN. Isolation and characterization of single chain bovine factor V. *J. Biol. Chem.* 254: 508–517, 1979.
449. NESHEIM, M. E., J. B. TASWELL, AND K. G. MANN. The contribution of bovine factor V and factor Va to the activity of prothrombinase. *J. Biol. Chem.* 254: 10952–10962, 1979.
450. NEUFELD, E. F., T. W. LIM, AND L. J. SHAPIRO. Inherited disorders of lysosomal metabolism. *Annu. Rev. Biochem.* 44: 357–376, 1975.
451. NIEWIAROWSKI, S., A. Z. BUDZYNSKI, AND B. LIPINSKI. Significance of the intact polypeptide chains of human fibrinogen in ADP-induced platelet aggregation. *Blood* 49: 635–644, 1977.
452. NIEWIAROWSKI, S., A. Z. BUDZYNSKI, T. A. MORINELLI, T. M. BRUDZYNSKI, AND G. J. STEWART. Exposure of fibrinogen receptor on human platelets by proteolytic enzymes. *J. Biol. Chem.* 256: 917–925, 1981.
453. NIEWIAROWSKI, S., A. Z. BUDZYNSKI, T. A. MORINELLI, AND M. JOHNSON. Deficient platelet-fibrinogen interaction in Glanzmann's thrombasthenia (Abstract). *Blood* 52, Suppl. 1: 285, 1978.
454. NIEWIAROWSKI, S., AND S. GOLDSTEIN. Interaction of cultured human fibroblasts with fibrin: modification by drugs and aging in vitro. *J. Lab. Clin. Med.* 82: 605–610, 1973.
455. NIEWIAROWSKI, S., AND E. KOWALSKI. Un novel anticoagulant dérivé du fibrinogène. *Rev. Hèmatol.* 13: 320–328, 1958.
456. NIEWIAROWSKI, S., E. REGOECZI, AND J. F. MUSTARD. Platelet interaction with fibrinogen and fibrin: comparison of the interaction of platelets with that of fibroblasts, leukocytes and erythrocytes. *Ann. NY Acad. Sci.* 201: 72–83, 1972.
457. NILSSON, I. M. Report of the working party on factor VIII-related antigens. *Thromb. Haemost.* 39: 511–520, 1978.
458. NILSSON, I. M., H. KROOK, N. H. STERNBY, E. SODERBERG, AND N. SODERSTROM. Severe thrombotic disease in a young man with bone marrow and skeletal changes and with a high content of an inhibitor of the fibrinolytic system. *Acta Med. Scand.* 169: 323–337, 1961.
459. NISHIBE, H., AND N. TAKAHASHI. The release of carbohydrate moieties from human fibrinogen by almond glycopeptidase without alteration in fibrinogen clottability. *Biochim. Biophys. Acta* 661: 274–279, 1981.
460. NORDENMAN, B., AND I. BJÖRK. Studies on the binding of heparin to prothrombin and thrombin and the effect of heparin-binding on thrombin activity. *Thromb. Res.* 12: 755–765, 1978.
461. NOSSEL, H. L. *The Contact Phase of Blood Coagulation.* Oxford, UK: Blackwell, 1964.
462. NOSSEL, H. L. Activation of factors XII (Hageman) and XI (PTA) by skin contact. *Proc. Soc. Exp. Biol. Med.* 122: 16–17, 1966.
463. NOSSEL, H. L. Relative proteolysis of the fibrinogen Bβ chain by thrombin and plasmin as a determinant of thrombosis. *Nature London* 291: 165–167, 1981.

464. NUSSENZWEIG, V., M. SELIGMANN, AND P. GRABAR. Les produits de dégradation du fibrinogène humain par la plasmine. II. Étude immunologique: mise en évidence d'anticorps anti-fibrinogène natif possédant des spécificités différentes. *Ann. Inst. Pasteur Paris* 100: 490–508, 1961.
465. NUSSENZWEIG, V., M. SELIGMANN, J. PELMONT, AND P. GRABAR. Le produits de dégradation du fibrinogène humain par la plasmine. I. Séparation et propriétés physico-chimiques. *Ann. Inst. Pasteur. Paris* 100: 377–389, 1961.
466. NYMAN, D. Interaction of collagen with the factor VIII antigen-activity-von Willebrand factor complex. *Thromb. Res.* 11: 433–438, 1977.
467. OFOSU, F., A. GILES, J. HIRSH, AND M. BLAJCHAM. Requirement of factor VIII for the generation of Xa in a purified system and in plasma. *Thromb. Haemost.* 42: 167–171, 1979.
468. OGREN, S., AND U. LINDAHL. Cleavage of macromolecular heparin by an enzyme from mouse mastocytoma. *J. Biol. Chem.* 250: 2690–2697, 1975.
469. OGSTON, D., B. BENNETT, R. J. HERBERT, AND A. S. DOUGLAS. The inhibition of urokinase by α_2-macroglobulin. *Clin. Sci.* 44: 73–79, 1973.
470. OLEXA, S. A., AND A. Z. BUDZYNSKI. Binding phenomena of isolated unique plasmic degradation products of human crosslinked fibrin. *J. Biol. Chem.* 254: 4925–4932, 1979.
471. OLEXA, S. A., AND A. Z. BUDZYNSKI. Primary soluble plasmic degradation product of human cross linked fibrin. Isolation and stoichiometry of the (DD)E complex. *Biochemistry* 18: 991–995, 1979.
472. OLEXA, S. A., AND A. Z. BUDZYNSKI. The effects of fibrinopeptide cleavage on the plasmic degradation pathways of human crosslinked fibrin. *Biochemistry* 19: 647–651, 1980.
473. OLEXA, S. A., AND A. Z. BUDZYNSKI. Evidence for four different polymerization sites involved in human fibrin formation. *Proc. Natl. Acad. Sci. USA* 77: 1374–1378, 1980.
474. OLEXA, S. A., AND A. Z. BUDZYNSKI. Localization of a fibrin polymerization site. *J. Biol. Chem.* 256: 3544–3549, 1981.
475. ORSTAVIK, K. H., AND K. LAAKE. Factor IX in warfarin treated patients. *Thromb. Res.* 13: 207–218, 1978.
476. OSHIMA, G., T. SATO-OHMORI, AND T. SUZUKI. Proteinase, arginineester hydrolase and kinin releasing enzyme in snake venoms. *Toxicon* 7: 229–233, 1969.
477. OSMOND, D. H., K. LOE, A. Y. LOH, E. A. ZINGGI, AND A. H. HEDLIN. Kallikrein and plasmin as activators of inactive renin. *Lancet* 2: 1375–1376, 1978.
478. ØSTERUD, B., B. N. BOUMA, AND J. H. GRIFFIN. Human blood coagulation factor IX. Purification, properties, and mechanism of activation by activated factor XI. *J. Biol. Chem.* 253: 5946–5954, 1978.
479. ØSTERUD, B., AND S. I. RAPAPORT. Synthesis of intrinsic factor X activator. Inhibition of the function of formed activator by antibodies to factor VIII and to factor IX. *Biochemistry* 9: 1854–1861, 1970.
480. ØSTERUD, B., AND S. I. RAPAPORT. Activation of factor IX by the reaction product of tissue factor and factor VII: additional pathway for initiating blood coagulation. *Proc. Natl. Acad. Sci. USA* 74: 5260–5263, 1977.
481. ØSTERUD, B., S. I. RAPAPORT, S. SCHIFFMAN, AND M. M. Y. CHONG. Formation of intrinsic factor-X-activator activity, with special reference to the role of thrombin. *Br. J. Haematol.* 21: 643–660, 1971.
482. OTTO, J. C. An account of an haemorrhagic disposition existing in certain families. *Med. Repository* 6: 1–4, 1803.
483. OUYANG, C., AND T. F. HUANG. Purification and characterization of the fibrinolytic principle of *Agkistrodon acutus* venom. *Biochim. Biophys. Acta* 439: 146–153, 1976.
484. OUYANG, C., AND T. F. HUANG. The properties of the purified fibrinolytic principle from *Agkistrodon acutus* snake venom. *Toxicon* 15: 161–167, 1977.
485. OUYANG, C., AND T. F. HUANG. α- and β-Fibrinogenases from *Trimeresurus gramineus* snake venom. *Biochim. Biophys. Acta* 571: 270–283, 1979.
486. OUYANG, C., AND C. TENG. Fibrinogenolytic enzymes of *Tri-*

meresurus mucrosquamatus venom. *Biochim. Biophys. Acta* 420: 298–308, 1976.

487. OUYANG, C., C. TENG, AND Y. CHEN. Physicochemical properties of α- and β-fibrinogenases of *Trimeresurus mucrosquamatus* venom. *Biochim. Biophys. Acta* 481: 622–630, 1977.

488. OWEN, C. A., JR., E. J. W. BOWIE, AND D. N. FASS. Generation of factor VIII coagulant activity by isolated, perfused neonatal pig livers and rat livers. *Br. J. Haematol.* 43: 307–315, 1979.

489. OWEN, W. G. Evidence for the formation of an ester between thrombin and heparin cofactor. *Biochim. Biophys. Acta* 405: 380–387, 1975.

490. OWEN, W. G., C. T. ESMON, AND C. M. JACKSON. The conversion of prothrombin to thrombin. I. Characterization of the reaction products formed during the activation of bovine prothrombin. *J. Biol. Chem.* 249: 594–605, 1974.

491. PALASCAK, J. E., AND J. MARTINEZ. Dysfibrinogenemia associated with liver disease. *J. Clin. Invest.* 60: 89–95, 1977.

492. PANDOLFI, M., S. ISACSON, AND I. M. NILSSON. Low fibrinolytic activity in the walls of veins of patients with thrombosis. *Acta Med. Scand.* 186: 1–5, 1969.

493. PANDOLFI, M., I. M. NILSSON, B. ROBERTSON, AND S. ISACSON. Fibrinolytic activity of human veins. *Lancet* 2: 127–128, 1967.

494. PANDYA, B. V., A. Z. BUDZYNSKI, R. N. RUBIN, AND S. A. OLEXA. Anticoagulant proteases from western diamondback rattlesnake venom (Abstract). *Federation Proc.* 40: 1790, 1981.

495. PAOLETTI, R., AND S. SHERRY (editors). *Thrombosis and Urokinase.* London: Academic, 1977.

496. PAPAHADJOPOULOS, D. P., AND D. J. HANAHAN. Observations on the interaction of phospholipids and certain clotting factors in prothrombin activator formation. *Biochim. Biophys. Acta* 90: 436–439, 1964.

497. PAPAHADJOPOULOS, D. P., C. HOUGIE, AND D. J. HANAHAN. Influence of surface charge of phospholipids on their clot-promoting activity. *Proc. Soc. Exp. Biol. Med.* 111: 412–416, 1962.

498. PARKER, K. R., AND M. J. MANT. Effects of tsetse (*Glossina morsitans morsitans* Westw.) (*Diptera: Glossinidae*) salivary gland homogenate on coagulation and fibrinolysis. *Thromb. Haemost.* 42: 743–751, 1979.

499. PASQUINI, R., AND E. J. HERSHGOLD. Effects of plasmin on human factor VIII(AHF). *Blood* 41: 105–111, 1973.

500. PATEK, A. J., AND F. H. L. TAYLOR. Hemophilia II. Some properties of a substance obtained from normal plasma effective in accelerating the clotting of hemophilic blood. *J. Clin. Invest.* 16: 113–124, 1937.

501. PAVLOVSKY, A. Contribution to the pathogenesis of hemophilia. *Blood* 2: 185–189, 1947.

502. PEABODY, R. A., M. J. TSAPOGAS, AND K. T. WU. Altered endogenous fibrinolysis and biochemical factors in atherosclerosis. *Arch. Surg. Chicago* 109: 309–313, 1974.

503. PEAKE, I. R., AND A. L. BLOOM. The dissociation of factor VIII by reducing agents, high salt concentration and affinity chromatography. *Thromb. Haemost.* 35: 191–201, 1976.

504. PEAKE, I. R., A. L. BLOOM, J. C. GIDDINGS, AND C. A. LUDLAM. An immunoradiometric assay for procoagulant factor VIII antigen: results in haemophilia, von Willebrand's disease and fetal plasma and serum. *Br. J. Haematol.* 42: 269–281, 1979.

505. PEERSCHKE, E. I., R. A. GRANT, AND M. B. ZUCKER. Relationship between aggregation and binding of ^{125}I-fibrinogen and 45-calcium to human platelets (Abstract). *Thromb. Haemost.* 42: 358, 1979.

506. PEERSCHKE, E. I., M. B. ZUCKER, R. GRANT, J. J. EGAN, AND M. M. JOHNSON. Correlation between fibrinogen binding to human platelets and platelet aggregability. *Blood* 55: 841–847, 1980.

507. PERLIN, A. S., D. M. MACKIE, AND C. P. DIETRICH. Evidence for a (1→4)-linked 4-O-(α-L-idopyranosyluronic acid 2-sulfate)-(2-deoxy-2-sulfamino-D-glucopyranosyl-6-sulfate) sequence in heparin. *Carbohydr. Res.* 18: 185–194, 1971.

508. PETERSON, C., R. KELLY, B. MINARD, AND L. P. CAWLEY. Antithrombin III. Comparison of functional and immunologic assays. *Am. J. Clin. Pathol.* 69: 500–504, 1978.

509. PFLEIDERER, G., AND G. SUMYK. Investigation of snake venom proteinases by cellulose ion-exchange chromatography. *Biochim. Biophys. Acta* 51: 482–493, 1961.

510. PHILLIPS, H. M., AND J. L. YORK. Bovine fibrinogen. I. Effects of amidination on fibrin-monomer aggregation. *Biochemistry* 12: 3637–3642, 1973.

511. PHILLIPS, H. M., AND J. L. YORK. Bovine fibrinogen. II. Effects of tyrosine modification on fibrin monomer aggregation. *Biochemistry* 12: 3642–3647, 1973.

512. PIERCE, J. V., AND J. A. GUIMARAES. Further characterization of highly purified human plasma kininogens. In: *Chemistry and Biology of the Kallikrein-Kinin System in Health and Disease*, edited by J. J. Pisano and K. F. Austen. Washington, DC: US Govt. Printing Office, 1974, p. 121–128. (Fogarty Int. Ctr. Proc. 27.)

513. PILGERAM, L. O. Abnormalities in clotting and thrombolysis as a risk factor for stroke. *Thromb. Diath. Haemorrh.* 31: 245–264, 1974.

514. PILLEMER, L., O. D. RATNOFF, L. BLUM, AND I. H. LEPOW. The inactivation of complement and its components by plasmin. *J. Exp. Med.* 97: 573–589, 1953.

515. PISANO, J. J., J. S. FINLAYSON, AND M. P. PEYTON. Cross-link in fibrin polymerized by factor XIII: ε-(γ-glutamyl)lysine. *Science* 160: 892–893, 1968.

516. PISANO, J. J., J. S. FINLAYSON, AND M. P. PEYTON. Chemical and enzymic detection of protein cross-links. Measurement of ε-(γ-glutamyl)lysine in fibrin polymerized by factor XIII. *Biochemistry* 8: 871–876, 1969.

517. PITLICK, F. A., AND Y. NEMERSON. Binding of the protein component of tissue factor to phospholipids. *Biochemistry* 9: 5105–5112, 1970.

518. PIZZO, S. V., M. L. SCHWARTZ, R. L. HILL, AND P. A. MCKEE. The effect of plasmin on the subunit structure of human fibrinogen. *J. Biol. Chem.* 247: 636–645, 1972.

519. PIZZO, S. V., M. L. SCHWARTZ, R. L. HILL, AND P. A. MCKEE. Mechanism of ancrod anticoagulation. A direct proteolytic effect on fibrin. *J. Clin. Invest.* 51: 2841–2850, 1972.

520. PIZZO, S. V., M. L. SCHWARTZ, R. L. HILL, AND P. A. MCKEE. The effect of plasmin on the subunit structure of human fibrin. *J. Biol. Chem.* 248: 4574–4583, 1973.

521. PIZZO, S. V., L. M. TAYLOR, JR., M. L. SCHWARTZ, R. L. HILL, AND P. A. MCKEE. Subunit structure of Fragment D from fibrinogen and cross-linked fibrin. *J. Biol. Chem.* 248: 4584–4590, 1973.

522. PLOW, E. F., C. BIRDWELL, AND M. H. GINSBERG. Identification and quantitation of platelet-associated fibronectin antigen. *J. Clin. Invest.* 63: 540–543, 1979.

523. PLOW, E. F., AND T. S. EDGINGTON. An alternative pathway for fibrinolysis. I. The cleavage of fibrinogen by leukocyte proteases at physiologic pH. *J. Clin. Invest.* 56: 30–38, 1975.

524. PLOW, E. F., AND G. A. MARGUERIE. Induction of the fibrinogen receptor on human platelets by epinephrine and the combination of epinephrine and ADP. *J. Biol. Chem.* 255: 10971–10977, 1980.

525. POLLEY, M. J., L. K. L. LEUNG, F. Y. CLARK, AND R. L. NACHMAN. Thrombin-induced platelet membrane glycoprotein IIb and IIIa complex formation. *J. Exp. Med.* 154: 1059–1068, 1981.

526. POUIT, L., G. MARCILLE, M. SUSCILLON, AND D. HOLLARD. Etude en microscopie électronique de différentes étapes de la fibrinoformation. *Thromb. Diath. Haemorrh.* 27: 559–572, 1972.

527. PROCTOR, R. R., AND S. I. RAPAPORT. The partial thromboplastin time with kaolin: a simple screening test for first stage plasma clotting deficiencies. *Am. J. Clin. Pathol.* 35: 212–219, 1961.

528. PURVES, L. R., G. G. LINDSEY, G. BROWN, AND J. FRANKS. Stabilization of the plasmin digestion products of fibrinogen and fibrin by calcium ions. *Thromb. Res.* 12: 473–484, 1978.

529. RABINER, S. F., I. D. GOLDFINE, A. HART, L. SUMMARIA, AND

K. C. Robbins. Radioimmunoassay of human plasminogen and plasmin. *J. Lab. Clin. Med.* 74: 265–273, 1969.
530. Radcliffe, R., A. Bagdasarian, R. Colman, and Y. Nemerson. Activation of bovine factor VII by Hageman factor fragments. *Blood* 50: 611–617, 1977.
531. Radcliffe, R., and Y. Nemerson. Activation and control of factor X and thrombin. Isolation and characterization of a single chain form of factor VII. *J. Biol. Chem.* 250: 388–395, 1974.
532. Radcliffe, R., and Y. Nemerson. Mechanism of action of bovine factor VII: products of cleavage by factor X. *J. Biol. Chem.* 251: 4797–4802, 1976.
533. Rakoczi, I., B. Wiman, and D. Collen. On the biological significance of the specific interaction between fibrin, plasminogen and antiplasmin. *Biochim. Biophys. Acta* 540: 295–300, 1978.
534. Rapaport, S. I., S. Schiffman, M. J. Patch, and B. S. Ames. The importance of activation of antihemophilic globulin and proaccelerin by traces of thrombin in the generation of intrinsic prothrombinase activity. *Blood* 21: 221–235, 1963.
535. Ratnoff, O. D. The biology and pathology of the initial coagulation. In: *Progress in Hematology*, edited by E. B. Brown and C. V. Moore. New York: Grune & Stratton, 1966, vol. V, p. 204–245.
536. Ratnoff, O. D. Activation of Hageman factor by L-homocysteine. *Science* 162: 1007–1009, 1968.
537. Ratnoff, O. D. The molecular basis of hereditary clotting disorders. In: *Progress in Hemostasis and Thrombosis*, edited by T. H. Spaet. New York: Grune & Stratton, 1972, vol. I, p. 39–74.
538. Ratnoff, O. D., and J. E. Colopy. A familial hemorrhagic trait associated with deficiency of clot-promoting fraction of plasma. *J. Clin. Invest.* 34: 601–613, 1955.
539. Ratnoff, O. D., E. W. Davie, and D. L. Mallett. Studies on the action of Hageman factor. Evidence that activated Hageman factor in turn activates plasma thromboplastin antecedant. *J. Clin. Invest.* 40: 803–819, 1961.
540. Ratnoff, O. D., and J. M. Rosenblum. Role of Hageman factor in the initiation of clotting by glass: evidence that glass frees Hageman factor from inhibition. *Am. J. Med.* 25: 160–168, 1958.
541. Ratnoff, O. D., and H. Saito. Amidolytic properties of single-chain activated Hageman factor. *Proc. Natl. Acad. Sci. USA* 76: 1461–1463, 1979.
542. Ratnoff, O. D., C. C. Slover, and M. C. Poon. Immunologic evidence that the properties of human antihemophilic factor (factor VIII) are attributes of a single molecular species. *Blood* 47: 657–667, 1976.
543. Rawala, R., S. Saraswathi, S. Niewiarowski, and R. W. Colman. Molecular changes during the activation of bovine factor V by snake venom proteases. *Circulation* 58: II-209, 1978.
544. Regañón, E., V. Vila, and J. Aznar. Identification of high-molecular weight derivatives of plasmic digests of cross-linked human fibrin. *Thromb. Haemost.* 40: 368–376, 1978.
545. Reich, E. Plasminogen activator: secretion by neoplastic cells and macrophages. In: *Proteases and Biological Control*, edited by E. Reich, D. B. Rifkin, and E. Shaw. New York: Cold Spring Harbor, 1975, vol. 2, p. 333–341. (Cold Spring Harbor Conf. Cell Proliferation.)
546. Reid, H. A., K. E. Chan, and P. C. Thean. Prolonged coagulation defect (defibrination syndrome) in Malayan viper bite. *Lancet* 1: 621–626, 1963.
547. Reisner, H. M., E. S. Barrow, and J. B. Graham. Radioimmunoassay for coagulant factor VIII-related antigen (VIII:CAg). *Thromb. Res.* 14: 235–239, 1979.
548. Revak, S. D., C. G. Cochrane, B. N. Bouma, and J. H. Griffin. Surface and fluid phase activities of two forms of activated Hageman factor produced during contact activation of plasma. *J. Exp. Med.* 147: 719–729, 1978.
549. Revak, S. D., C. G. Cochrane, and J. H. Griffin. The binding and cleavage characteristics of human Hageman factor during contact activation. A comparison of normal plasma with plasma deficient in factor XI, prekallikrein, or high molecular weight kininogen. *J. Clin. Invest.* 58: 1167–1173, 1977.
550. Revak, S. D., C. G. Cochrane, A. Johnston, and T. Higli. Structural changes accompanying enzymatic activation of Hageman factor. *J. Clin. Invest.* 54: 619–627, 1974.
551. Rick, M. E., and L. W. Hoyer. Immunologic studies of antihemophilic factor (AHF, factor VIII). V. Immunologic properties of AHF subunits produced by salt dissociation. *Blood* 42: 737–747, 1973.
552. Rick, M. E., and L. W. Hoyer. Activation of low molecular weight fragment of antihaemophilic factor (factor VIII) by thrombin. *Nature London* 252: 404–405, 1974.
553. Rickli, E. E., and W. I. Otavsky. A new method of isolation and some properties of the heavy chain of human plasmin. *Eur. J. Biochem.* 59: 441–447, 1975.
554. Risberg, B., H. I. Peterson, and L. Zettergren. Localization of plasminogen activator in the human lung. *Bibl. Anat.* 13: 279–280, 1975.
555. Robbins, K. C., P. Bernabe, L. Arzadon, and L. Summaria. NH_2-terminal sequences of mammalian plasminogens and plasmin S-carboxymethyl heavy (A) and light (B) chain derivatives. A reevaluation of the mechanism of activation of plasminogen. *J. Biol. Chem.* 248: 7242–7246, 1973.
556. Robbins, K. C., I. G. Boreisha, L. Arzadon, and L. Summaria. Physical and chemical properties of the NH_2-terminal glutamic acid and lysine forms of human plasminogen and their derived plasmins with an NH_2-terminal lysine heavy (A) chain. *J. Biol. Chem.* 250: 4044–4047, 1975.
557. Robbins, K. C., L. Summaria, B. Hsieh, and R. J. Shah. The peptide chains of human plasmin. Mechanism of activation of human plasminogen to plasmin. *J. Biol. Chem.* 242: 2333–2342, 1967.
558. Roberts, R. C., W. A. Riesen, and P. K. Hall. Studies on the quaternary structure of human serum α_2-macroglobulin. In: *Proteinase Inhibitors. Proc. Proteinase Conf., 2nd, Cologne, Germany, 1973*, edited by H. Fritz, H. Tschesche, L. J. Greene, and E. Truscheit. Berlin: Springer-Verlag, 1973, p. 63–71. (Bayer Symp. 5th.)
559. Roden, L., and M. I. Horowitz. Structure and biosynthesis of connective tissue proteoglycans. In: *The Glycoconjugates*, edited by M. D. Horowitz and W. Pigman. New York: Academic, 1977, vol. II, p. 3–15.
560. Rosenberg, R. D. Mechanism of antithrombin action and the structural basis of heparin's anticoagulant function. In: *The Chemistry and Physiology of the Human Plasma Proteins*, edited by D. H. Bing. New York: Pergamon, 1979, p. 353–368.
560a. Rosenberg, R. D. Hemorrhagic disorders. I. Protein interactions in the clotting mechanism. In: *Hematology*, edited by W. S. Beck. Cambridge, MA: MIT Press, 1981, chapt. 26, p. 373–400.
561. Rosenberg, R. D., G. Armand, and L. H. Lam. Structure-function relationships of heparin species. *Proc. Natl. Acad. Sci. USA* 75: 3065–3069, 1978.
562. Rosenberg, R. D., and P. S. Damus. The purification and mechanism of action of human antithrombin-heparin cofactor. *J. Biol. Chem.* 248: 6490–6505, 1973.
563. Rosenberg, R. D., R. E. Jordan, L. V. Favreau, and L. H. Tam. Highly active heparin species with multiple binding sites for antithrombin. *Biochem. Biophys. Res. Commun.* 86: 1319–1324, 1979.
564. Rosenthal, R. H., O. H. Dreskin, and N. Rosenthal. New hemophilia-like disease caused by deficiency of a third plasma thromboplastin factor. *Proc. Soc. Exp. Biol. Med.* 82: 171–174, 1953.
565. Rosing, D. R., D. R. Redwood, P. Brakman, and T. Astrup. Impairment of the diurnal fibrinolytic response in man. Effects of aging, type IV hyperlipoproteinemia, and coronary artery disease. *Circ. Res.* 32: 752–758, 1973.

566. Rothman, J. E., and J. Leonard. Membrane asymmetry. *Science* 195: 743–753, 1977.
567. Saito, H., G. H. Goldsmith, M. Moroi, and N. Aolei. Inhibitory spectrum of α_2-plasmin inhibitor. *Proc. Natl. Acad. Sci. USA* 76: 2013–2017, 1979.
568. Saito, H., and O. D. Ratnoff. Inhibition of normal clotting and Fletcher factor activity by rabbit antikallikrein antiserum. *Nature London New Biol.* 248: 597–599, 1974.
569. Saito, H., O. D. Ratnoff, and V. H. Donaldson. Defective activation of clotting, fibrinolytic and permeability-enhancing systems in human Fletcher trait plasma. *Circ. Res.* 34: 641–651, 1974.
570. Saito, H., O. D. Ratnoff, and J. Pensky. Radioimmunoassay of human Hageman factor (factor XII). *J. Lab. Clin. Med.* 88: 506–514, 1976.
571. Saito, H., O. D. Ratnoff, R. Waldmann, and J. P. Abraham. Fitzgerald trait. Deficiency of a hitherto unrecognized agent, Fitzgerald factor, participating in surface-mediated reactions of clotting, fibrinolysis, generation of kinins, and the property of dilated plasma enhancing vascular permeability (PF/DIL). *J. Clin. Invest.* 55: 1082–1089, 1975.
572. Sakata, Y., and N. Aoki. Cross-linking of α_2-plasmin inhibitor to fibrin by fibrin-stabilizing factor. *J. Clin. Invest.* 65: 290–297, 1980.
573. Saraswathi, S., and R. W. Colman. Role of galactose in bovine factor V. *J. Biol. Chem.* 250: 8111–8118, 1975.
574. Saraswathi, S., R. Rawala, and R. W. Colman. Subunit structure of bovine factor V. Influence of proteolysis during blood collection. *J. Biol. Chem.* 253: 1024–1029, 1978.
576. Schapira, M., C. F. Scott, and R. W. Colman. High molecular weight kininogen protects human plasma kallikrein and factor XIa against inactivation by plasma protease inhibitors. *Trans. Assoc. Am. Physicians* 94: 190–197, 1981.
577. Schapira, M., C. F. Scott, and R. W. Colman. Protection of human plasma kallikrein from inactivation by C1 inhibitor and other protease inhibitors. The role of high molecular weight kininogen. *Biochemistry* 20: 2738–2743, 1981.
578. Schapira, M., C. F. Scott, A. James, L. D. Silver, F. Kueppers, H. L. James, and R. W. Colman. High molecular weight kininogen or its light chain protects human plasma kallikrein from inactivation by plasma protease inhibitor. *Biochemistry* 21: 567–572, 1982.
579. Scheraga, H. A. Active site mapping of thrombin. In: *The Chemistry and Biology of Thrombin*, edited by R. L. Lundblad, J. W. Fenton II, and K. G. Mann. Ann Arbor, MI: Ann Arbor Science, 1977, p. 145–158.
580. Schick, L. A., and F. J. Castellino. Direct evidence for the generation of an active site in the plasminogen moiety of the streptokinase-human plasminogen activator complex. *Biochem. Biophys. Res. Commun.* 57: 47–54, 1974.
581. Schiffman, S., and P. Lee. Preparation, characterization, and activation of a highly purified factor XI: evidence that a hitherto unrecognized plasma activity participates in the interaction of factors XI and XII. *Br. J. Haematol.* 27: 101–114, 1974.
582. Schiffman, S., and P. Lee. Partial purification and characterization of control activation cofactor. *J. Clin. Invest.* 56: 1082–1092, 1975.
583. Schiffman, S., S. I. Rapaport, and M. M. Y. Chong. The mandatory role of lipid in the interaction of factors VIII and IX. *Proc. Soc. Exp. Biol. Med.* 123: 736–740, 1966.
584. Schreiber, A. D., and K. F. Austen. Hageman factor-independent fibrinolytic pathway. *Clin. Exp. Immunol.* 17: 587–600, 1974.
585. Schreiber, A. D., A. P. Kaplan, and K. F. Austen. Inhibition by C$\overline{1}$INH of Hageman factor fragment activation of coagulation, fibrinolysis, and kinin generation. *J. Clin. Invest.* 52: 1402–1409, 1973.
586. Schwartz, M. L., S. V. Pizzo, R. L. Hill, and P. A. McKee. Human factor XIII from plasma and platelets. Molecular weights, subunit structures, proteolytic activation, and cross-linking of fibrinogen and fibrin. *J. Biol. Chem.* 248: 1395–1407, 1973.
587. Scott, C. F., and R. W. Colman. Function and immunochemistry of prekallikrein-high molecular weight kininogen complex in plasma. *J. Clin. Invest.* 65: 413–421, 1980.
588. Scott, C. F., E. Kirby, P. Schick, and R. W. Colman. Effect of surfaces on fluid-phase prekallikrein activation. *Blood* 57: 553–560, 1981.
589. Scott, C. F., C. Y. Liu, and R. W. Colman. Human plasma prekallikrein: a rapid high-yield method for purification. *Eur. J. Biochem.* 100: 77–83, 1979.
589a. Scott, C. F., M. Schapira, and R. W. Colman. Effect of heparin on the inactivation rate of human factor XIa by antithrombin III. *Blood* 60: 940–947, 1982.
589b. Scott, C. F., M. Schapira, H. L. James, A. B. Cohen, and R. W. Colman. Inactivation of factor XIa by plasma protease inhibitors: predominant role of α_1-protease inhibitor and protective effect of high molecular weight kininogen. *J. Clin. Invest.* 69: 844–852, 1982.
589c. Scott, C. F., L. D. Silver, M. Schapira, and R. W. Colman. Cleavage of human high molecular weight kininogen markedly enhances its coagulant activity: evidence that this molecule exists as a procofactor. *J. Clin. Invest.* 73: 954–962, 1984.
589d. Scott, C. F., D. Sinha, F. S. Seaman, P. N. Walsh, and R. W. Colman. Amidolytic assay of factor XI in plasma: comparison with a coagulant assay and a new rapid radioimmunoassay. *Blood* 63: 42–50, 1984.
590. Sealey, J. E., S. A. Atlas, J. H. Laragh, M. Silverberg, and A. P. Kaplan. Initiation of plasma prorenin activation by Hageman factor-dependent conversion of plasma prekallikrein to kallikrein. *Proc. Natl. Acad. Sci. USA* 76: 5914–5918, 1979.
591. Seegers, W. H. Multiple protein interactions as exhibited by the blood clotting mechanism. *J. Phys. Colloid Chem.* 51: 198–206, 1947.
592. Seegers, W. H. Inactivation of thrombin. In: *Prothrombin*. Cambridge, MA: Harvard Univ. Press, 1962, p. 285–319.
593. Seegers, W. H., and C. Ouyang. Snake venoms and blood coagulation. In: *Handbook of Experimental Pharmacology. Snake Venoms*, edited by C. Y. Lee. Berlin: Springer-Verlag, 1979, vol. 52, p. 684–750.
594. Shafrir, E., and A. De Vries. Studies on the clot-promoting activity of glass. *J. Clin. Invest.* 35: 1183–1190, 1956.
595. Shainoff, J. R., and B. N. Dardik. Fibrinopeptide B and aggregation of fibrinogen. *Science* 204: 200–202, 1979.
596. Shainoff, J. R., B. Lahiri, and F. M. Bumpus. Ultracentrifuge studies on the reaction between thrombin and plasminized fibrinogen. *Thromb. Diath. Haemorrh.* 39: 302–317, 1970.
597. Shainoff, J. R., and I. H. Page. Cofibrins and fibrin-intermediates as indicators of thrombin activity, in vivo. *Circ. Res.* 8: 1013–1022, 1960.
598. Shapiro, S. S., and D. B. Anderson. Thrombin inhibition in normal plasma. In: *The Chemistry and Biology of Thrombin*, edited by R. L. Lundblad, J. W. Fenton II, and K. G. Mann. Ann Arbor, MI: Ann Arbor Science, 1977, p. 361–365.
599. Sherman, L. A., M. W. Mosesson, and S. Sherry. Isolation and characterization of the clottable low molecular weight fibrinogen derived by limited plasmin hydrolysis of human fraction I-4. *Biochemistry* 8: 1515–1523, 1969.
600. Sherry, S., and W. Troll. The action of thrombin on synthetic substrates. *J. Biol. Chem.* 208: 95–105, 1954.
601. Shively, J. E., and H. E. Conard. Formation of anhydrosugars in the chemical depolymerization of heparin. *Biochemistry* 15: 3932–3942, 1976.
602. Shotton, D. M., and H. C. Watson. Three-dimensional structure of tosyl-elastase. *Nature London* 225: 811–816, 1970.
603. Shulman, S. The size and shape of bovine fibrinogen. Studies of sedimentation, diffusion and viscosity. *J. Am. Chem. Soc.* 75: 5846–5852, 1953.
604. Shuman, M. A., and P. W. Majerus. The measurement of thrombin in clotting blood by radioimmunoassay. *J. Clin.*

Invest. 58: 1249-1258, 1976.
605. SIGLER, P. B., D. M. BLOW, B. W. MATTHEWS, AND R. HENDERSON. Structure of crystalline α-chymotrypsin. II. A preliminary report including a hypothesis for the activation mechanism. *J. Mol. Biol.* 35: 143-164, 1968.
606. SILVERTON, E. W., M. A. NAVIA, AND D. R. DAVIES. Three-dimensional structure of an intact human immunoglobulin. *Proc. Natl. Acad. Sci. USA* 74: 5140-5144, 1977.
607. SIZER, I. W., AND P. F. WAGLEY. The action of tyrosinase on thrombin, fibrinogen and fibrin. *J. Biol. Chem.* 192: 213-222, 1951.
608. SMITH, C. M., AND D. J. HANAHAN. The activation of factor V by factor Xa or alpha-chymotrypsin and comparison with thrombin and RVV-V action. An improved factor V isolation procedure. *Biochemistry* 15: 1830-1838, 1976.
609. SMITH, G. F., AND N. U. BANG. Formation of soluble fibrin polymers. Fibrinogen degradation fragments D and E fail to form soluble complexes with fibrin monomer. *Biochemistry* 11: 2958-2966, 1972.
610. SOBEL, G. W., S. R. MOHLER, N. W. JONES, A. B. C. DOWDY, AND M. M. GUEST. Urokinase: an activator of plasma profibrinolysin extracted from urine (Abstract). *Am. J. Physiol.* 171: 768-769, 1952.
611. SOLUM, N. O., AND H. STORMORKEN. Influence of fibrinogen on the aggregation of washed human platelets induced by adenosine diphosphate, thrombin, collagen, and adrenaline. *Scand. J. Clin. Lab. Invest. Suppl.* 84: 170-182, 1965.
612. SOTTRUP-JENSEN, L., H. CLAEYS, M. ZAJDEL, T. E. PETERSEN, AND S. MAGNUSSON. The primary structure of human plasminogen: isolation of two lysine-binding fragments and one "mini"-plasminogen (M. W. 38,000) by elastase-catalyzed-specific limited proteolysis. In: *Progress in Chemical Fibrinolysis and Thrombolysis*, edited by J. F. Davidson, R. M. Rowan, M. M. Samama, and P. D. Desnoyers. New York: Raven, 1978, vol. 3, p. 191-209.
613. SPARROW, J. T., H. J. POWNALL, F.-J. HSU, L. D. BLUMENTHAL, A. R. CULWELL, AND A. M. GOTTO. Lipid binding by fragments of apolipoprotein C-III-1 obtained by thrombin cleavage. *Biochemistry* 16: 5427-5431, 1977.
614. STATHAKIS, N. E., AND M. W. MOSESSON. Interactions among heparin, cold-insoluble globulin and fibrinogen in formation of the heparin-precipitable fraction of plasma. *J. Clin. Invest.* 60: 855-865, 1977.
615. STEAD, N. W., A. P. KAPLAN, AND R. D. ROSENBERG. The inhibition of human activated Hageman factor (HF) by human antithrombin-heparin cofactor (AT). *J. Biol. Chem.* 251: 6481-6488, 1976.
616. STENFLO, J. Vitamin K and the biosynthesis of prothrombin. IV. Isolation of peptides containing prosthetic groups from normal prothrombin and the corresponding peptides from dicoumarol-induced prothrombin. *J. Biol. Chem.* 249: 5527-5535, 1974.
617. STENFLO, J. Structural comparison of normal and dicoumarol-induced prothrombin in prothrombin and related coagulation factors. *Boerhaave Ser.* 10: 152-158, 1975.
618. STENFLO, J., AND P. O. GANROT. Vitamin K and the biosynthesis of prothrombin. I. Identification and purification of a dicoumarol-induced abnormal prothrombin from bovine plasma. *J. Biol. Chem.* 247: 8160-8166, 1972.
619. STENN, K. S., AND E. R. BLOUT. Mechanism of bovine prothrombin activation by an insoluble preparation of bovine factor S_a (thrombokinase). *Biochemistry* 11: 4502-4515, 1972.
620. STEWART, G. J., AND S. NIEWIAROWSKI. Nonenzymatic polymerization of fibrinogen by protamine sulfate: an electron microscope study. *Biochim. Biophys. Acta* 194: 462-469, 1969.
621. STEWART, G. J., AND S. NIEWIAROWSKI. Polymerization of fibrinogen and its derivatives by basic proteins: an electron microscope study. *Thromb. Diath. Haemorrh.* 25: 566-579, 1971.
622. STIVALA, S. S., L. YUAN, J. EHRLICH, AND P. A. LIBERTI. Physiochemical studies of fractionated bovine heparin. III. Some physical parameters in relation to biological activity. *Arch. Biochem. Biophys.* 122: 32-39, 1967.
623. STOCKER, K. Defibrinogenation with thrombin-like snake venom enzymes. In: *Handbook of Experimental Pharmacology. Snake Venoms*, edited by C. Y. Lee. Berlin: Springer-Verlag, 1979, vol. 52, p. 452-484.
624. STRICKLAND, S. Studies on the role of plasminogen activator in ovulation and early embryogenesis. In: *Regulatory Proteolytic Enzymes and Their Inhibitors*, edited by S. Magnusson, M. Ottesen, B. Foltman, K. Dano, and H. Neurath. Oxford, UK: Pergamon, 1978, p. 181-185.
625. STROUD, R. M., M. KRIEGER, R. E. KOEPPE, A. A. KOSSIAKOFF, AND J. L. CHAMBERS. Structure-function relationships in the serine proteases. In: *Proteases and Biological Control*, edited by E. Reich, D. B. Rifkin, and E. Shaw. New York: Cold Spring Harbor, 1975, vol. 2, p. 13-32. (Cold Spring Harbor Conf. Cell Proliferation.)
626. STUDER, A. Contribution a l'etude de la thrombokinase. In: *Jubilee Volume Dedicated to Emile Chrystophe Barell*. Basel: Roche, 1946, p. 229-237.
627. STURTEVANT, J. M., M. LASKOWSKI, T. H. DONNELLY, AND H. A. SCHERAGA. Equilibria in the fibrinogen-fibrin conversion. III. Heats of polymerization and clotting of fibrin monomer. *J. Am. Chem. Soc.* 77: 6168-6172, 1955.
628. SUMMARIA, L., L. ARZADON, P. BERNABE, AND K. C. ROBBINS. The activation of plasminogen to plasmin by urokinase in the presence of plasmin inhibitor Trasylol. The preparation of plasmin with the same NH_2-terminal heavy (A) chain sequence as the parent zymogen. *J. Biol. Chem.* 250: 3988-3995, 1975.
629. SUMMARIA, L., I. G. BOREISHA, L. ARZADON, AND K. C. ROBBINS. Activation of human Glu-plasminogen to Glu-plasmin by urokinase in the presence of plasmin inhibitors. Streptomyces leupeptin and human plasma $α_1$-antitrypsin and antithrombin III (plus heparin). *J. Biol. Chem.* 252: 3945-3951, 1977.
630. SUMMARIA, L., B. HSIEH, W. R. GROSKOPF, W. R. ROBBINS, AND G. H. BARLOW. The isolation and characterization of the S-carboxymethyl β (light) chain derivative of human plasmin. The localization of the active site on the β (light) chain. *J. Biol. Chem.* 242: 5046-5052, 1967.
631. SUSSMAN, I. I., AND H. J. WEISS. Spontaneous aggregation of low molecular weight factor VIII and its prevention by 2 mM $CaCl_2$. *Thromb. Res.* 9: 267-276, 1976.
632. SVENDSEN, L., B. BLOMBÄCK, M. BLOMBÄCK, AND P. I. OLSSON. Synthetic chromogenic substrates for determination of trypsin, thrombin and thrombin-like enzymes. *Thromb. Res.* 1: 267-278, 1972.
633. TAKAGI, T., AND R. F. DOOLITTLE. Amino acid sequence studies on factor XIII and the peptide released during its activation by thrombin. *Biochemistry* 13: 750-756, 1974.
634. TAKAGI, T., AND R. F. DOOLITTLE. Amino acid sequence studies on the α chain of human fibrinogen. Location of four plasmin attack points and a covalent cross-linking site. *Biochemistry* 14: 5149-5156, 1975.
635. TAKAGI, T., AND T. KAWAI. A simple and practical method for isolation of an early plasmin degradation product of human fibrinogen. *Thromb. Haemost.* 37: 464-470, 1977.
636. TANGEN, O., H. J. BERMAN, AND P. MURPHY. Gel filtration. A new technique for separation of blood platelets from plasma. *Thromb. Diath. Haemorrh.* 25: 268-287, 1971.
637. TAYLOR, F. B., JR., AND J. BOTTS. Purification and characterization of streptokinase with studies of streptokinase activation of plasminogen. *Biochemistry* 7: 237-242, 1968.
638. TAYLOR, F. B., JR., R. C. CARROLL, J. GERRARD, C. T. ESMON, AND R. D. RADCLIFFE. Lysis of clots prepared from whole blood and plasma. *Federation Proc.* 40: 2092-2098, 1981.
639. TAYLOR, R. L., J. E. SHIVELY, H. E. CONRAD, AND J. A. CIFONELLI. Uronic acid composition of heparins and heparan sulfates. *Biochemistry* 12: 3633-3636, 1973.
640. THOMPSON, A. R., D. L. ENFIELD, L. H. ERICSSON, M. E. LEGAZ, AND J. W. FENTON II. Human thrombin partial pri-

mary structure. *Arch. Biochem. Biophys.* 178: 356–367, 1977.
641. THOMPSON, R. E., R. MANDLE, JR., AND A. P. KAPLAN. Association of factor XI and high-molecular-weight kininogen in human plasma. *J. Clin. Invest.* 60: 1376–1380, 1977.
642. THOMPSON, R. E., R. MANDLE, JR., AND A. P. KAPLAN. Characterization of human high molecular weight kininogen. Procoagulant activity associated with the light chain of kinin-free high molecular weight kininogen. *J. Exp. Med.* 147: 488–499, 1978.
643. THORSEN, S. Differences in the binding to fibrin of native plasminogen and plasminogen modified by proteolytic degradation. Influence of omega-amino-carboxylic acids. *Biochim. Biophys. Acta* 393: 55–65, 1975.
644. THORSEN, S., AND S. MULLERTZ. Rate of activation and electrophoretic mobility of unmodified and partially degraded plasminogen. Effects of 6-aminohexanoic acid and related compounds. *Scand. J. Clin. Lab. Invest.* 34: 167–176, 1974.
645. TITANI, K., K. FUKIKAWA, D. L. ENFIELD, L. H. ERICSSON, K. A. WALSH, AND H. NEURATH. Bovine factor X_1 (Stuart Factor): amino-acid sequence of heavy chain. *Proc. Natl. Acad. Sci. USA* 72: 3082–3086, 1975.
646. TOLLEFSEN, D. M., J. R. FEAGLER, AND P. W. MAJERUS. The binding of thrombin to the surface of human platelets. *J. Biol. Chem.* 249: 2646–2651, 1974.
647. TOLLEFSEN, D. M., AND P. W. MAJERUS. Inhibition of human platelet aggregation by monovalent antibody fragment. *J. Clin. Invest.* 55: 1259–1268, 1975.
648. TOONEY, N. M., AND C. COHEN. Crystalline states of a modified fibrinogen. *J. Mol. Biol.* 110: 363–385, 1977.
649. TRIANTAPHYLLOPOULOS, D. C. Anticoagulant effect of incubated fibrinogen. *Can. J. Biochem. Physiol.* 36: 249–259, 1958.
650. TUDDENHAM, E. G. D., N. C. TRABOLD, J. A. COLLINS, AND L. W. HOYER. The properties of factor VIII coagulant activity prepared by immunoadsorbent chromatography. *J. Lab. Clin. Med.* 93: 40–53, 1979.
651. VAHERI, A., AND D. F. MOSHER. High molecular weight, cell surface-associated glycoprotein (fibronectin) lost in malignant transformation. *Biochim. Biophys. Acta* 516: 1–25, 1978.
652. VEHAR, G. A., AND E. W. DAVIE. Bovine factor VIII: purification of the procoagulant protein. *Thromb. Haemost.* 42: 342–347, 1979.
653. VERMEER, C., J. W. P. GOVERS-RIEMSLAG, B. A. M. SOUTE, M. J. LINDHOUT, J. KOP, AND H. C. HEMKER. The role of blood clotting factor V in the conversion of prothrombin and a decarboxy prothrombin into thrombin. *Biochim. Biophys. Acta* 538: 521–533, 1978.
654. VERSTRAETE, M. A far stretched program: rapid, safe and predictable thrombolysis in man. In: *Fibrinolysis*, edited by D. L. Kline and N. N. Reddy. Cleveland, OH: CRC, 1980, p. 185–200.
655. VERSTRAETE, M., J. VERMYLEN, A. AMERY, AND C. VERMYLEN. Thrombolytic therapy with streptokinase using a standard dosage scheme. *Br. Med. J.* 5485: 454–456 1966.
656. VOKE, J. Location of factor VIII coagulant activity in relation to factor VIII related antigen after rapid two-dimensional immunoelectrophoresis. *Thromb. Res.* 13: 53–60, 1978.
657. WALDMAN, R., AND J. ABRAHAM. Fitzgerald factor: a heretofore unrecognized coagulation factor. *Blood* 46: 761–768, 1975.
658. WALLÉN, P. Activation of plasminogen with urokinase and tissue activator. In: *Thrombosis and Urokinase*, edited by R. Paoletti and S. Sherry. London: Academic, 1977, p. 91–102.
659. WALLÉN, P., P. KOK, AND M. RANBY. The tissue activator of plasminogen. *FEBS Proc. Meet., 11th, Copenhagen* 47: 127–135, 1977.
660. WALTHER, P. J., R. L. HILL, AND P. A. MCKEE. The importance of the preactivation peptide in the two-stage mechanism of human plasminogen activation. *J. Biol. Chem.* 250: 5926–5933, 1975.
661. WALTHER, P. J., H. M. STEINMAN, R. L. HILL, AND P. A. MCKEE. Activation of human plasminogen by urokinase. Partial characterization of a preactivation peptide. *J. Biol. Chem.* 249: 1173–1181, 1974.
662. WALZ, D. A., D. HEWETT-EMMITT, AND W. H. SEEGERS. Amino acid sequence of human prothrombin fragments 1 and 2. *Proc. Natl. Acad. Sci. USA* 74: 1969–1972, 1977.
663. WALZ, D. A., AND W. H. SEEGERS. Amino acid sequence of human thrombin A chain. *Biochem. Biophys. Res. Commun.* 60: 717–721, 1974.
664. WALZ, D. A., W. H. SEEGERS, J. REUTERBY, AND L. E. MCCOY. Proteolytic specificity of thrombin. *Thromb. Res.* 4: 713–717, 1974.
665. WATT, K. W. K., T. TAKAGI, AND R. F. DOOLITTLE. Amino acid sequence of the β chain of human fibrinogen. *Biochemistry* 18: 68–76, 1979.
666. WAUGH, D. F., AND M. A. FITZGERALD. Quantitative aspects of antithrombin and heparin in plasma. *Am. J. Physiol.* 184: 627–639, 1956.
667. WEBSTER, M. E. Human plasma kallikrein, its activation and pathological role. *Federation Proc.* 27: 84–89, 1968.
668. WEBSTER, M. E., J. A. GUIMARAES, A. P. KAPLAN, R. W. COLMAN, AND J. V. PIERCE. Activation of surface bound Hageman factor: pre-eminent role of high molecular weight kininogen and evidence for a new factor. In: *Kinins: Pharmacodynamics and Biological Roles*, edited by F. Sicuteri, N. Black, and G. L. Haberland. New York: Plenum, 1976, p. 285–299.
669. WEBSTER, M. E., AND J. V. PIERCE. Activators of Hageman factor (factor XII): identification and relationship to kallikrein-kinin system (Abstract). *Federation Proc.* 32: 845, 1973.
670. WEINTRAUB, B. U., J. S. COBLYN, C. E. KAEMPFER, AND K. F. AUSTEN. Cleavage of fibrinogen by the human neutrophil neutral peptide-generating protease. *Proc. Natl. Acad. Sci. USA* 77: 5448–5452, 1980.
671. WEISEL, J. W., S. G. WARREN, AND C. COHEN. Crystals of modified fibrinogen: size, shape, and packing of molecules. *J. Mol. Biol.* 126: 159–183, 1978.
672. WEISS, A. S., J. I. GALLIN, AND A. P. KAPLAN. Fletcher factor deficiency: a diminished rate of Hageman factor activation caused by absence of prekallikrein with abnormalities of coagulation, fibrinolysis, chemotactic activity and kinin generation. *J. Clin. Invest.* 53: 622–633, 1974.
673. WEISS, H. J. A study of the cation- and pH-dependent stability of factors V and VIII in plasma. *Thromb. Diath. Haemorrh.* 14: 32–51, 1965.
674. WEISS, H. J., AND L. W. HOYER. Von Willebrand factor: dissociation from antihemophilic factor procoagulant activity. *Science* 182: 1149–1151, 1973.
675. WEISS, H. J., L. L. PHILLIPS, AND W. ROSNER. Separation of sub-units of antihemophilic factor (AHF) by agarose gel chromatography. *Thromb. Diath. Haemorrh.* 27: 212–219, 1972.
676. WEISS, H. J., AND J. ROGERS. Fibrinogen and platelets in primary arrest of bleeding. Studies in two patients with congenital afibrinogenemia. *N. Engl. J. Med.* 285: 369–374, 1971.
677. WEISS, H. J., I. I. SUSSMAN, AND L. W. HOYER. Stabilization of factor VIII in plasma by the von Willebrand factor. *J. Clin. Invest.* 60: 390–404, 1977.
678. WHITE, G. C., E. F. WORKMAN, AND R. L. LUNDBLAD. Platelet-thrombin interactions: the platelet as a substrate for thrombin. In: *The Chemistry and Biology of Thrombin*, edited by R. L. Lundblad, J. W. Fenton II, and K. G. Mann. Ann Arbor, MI: Ann Arbor Science, 1977, p. 479–498.
679. WHITE, W. F., G. H. BARLOW, AND M. M. MOZEN. The isolation and characterization of plasminogen activators (urokinase) from human urine. *Biochemistry* 5: 2160–2169, 1966.
680. WIGGINS, R. C., B. N. BOUMA, C. G. COCHRANE, AND J. H. GRIFFIN. Role of high-molecular-weight kininogen in surface binding and activation of coagulation factor XI and prekallikrein. *Proc. Natl. Acad. Sci. USA* 74: 4636–4640, 1977.
681. WIGGINS, R. C., AND C. C. COCHRANE. The autoactivation of rabbit Hageman factor. *J. Exp. Med.* 150: 1122–1132, 1979.
682. WILLIAMS, R. C. Morphology of bovine fibrinogen monomers and fibrin oligomers. *J. Mol. Biol.* 150: 399–408, 1981.

683. WILSON, S. J. Quantitative studies on antithrombin. *Arch. Intern. Med.* 69: 647–661, 1942.
684. WIMAN, B., AND D. COLLEN. Purification and characterization of human antiplasmin, the fast-acting plasmin inhibitor in plasma. *Eur. J. Biochem.* 78: 19–26, 1977.
685. WIMAN, B., AND D. COLLEN. Molecular mechanism of physiological fibrinolysis. *Nature London* 272: 549–550, 1978.
686. WIMAN, B., AND P. WALLEN. Activation of human plasminogen by an insoluble derivative of urokinase. Structural changes of plasminogen in the course of activation to plasmin and demonstration of a possible intermediate compound. *Eur. J. Biochem.* 36: 25–31, 1973.
687. WOHL, R. C., L. SUMMARIA, L. ARZADON, AND K. C. ROBBINS. Steady state kinetics of activation of human and bovine plasminogens by streptokinase and its equimolar complexes with various activated forms of human plasminogen. *J. Biol. Chem.* 253: 1402–1407, 1978.
688. WOHL, R. C., L. SUMMARIA, AND K. C. ROBBINS. Physiological activation of the human fibrinolytic system. Isolation and characterization of human plasminogen variants, Chicago I and Chicago II. *J. Biol. Chem.* 254: 9063–9069, 1979.
689. WOLF, P. Studies of temperature and pH stability of human antihaemophilic factor (AHF) in plasma and in a concentrate. *Br. J. Haematol.* 5: 169–176, 1959.
690. WOLFENSTEIN-TODEL, C., AND M. W. MOSESSON. Human plasma fibrinogen heterogeneity: evidence for an extended carboxyl-terminal sequence in a normal γ chain variant (γ'). *Proc. Natl. Acad. Sci. USA* 77: 5069–5073, 1980.
691. WORKMAN, E. F., JR., G. C. WHITE II, AND R. L. LUNDBLAD. Structure-function relationships in the interaction of α-thrombin with blood platelets. *J. Biol. Chem.* 252: 7118–7123, 1977.
692. WRIGHT, I. S. Nomenclature of blood clotting factors. *J. Am. Med. Assoc.* 170: 325–328, 1959.
693. WUEPPER, K. D. Biochemistry and biology of components of plasma kinin-forming system. In: *Inflammation: Mechanism and Control*, edited by I. H. Lepow and P. W. Ward. New York: Academic, 1972, p. 93–117.
694. WUEPPER, K. D. Precursor plasma thromboplastin antecedent (PTA, clotting factor XI) (Abstract). *Federation Proc.* 31: 624, 1972.
695. WUEPPER, K. D. Prekallikrein deficiency in man. *J. Exp. Med.* 138: 1345–1355, 1973.
696. YURT, R. W., R. W. LEID, K. F. AUSTEN, AND J. E. SILBERT. Native heparin from rat peritoneal mast cells. *J. Biol. Chem.* 252: 518–521, 1977.
697. ZIMMERMAN, T. S., AND T. S. EDGINGTON. Factor VIII coagulant activity and factor VIII-like antigen: independent molecular entities. *J. Exp. Med.* 138: 1015–1020, 1973.
698. ZIMMERMAN, T. S., O. D. RATNOFF, AND A. E. POWELL. Immunologic differentiation of classic hemophilia (factor VIII deficiency) and von Willebrand's disease, with observations on combined deficiencies of antihemophilic factor and proaccelerin (factor V) and on an acquired circulating anticoagulant against antihemophilic factor. *J. Clin. Invest.* 50: 244–254, 1971.
699. ZOLTON, R. P., E. T. MERTZ, AND H. T. RUSSELL. Assay of human plasminogen in plasma by affinity chromatography. *Clin. Chem. Winston-Salem, NC* 18: 654–657, 1972.
700. ZUCKER, M. B., M. W. MOSESSON, M. J. BROEKMAN, AND K. L. KAPLAN. Release of platelet fibronectin (cold-insoluble globulin) from alpha granules induced by thrombin or collagen: lack of requirement for plasma fibronectin in ADP-induced platelet aggregation. *Blood* 54: 8–12, 1979.
701. ZUR, M., AND Y. NEMERSON. The esterase activity of coagulation factor VII. Evidence for intrinsic activity of the zymogen. *J. Biol. Chem.* 253: 2203–2209, 1977.
702. ZWAAL, R. F. A. Membrane and lipid involvement in blood coagulation. *Biochim. Biophys. Acta* 515: 163–205, 1978.
703. ZWAAL, R. F. A., P. COMFURIUS, AND L. L. VAN DEENEN. Membrane asymmetry and blood coagulation. *Nature London* 268: 358–360, 1977.

CHAPTER 17

Platelet–blood vessel interactions

RUSSELL ROSS
STEPHEN M. SCHWARTZ

Department of Pathology, University of Washington, Seattle, Washington

CHAPTER CONTENTS

Morphological Models of Capillary Endothelium
Transport Across Endothelium
Cell Turnover
Endothelial Cell Culture
Endothelial Function
Endothelial Injury
Platelets
  Morphology and content
  Platelet function
  Platelet-derived growth factor
Endothelium–Smooth Muscle Interactions
Platelet–Endothelial Cell Interactions
Summary

TEN YEARS AGO investigators had only vague ideas concerning the noncoagulative and antithrombotic properties of endothelium. At that time, however, it seemed that this tissue was a semipermeable tube able to contain blood. This changed in 1973 with the advent of culture systems able to propagate endothelial cells (9, 16, 40, 54, 55, 59, 76, 82, 83, 120) and the recognition that endothelial damage could lead to smooth muscle proliferation (138). Since that time our understanding of the endothelium as a metabolically active tissue has greatly increased (16–18, 25, 27, 30, 32, 41, 42, 49, 52, 54, 59, 71, 74, 80, 91, 97, 117, 119, 124, 137, 145). This delicate, single-cell layer can no longer be considered simply a permeability barrier and a nonthrombogenic surface. Of particular interest is how endothelial integrity is maintained and how products derived from the endothelium affect adjacent cells, cells in the circulation, and distant target tissues. This synthesis of morphology and function forms the basis for this chapter: a dynamic picture of the endothelium and, where possible, an emphasis on the endothelium of the pulmonary vessels.

MORPHOLOGICAL MODELS OF CAPILLARY ENDOTHELIUM

In 1965 Majno (86) classified endothelia according to the continuity of the cellular layer (Table 1).

Pulmonary endothelium is classified as a "continuous endothelium together with cells that line the microvascular beds of striated muscle, small vessels in the central nervous system, and the large arteries" (135). Of all the endothelia the capillary endothelium of muscle has been the most extensively studied with physiological techniques. These studies imply that the endothelium is a continuous membrane system containing two sets of pores. In this model there are a large number of small pores that pass molecules with molecular weights of 10,000–100,000 and a small number of large pores that freely pass solutes without regard to their molecular weight. Flux through the large-pore system is limited because the total area of such pores is quite small. Most flux of water occurs either directly across cell membranes or via the small-pore system (14, 79).

Electron microscopists have made a major effort to identify the morphological sites equivalent to those predicted by the physiologists' model. This has led to the identification of at least five functionally distinct routes for the passage of macromolecules across the endothelium. These are shown schematically in Figure 1. Again it should be noted that whereas some permeation may occur by the direct passage of solutes across cell membranes, physiological studies require routes for the actual transport of plasma across the cell itself.

TRANSPORT ACROSS ENDOTHELIUM

Unlike movement via the other routes, vesicular transport is discontinuous. Vesicles function as a transport system by a series of steps involving endocytosis, transport, and exocytosis. Most of the evidence, including serial reconstructions of a small segment of one vessel and studies of the penetration of fixed endothelium with ruthenium red or lanthanum, indicates that the majority of vesicles and caveolae are discontinuous quanta of external space surrounded by the plasma membrane. Other vesicles fuse to form continuous, but tortuous, channels through the endothelium (13, 128, 131). Evidence from studies of the

TABLE 1. *Classification and Location of Endothelia*

Continuous	Fenestrated	Discontinuous
Capillaries	Capillaries	Sinusoids
Skeletal muscle	Endocrine glands	Liver
Myocardium	Glomeruli	Spleen
Lung	Ciliary bodies	Bone marrow
Central nervous system	Choroid plexus	Lymphatics
Smooth muscle of gastrointestinal tract	Exocrine pancreas	
Subcutaneous tissue	Salivary glands	
Placenta	Intestinal villi	
Veins, venules		
Small arteries		
Muscular arteries		
Aorta		

Data from Majno (86).

permeability of muscle capillaries to dextrans with molecular weights >100,000 suggests that restricted diffusion occurs in a molecular-weight range consistent with the size of the openings of the caveolae seen with electron microscopy (106, 128).

The major morphological evidence that these structures can transport aqueous solutes is based on studies with a wide variety of electron-dense tracer molecules. When endothelium exposed to these tracers is examined in the electron microscope, a consistent pattern of events is demonstrated. Tracer molecules enter the surface invaginations (caveolae), appear in enclosed vesicles within the cytoplasm, and finally appear on the abluminal side either in caveolae or free in the subendothelial connective tissue (14, 78, 128–130).

Vesicular transport can account for at least part of the large-pore system. Vesicles and caveolae, however, no matter how frequent, cannot account for the known ability of the endothelium to filter plasma. Filtration (flux driven by a pressure gradient) requires true pores or channels across the endothelium (106). According to physiologists, these channels should represent the small-pore system. Unfortunately the morphological location of the small-pore system remains a matter of considerable debate (14). The approach of morphologists has been to demonstrate permeation by direct visualization of molecules passing through the small-pore system. Most of the tracer molecules used to study vesicular transport are too large to enter pores of the size predicted for the small-pore system.

The exception to this is a series of peroxidatic enzymes that can be demonstrated histochemically. Karnovsky (78) introduced the most widely used of these enzymes, horseradish peroxidase (HRP) (151).

When HRP is injected intravenously and the animals are killed at intervals of 1–5 min, it is possible to demonstrate the presence of reaction product in the intercellular junctions and the vesicles and caveolae. The subendothelium is not labeled after these short intervals, so the localization of the reaction product is taken as evidence that the enzyme has both traversed the space between the endothelial cells and has been carried by vesicular transport. Using high magnification, Karnovsky (78) found a gap ~40 Å wide between the cells at the intercellular junctions. There were only small spots where the space between cells was completely occluded. Studies of fixed tissue with colloidal lanthanum also demonstrated this 40-Å gap between cells. In contrast to these studies of cell junctions in the endothelium of muscle capillaries, cell junctions in the endothelium of capillaries in the central nervous system were shown to be closed by tight junctions impermeable to lanthanum, HRP, and the extremely small (M_r = 1,900) microperoxidase (130). These observations are consistent with physiological measurements of the blood-brain barrier (72).

These observations contrast with more recent data from freeze-fracture experiments. Simionescu et al. (128) found that the structure of cell junctions in continuous endothelium depends on the size and type of the vessel. The aortic endothelium contains extensive arrays of tight occluding junctions, suggesting that it is not a route for permeation. The endothelial junctions become less complex as one proceeds toward the venular end. Extensive tight-junctional complexes are also seen at the capillary level, but these are simplified and discontinuous at the level of the postcapillary venule. This may be consistent with Majno's finding (86) that histamine stimulates the separation of these cell junctions. Using probes as small as microperoxidase, Simionescu et al. (129) found permeation only in vesicles. They concluded that even junctional transport of small microperoxidase fragments is unlikely except at the postcapillary level. This suggests that open junctions do not exist at the capillary level and are therefore too rare to account for the small-pore system. They propose that the small-pore system consists of connected chains of vesicles. The caveolae, however, are too wide to account for the effect of molecular weight on permeation of the endothelium by low-molecular-weight solutes. Simionescu and co-workers (131) point out that the narrow "neck" where the caveolae and plasmalemma join might function as a pore. Furthermore porosity may (in some cases) be modified by tenuous diaphragms at

FIG. 1. Mechanisms of permeation across endothelium. *A*, passage through cell junctions; *B*, passage through fenestrae; *C*, direct passage through cell across plasmalemma; *D*, passage through connected chains of vesicles; *E*, vesicular transport; and *F*, high-affinity endocytosis.

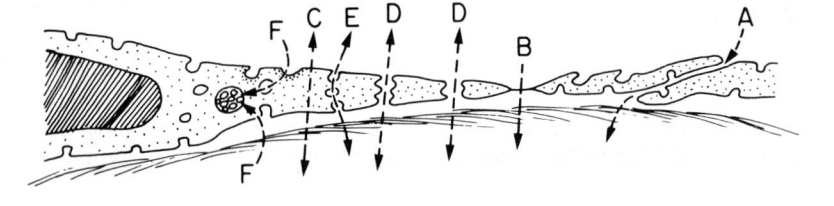

the opening of a transendothelial channel. This leaves two possible routes for the filtration of plasma across the endothelium: the connected chains of vesicles and openings located at cell junctions.

These data have limitations, however (131). Morphological studies assume that measurements of fixed and embedded tissues are accurate estimates of dimensions in vivo. In structures as small as a 40-Å gap, however, this may not be true. Furthermore this view is static; not only are membranes dynamic fluid structures, but, at least in the case of the postcapillary venule, the endothelial junction can open and close (86). Quantitative morphological studies with tracers are subject to problems with proving the absence of the tracer (151). Very little is known about the effects of fixation itself, and substantial changes in tracer concentration may occur during the fixation process. For example, Casley-Smith (20) has presented evidence that connected-vesicle chains may result from fixation. In addition very little is known about the effects of plasma macromolecules, although there is evidence that albumin can occupy a portion of the radius of the small pore (79). Most importantly, this analysis treated the endothelium as if it were a sheet of neutral material pierced by holes, a view that is no longer valid. Recent studies have shown that endothelial transport is also dependent on charge. The luminal surface contains discrete regions of differing charge and differing binding capacity for glycosylated lectins (100, 131, 147). For example, one form of endothelium, although composed of a continuous cell sheet, is made up of cells with a large number of channels or fenestrae through their cytoplasm. These fenestrae serve as sites for water filtration; they are, however, strongly charged with anionic groups derived from heparan sulfate. Thus the endothelium may be a selective filtration barrier, allowing the passage of neutral water but repelling the passage of anionic serum proteins. In contrast, the openings of surface caveolae, including those forming chains across the endothelium, are not strongly negatively charged (100, 129, 130, 131, 147).

Finally, it is also known that the endothelium, at least in culture, contains high-affinity receptors for plasma molecules including lipoproteins (25, 42, 136, 137, 145), thrombin (3), and a variety of neurotransmitters and other hormones (18, 27, 114). On cells other than the endothelia, receptors have been shown to be associated with coated pits and to be transported in the cytoplasm to the lysosomes (12). This form of endocytosis occurs in the endothelium in vitro as well, but it remains to be seen whether it occurs in vivo and whether it can transport substances across the endothelium.

CELL TURNOVER

Like other tissues, endothelium is subject to wear and tear. Evidence for endothelial cell turnover comes from studies that use the daily rate of cell replication as an indirect measure of endothelial turnover. The conclusions of these studies are remarkably consistent: cell turnover in the aortic endothelium is low (10^{-3} cells/day) except in focal areas (123). The presence of these focal areas of turnover indicates that spontaneously denuded areas might occur. Some evidence indicates that the permeability of these areas is altered, but studies of similar areas by scanning electron microscopy and transmission electron microscopy have not demonstrated such discontinuities in normal animals. Data for the microvascular endothelium is similar, though less extensive. Meyrick and Reid (90) provided data on endothelial cell replication in the rat lung. They found a replication frequency of 0.3%–1.4%, depending on the vessel studied. These values are probably low estimates of the daily frequency of labeling because they are based on only one dose of [^{3}H]thymidine. Based on endothelial cell-cycle parameters, the daily frequency of labeling cell replication is probably about three times these values (123). On the other hand, Meyrick and Reid (90) presented these values in terms of turnover but do not have evidence that the cell population in the pulmonary vascular tree has reached a steady state. Thus part of the replication values may represent continued growth or remodeling.

An indirect source of evidence suggesting spontaneous turnover of endothelium comes from studies of atherosclerotic lesion formation. Rheological data predict the occurrence of higher shear forces at sites known to have a predilection for atherosclerotic lesion formation (123). It is difficult, however, to design experiments to predict the amount of shear actually necessary to produce denudation. Both hyperlipidemia and hypertension have been reported to accelerate endothelial cell turnover (43, 51, 122, 125) as well as to produce or exacerbate atherosclerosis in nonhuman primates (102, 111) or swine (141). There is no compelling evidence, however, that the endothelium is actually denuded during the early phases (1–2 mo) of hypercholesterolemia in these studies. In contrast, Ross and Harker (111) observed endothelial denudation in the aortas of monkeys after they had been fed a hypercholesterolemic diet for 2 yr. The increase in plasma cholesterol in these monkeys was correlated with a decrease in platelet survival and a loss of 1% of the endothelium of the aorta at several sites. These sites were particularly seen at bifurcations and branches and had adherent platelets that were degranulated. In such regions the platelets tend to form a type of pseudoendothelium in which a layer of platelets adheres, degranulates, and is often covered by a second layer of less-adherent platelets (Fig. 2). Such platelet interactions are similar to those described by Stemerman and Ross (138) after mechanical de-endothelialization with an intra-arterial balloon catheter; 3–5 days after balloon catheter injury, smooth

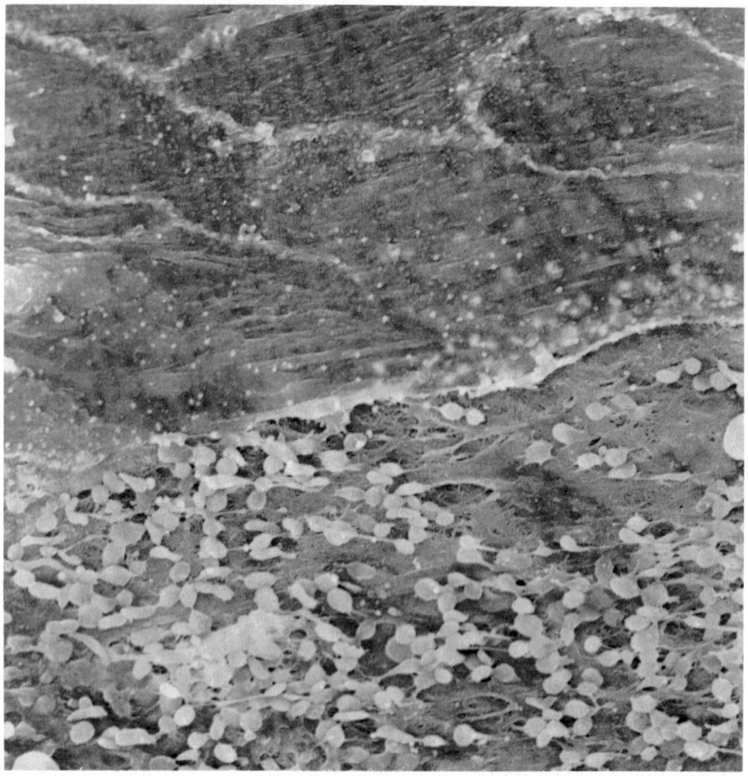

FIG. 2. Region of endothelial desquamation in thoracic aorta of a 2-yr-old pigtail monkey fed a hypercholesterolemic diet for 2 yr. Platelets have adhered to exposed subendothelial collagen. *Top*, intact endothelium. × 2,040.

muscle cells migrate from the media into the intima and develop into fibromusculoproliferative lesions.

The basis for the smooth muscle migration and proliferation at such sites of injury may be explained by the finding that platelets can release a hormone, the platelet-derived growth factor (PDGF), that can act both as a chemoattractant and as a mitogen (61). These latter observations are based on experiments on cell cultures. Although it remains to be determined whether this factor is active in vivo, some reports demonstrate that the proliferative response elicited after endothelial denudation requires platelet interactions at injury sites (46, 50, 64, 92).

Although most of the interest in these phenomena has been at the level of large arteries, evidence indicates that platelet–vessel wall interactions are also important in the responses of small vessels to injury. For example, Meyrick and Reid (90) reported increased endothelial cell replication in association with smooth muscle hyperplasia in response to hypoxia in the lung. Interestingly endothelial cell replication increases prior to smooth muscle replication and is seen only in those vessels that undergo smooth muscle hyperplasia. Meyrick and Reid (90) propose that some sort of mediator released by damaged endothelial cells stimulates smooth muscle replication. These events are similar to the sequence of events seen in the response of the peripheral arterial endothelium to hypertension. We have also proposed that the smooth muscle replication seen in peripheral hypertension may be the result of endothelial injury, exposure of the subendothelium, and the release of mitogens from cells, e.g., platelets or macrophages (109, 120).

ENDOTHELIAL CELL CULTURE

Over the last 10 years a large number of metabolic functions have been described for the endothelium, including interacting with clotting factors (41), acting as binding sites for lipoproteins (25, 42), responding to neurotransmitters (14), binding of lipoprotein lipase (126), converting angiotensin I to angiotensin II (114), and producing prostaglandins (65, 74, 119). Some of these functions were previously suspected, but their actual elucidation depended on the availability of endothelial cells in culture.

Our understanding of these functions began with the description of cultures of cells isolated from the human umbilical vein endothelium (HUVE). Little work was done with these cells, however, until improved culturing techniques were introduced (54, 76, 83). These methods all involve the use of either collagenase or trypsin to preferentially remove the endothelium by enzymatic dissociation from its underlying connective tissue matrix. Primary cultures of HUVE require relatively high concentrations of serum for optimal growth (20%–30%). In most cases the life span of HUVE cultures has been limited to 2–3 passages before the cells appear to be senescent or are overgrown by smooth muscle cells. Maciag et al. (85)

reported techniques that could be used to sustain endothelial cell viability through multiple passages by using a medium supplemented with a brain extract, termed *endothelial cell–derived growth factor* (ECDGF).

Several types of endothelial cells have been derived from bovine sources. Unlike human cells, bovine or porcine cells are relatively easy to grow (8, 121, 132), as are cells from pulmonary arterial endothelium (114, 115). Bovine aortic endothelial (BAE) cells show virtually the same extent of growth in concentrations of fetal calf serum ranging from 5% to 30%, and some growth can be seen in concentrations as low as 1%. The cells are readily passed, with reported life spans of from 40 to 90 doublings (40, 108, 124). The major difficulty in growing these cells has been the need to prevent smooth muscle cell overgrowth. Solutions for this include carefully selecting primary cultures, cloning, killing smooth muscle cells with [^{3}H]thymidine, or using a medium lacking PDGF (28, 108, 124).

One important observation is that both HUVE and BAE cells can be routinely grown in the absence of exogenous growth factors. This has been somewhat confusing because of assertions that one factor or another is required for endothelial growth. For example, Gospodarowicz and colleagues (58) reported that fibroblast growth factor (FGF) was required for clonal growth, growth at low densities, and prolonged replicative life span of BAE. In contrast, data from other groups show that endothelial cells can be cloned at low densities without FGF. The observation of an apparently unlimited life span, however, appears to be restricted to those cells propagated in FGF (28, 40, 74, 82, 108, 124). Thus the effects of FGF may be related just to cloning and prolonging the life span rather than to growth in a more general sense. Related reports indicate that several polypeptide growth factors stimulate growth of HUVE. As noted above, Maciag et al. (85) used this approach to increase the number of passages of human cells.

The most important growth factors to consider in the context of this review are epidermal growth factor (EGF) (26) and PDGF (112). These polypeptides are potentially available to arterial tissue in vivo. Epidermal growth factor is present in plasma and is thus available to the endothelium at concentrations near those needed to stimulate the growth of other cell types in vitro. Gospodarowicz et al. (58) have shown that EGF, either alone or in combination with thrombin, stimulates HUVE cell proliferation. Unlike HUVE, BAE cell proliferation is not stimulated by EGF, and BAE cells apparently lack EGF receptors.

The role of platelet-derived factors in endothelial cell growth is confusing. The levels of PDGF in plasma are relatively low, but they increase because of platelet release at sites of endothelial injury. Davies and Ross (32), Thorgeirsson et al. (142), and Wall et al. (146) stated that HUVE and BAE cells proliferate readily in plasma lacking PDGF and other platelet factors. In contrast D'Amore and Shepro (31) found that BAE cells responded to platelet-derived factors and whole platelets with increased cell proliferation rates. Similar reports have appeared for rabbit marginal vein endothelial cells (35). These differences could be due to short-lived platelet components other than PDGF or to impurities in PDGF preparations. Most recently Zetter and Antoniades (152) reported a migratory response to impure (but not to pure) preparations of the PDGF. This confusion was partly relieved by the availability of pure PDGF and the identification of PDGF receptors. Arterial endothelial cells derived from umbilical vein, bovine aorta, and monkey aorta (to name a few) do not mitogenically respond to PDGF, as do smooth muscle cells. Bowen-Pope and Ross (10) examined the binding characteristics of highly purified ^{125}I-labeled PDGF and found that cells such as smooth muscle and fibroblasts bind with a very high affinity (dissociation constant = 10^{-11} M) to PDGF. The number of receptors in these cells ranges from 600,000/cell (a high receptor line of Swiss 3T3 mouse embryo cells) to 50,000/cell (monkey arterial smooth muscle). In striking contrast, arterial endothelial cells have no PDGF receptors, which correlates with their lack of response to this growth factor.

One variable that may explain the different growth requirements of endothelium reported by various laboratories is the ability of endothelial cells to condition their own medium. Greenburg et al. (60) reported that conditioned medium aids the survival of endothelial cells plated at low densities. Gajdusek and Schwartz (53) found that conditioned medium supplemented with low concentrations of plasma-derived serum supports the growth of BAE in the absence of other growth factors. The fraction in conditioned medium supporting endothelial cell growth includes material with a molecular weight (based on dialysis) of 1,000–8,000. Reports by Castellot et al. (22), Birdwell et al. (5), and Wall et al. (146) indicate that conditioned media from other cell sources can also support BAE cell proliferation at either low or high serum concentrations in the absence of FGF. The relevance of these observations to the growth of endothelium in the high concentrations of serum or plasma seen in vivo is not clear.

Although most of our recent knowledge comes from studies of HUVE or BAE, several other methods for culturing microvascular endothelia exist (18, 34, 35, 37, 38, 44, 45, 94, 98, 99, 101, 127, 133). Of particular interest among these is a study of capillary endothelium from the mouse. Debault and co-workers (36, 37) reported the establishment of an immortal cell line of mouse brain capillary endothelium. This is a promising development for immunological studies because of the highly defined genetics of the parental mouse strain. Folkman and co-workers (44) reported multiple passages of capillary endothelium from human and bovine sources. This required the use of tumor-conditioned media. There are also reports of a clonal culture of rat lung endothelium, possibly of microvascular origin (98).

Finally, endothelial cell culture methods have been developed for a wide range of species, including dog, pig, guinea pig, and rabbit. The latter is particularly interesting because in vivo and in vitro results can be compared. Establishment of primary cultures of rabbit endothelium began with reports by Pollack and Kasai (103). These cultures, however, were rapidly overgrown by smooth muscle cells or fibroblasts. Buonassisi (16) succeeded in establishing a clonal line of rabbit aorta endothelium, and these cells apparently represent an immortal cell line but have not been used by other investigators to any great extent, perhaps because of concern that immortal cells may have altered properties. Rabbit marginal vein endothelium has also recently been grown in culture (34).

ENDOTHELIAL FUNCTION

Endothelial tissue is unique because of its location. An example of the importance of location is the endothelium's capacity to produce the prostaglandin derivative prostacyclin (PGI_2) (see the chapter by Bakhle and Ferreira in this *Handbook*). Prostacyclin is a potent antithrombotic and smooth muscle relaxing agent (65, 119). Other cell types produce PGI_2, but those tissues do not interface with vascular smooth muscle and the blood. The endothelium is an important site for the prevention of platelet interactions and thrombosis because of this location. Levin et al. (81) showed that nitroglycerin stimulates PGI_2 production. It is not clear whether this partially accounts for this vasoactive compound's ability to relax smooth muscle. Thrombin also stimulates PGI_2 production, allowing some form of feedback inhibition of thrombosis at sites where the endothelial integrity is lost (76, 150).

Prostacyclin is one of a growing list of endothelial cell metabolites that appear to have a hormonelike action on adjacent cells. Furchgott and Zawadzki (49) described another unidentified smooth muscle relaxant produced by the endothelium. Apparently this material is neither adenosine (a cyclic nucleotide) nor a prostaglandin but may instead be related to the leukotrienes.

The most-studied metabolic effects of the endothelium relate to its production of kininase II, or angiotensin-converting enzyme (see the chapter by Ryan in this *Handbook*). This enzyme is required for angiotensin II formation and probably plays a critical role in the regulation of vascular tone and in aldosterone metabolism (113). The plasma level of angiotensin-converting enzyme, however, appears to be too low to account for the known rates of conversion of the decapeptide angiotensin I to the active octapeptide angiotensin II (95). The resolution of this paradox came after the enzyme was localized in the pulmonary endothelium and other vascular beds, both in vivo and in vitro. Little is known about this enzyme's role in endothelial injury, but there are intriguing reports of its suppression in vitro by hypoxia (96, 134).

In addition to their ability to induce smooth muscle contractility, endothelial cells may also stimulate or inhibit smooth muscle proliferation by producing other growth factors or inhibitors (see ENDOTHELIUM–SMOOTH MUSCLE INTERACTIONS, p. 553).

Endothelial cell metabolic functions also depend on their interaction with plasma solutes that have specific activities. In addition to angiotensin, endothelial cells also bind lipoprotein lipase and therefore have a major role in fatty acid metabolism (126). (See the chapter by Hamosh and Hamosh in this *Handbook*.) Interactions between the endothelium and the enzymes of the clotting cascade are particularly interesting. Thrombin bound to endothelial cells can both stimulate platelet thrombosis and inhibit it, the latter by stimulating endothelial cells to produce PGI_2 (3, 48, 150). The thrombin-receptor complex apparently also activates protein C, a protease that digests certain clotting factors. Thus when thrombin binds to intact endothelium, it sets up a negative feedback loop for coagulation (41, 97). Similarly endothelial cells synthesize a urokinaselike and tissue factor–like plasminogen activator, as well as an inhibitor of the plasminogen activator (80).

Endothelial cells also synthesize connective tissue matrix components of the vessel wall (117). The location of the endothelium may make this activity significant. For example cell-surface heparan sulfate may play a role in the selective permeability of the endothelium. Endothelial cell production of large amounts of heparan sulfate (17) may also explain some of the cells' noncoagulant and antithrombotic properties. The antithrombogenicity of the vessel wall probably depends on the polarity of endothelial cell deposition of collagen, rather than on the spectrum of connective tissue proteins made by these cells (6). In culture, endothelial cells make fibronectin and types III, IV, and V collagen. Collagen is highly thrombogenic, however, and endothelial cells form collagen layers only on their under surfaces, both in vivo and in vitro (117). In contrast, transformed endothelial cells lose this polarity and are thrombogenic on their upper surface as well (30, 153). Endothelial cells have also been characterized by their capacity to synthesize factor VIII antigen, or von Willebrand's factor, which is present in both the circulation and the subendothelium and plays an important role in the binding of platelets to surfaces denuded of endothelium (77, 93, 105, 118, 149).

Finally, endothelial cells share three special properties of monocytes: *1*) the presence of converting enzyme (113), 2) the presence of receptors for modified low-density lipoprotein (LDL) (137), and 3) the ability to serve as accessory cells in the T-cell immune response (2, 71). Endothelial cells and monocytes both have large numbers of receptors for acetylated LDL and smaller numbers of receptors for native LDL (137). This may be an important route for the transport of LDL modified by interaction with the end products of free-radical metabolism. Both cell types can also process antigens in a mixed lymphocyte system (2, 71). The significance of this observation for the endothelial cell is not clear. Macrophages (like endothelial cells) also produce a mitogen, the macrophage-derived growth factor (57, 88).

ENDOTHELIAL INJURY

A wide range of morphological changes accompany endothelial cell injury. Mason and Balis (89) reviewed these changes. In most cases the functional significance of the observed changes is not understood; in some cases, however, they may be due to cell death. Episodic reports suggest that intact endothelium may contain dead cells. Studies with the transmission electron microscope show a variety of changes that might be evidence of cell death. These include the presence of "dark cells" or "light cells," the loss of plasma membrane integrity, and the formation of blebs. In addition, when the endothelium is exposed to permeability tracers, occasional cells stain with HRP, ruthenium red, or lanthanum oxide. A related postmortem staining procedure with Alcian blue correlates with traditional trypan blue uptake (143).

Bondjers et al. (7) directly approached this question when they reported that the endothelium of arteries in short-term organ culture contains cells able to take up trypan blue. Such injury may have been artifactual, so Hansson et al. (63) confirmed these studies by demonstrating specific immunofluorescence for immunoglobulin G (IgG) in the cytoplasm of endothelial cells. Rabbit IgG is only present in vivo; therefore these experiments argue for a change in the intact animal. A cell permeable to IgG is likely to be necrotic. Nothing is known about the line between cell death and cell detachment, so it is reasonable to believe that dead cells may remain as part of a continuous endothelium for some time. The possible role of such cells in the responses of vessels to injury is open to speculation.

Relatively few attempts have been made to use an endothelial cell culture to define mechanisms of endothelial cell death. Sacks et al. (116) and Weiss et al. (149) studied mechanisms of oxygen radical–mediated endothelial damage caused by activated leukocytes. Harlan et al. (66) presented evidence for sublethal endothelial detachment by granule proteases as another major mechanism of leukocyte-mediated injury. Evidence indicates that thrombin can cause endothelial cells to retract from one another and that endotoxin can cause cell detachment (65). Cell detachment may be of particular interest in the lung. There are also reports that LDL from hyperlipemic serum can directly injure endothelial cells as demonstrated by chromium release, cell detachment, or decreased cell number. Effects are only seen in these studies in serum free of high-density lipoprotein and at lipoprotein concentrations well below their physiological range (69, 70, 139).

In terms of pulmonary pathology, the most important forms of cell injury are those related to inflammatory disease. A recent development in this area is that injury induces the development of FC and C3 receptors on endothelium (115). Viral infection also increases the adherence of viruses to the endothelium in vitro (84). Chemotactic peptides increase the adherence of neutrophils to endothelium, and sickle cell or malaria-infected erythrocytes show an abnormal adherence to endothelial cells (29, 73, 75, 144). More recently, Wedmore and Williams (148) showed that neutrophils are required for the chronic phase of edema formation. Their data suggest that this form of edema may require a vasodilator to allow leukocytes access and a chemotactic factor to stimulate the interaction of leukocytes with endothelium. These in vivo observations have been extended to in vitro systems that have monolayers of endothelium grown on filters and time-lapse microscopy to study the interaction of the two cell types (4, 140).

PLATELETS

Morphology and Content

Platelets contain several discrete populations of granules, as well as a series of vesicles and tubular profiles, whose contents have mainly been determined. The granules fall into two populations: the α-granules and the dense granules. The α-granules contain a number of proteins including PDGF, platelet factor 4, β-thromboglobulin, platelet-activating protein, and possibly some hydrolytic or lysosomal enzymes (although the latter have not been clearly determined) (110, 112). The dense granules contain calcium, ADP, serotonin, and possibly other substances; the vesicular structures contain lysosomal enzymes. The tubular system may be related to modes of transit and release of these granule-containing materials to the exterior of the cell. Platelets in the circulation have a discoid shape maintained by a peripheral ring of microtubules (110, 154). On exposure to an appropriate substrate (e.g., collagen or thrombin) this microtubular ring disaggregates, the platelet changes shape and contracts, and the surface of the platelet becomes "sticky." These changes result in the increased adherence of platelets to available surfaces and to one another. Adherence occurs concomitantly with platelet degranulation and causes the platelet-release reaction (154).

Platelet Function

Platelets play two principal roles in blood coagulation. Their most important role is their well-known ability to form a hemostatic plug. After the appropriate stimulation, the increased platelet adherence (as discussed above) causes the rapid formation of a massive three-dimensional meshwork or platelet plug that can, if the injury is small enough, induce hemostasis (154). When the platelets degranulate, a host of substances are released, including materials that can accelerate the cascade of coagulation factors present with the plasma. In addition, platelets can concentrate low-molecular-weight substances (e.g., serotonin and possibly others) from the plasma. Platelets can also release potent vasoactive agents (e.g., thromboxane), which may be important in hemostasis (154).

A second potentially important function of platelets may be to provide PDGF, a mitogenic substance, at sites of wounds or injury in order to initiate a proliferative response; this response is important in the connective tissue formation that eventually leads to healing and scar formation. This might happen in both normal wound repair and in abnormal wounding responses that may be progenitors of disease (particularly atherosclerosis) (109, 112). The PDGF is a potent mitogen, has been purified to a high degree, and has a number of effects on susceptible cells, among them the stimulation of DNA synthesis (Fig. 3).

Platelet-Derived Growth Factor

This growth factor's discovery resulted from the observation that serum made from cell-free plasma contained no mitogenic activity for fibroblasts or smooth muscle cells, whereas whole blood serum was well known to be important for mitogenesis and the maintenance of the cell's viability in culture. A systematic analysis of the blood cells that are responsible for whole blood serum's mitogenic capacity and that are absent in cell-free plasma-derived serum showed that the platelet was responsible for most of the activity in the whole blood serum.

Several laboratories have pursued the purification and characterization of PDGF (1, 39, 67, 104). This factor has been highly purified (>500,000-fold) and in pure form is somewhat heterogeneous, because it appears to contain four closely related proteins with molecular weights ranging from 27,000 to 31,000. Raines and Ross (104) used two-dimensional gels of proteolytic digests of each of these components to demonstrate that the four proteins are essentially identical, with only minor differences among them. This is presumably due to proteolytic cleavage, which may have occurred at the time of PDGF release, and the hydrolytic enzymes present when platelets aggregate and degranulate. The PDGF contains disulfide bonds and on reduction of these bonds, two inactive peptides of ~17,000 M_r and ~14,000 M_r form. Once formed they cannot reassociate into an active moiety.

Platelet-derived growth factor has been radioiodinated and the labeled factor retains all of its mitogenic activity (10, 68). Studies with radioiodinated PDGF have demonstrated that it binds selectively to a high-affinity receptor on the surface of susceptible cells, including skin fibroblasts, human and monkey arterial smooth muscle cells, Swiss 3T3 cells, and glial cells. Bowen-Pope and Ross (10) observed that the mitogenic capacity of PDGF correlates closely with its ability to bind to the high-affinity receptors on these cells. Of particular interest is the fact that vascular endothelial cells have no PDGF receptors (10).

Glenn et al. (56) identified the PDGF receptor as an ~167,000-M_r protein that binds specifically to PDGF; they also noted that PDGF competes for this binding, whereas other purified growth factors, e.g.,

FIG. 3. Hemostatic plug formation. Platelets are normally nonreactive to intact vascular endothelium. Vessel injury initiates platelet adherence with von Willebrand's factor (vWF) as essential plasma co-factor. Adherent platelets release dense-granule contents, including ADP, and α-granule contents, including platelet factor 4 (PF4), β-thromboglobulin (βTG), and platelet-derived growth factor (PDGF). Thrombin is generated locally through tissue factor (XII$_a$) and platelet procoagulant activity. Thromboxane A$_2$ (TXA$_2$) is synthesized from arachidonic acid liberated by membrane phospholipases. Released ADP, TXA$_2$, and thrombin recruit additional circulating platelets to the enlarging platelet mass. Thrombin-generated fibrin stabilizes the platelet mass. Prostacyclin (PGI$_2$) released by the vessel wall in response to thrombin limits thrombus formation by inhibiting further platelet aggregation. [From Harlan and Harker (64).]

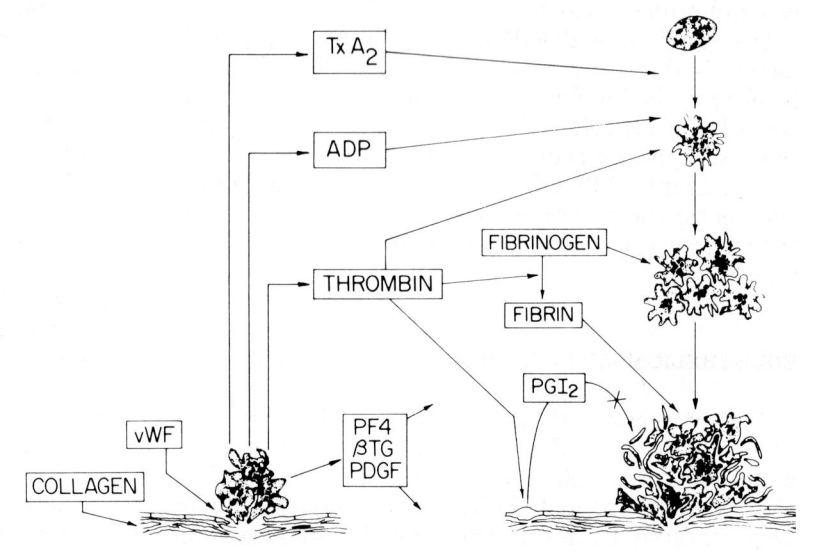

EGF, FGF, insulin, and LDL, cannot compete for it. Further studies of this receptor, its reaction with PDGF, and the subsequent effects of receptor binding by PDGF on susceptible cells should expand the understanding of its many biological effects.

Other effects besides mitogenesis occur in cells that bind to PDGF. Many of these changes occur before DNA synthesis, which requires 16–20 h before an increase in thymidine incorporation can be detected. Habenicht et al. (62) demonstrated a marked increase in phospholipid metabolism within minutes after the exposure of cells to PDGF. Phosphatidylinositol breakdown begins shortly after the exposure of 3T3 cells to PDGF, resulting in a rapid increase of intracellular diglyceride levels and the activation of a diglyceride lipase within the cells. The diglyceride lipase causes the release of monoglycerides and free arachidonic acid, which is a substrate for prostaglandins and leukotrienes. This activity may explain observations suggesting that the interaction of cells such as smooth muscle with PDGF leads to the formation of PGI_2.

In addition to increases in phospholipid metabolism, smooth muscle cells show increased binding of LDL and an increased degradation of LDL after exposure to PDGF (21). Smooth muscle cells also exhibit a marked increase in their rate of endogenous cholesterol synthesis after exposure to PDGF (in the absence of an exogenous source of cholesterol, like LDL). Therefore the exposure of smooth muscle cells to PDGF leads not only to augmented phospholipid metabolism but also to increased cholesterol metabolism, based on the availability of exogenous sources of cholesterol (e.g., LDL) and its effects on hydroxymethylglutaryl-CoA reductase, the rate-limiting enzyme of endogenous cholesterol synthesis.

Davies and Ross (32) observed that the capacity of cells to endocytose substances in culture is rapidly augmented by exposure to PDGF. In addition to increases in the rate of endocytosis, susceptible cells show increased synthesis of proteins, including collagen and proteoglycans.

One function of PDGF unobserved in other growth factors is that (in contrast to purified EGF, FGF, or insulin) it is highly chemotactic for fibroblasts or smooth muscle cells (61). This chemotactic property (ability to induce cells to migrate along a concentration gradient of PDGF) may have important ramifications for the accumulation of cells at sites of endothelial injury where platelet aggregation and release may occur.

ENDOTHELIUM–SMOOTH MUSCLE INTERACTIONS

The interactions that may take place between cells as closely juxtaposed as the endothelium and smooth muscle are not well understood. Minick et al. (91) observed that intimal thickening is much greater in areas covered by regenerated endothelium than in areas devoid of endothelium after balloon catheterization of an artery in a lipid-fed animal. The endothelium can synthesize a growth factor that stimulates the proliferation of smooth muscle cells in vitro. There is no evidence for such a factor existing in vivo, however. There is evidence for increased connective tissue and lipid synthesis at sites of endothelial injury. The critical factor may be the mechanisms controlling connective tissue synthesis at the sites of injury, particularly because glycosaminoglycans may be able to bind lipoproteins (107).

The endothelium is characteristically separated from the underlying smooth muscle by a basement membrane to which the endothelial cells are apparently loosely attached (47) and which serves as a crude filter for substances transported from the plasma into the subendothelial space. The endothelium is the first barrier determining which substances shall have access (and at what rate) to the underlying smooth muscle cells. Removing this barrier could alter transport rates, the interaction of platelets with the subendothelium, and the possibility that other blood cells (e.g., monocytes) might be attracted into the subendothelium. Thus the endothelium's capacity to withstand these various forces may be important in disease prevention and homeostatic maintenance.

The discovery that the endothelial cells make a potent growth factor (ECDGF) has stimulated the development of a new view of the endothelium. Gajdusek et al. (52) discovered ECDGF and found that medium lacking PDGF markedly stimulated the growth of smooth muscle cells and 3T3 cells, provided the medium had either been conditioned by endothelial cells or the endothelial cells and the other cells were co-cultured. They observed that ECDGF was also formed in serum-free medium. Endothelial cells maintained in serum-free medium for prolonged periods of time (up to 72 h) continued to form increasing amounts of ECDGF in culture. P. E. DiCorleto, D. Bowen-Pope, and R. Ross (unpublished observations) partially purified ECDGF and found that it and PDGF differed in several ways. They found that ECDGF binds to ion exchange resins under conditions in which PDGF does not bind and vice versa. However, ECDGF is similar to PDGF in that it appears to partially compete with PDGF in binding to smooth muscle cells, for example. It is not clear how these two substances are related to one another, if they are at all. Every type of arterial endothelium thus far studied (human, nonhuman primate, swine, bovine, and rabbit) forms ECDGF. No information as to whether capillary endothelial cells form a similar substance is available.

In contrast, Castellot et al. (21) described a growth inhibitor produced by endothelial cells. Apparently this material is a form of heparan sulfate. Consistent with this observation, Chamley-Campbell et al. (24) found that endothelial cell conditioned medium can maintain freshly dispersed smooth muscle cells in a contractile state. In the absence of endothelial cells they found that smooth muscle cells undergo a change to a synthetic phenotype capable of proliferation but not contractility.

In addition to producing growth factors, endothelial cells provide some means of entry for other blood cells, including platelets and monocytes, into the subjacent tissue. The monocyte is a well-known source of tissue macrophages. Pulmonary capillary endothelium somehow permits monocytes to enter the pulmonary interstitial connective tissue via junctional complexes between the endothelial cells. Factors that are chemotactic for monocytes and bring them into these tissues have only been partially identified. The monocyte's ability to enter the alveolar connective tissue is important in relation to this cell's role in inflammation in the lung. Furthermore intimal accumulation of macrophages in medium and large arteries may in some cases lead to the formation of early atherosclerotic lesions, the "fatty streak," and possibly more-advanced lesions as well. Under these circumstances the endothelium plays a key role either by permitting monocyte entry or by actively promoting monocyte movement into the underlying connective tissue. After it becomes an activated macrophage the monocyte can have long-term effects on the connective tissue because it can also produce a growth factor, the macrophage-derived growth factor, which is an extraordinarily potent mitogen with various effects on the surrounding cells and tissues (57). Although the macrophage-derived growth factor (together with ECDGF and PDGF) may be important in the fibroproliferative responses of reactions ranging from inflammation and wound repair to atherogenesis, its function is not discussed in this review.

PLATELET-ENDOTHELIAL CELL INTERACTIONS

By design endothelial cells characteristically form a nonthrombogenic or thromboresistant surface. Apparently two principal mechanisms are involved in this. The first of these mechanisms is the endothelial cell's capacity to produce PGI_2. Prostacyclin is one of the most potent antiaggregatory substances known and is also a strong vasodilator. Endothelial cells exposed to arachidonic acid form PGI_2 via a cyclooxygenase enzyme pathway that is also used in the formation of thromboxane A_2 (65, 119). Platelets can apparently act as a source of arachidonic acid for the endothelium, and the endothelium's formation of PGI_2 may be particularly important in preventing thrombus formation (87). Endothelial cells also contain a surface coat that interferes with platelet-endothelial cell interactions and that may be important in preventing platelet adherence (100, 131, 147). It has been postulated that when endothelial cells are injured or altered, this surface coat's capacity to prevent platelet interactions may be altered. Therefore it is possible that platelet adherence and perhaps monocyte adherence at sites of such injured endothelium may be important first steps in the entry of platelets and monocytes into the underlying connective tissue.

SUMMARY

The major advance in our understanding of platelet-endothelial cell interactions has been the recognition that the endothelium is more than just a passive cell layer. It is a metabolically active tissue, with hormonal and synthetic activities comparable to a major organ. Some of those properties, particularly the synthesis of prostaglandins and of thrombogenic and antithrombogenic connective tissue materials, relate directly to the interaction of the platelet with sites of endothelial injury. The endothelium may produce substances that modulate the behavior of the underlying smooth muscle cells and may, in this way, modulate the effects of platelets and platelet products on the vessel wall. Evidence also shows that the endothelium plays an active role in coagulation and that it secretes both procoagulant and anticoagulant macromolecules. Finally, advances have been made in our understanding of the metabolic interactions of the endothelial cells with lymphocytes and monocytes in the immune response. Whether similar phenomena occur in the endothelial cells' relationships with leukocytes and platelets remains unexplored.

REFERENCES

1. ANTONIADES, H. N., C. D. SCHER, AND C. D. STILES. Purification of human platelet-derived growth factor. *Proc. Natl. Acad. Sci. USA* 76: 1809-1813, 1979.
2. ASHIDA, E. R., A. R. JOHNSON, AND P. E. LIPSKY. Human endothelial cell-lymphocyte interaction. Endothelial cells function as accessory cells necessary for mitogen-induced human T lymphocyte activation in vitro. *J. Clin. Invest.* 67: 1490-1499, 1981.
3. AWBREY, B. J., S. C. HOAK, AND W. G. OWEN. Binding of human thrombin to cultured human endothelial cells. *J. Biol. Chem.* 254: 4092-4095, 1979.
4. BEESELEY, J. E., J. D. PEARSON, A. HUTCHINGS, J. S. CARLETON, AND J. GORDON. Granulocyte migration through endothelium in culture. *J. Cell Sci.* 38: 237-248, 1979.
5. BIRDWELL, C. R., D. GOSPODAROWICZ, AND G. L. NICOLSON. Factors from 3T3 cells stimulate proliferation of cultured vascular endothelial cells. *Nature London* 268: 528-531, 1977.
6. BIRDWELL, C. R., D. GOSPODAROWICZ, AND G. L. NICOLSON. Identification, localization, and role of fibronectin in cultured bovine endothelial cells. *Proc. Natl. Acad. Sci. USA* 75: 3273-3277, 1978.
7. BONDJERS, G., S. BJORKERUD, R. BRATTSAND, A. BYLOCK, G. HANSSON, AND H.-A. HANSSON. Endothelial injury in normocholesterolemic and hypercholesterolemic rabbits. In:

International Conference on Atherosclerosis, edited by L. A. Carlson, R. Paoletti, and C. R. Weber. New York: Raven, 1978, p. 567-573.

8. BOOYSE, F. M., A. J. QUARFOOT, S. BELL, D. N. FASS, J. C. LEWIS, AND K. MANN. Cultured von Willebrand porcine aortic endothelial cells: an in vitro model for studying the molecular defects of the disease. *Proc. Natl. Acad. Sci. USA* 74: 5702-5750, 1977.

9. BOOYSE, F. M., B. J. SEDLAK, AND M. J. RAFELSON, JR. Culture of arterial endothelial cells. Characterization and growth of bovine aortic cells. *Thromb. Diath. Haemorrh.* 34: 825-839, 1975.

10. BOWEN-POPE, D., AND R. ROSS. Platelet-derived growth factor. II. Specific binding on cultured cells. *J. Biol. Chem.* 257: 5161-5171, 1982.

11. BOWMAN, P. D., A. L. BETZ, D. AR, J. S. WOLINSKY, J. B. PENNEY, R. R. SHIVERS, AND G. W. GOLDSTEIN. Primary culture of capillary endothelium from rat brain. *In Vitro* 17: 353-362, 1981.

12. BROWN, M. S., R. G. W. ANDERSON, AND J. L. GOLDSTEIN. Role of the coated endocytic vesicle in the uptake of receptor-bound low density lipoprotein in human fibroblasts. *Cell* 10: 351-364, 1977.

13. BRUNS, R. R., AND G. E. PALADE. Studies on blood capillaries. I. General organization of blood capillaries in muscle. *J. Cell Biol.* 37: 244-276, 1969.

14. BUNDGAARD, M. Transport pathways in capillaries—in search of pores. *Annu. Rev. Physiol.* 42: 325-336, 1980.

15. BUNDGAARD, M., J. FRØKJAER-JENSEN, AND C. CRONE. Endothelial plasmalemmal vesicles as elements in a system of branching invaginations from the cell surface. *Proc. Natl. Acad. Sci. USA* 76: 6439-6442, 1979.

16. BUONASSISI, V. Sulfated mucopolysaccharide synthesis and secretion in endothelial cell cultures. *Exp. Cell Res.* 76: 363-368, 1973.

17. BUONASSISI, V., AND M. ROOT. Enzymatic degradation of heparin-related mucopolysaccharides from the surface of endothelial cell cultures. *Biochim. Biophys. Acta* 385: 1-10, 1975.

18. BUONASSISI, V., AND J. C. VENTER. Hormone and neurotransmitter receptors in an established vascular endothelial cell line. *Proc. Natl. Acad. Sci. USA* 73: 1612-1616, 1976.

19. BUZNEY, S. M., AND S. J. MASSICOTTE. Retinal vessels: proliferation of endothelium in vitro. *Invest. Ophthalmol. Visual Sci.* 18: 1191-1195, 1979.

20. CASLEY-SMITH, J. R. Freeze-substitution of capillary endothelium—the artefactual nature of transendothelial channels and the forms of attached vesicles. *Micron* 11: 461-462, 1980.

21. CASTELLOT, J. J., M. L. ADDONIZIO, R. ROSENBERG, AND M. J. KARNOVSKY. Cultured endothelial cells produce heparin-like inhibitor of smooth muscle cell growth. *J. Cell Biol.* 90: 372-379, 1981.

22. CASTELLOT, J. J., M. J. KARNOVSKY, AND B. M. SPIEGELMAN. Potent stimulation of vascular endothelial cell growth by differentiated 3T3 adipocytes. *Proc. Natl. Acad. Sci. USA* 77: 6007-6011, 1980.

23. CHAIT, A., R. ROSS, J. J. ALBERS, AND E. L. BIERMAN. Platelet-derived growth factor stimulates activity of low density lipoprotein receptors. *Proc. Natl. Acad. Sci. USA* 77: 4084-4088, 1980.

24. CHAMLEY-CAMPBELL, J. H., G. R. CAMPBELL, AND R. ROSS. Phenotype-dependent response of cultured aortic smooth muscle to serum mitogens. *J. Cell Biol.* 89: 379-383, 1981.

25. COETZEE, G. A., O. STEIN, AND Y. STEIN. Uptake and degradation of low density lipoproteins (LDL) by confluent, contact-inhibited bovine and human endothelium cells exposed to physiological concentrations of LDL. *Atherosclerosis* 33: 425-431, 1979.

26. COHEN, S., G. CARPENTER, AND K. J. LEMBACH. Interaction of epidermal growth factor (EGF) with cultured fibroblasts. In: *Advances in Metabolic Disorders*, edited by R. Luft and K. Hall. New York: Academic, 1975, p. 265-284.

27. COLBURN, P., AND V. BUONASSISI. Estrogen-binding sites in endothelial cell cultures. *Science* 201: 817-819, 1978.

28. COTTA-PEREIRA, G., H. SAGE, P. BORNSTEIN, R. ROSS, AND S. SCHWARTZ. Studies of morphologically atypical ("sprouting") cultures of bovine aortic endothelial cells. Growth characteristics and connective tissue protein synthesis. *J. Cell. Physiol.* 102: 183-191, 1980.

29. CRADDOCK, P. R., J. FEHR, K. L. BRIGHAM, R. S. KRONENBERG, AND H. S. JACOB. Complement and leukocyte-mediated pulmonary dysfunction in hemodialysis. *N. Engl. J. Med.* 296: 769-774, 1977.

30. CURWEN, K. D., M. A. GIMBRONE, JR., AND R. I. HANDIN. In vitro studies of thromboresistance: the role of prostacyclin (PGI_2) in platelet adhesion to cultured normal and virally transformed human vascular endothelial cells. *Lab. Invest.* 42: 366-374, 1980.

31. D'AMORE, P. A., AND D. SHEPRO. Stimulation of growth and calcium influx in cultured bovine aortic endothelial cells by platelets and vasoactive substances. *J. Cell. Physiol.* 92: 177-184, 1977.

32. DAVIES, P., AND R. ROSS. Mediation of pinocytosis in cultured arterial smooth muscle and endothelial cells by platelet-derived growth factor. *J. Cell Biol.* 79: 663-671, 1978.

33. DAVIES, P., AND R. ROSS. Growth-mediated, density-dependent inhibition of endocytosis in cultured arterial smooth muscle cells. *Exp. Cell Res.* 129: 329-336, 1980.

34. DAVISON, P. M., K. BENSCH, AND M. A. KARASEK. Growth and morphology of rabbit marginal vessel endothelium in cell culture. *J. Cell Biol.* 85: 187-198, 1980.

35. DAVISON, P. M., K. BENSCH, AND M. A. KARASEK. Isolation and growth of endothelial cells from the microvessels of the newborn human foreskin in cell culture. *J. Invest. Dermatol.* 75: 316-321, 1980.

36. DEBAULT, L. E., E. HENRIQUEZ, M. N. HART, AND C. A. CANCILLA. Cerebral microvessels and derived cells in tissue culture. II. Establishment, identification, and preliminary characterization of an endothelial cell line. *In Vitro* 17: 480-494, 1981.

37. DEBAULT, L. E., L. E. KAHN, S. P. FROMMES, AND P. A. CANCILLA. Cerebral microvessels and derived cells in tissue culture: isolation and preliminary characterization. *In Vitro* 15: 437-440, 1979.

38. DELVECCHIO, P. J., U. S. RYAN, AND J. W. RYAN. Isolation of capillary segments from rat adrenal gland (Abstract). *J. Cell Biol.* 75: 73A, 1977.

39. DEUEL, T. F., J. S. HUANG, R. T. PROFFITT, J. U. BAENZIGER, D. CHANG, AND B. B. KENNEDY. Human platelet-derived growth factor. Purification and resolution into two active protein fractions. *J. Biol. Chem.* 256: 8896-8899, 1981.

40. DUTHU, G. S., AND J. R. SMITH. In vitro proliferation and lifespan of bovine aorta endothelial cells: effects of culture conditions and fibroblast growth factor. *J. Cell. Physiol.* 103: 385-392, 1980.

41. ESMON, C. T., AND W. G. OWEN. Identification of an endothelial cell cofactor for thrombin-catalyzed activation of protein C. *Proc. Natl. Acad. Sci. USA* 78: 2249-2252, 1981.

42. FIELDING, C. J., I. VLODAVSKY, P. E. FIELDING, AND D. GOSPODAROWICZ. Characteristics of chylomicron binding and lipid uptake by endothelial cells in culture. *J. Biol. Chem.* 254: 8861-8868, 1979.

43. FLORENTIN, R. A., S. C. NAM, K. T. LEE, AND W. A. THOMAS. Increased ^{3}H-thymidine incorporation into endothelial cells of swine fed cholesterol for 3 days. *Exp. Mol. Pathol.* 10: 250-255, 1969.

44. FOLKMAN, J., C. C. HAUDENSCHILD, AND B. R. ZETTER. Long-term culture of capillary endothelial cells. *Proc. Natl. Acad. Sci. USA* 76: 5217-5221, 1979.

45. FRANK, R. N., V. E. KINSEY, K. W. FRANK, K. P. MIKUS, AND A. RANDOLPH. In vitro proliferation of endothelial cells from kitten retinal capillaries. *Invest. Ophthalmol. Visual Sci.* 18: 1195-1200, 1979.

46. FRIEDMAN, R. J., M. B. STEMERMAN, B. WENZ, S. MOORE, J. GAULDIE, M. GENT, M. L. TIELL, AND T. H. SPAET. The effect of thrombocytopenia on experimental atherosclerotic lesion formation in rabbits. Smooth muscle cell proliferation and re-endothelialization. *J. Clin. Invest.* 60: 1191–1201, 1977.
47. FRY, D. I. Acute vascular endothelial changes associated with increased blood velocity gradients. *Circ. Rev.* 22: 165–197, 1968.
48. FRY, G. L., R. L. CZERVIONKE, J. C. HOAK, J. B. SMITH, AND D. L. HAYCRAFT. Platelet adherence to cultured vascular cells: influence of prostacyclin PGI_2. *Blood* 55: 271–275, 1980.
49. FURCHGOTT, R. F., AND J. V. ZAWADZKI. The obligatory role of endothelial cells in the relaxation of arterial smooth muscle by acetylcholine. *Nature London* 288: 373–376, 1980.
50. FUSTER, W., E. J. BOWIE, J. C. LEWIS, D. N. FASS, C. A. OWEN, JR., AND A. L. BROWN. Resistance to arteriosclerosis in pigs with von Willebrand's disease. Spontaneous and high cholesterol diet-induced arteriosclerosis. *J. Clin. Invest.* 61: 722–730, 1978.
51. GABBIANI, G., G. ELEMER, C. GUELPA, M. B. VALLOTTAN, M. C. BADONNEL, AND I. HÜTTNER. Morphologic and functional changes of the aortic intima during experimental hypertension. *Am. J. Pathol.* 96: 399–422, 1979.
52. GAJDUSEK, C., P. DICORLETO, R. ROSS, AND S. SCHWARTZ. An endothelial cell-derived growth factor. *J. Cell Biol.* 85: 467–472, 1980.
53. GAJDUSEK, C. M., AND S. M. SCHWARTZ. Ability of endothelial cells to condition culture medium. *J. Cell. Physiol.* 110: 35–42, 1982.
54. GIMBRONE, M. A., JR. Culture of vascular endothelium. In: *Progress in Hemostasis and Thrombosis*, edited by T. H. Spaet. New York: Grune & Stratton, 1976, vol. 3, p. 1–28.
55. GIMBRONE, M. A., JR., R. S. COTRAN, AND J. FOLKMAN. Human vascular endothelial cells in culture. Growth and DNA synthesis. *J. Cell Biol.* 60: 673–684, 1974.
56. GLENN, K., D. F. BOWEN-POPE, AND R. ROSS. Platelet-derived growth factor. III. Identification of a platelet-derived growth factor receptor by affinity labeling. *J. Biol. Chem.* 257: 5172–5176, 1982.
57. GLENN, K. C., AND R. ROSS. Human monocyte-derived growth factor(s) for mesenchymal cells: activation of secretion by endotoxin and concanavalin A. *Cell* 25: 603–615, 1981.
58. GOSPODAROWICZ, D., G. GREENBURG, H. BIALECKI, AND B. R. ZETTER. Factors involved in the modulation of cell proliferation in vivo and in vitro: the role of fibroblast and epidermal growth factors in the proliferative response of mammalian cells. *In Vitro* 14: 85–118, 1978.
59. GOSPODAROWICZ, D., AND C. ILL. Extracellular matrix and control of proliferation of vascular endothelial cells. *J. Clin. Invest.* 65: 1351–1364, 1980.
60. GREENBURG, G., I. VLODAVSKY, J. M. FOIDART, AND D. GOSPODAROWICZ. Conditioned medium from endothelial cell cultures can restore the normal phenotypic expression of vascular endothelium maintained in vitro in the presence of fibroblast growth factor. *J. Cell. Physiol.* 103: 333–347, 1980.
61. GROTENDORST, G. R., H. SEPA, H. K. KLEINMAN, AND G. R. MARTIN. Attachment of smooth muscle cells to collagen and their migration toward platelet-derived growth factor. *Proc. Natl. Acad. Sci. USA* 78: 3669–3672, 1981.
62. HABENICHT, H. J. R., J. A. GLOMSET, W. C. KING, C. NIST, C. D. MITCHELL, AND R. ROSS. Early changes in phosphatidylinositol and arachidonic acid metabolism in quiescent Swiss 3T3 cells stimulated to divide by platelet-derived growth factor. *J. Biol. Chem.* 256: 12329–12335, 1981.
63. HANSSON, G. K., T. BJÖRNHEDEN, A. BYLOCK, AND G. BONDJERS. Fc-dependent binding of monocytes to areas with endothelial injury in the rabbit aorta. *Exp. Mol. Pathol.* 34: 264–280, 1981.
64. HARKER, L., R. ROSS, S. SLICHTER, AND C. SCOTT. Homocystine-induced arteriosclerosis: the role of endothelial cell injury and platelet response in its genesis. *J. Clin. Invest.* 58: 731–741, 1976.
65. HARLAN, J. M., AND L. A. HARKER. Hemostasis, thrombosis, and thromboembolic disorders. The role of arachidonic acid metabolites in platelet-vessel wall interactions. *Med. Clin. North Am.* 65: 855–880, 1981.
66. HARLAN, J. M., P. D. KILLEN, L. A. HARKER, G. E. STRIKER, AND D. G. WRIGHT. Neutrophil-mediated endothelial injury in vitro: mechanisms of cell detachment. *J. Clin. Invest.* 68: 1394–1403, 1981.
67. HELDIN, C.-H., B. WESTERMARK, AND A. WASTESON. Platelet-derived growth factor. Purification and partial characterization. *Proc. Natl. Acad. Sci. USA* 76: 3722–3726, 1979.
68. HELDIN, C.-H., B. WESTERMARK, AND A. WASTESON. Specific receptors for PDGF on cells derived from connective tissue. *Proc. Natl. Acad. Sci. USA* 78: 3664–3668, 1981.
69. HENRIKSEN, T., S. A. EVENSEN, AND B. CARLANDER. Injury to human endothelial cells in culture induced by low density lipoproteins. *Scand. J. Clin. Lab. Invest.* 39: 361–368, 1979.
70. HESSLER, J. R., A. L. ROBERTSON, AND G. M. CHISOLM. LDL-induced cytotoxicity and its inhibition by HDL in human vascular smooth muscle and endothelial cells in culture. *Atherosclerosis* 32: 213–229, 1979.
71. HIRSCHBERG, H., O. T. BERGH, AND E. THORSHY. Antigen presenting properties of human vascular endothelial cells. *J. Exp. Med.* 152: 249–255, 1980.
72. HJELLE, J. T., J. BAIRD-LAMBERT, G. CARDINALE, S. SPECOR, AND S. UDENFRIEND. Isolated microvessels: the blood-brain barrier in vitro. *Proc. Natl. Acad. Sci. USA* 75: 4544–4548, 1978.
73. HOOVER, R. L., R. T. BRIGGS, AND M. J. KARNOVSKY. The adhesive interaction between polymorphonuclear leukocytes and endothelial cell in vitro. *Cell* 14: 423–428, 1978.
74. INGERMAN-WOJENSKI, C., M. J. SILVER, J. B. SMITH, AND E. MACARAK. Bovine endothelial cells in culture produce thromboxane as well as prostacyclin. *J. Clin. Invest.* 67: 1292–1296, 1981.
75. JACOBS, H. S., R. P. HEBBEL, O. YAMADA, AND C. F. MOLDOW. Abnormal adherence of sickle erythrocytes to cultured vascular endothelium. *J. Clin. Invest.* 65: 154–160, 1980.
76. JAFFE, E. A., R. L. NACHMAN, C. G. BECKER, AND C. R. MINICK. Culture of human endothelial cells derived from umbilical veins. *J. Clin. Invest.* 52: 2745–2756, 1973.
77. JONES, T. R., K. J. KAO, S. V. PIZZO, AND D. D. BIGNER. Endothelial cell surface expression and binding of factor VIII/von Willebrand's factor. *Am. J. Pathol.* 103: 304–308, 1981.
78. KARNOVSKY, M. J. The ultrastructural basis of capillary permeability studied with peroxidase as a tracer. *J. Cell Biol.* 35: 213–236, 1967.
79. LANDIS, E. M., AND J. R. PAPPENHEIMER. Exchange of substances through the capillary walls. In: *Handbook of Physiology. Circulation*, edited by W. F. Hamilton. Washington, DC: Am. Physiol. Soc., 1963, sect. 2, vol. II, chapt. 29, p. 961–1034.
80. LEVIN, E. G., AND D. J. LOSKUTOFF. Serum mediated suppression of cell associated plasminogen activator in cultured endothelial cells. *Cell* 22: 701–707, 1980.
81. LEVIN, R. I., E. A. JAFFE, B. B. WEKSLER, AND K. TACK-GOLDMAN. Nitroglycerin stimulates synthesis of prostacyclin by cultured human endothelial cells. *J. Clin. Invest.* 67: 762–769, 1981.
82. LEVINE, E. M., AND S. N. MUELLER. Cultured vascular endothelial cells as a model system for the study of cellular senescence. *Int. Rev. Cytol. Suppl.* 10: 67–76, 1979.
83. LEWIS, L. J., J. C. HOAK, R. D. MACA, AND G. L. FRY. Replication of human endothelial cells in culture. *Science* 181: 453–454, 1973.
84. MACGREGOR, R. R., H. M. FRIEDMAN, E. J. MACARAK, AND N. A. KEFALIDES. Virus infection of endothelial cells increases granulocyte adherence. *J. Clin. Invest.* 65: 1469–1477, 1980.
85. MACIAG, T., J. CERUNDOLO, S. ILSLEY, P. R. KELLEY, AND R. FORAND. An endothelial cell growth factor from bovine hypothalamus: identification and partial characterization. *Proc. Natl. Acad. Sci. USA* 76: 5674–5678, 1979.

86. MAJNO, G. Ultrastructure of the vascular membrane. In: *Handbook of Physiology. Circulation*, edited by W. F. Hamilton. Washington, DC: Am. Physiol. Soc., 1965, sect. 2, vol. III, chapt. 64, p. 2293-2375.
87. MARCUS, A. J., B. B. WEKSLER, E. A. JAFFE, AND M J. BROEKMAN. Synthesis of prostacyclin from platelet-derived endoperoxides by cultured human endothelial cells. *J. Clin. Invest.* 66: 979-986, 1980.
88. MARTIN, B. M., M. A. GIMBRONE, JR., G. R. MAJEAU, E. R. UNANUE, AND R. S. COTRAN. Monocyte/macrophage-derived growth factor production: modulation by cold-insoluble globulin and extracellular matrix (Abstract). *Circulation* 64, Suppl. 4: 214, 1981.
89. MASON, R. G., AND J. U. BALIS. Pathology of the endothelium. *Pathobiol. Cell Membr.* 2: 425-471, 1980.
90. MEYRICK, B., AND L. REID. Endothelial and subintimal changes in rat hilar pulmonary artery during recovery from hypoxia. A quantitative ultrastructural study. *Lab. Invest.* 42: 603-615, 1980.
91. MINICK, C. R., M. B. STEMERMAN, AND W. INSULL, JR. Effect of regenerated endothelium on lipid accumulation in the arterial wall. *Proc. Natl. Acad. Sci. USA* 74: 1724-1728, 1977.
92. MOORE, A., R. J. FRIEDMAN, D. P. SINGAL, J. GAULDIE, AND M. A. BLAJCHMAN. Inhibition of injury induced thromboatherosclerotic lesions by antiplatelet serum in rabbits. *Thromb. Diath. Haemorrh.* 35: 70-81, 1976.
93. NACHMAN, R. L., E. A. JAFFE, AND B. FERRIS. Multiple forms of endothelial cell factor VIII related antigen. *Biochim. Biophys. Acta* 667: 361-369, 1981.
94. NEES, S., A. L. GERBES, E. GERLACH, AND J. STAUBESAND. Isolation, identification, and continuous culture of coronary endothelial cells from guinea pig hearts. *Eur. J. Cell Biol.* 24: 287-297, 1981.
95. NG, K. K. F., AND J. R. VANE. Conversion of angiotensin I to angiotensin II. *Nature London* 216: 762-766, 1967.
96. O'BRODOVICH, H. M., S. A. STALCUP, L. M. PANG, J. S. LIPSET, AND R. B. MELLINS. Bradykinin production and increased pulmonary endothelial permeability during acute respiratory failure in unanesthetized sheep. *J. Clin. Invest.* 67: 514-522, 1981.
97. OWEN, W. G., AND C. T. ESMON. Functional properties of an endothelial cell cofactor for thrombin-catalyzed activation of protein C. *J. Biol. Chem.* 256: 5532-5535, 1981.
98. PARSHLEY, M. S., J. M. CERRETA, I. MANDL, J. A. FIERER, AND G. M. TURINO. Characteristics of a clone of endothelial cells derived from a line of normal adult rat lung cells. *In Vitro* 15: 709-722, 1979.
99. PAULI, B. U., S. N. ANDERSON, V. A. MEMOLI, AND K. Z. KUETTNER. The isolation and characterization in vitro of normal epithelial cells, endothelial cells and fibroblasts from rat urinary bladder. *Tissue Cell* 12: 419-436, 1980.
100. PELIKAN, P., M. A. GIMBRONE, JR., AND R. S. COTRAN. Distribution and movement of anionic cell surface sites in cultured human vascular endothelial cells. *Atherosclerosis* 32: 69-80, 1979.
101. PHILLIPS, P., P. KUMAR, S. KUMAR, AND M. WAGHE. Isolation and characterization of endothelial cells from rat and cow brain white matter. *J. Anat.* 129: 261-272, 1979.
102. PICK, R., P. J. JOHNSON, AND G. GLICK. Deleterious effects of hypertension on the development of aortic and coronary atherosclerosis in stumptail macaques (*Macaca speciosa*) on an atherogenic diet. *Circ. Res.* 35: 472-482, 1974.
103. POLLACK, O. J., AND T. KASAI. Appearance and behavior of aortic cells in vitro. *Am. J. Med. Sci.* 248: 71-78, 1964.
104. RAINES, E. W., AND R. ROSS. Platelet-derived growth factor. I. High yield purification and evidence for multiple forms. *J. Biol. Chem.* 257: 5154-5160, 1982.
105. RAND, J. H., J. J. SUSSMAN, R. E. GORDON, S. V. CHU, AND V. SOLOMAN. Localization of factor-VIII-related antigen in human vascular subendothelium. *Blood* 55: 752-756, 1980.
106. RENKIN, E. M. Transport pathways through capillary endothelium. *Microvasc. Res.* 15: 123-135, 1978.
107. RICHARDSON, M., I. IHNATOWYCZ, AND S. MOORE. Glycosaminoglycan distribution in rabbit aortic wall following balloon catheter deendothelialization. An ultrastructural study. *Lab. Invest.* 43: 509-516, 1980.
108. ROSEN, E. M., S. N. MUELLER, J. P. NOVERAL, AND E. M. LEVINE. Proliferative characteristics of clonal endothelial cell strains. *J. Cell. Physiol.* 107: 123-137, 1981.
109. ROSS, R. George Lyman Duff Memorial Lecture. Atherosclerosis: a problem of the biology of arterial wall cells and their interaction with blood components. *Arteriosclerosis* 1: 293-311, 1981.
110. ROSS, R. The platelet-derived growth factor. In: *Tissue Growth Factors*, edited by R. Baserga. Heidelberg, West Germany: Springer-Verlag, 1981, p. 133-159.
111. ROSS, R., AND L. HARKER. Hyperlipidemia and atherosclerosis. Chronic hyperlipidemia initiates and maintains lesions by endothelial cell desquamation and lipid accumulation. *Science* 193: 1094-1100, 1976.
112. ROSS, R., AND A. VOGEL. The platelet-derived growth factor. *Cell* 14: 203-210, 1978.
113. RYAN, U. S. Structural basis for metabolic activity. *Annu. Rev. Physiol.* 44: 223-239, 1982.
114. RYAN, U. S., E. CLEMENT, D. HABILSTAN, AND J. W. RYAN. Isolation and culture of pulmonary artery endothelial cells. *Tissue Cell* 10: 535-554, 1978.
115. RYAN, U. S., D. R. SCHULTZ, AND J. W. RYAN. Fc and C3b receptors on pulmonary endothelial cells: induction by injury. *Science* 214: 557-558, 1981.
116. SACKS, T., C. F. MOLDOW, P. R. CRADDOCK, T. K. BOWERS, AND H. S. JACOB. Oxygen radicals mediate endothelial cell damage by complement-stimulated granulocytes. *J. Clin. Invest.* 61: 1161-1167, 1978.
117. SAGE, H., P. PRITZL, AND P. BORNSTEIN. Characterization of cell matrix associated collagens synthesized by aortic endothelial cells in culture. *J. Biol. Chem.* 20: 436-442, 1981.
118. SAKARIASSEN, K. S., P. A. BOLHUIS, AND J. J. SIXMA. Human blood platelet adhesion to artery subendothelium is mediated by factor VIII-von Willebrand factor bound to the subendothelium. *Nature London* 279: 636-638, 1979.
119. SAMUELSSON, B., G. FOLCO, E. GRANSTRÖM, H. KINDAHL, AND C. MALMSTEN. Prostaglandins and thromboxanes: biochemical and physiological considerations. *Adv. Prostaglandin Thromboxane Res.* 4: 1-25, 1978.
120. SCHWARTZ, S. M. Hypertension, endothelial injury, and atherosclerosis. *Cardiovasc. Med.* 2: 991-1002, 1977.
121. SCHWARTZ, S. M. Selection and characterization of bovine aortic endothelial cells. *In Vitro* 14: 966-980, 1978.
122. SCHWARTZ, S. M., AND E. P. BENDITT. Aortic endothelial cell replication. I. Effects of age and hypertension in the rat. *Circ. Res.* 41: 248-255, 1977.
123. SCHWARTZ, S. M., C. M. GAJDUSEK, M. A. REIDY, S. C. SELDEN III, AND C. C. HAUDENSCHILD. Maintenance of integrity in aortic endothelium. *Federation Proc.* 39: 2618-2625, 1980.
124. SCHWARTZ, S. M., S. C. SELDEN III, AND P. BOWMAN. Growth control in aortic endothelium at wound edges. In: *Hormones and Cell Culture*, edited by R. Ross and G. Sato. Cold Spring Harbor, NY: Cold Spring Harbor Lab., 1979, p. 593-610. (Cold Spring Harbor Conf. Cell Proliferation, 3rd, 1979.)
125. SCHWARTZ, S. M., AND D. M. STANDAERT. Endothelial cell turnover in rats: effects of angiotensin, age and chronic hypertension. *Atheroscler. Rev.* 9: 109-121, 1982.
126. SCOW, R., E. J. BLANCHETTE-MACKIE, AND L. C. SMITH. Role of capillary endothelium on the clearance of chylomicrons. *Circ. Res.* 39: 149-162, 1976.
127. SHERER, G. K., T. P. FITZHARRIS, W. P. FAULK, AND E. C. LEROY. Cultivation of microvascular endothelial cells from human preputial skin. *In Vitro* 16: 675-684, 1980.
128. SIMIONESCU, N., M. SIMIONESCU, AND G. E. PALADE. Permeability of intestinal capillaries. Pathway followed by dextrans

and glycogens. *J. Cell Biol.* 53: 365–392, 1972.

129. SIMIONESCU, M., N. SIMIONESCU, AND G. E. PALADE. Segmental differentiations of cell junctions in the vascular endothelium. The microvasculature. *J. Cell Biol.* 67: 863–885, 1975.

130. SIMIONESCU, N., M. SIMIONESCU, AND G. E. PALADE. Structural-functional correlates in the transendothelial exchange of water-soluble macromolecules. *Thromb. Res.* 8, Suppl. 11: 257–269, 1976.

131. SIMIONESCU, N., M. SIMIONESCU, AND G. E. PALADE. Differentiated microdomains on the luminal surface of capillary endothelium. I. Preferential distribution of anionic sites. *J. Cell Biol.* 90: 605–613, 1981.

132. SLATER, D. N., AND J. M. SLOAN. The porcine endothelial cell in tissue culture. *Atherosclerosis* 21: 259–274, 1975.

133. SPATZ, M., J. BEMBRY, R. DODSON, H. HERVONEN, AND M. R. MURRAY. Endothelial cell cultures derived from isolated cerebral microvessels. *Brain Res.* 191: 577–582, 1980.

134. STALCUP, S. A., J. S. LIPSET, J.-M. WOAN, P. LEUONBERGER, AND R. B. MELLINS. Inhibition of angiotensin converting enzyme activity in cultured endothelial cells by hypoxia. *J. Clin. Invest.* 63: 966–976, 1979.

135. STAUB, N. C. Brief reviews: pulmonary edema due to increased microvascular permeability to fluid and protein. *Circ. Res.* 43: 143–151, 1978.

136. STEIN, O., AND Y. STEIN. High density lipoproteins reduce the uptake of low density lipoproteins by human endothelial cells in culture. *Biochim. Biophys. Acta* 431: 363–368, 1976.

137. STEIN, O., AND Y. STEIN. Bovine aortic endothelial cells display macrophage-like properties towards acetylated ^{125}I-labeled low density lipoprotein. *Biochim. Biophys. Acta* 620: 631–635, 1980.

138. STEMERMAN, M. B., AND R. ROSS. Experimental arteriosclerosis. I. Fibrous plaque formation in primates. An electron microscopic study. *J. Exp. Med.* 136: 769–789, 1972.

139. TAUBER, J. P., J. CHENG, AND D. GOSPODAROWICZ. Effect of high and low density lipoproteins on proliferation of cultured bovine vascular endothelial cells. *J. Clin. Invest.* 66: 696–708, 1980.

140. TAYLOR, R. F., T. H. PRICE, S. M. SCHWARTZ, AND D. C. DALE. Neutrophil-endothelial cell interactions on endothelial monolayers grown on micropore filters. *J. Clin. Invest.* 67: 584–587, 1981.

141. THOMAS, W. A., J. M. REINER, R. A. FLORENTIN, AND R. F. SCOTT. Population dynamics of arterial cells during atherogenesis. VIII. Separation of the roles of injury and growth stimulation in early aortic atherogenesis in swine originating in pre-existing intimal smooth muscle cell masses. *Exp. Mol. Pathol.* 31: 124–144, 1979.

142. THORGEIRSSON, G., A. L. ROBERTSON, JR., AND D. H. LOWDAN. Migration of human vascular endothelial and smooth muscle cells. *Lab. Invest.* 41: 51–62, 1979.

143. THORNTHWAITE, J. T., AND R. C. LEIF. A permanent cell viability assay using alcian blue. *Stain Technol.* 53: 199–204, 1978.

144. UDEINYA, I. J., J. A. SCHMIDT, M. AIKAWA, L. H. MILLER, AND I. GREEN. Falciparum malaria-infected erythrocytes specifically bind to cultured human endothelial cells. *Science* 312: 555–557, 1981.

145. VLODAVSKY, I., P. E. FIELDING, C. J. FIELDING, AND D. GOSPODAROWICZ. Role of contact inhibition in the regulation of receptor mediated uptake of low density lipoprotein in cultured vascular endothelial cells. *Proc. Natl. Acad. Sci. USA* 75: 356–360, 1978.

146. WALL, R. T., L. A. HARKER, L. J. QUADRACCI, AND G. E. STRIKER. Factors influencing endothelial cell proliferation in vitro. *J. Cell. Physiol.* 96: 203–214, 1978.

147. WEBER, G., P. FABBRINI, L. RESI, AND P. TOTI. Aortic surface coat scanning electron-microscopic modifications after short-term hypercholesterolic diet, visualized in rabbits by con A-haemocyanin reaction. *Atherosclerosis* 27: 141–145, 1977.

148. WEDMORE, C. V., AND T. J. WILLIAMS. Control of vascular permeability by polymorphonuclear leukocytes in inflammation. *Nature London* 289: 646–650, 1981.

149. WEISS, H. J., H. R. BAUMGARTNER, T. B. TSCHOPP, D. COHEN, AND V. T. TURITTO. Correction by factor VIII of the impaired platelet adhesion to subendothelium in von Willibrand disease. *Blood* 51: 267–279, 1978.

150. WEKSLER, B. B., C. W. LEY, AND E. A. JAFFE. Stimulation of endothelial cell prostacyclin production of thrombin, trypsin, and the ionophore A 23187. *J. Clin. Invest.* 62: 923–930, 1978.

151. WILLIAMS, M. C., AND S. L. WISSIG. The permeability of muscle capillaries to horseradish peroxidase. *J. Cell Biol.* 66: 531–555, 1975.

152. ZETTER, B. R., AND H. N. ANTONIADES. Stimulation of human vascular endothelial cell growth by a platelet-derived growth factor and thrombin. *J. Supramol. Struct.* 11: 361–370, 1979.

153. ZETTER, B. R., L. K. JOHNSON, M. A. SHUMAN, AND D. GOSPODAROWICZ. The isolation of vascular endothelial cell lines with altered cell surface and platelet binding properties. *Cell* 14: 501–509, 1978.

154. ZUCKER, M. B. The functioning of blood platelets. *Sci. Am.* 242: 86–103, 1980.

INDEX

Index

Acetylcholine
  effects on pulmonary circulation, 127
Acidosis, respiratory
  effects on pulmonary circulation, 142
Adaptation, physiological
  adaptive growth of gas-exchange apparatus, 26–31
    exposure to hypoxia, 26–27
    increased O_2 consumption, 27–28
    lung tissue resection, 28–30
Adenine nucleotides
  lung energy production, 269–270
    nucleotide pools, 270
    O_2 as substrate, 270
    substrates, 270
Adenosine triphosphate
  biosynthesis in lung in relation to energy state, 237–239
  biosynthesis of, control of, 235–236
Adrenal cortex hormones
  influence on production of pulmonary surfactant, 36–37
Aging
  effects on distribution of pulmonary blood flow, 98
Altitude, high
  pulmonary edema at, 210–211
Alveoli: see Pulmonary alveoli
Alveolitis, fibrosing: see Pulmonary fibrosis
Amiloride
  effects on sodium absorption in airway epithelia, 434–435
Amines
  basic amines, uptake by lungs, 345–346
Amino acids
  compartmentation for protein synthesis in perfused lung, 283–284
  composition of lipoprotein lipase and hepatic lipase, 399
  exogenous, in regulation of protein degradation in lung, 287–288
    interaction between exogenous amino acids and hypoxia, 289–290
    potential physiological importance of interaction between amino acids and hypoxia, 290
  precursor pools for protein synthesis, 280–282
    in pulmonary macrophages, 299
Aminorex
  causing pulmonary hypertension, 149–150
Anaphylaxis
  eicosanoid production in lungs after, 375–376
Anesthetics
  effects on mucociliary clearance in respiratory tract, 489
  effects on norepinephrine uptake by lungs, 342
Angiotensin-converting enzyme
  activity in lungs, 356
  synthesis by pulmonary endothelial cells, 357–358
Angiotensins
  effects on lungs, 358–359
    interactions among vasoactive agents and their target cells, 359
    interdependence of endothelial cells and smooth muscle cells, 359
  effects on pulmonary circulation, 126
    II, as intrinsic chemical mediator of circulatory response to acute hypoxia, 133–134
  processing by lung, 353–359
    angiotensin-converting enzyme: kininase II, 356
    angiotensin I, 354
    angiotensin II, 355
    angiotensin III, 355–356
    cellular and subcellular sites of relevant pulmonary enzymes, 356
    clinical implications, 358
    immunocytochemistry, 356
    pulmonary endothelial cells as model system, 356–358
Animals, newborn
  normal postnatal growth of respiratory tissue in, 21–24
  postnatal development of respiratory tissue in, alveolar stage, 16–20
  pulmonary circulation in, 145–148
    postnatal pulmonary vasodilation, 148
Anoxia
  acute hypoxia, effects on pulmonary circulation, 129–138
    cellular events in vascular smooth muscle, 134–137
    extrinsic nerves and reflexes, 131
    hypoxia in atelectasis, 138
    intrinsic chemical mediators, 132–134
    intrinsic pulmonary mechanisms, 131–132
    local reflexes, 132
    overview of pressor responses, 138
    sites of pulmonary vasoconstriction, 137–138
  chronic hypoxia, effects on pulmonary circulation, 138–142
    functional component of increased pulmonary vascular resistance, 141–142
    site of increased pulmonary vascular resistance, 141
    teleological considerations, 142
  exposure to hypoxia and adaptive growth of lungs, 26–27
  hypoxic model of experimental chronic pulmonary hypertension, 149
  influence on protein degradation in lung, 288–289
    interaction between exogenous amino acids and hypoxia, 289–290
    potential physiological importance of interaction between amino acids and hypoxia, 290
  regulatory effect on pulmonary carbohydrate metabolism, 263–264
Antioxidants
  defenses of cell against O_2 toxicity, 246–249
    enzymatic defenses, 246–247
    nonenzymatic defenses, 247–248
Antithrombin III
  properties and interactions of, 509–511
Apolipoproteins
  metabolism of, role of lung lipoprotein lipase in, 407–408
  of pulmonary surfactant, 315–318
    composition, 315–317
    lipid-protein interactions, 317–318
    relationship between protein and lipid metabolism, 328–330
  role in hydrolysis of circulating triglycerides by lipoprotein lipase, 401–404
    apoprotein C-II, 401
    apoprotein E, 401–404
Arachidonic acid
  effects on pulmonary circulation, 127–129

Arachidonic acid (*continued*)
  endogenous, as source for biosynthesis of eicosanoids by lungs, 375–378
    release of eicosanoids after anaphylactic reactions, 375–376
    release of eicosanoids by endogenous mediators, 377–378
    release of eicosanoids by mechanical stimulation, 377
  exogenous, as source for biosynthesis of eicosanoids by lungs, 373–375
Ascorbic acid
  as defense against O_2 toxicity, 247–248
Atelectasis
  hypoxia in, effects on pulmonary circulation, 138

Bioenergetics: *see* Energy metabolism
Biological transport
  see also Ion transport
  glucose transport by lung tissue, 261
Blood cells
  see also Blood platelets; Granulocytes
  interaction of fibrinogen with, 519–520
Blood circulation
  see also Microcirculation; Pulmonary circulation
  bronchial circulation, 142–145
    determination of blood flow, 144–145
    in disease, 145
    in normal lung, 145
    normal levels of blood flow, 145
Blood coagulation
  clot formation and lysis, role of fibrin in, 522–523
  conversion of fibrinogen to fibrin clot, 514–516
  cross-linking of fibrin, 517–518
  intrinsic and extrinsic coagulation, relationship of, 503–504
    factor VII, 504
    factor X, 503–504
    thromboplastin, 504
  polymerization sites in fibrin formation, 516–517
  review of, 495–544
Blood coagulation factors
  congenital deficiencies in initiation of blood coagulation, 495–503
    factor VIII, 501–503
    factor IX, 500–501
    factor XI, 499–500
    factor XII, 496–497
    interaction of contact-system proteins, 498–499
    plasma kininogens, 498
    plasma prekallikrein, 497–498
Blood platelets
  function of, 552
  morphology and content, 551–553
  platelet–blood vessel interactions, 545–558
    platelet–endothelial cell interactions, 554
  platelet-derived growth factor, 552–553
  platelet-lung relationships in serotonin uptake by lung, 340
Blood pressure
  see also Capillary pressure; Hypertension
  pressure-volume and pressure-flow relationships in pulmonary circulation, 116–122
    distensibility, 116
    pulmonary vascular impedance, 121–122
    pulmonary vascular resistance, 116–121
  pulmonary blood flow and pressure waves, 98–99
    changes in patterns of propagation, 98–99
    propagation of flow and pressure waves, 98
  pulmonary vascular pressures, 107–113
    effects of exercise, 112–113
    effects of mechanical ventilation, 112
    influence of intrathoracic pressure on, 111
    pulmonary arteriovenous pressure differences, 109–110
    pulmonary artery, 108
    pulmonary microcirculation, 108–109
    pulmonary veins and left atrium, 109
    pulmonary wedge pressure, 110–111
    transmural vs. luminal pressures, 111–112
Blood proteins
  see also Fibrinogen
  colloid osmotic pressure gradient in pulmonary interstitial spaces and lymphatics, 194–200
    effect of increasing capillary pressure on, 198–200
    equilibration times of proteins between plasma and lymph, 200
    measurement of capillary selectivity to plasma proteins, 195–198
Blood vessels
  see also Capillaries; Microcirculation; Muscle, smooth, vascular; Pulmonary artery; Pulmonary veins; Vascular resistance
  platelet–blood vessel interactions, 545–558
Blood volume
  pulmonary, 113–116
    changes, 114–115
    measurement, 114
    normal values, 115
    partition, 115–116
Bradykinin
  effects on pulmonary circulation, 127
  processing by lung, 354–355, 359–360
Bronchi
  blood circulation in, 142–145
    determination of blood flow, 144–145
    in disease, 145
    in normal lung, 145
    normal levels of blood flow, 145
Bronchitis
  chronic bronchitis, study using experimental hypertrophy of mucus-secreting cells as model for, 429–430

Calcium
  Ca^{2+} concentration around cilia, control by ciliary membrane, 484
  Ca^{2+} role in ciliary arrest, 484
  Ca^{2+} role in regulation of prothrombin activation, 506–507
Calmodulin
  role in control of ciliary sliding, 484–485
Capillaries
  capillary endothelium, morphological models of, 545
  capillary endothelium of lungs, structure of, 73–74
Capillary permeability
  abnormal permeability to plasma proteins in pulmonary edema, causative factors, 207–214
    hemorrhagic shock, 208–209
    high-altitude edema, 210–211
    histamine, 210
    hydrochloric acid aspiration, 208
    microembolic vascular damage, 211
    α-naphthylthiourea, 207–208
    neurogenic pulmonary edema, 211
    other compounds, 212
    O_2 toxicity, 211–212
    septic shock, 209–210
    superoxide system as possible mechanism, 212–214
Capillary pressure
  increased capillary pressure, effect on lymph flow in pulmonary interstitial spaces, 202–203
  increasing capillary pressure in pulmonary interstitial spaces, effect on colloid osmotic gradient, 198–200
  pulmonary, in Starling equation, 179–182
Carbohydrates
  lung metabolism of, methods of study, 258–261
    compartmentation, 258–259
    isolated lung mitochondria, 259–261
    isotopic tracer techniques, 258

lung metabolism of, physiological significance, 257–258
lung metabolism of, regulation of, 263–265
  hypoxia, 263–264
  insulin and diabetes, 264–265
  nutrition, 264
Carbon radioisotopes
  use in study of lung carbohydrate metabolism, 258
β-Carotene
  as defense against O_2 toxicity, 247–248
Catecholamines
  see also Norepinephrine
  as intrinsic chemical mediators of pulmonary circulatory responses to acute hypoxia, 132–133
  naturally occurring catecholamines, uptake by lungs, 343–344
    dopamine, 344
    epinephrine, 344
    octopamine, 344
    β-phenylethylamine, 343–344
Cell membrane
  review of, 52–53
Cell nucleus
  review of, 48
Cells
  see also Lung cells; names of specific cells
  basic plan of, 47–53
    cell nucleus, 48
    cytoplasmic membrane systems and granules, 48–51
    ground substance, and cytoskeleton, 51–52
    mitochondria, 51
    plasma membrane, 52–53
Cells, cultured
  endothelial cells, 548–550
  in vitro methods for measuring phagocytic properties of pulmonary macrophages, 462–464
    monolayer assays, 463
    suspension assays, 463–464
  pulmonary endothelial cells as model system for study of processing of angiotensins and bradykinin, 356–358
  vascular endothelial cells, serotonin uptake in, 340
Central nervous system
  neurogenic pulmonary edema, mechanism of, 211
Chlorcyclizine
  uptake by lungs, 345–346
Chlorides
  secretion by dog tracheal epithelium, 430–434
Choline kinase
  in lipid synthesis in lungs, 321
Cholinephosphate cytidyltransferase
  in lipid synthesis in lungs, 321–322
Cholinephosphotransferase
  in lipid synthesis in lungs, 322
Chylomicrons: see Lipoproteins
Cilia
  in respiratory system of mammals, function-structure correlations in, 473–494
    axoneme, 476–477
    ciliary beat, 485
    ciliary crown, 477
    ciliary dysfunction in humans, 490–491
    ciliary membrane, 477–480
    ciliary necklace, 478–480
    ciliogenesis, 474–476
    distribution and general organization, 473–474
    freeze-fracture studies and membrane organization, 478
    function of metachronism, 486–487
    mucociliary clearance, influencing factors, 487–489
    mucociliary transport, 485–486
    mucous layer in mucociliary transport, 486
    periciliary fluid in mucociliary transport, 485–486
  sliding-microtubule mechanism of motion of, 480–483
    direct examination of sliding, 481–482
    geometry of sliding, 480–481
    human dynein, 483
    structure and function of dynein arm, 482–483
  sliding of, control of, 483–485
    Ca^{2+} and ciliary arrest, 484
    calmodulin role, 484–485
    membrane control of Ca^{2+} concentration, 484
    mutant studies, 483
    sliding and switching mechanisms, 484
Ciliary motility disorders
  in humans, 490–491
  genetic and structural implications of, 491
Coenzymes
  pyridine nucleotides in generation of reducing equivalents during lung glucose metabolism, 267–269
  reduced pyridine and flavin nucleotides, generation in conservation of energy released from biological oxidations, 231–232
Collagen
  in lung, 290–293, 295
    changes in collagen content, 292–293
    composition and synthesis of, 291–292
    relation to development of pulmonary fibrosis, 295
  O_2-dependent synthesis by lung tissues, 242–243
Connective tissue
  components of, O_2-dependent synthesis by lung tissue, 242–243
  of lungs, cells related to, 75–77
  proteins of lung, 290–295
    collagen, 290–293
    elastin, 293–295
  pulmonary interstitial connective tissues, composition, structure, and function of, 168–170
Cyclooxygenase: see Prostaglandin synthase
Cytochrome P-450
  P-450–linked monooxygenase activity in lung, 241–242
Cytoplasmic granules
  review of, 48–51

Diabetes mellitus
  influence on pulmonary carbohydrate metabolism, 264–265
  lung lipoprotein lipase activity in, 405–406
Diet
  dietary model of experimental chronic pulmonary hypertension, 149–151
  effects on lipoprotein lipase activity, 395–396
  regulation of general protein turnover, 285–286
Dopamine
  uptake by lungs, 344

Eicosanoids
  see also Leukotrienes; Prostaglandins; Thromboxanes
  antagonists of eicosanoids and inhibitors of their synthesis, 367–369
  biosynthesis by lungs from endogenous arachidonic acid, 375–378
    release of eicosanoids after anaphylactic reactions, 375–376
    release of eicosanoids by endogenous mediators, 377–378
    release of eicosanoids by mechanical stimulation, 377
  biosynthesis by lungs from exogenous arachidonic acid, 373–375
  biosynthesis of, overview, 366–367
  effects on lungs, 369–370
  history of, 365–366
  inactivation in lungs, 370–373
  metabolism by lungs, 365–386
Elastin
  in lung, 293–295
    content of, 294
    turnover of, 294–295
  O_2-dependent synthesis by lung tissues, 242–243

Embryo
    lung development in humans, 8–10
        airways, 8–9
        blood vessels, 9–10
Emphysema, pulmonary: *see* Pulmonary emphysema
Endocrine glands
    endocrine cells in airway epithelium, 61–62
Endoplasmic reticulum
    review of, 48–51
Endothelium
    capillary, morphological models of, 545
    cell turnover in, 547–548
    classification and location of, 546
    endothelial cell culture, 548–550
    endothelial pathways for lung interstitial fluid, 174–176
    endothelium-dependent pulmonary vasodilation, mechanisms in, 152–153
    function of, 550–551
    injury to, 551
    interactions with smooth muscle, 553–554
    lipoprotein lipase binding to, mechanism of, 400–401
    lipoprotein lipase in and relation to hydrolysis of circulating triglycerides, 400
    lipoprotein lipase in, origin of, 400
    platelet–endothelial cell interactions, 554
    transport across, 545–547
    vascular endothelium of lungs, 73–74
        as model system for study of processing of angiotensins and bradykinin, 356–358
        interdependence with smooth muscle cells in actions of angiotensins on lungs, 359
        isolated and cultured cells, serotonin uptake in, 340
        isolated cells, norepinephrine uptake by, 342
        metabolic functions of endothelial cells, 74
        monoamine oxidases of, role in serotonin uptake, 339
        structure of arterial and venous endothelium, 74
        structure of capillary endothelium, 73–74
        synthesis of angiotensin-converting enzyme, 357–358
Endotoxins
    sepsis model of experimental pulmonary hypertension, 151
Energy metabolism
    bioenergetics of O_2 utilization, general concepts, 231–236
        control of ATP synthesis, 235–236
        electron-transport chain, 232–233
        energy conservation, 231
        generation of reduced pyridine and flavin nucleotides, 231–232
        inhibitors and uncouplers of mitochondrial bioenergetics, 234–235
        oxidative phosphorylation, 233–234
        substrate-level phosphorylation, 232
    lung bioenergetics, 236–240
    lung energy production, 269–270
        nucleotide pools, 270
        O_2 as substrate, 270
        substrates, 270
Epinephrine
    see also Norepinephrine
    uptake by lungs, 344
Epithelium
    see also Endothelium
    mesothelial cells of pleura, 86
    of airways and air spaces, 55–73
    of alveoli, 63–73
        brush cells: type III pneumocytes, 71
        cell kinetics in, 71–73
        lining cells: type I pneumocytes, 63–65
        secretory cells: type II pneumocytes, 65–71
    of conducting airways, 56–63
        cell kinetics in, 62–63
        ciliated cells, 57–60

    endocrine and other cells, 61–62
    exocrine cells, 60–61
    of trachea, chloride secretion in dog, 430–434
    of trachea, sodium absorption in dog, 434–435
Eukaryotic cells: *see* Cells
Exertion
    effects on pulmonary blood flow, 96–97

Factor V
    role in regulation of prothrombin activation, 506
Factor VII
    role in intrinsic and extrinsic blood coagulation, 504
Factor VIII
    congenital deficiency and disorder in blood coagulation, 501–503
Factor IX
    congenital deficiency and disorder in blood coagulation, 500–501
Factor X
    role in intrinsic and extrinsic blood coagulation, 503–504
Factor XI
    congenital deficiency and disorder in blood coagulation, 499–500
Factor XII
    congenital deficiency and disorder in blood coagulation, 496–497
Fasting
    effect on pulmonary carbohydrate metabolism, 264
Fetus
    lung structural development in human, 10–16
        canalicular stage, 12–13
        pseudoglandular stage, 10–12
        terminal sac stage, 13–16
    lung surfactant in, pathways of biosynthesis of, 33–35
    pulmonary circulation in, 145–148
        morphologic changes, 147
        regulation of, 147–148
Fibrin
    clot formation from fibrinogen, 514–516
    cross-linking of, 517–518
    degradation by plasmin, 521–523
    degradation by proteases other than plasmin, 520–521
    interaction with thrombin, 511
    role in clot formation and lysis, 522–523
Fibrinogen
    degradation by plasmin, 521–523
    degradation by proteases other than plasmin, 520–521
    electron microscopy of, 512
    interaction with cells, 519–520
    interaction with plasma proteins, 518–519
    structure of, 512–518
        conversion of fibrinogen to fibrin clot, 514–516
        cross-linking of fibrin, 517–518
        model of fibrinogen molecules, 514
        polymerization sites, 516–517
Fibrinolysin: *see* Plasmin
Fibrinolysis
    physiological, 526–527
    review of, 495–544
Fibroblasts
    in lungs, 75–77
    myofibroblasts in lungs, 79–81
Fibronectins
    interaction of fibrinogen with, 518–519
Free radicals
    production of, implication as mechanism of O_2 toxicity, 244–245

Gluconeogenesis
    in lung, 263
Glucose
    and intermediary metabolism of lungs, 255–275
        oxidants and carbohydrate metabolism, 270–271
        pathophysiology and toxicology of, 270–272
    consumption by lung tissue, 262–263

during pulmonary edema, 271–272
  effect on protein degradation in lung, 290
  metabolism by lung, major products of, 265–269
    generation of reducing equivalents, 267–269
    lactate, 265–266
    lactate production by isolated perfused lung, 267
    lactate production in vivo, 266–267
    pentose phosphate pathway, 269
  metabolism of, major pathways, 255–257
    cellular respiration, 257
    glycolysis, 255–257
  transport by lung tissue, 261
Glycogen
  glycogenesis in lung, 263
Granulocytes
  in pulmonary defense system, 86

Heart
  left atrium blood pressure, 109
Hemodynamics
  see also Blood pressure; Blood volume; Vascular resistance
  pulmonary hemodynamics, 96–122
    general aspects of pulmonary blood flow, 96–98
    mechanical influences on pulmonary blood flow, 99–107
    pressure-volume and pressure-flow relationships, 116–122
    pulmonary blood flow and pressure waves, 98–99
    pulmonary blood volume, 113–116
    pulmonary vascular pressures, 107–113
Heparin
  properties and interactions of, 509–511
High-density lipoproteins: see Lipoproteins
Histamine
  as intrinsic chemical mediator of pulmonary circulatory response to acute hypoxia, 133
  causing abnormal capillary permeability to plasma proteins (leaky lung syndromes), 210
  effects on pulmonary circulation, 126–127
  loss and uptake in lungs, 345
Hormones
  effects on lipoprotein lipase activity, 395–396
  regulation of protein turnover in lungs, 286
Hydrochloric acid
  aspiration causing lung damage and pulmonary edema, 208
Hypercapnia
  acute hypercapnia, effects on pulmonary circulation, 142
Hyperlipoproteinemia
  lung lipoprotein lipase activity in, 406–407
Hyperoxia: see Oxygen
Hypertension
  spontaneous hypertension in rats, lung uptake of serotonin and norepinephrine in, 343
Hypoxia: see Anoxia

Imipramine
  uptake by lungs, 345–346
Immotile cilia syndrome: see Ciliary motility disorders
Infant, newborn
  normal postnatal growth of respiratory tissue in, 24–26
    airways, 24–25
    pulmonary arteries, 25–26
    pulmonary veins, 26
  postnatal development of respiratory tissue in, alveolar stage, 20–21
Insulin
  effect on protein degradation in lung, 290
  effect on pulmonary carbohydrate metabolism, 264–265
Interstitial spaces of lung: see Lung interstitial spaces
Intracellular membranes
  cytoplasmic membrane systems, review of, 48–51

Ion transport
  in respiratory system, 430–440
    chloride secretion by dog tracheal epithelium, 430–434
    mechanisms of, 430–435
    other ion-transport processes, 435
    regulation of, 435–438
    relationship between ion transport and water movement, 438–440
    sodium absorption, 434–435
Irritants
  effects on airway mucous secretion, 423
Isoproterenol
  effects on pulmonary circulation, 127
  uptake by lungs, 344–345

Kininase II: see Angiotensin-converting enzyme
Kininogens
  congenital deficiencies and disorders in blood coagulation, 498

Lactates
  as product of lung glucose metabolism, 265–267
    lactate production by isolated perfused lung, 267
    lactate production in vivo, 266–267
Leukotrienes
  O_2-dependent synthesis by lung tissues, 243
Levonorepinephrine: see Norepinephrine
Lipase
  see also Lipoprotein lipase
  hepatic, amino acid composition of, 399
Lipids
  see also Phospholipids
  composition of lung tissue, 309–318
    alveolar type II cells, 310–311
    apolipoproteins of surfactant, 315–318
    extracellular surfactant lipids, 311–314
    lamellar bodies, 314–315
    parenchyma, 309–310
    pulmonary surfactant, 311–318
  metabolic pathways in lung tissue, 318–322
    other lipids in surfactant, 320–321
    phosphatidylcholine, 318–319
    phosphatidylglycerol, 319–320
  metabolism of, role of lung lipoprotein lipase in, 407
  peroxidation as mechanisms of O_2 toxicity, 245
  synthesis and surfactant turnover in lungs, 309–336
    enzymes of, 321–322
    regulation of clearance of surfactant components, 326–328
    regulation of secretion of surfactant components, 324–326
    regulation of synthesis and storage of surfactant components, 322–324
    relationship between protein and lipid metabolism, 328–330
Lipoprotein lipase
  characteristics of, 397, 398–399
    amino acid composition, 399
  distribution of, 395
  history of, 394–395
  hydrolysis of circulating triglycerides, mechanisms of, 399–404
    endothelial lipoprotein lipase, 400
    mechanism of binding to endothelium, 400–401
    origin of endothelial lipoprotein lipase, 400
    role of apoprotein C-II, 401
    role of apoprotein E, 401–404
  in lung, 404–408
    functions of, 407–408
    in diabetes, 405–406
    in severe lipemia, 406–407
    in trauma, 406
    origin of, 407
    role in apoprotein metabolism, 407–408
    role in lipid metabolism, 407

Lipoprotein lipase (continued)
    tissue distribution and regulation of its activity, 405
  lipolytic activity of, characteristics of, 404
  ontogeny of, 397–398
  regulation of its activity, 395–397
    cellular regulation, 396–397
    intracellular regulation of its synthesis, 397
    nutritional and hormonal effects, 395–396
    substrate affinity, 396
  review of, 393–404

Lipoproteins
  see also Apolipoproteins; Hyperlipoproteinemia
  review of, 387–393
    chylomicrons, 388
    high-density lipoproteins, 392–393
    low-density lipoproteins, 391–392
    very-low-density lipoproteins, 389–391

Liver
  lipase of, amino acid composition of, 399

Low-density lipoproteins: *see* Lipoproteins

Lung
  see also Bronchi; Lung cells; Lung interstitial spaces; Pulmonary alveoli; Pulmonary surfactant
  adaptive growth of gas-exchange apparatus, 26–31
    exposure to hypoxia, 26–27
    increased O_2 consumption, 27–28
    lung tissue resection, 28–30
    structural features of adaptive response, 31
  bioenergetics of, 236–240
    energy state and ATP generation, 237–239
    lung mitochondria, 239–240
    O_2 uptake, 236–237
  biosynthesis of eicosanoids from endogenous arachidonic acid, 375–378
    release of eicosanoids after anaphylactic reactions, 375–376
    release of eicosanoids by endogenous mediators, 377–378
    release of eicosanoids by mechanical stimulation, 377
  biosynthesis of eicosanoids from exogenous arachidonic acid, 373–375
  carbohydrate metabolism in, methods of study, 258–261
    compartmentation, 258–259
    isolated lung mitochondria, 259–261
    isotopic tracer techniques, 258
  carbohydrate metabolism in, physiological significance of, 257–258
  carbohydrate metabolism in, regulation of, 263–265
    hypoxia, 263–264
    insulin and diabetes, 264–265
    nutrition, 264
  collagen in, 290–293, 295
    changes in collagen content, 292–293
    composition and synthesis of, 291–292
    relation to development of pulmonary fibrosis, 295
  connective tissue proteins of, 290–295
  defense system of, cells of, 82–86
  development and growth in humans, 1–46
  effects of eicosanoids on, 369–370
  effects of peptide hormones on, 358–359
    interactions among vasoactive agents and their target cells, 359
    interdependence of endothelial cells and smooth muscle cells, 359
  elastin in, 293–295
    content of, 294
    turnover of, 294–295
  embryonic development in humans, 8–10
    airways, 8–9
    blood vessels, 9–10
  energy production by, 269–270
    nucleotide pools, 270
    O_2 as substrate, 270
    substrates, 270
  fetal period of development in humans, 10–16
    canalicular stage, 12–13
    pseudoglandular stage, 10–12
    terminal sac stage, 13–16
  final dimensions in humans, 31
  glucose and intermediary metabolism of, 255–275
    oxidants and carbohydrate metabolism, 270–271
    pathophysiology and toxicology of, 270–272
  glucose consumption by, 262–263
    during pulmonary edema, 271–272
  glucose metabolism in, major products of, 265–269
    generation of reducing equivalents, 267–269
    lactate, 265–266
    lactate production by isolated perfused lung, 267
    lactate production in vivo, 266–267
    pentose phosphate pathway, 269
  glucose transport by, 261
  glycogenesis and gluconeogenesis in, 263
  growth of, 21–31
  histamine loss and uptake in, 345
  histogenetic origin of, 53–54
  lipid composition of, 309–318
    alveolar type II cells, 310–311
    lamellar bodies, 314–315
    lipid-protein interactions, 317–318
    parenchyma, 309–310
    pulmonary surfactant pools, 311–318
  lipid metabolic pathways in, 318–322
    other lipids in surfactant, 320–321
    phosphatidylcholine, 318–319
    phosphatidylglycerol, 319–320
  lipid synthesis in, 309–336
    enzymes of, 321–322
  lipoprotein lipase in, 404–408
    functions of, 407–408
    in diabetes, 405–406
    in severe lipemia, 406–407
    in trauma, 406
    origin of, 407
    role in apoprotein metabolism, 407–408
    role in lipid metabolism, 407
    tissue distribution and regulation of its activity, 405
  lymphatic capillaries in, 81
  lymphatics of, 167–230
  metabolism of eicosanoids, 365–386
    inactivation in lungs, 370–373
  morphology of, 1–8
    airways, 5–7
    blood vessels, 7–8
    gas-exchange region, 1–5
  norepinephrine uptake by, 340–342
    characterization of uptake process, 340–341
    effects of anesthesia on, 342
    effects of hyperoxia on, 343
    effects of monocrotaline on, 342
    in spontaneously hypertensive rats, 343
    localization of, 341–342
    measurement in human clinical problems, 343
    neuronal and extraneuronal uptake, 342
    uptake by isolated endothelial cells, 342
  normal postnatal growth in animals, 21–24
  normal postnatal growth in humans, 24–26
    airways, 24–25
    pulmonary arteries, 25–26
    pulmonary veins, 26
  O_2-dependent metabolic reactions in, 241–243
    bactericidal activity, 243
    cytochrome P-450–linked monooxygenase, 241–242
    inactivation of vasoactive amines, 242
    synthesis of connective tissue components, 242–243
    synthesis of eicosanoids, 243
  O_2 toxicity for, 243–244, 248–249

INDEX

causing abnormal capillary permeability to plasma proteins (leaky lung syndromes), 211–212
    protection against, 248–249
O₂ utilization and toxicity in, 231–254
postnatal development of, alveolar stage, 16–21
    experimental studies, 16–20
    human observations, 20–21
processing of angiotensin and other peptides by, 351–364
    angiotensin-converting enzyme, 356
    angiotensin I, 354
    angiotensin II, 355
    angiotensin III, 355–356
    bradykinin, 354–355
    cellular and subcellular sites of relevant pulmonary enzymes, 356
    clinical implications, 358
    historical background, 351–353
    immunocytochemistry, 356
    other peptides, 359–360
    pulmonary endothelial cells as model system, 356–358
protein degradation in, 286–287
protein degradation in, regulation of, 287–290
    exogenous amino acids, 287–288
    glucose and insulin, 290
    hypoxia, 288–289
    interaction between exogenous amino acids and hypoxia, 289–290
    potential physiological importance of interaction between amino acids and hypoxia, 290
protein synthesis in, effect of hyperoxia, 297–298
protein turnover in, 277–308
    amino acid compartmentation in perfused lung, 283–284
    dietary regulation of, 285–286
    hormonal regulation of, 286
    in pulmonary macrophages, 298–301
    methods of studying, 279–280
    role of proteases and protease inhibitors, 295–297
    turnover rates, 284–285
resection of, adaptive response of remaining tissue to, 28–30
serotonin and other amines in, 337–349
serotonin uptake by, 338–340, 342–343
    and pharmacological action of serotonin on pulmonary circulation, 340
    and platelet–lung relationships, 340
    characterization of uptake process, 338–339
    effects of cigarette smoke, 343
    effects of hyperoxia on, 343
    effects of monocrotaline on, 342
    effects of α-naphthylthiourea on, 342–343
    effects of paraquat on, 342
    efflux of accumulated serotonin, 340
    in spontaneously hypertensive rats, 343
    localization of, 339
    measurement in human clinical problems, 343
    monoamine oxidases of pulmonary endothelial cells, 339
    pharmacological inhibition of uptake process, 339
    uptake in isolated and cultured endothelial cells, 340
structural development in humans, 8–21
uptake of basic amines, 345–346
uptake of other naturally occurring catecholamines, 343–344
    dopamine, 344
    epinephrine, 344
    octopamine, 344
    β-phenylethylamine, 343–344
uptake of sympathomimetic drugs, 344–345
    isoproterenol, 344–345
    mescaline, 345
    metaraminol, 344
Lung cells
    alveolar epithelium, 63–73
        brush cells; type III pneumocytes, 71
        cell kinetics in, 71–73

        lining cells: type I pneumocytes, 63–65
        secretory cells: type II pneumocytes, 65–71
    alveolar type II cells, lipid composition of, 310–311
    biology of, 47–91
    cells of pulmonary defense system, 82–86
        alveolar and interstitial macrophages, 82–85
        cells of immune defense system, 85–86
        granulocytes, 86
    epithelium of conducting airways, 56–63
        cell kinetics in, 62–63
        ciliated cells, 57–60
        endocrine and other cells, 61–62
        exocrine cells, 60–61
    interstitial cells, 74–82
        cells related to connective tissue fibers, 75–77
        cells with contractile properties, 77–81
        fibroblasts, 75–77
        lymphatics and free cells, 81
        myofibroblasts and pericytes, 79–81
        nerves, 81–82
        smooth muscle cells, 77–79
    macrophages, 447–471
        classes of, 447–449
        fate of, 452
        harvesting of, 452–455
        in emphysema, 465–466
        in fibrosis, 466–467
        mucociliary transport function, 457–459
        origin of, 449–451
        particle clearance by, 455–457
        pathophysiology of, 464–467
        phagocytic properties of, measurement, 460–464
        role of, 455–460
        secreted products of, 460
        secretion and regulation functions, 459–460
    macrophages, protein turnover in, 298–301
        choice of precursor amino acid, 298–299
        other factors affecting turnover, 301
        phagocytosis and protein turnover, 300–301
        precursor pools, 299
        protein degradation, 300
        substrates and protein turnover, 301
    mesothelial cells of pleura, 86
    organization of, 53–55
        differentiation of functional zones, 54
        histogenetic origin of lung cells and tissues, 53–54
        morphometry of cell population, 54–55
    vascular endothelium, 73–74
        as model system for study of processing of angiotensins and bradykinin, 356–358
        interdependence with smooth muscle cells in actions of angiotensins on lungs, 359
        isolated and cultured cells, serotonin uptake in, 340
        isolated cells, norepinephrine uptake by, 342
        metabolic functions of endothelial cells, 74
        monoamine oxidases of, role in serotonin uptake, 339
        structure of arterial and venous endothelium, 74
        structure of capillary endothelium, 73–74
        synthesis of angiotensin-converting enzyme, 357–358
Lung diseases
    see also Atelectasis; Bronchitis; Pulmonary edema; Pulmonary emphysema; Pulmonary fibrosis; Pulmonary hypertension
    bronchial circulation in, 145
Lung interstitial spaces
    review of, 167–230
    Starling forces and lymph flow, 173–207
        analyses of force changes during formation of alveolar edema: edema safety factor, 206–207
        average interstitial fluid pressure, estimation by analysis of transcapillary forces, 183–185
        average interstitial pressure, measurement of, 182–183

Lung interstitial spaces (*continued*)
    capillary pressure, 179–182
    colloid osmotic pressure gradient, 194–200
    effect of airway pressure on capillary filtration, 204–206
    effect of increased capillary pressure on lymph flow, 202–203
    effect of lymphatic obstruction, 203–204
    endothelial pathways, 174–176
    filtration coefficient, 176–179
    formation of lymph, 200–202
    hilar perivascular fluid pressure, measurement of, 186–187
    interstitial compliance, 189–192
    interstitial fluid pressure, effect of interdependence on, 188–189
    interstitial fluid pressure gradients, 192–194
    intra-alveolar fluid pressure, estimation by analysis of structure, 188
    measurement theories for tissue fluid pressure, 182
    mechanisms of lymph propulsion, 203
    perivascular pressure, calculation with mechanical stress analyses, 185–186
    septal perivascular fluid pressure, measurement of, 187–188
    theoretical considerations, 173–174
    tissue fluid pressure, 182–189
  structure and composition of, 168–173
    effect of increased hydration on tissue fluid compartments, 172–173
    interstitial connective tissues, 168–170
    physicochemical properties of intersititial matrix, 170–171
    vascular and extravascular fluid compartments in lung, 171–172
Lymphatic system
  of lung, 167–230
    effect of airway pressure on capillary filtration, 204–206
    effect of increased capillary pressure on lymph flow, 202–203
    effect of lymphatic obstruction, 203–204
    formation of lymph, 200–202
    lymphatic capillaries, 81
    mechanisms of lymph propulsion, 203

Macrophages
  alveolar and interstitial macrophages of nonimmune defense system of lungs, 82–85
  of lung, 447–471
    classes of, 447–449
    fate of, 452
    harvesting of, 452–455
    in emphysema, 465–466
    in fibrosis, 466–467
    mucociliary transport function, 457–459
    origin of, 449–451
    particle clearance by, 455–457
    pathophysiology of, 464–467
    phagocytic properties of, measurement, 460–464
    role of, 455–460
    secreted products of, 460
    secretion and regulation functions, 459–460
  of lung, protein turnover in, 298–301
    choice of precursor amino acid, 298–299
    other factors affecting turnover, 301
    phagocytosis and protein turnover, 300–301
    precursor pools, 299
    protein degradation, 300
    substrates and protein turnover, 301
Mechanical ventilation: *see* Respiration, artificial
Mescaline
  uptake by lungs, 345
Mesothelium: *see* Epithelium
Metaraminol
  uptake by lungs, 344
Methadone
  uptake by lungs, 345–346

Microcirculation
  see also Capillaries
  pulmonary microcirculation, pressures in, 108–109
Microscopy, electron
  of fibrinogen, 512
Mitochondria
  isolated lung mitochondria in study of lung carbohydrate metabolism, 259–261
  of lung, substrate utilization and O_2 consumption in, 239–240
  review of, 51
Monoamine oxidase
  pulmonary endothelial cells, role in uptake of serotonin, 339
Monocrotaline: *see* Pyrrolizidine alkaloids
Muscle, smooth
  smooth muscle cells in lungs, 77–79
    interdependence with pulmonary endothelial cells in actions of angiotensins on lungs, 359
Muscle, smooth, vascular
  cellular events involved in pulmonary circulatory response to acute hypoxia, 134–137
    electrical activity and electrical-mechanical coupling, 136–138
    metabolic effects, 136
  endothelium–smooth muscle interactions, 553–554

α-Naphthylthiourea
  causing abnormal capillary permeability to plasma proteins (leaky lung syndromes), 207–208
  effects on serotonin uptake by lungs, 342–343
Nerve fibers
  in lungs, 81–82
  nonadrenergic, noncholinergic nerves of airway submucosal glands, 425
Neurons
  neuronal and extraneuronal uptake of norepinephrine by lung, 342
Norepinephrine
  O_2-dependent inactivation by pulmonary endothelium, 242
  uptake by lungs, 340–342
    characterization of uptake process, 340–341
    effects of anesthesia on, 342
    effects of hyperoxia on, 343
    effects of monocrotaline on, 342
    in spontaneously hypertensive rats, 343
    localization of, 341–342
    measurement in human clinical problems, 343
    neuronal and extraneuronal uptake, 342
    uptake by isolated endothelial cells, 342
Nucleotides
  nucleotide pools in lung energy metabolism, 270
  pyridine nucleotides in generation of reducing equivalents during lung glucose metabolism, 267–269
  reduced pyridine and flavin nucleotides, generation in conservation of energy released from biological oxidations, 231–232

Octopamine
  uptake by lungs, 344
Osmotic pressure
  colloid osmotic pressure gradient in pulmonary interstitial spaces and lymphatics, 194–200
    effect of increasing capillary pressure on, 198–200
    equilibration times of proteins between plasma and lymph, 200
    measurement of capillary selectivity to plasma proteins, 195–198
Oxidation-reduction
  generation of reducing equivalents during lung glucose metabolism, 267–269
  oxidation of tissue components as mechanism of O_2 toxicity, 245–246
    lipid peroxidation, 245
    oxidation of other components, 245–246
    protein oxidation, 245

INDEX

Oxygen
    acute hyperoxia, effects on pulmonary circulation, 142
    as substrate in lung energy metabolism, 270
    hyperoxia, effects on lung uptake of serotonin or norepinephrine, 343
    hyperoxia, effects on protein synthesis in lung, 297–298
    pathological effects of, 243–244
    superoxide system as possible mechanism of pulmonary edema, 212–214

Oxygen consumption
    bioenergetics of, general concepts, 231–236
        control of ATP synthesis, 235–236
        electron-transport chain, 232–233
        energy conservation, 231
        generation of reduced pyridine and flavin nucleotides, 231–232
        inhibitors and uncouplers of mitochondrial bioenergetics, 234–235
        oxidative phosphorylation, 233–234
        substrate-level phosphorylation, 232
    conditions causing increased consumption, adaptive growth of lungs in response to, 27–28
    of lung, 236–240
        energy state and ATP generation, 237–239
        lung mitochondria, 239–240
        O_2 uptake, 236–237
    O_2-dependent metabolic reactions, 240–243
        in lung, 241–243
        pathways of O_2 utilization, 240–241

Oxygen toxicity
    antioxidant defenses against, 246–249
        enzymatic defenses, 246–247
        nonenzymatic defenses, 247–248
    general aspects, 243
    mechanisms of, 244–246
        alterations of metabolic function, 246
        free-radical production, 244–245
        oxidation of tissue components, 245–246
    pulmonary, 243–244, 248–249
        causing abnormal capillary permeability to plasma proteins (leaky lung syndromes), 211–212
        protection against, 248–249

Paraquat
    effects on serotonin uptake by lungs, 342
Parasympathetic nervous system
    innervation of airway submucosal glands, 424
Parasympathomimetics
    effects on mucociliary clearance in respiratory tract, 489
Pentose phosphate pathway
    in lung glucose metabolism, 269
Peptide hydrolases
    other than plasmin, degradation of fibrinogen by, 520–521
    role in protein turnover in lungs, 295–297
    thrombinlike enzymes in snake venoms, 511–512
Peptides
    processing by lungs, 351–364
Peroxides
    lipid peroxidation as mechanism of O_2 toxicity, 245
Phagocytosis
    and protein turnover in pulmonary macrophages, 300–301
    phagocytic properties of pulmonary macrophages, measurement of, 460–464
        in situ, 460–462
        in vitro, 462–464
        monolayer assays, 463
        suspension assays, 463–464
Phenylalanine
    as choice precursor amino acid in study of protein turnover in pulmonary macrophages, 298–299
β-Phenylethylamine
    uptake by lungs, 343–344

Phosphatidate phosphatase
    in lipid synthesis in lungs, 322
Phosphatidylcholines
    biosynthetic pathways in adult and fetal lungs, 33–35
    metabolic pathways in lung tissue, 318–319
    remodeling enzymes in lipid synthesis in lungs, 322
Phosphatidylglycerols
    biosynthetic pathways in adult and fetal lungs, 33–35
    metabolic pathways in lung tissue, 319–320
Phospholipids
    coagulant phospholipid surfaces, role in regulation of prothrombin activation, 506
Plasma membrane: *see* Cell membrane
Plasma proteins: *see* Blood proteins
Plasmin
    degradation of fibrinogen and fibrin, 521–523
    inhibitors of, 525–526
    properties of, 523–527
Plasminogen
    activators of, 523–525
    inhibitors of, 525–526
    properties of, 523–527
Platelets: *see* Blood platelets
Pleura
    mesothelial cells of, 86
Posture
    effects on pulmonary blood flow, 97
Prekallikrein
    congenital deficiency and disorder in blood coagulation, 497–498
Propranolol
    uptake by lungs, 345–346
Prostacyclin: *see* Prostaglandins
Prostaglandin synthase
    products of, synthesis by lungs, 373–378
        from endogenous arachidonic acid, 375–378
        from exogenous arachidonic acid, 373–375
Prostaglandins
    as intrinsic chemical mediators of pulmonary circulatory responses to acute hypoxia, 134
    effects on pulmonary circulation, 127–129
    O_2-dependent synthesis by lung tissues, 243
Protease inhibitors
    role in protein turnover in lungs, 295–297
Proteases: *see* Peptide hydrolases
Proteins
    see also Blood proteins; Lipoproteins
    degradation in lungs, 286–287
    degradation in lungs, regulation of, 287–290
        exogenous amino acids, 287–288
        glucose and insulin, 290
        hypoxia, 288–289
        interaction between exogenous amino acids and hypoxia, 289–290
        potential physiological importance of interaction between amino acids and hypoxia, 290
    oxidation as mechanism of O_2 toxicity, 245
    turnover of, 277–308
        amino acid compartmentation in perfused lung, 283–284
        dietary regulation of, 285–286
        effect of proteolysis on extracellular specific radioactivity, 282–283
        elastin turnover in lung, 294–295
        hormonal regulation of, 286
        in lung, role of proteases and protease inhibitors, 295–297
        in lung, study methods, 279–280
        in nonpulmonary tissues and cells, 278
        in pulmonary macrophages, 298–301
        physiological importance of, 278–279
        precursor pools, 280–282
        turnover rates in various tissues, 284–285
Prothrombin
    activation of, regulation of, 504–512

Prothrombin (*continued*)
    Ca^{2+}, 506–507
    coagulant phospholipid surfaces, 506
    factor V, 506
    heparin and antithrombin III, 509–511
    interaction of thrombin with fibrin, 511
    nonmammalian inhibitors of thrombin, 511
    prothrombin, 504–506
    regulation of thrombin activity, 508–509
    thrombin formation, 507
    thrombin specificity, 507–508
  regulation of prothrombin activation, 504–506
Pulmonary alveoli
  epithelium of, 63–73
    brush cells: type III pneumocytes, 71
    cell kinetics in, 71–73
    lining cells: type I pneumocytes, 63–65
    secretory cells: type II pneumocytes, 65–71
  intra-alveolar fluid pressure, estimation by analysis of structure, 188
  macrophages of nonimmune defense system, 82–85
  type II cells of, lipid composition of, 310–311
Pulmonary artery
  endothelium of, structure, 74
  normal postnatal growth in humans, 25–26
  pressure in, 108
Pulmonary circulation
  effects of acute acidosis on, 142
  effects of acute hypercapnia on, 142
  effects of acute hyperoxia on, 142
  effects of acute hypoxia on, 129–138
    cellular events in vascular smooth muscle, 134–137
    extrinsic nerves and reflexes, 131
    hypoxia in atelectasis, 138
    intrinsic chemical mediators, 132–134
    intrinsic pulmonary mechanisms, 131–132
    local reflexes, 132
    overview of pressor responses, 138
    sites of pulmonary vasoconstriction, 137–138
  effects of chronic hypoxia on, 138–142
    functional component of increased pulmonary vascular resistance, 141–142
    site of increased pulmonary vascular resistance, 141
    teleological considerations, 142
  effects of serotonin on, relation to serotonin uptake by lung, 340
  effects of vasoactive prostaglandins and their precursors, 127–129
  effects of vasoconstrictors on, 126–127
    angiotensin II, 126
    histamine, 126–127
    serotonin, 127
  effects of vasodilators on, 127
    acetylcholine, 127
    bradykinin, 127
    isoproterenol, 127
  general aspects of, 96–98
    at rest, 96
    distribution of blood flow, 98
    effects of aging, 98
    effects of exercise, 96–97
    effects of posture, 97
    effects of respiration, 97–98
  in fetus and newborn, 145–148
    morphologic changes, 147
    postnatal pulmonary vasodilation, 148
    regulation in fetus, 147–148
  mechanical influences on blood flow, 99–107
    alveolar vessels, 104–106
    corner vessels, 106–107
    distension and recruitment, 104
    extra-alveolar vessels, 107
    extrapulmonary vessels, 104
    inflation, 107
    intrapulmonary vessels, 104
    vascular waterfall, 100–101
    zones of lungs, 101–104
  pressure-volume and pressure-flow relationships of, 116–122
    distensibility, 116
    pulmonary vascular impedance, 121–122
    pulmonary vascular resistance, 116–121
  pulmonary blood flow and pressure waves, 98–99
    changes in patterns of propagation, 98–99
    propagation of flow and pressure waves, 98
  pulmonary blood volume, 113–116
    changes, 114–115
    measurement, 114
    normal values, 115
    partition, 115–116
  pulmonary hemodynamics, 96–122
  pulmonary vascular pressures, 107–113
    effects of exercise, 112–113
    effects of mechanical ventilation, 112
    influence of intrathoracic pressure on, 111
    pulmonary arteriovenous pressure differences, 109–110
    pulmonary artery, 108
    pulmonary microcirculation, 108–109
    pulmonary veins and left atrium, 109
    pulmonary wedge pressure, 110–111
    transmural vs. luminal pressures, 111–112
  pulmonary vascular resistance, 116–121, 141–142
    calculation of, 116–117
    critical closure, 120
    interpretation of change in, 117–118
    modifiers of, 118–119
    sites of vascular resistance, 120–121
    zones of lungs and calculated resistance, 119–120
  review of, 93–165
  vascular endothelium of, 73–74
    metabolic functions of endothelial cells, 74
    structure of arterial and venous endothelium, 74
    structure of capillary endothelium, 73–74
  vascular fluid compartments in lung, 171–172
  vasomotor regulation of, 122–142
    chemical control, 126–142
    detection of vasomotor response, 123
    level of initial tone, 123
    nervous control, 124–126
    sites of pulmonary vasoconstriction, 123–124
    vasomotor mechanisms, 124–142
    vasomotor reflexes, 125–126
Pulmonary edema
  abnormal capillary permeability to plasma proteins in, causative factors, 207–214
    hemorrhagic shock, 208–209
    high-altitude edema, 210–211
    histamine, 210
    hydrochloric acid aspiration, 208
    microembolic vascular damage, 211
    α-naphthylthiourea, 207–208
    neurogenic pulmonary edema, 211
    other compounds, 212
    O_2 toxicity, 211–212
    septic shock, 209–210
    superoxide system as possible mechanism, 212–214
  alveolar edema, analyses of Starling force changes during formation of, 206–207
  formation of, sequence and pathways for, 214–215
  glucose consumption by lung during, 271–272
  role of pulmonary interstitial spaces and lymphatics in, 167–230
Pulmonary emphysema
  role of pulmonary macrophages in, 465–466

INDEX

Pulmonary fibrosis
  relation to lung collagen content and type, 295
  role of pulmonary macrophages in, 466–467
Pulmonary hypertension
  endothelium-dependent pulmonary vasodilation, 152–153
  experimental chronic, 148–151
    blood component model, 151
    dietary model, 149–151
    hypoxic model, 149
    other models, 151
    sepsis model, 151
  pathogenesis of, 148
  vasodilator therapy of, 151–152
Pulmonary surfactant
  apolipoproteins of, 315–318
    composition, 315–317
    lipid-protein interactions, 317–318
  biochemistry of, 32–35
    composition, 32–33
    pathways of phosphatidylcholine and phosphatidylglycerol synthesis in adult and fetal lungs, 33–35
    start of surfactant synthesis during canalicular stage of fetal period, 13
    surfactant turnover, 35
  development of surfactant system, 31–38
  historical background and function of, 32
  lipid composition of, 311–318
    extracellular surfactant lipids, 311–314
    lamellar bodies, 314–315
    lipid-protein interactions, 317–318
  lipid metabolic pathways in, 318–322
    other lipids, 320–321
    phosphatidylcholine, 318–319
    phosphatidylglycerol, 319–320
  lipid synthesis in, enzymes of, 321–322
    choline kinase, 321
    cholinephosphate cytidyltransferase, 321–322
    cholinephosphotransferase, 322
    phosphatidic acid phosphohydrolase, 322
    phosphatidylcholine remodeling enzymes, 322
  metabolism of, regulation of, 322–330
    regulation of clearance of surfactant components, 326–328
    regulation of secretion of surfactant components, 324–326
    regulation of synthesis and storage of surfactant components, 322–324
    relationship between protein and lipid metabolism, 328–330
  turnover of, 309–336
    compartmental analysis in studies of, 330–331
  type II cells, and regulation of production of, 35–38
    influence of corticosteroids, 36–37
    influence of thyroid hormones, 37–38
    lamellar bodies, and surfactant production, 35
Pulmonary veins
  endothelium of, structure, 74
  normal postnatal growth in humans, 26
  pressure in, 109
Pyrrolizidine alkaloids
  monocrotaline, effects on serotonin and norepinephrine uptake by lungs, 342

Receptors, endogenous
  role in hormonal regulation of protein turnover in lungs, 286
Reduction: see Oxidation-reduction
Reflex
  local reflexes in pulmonary circulatory responses to acute hypoxia, 132
  role in pulmonary circulatory responses to acute hypoxia, 131
  vasomotor reflexes and pulmonary circulation, 125–126
Respiration
  effects on pulmonary blood flow, 97–98

Respiration, artificial
  effects on pulmonary vascular pressures, 112
Respiratory system
  see also Lung; Pleura; Trachea
  airway secretions, regulation of, 419–445
    effects of drugs and mediators on, 425–426
  cilia in, function-structure correlations in, 473–494
    axoneme, 476–477
    ciliary beat, 485
    ciliary crown, 477
    ciliary dysfunction in humans, 490–491
    ciliary membrane, 477–480
    ciliary necklace, 478–480
    ciliogenesis, 474–476
    control of sliding, 483–485
    distribution and general organization, 473–474
    freeze-fracture studies and membrane organization, 478
    function of metachronism, 486–487
    mucociliary clearance, influencing factors, 487–489
    mucous layer in mucociliary transport, 486
    periciliary fluid in mucociliary transport, 485–486
    sliding-microtubule mechanism, 480–483
  conducting airways, epithelium of, 56–63
    cell kinetics in, 62–63
    ciliated cells, 57–60
    endocrine and other cells, 61–62
    exocrine cells, 60–61
  ion transport and water movement in, 430–440
    chloride secretion by dog tracheal epithelium, 430–434
    mechanisms of, 430–435
    other ion-transport processes, 435
    regulation of, 435–438
    relationship between ion transport and water movement, 438–440
    sodium absorption, 434–435
  macrophages in, 447–471
  mucociliary transport in, 457–459
  mucus-secreting cells, hypertrophy of, 426–430
    animal studies, 427–430
    experimental hypertrophy as model for chronic bronchitis, 429–430
    human studies, 426–427
    mechanism of, 428–429
  submucosal glands of, 423–425
    anatomy of, 423–424
    human studies on hypertrophy of, 426–427
    nonadrenergic, noncholinergic nerves of, 425
    parasympathetic innervation of, 424
    physiology of, 424–425
    sympathetic innervation of, 424–425
  surface mucus of, 419–423
    anatomy of, 419–422
    ciliated cells, 421–422
    Clara cells, 421
    effects of irritants on, 423
    epithelial serous cells, 420–421
    goblet cell hypertrophy in humans, 427
    goblet cells, 420
    innervation, 422
    neurohumoral control of, 422–423
    physiology of, 422–423

Serotonin
  effects on pulmonary circulation, 127
    relation to its uptake by lung, 340
  O_2-dependent inactivation by pulmonary endothelium, 242
  uptake by lungs, 338–340
    and pharmacological action of serotonin on pulmonary circulation, 340
    and platelet-lung relationships, 340

Serotonin (continued)
    characterization of uptake process, 338–339
    effects of cigarette smoke, 343
    effects of hyperoxia on, 343
    effects of monocrotaline on, 342
    effects of α-naphthylthiourea on, 342–343
    effects of paraquat on, 342
    efflux of accumulated serotonin, 340
    in spontaneously hypertensive rats, 343
    localization of, 339
    measurement in human clinical problems, 343
    monoamine oxidases of pulmonary endothelial cells, 339
    pharmacological inhibition of uptake process, 339
    uptake in isolated and cultured endothelial cells, 340
Shock
    hemorrhagic and septic, causing abnormal capillary permeability to plasma proteins (leaky lung syndromes), 208–210
Smoke
    cigarette smoke, effects on serotonin uptake by lungs, 343
Snake venoms
    thrombinlike enzymes in, 511–512
Sodium
    absorption by dog tracheal epithelium, 434–435
Surfactant, pulmonary: see Pulmonary surfactant
Sympathetic nervous system
    see also Vasomotor system
    innervation of airway submucosal glands, 424–425
Sympathomimetics
    effects on mucociliary clearance in respiratory tract, 489
    uptake by lungs, 344–345
        isoproterenol, 344–345
        mescaline, 345
        metaraminol, 344

Thorax
    intrathoracic pressure, influence on pulmonary vascular pressures, 111
Thrombin
    activity of, regulation of, 508–509
    formation in prothrombin activation, 507
    interaction with fibrin, 511
    nonmammalian inhibitors of, 511
    specificity in relation to prothrombin activation, 507–508
    thrombinlike enzymes in snake venoms, 511–512
Thromboplastin
    role in intrinsic and extrinsic blood coagulation, 504
Thromboxanes
    O_2-dependent synthesis by lung tissues, 243
Thyroid hormones
    influence on production of pulmonary surfactant, 37–38
Tobacco
    cigarette smoke, effects on serotonin uptake by lungs, 343

Tocopherol: see Vitamin E
Trachea
    epithelium of, chloride secretion in dog, 430–434
    epithelium of, sodium absorption in dog, 434–435
Trauma: see Wounds and injuries
Triglycerides
    circulating, mechanisms of hydrolysis by lipoprotein lipase, 399–404
        endothelial lipoprotein lipase, 400
        mechanism of binding to endothelium, 400–401
        origin of endothelial lipoprotein lipase, 400
        role of apoprotein E, 401–404

Vascular resistance
    pulmonary, 116–121, 141–142
        calculation of, 116–117
        critical closure, 120
        functional component of increased vascular resistance in chronic hypoxia, 141–142
        interpretation of change in, 117–118
        modifiers of, 118–119
        site of increased vascular resistance in chronic hypoxia, 141
        sites of vascular resistance, 120–121
        zones of lungs and calculated resistance, 119–120
Vasoconstrictor agents
    effects on pulmonary circulation, 126–127
Vasodilator agents
    effects on pulmonary circulation, 127
    therapy of pulmonary hypertension, 151–152
Vasomotor system
    regulation of pulmonary circulation, 122–142
        chemical control, 126–142
        detection of vasomotor response, 123
        effects of acute hypoxia, 129–138
        effects of chronic hypoxia, 138–142
        level of initial tone, 123
        nervous control, 124–126
        sites of pulmonary vasoconstriction, 123–124
        vasomotor mechanisms, 124–142
        vasomotor reflexes, 125–126
Ventilation, mechanical: see Respiration, artificial
Very-low-density lipoproteins: see Lipoproteins
Vitamin C: see Ascorbic acid
Vitamin E
    as defense against O_2 toxicity, 247–248

Water
    movement and ion transport in airways, 430–440
        mechanisms of, 430–435
        regulation of, 435–438
        relationship between ion transport and water movement, 438–440
Wounds and injuries
    lung lipoprotein lipase activity in, 406

Respiratory Mechanics

Main Symbols

C	compliance (capacity in symbols for subdivisions of lung volume)
E	elastance
f	frequency
G	conductance
I	inertance
P	pressure
R	resistance
sG	specific conductance
t	time
V	volume
W	work
$\dot{W}$	power
Z	impedance
$\dot{X}$	dot above any symbol indicates first time derivative; e.g., $\dot{V}$ is flow of gas
$\ddot{X}$	two dots above symbol indicate second time derivative; e.g., $\ddot{V}$ is acceleration of volume

Modifiers

A	alveolar
ab	abdomen
am	ambient
ao	airway opening
aw	airway
B	barometric
bs	body surface
ca	convective acceleration
di	diaphragm
ds	downstream
dyn	dynamic
E	expiratory
el	elastic
es	esophageal
fr	frictional or flow resistive
ga	gastric
I	inspiratory
ia	intercostal/accessory muscles
L	transpulmonary or lung or pulmonary
lam	laminar
m	mouth
max	maximum
mus	muscle
pl	pleural
rc	rib cage
rel	relaxed or relaxation
rs	respiratory system
st	static
ti	tissue
tm	transmural
tur	turbulence
us	upstream
w	chest wall

Subdivisions of Lung Volume

CC	closing capacity
CV	closing volume
ERV	expiratory reserve volume
FRC	functional residual capacity
IC	inspiratory capacity
IRV	inspiratory reserve volume
RV	residual volume
TLC	total lung capacity
VC	vital capacity
V_T	tidal volume

Measurements on Forced Respiratory Maneuvers

EPP	equal pressure points
FEF_{x-y}	mean forced expiratory flow between two designated volume points in FVC = $(V_x - V_y)/t$
FET_x	time required to forcibly expire percent of VC, x, from TLC
FEV_t	forced expiratory volume in time interval t
$FEV_t/FVC\%$	percent of FVC expired in time interval t
FVC	forced vital capacity
IVPF curve	isovolume pressure-flow curve
MEFV curve	maximum expiratory flow-volume curve
MFSR curve	maximum flow–static recoil curve
MIFV curve	maximum inspiratory flow-volume curve
MVV	maximum voluntary ventilation
MVV_t	maximum voluntary ventilation in time interval t
PEF	peak expiratory flow
PEFV curve	partial expiratory flow-volume curve
$\dot{V}max_{xx}$	maximum expiratory flow at xx% of VC (note: 100% VC is at TLC; 0% VC is at RV)
$\dot{V}max_{xx,TLC}$	maximum expiratory flow at xx% of TLC

Examples of Combinations

C_L	lung compliance
$C_{st,L}$	static lung compliance
P_A	alveolar pressure
Pao	pressure at the airway opening
$P_{E,m,max_{xx,TLC}}$	maximum expiratory mouth pressure at xx% of TLC
sGaw	specific airway conductance
$\dot{W}di$	diaphragmatic power
$W_{I,el,L}$	elastic work performed on the lung during inspiration